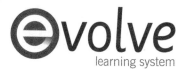

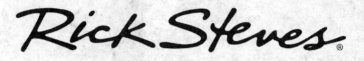

NORTHERN
EUROPEAN
CRUISE PORTS

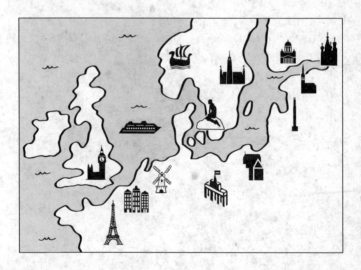

AVALON
TRAVEL

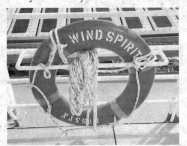

INTRODUCTION

Imagine yourself lazing on the deck of a floating city as you glide past the spiny skylines of Tallinn, Copenhagen, or St. Petersburg; the jagged fjords of Norway's west coast; or the thousands of picture-perfect islands topped by quaint red vacation cottages in the archipelago between Stockholm and Helsinki. Each day, stepping off the gangway, you're immersed in the vivid life of a different European city. Tour some of the world's top museums, take a Scandinavian-style coffee break while you people-watch from a prime sidewalk café, bask on a surprisingly sunny and sandy Baltic beach, and enjoy some of Europe's most expensive cities on the cheap. After a busy day in port, you can head back to the same cozy bedroom each night, without ever having to pack a suitcase or catch a train. As the sun sets and the ship pulls out of port, you have your choice of dining options—from a tuxedo-and-evening-gown affair to a poolside burger—followed by a world of nightlife. Plying the Baltic and North Sea waters through the night, you wake up refreshed in a whole new city—ready to do it all again.

Cruising in Europe is more popular today than ever before. And for good reason. Taking a cruise can be a fun, affordable way to experience Europe—*if* you choose the right cruise, keep your extra expenses to a minimum... and use this book to make the absolute most of your time in port.

Unlike most cruising guidebooks, which dote on details about this ship's restaurants or that ship's staterooms, *Rick Steves Northern European Cruise Ports* focuses on the main attraction: some of the

Map Legend

⅄ Viewpoint	🚢 Cruise Port/Dock	) (Tunnel
✦ Entrance	✈ Airport	▭▭ Pedestrian Zone
❶ Tourist Info	Ⓣ Taxi Stand	‒ ‒ ‒ ‒ Railway
Ⓦ🅒 Restroom	Ⓣ Tram Stop	·········· Ferry/Boat Route
🏰 Castle	Ⓑ Bus Stop	├─┼─┤ Tram
▪ Statue/Point of Interest	Ⓜ Metro Stop	▥▥▥▥ Stairs
▦ Building	Ⓣ T-Bana Stop (Oslo & Stockholm)	▪ ▪ ▪ ▪ Walk/Tour Route
⬆ Church	Ⓢ S-Tog Station (Copenhagen)	‑ ‑ ‑ ‑ Trail
✡ Synagogue	🄷 Harbor Bus (Copenhagen)	O╫╫╫╫O Funicular
◎ Fountain	🅿 Parking	⬚⬚⬚ Park

Use this legend to help you navigate the maps in this book.

grandest cities in Europe. Even if you have just eight hours in port, you can still ride a red double-decker bus through London, paddle a kayak on a Norwegian fjord, stroll Berlin's Unter den Linden or Copenhagen's Strøget, and walk in Lech Wałęsa's footsteps at the Solidarity shipyards in Gdańsk.

Yes, you could spend a lifetime in any of these places. But you've got a few hours...and I have a plan for you. Each of this book's destination chapters is designed as a mini-vacation of its own, with advice about what to do and detailed sightseeing information for each port. And, to enable you to do it all on your own, I've included step-by-step instructions for getting into town from the cruise terminal.

For each major destination, this book offers a balanced, comfortable mix of the predictable biggies and a healthy dose of "Back Door" intimacy. Along with marveling at masterpieces in the Louvre, Hermitage, and Rijksmuseum, you can sip a pint in a trendy London pub and sweat with the Finns in a working-class sauna.

In each port, you'll get all the specifics and opinions necessary to wring the maximum value out of your limited time and money. The best options in each port are, of course, only my opinion. But after spending half my adult life researching Europe, I've developed a sixth sense for what travelers enjoy.

ABOUT THIS BOOK

The book is divided into three parts: First, I'll suggest strategies for choosing which cruise to take, including a rundown of the major cruise lines, and explain the procedure for booking a cruise.

Please Tear Up This Book!

There's no point in hauling around 60 pages on Copenhagen for a day in Oslo. That's why I've designed this book to be

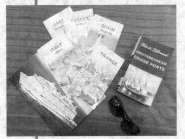

ripped apart. Before your cruise, attack this book with a utility knife to create an army of pocket-sized mini-guidebooks—one for each port of call.

I love the ritual of trimming down the size of guidebooks I'll be using: Fold the pages back until you break the spine, neatly slice apart the sections you want with a utility knife, then pull them out with the gummy edge intact. If you want, finish each one off with some clear, heavy-duty packing tape to smooth and reinforce the spine, or use a heavy-duty stapler along the edge to prevent the first and last pages from coming loose.

To make things even easier, I've created guidebook-page binders that have laminated covers with slide-on binders. Every evening, you can make a ritual of swapping out today's pages for tomorrow's. (For more on these binders, see www.ricksteves.com.)

As I travel in Europe, I meet lots of people with even more clever book treatments. This couple was proud of the job they did in the name of packing light: cutting out only the pages they'd be using and putting them into a spiral binding.

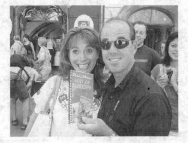

While you may be tempted to keep this book intact as a souvenir of your travels, you'll appreciate even more the footloose freedom of traveling light while you're in port.

Next, I'll give you a "Cruising 101"-type travel-skills briefing, with advice about what you should know before you go, and strategies for making the most of your time both on and off the ship. And finally, the vast majority of this book is dedicated to the European ports you'll visit, with complete plans for packing each day full of unforgettable experiences.

I haven't skimped on my coverage of the sights in this book—which is why it's a bricklike tome. To get the most out of the book, please don't hesitate to tear out just the pages that you need for each day in port (see sidebar).

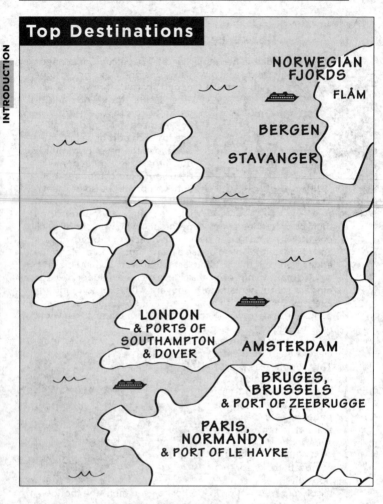

Top Destinations

NORWEGIAN FJORDS

FLÅM

BERGEN

STAVANGER

LONDON
& PORTS OF
SOUTHAMPTON
& DOVER

AMSTERDAM

BRUGES,
BRUSSELS
& PORT OF ZEEBRUGGE

PARIS,
NORMANDY
& PORT OF LE HAVRE

IS A EUROPEAN CRUISE RIGHT FOR YOU?

I'm not going to try to convince you to cruise or not to cruise. If you're holding this book, I assume you've already made that decision. But if you're a cruise skeptic—or even a cruise cynic—and you're trying to decide whether cruising suits your approach to experiencing Europe, I'll let you in on my own process for weighing the pros and cons of cruising.

I believe this is the first and only cruising guidebook written by someone with a healthy skepticism about cruises. When I was

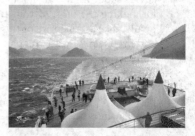

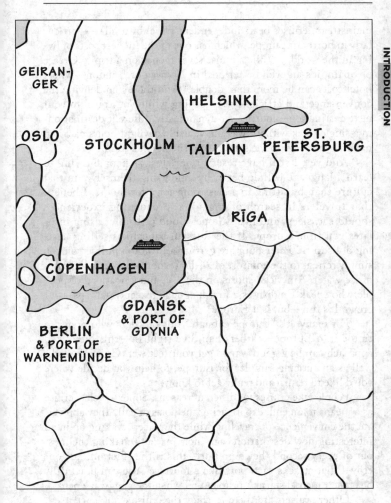

growing up, cruising was a rich person's hobby. I used to joke that for many American cruisers, the goal was not travel but hedonism (how many meals can you eat in a day?).

But now I understand that cruising can be cost-effective if done smartly. After three decades of exploring and writing about Europe, I haven't found a more affordable way to see certain parts of the continent than cruising (short of sleeping on a park bench).

For a weeklong European cruise that includes room, board, transportation, tips, and port fees, a couple can pay as little as $100 per night—that's as much as a budget hotel room in many cities. To link all the places on an exciting one-week European cruise on your own, the hotels, rail passes, boat tickets, taxi transfers, restaurants, and so on would add up fast. The per-day base cost for mainstream cruises beats independent travel by a mile—particularly in northern Europe, which has one of the highest costs of living in the world. (While a cruise saves money on a trip to Greece or Spain, it's an even better deal in Norway or London—where hotel costs can be more than double.) And there's no denying the convenience and efficiency of sleeping while you travel to your next destination—touring six dynamically different destinations in a single week without wasting valuable daylight hours packing, hauling your bags to the station, and sitting on a train.

And yet, I still have reservations. Just as people trying to learn a language will do better by immersing themselves in that culture than by sitting in a classroom for a few hours, I believe that travelers in search of engaging, broadening experiences should eat, sleep, and live Europe. Good or bad, cruising insulates you from Europe. If the Russian babushkas selling nesting dolls in St. Petersburg are getting a little too pushy, you can simply retreat to the comfort of 24-hour room service, tall glasses of ice water, American sports on the TV, and a boatload of people who speak English as a first language (except, perhaps, your crew). It's fun—but is it Europe?

For many, it's "Europe enough." For travelers who prefer to tiptoe into Europe—rather than dive right in—this bite-sized approach can be a good way to get your feet wet. Cruising works well as an enticing sampler for Europe, to help you decide where you'd like to return and really get to know.

People take cruises for different reasons. Some travelers cruise as a means to an end: experiencing the ports of call. They appreciate the convenience of traveling while they sleep, waking up in an interesting new destination each morning, and making the most out of every second they're in port. This is the "first off, last on" crowd that attacks each port like a footrace. You can practically hear their mental starter's pistol go off when the gangway opens.

Other cruisers are there to enjoy the cruise experience itself. They enjoy lying by the pool, taking advantage of onboard activities, dropping some cash at the casino, ringing up a huge bar tab, napping, reading, and watching ESPN on their stateroom TVs. If the *Mona Lisa* floated past, they might crane their necks, but wouldn't strain to get out of their deck chairs.

With all due respect to the latter group, I've written this book primarily for the former. But if you really want to be on vacation, aim for somewhere in the middle: Be sure to experience the ports that really tickle your wanderlust, but give yourself a "day off" every now and again in the less-enticing ports to sleep in or hit the beach.

Another advantage of cruising is that it can accommodate a family or group of people with vastly different travel philosophies. It's possible for Mom to go to the museum, Dad to lie by the pool, Sally to go for a bike ride, Bobby to go shopping, Grandma and Grandpa to take in a show...and then all of them can have dinner together and swap stories about their perfect days. (Or, if they're really getting on each other's nerves, there's plenty of room on a big ship to spread out.)

Cruising is especially popular among retirees, particularly those with limited mobility. Cruising rescues you from packing up your bags and huffing to the train station every other day. Once on land, accessibility for wheelchairs and walkers can vary dramatically—though some cruise lines offer excursions specifically designed for those who don't walk well. A cruise aficionado who had done the math once told me that, if you know how to find the deals, it's theoretically cheaper to cruise indefinitely than to pay for a retirement home.

On the other hand, the independent, free-spirited traveler may not appreciate the constraints of cruising. For some, seven or eight hours in port is a tantaliz-

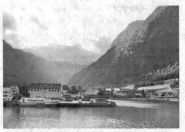

ing tease of a place where they'd love to linger for the evening— and the obligation to return to the ship every night is frustrating. Cruisers visiting Paris will never experience the City of Light after dark. If you're antsy, energetic, and want to stroll the cobbles of Europe at all hours, cruising may not be for you. However, even some seasoned globetrotters find that cruising is a good way to travel in Europe on a shoestring budget, yet still in comfort.

One cruise-activities coordinator told me that cruisers can be divided into two groups: Those who stay in their rooms, refuse to try to enjoy the dozens of activities offered to them each day, and complain about everything; and those who get out and try to get to know their fellow passengers, make the most of being at sea, and have the time of their lives. Guess which type (according to him) enjoys the experience more?

Let's face it: Americans take the shortest vacations in the rich world. Some people choose to dedicate their valuable time off to an all-inclusive, resort-style vacation in Florida, Hawaii, or Mexico: swimming pools, song-and-dance shows, shopping, and all-you-can-eat buffets. Cruising gives you much the same hedonistic experience, all while you learn a lot about Europe—provided you use your time on shore constructively. It can be the best of both worlds.

UNDERSTANDING THE CRUISE INDUSTRY

Cruising is a $37 billion-a-year business. Approximately one out of every five Americans has taken a cruise, and each year about 17 million people take one. In adjusted dollars, cruise prices haven't risen in decades. This, partly, has sparked a huge growth in the cruise industry in recent years. The aging baby boomer population has also boosted sales, as older travelers discover that a cruise is an easy way to see the world. While the biggest growth has come from the North American market, cruise lines have also started marketing more internationally.

The industry has changed dramatically over the last generation. For decades, cruise lines catered exclusively to the upper crust—people who expected top-tier luxury. But with the popularity of *The Love Boat* television series in the 1970s and 1980s, then the one-upmanship of increasingly bigger megaships in the early 1990s, cruising went mainstream. Somebody had to fill all the berths on those gargantuan vessels, and cruise lines lowered their prices to attract middle-class customers. The "newlyweds and nearly deads" stereotype about cruise clientele is now outmoded. The industry has made bold efforts to appeal to an ever-broader customer base, representing a wide spectrum of ages, interests, and income levels.

In order to compete for passengers and fill megaships, cruise lines offer fares that can be astonishingly low. In fact, they make little or no money on ticket sales—and some "loss-leader" sailings actually lose money on the initial fare. Instead, the cruise lines' main income comes from three sources: alcohol sales, gambling (onboard casinos), and excursions. So while cruise lines are in the business of creating an 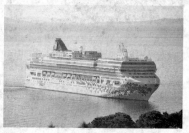 unforgettable vacation for you, they're also in the business of separating you from your money (once on the ship) to make up for their underpriced fares.

Just as airlines have attempted to bolster their bottom lines by "unbundling" their fares and charging more "pay as you go" fees (for food, checking a bag, extra legroom, and so on), cruise lines are now charging for things they used to include (such as "specialty restaurants"). The cruise industry is constantly experimenting with the balance between all-inclusive luxury and nickel-and-dime, à la carte, mass-market travel. (For tips on maximizing your experience while minimizing your expenses, see the sidebar on page 80.)

It's also worth noting that cruise lines are able to remain profitable largely on the backs of their low-paid crew, who mostly hail from the developing world. Working 10 to 14 hours a day, 7 days a week—almost entirely for tips—the tireless crew are the gears that keep cruises spinning. (For more, see page 73.)

Understanding how the cruise industry works can help you take advantage of your cruise experience...and not the other way around. Equipped with knowledge, you can be the smart consumer who has a fantastic time on board and in port without paying a premium. That's what this book is all about.

TRAVELING AS A TEMPORARY LOCAL

Most travelers tramp through Europe as if they're visiting the cultural zoo. "Oooh, that Norwegian fisherman is mending his nets! Excuse me, could you do that in the sunshine with my wife next to you so I can take a snapshot?" This is fun. It's a part of travel. But a camera bouncing on your belly tells locals you're hunting cultural peacocks. When I'm in Europe, I try to be the best Swede or Dane or Estonian I can be.

Europeans generally like Americans. But if there is a negative aspect to their image of Americans, it's that we are loud, wasteful, ethnocentric, too informal (which can seem disrespectful), and a bit naive.

Even if you believe American ways are best, your trip will go more smoothly if you don't compare. Enjoy doing things the European way, and you'll experience a more welcoming Europe.

We travel all the way to Europe to enjoy differences—to become temporary locals. You'll experience frustrations. Certain truths that we find "God-given" or "self-evident," such as cold beer, ice in drinks, bottomless cups of coffee, and bigger being better, are suddenly not so true. One of the benefits of travel is the eye-opening realization that there are logical, civil, and even better alternatives. A willingness to go local ensures that you'll enjoy a full dose of European hospitality.

While Europeans look bemusedly at some of our Yankee excesses—and worriedly at others—they nearly always afford us individual travelers all the warmth we deserve.

Judging from all the happy feedback I receive from travelers who have used my books, it's safe to assume you'll enjoy a great, affordable vacation—with the finesse of an independent, experienced traveler.

Thanks, and bon voyage!

Back Door Travel Philosophy
From *Rick Steves Europe Through the Back Door*

Travel is intensified living—maximum thrills per minute and one of the last great sources of legal adventure. Travel is freedom. It's recess, and we need it.

Experiencing the real Europe requires catching it by surprise, going casual..."through the Back Door."

In many ways, spending a lot of money on sightseeing and excursions only builds a thicker wall between you and what you came to see. Europe is a cultural carnival, and, time after time, you'll find that its best acts are free and the best seats are the cheap ones.

A tight budget forces you to travel close to the ground, meeting and communicating with the people, not relying on service with a purchased smile.

Connecting with people carbonates your experience. Extroverts have more fun. If your trip is low on magic moments, kick yourself and make things happen. If you don't enjoy a place, maybe you don't know enough about it. Seek the truth. Recognize tourist traps. Give a culture the benefit of your open mind. See things as different but not better or worse. Any culture has much to share.

Of course, travel, like the world, is a series of hills and valleys. Be fanatically positive and militantly optimistic. If something's not to your liking, change your liking.

Travel can make you a happier American as well as a citizen of the world. Our Earth is home to seven billion equally precious people. It's humbling to travel and find that people don't have the "American Dream"—they have their own dreams. Europeans like us, but, with all due respect, they wouldn't trade passports.

Thoughtful travel—even from the comfortable springboard of a cruise ship—engages us with the world. In tough economic times, it reminds us what is truly important. By broadening perspectives, travel teaches new ways to measure quality of life.

Globe-trotting destroys ethnocentricity, helping you understand and appreciate different cultures. Rather than fear the diversity on this planet, celebrate it. Among your prized souvenirs will be the strands of different cultures you choose to knit into your own character. The world is a cultural yarn shop, and Back Door travelers are weaving the ultimate tapestry. Join in!

CHOOSING AND BOOKING A CRUISE

CHOOSING A CRUISE

Each cruise line has its own distinct personality, quirks, strengths, and weaknesses. Selecting a cruise that matches your travel style and philosophy can be critical for the enjoyment of your trip. On the other hand, some cruisers care only about the price, go on any line that offers a deal, and have a great time.

Still, the more your idea of "good travel" meshes with your cruise line's, the more likely you are to enjoy both your trip and your fellow passengers. For information on booking a cruise, see the next chapter.

GATHERING INFORMATION

Comparison-shopping can be a fun part of the cruise experience. Read the cruise-line descriptions in this chapter, then browse the websites of the ones that interest you. Ask your friends who've cruised, and who share your interests, about the lines they've used, and what they thought of each one. Examine the cruise lines' glossy brochures (view online, request them, or get them from your local travel agent)—how the line markets itself says a lot about what sort of clientele it attracts. Tune into the ubiquitous TV commercials for cruise lines. Photos of individual ships' staterooms and amenities—which you'll also find on the cruise lines' websites—can be worth a thousand words in getting a sense of the vibe of each vessel.

Once you've narrowed down the choices, read some impartial online reviews. The most popular site, www.cruisecritic.com, has reviews of cruise lines, specific ships, tips for visiting each port, and more. Other well-respected websites are www.cruisediva.com, www.cruisemates.com, and www.avidcruiser.com. If you feel that cruising is all about the ship, check www.shipparade.com, which delves into details about each vessel.

Cruising the Internet

While there are many cruise-related websites, Cruise Critic (www.cruisecritic.com) dominates cyberspace. Not only are its forums crammed with reviews about ships, excursions, local guides, and ports of call, but it's also a nifty networking tool. By signing up on its Roll Call page for your cruise, you can introduce yourself to others on the same ship and look for partners to share taxis or local guides. Some cruise lines—such as Azamara, Celebrity, Crystal, and Royal Caribbean—even sponsor a social gathering of Cruise Critic members early in the cruise, often with complimentary food and drinks.

Many travel agencies that sell cruises have surprisingly informative websites. One of the best, www.vacationstogo.com, not only sorts different cruise options by price and destination, but also has useful facts, figures, and photos for each ship and port.

Most cruising guidebooks devote more coverage to detailed reviews of specific ships and their amenities than to the destinations—which make them the perfect complement to this book. Look for *The Unofficial Guide to Cruises*, *Frommer's European Cruises and Ports of Call*, *Fodor's Complete Guide to European Cruises*, and others. (For destination-specific guidebooks, see the list on page 1149.)

As you compare cruises, decide which of the factors in the following section matter the most to you, then find a cruise line that best matches what you're looking for.

Cruise Considerations

In the next few pages you'll find a wide range of issues, big and small, to take into account when selecting your cruise. Of these, the three main factors—which should be weighted about equally—are **price, itinerary** (length, destinations, and time spent in each port), and **cruise line** (personality and amenities).

If you've cruised in the Caribbean but not Europe, be aware that there are some important differences. In general, European cruises are more focused on the destinations, while Caribbean cruises tend to be more focused on the ship (passengers spend more time on the ship, and therefore the shipboard amenities are more important). People choosing among European cruises usually base their decision on the places they'll be visiting: Which cities—St. Petersburg, London, Oslo, Copenhagen—appeal? Is the focus more on urban sights or on natural wonders (such as fjords and islands)? In contrast, on a Caribbean cruise the priority is simply hedonistic fun in the sun.

CRUISE LINE

This chapter will give you a quick overview of some of the major lines to help you find a good match. For example, some cruise lines embrace cruising's nautical heritage, with decor and crew uniforms that really let you know you're on a ship. Others are more like Las Vegas casinos at sea. An armchair historian will be disappointed on a hedonistic pleasure boat, and a young person who's in a mood to party will be miserable on the *SS Septuagenarian*. Do you want a wide range of dining options on the ship, or do you view mealtime as a pragmatic way to fill the tank? After dinner, do you want to get to bed early, or dance in a disco until dawn?

American vs. European: While most US travelers opt for an American cruise line, doing so definitely Americanizes your travel experience. When you're on board, it feels almost as if you'd never left the good old U. S. of A.—with American shows on the TV, Heinz ketchup in the buffet line, and fellow Yanks all around you. If you'd rather leave North America behind, going with a European-flavored cruise line can be an interesting cultural experience in itself. While Europeans are likely to be among the passengers on any cruise line, they represent a larger proportion on European-owned or -operated boats. Surrounded by Germans who enthusiastically burp after a good meal, Italians who nudge ahead of you in line, and French people who enjoy sunbathing topless—and listening to every announcement translated into six different languages—you'll definitely know you're in Europe. I recently cruised for a week in Norway as one of just 13 Americans on a budget ship with more than 2,000 passengers. I never saw another Yank, spent my time on board and in port with working-class Italians and Spaniards from towns no tourist has ever heard of, and had what was quite possibly the most truly "European" experience of my life.

Environmental Impact: Most forms of travel come with a toll on the environment. And cruise ships are no exception—they gulp fuel as they ply scenic seas, struggling to find waste-disposal methods that are as convenient as possible while still being legal. Some cruise lines are more conscientious about these issues than others. If environmental impact is a major concern of yours, you can compare the records for all the major cruise lines at www.foe.org/cruise-report-card.

DURATION

European cruises can range in length from a few days to a few weeks. The typical cruiser sails for 7 days, but some travelers enjoy taking a 10-, 12-, or 14-day cruise, then adding a few days on land at either end to stretch their trip to 2 weeks or more. A cruise of seven days or shorter tends to focus on one "zone" of northern

Europe (Norwegian fjords, Baltic highlights, Western Europe); a longer cruise is more likely to provide you with a sampler of the whole area.

WHEN TO GO

Due to the chilly weather at these latitudes, the tourist season in northern Europe is extremely brief: June, July, and August. While a few straggler cruises may be offered outside that three-month window, I'd think twice before heading to Oslo, Helsinki, or St. Petersburg in other months (and if you do, be prepared for rainy and cold weather). For a month-by-month climate chart that includes various ports, see page 1153.

Fortunately, even though tourists bombard the region during those key months, northern European destinations are still typically less crowded than Mediterranean hot spots like Venice or Barcelona. (There are exceptions: Any day during cruise season, the crowds inside St. Petersburg's Hermitage museum are next to unbearable.)

PRICE

If you're on a tight budget and aren't fussy, look for the best deals. From the Mass-Market to the Ultra-Luxury categories, the per-person price can range from $100 to $700+ per day. Sales can lower those prices. (For more on cruise pricing, see the next chapter.)

While going with the cheapest option is tempting, it may be worth paying a little extra for an experience that better matches your idea of a dream cruise. If you're hoping for glitzy public spaces and sparkling nightly revues, you'll kick yourself later if you saved $40 a day—but ended up on a musty ship with stale shows. If you want to maximize time exploring European destinations, it can be worth paying an extra $20 a day for an itinerary with two more hours at each port—that translates to just 10 bucks an hour, a veritable steal compared to the extra experiences it'll allow you to cram in. Don't be penny-wise and pound-foolish in this regard.

On the other hand, in my (admittedly limited) cruise experience, I've noticed a trend: The more people pay for the cruise, the higher their expectations—and, therefore, the more prone they are to disappointment. I've cruised on lines ranging from bargain-basement to top-end, and I've noticed an almost perfect correlation between how much someone pays and how much they enjoy complaining. In my experience, folks who pay less are simply more fun to cruise with. When considering the people I'll wind up dining and going on shore excursions with, price tag aside, I'd rather go with a midrange cruise line than a top-end one.

When evaluating prices and making a budget, remember to take into account all of the "extras" you might wind up buying from the cruise line: alcoholic drinks, meals at specialty restaurants, the semi-mandatory "auto-tip" (about $10-12 per day per person), shore excursions, and your gambling tab from the casino, just to name a few. (For more details on these hidden costs, see page 78.)

SHIP SIZE AND AMENITIES

When it comes to cruise ships, bigger is not necessarily better... although it can be, depending on your interests.

The biggest ships offer a wide variety of restaurants, activities, entertainment, and other amenities (such as resources for kids). The main disadvantage of a big ship is the feeling that you're being herded along with thousands of other passengers—3,000 tourists piling off a ship into a small port town definitely changes the character of the place.

Smaller ships enjoy fewer crowds, access to out-of-the-way ports, and less hassle when disembarking (especially when tendering—see page 116). If you're focusing your time and energy on the destinations anyway, a smaller ship can be more relaxing to "come home" to. On the other hand, for all of the above reasons, cruises on the smallest ships are typically much more expensive. Small ships also physically can't offer the wide range of eateries and activities as the big vessels; intimate, yacht-like vessels have no room for a climbing wall or an ice rink. And finally, on a small ship, you may feel the motion of the sea more than on a big ship (though because of the stabilizers used by small ships, this difference isn't that dramatic).

Think carefully about which specific amenities are important to you, and find a cruise line that offers those things. Considerations include:

Food, both in terms of quality and variety (some cruise lines offer a wide range of specialty restaurants—explained on page 99; generally speaking, the bigger the ship, the more options are available);

Entertainment, such as a wide range of performers (musicians, dancers, and so on) in venues both big and small;

Athletic facilities, ranging from a running track around the deck, to a gym with equipment and classes, to swimming pools and hot tubs, to a simulated surf pool and bowling alley, to a spa with massage and other treatments;

Children's resources, with activities and spaces designed for teens and younger kids, and a babysitting service (for more on cruising with kids, see page 93);

Other features, such as a good library, lecturers, special events, a large casino, wheelchair accessibility, and so on.

Some first-time cruisers worry they'll get bored while they're on board. Don't count on it. You'll be bombarded with entertainment options and a wide range of activities—particularly on a big ship.

DESTINATIONS

If you have a wish list of ports, use it as a starting point when shopping for a cruise. It's unlikely you'll find a cruise that visits every one of your desired destinations, but you can usually find one that comes close.

Most itineraries of a week or more include a day "at sea": no stops at ports—just you and the open sea. These are usually included for practical reasons. Most often a day at sea is needed to connect far-flung destinations with no worthwhile stop in between...but cruise lines also don't mind keeping passengers on board, hoping they'll spend more money. Because cruise ships generally travel at around 20 knots—that's only about 23 land miles per hour—they take a long time to cover big distances. For some cruise aficionados, days at sea are the highlight of the trip; for other passengers, they're a boring waste of time. If you enjoy time on the ship, try to maximize days at sea; if you're cruising mainly to sightsee on land, try to minimize them.

TIME SPENT IN PORT

If exploring European destinations is your priority, look carefully at how much time the ship spends in each port. Specific itinerary rundowns on cruise-line websites usually show the scheduled times of arrival and departure. Typical stops can range anywhere from 6 to 12 hours, with an average of around 8 or 9 hours. At the same port—or even on the same cruise line—the difference in port time from one cruise ship to another can vary by hours. On a recent cruise, I was on one of two ships pulling into Stavanger, Norway, at about the same time. Five hours later, I trudged back to my ship, noticing that the other ship had three more hours before embarkment...giving those passengers (unlike me) just enough time for a visit to the Lysefjord's renowned Pulpit Rock.

Most cruise lines want you on the ship as long as possible— the longer you're aboard, the more likely you are to spend money there (and for legal reasons, they can't open their lucrative casinos and duty-free shops until they're at sea).

In general, the more expensive Luxury- and Ultra-Luxury-class lines offer longer stays in port. However, even if you compare cheaper lines that are similar in price, times can vary. For example, Norwegian, Costa, and MSC tend to have shorter times in port, while Royal Caribbean lingers longer.

REPOSITIONING CRUISES

Ships that cruise in Europe are usually based in the Caribbean during the winter, so they need to cross the Atlantic Ocean each spring and fall. This journey, called a "repositioning cruise," includes a lengthy (5-7 days) stretch where the ship is entirely at sea. Also called a "crossing" or a "transatlantic crossing," these are most common in early April (to Europe), or late October and November (from Europe).

If you really want to escape from it all, and just can't get enough of all the shipboard activities, these long trips can be a dream come true; if you're a fidgety manic sightseer, they're a nightmare. Before committing to a repositioning cruise, consider taking a cruise with a day or two at sea just to be sure you really, really enjoy being on a ship that much. Several notes of warning: The seas can be rougher on transatlantic crossings than in the relatively protected waters closer to land; the weather will probably be cooler; and there are a couple of days in the middle of the voyage where most ships lose all satellite communication—no shipboard phones, Wi-Fi, or cable channels. While the officers are in touch with land in the event of emergencies, your own day-to-day contact with the outside world will disappear.

If you're considering a repositioning cruise, don't be misled by the sometimes astonishingly low sticker price. (These typically don't sell as well as the more destination-oriented cruises, so they're perennially on the push list.) You'll only need a one-way plane ticket between the US and Europe—but that may exceed the cost of a round-trip ticket (don't expect to simply pay half the round-trip price).

Cruise Lines

I don't pretend to be an expert on all the different cruise lines—the focus of this book is on the destinations rather than the ships. But this section is designed to give you an overview of options to get you started. (To dig deeper, consider some of the sources listed under "Gathering Information," at the beginning of this chapter.)

While nobody in the cruise industry formally recognizes different "classes" of companies, just about everybody acknowledges that cruise lines fall into four basic categories, loosely based on the price range (estimated per-person prices given here are based on double occupancy in the cheapest cabin, and don't include taxes, port fees, or additional expenses): **Mass-Market** ($100-200/day), **Premium** ($200-350/day), **Luxury** (sometimes called "**Upper Premium**"; $350-700/day), and **Ultra-Luxury** ($700 or more/day). Of course, a few exceptions straddle these classifications and buck the trends, and some cruise lines are highly specialized—such as

Disney Cruise Line (very kid-friendly and experience-focused) and Star Clippers (an authentic tall-ship experience with a mainsail that passengers can help hoist).

Most cruise lines are owned by the same handful of companies. For example, Carnival Corporation owns Carnival, Costa, Cunard, Holland America, Princess, Seabourn, and four other lines (representing about half of the worldwide cruise market). Royal Caribbean owns Celebrity and Azamara Club Cruises. Within these groups, each individual line may be, to varying degrees, operated by a different leadership, but they do fall under the same umbrella and tend to have similar philosophies and policies.

In assembling the following information, I've focused exclusively on European itineraries. The average hours in port are based on a selection of each line's sailings; your cruise could be different, so check carefully.

MASS-MARKET LINES

The cheapest cruise lines, these huge ships have a "resort-hotel-at-sea" ambience. Prices are enticingly low, but operators try to make up the difference with a lot of upselling on board (specialty restaurants, borderline-aggressive photographers, constant pressure to shop, and so on). The clientele is wildly diverse (including lots of families and young people) and, generally speaking, not particularly well-traveled; they tend to be more interested in being on vacation and enjoying the ship than in sightseeing. Mass-Market lines provide an affordable way to sample cruising.

Costa

Contact Information: www.costacruise.com, tel. 800-247-7320
Number and Capacity of Ships: 17 ships, ranging from 800 to 4,947 passengers
Average Hours in Port: 6-7 hours
Description: With frequent sales that can drive its prices lower, Costa is one of the cheapest lines for European cruises. It also has the largest fleet and the most seven-day cruises in the region. Although owned by the American- and UK-based Carnival

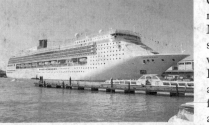

Corporation, Costa proudly retains its Italian identity. Most of your fellow passengers will be Europeans, with large contingents of Italians, French, Spanish, and Germans. (Only a small fraction of Costa passengers are from the US or Canada.)

North American cruisers find both pros and cons about traveling with a mostly European crowd: While some relish the fact that it's truly European, others grow weary of the time-consuming multilingual announcements, and have reported "rude" behavior from some fellow passengers (some Europeans are not always polite about waiting in line). The ships' over-the-top, wildly colorful decor borders on gaudy—it can be either appealing or appalling, depending on your perspective. Onboard activities also have an Italian pizzazz, such as singing waiters or heated international bocce-ball tournaments. Outrageous ambience aside, the cruising experience itself is quite traditional (there's no open seating in the dining room, and formal nights are taken seriously). Dining options are limited to the main dining room (serving reliably well-executed, if not refined, Italian fare); huge buffets serving disappointing cafeteria fare; and sparse, overpriced, and underwhelming specialty restaurants.

Costa attracts a wide demographic—from twentysomethings to retirees—and you can expect families during the summer and school breaks. The short hours in port draw criticism—and Costa's shore excursion packages are relatively expensive.

The January 2012 *Costa Concordia* disaster took more than 30 lives and cast a pall over the cruise-ship industry—but it also resulted in new safety policies that many cruise lines, including Costa, voluntarily adopted in 2013.

MSC Cruises

Contact Information: www.msccruises.com, tel. 877-655-4655
Number and Capacity of Ships: 12 ships, each carrying 1,560-4,345 passengers
Average Hours in Port: 6 hours
Description: Italian-owned MSC's tag line sums up its philosophy: the Mediterranean way of life. Even more so than the similar Costa (described earlier), this low-priced company caters mostly to Europeans—only about 5 percent of the passengers on their European cruises are from the US or Canada. This is a plus if you want to escape America entirely on your vacation, but can come with some language-barrier and culture-shock issues. Since children ride free, summer and school breaks tend to be dominated by families, while at other times passengers are mostly retirees.

The basic price is often a borderline-outrageous bargain (deep discounts are common), but MSC charges for amenities that are free on many other cruise lines—such

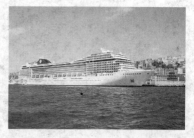

as basic drinks, room service, and snacks. In the dining room, you even have to pay for tap water. MSC has shorter hours in port than most cruise lines, and their shore excursions have a heightened emphasis on shopping. The food and entertainment are average; your choices at the breakfast and lunch buffets are the same for the entire cruise. Keep your expectations low—as one passenger noted, "It's not really a cruise—just a bus tour that happens on a nice boat."

Norwegian Cruise Line (NCL)

Contact Information: www.ncl.com, tel. 866-234-7350
Number and Capacity of Ships: 14 ships, ranging from 2,000 to 4,100 passengers
Average Hours in Port: 8-9 hours
Description: Norwegian was an industry leader in the now-widespread trend toward flexibility, and is known for its "Freestyle Cruising" approach. "Whatever" is the big word here (as in, "You're free to do...whatever"). For example, their ships typically have no assigned seatings for meals (though reservations are encouraged), and offer the widest range of specialty restaurants, which can include French, Italian, Mexican, sushi, steakhouse, Japanese teppanyaki, and more. Norwegian also has a particularly wide range of cabin categories, from very basic inside cabins to top-of-the-line, sprawling suites that rival the Luxury lines' offerings.

Norwegian has a Las Vegas-style glitz. On the newer ships, such as the gigantic, 4,100-passenger, much-publicized *Norwegian Epic*, the entertainment is ramped up, with world-class shows such as Cirque du Soleil—requiring advance ticket purchase. Their vessels tend to be brightly decorated—bold murals curl across the prows of their ships, and the public areas are colorful (some might say garish or even tacky). This approach, coupled with relatively low prices, draws a wide range of passengers: singles and families, young and old, American and European, middle-class and wealthy.

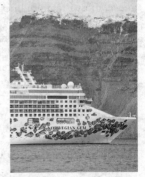

Onboard amenities cater to this passenger diversity; along with all of the usual services, some ships have climbing walls and bowling alleys. The crew is also demographically diverse, and the service is acceptable, but not as doting as on some cruise lines, making some passengers feel anonymous. Education and enrichment activities are a low priority—most lectures are designed to sell you something (excursions, artwork, and so on), rather than prepare you for the port.

Royal Caribbean International

Contact Information: www.royalcaribbean.com, tel. 866-562-7625

Number and Capacity of Ships: 23 ships—and growing, ranging from 1,800 to 5,400 passengers

Average Hours in Port: 10 hours

Description: Royal Caribbean is the world's second-largest cruise line (after Carnival). Similar to Norwegian, but a step up in both cost and (in their mind, at least) amenities, Royal Caribbean edges toward the Premium category.

Offering an all-around quintessential cruising experience, Royal Caribbean attracts first-time cruisers. The majority are from the US and Canada. The line likes to think of itself as catering to a more youthful demographic: couples and singles in their 30s to 50s on shorter cruises; 50 and up on cruises longer than seven nights. With longer hours in port and onboard fitness facilities (every ship has a rock-climbing wall, some have water parks and mini golf), they try to serve more active travelers.

The food on board is American cuisine, and its entertainment style matches other cruise lines in this category—expect Vegas-style shows and passenger-participation games. Even though some of its ships are positively gigantic, Royal Caribbean, which prides itself on service, delivers: Most of its passengers feel well-treated.

PREMIUM LINES

A step up from the Mass-Market lines both in price and in elegance, most Premium lines evoke the "luxury cruises" of yore. The ships can be nearly as big as the Mass-Market options, but are designed to feel more intimate. The upselling is still there, but it's more restrained, and the clientele tends to be generally older, better-traveled, and more interested in sightseeing. While the Mass-Market lines can sometimes feel like a cattle call, Premium lines ratchet up the focus on service, going out of their way to pamper their guests.

Celebrity

Contact Information: www.celebritycruises.com, tel. 800-647-2251

Number and Capacity of Ships: 11 ships, ranging from 98 to 3,046 passengers

Average Hours in Port: 10-11 hours

Description: Originally a Greek company, Celebrity was bought by Royal Caribbean in 1997 and operates as its upscale sister cruise line. (The "X" on the smokestack is the Greek letter "chi," which stands for Chandris—the founder's family name.) Celebrity distinguishes itself from the other Premium category lines with bigger ships and a slightly younger demographic. The company likes to point out that its larger ships have more activities and restaurants than the smaller Premium (or even Luxury category) ships. Most of its passengers are from the US or Canada, and it's reportedly popular with baby boomers, seniors, gay cruisers, and honeymooners. Among the Premium lines, Celebrity offers some of the best amenities for kids (aside from Disney, of course).

Celebrity's smallest stateroom is quite spacious compared with those on other lines in this category. On its European cruises, the main dining room cuisine seems more European than American (with some high-end options—a plus for many travelers), but there are plenty of specialty restaurants, ranging from Asian-fusion to a steakhouse. Most ships are decorated with a mod touch—with all the bright lights and offbeat art, you might feel like you're in Miami Beach. Adding to the whimsy, some ships even come with a real grass lawn on the top deck. Celebrity's service consistently gets high marks, and the onboard diversions include the usual spas, enrichment lectures, Broadway revues, cabarets, discos, theme parties, and casinos.

Cunard Line

Contact Information: www.cunard.com, tel. 800-728-6273
Number and Capacity of Ships: *Queen Elizabeth* carries 2,092 passengers, *Queen Mary 2* carries 2,620, and *Queen Victoria* carries 2,014
Average Hours in Port: 10 hours
Description: Cunard Line plays to its long, historic tradition and caters to an old-fashioned, well-traveled, and well-to-do clientele in their 50s and older. Passengers on their European itineraries tend to be mostly British, along with some Americans and other Europeans. Although the line is suitable for families (kids' programs are staffed by trained British nannies), it's not seriously family-friendly. This line features large ships and offers a pleasantly elegant experience with a British bent—you can even have afternoon tea or enjoy bangers and mash in a pub.

About a sixth of the passengers book suites and have access to specialty restaurants—a remnant of the traditional class distinctions in jolly olde England. The entertainment and lecture programs tend to be more "distinguished"; there's a good library; and activities include ballroom dancing, croquet, tennis, fencing, and lawn bowling. Each ship has a viewable collection of historic Cunard artifacts. The famously refined Cunard dress code seems to be more of a suggestion these days, as many show up in relatively casual dress at formal dining events. Passengers give mixed reviews—some feel that the experience doesn't quite live up to the line's legacy.

Disney Cruise Line

Contact Information: www.disneycruise.com, tel. 800-951-3532

Number and Capacity of Ships: 4 ships, ranging from 2,700 to 4,000 passengers

Average Hours in Port: 10-11 hours

Description: Disney is the gold standard for family cruise vacations. Passengers are families and multigenerational—expect at least a third to be kids. There'll be plenty of Disney flicks, G-rated floor shows, and mouse ears wherever you turn. Like its amusement parks, Disney's ships have high standards for service and cleanliness. The food is kid-friendly, but the ships also have a high-end Italian restaurant for parents. While your kids will never be bored, there are a few adult diversions as well (including nightclubs and an adults-only swimming pool)—but no casino. Disney cruises may be the best option if you're taking along your kids or grandkids. Be warned: Parents who think a little Disney goes a long way might overdose on this line.

Holland America Line (HAL)

Contact Information: www.hollandamerica.com, tel. 877-932-4259

Number and Capacity of Ships: 15 ships, ranging from 835 to 2,100 passengers

Average Hours in Port: 9-10 hours

Description: Holland America, with a history dating back to 1873 (it once carried immigrants to the New World), prides itself on tradition. Generally, this line has one of the most elderly clienteles in the business, though they're trying to promote their cruises to a wider demographic (with some success). Cruisers appreciate the line's delicate balance between a luxury and a casual vacation—it's formal, but not *too* formal.

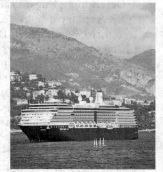

Ship decor emphasizes a connection to the line's nautical past, with lots of wood trim and white railings; you might feel like you're on an oversized yacht at times. That's intentional: When building their biggest ships, Holland America designers planned public spaces to create the illusion that passengers are on a smaller vessel (for example, hallways bend every so often so you can't see all the way to the far end). This line also has high service standards; they operate training academies in Indonesia and the Philippines, where virtually all of their crew hails from. These stewards are trained to be good-natured and to make their guests feel special. Dining options on board tend to be limited; there isn't a wide range of specialty restaurants.

Holland America takes seriously the task of educating their passengers about the ports; most ships have a "Travel Guide" who lectures on each destination and is available for questions, and some excursions—designated "Cruise with Purpose"—are designed to promote a more meaningful, participatory connection with the destinations (though these are relatively rare in Europe).

Princess

Contact Information: www.princess.com, tel. 800-774-6237
Number and Capacity of Ships: 18 ships, ranging from 670 to 3,080 passengers
Average Hours in Port: 9-10 hours
Description: Princess appeals to everyone from solo travelers to families, with most passengers over 50. Because their market reach is so huge, expect many repeat cruisers enjoying their mainstream cruise experience. While Princess has long been considered a Premium-category line, many cruise insiders suggest that the line has been lowering its prices—and, many say, its standards—so these days it effectively straddles the Premium and Mass-Market categories. Still, Princess passengers tend to be very loyal.

Princess got a big boost when the 1970s *Love Boat* TV series featured two Princess ships. Those "love boats" have now been

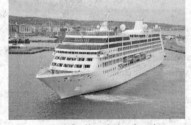

retired, and the Princess fleet is one of the most modern in the industry—half of its ships have been launched in the last 10 years. It's known for introducing innovative features such as a giant video screen above the main swimming pool showing movies and sports all day...and into the night. Still, while the ships are new, the overall experience is traditional compared with some of the bold and brash Mass-Market lines. The line has the usual activities, such as trivia contests, galley tours, art auctions, and middle-of-the-road musical revues—though some passengers report that they found fewer activities and diversions on Princess ships than they expected for vessels of this size. While its service gets raves and the food is fine, there is some repetition in the main dining room—expect the same dessert choices each night.

LUXURY LINES

While some purists (who reserve the "Luxury" label for something really top-class) prefer to call this category "Upper Premium," it's certainly a notch above the lines listed previously. Luxury lines typically use smaller ships, offer better food and service, command higher prices, and have a more exclusive clientele. You get what you pay for—this is a more dignified experience, with longer days in port and less emphasis on selling you extras. In general, while Luxury ships are very comfortable, the cruise is more focused on the destinations than the ship.

Once you're in this price range, you'll find that the various lines are variations on a theme (though there are a few notable exceptions, such as the unique casual-sailboat ambience of Windstar, or the opportunity to actually rig the sails on Star Clippers). It can be hard to distinguish among the lines; within the Luxury category, passengers tend to go with a cruise line recommended to them by a friend.

Note: Luxury and Ultra-Luxury lines (described later) generally run smaller ships, which can visit out-of-the-way ports that larger cruise ships can't. However, remember the drawbacks of smaller ships: fewer onboard activities, a narrower range of restaurants, and—for some travelers prone to seasickness—a slightly rougher ride.

Azamara Club Cruises

Contact Information: www.azamaraclubcruises.com, tel. 877-999-9553

Number and Capacity of Ships: *Journey* and *Quest* each carry 686 passengers

Average Hours in Port: 11-12 hours

Description: Azamara Club Cruises attracts a moderately affluent, educated, and active middle-age to retirement-age traveler. Their stated aim is to allow their customers to immerse themselves in each destination. Azamara passengers want value and are interested in more unusual destinations and longer port stays—their itineraries include more frequent overnight stops. The clientele is mainly American and British, along with a few Germans and other nationalities. There are no programs or facilities for children.

The atmosphere is casual, with open seating at meals and a focus on good food and wine; the cuisine is Mediterranean-influenced with other international dishes and healthy options. With a high crew-to-passenger ratio, the service is attentive. Live entertainment is more limited than on larger ships; the types of programs encourage meeting other guests, which contributes to a cozier, more social experience.

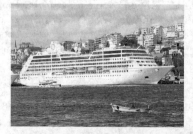

Cabins and bathrooms can be small, but are well laid-out. The company's good-value, all-inclusive pricing covers many amenities you'd pay extra for on other lines, such as good house wine, specialty coffees, bottled water and sodas, basic gratuities (for cabin stewards, bar, and dining), self-service laundry, and shuttle buses in some ports.

Oceania Cruises

Contact Information: www.oceaniacruises.com, tel. 855-OCEANIA

Number and Capacity of Ships: *Marina* and *Riviera* each carry 1,250 passengers; *Insignia, Nautica,* and *Regatta* each carry 684

Average Hours in Port: 9-10 hours

Description: Oceania Cruises appeals to well-traveled, well-heeled baby boomers and older retirees who want fine cuisine, excellent service, and a destination-oriented experience—toeing the fine line between upscale and snooty. The atmosphere is casually sophisticated—tastefully understated elegance. Although the line does not discourage children, kids' amenities (and young passengers) are sparse. Oceania's itineraries tend to be on the longer side; European sailings under 10 days are rare.

Staterooms are particularly well-equipped, reminiscent of stylish boutique hotels, with a cozy and intimate atmosphere. On the smaller ships, the staterooms and bathrooms are smaller than on most Luxury ships—but with great beds and fine linens. Oceania touts its cuisine; some of their menus were designed by celebrity chef Jacques Pépin, and their ships have a variety of specialty restaurants—French, Italian, steakhouse, and so on—for no extra charge (but reserve ahead). The larger ships have a culinary arts center with hands-on workshops (for a fee).

Oceania is noted for courting experienced crew members and for low crew turnover. The ships offer extensive onboard libraries, but relatively few organized activities, making these cruises best for those who can entertain themselves (or who make the most of time in port). While a few extras (such as specialty coffee drinks) are included, others are still à la carte; these, and Oceania's excursions, are a bit pricier than average.

Star Clippers

Contact Information: www.starclippers.com, tel. 800-442-0551

Number and Capacity of Ships: *Royal Clipper* carries 227 passengers; *Star Clipper* and *Star Flyer* each carry 170

Average Hours in Port: 8-9 hours

Description: Star Clippers takes its sailing heritage very seriously, and its three ships are among the world's largest and tallest sailing vessels (actual "tall ships," with diesel engines for backup power).

While the Windstar ships (described next) also have sails, those are mostly for show—Star Clippers' square-riggers are real sailboats. Passengers with nautical know-how are invited to pitch in when sails are hoisted or lowered. If the weather is right during the trip, you can even climb the main mast up to the crow's nest (wearing a safety harness, of course). There's a goose-bump-inducing ceremony every time you leave port: The crew raises the sails while haunting music plays over the loudspeakers.

With its sailing focus, Star Clippers draws more active, adventurous customers, ranging in age from 30s to 70s, who don't need to be pampered. Passengers are primarily Europeans (one recent sailing had passengers from 38 countries), and almost 60 percent are repeat customers. People who choose Star Clippers love the simple life on board a sailboat; enjoy a casual, easygoing cruise experience; and don't want the nightclubs and casinos offered by mainstream cruise lines. Kids are welcome, but there are no children's programs, counselors, or video-game parlors. Given the constraints of a small vessel, the cabins are not as big or luxurious as you might expect at this price range (for example, none have verandas).

The food, while adequate, comes in modest (European-size) portions. There's open seating in the dining room, the dress code is casual, and there are no rigid schedules. Activities include beach barbecues, crab races, scavenger hunts, talent nights, fashion shows, and performances by local musicians. You'll also have access to complimentary water activities, including snorkeling, kayaking, and sailing.

Windstar Cruises

Contact Information: www.windstarcruises.com, tel. 800-258-7245

Number and Capacity of Ships: *Wind Surf* carries 310 passengers, *Wind Star* and *Wind Spirit* each carry 148, and *Star Pride*, *Star Breeze*, and *Star Legend* each carry 212

Average Hours in Port: 10 hours

Description: Windstar's gimmick is its sails—each of its ships has four big, functional sails that unfurl dramatically each time the ship leaves port. (While the sails are capable of powering the ship in strong winds, they're more decorative than practical—although they do reduce the amount of fuel used by the engines.) This line provides an enticing bridge between the more rough-around-the-edges sailboat experience of Star Clippers (described above) and the comforts of mainstream lines. For many, it's an ideal combination—the romance of sails plus the pampering of a Luxury cruise. For this price range, it has a relatively casual atmosphere, with no formal nights.

Windstar passengers are professionals and experienced independent-minded travelers who range in age from 40s to 70s. First-time cruisers, honeymooners, and anniversary celebrants are enticed by Windstar's unique approach. The smaller ships favor more-focused itineraries and smaller ports, with generous time ashore. Passengers are more "travelers" than "cruisers"— they're here to spend as much time as possible exploring the port towns.

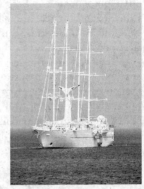

The small vessels also mean fewer on-ship activities. The casino and swimming pool are minuscule, the smaller ships have only one specialty restaurant, and nightlife is virtually nonexistent. However, the lounge hosts talented musicians, and each stateroom has a DVD player (there's a free DVD library). On some days when the ship is tendered, they lower a platform from the stern, allowing passengers to enjoy water-sports activities right off the back of the vessel. The food is high-quality, and there's a barbecue night on the open deck. Windstar also touts its green-ness (thanks to those sails) and its rare open-bridge policy, whereby passengers can visit the bridge during certain times to see the instruments and chat with the captain and officers.

ULTRA-LUXURY
You'll pay top dollar for these cruises, but get an elite experience in return. The basic features of the previously described Luxury cruises apply to this category as well: small ships (with the exception of Crystal), upscale clientele, a classier atmosphere, less emphasis on onboard activities, and a more destination-focused experience. There's less focus on selling you extras—at these prices, you can expect more and more extras to be included (ranging from alcoholic drinks to shore excursions).

Crystal Cruises
Contact Information: www.crystalcruises.com, tel. 888-722-0021
Number and Capacity of Ships: *Serenity* carries 1,070 passengers; *Symphony* carries 922 passengers
Average Hours in Port: 10 hours
Description: While most Luxury and Ultra-Luxury lines have smaller ships, Crystal Cruises distinguishes itself by operating larger ships, closer in size to the less-expensive categories. This allows it to offer more big-ship activities and amenities, while still fostering a genteel, upper-crust ambience (which some may

consider "stuffy"). Crystal attracts a retired, well-traveled, well-heeled crowd (although there are also a fair number of people under 50). Approximately 75 percent of the travelers are from the US and Canada, and the rest are mainly British. There are basic programs for children (most kids seem to come with multigenerational family groups) that are better than those on most Ultra-Luxury lines.

The food and the service are both well-regarded (and their seafood comes from sustainable and fair-trade sources). Their acclaimed enrichment programs are noted for having a wide range of minicourses in everything from foreign languages to computer skills, and excursions include opportunities for passengers to participate in a local volunteering effort.

Note: Crystal Cruises are sold exclusively through travel agents.

Regent Seven Seas Cruises (RSSC)

Contact Information: www.rssc.com, tel. 1-844-4Regent
Number and Capacity of Ships: *Voyager* and *Mariner* each carry 700 passengers; *Navigator* carries 490
Average Hours in Port: 10-11 hours
Description: Regent Seven Seas Cruises appeal to well-educated, sophisticated, and affluent travelers—generally from mid-40s to retirees—looking for a destination-oriented experience. Their exclusive, clubby, understatedly elegant atmosphere attracts many repeat cruisers (the *Voyager* seems especially popular). Most passengers are from North America, with the rest from Great Britain, New Zealand, and Australia. The line welcomes families during summer and school breaks, when it offers a children's program; the rest of the year, there's little to occupy kids.

Their "ultra-inclusive" prices are, indeed, among the most inclusive in the industry, covering premium soft drinks, house wines, tips, ground transfers, round-trip airfare from the US, one night's pre-cruise hotel stay, and unlimited excursions. The ships are known for their spacious, elegantly appointed suites (all with verandas). This line has some of the industry's highest space-per-guest and crew member-per-guest ratios, and customers report outstanding service. The French-based cuisine has an international flair, and also attempts to mix in local fare from the ships' ports of call. Passengers tend to be independent-minded and enjoy making their own plans, rather than wanting to be entertained by the cruise line (the entertainment is low-key, and notably, there is no onboard photography service). The crew tries to incorporate the ship's destinations into the entertainment, events, and lectures. Excursions include private tours, strenuous walking tours, and some soft-adventure offerings such as kayaking.

Seabourn Cruise Line

Contact Information: www.seabourn.com, tel. 866-755-5619
Number and Capacity of Ships: *Odyssey, Sojourn,* and *Quest* each carry 450 passengers
Average Hours in Port: 10 hours
Description: Seabourn Cruise Line attracts affluent, well-traveled couples in their late 40s to late 60s and older, who are not necessarily cruise aficionados but are accustomed to the "best of the best." Deep down, Seabourn passengers want to be on a yacht, but don't mind sharing it with other upper-class travelers—who, as the line brags, are "both interesting and interested." The focus is on exploring more exotic destinations rather than just relaxing on the ship. Most passengers are American, and the onboard atmosphere is classically elegant. Kids are present in summer and during school vacations, usually with multigenerational groups.

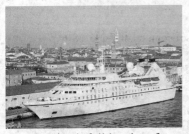

These ships feel like private clubs, with pampering as a priority. The extremely high crew member-to-guest ratio is about 1:1, and the crew addresses guests by name. Activities are designed for socializing with other passengers. Most of the ships offer a stern platform for swimming and kayaking right off the back of the ship. The line's all-inclusive pricing includes freebies like a welcome bottle of champagne, an in-suite bar (with full bottles of your preselected booze), and nearly all drinks, including decent wines at mealtime (you pay extra only for premium brands). Also included are tips, some excursions, poolside mini-massages, and activities such as exercise classes and wine-tasting seminars.

SeaDream Yacht Club

Contact Information: www.seadream.com, tel. 800-707-4911
Number and Capacity of Ships: *SeaDream I* and *SeaDream II* each carry 110 passengers
Average Hours in Port: 12+ hours
Description: SeaDream's tiny, intimate ships—the smallest of all those described here—are essentially chic, Ultra-Luxury megayachts. This line appeals to active travelers who are well-heeled and well-traveled, ranging in age from 40s to 70s (the shorter itineraries appeal to those still working). Passengers are primarily from North America and Europe, the atmosphere is laid-back, and the dress code is country-club casual (with no formal nights). There are no kids' facilities or services on board.

The attentive crew anticipates guests' needs without fawning.

The unstructured environment is best for independent-minded passengers, as you're pretty much on your own for entertainment. The line is perfect for those who want to relax on deck and be outdoors as much as possible. In fact, a unique—and extremely popular—activity is sleeping out under the stars on double loungers. Itineraries include overnight stays in port (allowing guests the option to experience local nightlife) and are somewhat flexible, allowing the captain to linger longer in a port or depart early. Rather than hiring local guides for all their shore excursions, some trips are led by the ship's officers or other crew members. (Note that organized excursions may be canceled if the quota isn't reached, which can happen, given the small number of passengers.) The ships have a sports platform off the stern with water-sports toys such as kayaks and water skis, and there's a fleet of mountain bikes for exploring the destinations. Prices include decent house wines, cocktails, tips, water-sports equipment, DVDs, and shore excursions.

Silversea Cruises
Contact Information: www.silversea.com, tel. 877-276-6816
Number and Capacity of Ships: *Silver Spirit* carries 540 passengers, *Silver Whisper* carries 382, *Silver Wind* and *Silver Cloud* each carry 296, and *Silver Shadow* carries 382
Average Hours in Port: 11 hours
Description: The Italian-owned, Monaco-based Silversea Cruises is popular with well-educated, well-traveled, upper-crust cruisers, generally ranging in age from late 40s to 80s (with many in their 70s). Most passengers are accustomed to the finest and are very discriminating. The ships' Art Deco design lends an elegant 1930s ambience, and the atmosphere on board is clubby. Half of their clientele is from North America, with the other half predominantly from the UK, Europe, and Australia. There are no organized children's programs, and you'll see few children on board.

The cuisine is very good, and the service excellent; the spacious suites even have an assigned butler. Partly as a function of the ships' small size and fewer passengers, the events and entertainment are low-key.

BOOKING A CRUISE

Once you've narrowed down your cruise-line options, it's time to get serious about booking. This chapter covers where, when, and how to book your cruise, including pointers on cruise pricing, cabin assignments, trip insurance, pre- and post-cruise plans, and other considerations.

Where to Book a Cruise

While plane tickets, rental cars, hotels, and most other aspects of travel have gradually migrated to do-it-yourself, cruises are the one form of travel that is still booked predominantly through a travel agent.

While it's possible to book a cruise directly with the cruise line, most lines actually prefer that you go through an intermediary. That's because their customers are rarely just booking a cruise—while they're at it, they want to look into airfares, trip insurance, maybe some hotels at either end of the cruise, and so on. That's beyond the scope of what cruise lines want to sell—their booking offices mainly take orders, they don't advise—so they reduce their overhead by letting travel agents do all that hard work (and hand-holding).

It can also be cheaper to book through a travel agent. Some cruise lines discount fares that are sold through their preferred agents; because they've built up relationships with these agents over the years, they don't want to undersell them. In other cases, the travel agency reserves a block of cabins to secure the lowest possible price, and then passes the savings on to their customers.

There are, generally speaking, two different types of cruise-sales agencies: your neighborhood travel agent, where you can get in-person advice; or a giant company that sells most of its inventory online or by phone. Because cruise prices vary based on volume, a big agency can usually undersell a small one. Big agencies are also more likely to offer incentives (such as onboard credit or cabin upgrades) to sweeten the pot. However, some small agencies belong to a consortium that gives them as much collective clout as a big agency. And some travelers figure the intangible value of personal service they get at a small agency is worth the possibility of paying a little extra. (Although most travel agents don't charge a fee, their commission is built into the cruise price.)

The big cruise agencies often have websites where you can easily shop around for the best price. These include www.vacationstogo.com, www.cruisecompete.com, and www.crucon.com. One site, www.cayole.com, tries to predict when prices for a particular departure may be lowest—giving you advice about how soon you should book.

I use the big websites to do some comparison-shopping. But—call me old-fashioned—when it comes time to book, I prefer to sit down with a travel agent to make my plans in person. Ideally, find a well-regarded travel agent in your community who knows cruising and will give you the personal attention you need to sort through your options. Tell them the deals you've seen online, and ask if they can match or beat them. A good travel agent knows how to look at your whole travel picture (airfare, hotels, and so on), not just the cruise component. And they can advise you about "insider" information, such as how to select the right cabin. Keep in mind that if you do solicit the advice of a travel agent, you should book the cruise through them—that's the only way they'll get their hard-earned commission. Once you've booked your cruise, you can arrange airfare through your travel agent, or you may choose to do that part on your own; for hotels, I always book direct.

When to Book a Cruise

Most cruise lines post their schedules a year or more in advance. A specific departure is called a "sailing." If you want to cruise in the summertime, and your plans are very specific (for example, you have your heart set on a certain sailing, or a particular cabin setup, such as adjoining staterooms), it's best to begin looking the preceding November. (For cruises in shoulder season—spring and fall—you may have a little more time to shop around.) Because the cruise lines want to fill up their ships as fast as possible, they typically offer early-booking discounts if you buy your cruise well in advance (at least 6-12 months, depending on the company).

Meanwhile, the most popular time of year to book a cruise is during the first few weeks of January. Dubbed "wave season" by industry insiders, this is when a third of all cruises are booked. If

Sample Pretrip Timeline

While this can vary, here's a general timeline for what to do and when—but be sure to carefully confirm with your specific cruise line.

What to Do	Time Before Departure
Book cruise and pay initial deposit	8-10 months (for best selection)
Buy trip insurance, if desired	At time of booking (if through cruise line); within about 2 weeks of booking (if through a third party)
Full payment due	45-60 days
Online check-in	Between booking and full payment (check with cruise line)
Fly to meet your cruise	1-2 days ahead (remember you lose one day when flying from the US to Europe)

you wait until this time, you'll be competing with other travelers for the deals. The sooner you book, the more likely you are to have your choice of sailing and cabin type—and potentially an even better price.

If a cruise still has several cabins available 90 days before departure, they're likely to put them on sale—but don't count on it. People tend to think the longer they wait, the more likely it is they'll find a sale. But this isn't always the case. Last-minute sales aren't as likely for Europe as they are for some other destinations, such as the Caribbean. Unlike the Caribbean market, the European market has a much shorter season and fewer ships, which means fewer beds to fill...and fewer deals to fill them. And even if you do find a last-minute deal, keep in mind that last-minute airfares to Europe can be that much more expensive.

If you're unsure of when to book, consult your travel agent.

How to Book a Cruise

Once you find the cruise you want, your travel agent may be able to hold it for you for a day or two while you think it over. When you've decided, you'll secure your passage on the cruise by paying a deposit. While this varies by cruise line, it averages about $500 per person (this becomes nonrefundable after a specified date, sometimes immediately—ask when you book). No matter how far ahead you book, you generally won't have to pay the balance until 45-60 days before departure. After this point, cancellation comes at a heftier price; as the departure date approaches, your cruise becomes effectively nonrefundable. In general, read the fine print of your cruise ticket carefully.

CRUISE PRICING

Like cars or plane tickets, cruises are priced very flexibly. Some cruise lines don't even bother listing prices in their brochures—they just send customers to the Web. In general, for a Mass-Market cruise, you'll rarely pay the list price. Higher-end cruises are less likely to be discounted.

The main factor that determines the actual cost of a cruise is demand (that is, the popularity of the date, destination, and specific ship), but other factors also play a role.

Cruise lines and travel agencies use **sales and incentives** to entice new customers. With the recent proliferation of megaships, there are plenty of cabins to fill, and cruise industry insiders rigidly follow the mantra, "Empty beds are not tolerated!" The obvious approach to filling up a slow-selling cruise is to reduce prices. But they may also offer "onboard credit," which can be applied to your expenses on the ship (such as tips, alcoholic drinks, or excursions). In other cases, they may automatically upgrade your stateroom ("Pay for Category C, and get a Category B cabin for no extra charge!"). To further entice you, they might even throw in a special cocktail reception with the captain, or a night or two at a hotel at either end of your cruise. Your travel agent should be aware of these sales; you can also look online, or—if you're a fan of a particular cruise line—sign up to get their email offers.

Some cruise lines offer **discounts** for seniors (including AARP members), AAA members, firefighters, military, union workers, teachers, those in the travel industry, employees of certain corporations, and so on. It never hurts to ask.

Keep in mind that you'll pay a premium for **novelty.** It usually costs more to go on the cruise line's newest, most loudly advertised vessel. If you go on a ship that's just a few years older—with most of the same amenities—you'll likely pay less.

If you are a **repeat cruiser**—or think you may become one—sign up for the cruise line's "frequent cruiser" program. Like the airlines' mileage-rewards programs, these offer incentives, upgrades, and access to special deals.

No matter who you book your cruise through, use a **credit card** to give yourself a measure of consumer protection. A credit-card company can be a strong ally in resolving disputes.

If the **price drops after you book** your cruise, try asking for the new price. A good time to ask is just before or when you make the final payment. They don't have all your money yet and tend to be more eager to look for specials that will reduce your bottom line. You'll often be given a discount, or possibly an upgrade.

Taxes, Port Fees, and Other Hidden Charges

The advertised price for your cruise isn't all you'll have to pay. All the miscellaneous taxes, fees, and other expenses that the ship incurs in port are divvied up and passed on to passengers, under the category **"taxes and port fees."** While this can vary dramatically from port to port, it'll run you a few hundred dollars per person. These amounts are not locked in at the time you book; if a port increases its fees, you'll pay the difference.

Like airlines, cruise lines reserve the right to tack on a **"fuel surcharge"** in the event that the price of oil goes over a certain amount per barrel. This can be added onto your bill even after you book the cruise.

Once you're on the cruise, most lines automatically levy an **"auto-tip"** of around $10-12/day per person (which you can adjust upward or downward once on board). While this won't be included in your up-front cruise cost, you should budget for it. Many cruisers also choose to give excellent crew members an additional cash tip. For more details on tipping, see page 79.

SPECIAL CONSIDERATIONS

Families, singles, groups, people celebrating milestones, and those with limited mobility are all special in my book.

If you're traveling with a family, note that fares for **kids** tend to be more expensive during spring break and summertime, when they're out of school and demand is high; it can be cheaper to bring them off-season. Adjoining staterooms (also called "connecting" rooms) that share an inside door tend to book up early, particularly in the summertime. If those are sold out, consider an inside cabin across from an outside cabin. Some rooms have fold-down bunk beds (or "upper berths"), so a family of three or four can cram into one room (each passenger after the second pays a reduced fare)—but the tight quarters, already cramped for two people, can be challenging for the whole clan. Like connecting staterooms, these triple or quad cabins sell out early. Note that women who are more than six months **pregnant**—and **babies** who are younger than six months—are typically not allowed on a cruise.

Single cabins are rare on cruise ships; almost all staterooms are designed with couples in mind. Therefore, cruise rates are quoted per person, based on double occupancy. If you're traveling solo, you'll usually have to pay a "single supplement." This can range from reasonable (an additional 10 percent of the per-person double rate) to exorbitant ("100 percent" of the double rate—in other words, paying as much as two people would). On average, figure paying about 50 percent above the per-person double rate for your own single cabin. Sometimes it's possible to avoid the single supplement by volunteering to be assigned a random roommate by the cruise line, but this option is increasingly rare.

Groups taking eight or more cabins may be eligible for

discounts if they're booked together—ask. The discounts often don't add up to much, but you may wrangle a shipboard credit or a private cocktail party.

If you'll be celebrating a **special occasion**—such as a birthday or anniversary—on board, mention it when you book. You may get a special bonus, such as a fancy dessert or cocktails with the captain.

If you have **limited mobility,** cruising can be a good way to go—but not all cruise lines are created equal. Some ships are wheelchair-accessible, including fully adapted cabins; others (especially small vessels) may not even have an elevator. When shopping for your cruise, ask the cruise line about the features you'll need, and be very specific. Unfortunately, once you reach port, all bets are off. While some cities are impressively accessible, others (especially smaller towns) may have fewer elevators than the ship you arrived on. The creaky and cobbled Old World doesn't accommodate wheelchairs or walkers very well. Taking a shore excursion can be a good way to see a place with minimum effort; cruise lines can typically inform you of the specific amount of walking and stairs you'll need to tackle for each excursion.

CABIN CLASSES

Each cruise ship has a variety of staterooms. In some cases, it can be a pretty narrow distinction ("Category A" and the marginally smaller "Category B"). On other ships, it can be the difference between a "Class 1" suite with a private balcony and a "Class 10" windowless bunk-bed closet below the waterline. On its website, each cruise line explains the specific breakdown of its various categories, along with the amenities in each one. In general, the highest demand is for the top-end and bottom-end cabins. Also, as verandas are increasingly popular, the most affordable rooms with verandas are often the first fares to sell out.

You'll see these terms:

Inside/Interior: An inside cabin has no external windows (though there's often a faux porthole to at least create the illusion of outside light). While these terrify claustrophobes, inside cabins offer a great value that tempts budget travelers. And many cruisers figure that with a giant ship to explore—not to mention Europe at your doorstep each morning—there's not much point hanging out in your room anyway.

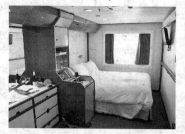

Outside: With a window to the sea, an outside cabin costs more—but for some travelers, it's worth the splurge to be able to see the world go by. But be aware that you're rarely able to open those windows (for that, you need a veranda). If your view is blocked (by a lifeboat, for example), it should be classified as "obstructed."

Veranda: Going one better than an outside cabin, a "veranda" is cruise jargon for a small outdoor balcony attached to your

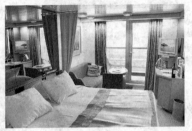

room. Because windows can't be opened, one big advantage of a veranda is that you can slide open the door to get some fresh air. The size and openness of verandas can vary wildly; for wind-shear reasons, some verandas can be almost entirely enclosed, with only a big picture window-sized opening to the sea. Sitting on the veranda while you cruise sounds appealing, but keep in mind that most of the time you're sailing, it'll be dark outside.

Suite: A multiroom suite represents the top end of cruise accommodations. These are particularly handy for families, but if you can't spring for a suite, ask about adjoining staterooms (see earlier).

Location Within Ship: In general, the upper decks (with better views, and typically bigger windows and more light) are more desirable—and more expensive—than the lower decks. Cabins in the middle of the ship (where the "motion of the ocean" is less noticeable) are considered better than those at either end. And cabins close to the engines (low and to the rear of the ship) can come with extra noise and vibrations.

Look for the **deck plan** on your cruise line's website. If you have a chance to select your own cabin (see next section), study the deck plan carefully to choose a good location. You'd want to avoid a cabin directly below a deck that has a lot of noisy foot traffic (such as the late-night disco or stewards dragging pool chairs across the deck).

Cabin Assignments and Upgrades

Cruise lines handle specific cabin assignments in different ways. While some cruise lines let you request a specific stateroom when you book, others don't offer that option; they'll assign your stateroom number at a future date. In other cases, you can request a "guarantee"—you pay for a particular class and are guaranteed that class of cabin (or better), but are not yet assigned a specific stateroom. As time passes and the cruise line gets a better sense of the occupancy on your sailing, there's a possibility that they will upgrade you to a better cabin for no extra charge. There's no way of predicting when you'll find out your specific cabin assignment—it can be months before departure, or days before. (Cabin assignments seem to favor repeat cruisers, rewarding customers for their loyalty.)

If you need a specific type of stateroom—for instance, you have limited mobility and need to be close to the elevator, or you're traveling with a large family and want to be as close together as possible—opt for a specific cabin assignment as early as you can.

If you don't have special needs, you might as well take your chances with a "guarantee"; you're assured of getting the class of cabin that you paid for...and you could wind up with a bonus veranda.

Assigned Dining: Traditionally, cruisers reserved not only their stateroom, but also which table and at what time they'd like to have dinner each night. Called a "seating," this tradition is fading. It's still mandatory on a few lines, but most lines either make it optional or have done away with it entirely. If your cruise line requires (or you prefer) a specific seating, reserve it when you book your cruise or cabin. (For more on assigned dining, see page 96.)

TRAVEL INSURANCE

Travel insurance can minimize the considerable financial risks of traveling: accidents, illness, cruise cancellations due to bad weather, missed flights, lost baggage, medical expenses, and emergency evacuation. If you anticipate any hiccups that may prevent you from taking your trip, travel insurance can protect your investment.

Trip-cancellation insurance lets you bail out without losing all of the money you paid for the cruise, provided you cancel for an acceptable reason, such as illness or a death in the family. This insurance also covers trip interruptions—if you begin a journey but have to cut it short for a covered reason, you'll be reimbursed for the portion of the trip that you didn't complete.

Travel insurance is also handy in the unlikely event that your ship breaks down midtrip. Though the cruise line should reimburse you for the cruise itself, travel insurance provides more surefire protection and can cover unexpected expenses, such as hotels or additional transportation you might need once you've gotten off the ship.

Travel insurance also includes basic medical coverage—up to a certain amount. If you have an accident or come down with a case of the "cruise-ship virus," your policy will cover doctor visits, treatment, and medication (though you'll generally have to pay a deductible). This usually includes medical evacuation—in the event that you become seriously ill and need to be taken to the nearest adequate medical care (that is, a big, modern hospital).

Baggage insurance, included in most comprehensive policies

(and in some homeowner or renter insurance policies), reimburses you for luggage that's lost, stolen, or damaged. However, some items aren't covered (ask for details when you buy). When you check a bag on a plane, it's covered by the airline (though, again, there are limits—ask).

Insurance prices vary dramatically, but most packages cost between 5 and 12 percent of the price of your trip. Two factors affect the price: the trip cost and your age at the time of purchase (rates go up dramatically for every decade over 50). For instance, to insure a 70-year-old traveler for a $3,000 cruise, the prices can range from about $150 to $430, depending on the level of coverage. To insure a 40-year-old for that same cruise, the cost can be about $90-215. Coverage is generally inexpensive or even free for children 17 and under. To ensure maximum coverage, it's smart to buy your insurance policy within a week of the date you make the first payment on your trip. Research policies carefully; if you wait too long to purchase insurance, you may be denied certain kinds of coverage, such as for pre-existing medical conditions.

Cruise lines offer their own travel insurance, but these policies generally aren't as comprehensive as those from third-party insurance companies. For example, a cruise-line policy only covers the cruise itself; if you book your airfare and pre- and post-cruise hotels separately, they will not be covered. And if your cruise line ceases operations, their insurance likely won't cover it. On the other hand, many cruise-line policies are not tied to age—potentially making them attractive to older passengers who find third-party policies prohibitively expensive.

Reputable independent providers include Betins (www.betins. com, tel. 866-552-8834 or 253/238-6374), Allianz (www.allianz travelinsurance.com, tel. 866-884-3556), Travelex (www.travelex insurance.com, tel. 800-228-9792), Travel Guard (www.travel guard.com, tel. 800-826-4919), and Travel Insured International (www.travelinsured.com, tel. 800-243-3174). InsureMyTrip allows you to compare insurance policies and costs among various providers (they also sell insurance; www.insuremytrip.com, tel. 800-487-4722).

Some credit-card companies may offer limited trip-cancellation or interruption coverage for cruises purchased with the card—it's worth checking before you buy a policy. Also, check whether your existing insurance (health, homeowners, or renters) covers you and your possessions overseas. For more tips, see www. ricksteves.com/insurance.

AIRFARE AND PRE- AND POST-CRUISE TRAVEL

When booking your airfare, think carefully about how much time you want before and after your cruise. Remember that most

Europe-bound flights from the US travel overnight and arrive the following day. The nearest airport is often far from the cruise port; allow plenty of time to get to your ship. You'll need to check in at least two hours before your cruise departs (confirm with your cruise line; most passengers show up several hours earlier).

If your travel plans are flexible, consider arriving a few days before your cruise and/or departing a few days after it ends—particularly if the embarkation and disembarkation points are places you'd like to explore. Remember, if you arrive just hours before (or depart just hours after) your cruise, you won't actually have any time to see the beginning and ending ports at all. Common starting and ending points include Copenhagen, Stockholm, Amsterdam, and ports near London (Southampton and Dover)—all of which merit plenty of time (and are covered a little more thoroughly in this book for that reason).

Arriving at least a day early makes it less likely that you'll miss the start of your cruise if your flight is delayed. If you miss the ship, you're on your own to catch up with it at its next port. In talking with fellow cruisers, while I've rarely heard of people missing the boat at a port of call, I've heard many horror stories about flight delays causing passengers to miss the first day of the cruise—and often incurring a time-consuming, stressful, and costly overland trip to meet their ship at the next stop.

In the past, most cruises included what they called "free air" (or "air/sea"), but these days your airfare to and from Europe costs extra—and you're usually best off booking it yourself. (Relatively few cruise passengers book airfare through their cruise line.) If you book your airfare through the cruise line, you'll typically pay more, but in case of a flight delay, the cruise line will help you meet the cruise at a later point. However, booking your airfare this way has its disadvantages—the cruise line chooses which airline and routing to send you on. They'll select an airline they have a contract with, regardless of whether it's one you want to fly (though it's sometimes possible to pay a "deviation fee" to switch to an airline and routing of your choice).

If you decide to add some days on either end of your trip, it's best to make your own arrangements for hotels and transfers. While most cruise lines offer pre- and post-tour packages (that include the hotel, plus transfers to and from the airport and the cruise port), they tend to be overpriced. For each of the arrival and departure cities in this book, I've recommended a few hotels for you to consider.

Some embarkation ports are quite distant from town (for example, Dover and Southampton are each about 80 miles from London). For these ports, a cruise-line airport transfer—which can save you a complicated journey through a big city's downtown—may be worth considering. You can often book a transfer even if you're booking your pre- or post-tour hotel on your own—ask.

In some rare circumstances, it's convenient for a cruise passenger to leave the ship before the cruise is completed—for example, you want to get off to have some extra time in Tallinn, rather than spend a day at sea to return to your starting point in Copenhagen. Cruise lines usually permit this, but you'll pay for the full cost of the cruise (including the portion you're not using), and you'll need to get permission in advance.

ONLINE CHECK-IN

At some point between when you book and when your final payment is due, you'll be invited to check in online for your cruise. This takes only a few minutes. You'll register your basic information and sometimes a credit-card number (for onboard purchases—or you can do this in person when you arrive at the ship). Once registered, you'll be able to print out e-documents (such as your receipt and boarding pass), access information about shipboard life, and learn about and prebook shore excursions.

TRAVEL SKILLS FOR CRUISING

BEFORE YOUR CRUISE

As any sailor knows, prepare well and you'll enjoy a smoother voyage. This chapter covers what you should know before you go (including red tape, money matters, and other practicalities), as well as pointers for packing.

Know Before You Go

RED TAPE

You need a **passport** to travel to the countries covered in this book. You may be denied entry into certain European countries if your passport is due to expire within three months of your ticketed date of return (Russia requires a six-month window). Get it renewed if you'll be cutting it close. It can take up to six weeks to get or renew a passport (for more on passports, see www.travel.state.gov).

If your itinerary includes **St. Petersburg, Russia,** you'll have to decide if you want a visa: You'll need one to explore the city on your own—but it's pricey and must be arranged well in advance. If you pay for cruise-line excursions, you don't need a visa but must stay with your guide at all times. For all the details, see page 352.

If you're traveling with **kids,** each minor must possess a passport. Grandparents or guardians can bring kids on board sans parents only if they have a signed, notarized document from the parent(s) to prove to authorities that they have permission to take the child on a trip. Even a single parent traveling with children has to demonstrate that the other parent has given approval. Specifically, the letter should grant permission for the accompanying adult to travel internationally with the child. Include your name, the name of your child, the dates of your trip, destination countries, and the name, address, and phone number of the parent(s) at home. If you have a different last name from your

Before-You-Go Checklist

Here are a few things to consider as you prepare for your cruise:

❑ Contact your **credit- and debit-card companies** to tell them you're going abroad and to ask about fees, limits, and more; see next page.

❑ Ask your **health insurance** provider about overseas medical coverage, both on the ship and on shore. For more on health care, see page 82.

❑ Consider buying **trip insurance.** For details, see page 40.

❑ For cruises with **assigned dining,** request your preference for seating time and table size when you reserve. See page 96.

❑ Vegetarians, those with food allergies, or anyone with a **special diet** should notify their cruise line at least 30 days before departure. See page 95.

❑ Your US **mobile phone** may work in Europe; if you want the option to use it while traveling, contact your mobile-phone service provider for details. See page 87.

❑ Be sure that you **know the PIN** for your credit and/or debit cards. You will likely encounter the chip-and-PIN payment system, which is widely used in Europe. For details on this system, see page 130.

❑ If you'll be visiting St. Petersburg, decide whether you want to get a visa, which will enable you to sightsee independently in the city. For details, see page 352.

❑ Some major sights in St. Petersburg, Berlin, Amsterdam, and Paris offer or require reservations, and some sights sell tickets online. It's a time-saver, allowing you to bypass long ticket-buying lines. For a list of sights to book in advance, see page 50.

❑ If you'll be going to Warnemünde (Germany), check the train schedules at www.bahn.com for the best connections to and from Berlin, to help you decide whether to take the train or pay for an excursion. See page 563.

❑ If you'll be going to Flåm (Norwegian fjords), check the schedules for the "Norway in a Nutshell" route for the day of your visit (see www.ruteinfo.net)—and compare them to your arrival and all-aboard time to be sure you can comfortably fit it in. See page 765.

❑ **Smokers,** or those determined to avoid smoke, can ask about their ship's smoking policy. See page 86.

❑ If you're prone to **seasickness,** ask your doctor for advice; certain medication requires a prescription. For a rundown of seasickness treatments, see page 82.

❑ If you're taking a child on a cruise without both parents, you'll need a signed, notarized document from the parent(s). See facing page.

child, it's smart to bring a copy of the birth certificate (with your name on it). For parents of adopted children, it's a good idea to bring their adoption decree as well.

Before you leave on your trip, make two sets of **photocopies** of your passport, tickets, and other valuable documents (front and back). Pack one copy and leave the other copy with someone at home—to email or fax to you in case of an emergency. It's easier to replace a lost or stolen passport if you have a photocopy proving that you really had what you lost. A couple of passport-type pictures brought from home can expedite the replacement process.

MONEY

At the start of your cruise, you must register your credit card (either at check-in or on board the ship). All purchases are made using your room number, and you'll be billed for onboard purchases when you disembark. Be aware that the cruise line may put a hold on your credit card during your trip to cover anticipated shipboard expenses; if you have a relatively low limit, you might come uncomfortably close to it. If you're concerned, ask the cruise line what the amount of the hold will be.

For your time on **land,** bring both a credit card and a debit card. You'll use the debit card at cash machines (ATMs) to withdraw local cash for most purchases, and the credit card to pay for larger items. Some travelers carry a third card as a backup, in case one gets demagnetized or eaten by a temperamental machine. As an emergency reserve, I also bring a few hundred dollars in hard cash (in easy-to-exchange $20 bills).

Cash

Most cruise ships are essentially cashless (though you may want to bring some US cash for tipping). But on land, cash is just as desirable as it is at home. Don't bother changing money before you leave home—ATMs in Europe are easy to find and use (for details, see page 128). And skip traveler's checks—they're not worth the fees or waits in line at slow banks.

Credit and Debit Cards

For maximum usability, bring cards with a Visa or MasterCard logo. You'll also need to know the PIN code for each card in numbers, as there are no letters on European keypads. Before your trip, contact the company that issued your debit or credit cards and ask them a few questions.

• Confirm your card will work overseas, and alert them that you'll be using it in Europe; otherwise, they may deny transactions if they perceive unusual spending patterns.

• Ask for the specifics on transaction **fees.** When you use your credit or debit card—either for purchases or ATM withdrawals—you'll typically be charged additional "international transaction" fees of up to 3 percent (1 percent is normal) plus $5 per transaction. If your card's fees seem high, consider getting a different card just for your trip: Capital One (www.capitalone.com) and most credit unions have low-to-no international fees.

• If you plan to withdraw cash from ATMs, confirm your daily **withdrawal limit,** and if necessary, ask your bank to adjust it. Some travelers prefer a high limit that allows them to take out more cash at each ATM stop (saving on bank fees), while others prefer to set a lower limit in case their card is stolen. Note that foreign banks also set maximum withdrawal amounts for their ATMs. Also, remember that you're withdrawing the local currency, not dollars. Many frustrated travelers have walked away from ATMs thinking their cards were rejected, when actually they were asking for more cash in euros than their daily limit allowed.

• Find out your card's **credit limit.** Some cruise lines put a hold on your credit card to cover anticipated onboard expenses; if this or your on-shore spending is likely to crowd your limit, ask for a higher amount or bring a second credit card.

• Get your bank's emergency **phone number** in the US (but not its 800 number, which isn't accessible from overseas) to call collect if you have a problem.

• Ask for your credit card's **PIN** in case you need to make an emergency cash withdrawal or encounter Europe's "chip-and-PIN" system (for details, see page 130). The bank won't tell you your PIN over the phone, so allow time for it to be mailed to you.

PRACTICALITIES

Time Zones: While Norwegian cruises stay within the same time zone, cruises on the Baltic are prone to crossing time zones with each sailing. Most of Western Europe—from France to Norway, Denmark, Sweden, and Poland—is in the Central European time zone, or CET (generally six/nine hours ahead of the East/West Coasts of the US). Moving farther east, the Baltic States (Estonia, Latvia, Lithuania) and Finland are in the Eastern European time zone—one hour ahead of CET. And St. Petersburg, Russia, is yet another hour ahead (i.e., two hours ahead of CET). Britain is one hour earlier than CET, so if your cruise begins in London and stops in Tallinn on its way to St. Petersburg before ending in Copenhagen, you'll change your watch five times. Confusing as it sounds, time changes are clearly noted in the daily program—and your cabin steward will usually leave a reminder on your bed the evening before.

The exceptions are the beginning and end of Daylight Saving Time: Europe "springs forward" the last Sunday in March (two

Rick Steves Audio Europe

If you're bringing a mobile device, be sure to check out **Rick Steves Audio Europe,** where you can download free audio tours and hours of travel interviews (via the Rick Steves Audio Europe app, www.ricksteves.com/audioeurope, Google Play, or iTunes).

My self-guided **audio tours** are user-friendly, easy to follow, fun, and informative, covering the major sights and neighborhoods in London, Paris, Amsterdam, and Berlin. Compared to live tours, my audio tours are hard to beat: Nobody will stand you up, the quality is reliable, you can take the tour exactly when you like, and they're free.

Rick Steves Audio Europe also offers a far-reaching library of intriguing **travel interviews** with experts from around the globe.

weeks after most of North America), and "falls back" the last Sunday in October (one week before North America). For a handy online time converter, see www.timeanddate.com/worldclock.

Watt's Up? Virtually all cruise ships have American-style outlets, so you don't need an adapter or converter to charge your phone or blow-dry your hair. (If you're cruising with a European line, you may want to confirm the outlet type.)

But if you're staying at a hotel before or after the cruise, you'll need to adapt to Europe's electrical system, which is 220 volts, instead of North America's 110 volts. Most newer electronics (such as hair dryers, laptops, and battery chargers) convert automatically, so you won't need a converter, but you will need an adapter plug with three square prongs for Britain or two round prongs for the rest of Europe (sold inexpensively at travel stores in the US). Avoid bringing older appliances that don't automatically convert voltage; instead, buy a cheap replacement appliance in Europe.

Driving in Europe: If you're planning on renting a car, bring your driver's license. An International Driving Permit—an official translation of your driver's license—is recommended in France, Germany, Britain, and Scandinavia, and required in the Netherlands (sold at your local AAA office for $15 plus the cost of two passport-type photos; see www.aaa.com). While that's the letter of the law, I've often rented cars in these countries without having this permit. If all goes well, you'll likely never be asked to show the permit—but it's a must if you end up dealing with the police.

Reservations and Advance Tickets for Major Sights: If you plan ahead, you can scoot right into the following sights, avoiding long ticket-buying lines.

In **St. Petersburg,** the famous Hermitage (palace and art museum) lets you purchase tickets on their website (see page 387), as does Tsarskoye Selo, the palace complex on the outskirts of town (see page 429).

In **Berlin,** reservations are required for climbing the Reichstag dome (see page 595) and highly recommended for entering the Pergamon and Neues museums on Museum Island (see page 614).

In **Amsterdam,** several key sights—including the Rijksmuseum, the Van Gogh Museum, and the Anne Frank House—sell tickets online (see page 800).

In **Paris,** it's essential to reserve tickets for the Eiffel Tower in advance (see page 1093).

Discounts: While this book does not list discounts for sights and museums, seniors (age 60 and over), students with International Student Identification Cards, teachers with proper identification, and youths under 18 often get discounts—but you have to ask. To get a teacher or student ID card, visit www.statravel.com or www.isic.org.

Online Translation Tip: You can use Google's Chrome browser (available free at www.google.com/chrome) to instantly translate websites. With one click, the page appears in (very rough) English translation. You can also paste the URL of the site into the translation window at www.google.com/translate.

Packing

One of the advantages of cruising is unpacking just once—in your stateroom. But don't underestimate the importance of packing light. Cruise-ship cabins are cramped, and large suitcases consume precious living space. Plus, you'll still need to get to the airport, on and off the plane, and between the airport and the cruise port. The lighter your luggage is, the easier your transitions will be. And when you carry your own luggage, it's less likely to get lost, broken, or stolen.

Consider packing just one carry-on-size bag (9" by 21" by 14"). I know—realistically, you'll be tempted to bring more. But cruising with one bag can be done without adversely impacting your trip (I've done it, and was happy I did). No matter how much you'd like to bring along that warm jacket or extra pair of shoes, be strong and do your best to pack just what you need.

Here's another reason to favor carry-on bags: If the airline loses your checked luggage and doesn't get it to your embarkation port by the time your ship sets sail, the bags are unlikely to catch up to you. If you booked air travel through the cruise line, the company will do what it can to reunite you with your lost bags. But if you arranged your own flights, the airline decides whether and how to help you—and rarely will it fly your bags to your next port of call. (If you purchase travel insurance, it may cover lost luggage—ask when you buy; for details on insurance, see page 40.) For this reason, even if you check a bag, be sure you pack essentials (medications, change of clothes, travel documents) in your carry-on.

If you're traveling as part of a couple, and the one-piece-per-person idea seems impossible, consider this compromise: Pack one bag each, as if traveling alone, then share a third bag for bulky cruise extras (such as formal wear). If traveling before or after the cruise, you can leave that third, nonessential bag at a friendly hotel or in a train-station luggage locker, then be footloose and fancy-free for your independent travel time.

Remember, packing light isn't just about the trip over and back—it's about your traveling lifestyle. Too much luggage marks you as a typical tourist. With only one bag, you're mobile and in control. You'll never meet a traveler who, after five trips, brags: "Every year I pack heavier."

BAGGAGE RESTRICTIONS

Baggage restrictions provide a built-in incentive for packing light. Some cruise lines limit you to two bags of up to 50 pounds apiece; others don't enforce limits (or request only that you bring "a reasonable amount" of luggage). But all airlines have restrictions on the number, size, and weight of both checked and carry-on bags. These days, except on intercontinental flights, you'll most likely pay for each piece of luggage you check—and if your bag is overweight, you'll pay even more. Check the specifics on your airline's website (or read the fine print on your airline eticket).

Knives, lighters, and other potentially dangerous items are not allowed in airplane carry-ons or on board your cruise. Large quantities of liquids or gels must be packed away in checked baggage. Because restrictions are always changing, visit the Transportation Security Administration's website (www.tsa.gov) for an up-to-date list of what you can bring on the plane with you...and what you must check.

If you plan to check your bag for your flight, mark it inside and out with your name, address, and emergency phone number. If you have a lock on your bag, you may be asked to remove it to accommodate increased security checks, or it may be cut off so the bag can be inspected (to avoid this, consider a TSA-approved lock). I've never locked my bag, and I haven't had a problem. Still, just in case, I wouldn't pack anything valuable (such as cash or a camera) in my checked luggage.

As baggage fees increase, more people are carrying on their luggage. Arrive early for aircraft boarding to increase the odds that you'll snare coveted storage space in the passenger cabin.

WHAT TO BRING

How do you fit a whole trip's worth of luggage into one bag? The answer is simple: Bring very little. You don't need to pack for the worst-case scenario. Pack for the best-case scenario and simply buy yourself out of any jams. Bring layers rather than pack a heavy coat. Think in terms of what you can do without—not what might be handy on your trip. When in doubt, leave it out. The shops on your cruise ship (or on shore) are sure to have any personal items you forgot or have run out of.

Use the "Packing Checklist" on page 58 to organize and make your packing decisions.

Clothing

Most cruisers will want two to three changes of clothes each day: comfortable, casual clothes for sightseeing in port; more formal evening wear for dinners on the ship; and sportswear, whether it's a swimsuit for basking by the pool or athletic gear for hitting the gym or running track. But that doesn't mean you have to bring along 21 separate outfits for a seven-day cruise. Think versatile. Some port wear can double as evening wear. Two pairs of dressy dinner slacks can be worn on alternating nights, indefinitely. As you choose clothes for your trip, a good rule of thumb is: If you're not going to wear an item more than three times, don't pack it. Every piece of clothing you bring should complement every other item or have at least two uses (for example, a scarf doubles as a shoulder wrap; a sweater provides warmth and dresses up a short-sleeve shirt). Accessories, such as a tie or scarf, can break the monotony and make you look snazzy.

First-time cruisers may worry about "formal nights." While most cruises do have a few formal nights with a dress code, they're not as stuffy as you might think. And those formal nights are optional—you can always eat somewhere other than the formal dining room. So dress up only as much as you want to (but keep in mind that most cruise lines forbid shorts or jeans in the dining room at dinnertime). For a general idea of what people typically wear on board, read the sidebar on the next page, then find out what your ship's dress code is.

When choosing clothes for days in port, keep a couple of factors in mind: Most Northern European cruises set sail during the best-weather months of June, July, and August. While you shouldn't expect scorching Mediterranean temperatures, summer heat waves can hit Oslo and Berlin. But at these northern latitudes, it can get quite chilly—especially after the sun goes down. The key here is versatility: Wear layers, and always carry a lightweight sweater or raincoat in case clouds roll in and temperatures drop. Also, a few Northern European churches (particularly

Cruise Ship Dress Code

First-time cruisers sometimes worry about the need to dress up on their vacation. Relax. Cruise ships aren't as dressy as they used to be. And, while on certain nights you may see your fellow cruisers in tuxes and gowns, there's usually a place to go casual as well. (In general, the more upscale a cruise is, the more formal the overall vibe—though some luxury lines, such as Windstar, have a reputation for relaxed dress codes.)

During the day, cruisers wear shorts, T-shirts, swimsuits with cover-ups, flip-flops, or whatever they're comfortable in. (On pricier cruises, you may see more passengers in khakis or dressy shorts and polo shirts.)

But in the evenings, a stricter dress code emerges. On most nights, dinner is usually "smart casual" in the main dining room and at some (or all) specialty restaurants. People generally aren't too dressed up—though jeans, shorts, and T-shirts are no-nos. For men, slacks and a button-down or polo shirt is the norm; most women wear dresses, or pants or skirts with a nice top. Plan to wear something a little nicer on the first evening; after you get the lay of the land, you can adjust your wardrobe for the rest of the meals.

Most cruises host one or two "formal" nights per week. On these evenings, men are expected to put on jackets (and sometimes ties), while women generally wear cocktail dresses—or pair a dressy skirt or pants with a silky or sparkly top. Basically, dress as you would for a nice church wedding or a night at the theater. A few overachievers show up wearing tuxedos or floor-length dresses. Note that formal nights will sometimes extend beyond the dining room into the ship's main theater venue.

For those who don't want to dress up at all, most cruise ships have dining venues that are completely informal—the buffet, the poolside grill, and so on. If you never want to put on a collared shirt, you can simply eat at these restaurants for the entire cruise.

To pack light for your cruise, bring multifunctional clothing that allows you to go minimally formal and also feel chic in port. Men can get by with slacks and a sports coat. (I got a lot of good use out of my summery sports coat.) Women can wear a casual dress and jazz it up with accessories, such as jewelry or a wrap.

If you want to get decked out without lugging excess clothing on board, ask if your cruise line has a tuxedo-rental program (some cruise lines also offer a rental program for women's formal wear). You may be able to borrow a jacket or rent a tux on the spot, but selection can be limited—so it's better to order in advance. Simply provide your measurements beforehand, and a tux will be waiting in your cabin when you board.

Orthodox ones, such as those in St. Petersburg) enforce a strict "no shorts or bare shoulders" dress code. Pants with zip-off/zip-on legs can be handy in these situations.

Laundry options vary from ship to ship. Most provide 24-hour laundry service (at per-piece prices), enabling those without a lot of clothing to manage fine. But self-service launderettes are rare on board—ask your cruise line in advance about available options. Remember that you can still bring fewer clothes and wash as needed in your stateroom sink. It helps to pack items that don't wrinkle, or look good wrinkled. You should have no trouble drying clothing overnight in your cabin (though it might take longer in humid climates).

It can be worth splurging a little to get just the right clothes for your trip. For durable, lightweight travel clothes, consider ExOfficio (www.exofficio.com), TravelSmith (www.travelsmith.com), Tilley Endurables (www.tilley.com), Eddie Bauer (www.eddiebauer.com), and REI (www.rei.com).

Ultimately—as long as you don't wear something that's outrageous or offensive—it's important to dress in a way that makes you comfortable. No matter how carefully you dress, your clothes probably will mark you as an American. And so what? To fit in and be culturally sensitive, I watch my manners, not the cut of my clothes.

Here are a few specific considerations:

Shirts/blouses. Bring short-sleeved or long-sleeved shirts or blouses in a cotton/polyester blend, ideally in a wrinkle- and stain-camouflaging pattern. Synthetic-blend fabrics (such as Coolmax or microfiber) often dry overnight. A sweater or lightweight fleece is good for cool evenings (warm and dark is best—for layering and dressing up). Indoor areas on the cruise ship can be heavily air-conditioned, so you may need a long-sleeved top, a sweater, or a wrap even in the height of summer.

Pants/skirts and shorts. Lightweight pants or skirts work well, particularly if you hit a hot spell (these are also handy for Orthodox churches with modest dress codes). Jeans typically work well in Northern Europe—but they can get hot in muggy weather, and many cruise lines don't consider them appropriate "smart casual" wear. Button-down wallet pockets are safest (though still not as thief-proof as a money belt, described later). Shorts are perfectly acceptable aboard your ship, but on land in Europe they're considered beachwear, mostly worn in coastal or lakeside resort towns. No one will be offended if you wear shorts, but you may be on the receiving end of some second glances.

Shoes. Bring one pair of comfortable walking shoes with good traction. Comfort is essential even on board, where you'll sometimes be walking considerable distances just to get to dinner.

And getting on and off tenders can involve a short hop to a pier—practical shoes are a must for port days. Sandals or flip-flops are good for poolside use or in case your shoes get wet. And don't forget appropriate footwear to go with your dinner clothes (though again, think versatile—for women, a stylish pair of sandals is nearly as good as heels).

Jacket. Bring a light and water-resistant windbreaker with a hood. Or—more versatile—bring a lightweight Gore-Tex raincoat; rain and cold weather are not uncommon, even in summer.

Swimsuit and cover-up. If you plan on doing a lot of swimming, consider bringing a second swimsuit so that you always have a dry one to put on. Most cruise lines forbid swimsuits anywhere beyond the pool area, so cover-ups are a necessity.

Packing Essentials

Money belt (or neck wallet). This flat, hidden, zippered pouch—worn around your waist (or like a necklace) and tucked under your clothes—is essential for the peace of mind it brings. You could lose everything except your money belt, and the trip could still go on. Lightweight and low-profile beige is best. Whenever you're in port, keep your **cash, credit cards, driver's license,** and **passport** secure in your money belt, and carry only a day's spending money in your front pocket.

Toiletries kit. Because sinks in staterooms come with meager countertop space, I prefer a kit that can hang on a hook or a towel

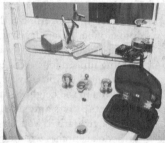

bar. For your overseas flight, put all squeeze bottles in sealable plastic baggies, since pressure changes in flight can cause even good bottles to leak. Pack your own bar of soap or small bottle of shampoo if you want to avoid using the ship-provided "itsy-bitsies" and minimize waste.

Bring any **medication** and vitamins you need (keep medicine in original containers, if possible, with legible prescriptions), along with a basic **first-aid kit.** If you're prone to motion sickness, consider some sort of **seasickness remedy.** (For various options, see page 82.) There are different schools of thought on **hand sanitizers** in preventing the spread of germs. Some cruise lines embrace them, others shun them (see page 84)—but they can come in handy when soap and water aren't readily available.

If you wear **eyeglasses** or **contact lenses,** bring a photocopy of your prescription—just in case. A strap for your glasses/sunglasses is handy for water activities or for peering over the edge of the ship in a strong breeze.

Sunscreen and sunglasses. Bring protection for your skin and your eyes. While you may think of Northern Europe as chilly, it can be bright and sunny in the summer—especially with the sun reflecting off all that water.

Laundry supplies (soap and clothesline). If you plan to wash your own clothes, bring a plastic squeeze bottle of concentrated, multipurpose, biodegradable liquid soap. For a spot remover, bring a few Shout wipes or a dab of Goop grease remover in a small plastic container. Some cruise-ship bathrooms have built-in clotheslines, but you can bring your own just in case (the twisted-rubber type needs no clothespins).

Packing aides. Packing cubes, clothes-compressor bags, and shirt-folding boards can help keep your clothes tightly packed and looking good.

Sealable plastic baggies. Bring a variety of sizes. In addition to holding your carry-on liquids, they're ideal for packing a picnic lunch, storing damp items, and bagging potential leaks before they happen. Some cruisers use baggies to organize their materials (cruise-line handouts, maps, ripped-out guidebook chapters, receipts) for each port of call. If you bring them, you'll use them.

Small daypack. A lightweight pack is great for carrying your sweater, camera, guidebook, and picnic goodies when you visit sights on shore. Don't use a fanny pack—they're magnets for pickpockets.

Fold-up tote bag. A large-capacity tote bag that rolls up into a pocket-size pouch can come in handy for bringing purchases home. It's also useful for the first and last days of your cruise, if you check your larger bags to be carried on or off the ship for you. During these times, you'll want to keep a change of clothes, any medications, and valuables with you.

Water bottle. If you bring one from home, make sure it's empty before you go through airport security (fill it at a drinking fountain once you're through). The plastic half-liter mineral water bottles sold throughout Europe are reusable and work great.

Guidebooks and maps. This book will likely be all you need. But if you want more in-depth coverage of the destinations or information on a place not covered in this book, consider collecting some other sources. (For suggestions, see page 1149.) I like to rip out appropriate chapters from guidebooks and staple them together, or use a slide-on laminated book cover. When I'm done, I give them away.

Address list. If you plan to send postcards, consider printing your mailing list onto a sheet of adhesive address labels before you leave.

Postcards from home and photos of your family. A small

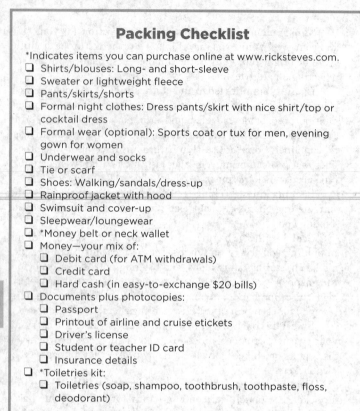

Packing Checklist

*Indicates items you can purchase online at www.ricksteves.com.

❑ Shirts/blouses: Long- and short-sleeve
❑ Sweater or lightweight fleece
❑ Pants/skirts/shorts
❑ Formal night clothes: Dress pants/skirt with nice shirt/top or cocktail dress
❑ Formal wear (optional): Sports coat or tux for men, evening gown for women
❑ Underwear and socks
❑ Tie or scarf
❑ Shoes: Walking/sandals/dress-up
❑ Rainproof jacket with hood
❑ Swimsuit and cover-up
❑ Sleepwear/loungewear
❑ *Money belt or neck wallet
❑ Money—your mix of:
  ❑ Debit card (for ATM withdrawals)
  ❑ Credit card
  ❑ Hard cash (in easy-to-exchange $20 bills)
❑ Documents plus photocopies:
  ❑ Passport
  ❑ Printout of airline and cruise etickets
  ❑ Driver's license
  ❑ Student or teacher ID card
  ❑ Insurance details
❑ *Toiletries kit:
  ❑ Toiletries (soap, shampoo, toothbrush, toothpaste, floss, deodorant)

collection of show-and-tell pictures (either printed or digital) is a fun, colorful conversation piece with fellow cruisers, your crew, and Europeans you meet.

Small notepad and pen. A tiny notepad in your back pocket or daypack is a great organizer, reminder, and communication aid.

Journal. An empty book to be filled with the experiences of your trip will be your most treasured souvenir. Attach a photo-copied calendar page of your itinerary. Use a hardbound type designed to last a lifetime, rather than a spiral notebook.

Electronics and Entertainment

As you're packing, try to go light with your electronic gear: You want to experience Europe, not interface with it. Of course, some devices are great tools for making your trip easier or better. As the functions of smartphones, tablets, cameras, GPS devices, and ereaders become more similar, think creatively about how you might pare down the number of gadgets you bring. Note that

- ❏ Medicines (including seasickness remedies, if needed)
- ❏ First-aid kit
- ❏ Hand sanitizer
- ❏ Glasses/contacts (with prescriptions)
- ❏ Sunscreen and sunglasses
- ❏ *Laundry soap and *clothesline
- ❏ Sealable plastic baggies
- ❏ *Daypack
- ❏ *Fold-up tote bag
- ❏ *Water bottle
- ❏ *Travel information (guidebooks and maps)
- ❏ Address list (for sending postcards)
- ❏ Postcards and photos from home
- ❏ *Notepad/journal and pen
- ❏ Electronics—your choice of:
  - ❏ Smartphone/mobile phone
  - ❏ Camera (and related gear)
  - ❏ Tablet/ereader/portable media player
  - ❏ Laptop
  - ❏ Chargers, headphones/earbuds, batteries, and plug adapters
- ❏ A good book
- ❏ Miscellaneous supplies (list on following page)

If you plan to carry on your luggage, note that all liquids must be in 3.4-ounce or smaller containers and fit within a single quart-size sealable bag. For details, see www.tsa.gov.

BEFORE YOUR CRUISE

many of these are big-ticket items; guard them carefully or look into insuring them (see page 40). Note that Wi-Fi aboard cruise ships can be slow and expensive—see page 86.

Consider bringing the following gadgets: **Smartphone/ mobile phone** (for details on using a US phone in Europe—or on a cruise ship—see page 87); **digital camera** (and associated gear); **other mobile devices** (laptop, tablet, portable media player, ereader); and **headphones/earbuds** (travel partners can bring a Y-jack for two sets of earphones). A small **auxiliary speaker** for your mobile device turns it into a better entertainment center. Bring each device's **charger,** or get a charger capable of charging multiple devices at once. Pack extra **batteries** (you can buy batteries on cruise ships and in Europe, but at a higher price).

Most cruises have limited TV offerings and charge a premium for pay-per-view movies (though you'll find DVD players in some staterooms). If you crave digital distraction, preload your mobile device with a selection of movies or TV shows. Cruise lines generally disable your stateroom TV's input jack, so you can't run a movie from your device on the TV.

For long days at sea, bring some leisure reading, whether on an ereader or just a good old paperback. Most ships also have free lending libraries and sell US paperbacks at reasonable prices.

Note: Most ships use North American electrical outlets, but if you're staying at a European hotel, you'll need an **adapter** to plug in electronics (for details, see "Watt's Up?" on page 50). Many staterooms have a limited number of outlets, so a lightweight **power strip** can be helpful if you have a lot of gadgets to charge at one time.

Miscellaneous Supplies

The following items are not necessities, but they generally take up little room and can come in handy in a pinch.

Basic **picnic supplies,** such as a Swiss Army-type knife and plastic cutlery, enable you to shop for a very European lunch at a market or neighborhood grocery store. Munch in port or in your stateroom (but remember not to pack a knife in your carry-on bag when flying).

Sticky notes (such as Post-it notes) are great for keeping your place in your guidebook. **Duct tape** cures a thousand problems. A **tiny lock** will keep the zippers on your checked baggage shut.

A small **flashlight** is handy for reading under the sheets while your partner snoozes, or for finding your way through an unlit passage (tiny-but-powerful LED flashlights—about the size of your little finger—are extremely bright and compact). **Small binoculars** are great for viewing scenery, sea life, and palace interiors.

Not every stateroom comes with an **alarm clock,** so bring a portable one just in case (or you can use the alarm on your watch or mobile phone). A **wristwatch** is handy for keeping track of important sailing and dinner times, especially if you'll be taking a break from your smartphone.

If night noises bother you, you'll love a good set of expandable foam **earplugs;** if you're sensitive to light, bring an **eye mask.** For snoozing on planes, trains, and automobiles, consider an inflatable **neck pillow.**

A **sewing kit** can help you mend tears and restore lost buttons. Because European restrooms are often not fully equipped, carry some toilet paper or **tissue packets** (sold at all newsstands in Europe).

WHAT NOT TO PACK

Don't bother packing **beach towels,** as these are provided by the cruise line.

Virtually every cruise-ship bathroom comes equipped with a

hair dryer (though if you need one for before or after your cruise, you may want to check with your hotels). The use of **flat irons, curlers,** or other hair-care appliances that heat up (and present a potential fire hazard) is discouraged, though most cruise lines tolerate their use.

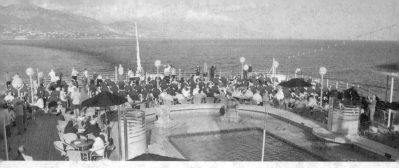

ON THE SHIP

Now that you've booked your cruise and packed your bags, it's time to set sail. This chapter focuses on helping you get to know your ship and adjust to the seafaring lifestyle.

Initial Embarkation

You've flown across the Atlantic, made your way to the port, and now finally you see your cruise ship along the pier, looming like a skyscraper turned on its side. The anticipation is palpable. But unfortunately, getting checked in and boarding the ship can be the most taxing and tiring part of the entire cruise experience. Instead of waltzing up a gangway, you'll spend hours waiting around as hundreds or even thousands of your fellow passengers are also processed. Add the fact that ports are generally in ugly and complicated, expensive-to-reach parts of town (not to mention that you're probably jet-lagged), and your trip can begin on a stressful note. Just go with the flow and be patient; once you're on the ship, you're in the clear.

ARRIVAL AT THE AIRPORT
Cruise lines offer hassle-free airport transfers directly to the ship. While expensive, these are convenient and much appreciated if you're jet-lagged or packing heavy. Taxis are always an option for easy door-to-door service but can be needlessly expensive (in many cities, taxis levy additional surcharges for both the airport and the cruise port). Public transportation can be a bit more complicated, and may be a drag with bags, but usually saves you plenty of money. For cities where cruises are likely to begin or end, I've included details on connecting to the airport on your own—either by taxi or by public transit—so you can easily compare the cost and

hassle with the transfer options offered by your cruise line. I've also included hotel recommendations.

Don't schedule your arrival in Europe too close to the departure of your cruise, as flights are prone to delays. Arriving on the same day your cruise departs—even with hours to spare—can be risky. And keep in mind that flights departing from the US to Europe generally get in the next calendar day. For more on these topics, see page 41.

Remember: Arriving in Europe a day or more before your cruise gives you the chance to get over jet lag, see your departure city, and avoid the potential stress of missing your cruise.

CHECKING IN AT THE PORT

Before you leave home, be clear on the exact location of the port for your ship (some cities have more than one port, and large embarkation ports typically have multiple terminals), as well as the schedule for checking in and setting sail. On their initial sailing, most ships depart around 17:00, but cruise lines usually request that passengers be checked in and on board by 15:30 or 16:00. (Like Europe, this book uses the 24-hour clock.) Better yet, arrive at the port at least an hour or two before that to allow ample time to find your way to the ship and get settled in. Most ships are open for check-in around 13:00. You might be able to drop off your bags even earlier—allowing you to explore your embarkation port (or your ship) baggage-free until your stateroom is available. Early check-in also helps you avoid the longest check-in lines of the day, which are typically in the midafternoon.

When you arrive at the terminal, cruise-line representatives will direct you to the right place. There are basically three steps to getting on the ship, each of which might involve some waiting: 1) dropping off bags; 2) check-in; and 3) embarkation (security checkpoint, boarding the ship, and finding your stateroom).

First, you have the option to **drop off your bags**—usually at a separate location from check-in. From here, your bags will be transported to your stateroom. If you're packing light, I recommend skipping the drop-off and carrying your own bags to the cabin, which allows you to dispense with formalities and potential delays (waiting to check the bags, and later, waiting for them to arrive in your cabin). But if you're packing heavy—or just want to be rid of your bags to do a little last-minute sightseeing before boarding—checking your bags typically works fine. Your cruise materials (mailed to you prior to your trip) likely included luggage tags marked with your cabin number; to save time, affix these to your bags before dropping them off (if you don't have these tags, baggage stewards can give you some on the spot). From here, the crew will deliver your bags to your stateroom. On a big ship, this

Cruising Terms Glossary

To avoid sounding like a naive landlubber, learn a few nautical terms: It's a "line," not a "rope." It's a "ship," not a "boat."

aft/stern: back of ship

all aboard: time that all passengers must be on board the ship (typically 30 minutes before departure)

astern: ahead of the stern (that is, in front of the ship)

beam: width of the ship at its widest point

bearing/course: direction the ship is heading (on a compass, usually presented as a degree)

berth: bed (in a cabin) or dock (at a port)

bridge: command center, where the ship is steered from

bulkhead: wall between cabins or compartments

colors: ship's flag (usually the country of registration)

deck: level or "floor" of the ship

deck plan: map of the ship

disembark: leave the ship

draft: distance from the waterline to the deepest point of the ship's keel

embark: board the ship

even keel: the ship is level (keel/mast at 90 degrees)

fathom: unit of nautical depth; 1 fathom = 6 feet

flag: ensign of the country in which a ship is officially registered (and whose laws apply on board)

fore/bow: front of the ship

funnel/stack: ship's smokestack

galley: kitchen

gangway: stairway between the ship and shore

gross registered tonnage: unit of a ship's volume; 1 gross registered ton = 100 cubic feet of enclosed space

hatch: covering for a hold

helm: steering device for the ship; place where steering device is located

HMS: His/Her Majesty's Ship (before the vessel name); British-flagged ships only

hold: storage area below decks

hotel manager: officer in charge of accommodations and food operations

hull: the body of the ship

keel: the "fin" of the ship that extends below the hull

knot: unit of nautical speed; 1 knot = 1 nautical mile/ hour = 1.15 land miles/hour

league: unit of nautical distance; 1 league = 3 nautical miles = 3.45 land miles

leeward: direction against the wind (that is, into the wind); downwind

lido (lido deck): deck with outdoor swimming pools, athletic area, and other amenities

line: rope

list/listing: tilt to one side

manifest: list of the ship's passengers, crew, and cargo

midship/amidships: a spot halfway between the bow and the stern

MS/MSY: motor ship/motorized sailing yacht (used before the vessel name)

muster station: where you go if there's an emergency and you have to board the lifeboats

nautical mile: unit of nautical distance; 1 nautical mile = 1.15 land miles

pilot: local captain who advises the ship's captain, or even steers the ship, on approach to a port

pitch/pitching: rise and fall of the ship's bow as it maneuvers through waves

port: left side of the ship (here's a mnemonic device: both "left" and "port" have four letters)

prow: angled front part of the ship

purser/bursar: officer in charge of finances, sometimes also with managerial responsibilities

quay: dock or pier (pron. "key")

rigging: cables, chains, and lines

roll/rolling: side-to-side movement of a ship

seating: assigned seat and time for dinner in the dining room (often optional)

stabilizer: fin that extends at an angle from the hull of the ship into the water to create a smoother ride

starboard: right side of the ship

stateroom/cabin: "hotel room" on the ship

stem: very front of the prow

steward: serving crew, including the cabin steward (housekeeping), dining steward (waiter), or wine steward (sommelier)

superstructure: parts of the ship above the main deck

swell: wave in the open sea

technical call: when the ship docks or anchors, but passengers are not allowed off (except, in some cases, when those passengers have bought an excursion)

tender: small boat that carries passengers between an anchored ship and the shore

tendered: when a ship is anchored (in the open water) rather than docked (at a pier); passengers reach land by riding tender boats

upper berth: fold-down bed located above another bed

veranda: private balcony off a stateroom

wake: trail of disturbed water that a ship leaves behind it

weigh: raise (for example, "weigh anchor")

windward: in the direction the wind is blowing (with the wind); upwind

ON THE SHIP

can take hours; if you'll need anything from your luggage soon after departure—such as a swimsuit, a jacket for dinner, or medication—keep it with you. Don't leave anything fragile in your bags. And be aware that your bags might be sitting in the hallway outside your room for quite some time, where passersby have access to them; while theft is rare, you shouldn't leave irreplaceable documents or other valuables in them. Pack as you would for bags being checked on an airline.

At **check-in,** you'll be photographed (for security purposes) and given a credit-card-like room key that you'll need to show whenever you leave and reboard the ship. Crew members will inspect your passport. They also may ask for your credit-card number to cover any onboard expenses (though some cruise lines ask you to do this after boarding, at the front desk). Remember that they may place a hold on your credit card to cover anticipated charges. If you're accompanying a child on board, see page 46 for the documentation you may need.

As part of check-in, you'll fill out a form asking whether you've had any flu-like symptoms (gastrointestinal or nose/throat) over the last several days, and you may also be asked about recent travel to areas with health epidemics. If you have, the ship's doctor will evaluate you free of charge before you are allowed to board. This is a necessary public-health measure, considering that contagious diseases spread like wildfire on a cruise ship (see page 83).

After check-in, you'll be issued a boarding number and asked to wait in a large holding area until your number is called. It could take minutes...or hours.

When your number comes up, you'll have to clear immigration control/customs (usually just a formality—you may not even have to flash your passport) and go through a **security check** to make sure you have no forbidden items, ranging from firearms to alcohol (many cruise lines won't let you BYOB on board, and others limit how much you can bring; for details, see page 101).

YOUR FIRST FEW HOURS ON BOARD

Once you're on the ship, head to your **stateroom** and unpack. (For more on your stateroom, see "Settling In," later.) During this time, your cabin steward will likely stop by to greet you. The cabin steward—who is invariably jolly and super-personable—is responsible for cleaning your room (generally twice a day, after breakfast and during dinner) and taking care of any needs you might have.

As soon as you step on board, you'll be very aware that you're on a seaborne vessel. You'll quickly remember the old truism about landlubbers having to find their **"sea legs."** At first, you may stagger around like you've had one too many. Hang onto handrails (on stairways and, if it's really rough, in the hallways) and step carefully. You'll eventually get used to it, and you might even discover when you return to shore that you'll need to find your "land legs" all over again. While you may worry that the motion of the ocean will interfere with sleep, many cruisers report exactly the opposite. There's something soothing about being rocked gently to sleep at night, with the white noise of the engines as your lullaby.

Just before departure, the crew holds an **emergency drill** (or **muster drill**) to brief you on the location of your lifejacket, how to put it on, and where to assemble in the event that the ship is

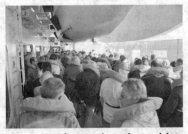

evacuated (called a muster station). After being given a lifeboat number, you must gather at your muster station, along with others assigned to the same lifeboat (though sometimes this drill is held elsewhere on the ship). This is serious business, and all are required to participate. For more

on safety on board—and how to prepare for the worst-case scenario—see the "Cruise-Ship Safety Concerns" sidebar on page 72.

It's traditional—and fun—for passengers to assemble on the deck while the ship **sets sail,** waving to people on shore and on other ships. On some lines, the ship's loudspeakers play melodramatic music as the ship glides away from land. Sometimes the initial departure comes with live musicians, costumed crew members, and a festive cocktail-party atmosphere.

You'll also get acquainted with the ship's **dining room** or other restaurants. If your ship has traditional "seatings"—an assigned time and seat for dinner each night—this first evening is an important opportunity to get to know the people you'll be dining with. If you have any special requests, you can drop by the dining room a bit before dinnertime to chat with the maître d'.

Memorize your **stateroom number**—you'll be asked for it constantly (when arriving at meals, disembarking, making onboard purchases, and so on). And be aware of not only your cruise line, but the name of your specific ship (e.g., Norwegian *Star,* Royal Caribbean *Serenade of the Seas,* Celebrity *Eclipse,* Holland America *Eurodam*)—people in the cruise industry (including those in port) refer to the ship name, not the company.

Various **orientation activities** are scheduled for your first evening; these may include a ship tour or a presentation about the various shore excursions that will be offered during the cruise. While this presentation is shamelessly promotional, it can be a good use of time to find out your options.

ON THE SHIP

Life on Board

Your cruise ship is your home away from home for the duration of your trip. This section provides an overview of your ship and covers many of the services and amenities that are offered on board.

SETTLING IN

From tiny staterooms to confusing corridors, it might take a couple of days to adjust to life on board a ship. But before long, you will be an expert at everything from getting to the dining room in the shortest amount of time to showering in tight spaces.

Your Stateroom

While smaller than most hotel rooms, your cabin is plenty big enough if you use it primarily as a place to sleep, spending the majority of your time in port and in the ship's public areas. As you unpack, you'll discover that storage space can be minimal. But—as sailors have done for centuries—cruise-ship designers are experts at cramming little pockets of storage into every nook and cranny. Remember where you

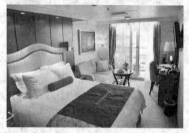

tuck things so you can find them when it's time to pack up at the end of your trip.

Unpack thoroughly and thoughtfully right away. Clutter makes a small cabin even smaller. I pack heavier when cruising than when traveling on land, so I make a point to unpack completely, establishing a smart system for keeping my tight little cabin shipshape. Deep-store items you won't need in your suitcase, which you can stow under your bed (or ask your steward to show you any hidden storage areas). Survey all storage areas and make a

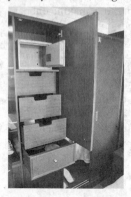

plan to use them smartly. For example, use one drawer for all things electronic, establish a pantry for all food items, and use the safe for some things even if you don't bother locking it. Unclutter the room by clearing out items the cruise line leaves for you (such as promotional materials). I have a ritual of toggling from shore mode to ship mode by putting my pocket change and money belt (neither of which are of any value on board) in a drawer or the safe when I return to the ship.

Staterooms usually have a safe, coffee maker, minifridge, phone for calling the front desk or other cabins, and television. TV channels include information about the ship, sales pitches for shore excursions and other cruises, various American programming (such as ESPN or CNN), and pay-per-view movies. Some lines even broadcast my TV shows. The beds are usually convertible—if you've got a double bed but prefer twins, your cabin steward can pull them apart and remake them for you (or vice versa). Inside the cabin is a lifejacket for each passenger. Make note of where these are stored, and the best route to your muster station, just as you would the locations of emergency exits on an airplane.

Cabin **bathrooms** are generally tight but big enough to take

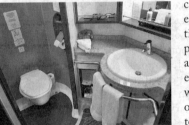

care of business. Bathrooms come equipped with hair dryers. First-time cruisers are sometimes surprised at the high water pressure and dramatic suction that powers each flush. Read and heed the warnings not to put any foreign objects down the toilet: Clogged toilets are not uncommon, and on a cruise ship, this can jam up the system for your whole hallway... not a good way to make friends.

Getting to Know Your Ship

After you're settled in your stateroom, start exploring. As you wander, begin to fill in your mental map of the ship with the things

you may want to find later: front desk, restaurants, theater, and so on. Many cruises offer a tour of the ship early on, which can help you get your bearings on a huge, mazelike vessel. Deck plans (maps of the ship) are posted throughout the hallways, and you can pick up a pocket-size plan to carry with you. If your ship has touchscreen activity schedules and deck plans on each floor, use them.

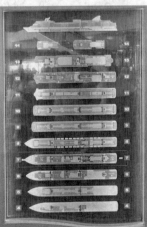

On my first day, I physically hike the entire ship, deck by deck, inside and out, to see what's where. Ships have peaceful outdoor decks that are rarely visited (perfect for sunsets). They have plenty of bars, cafés, and lounges, some of which may fit your style to a T. Crew members know about their ship's special little places, but many passengers never find them. Discover these on your first day rather than your last. Pop into each of the specialty restaurants for a chat with the maître d' and to survey the menu, cover charge, and seating.

As you walk down long hallways, it's easy to get turned around and lose track of whether you're headed for the front (fore)

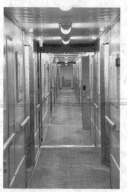

or the back (aft) of the ship. For the first couple of days, I carry around my ship deck plan and try to learn landmarks: For example, the restaurants (and my cabin) are near the back of the ship, while entertainment venues (casino, big theater) are at the front. Several banks of elevators are usually spread evenly throughout the ship. Before long, you'll figure out the most direct way between your stateroom and the places you want to go. It can also be tricky to find your room in a very long, anonymous hall

with identical doors. Consider marking yours in a low-profile way (for example, tape a small picture below your room number) to help you find it in a hurry.

ON THE SHIP

The double-decker main artery running through the middle of the ship, often called the **promenade deck,** connects several key amenities: theater, main dining room and other eateries, shopping area, library, Internet café, art gallery, photography sales point, and so on. Wrapping around the outside of the promenade deck is the namesake outdoor (but covered) deck, where you can go for a stroll.

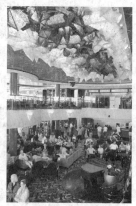

At the center of the promenade deck is the main **lobby** (often called the atrium). This area, usually done up with over-the-top decor, has bars, a big screen for occasional presentations, tables of stuff to buy, and not enough seating. If you

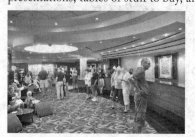

get lost exploring the ship, just find your way to the lobby and reorient yourself.

The lobby is also where the **guest services desk** is located. Like the reception desk of a hotel, this is your point of contact if you have concerns about your stateroom or other questions. Nearby you'll usually find the excursions desk (where you can get information about and book seats on shore excursions), a "cruise consultant" (selling seats on the line's future sailings), and the financial services desk (which handles any monetary issues that the guest services desk can't).

If the lobby is the hub of information, then the **lido deck** is the hub of recreation. Generally the ship's sunny top deck, the lido

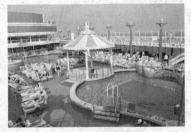 has swimming areas, other outdoor activities, and usually the buffet restaurant. With a variety of swimming pools (some adults-only, others for kids) and hot tubs; a casual poolside "grill" serving up burgers and hot dogs; ice-cream machines; long rows of sunbathing chairs; and "Margaritaville"-type live music at all hours, the lido deck screams, "Be on vacation!"

INFORMATION

Each evening, the **daily program** for the next day is placed inside your cabin or tucked under your door. These information-packed leaflets offer an hour-by-hour schedule for the day's events, from arrival and all-aboard times to dinner seatings, bingo games, and AA meetings. (They're also peppered with ads touting various spa specials, duty-free sales, and drink discounts.) With a staggering number of options each day, this list is crucial for keeping track of where you want to be and when. I tuck this in my back pocket and refer to it constantly. Bring it with you in port to avoid that moment of terror when you suddenly realize you don't remember what time you have to be back on the ship.

Most cruise lines also give you an **information sheet** about each port of call. These usually include a map and some basic historical and sightseeing information. But the dominant feature is a list of the cruise line's "recommended" shops in that port and discounts offered at each one. Essentially, these are the shops that pay the cruise line a commission. These stores can be good places to shop, but they aren't necessarily the best options. (For more details on shopping in port, see page 132.)

The daily program and/or information sheet usually lists your vessel's **port agent** for that day's stop. This is where you'd turn in the unlikely event that you miss your departing ship (for details, see page 139).

Most cruise lines offer **"port talks"**—lectures about upcoming destinations. The quality of these can vary dramatically, from educational seminars that will immeasurably deepen your

ON THE SHIP

Cruise-Ship Safety Concerns

The tragic grounding of the *Costa Concordia* in January of 2012 off the coast of Italy had some cruisers asking, "How safe is my cruise ship?"

Like any form of travel, cruising comes with risks. But statistically, even taking into account the *Concordia* disaster, cruising remains remarkably safe. While death statistics for cruise passengers aren't easy to find, the estimate of the number of deaths are quite low (for example, just 16 deaths related to marine casualties were reported from 2005 to 2010).

A set of laws called Safety of Life at Sea (SOLAS) has regulated maritime safety since the *Titanic* sank a century ago. After the *Concordia* disaster, regulations now require that a safety briefing and muster drill take place before departure. Still, the *Concordia* disaster underscores that cruisers should take responsibility for their own safety. Know where lifejackets are stowed (they're usually in your stateroom, but on very large ships, they may be kept at the muster station). If you are traveling with kids, ask the cruise line for child-size lifejackets to have on hand. Be clear on the location of your muster station, and know how to get there—not only from your stateroom, but from other parts of the ship. Pack a small flashlight, and keep it handy.

Legally, ships are required to have one lifeboat seat per person on board, plus an additional 25 percent. Aside from the primary lifeboats, large white canisters on the ship's deck contain smaller inflatable lifeboats, which can be launched if the normal lifeboats are disabled. In the event of an evacuation, crew members are responsible for providing instructions and for loading and operating the lifeboats. In theory, a cruise ship's evacuation procedure is designed to safely remove everyone on board within 30 minutes. However, actual full-ship evacuation is almost never practiced. The "women and children first" rule is nautical tradition, but not legally binding. The captain, however, is legally obligated to stay with the ship to oversee the evacuation.

Ultimately, the *Costa Concordia* disaster is a glaring exception to the otherwise sterling safety record of the cruise industry. But it is a cautionary tale that should encourage cruisers to take the initiative to protect themselves, in case the worst-case scenario becomes a reality.

appreciation for the destination, to thinly veiled sales pitches for shore excursions.

Better cruises have a **destination expert** standing by when you get off the ship to answer your questions about that port (usually near the gangway or in the lobby). Again, beware: While some are legitimate experts, and others work for the local tourist board, most are employees of local shops. They can give you some good sightseeing advice, but any shopping pointers they offer should be taken with a grain of salt.

English is generally the first **language** on the ship, though—especially on bigger ships—announcements are repeated in other languages as well (often French, German, Italian, and/or Spanish, depending on the clientele). Most crew members who interact with passengers speak English well—though usually it's their second language.

When passing important landmarks, especially on days at sea, the **captain** may periodically come over the loudspeaker to offer commentary. Or, if the seas are rough, the captain may try to soothe rattled nerves (and stomachs) with an explanation of the weather that's causing the turbulence.

Speaking of **announcements,** cruise lines have varying philosophies about these: Some lines barrage you with announcements every hour or so. On other lines, they're rare. On most ships, in-cabin speakers are only used for emergency announcements. If you can't make out a routine announcement from inside your cabin, crack the door to hear the hallway loudspeakers, or tune your TV to the ship-information channel, which also broadcasts announcements.

YOUR CREW

Your hardworking crew toils for long hours and low pay to make sure you have a great vacation. Whether it's the head waiter who remembers how you like your coffee; the cabin steward who cleans your room with a smile and shows you pictures of his kids back in Indonesia; or the unseen but equally conscientious workers who prepare your meals, wash your laundry, scrub the deck, or drive the tender boats, the crew is an essential and often unheralded part of your cruise experience.

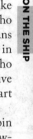

The all-purpose term for crew members is "steward"—cabin steward (housekeeping), wine steward (sommelier), dining steward (waiter), and so on. Your cabin steward can be very helpful if you have a basic question or request; for something more complicated, ask the front-desk staff or the concierge. In the dining room, the maître d' assigns tables and manages the dining room, the head waiter takes your order, and the assistant waiters bring your food and bus your dishes.

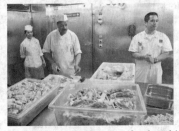

The ship's cruise director (sometimes called a host or hostess) is a tireless cheerleader, keeping you informed about the various activities and other happenings on board, usually via perky announcements over the ship's loudspeaker several times a day. The cruise director manages a (mostly American) "cruise staff" that leads activities throughout the ship. I have a lot of sympathy for these folks, partly because of my own background as a tour guide—I can't imagine the responsibility of keeping thousands of people informed and entertained 24/7. Experienced cruisers report that the more enthusiastic and energetic the cruise director and staff are, the more likely you are to enjoy your cruise. Gradually you'll come to feel respect, appreciation, and even affection for these people who really, really want you to have a great time on your vacation.

A great bonus for me is to make friends with members of the crew. They are generally hardworking, industrious, young, and fun-loving people from the developing world who, in spite of their required smiles, genuinely enjoy people. Many are avid travelers, and you'll see them enjoying time on shore (when they are given a break) just like you. While there are strict limits to how crew members can mingle with passengers, you are more than welcome to have real and instructive conversations with them about cruise life, their world back home, or whatever.

Befriending a crew member can also come with a bonus drink. If you see a crew member nursing a drink on their own at a shipboard bar, strike up a conversation. There's a good chance they'll offer to buy you a drink. That's because when drinking alone, they have to pay for their own drinks; but if they're "entertaining" a passenger, both their drink and yours are on the cruise line. It's a win-win.

Crew Wages

Other than the officers and cruise staff, a ship's crew is primarily composed of people from the developing world. With rare exceptions, these crew members are efficient, patient, and friendly (or, at least, always smiling).

It's clear that crew members work hard. But most passengers would be surprised to learn just how long they work—and for how

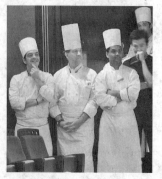

little. Because US labor laws don't apply to sailing vessels, cruise lines can pay astonishingly low wages for very long hours of work. Crew members who receive tips are paid an average base salary (before tips) of about $1 each day. This makes tips an essential part of the crew's income (see "Tipping" on page 79). After tips, the English-speaking service crew who interact with passengers make about

ON THE SHIP

$2,000-3,000 per month, while the anonymous workers toiling at entry-level jobs below decks can make less than $1,000 per month. While clear industry-wide numbers are hard to come by, the following monthly wages (after tips) are typical:

Cabin steward	$2,000
Waiter	$3,000
Bartender	$1,800
Cook	$1,500-2,100
Dishwasher	$600
Seaman (maintenance)	$1,500
Cruise staff	$2,000
Cruise director	$5,800
Captain	$10,000

These earnings don't seem unreasonable...until you factor in the long hours. Most crew members sign a nine- to ten-month contract, then get two or three months off. While they are under contract, they work 7 days a week, at least 10 hours a day; the international legal maximum is 14 hours a day, but according to insiders, some crew members put in up to 16 hours. The hours worked are rarely consecutive—for example, a crew member might work 6 hours, have 2 or 3 hours off, then work 7 more hours. They rarely if ever get a full day off during their entire months-long contract, though they get enough sporadic time off during the day to be able to rest and occasionally enjoy the ports of call. Do the math: If most crew members work an average of 12 hours a day, 30 days a month, that's 360 hours a month—more than double the 160 hours of a 9-to-5 worker.

Cruise lines do cover their crew's accommodations, food, medical care, and transportation (including a flight home once their contract is completed). This means the crew can pocket or send home most of their earnings. While income-tax laws do not apply on the ship, crew members are required to pay taxes in their home country.

ON THE SHIP

The Secret Lives of Crew Members

Most cruise lines have somewhere between 1.5 and 2 passengers per crew member. So a 3,000-passenger ship has around 2,000 crew members, who need to be housed and fed—in some ways, they are a vast second set of passengers. The crew's staterooms—the lowest (below the waterline, close to the rumbling engine noise) and smallest on the ship—are far more humble than your

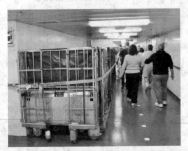

Running a Cruise Ship

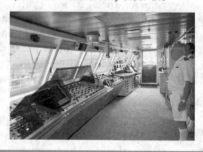

The business of running a ship is divided into three branches, which work together to create a smooth experience: the engine room; the hotel (rooms and food service); and the deck. This last branch includes the physical decks and railings as well as the bridge (the area from which the ship is navigated) and tendering (shore transport). Each department has its leader (chief engineer, hotel manager, and chief officer, respectively), with the captain overseeing the entire operation.

Of course, these days the captain doesn't actually steer the ship while standing at a big wooden wheel. Modern cruise ships are mostly computerized. The "watch"—responsibility for guiding the ship and dealing with any emergencies—rotates among the officers, who usually work four hours on, then eight hours off. The watch continues when the ship is at anchor or

own, and usually shared by two to six people. Some cruise staff may have nicer cabins in the passenger areas, but only officers get outside cabins.

While you may see officers eating in the passenger dining room or buffet, most of the crew dines in mess halls with menus that reflect the cuisine of their native lands. Working long hours and far from home, the crew expects to eat familiar comfort food—Southeast Asians want fish and rice; Italians get pasta; and so on. A well-fed crew is a happy crew, which leads to happy passengers—so substantial effort and resources go toward feeding the crew.

The more diverse the crew, the more complicated and expensive it can be to keep everyone satisfied. On some ships, each nationality has its own mess hall and menu that changes day to day. Some cruise lines have found it more efficient to hire employees predominantly from one or two countries. For example, on Holland America, the cabin crew is entirely Indonesian, while the kitchen and dining room crew is Filipino (to recruit employees, the cruise line operates training academies in those two countries).

ON THE SHIP

docked, when officers must keep an eye on moorings, make sure the ship is in the correct position, and so on.

The ship is dry-docked (taken out of the water) every two years or so to clean algae, barnacles, and other buildup from the hull and to polish the propeller. A very smooth propeller is crucial for a fluid ride—a dented or porous one can lead to lots of noise and bubbles. Sometimes a crew engineer will put on a wetsuit and dive down to polish the rudder underwater.

As you approach a port (or a challenging-to-navigate passage), a little boat zips out to your cruise ship, and a "pilot"—a local captain who's knowledgeable about that port—hops off.

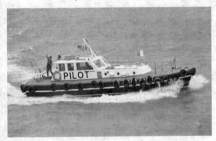

The pilot advises your ship's captain about the best approach to the dock and sometimes even takes the helm. Once the job is done, another boat might zip out to pick up the pilot.

If you're intrigued by the inner workings of your ship, ask about a behind-the-scenes tour. Many ships offer the opportunity to see the galley (kitchen), food stores, crew areas, and other normally off-limits parts of the ship (usually for a fee).

Many crew members have spouses back home who are raising their children; in port, they buy cheap phone cards or use Skype to keep in touch. In fact, most portside Internet cafés and calling shops target the crew rather than the passengers ("Cheap rates to the Philippines!"). If a café near the port offers free Wi-Fi for customers, you'll invariably see a dozen of your crew huddled over their laptops, deep in conversation.

While many crew members have families to feed, others are living the single life. The crew tends to party together (the crew bar is even more rollicking than the passenger bars), and inter-crew romances are commonplace—though fraternization between crew members and passengers is strictly forbidden.

Is It Exploitation?

The national and racial stratification of the entire crew evokes the exploitation and indentured servitude of colonial times: The officers and cruise staff are often Americans, Brits, or Europeans, while those in menial roles (kitchen, waitstaff, cleaning crew, engineers) are Indonesian, Filipino, or another developing-world nationality. It's a mark of a socially conscious company when Southeast Asian employees are given opportunities to rise through the ranks and take on roles with greater responsibility.

The cruise lines argue that their employees are making far more money at sea in glamorous locations—where they get occasional time off to leave the ship and explore the ports—than they would at menial jobs back home. What some see as exploitation, others see as empowerment. Another way to look at it is as "insourcing"—importing cheap labor from the lowest bidder. For better or worse, the natural gregariousness of the crew gives cruisers the impression that they can't be so terribly unhappy with their lives. And the remarkable loyalty of many crew members (working many, many years for the same cruise line)—especially on certain lines—is a testament to the success of the arrangement.

Is it wrong to employ Third World people at low wages to wait on First World, mostly white, generally wealthy vacationers? I don't know. But I do know that your crew members are some of the friendliest people on board. Get to know them. Ask about their families back home. And make sure they know how much you appreciate everything they're doing to make your trip more comfortable.

MONEY MATTERS

Most cruise ships are essentially cashless. Your stateroom key card doubles as a credit card. When buying anything on board, you'll simply provide your cabin number, then sign a receipt for the expense. You'll likely need cash on board only for tipping (explained later), paying a crew member to babysit, or playing the casino (most slot machines and table games take cash; you can use your onboard account to finance your gambling, but you'll pay a fee for the privilege). To avoid exorbitant cash-advance fees at the front desk, bring along some US cash for these purposes.

Most cruise lines price everything on board (from drinks to tips to souvenirs) in US dollars, regardless of the countries visited during the trip.

Onboard Expenses

First-time cruisers thinking they've paid up front for an "all-inclusive" trip are sometimes surprised by how many add-ons they are offered on board. Your cruise ticket covers accommodations, all the meals you can eat in the ship's main dining room and buffet (with some beverages included), and transportation from port to port. You can have an enjoyable voyage and not spend a penny more (except for expenses in port). But the cruise industry is adept at enticing you with extras that add up quickly. These include shore excursions, casino games, premium drinks (alcohol, name-brand soft drinks, and lattes), specialty restaurant surcharges (explained later, under "Eating"), duty-free shopping, fitness classes, spa treatments, photos, and many other goods and services.

It's very easy to get carried away—a round of drinks here, a night of blackjack there, a scuba dive, a castle tour, and more. First-timers—even those who think they're keeping a close eye on their bottom line—can be astonished when they get their final onboard bill, which can easily exceed the original cost of the trip (or so hope the cruise lines).

With a little self-control, you can easily limit your extra expenditures, making your seemingly "cheap" cruise actually cheap. It's a good idea to occasionally check your current balance (and look for mistaken charges) at the front desk or on your cabin TV. You don't have to avoid extras entirely. After all, you're on vacation—go ahead and have that "daily special" cocktail to unwind after a busy day of sightseeing, or stick a $20 bill into a slot machine. But you always have the right to say, "No, thanks." As long as you're aware of these additional expenses and keep your spending under control, a cruise can still be a great value.

Getting Local Cash on Board

While you don't need much cash on board the ship, you will need local money for your time in port, as many European vendors will not accept credit cards or dollars. It's possible to get local cash on board the ship—but it's expensive. At the front desk, you can exchange cash or traveler's checks into the local currency (at bad rates and often with high commissions), or you can get a cash advance on your credit card (at a decent exchange rate but typically with exorbitant fees).

You'll save money if you plan ahead and make use of ATMs near the cruise port. For each destination, I've noted the location of the nearest ATM, which can often be found inside the cruise terminal or close to it (for more on withdrawing money in port, see page 128).

Among the destinations in this book, the euro is used in Belgium, Estonia, Finland, France, Germany, Latvia, and the Netherlands. The other destinations have retained their traditional currencies—the Russian ruble, the Norwegian krone, the British pound, and so on. In certain places (as noted in each chapter), it can be tricky to get local funds near your ship. In these cases, it may be worth the added expense to change a small amount of cash on board the ship to finance your trip into town.

Tipping

Tipping procedures aboard cruise ships have changed dramatically over the last two decades. Through the late 1980s, cruising was a

Money-Saving Tips

Many people choose cruising because it's extremely affordable. When you consider that you're getting accommodations, food, and transportation for one low price, it's simply a steal. But reckless spending on a cruise can rip through a tight budget like a grenade in a dollhouse. If you're really watching your money, consider these strategies:

Buy as little on board as possible. Everything—drinks, Internet access, knickknacks—is priced at a premium for a captive audience. For most items, you're paying far more than you would off the ship. If you're shopping for jewelry, find a local boutique in port rather than patronize your ship's shop. On the other hand, be aware that northern Europe can be very expensive. You may find it's cheaper to buy a Coke from your stateroom minibar than at a Norwegian minimart.

Skip the excursions. While cruise-line excursions are easy and efficient, you may be charged $80-100/person for a transfer into town and a walking tour of the old center. But for the cost of a $2 bus ticket, you can get downtown yourself and join a $15 walking tour that covers most of the same sights. This book's destination chapters are designed to help you understand your options.

Stick with the main dining room. If your ship has specialty restaurants that levy a surcharge, skip them in favor of the "free" (included) meals in the main dining room—which are typically good quality.

Save some breakfast for lunch. If you're heading out for a long day in port, help yourself to a big breakfast and bag up the leftovers to keep you going until dinnertime. Some cruise lines will sell you a packed lunch for about $10.

pastime of the wealthy, and passengers enjoyed tipping the crew royally as part of the experience. Each crew member—cabin steward, maître d', head waiter, assistant waiter, and so on—expected to be tipped a specific amount per day. After the final passenger disembarked, the crew would meet and dump all their tip money into a communal pot, to be divided equally among themselves. But as cruising went mass-market, more frugal middle-class passengers began signing up. Having already paid for their trip, many resented the expectation to tip...so they simply didn't. The crew's take-home pay plummeted, and many workers quit, leaving the cruise lines in dire straits.

These days, cruise lines use a standard "auto-tip" system, in which a set gratuity (generally about $10-12/person per day) is automatically billed to each passenger's account and then divided among the crew (this system, started around 2000, effectively formalizes the process that had been going on for decades). About a

Minimize premium beverage purchases. Because alcohol, soda, and specialty coffee drinks all cost extra, drink tabs can add up fast. Since many cruise lines prohibit or limit bringing your own alcohol on board, you'll pay dearly for wetting your whistle.

Stay out of the casino. With a casino and slots on board, it's easy to fall into a gambling habit. Most cruise lines allow you to use your key card to get cash from your room account for gambling. But read the fine print carefully—you're paying a percentage for this convenience. Also, keep in mind that your odds of winning may be even less than at land-based casinos (see page 91).

Don't buy onboard photos. Come to think of it, don't even let them take your photo—so you won't be tempted to buy it later.

Don't use the shipboard mobile phone network or Wi-Fi. Shipboard Internet access and phone rates are very high. To check your email, use a Wi-Fi hot spot in port rather than on board. For phone options, see page 87.

Take advantage of free services on board. Rather than buy a book, check one out from the ship's library. Instead of ordering a pricey pay-per-view movie in your cabin, enjoy the cruise's free musical performances, classes, and activities. Read your daily program: There's something free going on, somewhere on the ship, virtually every minute of every day.

Don't cheap out at the expense of fun. If you're having a nice dinner, spring for a glass of wine—but keep a mental tally of all these little charges so you're not shocked by the final bill.

ON THE SHIP

third of this tip goes to your cabin steward, a third to the restaurant stewards, and a third to others, including people who worked for you behind the scenes (such as the laundry crew). While overall tips are still not what they were 20 years ago, auto-tipping has proven to be a suitable compromise for both passengers and crew.

Cruise lines explain that, with auto-tipping, additional tipping is "not expected." But it is still most certainly appreciated by the crew. This can cause stress for passengers who are unsure whom, how much, and when to tip; conscientious tippers miss the "good old days" when there was a clearly prescribed amount earmarked for each crew member. Even more confusing, with all the new alternative dining options, you likely won't be served by the same waiter every night—in fact, you might never eat at the same restaurant twice. In general, the rule of thumb is to give a cash tip at the end of the cruise to those crew members who have provided exceptional service (for specific guidelines, see page 103).

At any point, you can increase or decrease your auto-tip amount to reflect your satisfaction with the service you've received. So, if you don't have cash for your final tip, you can simply go to the front desk and increase the auto-tip amount instead (but try to do so before the final night, when accounts are being finalized).

In addition to a monetary tip, crew members appreciate it when you pass along positive feedback. Most cruise lines provide guests with comment cards for this purpose, and they can be taken very seriously when determining promotions. If someone has really gone above and beyond for you, fill out a comment card on their behalf.

HEALTH

Health problems can strike anywhere—even when you're relaxing on a cruise ship in the middle of the sea. Every ship has an onboard doctor (though he or she may not be licensed in the US). If you have to visit the shipboard physician, you will be charged. Before you leave home, ask your health insurance company if the cost is covered or reimbursable; if you buy travel insurance, investigate how it covers onboard medical care.

Fortunately, some of the most common health concerns on cruise ships, while miserable, are temporary and relatively easy to treat.

Seasickness

Naturally, one concern novice cruisers have is whether the motion of the ship will cause them to spend their time at sea with their head in the toilet. And, in fact, a small percentage of people discover (quickly and violently) that they have zero tolerance for life at sea. But the vast majority of cruisers do just fine.

The Baltic is a mostly enclosed sea with very little tide or turbulence; the North Sea can be rougher, but is still calmer than the open ocean. Remember that you're on a gigantic floating city—it takes a lot of agitation to really get the ship moving. Cruise ships are also equipped with stabilizers—wing-like panels that extend below the water's surface and automatically tilt to counteract rolling (side-to-side movement) caused by big swells.

But rough seas can occur, and when they do, waves and winds may toss your ship around quite noticeably. When this happens, chandeliers and other fixtures begin to jiggle and clink, motion sickness bags discreetly appear in the hallways, and the captain comes over the loudspeaker to comfortingly explain what's being done to smooth out the ride. Lying in bed, being rocked to sleep like a baby, you hear the hangers banging the sides of your closet. Some cruisers actually enjoy this experience; for others, it's pure misery.

If you're prone to motion sickness, visit your doctor before your cruise, and be prepared with a remedy (or several) in case you're laid low. Below are several options that veteran cruisers swear by.

Dramamine (generic name: Dimenhydrate) is easy to get over the counter but is highly sedating—not ideal unless you are desperate. Some cruisers prefer the less-drowsy formula, which is actually a different drug (called Meclozine, sometimes marketed as **Bonine**). **Marezine** (generic name: Cyclizine) has similar properties and side effects to Dramamine.

Scopolamine patches (sometimes called by the brand name Transderm) are small (dime-sized) and self-adhesive; just stick one on a hairless area behind your ear. They work well for many travelers (the only major side effect is dry mouth), but require a prescription and are expensive (figure $15 for a three-day dose). Some cruisers apply them prophylactically just before first boarding the ship (especially if rough weather is forecast). After removing one of these patches, wash your hands carefully—getting the residue in your eyes can cause dilated pupils and blurry vision.

Acupressure wristbands (such as **Sea-Bands**) have little buds that press on the pressure points on your wrist associated with nausea. You can buy them in any drugstore. They are easy to wear (if a bit goofy-looking—they look like exercise wristbands), and many people prefer them as a cheap and nonmedicinal remedy.

Every cruise aficionado has a favorite homegrown seasickness remedy. Some say that eating green apples or candied ginger can help settle a queasy stomach. Others suggest holding a peeled orange under the nose. Old sea dogs say that if you stay above deck, as close to the middle of the ship as possible, and keep your eyes on the horizon, it will reduce the effects of the motion.

Illness

Like a college dorm or a day-care center, a cruise ship is a veritable incubator for communicable disease. Think about everything that you (and several thousand other passengers) are touching: elevator buttons, railings, serving spoons in the buffet, and on and on. If one person gets sick, it's just a matter of time before others do, too.

The common cold is a risk. But perhaps even more likely are basic gastrointestinal upsets, most often caused by the norovirus (a.k.a. the Norwalk virus)—tellingly nicknamed the "cruise-ship virus." Most often spread through fecally contaminated food or person-to-person contact, the norovirus is your basic nasty stomach bug, resulting in nausea, diarrhea, vomiting, and sometimes fever or cramps. It usually goes away on its own after a day or two.

Because contagious maladies are a huge concern aboard a ship, the cruise industry is compulsive about keeping things clean.

Between cruises, ships are thoroughly disinfected with a powerful cleaning agent. When you check in, you'll be quizzed about recent symptoms to be sure you aren't bringing any nasty bugs on board. Some cruise lines won't allow passengers to handle the serving spoons at the buffet for the first two days—the crew serves instead. And, if you develop certain symptoms, the cruise line reserves the right to expel you from the ship at the next port of call (though, in practice, this is rare—more likely, they'll ask you to stay in your stateroom until you're no longer contagious).

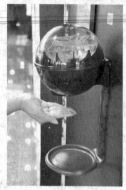

Many cruise lines douse their passengers with waterless hand sanitizers at every opportunity. Dispensers are stationed around the ship, and smiling stewards might squirt your hands from a spray bottle at the entrance to restaurants or as you reboard the ship after a day in port. Whether this works is up for debate. Several studies have demonstrated that using these sanitizers can actually be counterproductive. The US Centers for Disease Control (CDC) recommend them only as an adjunct to, rather than a replacement for, hand washing with soap and warm water. The gels work great against bacteria, but not viruses (such as the norovirus). Following the CDC's lead, some cruise lines have discontinued the use of waterless sanitizers—and have seen an immediate *decrease* in their rate of outbreaks. The logic is that hand sanitizers actually discourage proper hand-washing behavior. When people apply sanitizers, they assume their hands are clean—and don't bother to wash with soap and water. All the while, that spunky norovirus survives on their hands, gets transferred to the serving spoon at the buffet, and winds up on other people's hands while they're eating dinner.

On your stateroom TV, you might find a channel with instructions on how to wash your hands. Patronizing, yes. But not undeservedly. In a recent international study, Americans were found to be less diligent than other nationalities when it comes to washing their hands after using the bathroom. They then go straight to the buffet, and...you know the rest. It's disgusting but true. If you're a total germophobe, you have two options: Avoid the buffet entirely—or just get over it.

Staying Fit on Board

While it's tempting to head back to the buffet for a second dessert (or even a second dinner) at 11:00 p.m., file away this factoid: A typical cruise passenger gains about a pound a day. After two weeks at sea, you've put on the "Seafaring 15."

Water, Trash, and Poo:
The Inside Scoop

Wondering how cruise ships deal with passengers' basic functions? Here are the answers to some often-asked questions:

Is the water clean and drinkable? Drinking water is usually pumped into the ship at the point of embarkation. Throughout the duration of the cruise, this supply is what comes out of your bathroom tap and is used in restaurant drinks.

Larger ships also have the capacity to desalinize (remove salt from) seawater for use aboard. While perfectly safe to drink, this water doesn't taste good, so it's reserved primarily for cleaning. The water in your stateroom's toilet or shower might be desalinated.

Waste water from the ship is purified on board. While theoretically safe to drink, it's usually deposited into the sea.

Where does the trash go? Trash from shipboard restaurants is carefully sorted into garbage, recyclables, and food waste. Garbage is removed along with other solid waste in port. Cruise lines pay recycling companies to take the recyclables (interestingly, in the US it's the other way around; the companies pay the ship for their recyclables). Food waste is put through a powerful grinder that turns it into a biodegradable puree. This "fish food" is quietly piped out the end of the ship as it sails through the night.

What happens to poo? You may wonder whether shipboard waste is deposited into the sea as you cruise. These things are dictated by local and international law as well as by the policies of individual cruise lines. Most mainstream cruise lines do not dump solid waste into the sea. Instead it is collected, stored, and removed from the ship for proper disposal in port.

ON THE SHIP

Whether you're a fitness buff or simply want to stave off weight gain, cruise ships offer plenty of opportunities to get your body moving. Most ships have fitness centers with exercise equip-

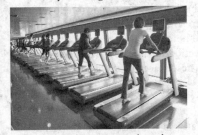

ment, such as bikes, treadmills, elliptical trainers, and weight machines. Some offer the services of personal trainers, plus classes like boot camp, spinning, Pilates, and yoga (newbies and yoga-heads alike will find it an interesting challenge to hold tree pose on a moving ship). These services usually cost extra, though some classes can be free (usually things like stretching or ab work).

If you're not the gym type, there are other ways to burn

calories. Besides swimming pools, many ships have outdoor running tracks that wrap around the deck, complete with fresh air and views. And some ships have more extreme-type sports, such as rock-climbing walls and surfing simulators.

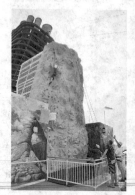

Even if you don't take advantage of sports-related amenities, simply staying active throughout your cruise will help keep those multicourse dinners from going straight to your hips. With multiple levels, your cruise ship is one giant StairMaster. Take the stairs instead of the elevator (which often saves time, too), or run down to the bottom floor and hike back up to the top a couple of times a day. Opt for a walking tour instead of a bus tour when you're in port. Hit the dance floor at night. But just in case, bring along your roomy "Thanksgiving pants."

Smoking

Smoking presents both a public health issue and a fire hazard for cruise lines. While policies are evolving, these days most cruise lines prohibit smoking in nearly all enclosed public spaces as well as in many outdoor areas, as well as in staterooms or on verandas. You may be able to smoke in certain bars or lounges and in dedicated outdoor spots. If you're a dedicated smoker or an adamant nonsmoker, research the various cruise lines' policies when choosing your vacation.

COMMUNICATING

Because phoning and Internet access are prohibitively expensive on board—and because the times you'll be in port are likely to coincide with late-night or early-morning hours back home (8:00-17:00 in most of Europe is 2:00-11:00 a.m. on the East Coast and 23:00-8:00 a.m. on the West Coast)—keeping in touch affordably can be tricky. Let the folks back home know not to expect too many calls, or figure out if there are any late evenings in ports when it might be convenient to call home.

Check the "Helpful Hints" section in each destination chapter for advice on the cheapest, easiest places in each port to get online.

Getting Online

It's useful to get online periodically as you travel—to confirm trip plans, get weather forecasts, catch up on email, or post status updates and photos from your trip. But with high prices and slow speeds, shipboard Internet is not the best option.

ON THE SHIP

Most cruise ships have an Internet café with computer terminals, and many also have Wi-Fi (some offer it in select areas of the ship, others provide it in staterooms). Either way, onboard Internet access is very expensive—figure $0.80-1/minute (the more minutes you buy, the cheaper they are, and special deals can lower the cost substantially). Before you pay for access, be warned that—since it's satellite-based rather than hard-wired—onboard Internet is tortoise-slow compared with high-speed broadband (remember dial-up?). And while an app such as Skype or FaceTime to make voice or video calls over a Wi-Fi connection is an excellent budget option on land, it's impractical on the ship. Onboard Internet access has such limited bandwidth that these services often don't work well—if at all.

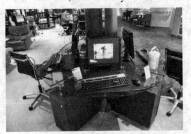

In short, shipboard Internet access is practical only for quick tasks, such as downloading email. Limit the time you need to spend online by reading and composing emails or social media posts offline, then going online periodically just to download/upload. You can also set up certain smartphone apps to do this; for example, some news apps let you download all of the day's top stories at once, rather than clicking to read them one at a time. When you're done, be sure that you properly log out of the shipboard network to avoid unwittingly running up Internet fees.

Ideally, wait until you're in port to get online. If you have a mobile device, find a café on shore where you can sit and download your email or log into Facebook over Wi-Fi while enjoying a cup of coffee—at a fraction of the shipboard cost. Or hop on a computer at an Internet café to quickly go online.

For more pointers on getting online in port, see page 126.

Phoning

If you want to make calls during your trip, you can do it either from land or at sea. It's much cheaper to call home from a pay phone on shore (explained on page 126) or from a mobile phone on a land-based network (explained later). Calling from the middle of the sea is pricey, but if you're in a pinch, you can dial direct from your stateroom telephone or use a mobile phone while roaming on the costly onboard network. For details on how to dial European phone numbers, see page 1146.

Stateroom Telephones: Calling **within the ship** (such as to the front desk or another cabin) is free on your stateroom telephone, or from phones hanging at strategic locations around the ship. Some ships provide certain crew members with an on-ship mobile phone and a four-digit phone number. If there's a crew member or service desk you want to contact, just remember their number and dial it toll-free.

Calling **to shore** (over a satellite connection) is usually possible, but expensive—anywhere from $6 to $20 a minute (if you prepay for a large block of calling time, it can be cheaper—for example, $25 for 12 minutes; ask for specifics at the front desk). Note: Similar charges apply if someone calls from shore to your stateroom.

Mobile Phones: Most people enjoy the convenience of bringing their own phone, and some cruise lines, such as Norwegian and Disney, even have their own apps with your ship's deck plans, menus, and booking services. Start by figuring out whether your phone works in Europe: Check your operating manual (look for "tri-band," "quad-band," or "GSM"). If you're not sure, ask your service provider. Also ask about roaming charges for voice calls, text messaging, and data, and consider an add-on plan that you can activate temporarily.

If you're worried about the added expense, before your trip, make sure you know how to use your phone cost-effectively. For more on using your phone in Europe, see www.ricksteves.com/phoning. Here are the basics:

1. Disable roaming. To prevent accidentally roaming on the sea-based network, simply disable roaming (or put your phone in "Airplane Mode") as soon as you board the ship. And be warned that receiving a call—even if you don't answer it—costs the same as making a call. You can re-enable Wi-Fi if you decide to pay the fee onboard your ship or when using Wi-Fi in port.

2. Use land networks. If you are using a mobile phone, it's essential to distinguish between land and sea networks. Because many European cruise itineraries stay fairly close to land, you can often roam on the cheaper **land-based networks,** even when you're at sea. Your phone will automatically find land-based networks if you're within several miles of shore. The **onboard network,** which doesn't even turn on until the ship is about 10 miles out, is far more expensive—about $2.50-5/minute (ask your mobile service provider for details about your ship).

Before placing a call or accessing a data-roaming network from your ship, carefully note which network you're on (this is displayed on your phone's readout, generally next to the signal bars). You might not recognize the various land-based network names; to be safe, learn the name of the cruise-line network (it's usually something obvious, such as "Phone at Sea")—then avoid making any calls or using data if that name pops up.

3. Turn off data or purchase a data plan. If you plan to use a service like Skype or Google+ for real-time communication, Wi-Fi is all you need. If you purchase a data plan from your cruise ship or phone-service provider, you will need to keep data turned on. In this case, it is recommended to reset your usage stats (if possible) to monitor how much data you are using during your travels (ask your phone carrier for further direction on this).

ONBOARD ACTIVITIES

Large cruise ships are like resorts at sea. In the hours spent cruising between ports, there's no shortage of diversions: swimming

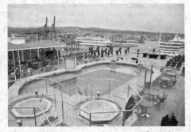

pools, hot tubs, and water slides; sports courts, exercise rooms, shuffleboard courts, giant chess-boards, and rock-climbing walls; casinos with slots and table games; shopping malls; art galleries with works for sale; children's areas with playground equipment and babysitting services; and spas where you can get a facial, massage, or other treatments. Many activities have an extra charge associated—always ask before you participate.

To avoid crowds, take advantage of shipboard activities and amenities at off times. The gym is quieter late in the evenings, when many cruisers are already in bed. Onboard restaurants are typically less crowded for the later seatings. If you're dying to try out that rock-climbing wall, drop by as soon as you get back on the ship in the afternoon; if you wait an hour or two, the line could get longer.

Days at sea are a good time to try all the things you haven't gotten around to on busy port days, but be warned that everyone else on the ship has the same idea. Services such as massages are particularly popular on sea days—book ahead and be prepared to pay full price (if you get a massage on a port day, you might get a discount). Premium restaurants and other activities also tend to fill up far earlier for days at sea, so don't wait around too long to book anything you have your heart set on.

Remember, the schedule and locations for all of these options—classes, social activities, entertainment, and more—are listed in your daily program.

Social Activities

Many ships offer a wide array of activities, ranging from seminars on art history to wine- and beer-tastings to classes on how to fold towels in the shape of animals (a skill, you'll soon learn, that your cabin steward has mastered). Quite a few of these are sales pitches in disguise, but others are just for fun and a great way to make friends. Bingo, trivia contests, dancing lessons, cooking classes, goofy poolside games, newlywed games, talent shows, nightly mixers for singles, scrapbooking sessions, high tea—there's something for everyone. Note that a few offerings might use code words or abbreviations: "Friends of Bill W" refers to a meeting of Alcoholics Anonymous; "Friends of Dorothy" or

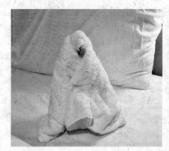

"LGBT" refers to a meeting of gay people. Ships have a community bulletin board where these and other meetings are posted. You can even post your own.

Entertainment and Nightlife

Most cruise ships have big (up to 1,000-seat) theaters with nightly shows. An in-house troupe of singers and dancers generally puts on

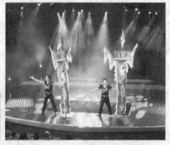

two or three schmaltzy revue-type shows a week (belting out crowd-pleasing hits). On other nights, the stage is taken up by guest performers (comedy acts, Beatles tribute bands, jugglers, hypnotists, and so on). While not necessarily Broadway-quality, these performances are a fun diversion; since they're

typically free and have open seating, it's easy to drop by for just a few minutes (or even stand in the back) to see if you like the show before you commit. On some of the biggest new megaships, the cruise lines are experimenting with charging a fee and assigning seats for more elaborate shows.

Smaller lounges scattered around the ship offer more intimate entertainment with just-as-talented performers—pianists, singers,

duos, or groups who attract a faithful following night after night. Some cruisers enjoy relaxing in their favorite lounge to cap their day.

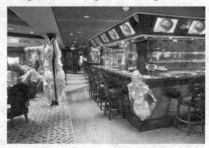

Cruises often screen second-run or classic movies for passengers to watch. Sometimes there's a dedicated cinema room; otherwise, films play in the main theater at off times.

Eating, always a popular pastime, is encouraged all hours of the day and night. While the main shipboard eateries tend to close by about midnight, large ships have one or two places that remain open 24 hours a day.

And if you enjoy dancing, you have plenty of options ranging from classy ballroom-dance venues to hopping nightclubs that pump dance music until the wee hours.

Shopping

In addition to touting shopping opportunities in port, cruise ships have their own shops on board, selling T-shirts, jewelry, trinkets,

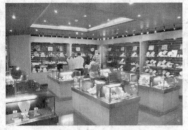

and all manner of gear emblazoned with their logo. At busy times, they might even set up tables in the lobby to lure in even more shoppers. In accordance with international maritime law, the ship's casino and duty-free shops can open only once the ship is seven miles offshore.

While shopping on board is convenient and saves on taxes, most of the items sold on the ship can be found at home or online—for less. If you like to shop, have fun doing it in port, seeking out locally made mementos in European shops. (If you enjoy both sightseeing and shopping, balancing your port time can be a challenge; I'd suggest doing a quick surgical shopping strike in destinations where you have something in particular you'd like to buy, so you won't miss out on the great sights.) You'll find more information on shopping in port on page 132. In the destination chapters, I've given some suggestions about specific local goods to shop for.

You'll find more information on shopping in port on page 132.

Casino

Cruise ships offer Vegas-style casinos with all the classic games, including slots, blackjack, poker, roulette, and craps. But unlike Vegas—where casinos clamor for your business with promises of the "loosest slots in town"—cruise ships know they have a captive audience. And that means your odds of winning are even worse than they are in Vegas.

Onboard casinos also offer various trumped-up activities to drum up excitement. Sure, a poker tournament can be exciting and competitive—but I can't for the life of me figure out the appeal of a slot tournament

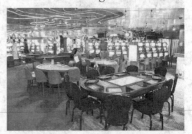

ON THE SHIP

(no joking). If you want to test your luck—but you're not clear on the rules of blackjack, craps, or other casino games—take advantage of the free gambling classes that many cruise lines offer early in the trip.

Art Gallery

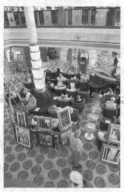

Many ships have an art gallery, and some even display a few genuinely impressive pieces from their own collection (minor works by major artists). But more often the focus is on selling new works by lesser-known artists. Your ship might offer lectures about the art, but beware: These often turn out to be sales pitches for "up-and-coming" artists whose works are being auctioned on board. While the artists may be talented, the "valuation" prices are dramatically inflated. Art auctions ply bidders with free champagne to drive up the prices...but no serious art collector buys paintings on a cruise ship.

Photography

Once upon a time, photographers snapped a free commemorative portrait of you and your travel partner as you boarded the ship. But when the cruise lines figured out that people were willing to shell out $8-15 for one of these pictures, they turned it into big business. Roving photographers snap photos of you at dinner, and makeshift studios with gauzy backgrounds suddenly appear in the lobby on formal night. As you disem-

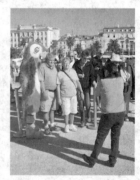

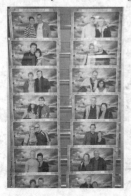

bark at each port, photographers ask you to pose with models in tacky costumes. Later that day, all those photos appear along one of the ship's hallways for everyone to see (perusing my fellow passengers' deer-in-the-headlights mug shots is one of my favorite onboard activities). While it's hard to justify spending 10 bucks on a cheesy snapshot, you might be able to bargain the price down toward the end of the trip. Repeat cruisers report that if you swing by the photography area on the last evening, the salespeople—eager to unload their inventory—may cut a deal if you pay cash.

Spa/Beauty Salon

Most cruise ships have spa facilities, where you can get a massage, facial, manicure, pedicure, and so on. There may also be a beauty salon where you can get your hair done. While convenient, these services are obviously priced at a premium—though specials are often available. These treatments often come with a sales pitch for related products. Tip as you would back home (either in cash or by adding a tip when you sign the receipt).

Library

The onboard library has an assortment of free loaner books, ranging from nautical topics to travel guidebooks to beach reading.

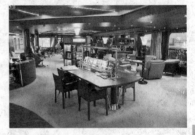

Usually outfitted with comfortable chairs and tables, this can also be a good place to stretch out and relax while you read. If the ship's staterooms are equipped with DVD players, the library may have DVDs for loan or rent.

Chapel

Many ships have a nondenominational chapel for prayer or silent reflection. If you're cruising during a religious holiday, the cruise line may invite a clergy member on board to lead a service.

CRUISING WITH KIDS

Cruises can be a great way to vacation with a family. But do your homework: Cruise lines cater to kids to varying degrees. For example, Disney, Celebrity, and Royal Caribbean are extremely kid-friendly, while other lines (especially the higher-end luxury ones) offer virtually nothing extra for children—a hint that they prefer you to leave the kiddos at home.

Kids' Programs and Activities

Family-friendly cruise lines have "kids clubs" that are open for most of the day. It's a win-win situation for both parents and children. Kids get to hang out with their peers and fill their time with games, story time, arts and crafts, and other fun stuff, while parents get to relax and enjoy the amenities of the ship.

Most kids clubs are for children ages three and older, and require your tots to be potty-trained. Kids are separated by age so that tweens don't have to be subjected to younger children. For older kids, there are teen-only hangouts. If you have kids under three, options are limited: You might find parent/baby classes (no drop-and-go) and, in rare cases, onboard day care.

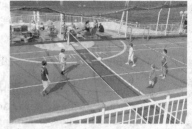

Rules for kids clubs differ across cruise lines. Some charge for the service, others include it. While kids clubs are generally open throughout the day (about 9:00–22:00), some close at mealtimes, so you'll have to collect your kids for lunch and dinner. Port-day policies vary—some kids clubs require a parent or guardian to stay on board (in case they need to reach you); others are fine with letting you off your parental leash.

There are also plenty of activities outside the kids club. All

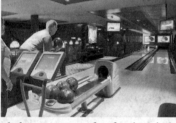

ships have pools, and some take it to the next level with rock-climbing walls, bowling alleys, and in-line skating. Arcades and movies provide hours of entertainment, and shows are almost always appropriate for all ages. Many scheduled activities are fun for the whole family, such as art classes, ice-carving contests, or afternoon tea.

Babysitting

Because cruise lines want you to explore the ship and have fun (and, of course, spend money at bars and the casino), many have babysitting services. On some ships, you can arrange for a babysitter to come to your stateroom, while others offer late-night group babysitting for a small fee.

To line up babysitting, ask at the front desk or the kids club. Or, if you and your child hit it off with one of the youth counselors at the kids club, you could consider asking her or him for some private babysitting. Oftentimes, crew members have flexible hours and are looking to earn extra money. Some have been separated from their families and even relish the opportunity to play with your kids—let them!

When hiring a babysitter, ask up front about rates; otherwise, offer the standard amount you pay at home. And remember to have cash on hand so you can compensate the babysitter at the end of the evening.

Food

Pizza parlors, hamburger grills, ice cream stands...thanks to the diverse dining options on ships, even the pickiest of eaters should be satisfied. Here are some tips for dining with children:

If you prefer to eat with your kids each night, choose the first dinner seating, which has more families and suits kids' earlier eating schedules. If your kids are too squirmy to sit through a five-course formal dinner every night, choose the buffet or a casual poolside restaurant (described later, under "Eating").

Don't forget about room service. This can be a nice option for breakfast, so you don't have to rush around in the morning. It's also an easy solution if you're cabin-bound with a napping child in the afternoon.

Set ground rules for sweets and soda ahead of time. If your kids have convinced you to let them drink soda (which costs extra on a cruise), buy a soft drink card for the week to save over ordering à la carte.

In Port

If you plan to take your kids off the ship and into town, remember that a lot of Europe's streets and sidewalks are old, cobbled, and uneven—not ideal for a stroller. If your kids can't walk the whole way themselves, consider bringing a backpack carrier rather than a stroller for more mobility.

While excursions are often not worth the expense, they make sense for some ports and activities, especially when you have kids in tow. You don't have to deal with transportation, nor do you have to worry about missing the boat. (For more on excursions, see page 105.)

If you do take your kids into port, consider draping a lanyard around their necks with emergency contact information in case you get separated. Include your name and mobile phone number, your ship's name, the cruise line, the itinerary, a copy of the child's passport, and some emergency cash.

Eating

While shipboard dining used to be open-and-shut (one restaurant, same table, same companions, same waitstaff, same time every night), these days you have choices ranging from self-service buffets to truly inspired specialty restaurants. On bigger ships, you could spend a week on board and never eat at the same place twice.

Note that if you have food allergies or a special diet—such as vegetarian, vegan, or kosher—most cruise lines will do their best to accommodate you. Notify them as far ahead as possible (when you book your cruise or 30 days before you depart).

DINING ONBOARD

Most cruise ships have a main dining room, a more casual buffet, a variety of specialty restaurants, and room service.

Main Dining Room

The main restaurant venue on your ship is the old-fashioned dining room. With genteel decor, formal waiters, and a rotating menu of

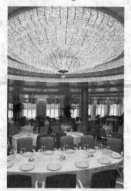

upscale cuisine, dining here is an integral part of the classic cruise experience.

Traditionally, each passenger was assigned a particular seating time and table for all dinners in the dining room. But over the last decade or so, this **"assigned dining"** policy has been in flux, with various cruise lines taking different approaches. Some lines (including Royal Caribbean, Costa, MSC, Celebrity, and Disney) still have assigned dining. Others (such as Holland America, Princess, and Cunard) make it optional: You can choose whether you want assigned seating (if you don't, just show up, and you'll be seated at whichever table is available next). Norwegian Cruise Line, along with several of the smaller luxury lines (Oceania, Silversea, Azamara, Windstar, Star Clippers, Seabourn, Regent Seven Seas), have no assigned dining—it's first-come, first-served, in any dining venue.

If you choose assigned dining, you'll eat with the same people every night (unless you opt to dine elsewhere on some evenings). Tables for two are rare, so couples will likely wind up seated with others. You'll really get to know your tablemates...whether you like it or not. Some cruisers prefer to be at a table that's as large as possible—if you are seated with just one other couple, you risk running out of conversation topics sooner than at a table with 10 or 12 people.

Diners are assigned either to an early seating (typically around 18:30) or a late seating (around 20:45). Avid sightseers might prefer the second seating, so they can fully enjoy the port without rushing back to the ship in time to change for dinner (on the other hand, the first seating lets you turn in early to rest up for the next day's port). In general, families and older passengers seem to opt for the first seating, while younger passengers tend to prefer the later one.

If your cruise line has assigned dining (whether mandatory or optional), you can request your seating preferences (time and table size) when you book your cruise. These assignments are first-come,

Formal Nights

Many cruises have one or two designated formal nights each week in the main dining room, when passengers get decked 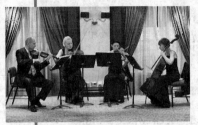 out for dinner in suits and cocktail dresses—or even tuxes and floor-length gowns (for tips on how to pack for formal night, see the sidebar on page 54). In general, on formal nights the whole ambience of the ship is upscale, with people hanging out in the bars, casinos, and other public areas dressed to the nines. And cruises like formal nights because passengers behave better and spend more money (for example, ordering a nicer bottle of wine or buying the posed photos).

Ships may also have semiformal nights (also one or two per week), which are scaled-down versions of the formal nights—for example, men wear slacks and a tie, but no jacket.

Some passengers relish the opportunity to dress up on formal nights. But if you don't feel like it, it's fine to dress however you like—as long as you stay out of the dining room. Skip the formal dinners and eat at another restaurant or the buffet, or order room service.

first-served, so the earlier you book and make your request, the better. If you don't get your choice, you can ask to be put on a waiting list.

If you're not happy with your assignment, try dropping by the dining room early on the first night to see if the maître d', who's in charge of assigning tables, can help you. He'll do his best to accommodate you (you won't be the only person requesting a change—there's always some shuffling around). If the maître d' is able to make a switch, it's appropriate to thank him with a tip.

Some people really enjoy assigned dining. It encourages you to socialize with fellow passengers and make friends. Tablemates sometimes team up and hang out in port together as well. And some cruisers form lasting friendships with people they were, once upon a time, randomly assigned to dine with. If, on the other hand, you're miserable with your dinner companions, ask the maître d' to reseat you. Be aware that the longer you wait to request a change, the more difficult (and potentially awkward) it becomes.

If you get tired of assigned dining, you can always find variety by eating at the buffet or a specialty restaurant, or by ordering room service. And if you have an early seating but decide to skip dinner one night to stay late in port, you can still dine at the other onboard restaurants. Since the various onboard eateries are all included (except for specialty-restaurant surcharges), money is no object. While I enjoy the range of people at my assigned dinner table, I usually end up dining there only about half the nights on a given cruise.

Note that the main dining room is typically also open for breakfast and lunch. At these times, it's generally open seating (no preassigned tables), but you'll likely be seated with others. The majority of travelers prefer to have a quick breakfast and lunch at the buffet (or in port). But some cruisers enjoy eating these meals in the dining room (especially on leisurely sea days) as a more civilized alternative to the mob scene at the buffet; it's also an opportunity to meet fellow passengers who normally sit elsewhere at dinner.

Dress Code: In the main dining room, most cruise lines institute a "smart casual" dress code. This means no jeans, shorts, or T-shirts. Men wear slacks and button-down or polo shirts; women wear dresses or nice separates. "Formal night" dress codes apply in the dining room (see sidebar, previous page).

Casual Dining: Buffet and Poolside Restaurants

Besides the main dining room, most ships have at least one additional restaurant, generally a casual buffet. This has much longer hours than the dining room, and the food is not necessarily a big step down: The buffet often has some of the same options as in the dining room, and it may even have some more unusual items, often themed (Greek, Indian, sushi, and so on). Most ships also have an even more casual "grill"

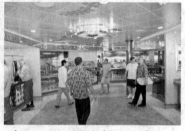

restaurant, usually near the pool, where you can grab a quick burger or hot dog and other snacks. These options are handy if you're in a hurry, or just want a break from the dining room.

When eating at the buffet, keep in mind that this situation—with hundreds of people handling the same serving spoons and tongs, licking their fingers, then handling more spoons and tongs—is nirvana for communicable diseases. Compound that with the fact that some diners don't wash their hands (incorrectly believing that hand sanitizer is protecting them from all illness), and you've got a perfect storm. At the risk of sounding like a germophobe, wash your hands before, during, and after your meal. For more on this cheerful topic, see page 83.

Dress Code: The buffet and "grill" restaurants have a casual dress code. You'll see plenty of swimsuits and flip-flops, though most cruise lines require a shirt or cover-up in the buffet.

Specialty Restaurants

Most ships (even small ones) have at least one specialty eatery, but some have a dozen or more. If there's just one specialty restau-

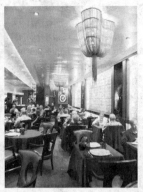

rant on board, it serves food (such as steak or seafood) that's a notch above what's available in the dining room. If there are several, they specialize in different foods or cuisines: steakhouse, French, sushi, Italian, Mexican, and so on.

Because specialty restaurants are more in demand than the traditional dining room, it's smart to make reservations if you have your heart set on a particular one. At the beginning of your cruise, scope out the dining room's menu for the week; if one night seems less enticing to you, consider

booking a specialty restaurant for that evening. Days at sea are also popular nights in specialty restaurants. I enjoy using the specialty restaurants when I want to dine with people I've met on the ship outside of my usual tablemates. Remember that if you want a window seat with a view, eat early. When darkness settles, the window becomes a pitch-black pane of glass, and that romantic view is entirely gone.

Occasionally these restaurants are included in your cruise price, but more often they require a special cover charge (typically $10-50). In addition to the cover charge, certain entrées incur a supplement ($10-20). A couple ordering specialty items and a bottle of wine can quickly ring up a $100 dinner bill. If you're on a tight budget, remember: Specialty restaurants are optional. You can eat every meal at the included dining room and buffet if you'd rather not spend the extra money. (By the way, if you order a bottle of wine and don't finish it, they can put your name on it and bring it to you in the main dining hall the next night.)

Some routine cruisers allege that the cruise lines are making the food in their dining room intentionally worse in order to steer passengers to the specialty restaurants that charge a cover. But from a dollars-and-cents perspective, this simply doesn't add up. The generally higher-quality ingredients used in specialty restaurants typically cost far more than the cover charge; for example, you might pay $20 to eat a steak that's worth $30. The cover charge is designed not to be a moneymaker, but to limit the number of people who try to dine at the specialty restaurants. It's just expensive enough to keep the place busy every night, but not cheap enough that it's swamped. So if cruise food is getting worse, it's not on purpose.

Dress Code: Specialty restaurants usually follow the same dress code as the main dining room (including on formal nights), though it depends on how upscale the menu is. The steakhouse might be more formal than the main dining room; the sushi bar could be less formal. If you're unsure, ask.

Room Service

Room service is temptingly easy and is generally included in the cruise price (no extra charge). Its menu appears to be much more limited than what you'd get in any of the restaurants, but you can often request items from the dining room menu as well. (If you don't want to dress up on formal night—but still want to enjoy the generally fancier fare on those evenings—ask in advance whether you can get those same meals as room service.) Either way, it's very convenient, especially on mornings when the ship arrives in port early. By eating breakfast in your room (place your order the night before), you can get ready at a more leisurely pace and avoid the crowd at the buffet. You can also arrange for room service to be waiting when you get back on the ship from exploring a port.

It's polite to thank the person who delivers your food with about a $2 tip; sometimes you can put this on your tab and sign for it, but not always, so it's smart to have cash ready.

Dress Code: From tuxes and gowns to your birthday suit, when you order room service, it's up to you.

CRUISE CUISINE

Reviews of the food on cruise ships range wildly, from raves to pans. It's all relative: While food snobs who love locally sourced bistros may turn up their noses at cruise cuisine, fans of chain restaurants are perfectly satisfied on board. True foodies should lower their expectations. High-seas cuisine is not exactly high cuisine.

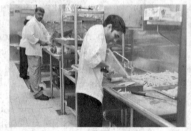

Cruise food is as good as it can be, considering that thousands of people are fed at each meal. Most cruise lines replenish their food stores about every two weeks, so everything you eat—including meat, seafood, and produce—may be less than fresh. Except on some of the top-end lines, the shipboard chefs are afforded virtually no room for creativity: The head office creates the recipes, then trains all kitchen crews to prepare each dish. To ensure cooks get it just right, cruise lines hang a photo in the galley (kitchen) of what each dish should look like. This is especially important since most of the cooks and servers come from countries where the cuisine is quite different.

Cruise-ship food is not local cuisine. Today's menu, dreamed

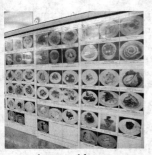

up months ago by some executive chef in Miami, bears no resemblance to the food you saw this afternoon in port. It can be frustrating to wander through a Norwegian fjordside market that sells freshly grilled salmon and herb-roasted potatoes, then go back to your ship for Caesar salad and prime rib.

On the other hand, cruise menus often feature famous but unusual dishes that would cost a pretty penny in a top-end restaurant back home. It can be fun to sample a variety of oddball items (such as frog legs, escargot, or foie gras) and higher-end meats (filet mignon, guinea fowl, lobster, crab)...with no expense and no commitment. (If you don't like it, don't finish it. Waiters are happy to bring you something else.)

Whether cruise food is good or bad, one thing's for sure: There's plenty of it. A ship with 2,500 passengers and 1,500 crew members might brag that they prepare "17,000 meals a day." Do the math: Someone's going back for seconds. A lot of someones, in fact. (If you're one of them, see "Staying Fit on Board" on page 84.)

All things considered, cruise lines do an impressive job of providing variety and quality. But cruise food still pales in comparison to the meals you can get in port, lovingly prepared with fresh ingredients and local recipes. Some travelers figure there's no point paying for food in port when you can just eat for free on the ship. But after a few days of cruise cuisine, I can't wait to sit down at a real European restaurant or grab some authentic street food... and I can really taste the difference.

DRINKS

In general, tap water, milk, iced tea, coffee and tea, and fruit juices are included. Other drinks cost extra: alcohol of any kind, name-brand soft drinks, fresh-squeezed fruit juices, and premium espresso drinks such as lattes and cappuccinos. You'll also pay for any drinks you take from your stateroom's minibar (generally the same price as in the restaurants). Beverages are priced approximately the same as in a restaurant on land (though in the most expensive Scandinavian countries—such as Norway—drink prices in port can exceed what you'll pay on board).

Early in your cruise, ask about special offers for reduced drink prices, such as discount cards or six-for-the-price-of-five beer offers. This also goes for soft drinks—if you guzzle Diet Coke, you can buy an "unlimited drink card" at the start of the cruise and order as many soft drinks as you want without paying more.

Cruise lines want to encourage alcohol sales on board, but

ON THE SHIP

without alienating customers. Before you set sail, find out your cruise line's policy on taking alcohol aboard so you can BYOB to save money. Some cruise lines ban it outright; others prohibit only hard liquor but allow wine and sometimes beer. On some ships, you may be able to bring one or two bottles of wine when you first board the ship. Keep in mind that if you bring aboard your own bottle of wine to enjoy with dinner on the ship, you'll most likely face a corkage fee (around $10-20).

To monitor the alcohol situation, cruise lines require you to go through a security checkpoint every time you board the ship. It's OK to purchase a souvenir bottle of booze in port, but you may have to check it for the duration of the cruise. Your purchases will be returned to you on the final night or the morning of your last disembarkation.

If you're a scofflaw who enjoys a nip every now and again, note that various cruising websites abound with strategies for getting around the "no alcohol" rules.

EATING ON PORT DAYS

For some travelers, port days present a tasty opportunity to sample the local cuisine. Others prioritize their port time for sightseeing or shopping rather than sitting at a restaurant waiting for their food to arrive. And still others economize by returning to the ship for lunch (which, to me, seems like a waste of valuable port time). For more tips on eating while in port, see page 135.

To save money, some cruise passengers suggest tucking a few items from the breakfast buffet into a day bag for a light lunch on the go. While this is, to varying degrees, frowned upon by cruise lines, they recognize that many people do it—and, after all, you are paying for the food. If you do this, do so discreetly. Some experienced cruisers suggest ordering room service for breakfast, with enough extra for lunch. Or you can get a room-service sandwich the evening before and tuck it into your minifridge until morning. To make it easier to pack your lunch, bring along sealable plastic baggies from home.

Final Disembarkation

When your cruise comes to an end, you'll need to jump through a few hoops before you actually get off the ship. The crew will give you written instructions, and you'll often be able to watch a presentation about the process on your stateroom TV. Many ships even have a "disembarkation talk" on the final day to explain the procedure. I keep it very simple: I review my bill for extra charges, accept the auto-tip, and carry my own bags off the ship any time after breakfast. While the specifics vary from cruise to cruise, most include the following considerations.

On your last full day on the ship, you'll receive an itemized copy of your **bill.** This includes the auto-tip for the crew (explained on page 79), drinks, excursions, shopping, restaurant surcharges, and any other expenses you've incurred. This amount will automatically be charged to the credit card you registered with the cruise line. If there are any mistaken charges, contest them as soon as you discover them (to avoid long lines just as everyone is disembarking).

If you'd like to give an additional cash **tip** to any crew members (especially those with whom you've personally interacted or who have given you exceptional service), it's best to do so on the final night in case you can't find the tippee in the morning. It's most common to tip cabin stewards and maybe a favorite waiter or two, particularly if they served you several times over the course of your cruise. There is no conventional amount or way to calculate tips; simply give what you like, but keep in mind that the crew has extremely low base wages (about $1/day). Some cruise lines provide envelopes (either at the front desk or in your stateroom on the final evening) for you to tuck a cash tip inside and hand it to the crew member.

The night before disembarking, leave any **bags** you don't want to carry off the ship (with luggage tags attached) in the hall outside your room. The stewards will collect these bags during the night, and they'll be waiting for you when you step off the ship. Be sure *not* to pack any items you may need before disembarking the next morning (such as medications, a jacket, or a change of clothes). I prefer to carry off my own bags—that way, I don't have to pack the night before and go without my personal items the last morning. Also, I can leave anytime I want, and I don't have to spend time claiming my bags after I've disembarked.

Before leaving your cabin, check all the drawers, other hidden stowage areas, and the safe—after a week or more at sea, it's easy to forget where you tucked away items when you first unpacked.

In the morning, you'll be assigned a **disembarkation time.** At that time, you'll need to vacate your cabin (so the crew can clean it for the passengers arriving in a few hours) and gather in a designated public area for further instructions on where to leave the ship and claim your luggage.

It's possible to get an **early disembarkation time**—particularly if you're in a hurry to catch a plane or train, or if you just want to get started on your sightseeing. Request early disembarkation near the start of your cruise, as there is a set number of slots, and they can fill up. Another option is to walk off with all your luggage (rather than leaving it in the hall overnight and reclaiming it once off the ship)—as this opportunity may be limited to a designated

ON THE SHIP

number of passengers, ask about it near the start of your cruise.

If you're hungry, you can have breakfast—your last "free" meal before re-entering the real world. Once you do leave the ship at the appointed time, the bags you left outside your room the night before will be waiting for you in the terminal building.

If you're sightseeing around town and need to **store your bags,** there is often a bag-storage service at or near the cruise terminal (I've listed specifics for certain ports in this book). If you're staying at a hotel after the cruise, you can take your bags straight there when you leave the ship; even if your room is not ready, the hotelier is usually happy to hold your bags until check-in time.

Most cruise lines offer a **transfer** service to take you to your hotel or the airport. Typically you'll do better arranging this on your own (taxis wait at the cruise terminal, and this book's destination chapters include detailed instructions for getting into town or to the airport). But if you book it through the cruise line, they may offer the option to let you pay a little extra to keep your stateroom and enjoy the pool until catching the airport shuttle for your afternoon flight. Some cruise lines also offer excursions at the end of the journey that swing by the city's top sights before ending at your hotel or the airport. This can be a good way to combine a sightseeing excursion with a transfer.

For **customs** regulations on returning to the US, see page 135.

ON THE SHIP

IN PORT

While some people care more about shipboard amenities than the actual destinations, most travelers who take a European cruise see it mainly as a fun way to get to the ports. This is your chance to explore some of Europe's most fascinating cities, characteristic seaside villages, and engaging regions.

Prior to reaching each destination, you'll need to decide whether you want to go on an excursion (booked on board through your cruise line) or see it on your own. This chapter explains the pros and cons of excursions and provides a rundown of which destinations are best by excursion—and which are easy to do independently (see the sidebar on page 110). It also fills you in on the procedure for getting off and back on the ship, and provides tips on how to make the most of your time on land.

Excursions

In each port, your cruise line offers a variety of shore excursions. While the majority involve bus tours, town walks (led by a local guide hired for the day by the cruise line), and guided visits to museums and archaeological sites, others are more active (biking, kayaking, hiking), and some are more passive (a trip to a beach, spa, or even a luxury-hotel swimming pool for the day). Most also include a shopping component (such as a visit to a Fabergé egg shop in St. Petersburg, a diamond-cutting demonstration in Amsterdam, or a glassblowing demonstration in Sweden). When shopping is involved, kickbacks are common. Local merchants may pay the cruise line or guide to bring the group to their shops, give them a cut of whatever's bought, or both. In extreme cases, shops even provide buses and drivers for excursions, so there's no risk the shopping stop will be missed. The prices you're charged are likely inflated to cover these payouts.

Excursions aren't cheap. On European cruises, a basic two-to three-hour town walking tour runs about $40-60/person; a half-day bus tour to a nearby sight can be $70-100; and a full-day bus-plus-walking-tour itinerary can be $100-150 or more. Extras (such as a boat ride or a lunch) add to the cost. There seems to be little dif-ference in excursion costs or qual-

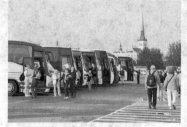

ity between a mass-market and a luxury line (in fact, excursions can be more expensive on a cheap cruise than on a pricey one).

On the day of your excursion, you'll gather in a large space (often the ship's theater, sometimes with hundreds of others), wait-ing for your excursion group to be called. You're given a sticker to wear with a number that corresponds to your specific group/bus number. Popular excursion itineraries can have several different busloads. Once called, head down the gangway—or to the tenders (small boats)—to meet your awaiting tour bus and local guide.

EXCURSION OPTIONS

The types of excursions you can book vary greatly, depending on the port. In a typical midsized port city, there might be two differ-ent themed walking tours of the city itself (for example, one focus-ing on the Old Town and art museum, and another on the New Town and architecture); a panoramic drive into the countryside for scenery, sometimes with stops (such as a wine-tasting, a restaurant lunch, or a folk-dancing show); and trips to outlying destinations, such as a neighboring village or an archaeological site.

Some ports have an even wider range of options. For example, if you dock at France's port of Le Havre, you'll be offered vari-ous trips into Paris, as well as guided visits to D-Day beaches and Impressionist sights closer to your ship. In these regions, excur-sions feature destinations bundled in different ways—look for an itinerary that covers just what you're interested in (see the "Excursions" sidebars in each destination chapter to help you sort through your options).

In some cases, there's only one worthy destination, but it takes some effort to reach it. For example, from the German port of Warnemünde, it's a three-hour bus or train ride into Berlin. It's possible—using this book—to get to these places by public trans-portation. But the cruise line hopes you'll pay them to take you instead.

Most excursions include a guided tour of town, but for those who want more freedom, cruise lines also offer "On Your Own" (a.k.a. "transfer-only" or "transportation-only") excursions: A bus will meet you as you disembark, and you might have a guide who narrates your ride into town. But once you reach the main destination, you're set free and given a time to report back to the bus. While more expensive than public transportation, these transfers cost less than fully guided excursions and are generally cheaper than hiring a taxi to take you into town (although you can split the cost of a taxi with other travelers).

Most cruise lines can also arrange a private driver or guide for you. While this is billed as an "excursion," you're simply paying the cruise line to act as a middleman. It's much more cost-effective to make these arrangements yourself (you can use one of the guides or drivers I recommend in this book).

BOOKING AN EXCURSION

The cruise lines make it easy to sign up for excursions. There's generally a presentation on excursions in the theater sometime during the first few days of your cruise (or during a day at sea), and a commercial for the different itineraries runs 24/7 on your stateroom TV. You can sign up at the excursions desk, through the concierge, or (on some ships) through the interactive menu on your TV. You can generally cancel from 24 to 48 hours before the excursion leaves (ask when you book); if you cancel with less notice—for any reason—you will probably have to pay for it.

You can also book shore excursions on the cruise line's website prior to your trip. But be warned: It's common to sign up in advance, then realize once on board that your interests have changed. Some cruise lines levy a cancellation fee; most waive that fee if you cancel the first day you're on board, while others will waive it if you upgrade to a more expensive excursion.

If you have to cancel because of illness, some cruise lines' excursions desks may be willing to try to sell your tickets to another passenger (and refund your money); if not, they can write you a note to help you recoup the money from your travel insurance.

Cruise lines use the words "limited space" to prod passengers to hurry up and book various extra services—especially excursions. (They're technically correct—if there's not room for every single passenger on board to join the excursion, then space is, strictly speaking, "limited," even if the excursion never sells out.) Sometimes excursions truly do fill up quickly; other times, you can sign up moments before departure. This creates a Chicken Little situation: Since they *always* claim "limited space," it's hard to know whether an excursion truly is filling up fast. If you have your heart set on a particular excursion, book it as far ahead as you can. But if you're on the fence, ask at the excursions desk how many seats are left and how soon they anticipate it filling up. If your choice is already booked when you ask, request to be added to the wait list—it's not unusual for the cruise line to have last-minute cancellations or to add more departures for popular excursions.

TAKE AN EXCURSION, OR DO IT ON MY OWN?

Excursions are (along with alcohol sales and gambling) the cruise lines' bread and butter. To sell you on them, they like to convey the "insurance" aspect of joining their excursion. They'll tell you that you can rest easy, knowing that you're getting a vetted local tour guide on a tried-and-true itinerary that will pack the best experience into your limited time—and you'll be guaranteed not to miss your ship when it leaves that evening.

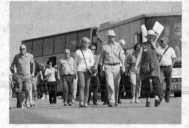

Some excursions are a great value, whisking you to top-tier and otherwise-hard-to-reach sights with an eloquent guide on a well-planned itinerary. But others can be disappointing time- and money-wasters, carting passengers to meager "sights" that are actually shopping experiences in disguise.

This book is designed not necessarily to discourage you from taking the cruise lines' excursions, but to help you make an informed decision, on a case-by-case basis, about whether a particular excursion is a good value for your interests and budget. In some situations (such as touring the D-Day beaches from Le Havre), I would happily pay a premium for a no-sweat transfer with a hand-picked, top-notch local guide. In other cases (such as the easy walk from Tallinn's cruise port to its atmospheric Old Town), the information in this book will allow you to have at least as good an experience, with more flexibility and freedom for a fraction of the price.

Pros and Cons of Excursions

Here are some of the benefits of taking an excursion, as touted by the cruise lines. Evaluate how these selling points fit the way you travel—and whether they are actually perks, or might cramp your style.

Returning to the Ship on Time: Cruise lines try to intimidate you into signing up for excursions by gravely reminding you that if you're on your own and fail to make it back to the ship on time, it could leave without you. If, however, a cruise-line excursion runs late for some reason, the ship will wait. In most places, provided that you budget your time conservatively (and barring an unforeseen strike or other crisis), there's no reason you can't have a great day in port and easily make it back on board in time. But if you don't feel confident about your ability to navigate back to the ship on time, or you have a chronic issue with lateness, an excursion may be a good option.

Getting Off First: Those going on excursions have priority for getting off the ship. This is especially useful when tendering (riding a small boat from your anchored ship to reach the shore), as tender lines can be long soon after arrival. But if you're organized and get a tender ticket as early as possible, you can make it off the ship almost as fast as the excursion passengers.

Optimizing Time in Port: Most excursions are well-planned by the cruise line to efficiently use your limited time in port. Rather than waiting around for a bus or train to your destination, you're whisked dockside-to-destination by the excursion bus. However, when weighing the "time savings" of an excursion, remember to account for how long it takes 50 people (compared to two people) to do everyday tasks: boarding a bus, walking through a castle, even making bathroom stops. If you're on your own and want to check out a particular shop, you can stay as long as you like—or just dip in and out; with a cruise excursion, you're committed to a half-hour, an hour, or however long the shopkeeper is paying your guide to keep you there. Every time your group moves somewhere, you're moving with dozens of other people, which always takes time. In many ports, you may actually reach the city center faster on your own than with an excursion, provided you are ready to hop off the ship as soon as you can, don't waste time getting to the terminal building, and know how, when, and where to grab public transport.

Many cruise lines schedule both morning and afternoon excursions. If you're a 30-minute bus ride from a major destination

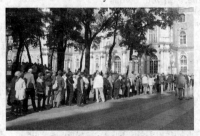

IN PORT

and select a morning excursion, your guide is instructed to bring you back to the ship (hoping that you'll join an afternoon excursion as well). If you prefer to spend your afternoon in town, it's perfectly acceptable to skip the return bus trip and make your way back to the ship, later, on your own (just be sure your guide knows you're splitting off).

Accessing Out-of-the-Way Sights: In most destinations, there's a relatively straightforward, affordable public-transportation option for getting from the cruise port to the major city or sight. But in a few cases, minor sights (or even the occasional major sight) are challenging, if not impossible, to reach without paying for a pricey taxi or rental car. For example, if your

Excursion Cheat Sheet

This simplified roundup shows which major ports are best by excursion and which are doable on your own (with this book in hand). For details, read the arrival information in each chapter.

Destination (Port)	Excursion?
COPENHAGEN	**No**

Bus #26 conveniently connects all three piers to downtown on weekdays. On weekends, take the shuttle to the train station, where you can take the train or bus #26 to the city center.

From Langelinie Pier: It's an easy 10-minute walk to see the *Little Mermaid*; from there, you can stroll all the way into town. For a faster trip, catch bus #26 from right in front of the ship or walk 15 minutes to Østerport train station.

From Frihavnen: On weekends, when the bus doesn't run, walk 10 minutes from your ship to the Nordhavn Station to ride the train into town. *From Oceankaj:* Depending on the terminal, it's a 15-minute or shorter walk to the #26 bus stop.

STOCKHOLM (Marseille/Toulon)	**No**

From Stadsgården: From some berths, you can walk to the Old Town (Gamla Stan) in about 20 minutes; from others, it's easier to catch the hop-on, hop-off boat to points around town.

From Frihamnen: Walk 5-10 minutes to the bus stop, and ride the public bus into town.

HELSINKI	**No**

From West Harbor: Ride public transportation downtown (bus #14 from Hernesaari terminal, tram #9 from West/Länsi terminal).

From South Harbor: You can walk into town from the Katajanokan and Olympia terminals in about 15 minutes (or hop on a tram).

ST. PETERSBURG	**Maybe**

Important: If you don't want to get a visa (expensive, must be arranged in advance—see page 354), you'll be allowed off the ship only if you pay your cruise line for an excursion. If you are on your own...

From Marine Facade: Ride a public bus-plus-metro connection downtown.

From Lieutenant Schmidt Embankment or English Embankment: Walk or catch a public bus or tram into downtown.

TALLINN	**No**

It's an easy 15-minute walk from the cruise port into town.

RĪGA	**No**

It's an easy 10- to 20-minute walk from the cruise port into town.

GDAŃSK (Gdynia)	**No**

From the port at Gydnia, make your way downtown to ride the train for 35 minutes to Gdańsk; once at Gdańsk's train station, it's a 15-minute walk to the scenic heart of town.

BERLIN (Warnemünde)	**Maybe**

Warnemünde's train station, a 5- to 10-minute walk from the cruise terminals, has frequent connections to nearby Rostock (21 minutes) and sparse connections to Berlin (3 hours, often with change in Rostock). If the Berlin train schedule doesn't work well with your cruise schedule (check www.bahn.com)—and maybe even if it does—a transportation-only "On Your Own" excursion from your cruise line can be the best way to get maximum time in Berlin.

Destination (Port)	Excursion?
OSLO	**No**

From Akershus or Revierkai: It's an easy walk downtown.
From Filipstad: This port is farther out and still walkable, but more convenient by cruise-line shuttle bus (worth paying for). Avoid expensive taxis.

STAVANGER	**Maybe**

It's an easy 5- to 15-minute walk into downtown. Consider an excursion only if you want to side-trip to Pulpit Rock and the Lysefjord.

BERGEN	**No**

From Skolten: You can walk into town from the port in about 10 minutes.
From Jekteviken/Dokken: Ride the free shuttle bus into downtown.

SOGNEFJORD (Flåm)	**Maybe**

It's possible to do the best part of the "Norway in a Nutshell" loop trip on your own (boat ride, twisty mountain bus, train ride, and another train steeply back down into the fjord). But this requires being organized, double-checking schedules (see page 780), and getting off the ship quickly.

GEIRANGERFJORD (Geiranger)	**Yes**

There's little to see in Geiranger town itself, and public transportation doesn't help you see much; it's smart to book a tour to local viewpoints and scenic roads—either through your cruise line or through a local tour operator.

AMSTERDAM	**No**

The cruise terminal is a 3-minute tram ride or 15-minute walk from the central train station, with connections to anywhere in the city.

BRUGES AND BRUSSELS (Zeebrugge)	**No**

Ride a shuttle bus to the port gate, then walk (10 minutes) to a tram stop. Ride the tram 10-15 minutes to the Blankenberge train station, where hourly trains zip to Bruges (15 minutes), Ghent (50 minutes), and Brussels (1.5 hours).

LONDON (Southampton or Dover)	**Maybe**

From Southampton: From the **Ocean** or **City Cruise Terminals,** you can walk into town and/or hop a free bus to the train station; from the **QEII** or **Mayflower Cruise Terminals,** spring for a taxi. From Southampton's station, trains go to London (1.25 hours, 2/hour) and Portsmouth (50 minutes, hourly).
From Dover: Ride a shuttle bus or taxi to the train station, where trains depart for London (1.5 hours, 2/hour) or Canterbury (20-30 minutes, 2/hour).

PARIS AND NORMANDY (Le Havre)	**Maybe**

Ride a cruise-line shuttle bus or walk about 35 minutes from the port to the train/bus station; from there, connect to Paris (2.25-hour train), Rouen (1-hour train), or Honfleur (30-minute bus). To see the D-Day beaches (about an hour's drive west), an excursion works best.

cruise is stopping at Le Havre, and you've always wanted to see the D-Day beaches, you'll find it nearly impossible to get there by public transportation—so the most reasonable choice is an excursion. This book is designed to help you determine how easy—or difficult—it is to reach the places you're interested in seeing.

Touring with Quality Guides: Most excursions are led by local guides contracted through the cruise line. While all guides have been vetted by the cruise line and are generally high-quality, a few oddball exceptions occasionally sneak through. The guide is the biggest wildcard in the success of your tour, but it's also something you have very little control over. You won't know which guide is leading your excursion until he or she shows up to collect you.

An alternative can be to hire a good local guide to show you around on a private tour. For two people, this can cost about as much as buying the excursion, but you get a much more personalized experience, tailored to your interests. And if you can enlist other passengers to join you to split the cost, it's even more of a bargain. I've recommended my favorite guides for most destinations; many of them are the same ones who are 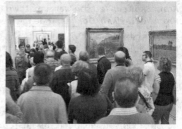 hired by the cruise lines to lead their excursions. Because local guides tend to book up when a big cruise ship is in town, it's smart to plan ahead and email these guides well before your trip.

Cruise lines keep track of which guides get good reviews, and do their best to use those guides in the future. If you do go on an excursion, take the time to give the cruise line feedback, good or bad, about the quality of your guide. They really want to know.

Beware of Crew Members' Advice

While most cruise lines understand that their passengers won't book an excursion at every port, there is some pressure to get you to take them. And if you ask crew members for advice on sightseeing (independent of an excursion), they may be less than forthcoming. Take crew members' destination advice with a grain of salt.

Philosophically, most cruise lines don't consider it their responsibility to help you enjoy your port experience—unless you pay them for an excursion. The longer you spend on the ship, the more likely you are to spend more money on board, so there's actually a financial disincentive for crew members to help you get off the ship and find your own way in the port. You're lucky if the best they offer is, "Take a taxi. I have no idea what it costs."

I have actually overheard excursion staff dispense misinformation about the time, expense, and difficulty involved in reaching downtown from a port ("The taxi takes 25 to 30 minutes, and I've never seen a bus at the terminal"—when in fact the taxi takes 10 minutes and there's an easy bus connection from the terminal). Was the crew being deceptive, or just ignorant? Either way, it was still misinformation.

The best plan is to get sightseeing information on your own. That's why detailed instructions for getting into town from the port are a major feature of this book. The local tourist office often sets up a desk or info tent right on the pier, in the terminal, or where shuttle buses drop you. Otherwise, you can usually find a tourist information office (abbreviated **TI** in this book) in the town center.

THE BOTTOM LINE ON EXCURSIONS

Some passengers are on a cruise because they simply don't want to invest the time and energy needed to be independent...they want to be on vacation. Time is money, and you spend 50 weeks a year figuring things out back home; on vacation, you want someone else to do the thinking for you. If that's you, excursions can be a good way to see a place.

But in many destinations, it honestly doesn't take that much additional effort or preparation to have a good experience without paying a premium for an excursion. And cost savings aside, if you have even a middling spirit of adventure, doing it on your own can be a fun experience in itself.

Planning Your Time

Whether you're taking an excursion, sightseeing on your own, or doing a combination of the two, it's important to plan your day on land carefully. Be sure to read this book's sightseeing information and walking tours the night before to make the most of your time, even if you're taking an excursion—many include free time at a sight or neighborhood, or leave you with extra time in port.

First, keep in mind that the advertised amount of time in port can be deceptive. If the itinerary says that the ship is in town from 8:00 to 17:00, mentally subtract an hour or two from that time. It can take a good half-hour to get off a big ship and to the terminal building (or even longer, if you're tendering), and from the terminal, you still have to reach the town center. At the end of the day, the all-aboard time is generally a half-hour before the ship departs. Not only do you have to be back on board by 16:30, but you must also build in the time it takes to get from downtown to the ship. Your nine-hour visit in port just shrank to seven hours...still plenty of time to really enjoy a place, but not quite as much time as you expected.

IN PORT

It's essential to realize that if you are late returning to the ship, you cannot expect them to wait for you (unless you're on one of the cruise line's excursions, and it's running late). The cruise line has the right to depart without you...and they will. While this seems harsh, cruise lines must pay port fees for every *minute* they are docked, so your half-hour delay could cost them more than your cruise ticket. Also, they have a tight schedule to keep and can't be waiting around for stragglers (for tips on what to do if this happens to you, see the end of this chapter).

To avoid missing the boat, work backward from the time you have to be back on board. Be very conservative, especially if you're going far—for example, riding a train or bus to a neighboring town. Public transportation can be delayed, and traffic can be snarled at rush hour—just when you're heading back to the ship. One strategy is to do the farthest-flung sights first, then gradually work your way back to the ship. Once you know you're within walking distance of the ship, you can dawdle to your heart's content, confident you can make it back on time.

If you're extremely concerned about missing the ship, just pretend it departs an hour earlier than it actually does. You'll still have several hours to enjoy that destination and be left with an hour to kill back at the cruise port (or on board).

Note that transportation strikes can be a problem in Europe (particularly in France). These can hit at any time, although they are usually publicized in advance. If you're going beyond the immediate area of the port, ask the local TI, "Are there any strikes planned for today that could make it difficult for me to return to my ship?" Even when there is a planned strike, a few trains and buses will still run—ask for the schedule.

If you're an early riser, you'll notice that your ship typically arrives at the port some time before the official disembarkation time. That's because local officials need an hour or more to "clear" the ship (process paperwork, passports, and so on) before passengers are allowed off. Even if you wake up early and find the ship docked, you'll most likely have to wait for the official disembarkation time to get off.

While you have to plan your time smartly, don't let anxiety paralyze you: Some travelers—even adventurous ones—get so nervous about missing the boat that they spend all day within view of the cruise port, just in case. Anyone who does that is missing out: In very few cities is the best sightseeing actually concentrated near the port. Cruise excursion directors have told me that entire months go by when they don't leave anyone behind. You have to be pretty sloppy—or incredibly unlucky—to miss your ship.

Managing Crowds

Unless you're on a luxury line, you can't go on a cruise and expect to avoid crowds. It's simply a fact of life. So be prepared to visit sights at the busiest possible time—just as your cruise ship funnels a few thousand time-pressed tourists into town (or, worse, when three or four ships simultaneously disgorge).

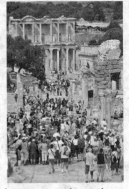

Keep in mind that my instructions for getting into town might sound easy—but when you're jostling with several hundred others to cram onto a public bus that comes once every 20 minutes, the reality check can be brutal. Be patient...and most important, be prepared. You'll be amazed at how many of your fellow cruisers will step off the ship knowing nothing about their options for seeing the place. By buying and reading this book, and doing just a bit of homework before each destination, you're already way ahead of the game.

Make a point of being the first person down the gangway (or in line for tender tickets) each day, and make a beeline for what you most want to see. While your fellow passengers are lingering over that second cup of coffee or puzzling over the bus schedule, you can be the first person on top of the city wall or on the early train to your destination. Yes, you're on vacation, so if you want to take it easy, that's your prerogative. But you can't be lazy and also avoid the crowds. Choose one.

Getting Off the Ship

Your ship has arrived at its destination, and it's time to disembark and enjoy Europe. This section explains the procedure for getting off the ship and also provides a rundown of the services you'll find at the port.

DOCKING VERSUS TENDERING

There are two basic ways to disembark from the ship: docking or tendering. On most European cruise itineraries, docking is far more common than tendering. (Of the ports covered in this book, the only ones where you may need to tender are on the Norwegian fjords.)

Docking

When your ship docks, it means that the vessel actually ties up to a pier, and you can simply walk off onto dry land. However, cruise

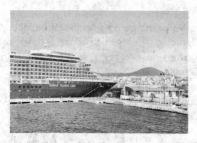

piers (like cruise ships) can be massive, so you may have to walk 10 to 15 minutes from the ship to the terminal building. Sometimes the port area is so vast, the cruise line will offer a shuttle bus between the ship and the terminal building.

Tendering

If your ship is too big or there's not enough room at the pier, the ship will anchor offshore and send passengers ashore using small boats called tenders. Passengers who have paid for excursions usually go first; then it goes in order of tender ticket (or tender number).

Tender tickets are generally distributed the night before or on the morning of arrival. Show up as early as you can to get your tender ticket (you may have to wait in line even before the official start time); the sooner you get your ticket, the earlier you can board your tender. Even then, you'll likely have to wait. (Sometimes passengers in more expensive staterooms are given a "VIP tender ticket," allowing them to skip the line whenever they want.)

The tenders themselves are usually the ship's lifeboats, but in some destinations, the port authority requires the cruise line to hire local tenders. Because tenders are small vessels prone to turbulence, transferring from the ship to the tender and from the tender to shore can be rough. Take your time, be sure of your footing, and let the tender attendants give you a hand—it's their job to prevent you from going for an unplanned swim.

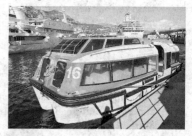

Tendering is, to many passengers, the scourge of cruising, as it can waste a lot of time. Obviously, not everyone on your big ship can fit on those little tenders all at once. Do the math: Your ship carries some 2,000 passengers. There are three or four tenders, which can carry anywhere from 30 to 150 people apiece, and it takes at least 20 minutes round-trip. This can all translate into a lot of waiting around.

There are various strategies for navigating the tender line: Some cruisers report that if you show up at the gangway, ready to go, before your tender ticket number is called, you might be able to slip on early. A crush of people will often jam the main

What Should I Bring to Shore?

- **Your room key card.** No matter how you leave the ship—tendering or docking, with an excursion or on your own—the crew must account for your absence. Any time you come or go, a security guard will swipe your room key. Your photo will flash onscreen to ensure it's really you. With this punch-in-and-out system, the crew knows exactly who's on board and who's on shore at all times.
- **Local cash.** After living on a cashless cruise ship, this is easy to forget. If you plan to withdraw local currency at an ATM, be sure to bring your debit card (and a credit card if you plan to make purchases).
- **Passport.** It's smart to carry your passport at all times (safely tucked away in a money belt—explained on page 56). While you typically won't have to show a passport when embarking or disembarking at each port (except the first and possibly the last), you may need it as a deposit for renting something (such as an audioguide or a scooter), or as ID when making a credit-card purchase or requesting a VAT refund. And you'll certainly want it in case you miss the boat and have to make your way to the next port. Some ships actually keep your passport until the end of the cruise. In that case, you'll go on shore without it; if you're one of the rare few who misses the ship, you'll find your passport with the port agent at the terminal office.
- **Weather-appropriate gear.** In chilly or rainy weather, bring a lightweight sweater or raincoat. If it's hot (less likely), that means sunscreen, a hat for shade, sunglasses, lightweight and light-colored clothing, and a water bottle (or buy one in port).
- **Long pants.** If you plan to visit any Orthodox churches (such as those in St. Petersburg, Helsinki, or Tallinn), you'll encounter a strict "no shorts, no bare shoulders" dress code.
- **Your cruise's destination information sheet (daily program).** At a minimum, jot down the all-aboard time and—if applicable—the time of the last tender or shuttle bus to the ship, along with contact details for the port agent (see page 119).
- **This guidebook,** or—better yet—tear out just the pages you need for today's port (see sidebar on page 3).

IN PORT

stairwells and elevators to the gangway. Some of these folks might block your passage despite having later tender tickets than yours. If you use a different set of stairs or elevators, then walk through an alternate hallway, you might be able to pop out near the gangway rather than get stuck in the logjam on the main stairwell. If you anticipate crowd issues while tendering, scope out the ship's layout in advance, when it's not busy.

Another strategy to avoid the crush of people trying to get off the ship upon arrival is to simply wait an hour or two, when you can waltz onto a tender at will. While you'll miss out on some valuable sightseeing time on shore, some cruisers figure that's a fair trade-off for avoiding the stress of tendering at a prime time.

If there's an advantage to tendering, it's that you're more likely to be taken to an arrival point that's close to the town's main points of interest. When you figure in the time it would take to get from the main cruise port to the city center, tendering might actually save you some time—provided you get an early tender ticket. In fact, on smaller ships, it

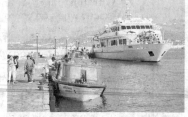

can even be an advantage to tender—there's little to no waiting, and you're deposited in the heart of town.

Strangely, crowds are rare on tenders returning to the ship; apparently passengers trickle back all through the day, so even the last tenders of the day are rarely jam-packed. (And if they are, the ship won't leave without you, provided you're waiting in the tender line.)

THE PORT AREA

In most destinations, the port is not in the city center; in some cases the port is actually in a separate town or city a lengthy train or bus ride away (for example, the port of Le Havre for Paris). In this book's destination chapters, I describe how near (or far) the port is from the town center. Be warned that the port area is, almost as a rule, the ugliest part of town—often an industrial and/or maritime area that had its historic charm bombed to bits in World War II. But once you're in the heart of town, none of that will matter.

Many ports have a terminal building, where you'll find pass-

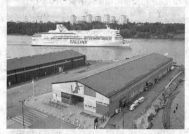

port check/customs control, and usually also ATMs, some duty-free shops, sometimes a travel agency and/or car-rental office, and (out front) a taxi stand and bus stop into town. Better terminals also have a TI that's staffed at times when cruise ships arrive. Most ports have lines painted on the pavement (often blue) that lead you from where you step off the ship or exit the port gate to services (such as TIs or terminal buildings) or transportation options (such as bus stops).

Note: Your passport will rarely be checked on a European cruise. Most of the destinations covered in this book belong to the open-borders Schengen Agreement, so you don't need to show a passport when crossing the border. Even in other countries, it likely won't be checked—they know you're on a cruise ship, that you'll be returning to the ship that evening, and that you're likely to spend a lot of money in port, so they want to make things easy for you. Of the destination countries in this book, only Russia requires a visa for those going ashore without an excursion (explained on page 354). So, while it's wise to carry your passport for identification purposes, don't be surprised if you never actually need it.

PORT AGENTS
In every port, your cruise line has an official port agent—a local representative who's designated to watch out for their passengers while they're in port. This person's name and contact information is listed on the port-of-call information sheet distributed by your cruise line and usually also in the daily program. Be sure to have this information with you when you go on shore; if you have an emergency and can't contact anyone from your ship, call the port agent for help. Likewise, if you're running late and realize that you won't make it back to the ship by the departure time, get in touch with your port agent, who will relay the information to the ship so they know you aren't coming. If you do miss the ship, sometimes the port agent can point you in the right direction for making your way to the next port of call on your own (for details, see "What If I Miss My Boat?" at the end of this chapter).

Sightseeing on Your Own

If you're planning to strike out on your own, you need to figure out in advance where you're going, how to get there, and what you want to do once you're there.

GETTING INTO TOWN
When it's a long distance from the ship to the cruise terminal, cruise lines usually offer a free shuttle bus to the terminal; if it's a short distance, you can walk. Either way, once you're at the terminal, you'll need to find your own way into town.

By Taxi
Exiting the terminal, you'll usually run into a busy taxi stand, with gregarious, English-speaking cabbies offering to take you for a tour around the area's main sights. While taxis are efficient, be aware that most cabbies' rates are ridiculously inflated to take

advantage of cruisers. You may be able to persuade them to just take you into town (generally at a hiked-up rate), though they usually prefer to find passengers willing to hire them for several hours. Sometimes just walking a block or two and hailing a cab on the street can save you half the rate.

To keep the fare reasonable, consider taking the taxi only as far as you need to (for example, to the nearest subway station to hop a speedy train into the city, rather than pay to drive all the way across town in congested traffic). Also keep in mind that there must be somebody on your ship who's going to the same place you are—strike up a conversation at breakfast or on the gangway to find someone to team up with and split the fare.

Remember: Taxis aren't just for getting from the port to town; they can also be wonderful time-savers for connecting sights within a big city. For more taxi tips, see the sidebar on the next page.

By Bus

Near the terminal, often just beyond the taxi stand, you'll usually find a **public bus** stop for getting into town. This is significantly cheaper than a taxi, and often not much slower. Even with an entire cruise ship emptying all at once, waiting in a long line for the bus is relatively rare. These buses usually take local cash only and sometimes require exact change. If you see a kiosk or ticket vending machine near the bus stop, try to purchase a bus ticket there, or at least buy something small to break big bills and get the correct change.

Occasionally, there's a **shuttle bus** into town; while handy, this happens mostly in ports that lack a good public-transit connection (such as Zeebrugge or Dover). If there is a shuttle, it's often your best option. The shuttle bus typically costs about $4-10 round-trip (buses run frequently when the ship arrives, then about every 15-20 minutes; pay attention to where the bus drops you downtown, as you'll need to find that stop later to return to the ship).

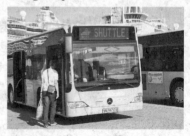

The shuttle bus can get very crowded when the ship first unloads—do your best to get off the ship and onto the bus quickly. At slower times, you might have to wait a little while for the bus to fill up before it departs. Note that the port shuttle sometimes doesn't start running until sometime after your ship actually docks (for example, you disembark at 7:00, but the bus doesn't start running until 8:30). This is a case when it can be worth springing for a taxi to avoid waiting around.

By Excursion

Cruise lines sometimes offer "On Your Own" excursions that include unguided transportation into town, then free time on your own. This may be worthwhile in places where the port is far from the main point of interest (such as the ports of Dover or Southampton for London, the port of Warnemünde for Berlin, or the port of Le Havre for Paris). While more expensive than public transportation—and sometimes even more expensive than a shared cab—this is a low-stress option that still allows you freedom to see the sights at your own pace. For details, see page 106.

SEEING THE TOWN

If you're touring a port on your own, you have several options for getting around town and visiting the sights (see the destination chapters for specifics).

On a Tour

It's easy to get a guided tour without having to pay excessively for an excursion. And there are plenty of choices, from walking to bus tours. Cruise Critic (www.cruisecritic.com) is a great resource for exploring these options.

At or near the terminal, you'll generally find travel agencies offering **package tours.** These tours are similar to the cruise-ship excursions but usually cost far less (half or even a third as much). However, what's offered can change from day to day, so they're not as reliable as the cruise line's offerings. It's possible to reserve these in advance, typically through a third party (such as a travel agency).

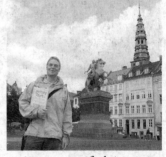

A great budget alternative is to join a regularly scheduled **local walking tour** (in English, departing at a specified time every day). Again, these are very similar to the cruise lines' walking tours and often use the same guides. Look for my walking tour listings in the destination chapters or ask at the local TI.

In a large city where sights are spread out, it can be convenient to join a **hop-on, hop-off bus tour.** These buses make a circle through town every 30 minutes or so, stopping at key points where passengers can hop on or off at will. While relatively expensive (figure around €25-30 for an all-day ticket), these tours are easier than figuring out public transportation, come with commentary (either recorded or from a live guide), and generally have a stop at or near the cruise port.

Taxi Tips

There's no denying that taxis are the fastest way to get from your ship to what you want to see. But you'll pay for that convenience. Regular fares tend to be high, and many cabbies are adept at overcharging tourists—especially cruise passengers—in shameless and creative ways. Here are some tips to avoid getting ripped off by a cabbie.

Finding a Cab: A taxi stand is usually right at the cruise terminal; if not (or if you're already in town), ask a local to direct you. Taxi stands are often listed prominently on city maps; look for the little Ts. Fly-by-night cabbies with a makeshift "Taxi" sign on the rooftop and no company logo or phone number on the door are less likely to be honest.

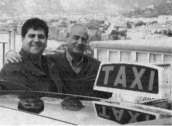

Establishing a Price: To figure the fare, you can either use the taxi meter or agree on a set price up front. In either case, it's important to know the going rate (the destination chapters include the prevailing rates for the most likely journeys from each port). Even if I'm using the taxi meter, I still ask for a rough estimate up front, so I know generally what to expect.

In most cities, it's best to use the **taxi meter**—and cabbies are legally required to do so if the passenger requests it. So insist. Cabbies who get feisty and refuse are probably up to no good. If you don't feel comfortable about a situation, just get out and find another taxi.

Even with the meter, cabbies can still find ways to scam you. For instance, they may try to set it to the pricier weekend tariff, even if it's a weekday—check the list of different meter rates (posted somewhere in the cab, often in English). If you're

Some cruisers hire a **private guide** to meet them at the ship and take them around town (see page 112). Book directly with the guide, using the contact information in this book; if you arrange the guide through a third party—such as a local travel agent or the cruise line—you'll pay a premium.

On Your Own

If you prefer to sightsee independently and are going to London, Paris, Amsterdam, or Berlin, take advantage of my free **audio tours,** which guide you through the most interesting neighborhoods and most famous sights in each of those cities. Audio tours allow your eyes to enjoy the wonders of the place while your ears learn its story. Before your trip, download the tours to your mobile device via the Rick Steves Audio Europe app, www.ricksteves.

confused about the tariff your cabbie has selected, ask for an explanation.

It's also possible (though obviously illegal) for cabbies to tinker with a taxi meter to make it spin like a pinwheel. If you glance away from the meter, then look back and see that it's mysteriously doubled, you've likely been duped. However, some extra fees are on the level (for instance, in most cities, there's a legitimate surcharge for picking you up at the cruise port). Again, these should be listed clearly on the tariff sheet. If you suspect foul play, following the route on your map or conspicuously writing down the cabbie's license information can shame him into being honest.

Agreeing to a **set price** for the ride is another option. While this is usually higher than the fair metered rate would be, sometimes it's the easiest way to go. Just be sure that the rate you agree to is more or less in the ballpark of the rate I've listed in this book. Consider asking a couple of cabbies within a block or two of each other for estimates. You may be surprised at the variation.

Many cabbies hire out for an hourly rate; if you want the taxi to take you to a variety of outlying sights and wait for you, this can be a good value. You can also arrange in advance to hire a driver for a few hours or the whole day (for some destinations, I've listed my favorite local drivers).

Settling Up: It's best to pay in small bills. If you use a large bill, state the denomination out loud as you hand it to the cabbie. They can be experts at dropping a €50 note and picking up a €20. Count your change. To tip a good cabbie, round up about 5 to 10 percent (to pay a €4.50 fare, give €5; for a €28 fare, give €30). But if you feel like you're being driven in circles or otherwise ripped off, skip the tip.

IN PORT

com/audioeurope, iTunes, or Google Play. These give all the information you'll want, while saving you lots of time and money—perfect for the thoughtful, independent cruiser.

It's possible to **rent a car** to see the sights. While this makes sense for covering a wide rural area (such as the D-Day beaches or the English countryside), I would never rent a car to tour a big city—public transportation is not only vastly cheaper, but it avoids the headaches of parking, unfamiliar traffic patterns, and other problems. In general, given the relatively short time you'll have in port and the high expense of renting a car for the day (figure €40-100/day, depending on the port), this option doesn't make much sense. However, if you're interested, you'll often find car-rental offices or travel agencies at or near the terminal that are accustomed to renting cars for short time periods to cruisers. You can also look for deals online (on rental companies' websites or travel-booking sites) in advance.

In some cities, renting a **bicycle** can be a good option. Northern European cities—especially Copenhagen and Amsterdam—are flat, laced with bike lanes, and bike-friendly. In these cities, you'll see locals using bikes more routinely than cars... join them.

With Fellow Passengers

The upside of traveling with so many other people is that you have ample opportunities to make friends. On a ship with thousands of people, I guarantee you'll find someone who shares your style of travel. If you and your traveling companion hit it off with others, consider teaming up for your shore time. This "double-dating" can save both money (splitting the cost of an expensive taxi ride) and stress (working together to figure out the best way into town). But be sure you're all interested in the same things before you head ashore—you don't want to end up in front of the Louvre, bickering about whether to tour Notre-Dame or saunter up the Champs-Elysées.

In-Port Travel Skills

Whether you're taking an excursion or tackling a port on your own, this practical advice will come in handy. This section includes tips on useful services, avoiding theft, using money, sightseeing, shopping, eating, and, in general, making the most of your time in port.

TRAVEL SMART

Europe is like a complex play—easier to follow and really appreciate on a second viewing. While no one does the same trip twice to gain that advantage, reading about the places you'll visit before you reach each destination accomplishes much the same thing.

Though you're bound to your ship's schedule, note the best times to visit various sights, and try to hit them as best as you can. Pay attention to holidays, festivals, and days when sights are closed. For example, many museums are closed on Mondays. Big sights and museums often stop admitting people 30 to 60 minutes before closing time.

Sundays have the same pros and cons as they do for travelers in the US (special events, limited hours, banks and many shops closed, limited public transportation, no rush hour). Saturdays are virtually weekdays with earlier closing times and no rush hour (though transportation connections can be less frequent than on weekdays).

When in port, visit the TI. Find a place to get online to research sights, make reservations (maybe book a guide or tour for your next destination), keep in touch with home, and so on. Then head for the sights you came so far to see.

Most important, connect with the culture. Set up your own quest to find the tastiest *kringle* in Denmark or the best *smörgåsbord* in Sweden. Slow down and be open to unexpected experiences. Enjoy the hospitality of the European people. Ask questions—most locals are eager to point you in their idea of the right direction. Wear your money belt, learn the currency, and figure out how to estimate prices in dollars. Those who expect to travel smart, do.

SERVICES

Tourist Information: No matter how well I know a town, my first stop is always the TI. TIs are usually located on the main square, in the city hall, or at the train station (just look for signs). Many cruise ports also have a temporary TI desk, which answers questions for arriving cruisers. Their job is to make sure your few hours in town are enjoyable, so you'll come back on your own later. At TIs, you can get information on sights and public transit, and pick up a city map and a local entertainment guide. Ask if guided walks, self-guided walking-tour brochures, or audioguides are available. If you need a quick place to eat, ask the TI staff where they go for lunch.

Medical Help: If you get sick or injured while in port—assuming you're not in need of urgent care—do as the Europeans do and go to a pharmacist for advice. European pharmacists diagnose and prescribe remedies for most simple problems. They are usually friendly and speak English, and some medications that are only available by prescription in the US are available over the counter (surprisingly cheaply) in Europe. If necessary, the pharmacist will send you to a doctor or the health clinic. For most destinations, I've listed pharmacies close to the cruise port.

Theft or Loss: To replace a **passport,** you'll need to go in person to a US embassy or consulate (neither of which is usually located in a port town) during their business hours, which are generally limited and restricted to weekdays. This can take a day or two. If you lose your passport, contact the port agent or the ship's guest services desk immediately—and be aware that you may not be able to continue your cruise if a replacement passport is not available before the ship sails. Having a photocopy of your passport and a backup form of ID such as your driver's license, as well as an extra passport photo, can speed up getting a replacement.

If your **credit and debit cards** disappear, cancel and replace them (see "Damage Control for Lost Cards" on page 130). File a police report on the spot for any loss (you'll need it to submit an insurance claim). For more info, see www.ricksteves.com/help.

Internet Cafés and Wi-Fi Hotspots: Finding an Internet café in Europe is a breeze. While these places don't always serve food or drinks—sometimes they're just big, functional, sweaty rooms filled with computers— they are an easy and affordable way to get online. It's even easier to find Wi-Fi with your smartphone, tablet, or laptop. There are hotspots at cafés and at other businesses. Sometimes Wi-Fi is free; other times you may have to pay by the minute or buy something in exchange for the network password.

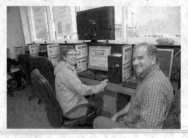

Public Phones: Because calling from the ship or a mobile phone can be costly (see page 87), you may want to seek out a pay phone in port to make calls. Coin-op phones are rare in Europe, so you'll need to purchase one of two types of prepaid phone cards. An **insertable phone card** can be used only at pay phones. Simply take the phone off the hook, insert the card, wait for a dial tone, and dial away. The phone displays your credit ticking down as you talk. Each European country has its own insertable phone card— so your German card won't work in a Polish phone. This type offers reasonable rates for domestic calls, and steeper but still acceptable rates for international calls (rarely exceeding $1/minute).

Prepaid **international phone cards** can be used to make inexpensive calls—within Europe, or to the US, for pennies a minute—from nearly any phone, including your hotel-room phone (for your hotel stays before or after your cruise). These cards come with a toll-free number and a scratch-to-reveal PIN code. If the voice prompts aren't in English, experiment: Dial your code, followed by the pound sign (#), then the phone number, then pound again, and so on, until it works. Be warned that in Germany and Britain the national telecom companies levy a hefty surcharge for using one of these cards from a pay phone—which effectively eliminates any savings. But you can still use them cheaply from a hotel-room phone.

OUTSMARTING THIEVES

In Europe, it's rare to encounter violent crime, but petty purse-snatching and pickpocketing are quite common. Thieves target Americans, especially cruise passengers—not because the thieves are mean, but because they're smart. Loaded down with valuables in a strange new environment, we stick out like jeweled thumbs. But being savvy and knowing what to look out for can dramatically reduce your risk of being targeted.

Pickpockets are your primary concern. To avoid them, be aware of your surroundings, don't keep anything valuable in your

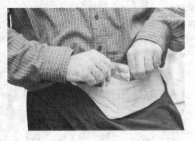

pockets, and wear a money belt (explained on page 56). In your money belt, carry your passport, credit and debit cards, and large cash bills. Keep just a day's spending money in your pocket—if you lose that, it's no big deal.

Many cruise lines hand out cloth bags emblazoned with their logo. Carrying these around town is like an advertisement for pickpockets and con artists (not to mention aggressive salesmen). Save them for supermarket runs back home.

Thieves thrive on tourist-packed public-transportation routes—especially buses that cover major sights. When riding the subway or bus, be alert at stops, when thieves can dash on and off with your day bag. Criminals—often dressed as successful professionals or even as tourists—will often block a bus or subway entry, causing the person behind you to "bump" into you.

Be wary of any unusual contact or commotion in crowded public places (especially touristy spots). For example, while being jostled at a crowded mar- 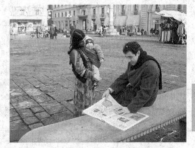 ket, you might end up with ketchup or fake pigeon poop on your shirt. The perpetrator then offers profuse apologies while dabbing it up—and pawing your pockets. Treat any disturbance (a scuffle breaking out, a beggar in your face, someone falling down an escalator) as a smokescreen for theft—designed to distract unknowing victims.

Europe also has its share of scam artists, from scruffy babushkas offering you sprigs of rosemary (and expecting money in return) to con artists running street scams, such as the shell game, in which players pay to guess which of the moving shells hides the ball (don't try it—you'll lose every time). Or somebody sells you an item, and turns around to put it in a box while you're getting out your money. Later on the ship, when you open the box, you find only...rocks. Always look inside the box before walking away.

The most rampant scams are more subtle, such as being overcharged by a taxi driver (see the "Taxi Tips" sidebar, earlier). Another common scam is the "slow count": A cashier counts

IN PORT

change back with odd pauses, in hopes the rushed tourist will gather up the money quickly without checking that it's all there. Waiters may pad the bill with mysterious charges—carefully scan the itemized bill and account for each item. If paying a small total with a large bill, clearly state the amount you're handing over, and be sure you get the correct change back. Don't be upset about these little scams—treat them as sport.

Nearly all crimes suffered by tourists are nonviolent and avoidable. Be aware of the pitfalls of traveling, but relax and have fun.

MONEY

Whenever you leave the ship, you must use local currency. Many of the countries in this book use the euro (specifically Belgium, Estonia, Finland, France, Germany, Latvia, and the Netherlands); stock up on euros early in your trip, and use them throughout the region.

The other destinations in this book don't officially use the euro (Denmark, Great Britain, Norway, Poland, Russia, and Sweden).

I've occasionally heard cruise-line employees tell their passengers, "We're only in the country for a day, and everyone takes euros, so you don't need to change money." That's true in many cases: Many merchants in non-euro countries do accept euros. But exchange rates are bad, and some vendors might flat-out refuse euros. Plus, euros often aren't accepted on public transportation or at major sights and museums. That's why it's better to get local cash, even if you're in town just for a few hours. In most port cities, ATMs are easy to find (I've listed the nearest locations for each destination). But in some of the more out-of-way ports, exchanging a small amount of money for local currency at the cruise ship's front desk can save you time looking for an ATM.

Because some countries have individual currencies, you'll likely wind up with leftover cash. Coins can't be exchanged once you leave the country, so try to spend them while you're in port. But bills are easy to convert to the "new" country's currency. When changing cash, use exchange bureaus rather than banks. The Forex desks (easy to find at major train stations) are considered reliable and fair.

Cash

Cash is just as desirable in Europe as it is at home. Small businesses (mom-and-pop cafés, shops, etc.) may prefer that you pay with cash. While most Northern European vendors take credit cards, American cards may not work properly (because they're not chip-and-PIN cards, described later), making cash a smart backup. Cash is the best—and sometimes only—way to pay for cheap food,

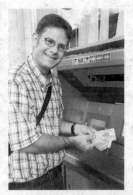

bus fare, taxis, and local guides.

Throughout Europe, ATMs are the standard way for travelers to get cash. In every port destination, I've tried to give directions for getting you (cash-free) to the nearest ATM. When possible, use ATMs located outside banks—a thief is less likely to target a cash machine near surveillance cameras, and if your card is munched by a machine, you can go inside for help. Stay away from "independent" ATMs such as Travelex, Euronet, Moneybox, Cardpoint, and Cashzone, which charge huge commissions, have terrible exchange rates, and may try to trick users with "dynamic currency conversion" (described at the end of "Credit and Debit Cards," next). Note that in many Scandinavian and Baltic countries, ATMs are relatively rare; in some ports, there may not be one right where you'll step off the ship. Fortunately, credit cards are widely accepted in this part of the world, even for small transactions.

Although you can use a credit card for an ATM transaction, it only makes sense in an emergency, because it's considered a cash advance (borrowed at a high interest rate) rather than a withdrawal.

Pickpockets target tourists. To safeguard your cash, wear a money belt—a pouch with a strap that you buckle around your waist like a belt and tuck under your clothes. Keep your cash, credit cards, and passport secure in your money belt, and carry only a day's spending money in your front pocket.

Credit and Debit Cards

For purchases, Visa and MasterCard are more commonly accepted than American Express. Just like at home, credit or debit cards work easily at larger restaurants, shops, and hotels. I typically use my debit card to withdraw cash to pay for most purchases. I use my credit card only in a few specific situations: to book hotel reservations by phone (when staying in Europe before or after a cruise), to buy advance tickets for events or sights, to cover major purchases, and to pay for things near the end of my trip (to avoid another visit to the ATM).

While you can use either a credit or a debit card for most purchases, using a credit card offers a greater degree of fraud protection (since debit cards draw funds directly from your bank account).

In most of Scandinavia, credit cards are widely accepted even for small purchases, as mentioned earlier. Danes, Swedes, and Norwegians rarely use cash. This can be a relief for cruisers in town who don't want to hassle with ATMs. But there's a catch: In these countries, most people use chip-and-PIN cards.

Chip and PIN: Europeans are increasingly using chip-and-PIN cards, which are embedded with an electronic security chip (in addition to the magnetic stripe found on American-style cards). To make a purchase with a chip-and-PIN card, the cardholder inserts the card into a slot in the payment machine, then enters a PIN (like using a debit card in the US) while the card stays in the slot. The chip inside the card authorizes the transaction; the cardholder doesn't sign a receipt.

Your magnetic-stripe-only card might not work at payment machines using this system, such as those at train and subway stations, toll roads, parking garages, luggage lockers, bike-rental kiosks, and self-serve gas pumps.

If you have problems using your American card in a chip-and-PIN machine, here are some suggestions: For either a debit card or a credit card, try entering that card's PIN when prompted. (Note that your credit-card PIN may not be the same as your debit-card PIN; you'll need to ask your bank for your credit-card PIN.) If your cards still don't work, look for a machine that takes cash, seek out a clerk who might be able to process the transaction manually, or ask a local if you can pay them cash to run the transaction on their card.

And don't panic. Many travelers who use only magnetic-stripe cards don't run into problems. Still, it pays to carry plenty of cash; remember that you can always use an ATM to withdraw cash with your magnetic-stripe debit card.

If you're still concerned, you can apply for a chip card in the US. One option is the no-fee GlobeTrek Visa, offered by Andrews Federal Credit Union in Maryland (open to all US residents; see www.andrewsfcu.org). With luck, by the time you travel, Visa and MasterCard chip cards will have become standard issue in the US.

Dynamic Currency Conversion: If merchants offer to convert your purchase price into dollars (called dynamic currency conversion, or DCC), refuse this "service." You'll pay even more in fees for the expensive convenience of seeing your charge in dollars. Some ATMs and retailers try to confuse customers by presenting DCC in misleading terms. If an ATM offers to "lock in" or "guarantee" your conversion rate, choose "proceed without conversion." Other prompts might state, "You can be charged in dollars: Press YES for dollars, NO for euros." Always choose the local currency in these situations.

Damage Control for Lost Cards: If you lose your credit, debit, or ATM card, you can stop people from using your card by reporting the loss immediately to the respective global customer-assistance centers. Call these 24-hour US numbers collect: Visa (tel. 303/967-1096), MasterCard (tel. 636/722-7111), and American Express (tel. 336/393-1111). European toll-free numbers (listed by country) can be found at the websites for Visa and MasterCard.

Providing the following information will allow for a quicker cancellation of your missing card: full card number, whether you are the primary or secondary cardholder, the cardholder's name exactly as printed on the card, billing address, home phone number, circumstances of the loss or theft, and identification verification (your birth date, your mother's maiden name, or your Social Security number—memorize this, don't carry a copy). If you are the secondary cardholder, you'll also need to provide the primary cardholder's identification-verification details. You can generally receive a temporary card within two or three business days in Europe (see www.ricksteves.com/help for more).

If you report your loss within two days, you typically won't be responsible for any unauthorized transactions on your account, although many banks charge a liability fee of $50.

SIGHTSEEING

Most cruise passengers are faced with far more to see and do than they have time for. That's why it's helpful to know what you can typically expect when visiting sights.

Perhaps the biggest challenge is **long lines.** At sights such as the Hermitage in St. Petersburg, the Eiffel Tower in Paris, and the Anne Frank House in Amsterdam, lines can be a real frustration. Study up, plan ahead, and use the information in this book to minimize time spent in line. For details on making **reservations** or **buying advance tickets** at major sights, see page 50.

Some important sights have a **security check,** where you must open your bag or send it through a metal detector. Some sights require you to check daypacks and coats. (If you'd rather not check your daypack, try carrying it tucked under your arm like a purse as you enter.)

A modest **dress code** (no bare shoulders, shorts, or above-the-knee skirts) is enforced at Orthodox churches you may want to enter in St. Petersburg, Tallinn, and Helsinki. If you are caught by surprise, you can improvise, using maps to cover your shoulders and a jacket tied around your waist to hide your legs.

If the museum's photo policy isn't clearly posted, ask a guard. Generally, **taking photos** without a flash or tripod is allowed. Some sights ban photos altogether.

Museums may have **special exhibits** in addition to their permanent collection. Some exhibits are included in the entry price, while others come at an extra cost (which you may have to pay even if you don't want to see that exhibit).

Expect changes—artwork can be on tour, on loan, out sick, or shifted at the whim of the curator. To adapt, pick up a floor plan as you enter, and ask museum staff if you can't find a particular item.

Many sights rent **audioguides,** which generally offer excellent

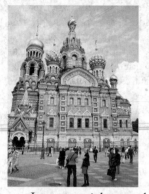

recorded descriptions in English. If you bring your own earbuds, you can enjoy better sound and avoid holding the device to your ear. To save money, bring a Y-jack and share one audioguide with your travel partner. Increasingly, museums are offering apps (often free) that you can download to your mobile device. And, as mentioned earlier, I've produced free downloadable **audio tours** of the major sights in Amsterdam, Paris, London, and Berlin; see page 50.

Important sights may have an **on-site café** or **cafeteria** (usually a handy place to rejuvenate during a long visit). The WCs at sights are free and generally clean.

Many places sell **postcards** that highlight their attractions. Before you leave a sight, scan the postcards and thumb through a guidebook to be sure you haven't overlooked something you'd like to see.

Be warned that you may not be allowed to enter if you arrive 30 to 60 minutes before **closing time.** And guards start ushering people out well before the actual closing time, so don't save the best for last.

Every sight or museum offers more than what's covered in this book. Use the information in this book as an introduction—not the final word.

IN PORT

SHOPPING

Shopping can be a fun part of any traveler's European trip. To have a good experience when you go ashore, be aware of the ins and outs of shopping in port.

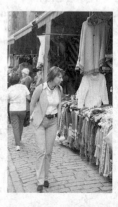

At every stop, your cruise line will give you an information sheet that highlights local shopping specialties and where to buy them. Remember that these shops commonly give kickbacks to cruise lines and guides. This doesn't mean that the shop (or what it sells) isn't good quality; it just means you're probably paying top dollar.

Regardless of whether a store is working

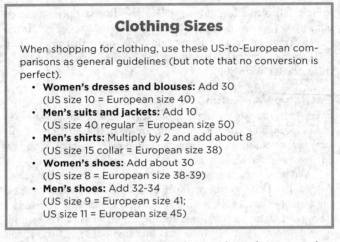

Clothing Sizes

When shopping for clothing, use these US-to-European comparisons as general guidelines (but note that no conversion is perfect).

- **Women's dresses and blouses:** Add 30
  (US size 10 = European size 40)
- **Men's suits and jackets:** Add 10
  (US size 40 regular = European size 50)
- **Men's shirts:** Multiply by 2 and add about 8
  (US size 15 collar = European size 38)
- **Women's shoes:** Add about 30
  (US size 8 = European size 38-39)
- **Men's shoes:** Add 32-34
  (US size 9 = European size 41;
  US size 11 = European size 45)

with the cruise line or not, many places jack up their rates when ships arrive, knowing they're about to get hit with a tidal wave of rushed and desperate shoppers. Remember: Northern Europe's cruise season lasts approximately three months—June, July, and August—and many people who live and work in that town must extract a year's worth of earnings from visitors during that period.

Finding Deals

So how can you avoid paying over-the-top, inflated prices for your treasured souvenirs? Go ahead and patronize the obvious tourist shops, but be sure to check out local shopping venues, too. Large department stores often have a souvenir section with standard knickknacks and postcards at prices way below those at cruise-recommended shops. These large stores generally work just like ours, and in big cities, most department-store staff are accustomed to wide-eyed foreign shoppers and can speak some English.

IN PORT

If you're adept at bargaining, head over to some of Europe's vibrant outdoor flea markets, where you can find local goods and soft prices. In Russia and at many street markets, haggling is the accepted (and expected) method of finding a compromise between the wishful thinking of both the merchant and the tourist.

Bargaining Tips: To be a successful haggler-shopper, first determine the item's value to you. Many tourists think that if they can cut the price by 50 percent they are doing great. So merchants quadruple their prices and the tourist happily pays double the fair value. The best way to deal with crazy prices is to ignore them. Show some interest in an item but say, "It's just too much money." You've put the merchant in a position to make the first offer.

Many merchants will settle for a nickel profit rather than lose a sale entirely. Work the cost down to rock bottom. When it seems to have fallen to a record low, walk away. That last price hollered out as you turn the corner is often the best price you'll get. If the price is right, go back and buy. And don't forget that prices often drop at the end of the day, when flea-market merchants have to think about packing up.

Getting a VAT Refund

Every year, tourists visiting Europe leave behind millions of dollars of refundable sales taxes. While for some, the headache of collecting the refund is not worth the few dollars at stake, if you do any serious shopping, it's hard cash—free and easy.

Wrapped into the purchase price of your souvenirs is a Value-Added Tax (VAT) of between 18 and 25 percent, depending on the country (for details, see www.ricksteves.com/vat). Almost all European countries require a minimum purchase for a refund, ranging from about $30 to several hundred dollars. If you spend that minimum at a store that participates in the VAT-refund scheme, you're entitled to get most of that tax back. Typically, you must ring up the minimum at a single retailer—you can't add up your purchases from various shops to reach the required amount.

Getting your refund is usually straightforward and, if you buy a substantial amount of souvenirs, well worth the hassle. If you're lucky, the merchant will subtract the tax when you make your purchase. (This is more likely to occur if the store ships the goods to your home.) Otherwise, you'll need to:

Get the paperwork. Have the merchant completely fill out the necessary refund document (either an official VAT customs form, or the shop or refund company's own version of it). You'll have to present your passport at the store. Get the paperwork done before you leave the store to ensure you'll have everything you need (including your original sales receipt).

Get your stamp at the border or airport. Process your VAT document at your last stop (for example, at the airport) with the customs agent who deals with VAT refunds. For purchases made in EU countries (in this book, everywhere but Russia and Norway), process your document when you leave the EU. It doesn't have to be the country where you made your purchases as long as you're still in the EU; if your flight connects through London's Heathrow airport, you can do it there. For non-EU countries such as Russia and Norway, process your VAT document at your last stop in that country (VAT refunds for tourists are a recent innovation in Russia; don't be surprised if the system still has a few kinks—or disappears). Arrive an additional hour before you need to check in for your flight to allow time to find the local customs office—and to stand in line. It's best to keep your purchases in your carry-on. If they're too large or dangerous to carry on (such as knives), pack them in your checked bags and alert the check-in agent. You'll be sent (with your tagged bag) to a customs desk outside security, where they'll examine your bag, stamp your paperwork, and put your bag on the belt. You're not supposed to use your purchased goods before you leave. If you show up at customs wearing your new Norwegian sweater, officials might look the other way—or deny you a refund.

Collect your refund. You'll need to return your stamped document to the retailer or its representative. Many merchants work with services, such as Global Blue or Premier Tax Free, that have offices at major airports, ports, or border crossings (either before or after security, probably strategically located near a duty-free shop). These services, which extract a 4 percent fee, can refund your money immediately in cash or credit your card (within two billing cycles). If the retailer handles VAT refunds directly, it's up to you to contact the merchant for your refund. You can mail the documents from home, or more quickly, from your point of departure (using an envelope you've prepared in advance or one that's been provided by the merchant). You'll then have to wait—it can take months.

Customs for American Shoppers

You are allowed to take home $800 worth of items per person duty-free, once every 30 days. You can take home many processed and packaged foods: vacuum-packed cheeses, dried herbs, jams, baked goods, candy, chocolate, oil, vinegar, mustard, and honey. Fresh fruits and vegetables and most meats are not allowed, with exceptions for some canned items. As for alcohol, you can bring in one liter duty-free (it can be packed securely in your checked luggage, along with any other liquid-containing items).

To bring alcohol (or liquid-packed foods) in your carry-on bag on your flight home, buy it at a duty-free shop at the airport. You'll increase your odds of getting it onto a connecting flight if it's packaged in a "STEB"—a secure, tamper-evident bag. But stay away from liquids in opaque, ceramic, or metallic containers, which usually cannot be successfully screened (STEB or no STEB).

For details on allowable goods, customs rules, and duty rates, visit www.cbp.gov.

EATING IN PORT

Eating in Europe is sightseeing for your taste buds. The memories of good meals can satisfy you for years. Even though most of your meals will be on the ship, you can still experience Europe's amazing cuisine while you're in port. Your options range from grabbing a lunch on the run to lingering over a leisurely meal at a sit-down restaurant. When deciding where to eat, be aware that table service in Europe is slow—sometimes painfully so—by American standards. Don't expect to dine and dash, but you can try explaining to the wait-staff that you're in a hurry.

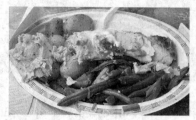

Lunch on the Go

You can eat quickly and still have a local experience. Every country has its own equivalent of the hot-dog stand, where you can grab a filling bite on the go: Danish *pølse* (sausage) carts and *smørrebrød* (open-face sandwich) shops, French *crêperies*, Berlin's *Currywurst* stands, and Russian *bliny* (potato pancake) shops. Or stop in a heavenly smelling bakery and buy a pastry or sandwich.

Ethnic eateries are usually cheap; eat in, or get your meal to go. Cafeterias, delis, and fast-food chains with salad bars are tourist-friendly and good for a quick meal.

Like businesspeople, cruise travelers have a lot on their day-time agendas and want to eat well but quickly. A good bet is to eat lunch at a place that caters to the local business clientele. You'll find many fine little restaurants advertising fast, two-course business lunches. These are inexpensive and served quickly. Each neighborhood is also likely to have a favorite deli/sandwich place where you'll see a thriving crowd of office workers spilling out onto the curb, eating fine, small meals or gourmet sandwiches—and often sipping a glass of top-end wine with their food.

Picnicking takes a little more time and planning but can be an even more exciting cultural experience: It's fun to dive into a marketplace and actually get a chance to do business there. Europe's colorful markets overflow with varied cheeses, meats, fresh fruits, vegetables, and still-warm-out-of-the-oven bread. Most markets are not self-service: You point to what you want and let the merchant weigh and bag it for you. The unit of measure throughout the Continent is a kilo, or 2.2 pounds. A kilo has 1,000 grams. One hundred grams is a common unit of sale for cheese or meat—and just the right amount to tuck into a chunk of French bread for a satisfying sandwich.

Keep an eye out for some of my favorite picnic treats: *Wasa* cracker bread (Sport is my favorite; *flatbrød* is ideal for munchies), packaged meat and cheese, brown "goat cheese" *(geitost)*, drinkable yogurt, freshly cooked or smoked fish from markets, fresh fruit and vegetables, lingonberries, and squeeze tubes of mustard and sandwich spreads (shrimp, caviar), which are perfect on rye bread.

Sit-Down Restaurants

For some cruisers, it's unimaginable to waste valuable port time lingering at a sit-down restaurant when they could be cramming their day with sightseeing. For others, a good European restaurant experience beats a cathedral or a museum by a mile.

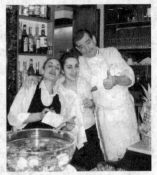

To find a good restaurant, head away from the tourist center and stroll around until you find a place with a happy crowd of locals. Look for menus handwritten in the native language (usually posted outside) and offering a small selection. This means they're cooking what was fresh in the market that morning for loyal return customers.

Restaurants in Europe usually do not serve meals throughout the day, so don't wait too long to find a place for lunch. Typically restaurants close from the late afternoon (about 14:00) until the dinner hour.

When entering a restaurant, feel free to seat yourself at any table that isn't marked "reserved." Catch a server's eye and signal to be sure it's OK to sit there. If the place is full, you're likely to simply be turned away: There's no "hostess" standing by to add your name to a carefully managed waiting list.

If no English **menu** is posted, ask to see one. What we call the menu in the US usually goes by some variation on the word "card" in Europe—for instance, *la carte* in French.

Be aware that the word "menu" can mean a fixed-price meal, particularly in France. Many small eateries offer an economical *"menu* of the day" (*plat du jour* in France)—a daily special with a fixed price. The "tourist *menu*" (*menu touristique* in France), popular in restaurants throughout Europe's tourist zones, offers visitors a no-stress, three-course meal for a painless price that usually includes service, bread, and a drink. You normally get a choice of several options for each course. Locals rarely order this, but if the options intrigue you, the tourist *menu* can be a convenient way to sample some regional flavors for a reasonable, predictable price. Particularly in Scandinavian countries, many restaurants offer cheap daily lunch specials *(dagens rett)* and buffets, popular with office workers.

In restaurants, Europeans generally drink bottled **water** (for taste, not health), served with or without carbonation. You can normally get free tap water, but you may need to be polite, patient, inventive, and know the correct phrase. There's nothing wrong with ordering tap water, and it is safe to drink in all the countries in this book, except for Russia.

One of the biggest surprises for Americans at Europe's restaurants is the service, which can seem excruciatingly slow when you're eager to get out and sightsee (or in a hurry to get back to your cruise ship). Europeans will spend at least two hours enjoying a good meal, and fast service is considered rude service. If you need to eat and run, make it very clear when you order.

To get the **bill,** you'll have to ask for it. Don't wait until you are in a hurry to leave. Catch the waiter's eye and, with raised hands, scribble with an imaginary pencil on your palm. Before it comes, make a mental tally of roughly how much your meal should cost. If the total is a surprise, ask to have it itemized and explained.

Tipping: At European restaurants, a base gratuity is already included in your bill. Virtually anywhere in Europe, if you're pleased with the service, you can round up a euro or more. In most restaurants, 5 percent is adequate and 10 percent is considered a big tip. Please believe me—tipping 15-20 percent in Europe is unnecessary, if not culturally insensitive. Tip only at restaurants with waitstaff; skip the tip if you order food at a counter. Servers prefer to be tipped in cash even if you pay with your credit card; otherwise the tip may never reach them (specifics on tipping are also provided in each country's introduction chapter).

Returning to the Ship

When it's time to head back to your ship, remember that the posted departure time is a bit misleading: The all-aboard time (when you absolutely, positively must be on your ship) is usually a half-hour before departure. And the last shuttle bus or tender back to the ship might leave an hour before departure...trimming your port time even more. If you want to max out on time ashore, research alternative options—such as a taxi or a public bus—that get you back to the ship even closer to the all-aboard time (but, of course, be cautious not to cut it *too* close). Before leaving the ship, make sure you understand when you need to be back on board, and (if applicable) when the last shuttle bus or tender departs.

All of that said, feel free to take every minute of the time you've got. If the last tender leaves at 16:30, don't feel you need to get back to the dock at 16:00. I make it a point to be the last person back on the ship at every port... usually five minutes or so before all-aboard time. I sometimes get

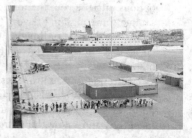

dirty looks from early birds who've been waiting for a few minutes on that last tender, but I didn't waste their time...they did.

WHAT IF I MISS MY BOAT?

You can't count on the ship to wait for you if you get back late. If you're cutting it close, call ahead to the port agent (the phone number is on your ship's port-of-call information sheet and/or daily program) and let them know you're coming. They will notify the ship's crew, so at least they know they didn't miscount the returning passengers. And there's a possibility (though a very slim one) that the ship could wait for you. But if it sets sail, and you're not on it, you're on your own to reach the next port. The cruise line will not cover any of your transportation or accommodations expenses, and you will not be reimbursed for any unused portion of your cruise.

You have approximately 24 hours to reach the ship before it departs from its next destination. Be clear on where the next stop is. If you're lucky, it's an easy two-hour train ride away, giving you bonus time in both destinations. If you're unlucky, it's a 20-hour overland odyssey or an expensive last-minute flight—or worse, the ship is spending the day at sea, meaning you'll miss out on two full cruising days.

First, ask the **port agent** for advice. The agent can typically give you a little help or at least point you in the right direction. Be aware that you'll be steered to the easiest, but not necessarily the most affordable, solution. For example, the agent might suggest hiring a private driver for hundreds of dollars, rather than taking a $50 bus ride. If your ship's policy is to hold passenger passports during the cruise, he'll have it waiting for you.

You can also ask for help from the **TI,** if it's still open. Local **travel agencies** should know most or all of your connection options and can book tickets for you (they'll charge you a small commission). Or—to do it yourself—find an **Internet café** and get online to research your train, flight, and bus options. German Rail's handy, all-Europe train timetables are a good place to start: www.bahn.com. Check the website of the nearest airport; these usually show the schedule of upcoming flights in the next day or two. To compare inexpensive flights within Europe, try www.skyscanner.com.

Don't delay in making your plans. The sooner you begin investigating your options, the more choices you may have. If you realize you've missed your ship at 20:00, there may be an affordable night train to the next stop departing from the train station across town at 21:00...and if you're not on it, you could pay through the nose for a last-minute flight instead.

Remember, most ships never leave anyone behind over the

IN PORT

course of the entire cruise. While the prospect of missing your ship is daunting, don't let it scare you into not enjoying your shore time. As long as you keep a close eye on the time and are conservative in estimating how long it'll take you to get back to the ship, it's easy to enjoy a very full day in port and be the last tired but happy tourist sauntering back onto the ship.

OVERNIGHTING IN PORT

At some major destinations (most often in St. Petersburg), the cruise ship might spend two days and an overnight in port. This allows you to linger in the evening and really feel like you've been to a place—treating your cruise ship like a hotel.

NORTHERN EUROPEAN CRUISE PORTS

NORTHERN EUROPEAN CRUISE PORTS

The rest of this book focuses on the specific cruise ports where you'll be spending your days. For each one, I've provided detailed instructions for getting from the port into town, and included my suggested self-guided tours and walks for the best one-day plan in that town.

Rick Steves Northern European Cruise Ports is a personal tour guide in your pocket, organized by destination. Each major destination is a mini-vacation on its own, filled with exciting sights, strollable neighborhoods, and memorable places to eat. You'll find the following sections in most of the destination chapters (although, because cruise port details can vary from place to place, not every destination will include all of these elements):

Planning Your Time suggests a schedule for how to best use your limited time in port. These plans are what I'd do with my time if I had only a few hours to spend in a particular destination. Be warned—I like to spend the maximum amount of time in port sightseeing, rather than relaxing, shopping, or dining. For each option, I've suggested the minimum amount of time you can reasonably expect to spend to get a good look at the highlights. If you find that my plan packs too much in, or shortchanges something you'd like to focus on, modify the plan by skipping one or two time-consuming options (read the descriptions in the chapters to decide which items interest you).

The **Excursions** sidebars help you make informed, strategic decisions about which cruise-line excursions to outlying destinations best match your interests.

The **Port** sections provide detailed, step-by-step instructions for getting from your cruise ship to wherever you're going (whether it's to the city center, or, in some cases, to a nearby town). Each one begins with a brief "Arrival at a Glance" section to help you get oriented to your options. I've also tracked down helpful services (such as ATMs and pharmacies) at or near each port.

Orientation includes specifics on public transportation, helpful hints, local tour options, easy-to-read maps, and tourist information.

Self-Guided Walks and Tours takes you through interesting neighborhoods and museums.

Sights describes the top attractions and includes their cost and hours. The "At a Glance" sections for bigger cities offer a quick overview of the sights.

Eating serves up a range of options, from inexpensive eateries to fancy restaurants.

Shopping offers advice on the most authentic local souvenirs and where to buy them.

The **What If I Miss My Boat?** section gives you a quick list of options for reaching your next port, in case you get stranded.

Starting or Ending Your Cruise info for the most common embarkation/disembarkation points (Copenhagen, Stockholm, Amsterdam, and London) spells out how to get from the airport to the cruise port, and lists a few of my favorite hotels.

A **practicalities** section for each country included in this book provides basic facts and figures, along with useful notes (such as the local currency, time zone, phone system, and tipping customs).

KEY TO THIS BOOK
Updates
This book is updated regularly—but things change. For the latest, visit www.ricksteves.com/update.

Abbreviations and Times
I use the following symbols and abbreviations in this book:

Sights are rated:

▲▲▲	**Don't miss**
▲▲	**Try hard to see**
▲	**Worthwhile if you can make it**
No rating	**Worth knowing about**

Tourist information offices are abbreviated as **TI,** and bathrooms are **WCs.**

Like Europe, this book uses the **24-hour clock.** It's the same through 12:00 noon, then keeps going: 13:00, 14:00, and so on. For anything over 12, subtract 12 and add p.m. (14:00 is 2:00 p.m.).

When giving **opening times,** I include both peak season and off-season hours if they differ. So, if a museum is listed as "May-Oct daily 9:00-16:00," it should be open from 9:00 a.m. until 4:00 p.m. from the first day of May until the last day of October (but expect exceptions).

For **transit** or **tour departures,** I first list the frequency, then the duration. So, a train connection listed as "2/hour, 1.5 hours" departs twice each hour, and the journey lasts an hour and a half.

Sleep Code

In each of the cities where you're likely to begin or end your trip, I list a few of my favorite accommodations. To help you easily sort through these listings, I've divided the accommodations into three categories, based on the highest price for a standard double room with bath during high season:

> **$$$ Higher Priced**
> **$$ Moderately Priced**
> **$ Lower Priced**

Prices can change without notice; verify the hotel's current rates online or by email. For the best prices, always book directly with the hotel.

To pack maximum information into minimum space, I use the following abbreviations to describe accommodations. Prices in this book are listed per room, not per person.

S = Single room (or price for one person in a double)
D = Double or twin room
T = Triple (generally a double bed with a single)
Q = Quad (usually two double beds)
b = Private bathroom with toilet and shower or tub

COPENHAGEN
Denmark

Denmark Practicalities

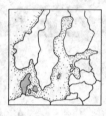

Denmark (Danmark), between the Baltic and the North Sea, is the smallest of the Scandinavian countries (16,600 square miles—roughly double the size of Massachusetts). But in the 16th century, it was the largest; at one time, Denmark ruled all of Norway and the three southern provinces of Sweden. Today's population is about 5.5 million; 10 percent are immigrants. The predominant religion is Protestant (mostly Evangelical Lutheran). The country consists of the largely flat, extensively cultivated Jutland peninsula, as well as over 400 islands (78 of which are inhabited, including Sjælland/Zealand, where Copenhagen is located).

Money: 6 Danish kroner (kr, officially DKK) = about $1. An ATM is called a *pengeautomat*. The local VAT (value-added sales tax) rate is 25 percent; the minimum purchase eligible for a VAT refund is 300 kr (for details on refunds, see page 134).

Language: The native language is Danish. For useful phrases, see page 229.

Emergencies: Dial 112 for police, medical, or other emergencies. In case of theft or loss, see page 125.

Time Zone: Denmark is on Central European Time (the same as most of the Continent, one hour ahead of Great Britain, and six/nine hours ahead of the East/West Coasts of the US).

Embassies in Copenhagen: The **US embassy** is at Dag Hammarskjölds Allé 24 (tel. 33 41 71 00, after-hours emergency tel. 33 41 74 00, http://denmark.usembassy.gov). The **Canadian embassy** is at Kristen Bernikowsgade 1 (tel. 33 48 32 00, www.canada.dk). Call ahead for passport services.

Phoning: Denmark's country code is 45; to call from another country to Denmark, dial the international access code (011 from the US/Canada, 00 from Europe, or + from a mobile phone), then 45, followed by the local number. For local calls within Denmark, dial the number as it appears in this book—whether you're calling from across the street or across the country. To place an international call from Denmark, dial 00, the code of the country you're calling (1 for US and Canada), and the phone number. For more help, see page 1146.

Tipping: Gratuity is included in the price of sit-down meals, so you don't need to tip further, though it's nice to round up your bill about 5-10 percent for great service. Tip a taxi driver by rounding up the fare a bit (pay 90 kr on an 85-kr fare). For more tips on tipping, see page 138.

Tourist Information: www.visitcopenhagen.com

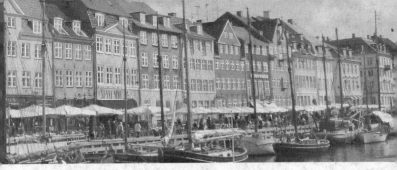

COPENHAGEN

København

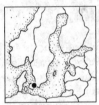

Copenhagen, Denmark's capital, is the gateway to Scandinavia. It's an improbable combination of corny Danish clichés, well-dressed executives having a business lunch amid cutting-edge contemporary architecture, and some of the funkiest counterculture in Europe. And yet, it all just works so tidily together. With the Øresund Bridge connecting Sweden and Denmark (creating the region's largest metropolitan area), Copenhagen is energized and ready to dethrone Stockholm as Scandinavia's powerhouse city.

PLANNING YOUR TIME

Copenhagen is spread out, with lots of sightseeing options. You can't squeeze everything into one day, so be selective. Below I've listed your most likely choices; I'd suggest starting with the first two, then choosing from the remaining list with whatever time you have left. If several of the later items appeal to you (or if the weather is dreary), skip the walk and cruise.

• **Copenhagen City Walk:** This self-guided stroll through town gives you your bearings in about two hours (longer if you tack on the extended route).

• **Harbor Cruise:** On a sunny day, this is well worth the hour it takes, as it gets you out on the water and shows you corners of the city that are otherwise hard to see. But if it's cold or rainy, I'd skip it.

• **Rosenborg Castle:** For a classic Renaissance castle experience right in the city center, plus a peek at the crown jewels, tour this palace. Allow 1.5 hours.

- **National Museum:** Offering an illuminating look at Danish history, this deserves at least 1.5 hours for the quickest visit (ideally longer).
- **Thorvaldsen's Museum** or **Ny Carlsberg Glyptothek:** For fans of Neoclassical sculpture or antiquities and paintings (respectively), each museum deserves an hour or more.
- **Christiana:** You can stroll through this unique hippie squatters' commune in about an hour, though it takes some time to get here.
- **Tivoli Gardens:** This quintessentially Danish amusement park is a delightful way to burn up whatever time you have remaining at the end of your busy Copenhagen day (allow at least an hour for strolling and Dane-watching). Conveniently located across the street from the main train station, Tivoli lets you hop right on bus #26 or an S-tog (suburban train) to hightail it back to your ship.

The Port of Copenhagen

Arrival at a Glance: Copenhagen's three main cruise ports are conveniently served by public bus #26, which delivers passengers to various spots around town. Both Langelinie and Frihavnen are about a 10- to 15-minute walk from a train station, with fast connections to downtown. Langelinie is also an easy 10-minute walk from *The Little Mermaid*. Other options include catching a tour bus, a cruise-ship shuttle bus, or a taxi.

Port Overview

As one of the primary cruise ports on the Baltic—and one of the most common places to begin or end a cruise—Copenhagen handles a vast volume of cruise traffic. Ships generally use one of three port areas:

Oceankaj: The city's newest cruise port is the farthest away—roughly 3.5 miles north of downtown. Its three terminals are expected to take the majority of cruise traffic.

Frihavnen ("Freeport"): This sprawling port area, about three miles north of downtown, is used by both industrial and cruise vessels. Most cruises use the piers closest to town: Sundkaj, Orientkaj, and Fortkaj. From these, it's an easy 5- to 10-minute walk to the port gate. Some cruises dock at the farther-out Levantkaj, to the north; as this is a much longer walk, the port provides a free shuttle bus to the port gate.

Langelinie: This pier juts out from the north end of Kastellet Park and is within long walking distance of downtown. It has two berths for big ships, but cruises do not typically begin or end here.

Excursions from Copenhagen

Most cruise lines offer a variety of bus and/or walking tours of **Copenhagen.** These often include guided tours of sights such as Tivoli Gardens, Rosenborg Castle, Amalienborg Palace, Christiansborg Palace, and Christianshavn. But all of these sights—and my self-guided walk through downtown Copenhagen—are easy to visit on your own and thoroughly covered in this book. Similarly, I wouldn't pay your cruise line for a harbor or canal tour, as these are much easier and cheaper to book direct once you arrive.

Excursions to a few out-of-town sights may be worth considering. Many cruise lines offer a tour combining two of the best castles just outside the city: **Frederiksborg** (with sumptuous rooms and an outstanding museum of Danish history) and **Kronborg** (less engaging inside, but very picturesque and with tentative ties to Hamlet). If you're not interested in Copenhagen itself, an excursion combining these two castles (tricky by public transit) could be a good choice. However, I'd skip the side-trip to the pretty but very touristy fishing village of **Dragør** (the much-touted view of the Øresund Bridge from here is only a bit closer than what you'll see from the deck of your ship).

Tourist Information: There is no TI at Copenhagen's cruise ports, though signs help you find your way to the nearest bus stop or train station. You'll also likely find free city maps at displays around the port area. Once in town, you can visit Copenhagen's official TI, near the main train station, but since it's mostly a promotional agency for local businesses, I wouldn't make a big effort to go there.

GETTING INTO TOWN
First I'll cover the options that work from all three ports: cruise-line shuttle buses, tours, taxis, and the public bus (cheap and easy). Then I'll give details for other options that are specific to Frihavnen and Langelinie.

By Cruise-Line Shuttle Bus
Many cruise lines run shuttle buses between the port and town, usually stopping at Kongens Nytorv (near Nyhavn) and/or Rådhuspladsen (City Hall Square). This can be pricey (varies by cruise line, but figure €12 round-trip)—though in this expensive city, that's not much more than the cost of round-trip public transit tickets. If it's available, I'd consider the shuttle for the convenience.

COPENHAGEN

By Tour

Cruise passengers arriving at Oceankaj or Frihavnen can take their cruise shuttle to *The Little Mermaid* and pick up a hop-on, hop-off bus at that sight. Those arriving at Langelinie can catch a hop-on, hop-off bus at the port. These bus tours are worth considering in order to get your bearings in this spread-out city. The same company owns City Sightseeing Copenhagen (red buses) and Open Top Tours (green buses); another outfit called Red Blue Bus Tours also runs hop-on, hop-off tours.

For other tour options—including the highly recommended harbor cruises and Richard Karpen's excellent group walking tours—see "Tours in Copenhagen" on page 163.

By Taxi

From Oceankaj and Frihavnen, taxis charge 200 kr or more for the ride into town. I'd skip this pricey option in favor of one of the fairly easy public transportation choices explained later—though with bags (i.e., if going to a hotel at the end of a tour), a taxi may be worth the splurge. Taxis also cluster along Langelinie's pier, offering a ride into downtown for about 160 kr, but given the ease of walking or public transportation, I wouldn't take a taxi.

By Public Bus #26

This made-for-cruisers bus is a handy way to connect any of Copenhagen's cruise ports to various points downtown. For details on taking bus #26, see the sidebar.

From Oceankaj: If your ship docks at Terminal 1, it's a short walk across the street, past a cluster of kiosks, and down the main road leading away from the cruise port to the stop for bus #26. If your ship arrives at the more distant Terminals 2 or 3, it's a 10- to 15-minute walk along the harborfront road to Terminal 1, where you'll turn right at the kiosks and go a short distance down the main road to the bus #26 stop.

From Frihavnen: Your first step will be making your way from your ship to the port gate. If your ship is at Sundkaj, Orientkaj, or Fortkaj, when you exit the terminal area, just look for the thick blue line painted in the sidewalk. Follow this to the port gate (5-10 minutes). If you're arriving at the farther-flung Levantkaj, a free shuttle bus will meet your ship for the quick ride to the port gate.

To find the stop for bus #26, exit straight from the port gate, and walk about 50 yards to the end of the street. You'll hit a T-intersection with a wide road (Sundkrogsgade). Turn right, walk along this road for about a half-block (passing the stop for bus #26 going *away* from town), then cross the street at the low-profile crosswalk (look for the blue-and-white arrow in the middle

Public Bus #26

Bus #26 is a convenient option for cruisers to get to downtown Copenhagen. It runs about every 10 minutes from stops near the ports, and the ride downtown takes about 20 minutes. On weekdays, bus #26 heads right into town. On Saturdays and Sundays, it runs as a "Cruise Ship Shuttle" from the ports to the Østerport train station and back. At Østerport you can either catch the S-tog train into the city center or board a regular bus #26 for the rest of the trip into town (be sure to ask for a transfer when you get on the #26 shuttle).

The bus costs 24 kr (or 80 kr for a 24-hour pass). The driver takes credit cards (you'll need your PIN) and euros (figure about €3 for a simple ticket; you'll get change back in Danish kroner).

Heading from the port into the city, be sure to take a bus going in the direction of Ålholm Plads. The bus makes several stops handy to downtown sightseeing. Stops are marked by a dark-blue post with a yellow top and the number *26*. Here are some of the major stops:

Østerport Stn: Østerport train station, for fast trains downtown

Kongens Nytorv: Big square near the colorful Nyhavn sailor's quarter

Holmenskirke: Church facing Slotsholmen Island and starting point for harbor cruises

Christiansborg: Palace on Slotsholmen Island

Stormboren, Nationalmuseet: National Museum

Rådhuspladsen: City Hall Square, at the start of my self-guided walk

Hoevdbanegården: Main train station, across the street from Tivoli amusement park

Returning to the Port: If you're riding bus #26 from downtown back to your ship, be sure to get on one going to the right place, because north of town, the bus splits into two different routes, heading either to Langelinie or to the Frihavnen and Oceankaj ports. Buses marked *Søndre Frihavn Indiakaj* return to Langelinie (get off at the stop at the entrance to the pier). Buses marked either *Faergehavn Nord* or *Faergehavn Nord UNICEF* head toward Frihavnen (get off at the Færgeterminalen Søndre Frihavn stop, a short walk from the port gate). Only buses marked *Faergehavn Nord UNICEF* go to Oceankaj (get off at the stop near Terminal 1). Even if a bus is marked, do as a bus driver once told me: "Always ask if you're getting on the right bus."

Services at the Ports

Expect few services at the piers. Several have money-exchange offices, but none has ATMs, so you'll need to head into town to withdraw money. You should be able to use your American credit card (or debit card) at public-transit ticket machines, but you'll need to know and use your four-digit PIN. Convenience stores such as 7-Eleven generally sell public transit tickets and take credit cards.

Here's an overview of what each port offers:

At **Oceankaj,** you'll find a cluster of kiosks across the street kitty-corner from Terminal 1, including a Ria Money Transfer (money exchange, phone cards, SIM cards, and Wi-Fi access), and shops selling tickets for bus #26, hop-on, hop-off bus tickets, and souvenirs. Oceankaj's three terminals have free Wi-Fi—look for instructions on how to access it.

At **Frihavnen,** you will find a small money-exchange office (Ria Money Transfer, huddled next to a red-brick building at the base of Sundkaj) that also sells cheap phone cards, SIM cards, and Internet access. The small souvenir kiosk (adjacent to the information post with free maps) has SIM cards and can answer questions about getting settled into Copenhagen. The port's terminal buildings are equipped with free Wi-Fi; look for posters with instructions on how to log on.

There's little at **Langelinie,** except a pier-front road with stops for taxis and hop-on, hop-off tour buses, and a row of cruise-oriented shops (duty-free, outlet stores).

of the street). Once across, you'll find the stop for bus #26 going into downtown Copenhagen.

From Langelinie: Bus #26 stops near the entrance to Langelinie. Leaving your ship, go left and walk down the pier (and under a pedestrian overpass) to its entrance at the roundabout, turn right on the street called Indiakaj, and walk a short distance to the bus stop (about 10 minutes from the far end of the pier).

Another Option from Frihavnen to Town

It's an easy 10-minute walk from Frihavnen's port gate to Nordhavn Station. From there, **trains** depart for downtown every couple of minutes.

After getting off the ship, follow the blue line, which directs cruisers out of the port and into the city. Cross the highway called Kalkbrænderihavnsgade and go under the railway underpass, then immediately turn left (on Østbanegade). Walk along this residential street, with the elevated train tracks on your left, until you reach the station. Find the station entrance by the 7-Eleven mini-market, which sells tickets (regular two-zone ticket or 24-hour pass) and accepts euros or credit cards. A ticket machine is located just up the stairs from the 7-Eleven on the track (credit cards work with a PIN). You can take any train on the track facing away from the cruise port area (on the left as you come up the stairs). Once on the track, confirm you're heading for the center (nearly everyone speaks English). Ride two stops to Nørreport (near Rosenborg Palace), or stay on four stops to København H—the main train station.

Another Option from Langelinie to Town

Arriving at Langelinie puts you within walking distance of most of Copenhagen's sights (10 minutes to *The Little Mermaid*, another 15 minutes to Amalienborg Palace, then another 10 minutes to Nyhavn). A good option could be to do my self-guided "Copenhagen City Walk" in reverse, starting at *The Little Mermaid* and ending at Rådhuspladsen.

To get to *The Little Mermaid*, turn left from your ship and walk the length of the pier, passing a row of shops on your right. At the entrance end of the pier, continue straight, passing the statue of the decidedly *not*-little mermaid, and cross the footbridge. Keep going straight, bearing uphill, slightly to your right, to walk with the sailboat harbor on your left.

Pass through the park with the angel monument. To reach *The Little Mermaid*, turn left from the park and head along the water to the commotion of tourists. From the *Mermaid*, you can keep walking along the waterfront past Kastellet Park and the Museum of Danish Resistance (currently closed) all the way to Amalienborg Palace (about 15 minutes beyond the *Little Mermaid*). From the palace, it's about another 10-minute walk to the colorful Nyhavn canal, at the edge of the town center.

RETURNING TO YOUR SHIP

You can ride **bus** #26 back to all three piers from various points downtown (including the train station, Holmenskirke near Slotsholmen island, or Kongens Nytorv near Nyhavn). Note: Because this bus line splits north of downtown to go to either Langelinie or the other two cruise ports, be sure to confirm with the driver that you're on the right one (see page 223 for details on taking this bus).

You can also take the S-tog **train** back to stations near Frihavnen and Langelinie, then walk (you can hop on any S-tog train from downtown in the directions of Hillerød, Holte, Farum, or Klampenborg).

For Frihavnen, ride the S-tog train to Nordhavn, then walk about 10 minutes. Exit the station to the right, then walk along the residential street (with the elevated tracks on your right) until you reach the railway underpass. Cross under it, then proceed straight across the street at the crosswalk, and turn left along the busy highway—walking with the port on your right. At the next intersection, turn right; at the intersection after that, the port gate is just to your right.

For Langelinie, ride the S-tog train to Østerport Station. Upon arrival, exit the station, turn left, and cross the busy street. Head down into the park, turn left, and walk around the moat of Kastellet Park. Exiting from the north end of the park, you're a short walk from Langelinie.

Copenhagen

Copenhagen is huge (with 1.2 million people), but for most visitors, the walkable core is the diagonal axis formed by the train station, Tivoli Gardens, Rådhuspladsen (City Hall Square), and the Strøget pedestrian street, ending at the colorful old Nyhavn sailors' harbor. Bubbling with street life, colorful pedestrian zones, and most of the city's sightseeing, the Strøget is fun. But also be sure to get off the main drag and explore. By doing things by bike or on foot, you'll stumble upon some charming bits of Copenhagen that many travelers miss. The city feels pretty torn up, as they are deep into a multiyear Metro expansion project, which will add 17 stations to their already impressive system.

Outside of the old city center are three areas of interest to tourists:

• To the north are Rosenborg Castle and Amalienborg Palace, with *The Little Mermaid* nearby.

• To the east, across the harbor, are Christianshavn (Copenhagen's "Little Amsterdam" district) and the alternative enclave of Christiania.

• To the west (behind the train station) is Vesterbro, a young and trendy part of town with lots of cafés, bars, and boutiques, and the hip Meatpacking District (Kødbyen).

All of these sights are walkable from the Strøget, but taking a bike, bus, or taxi is more efficient. I rent a bike (for about the cost of a single cab ride per day) and get anywhere in the town center literally faster than by taxi (nearly anything is within a 10-minute pedal). In good weather, the city is an absolute delight by bike (for more on biking in Copenhagen, see "Getting Around Copenhagen: By Bike," later).

Orientation to Copenhagen

TOURIST INFORMATION

Copenhagen's questionable excuse for a TI, which bills itself as "Wonderful Copenhagen," is actually a blatantly for-profit company. As in a (sadly) increasing number of big European cities, it provides information only about businesses that pay a hefty display fee of thousands of dollars each year. This colors the advice and information the office provides. While they can answer basic questions, the office is worthwhile mostly as a big rack of advertising brochures—you can pick up the free map at many hotels and other places in town (May-June Mon-Sat 9:00-18:00, Sun 9:00-14:00; July-Aug daily 9:00-19:00; Sept-April Mon-Fri 9:00-16:00, Sat 9:00-14:00, closed Sun; just up the street from train station—to the left as you exit the station—at Vesterbrogade 4A, good Lagkagehuset bakery in building, tel. 70 22 24 42, www.visitcopenhagen.com).

Copenhagen Card: This card includes entry to many of the city's sights (including expensive ones, like Tivoli and Rosenborg Castle) and all local transportation throughout the greater Copenhagen area. It can save busy sightseers some money; if you're planning on visiting a lot of attractions with steep entry prices, do the arithmetic to see if buying this pass adds up (339 kr/24 hours, 469 kr/48 hours, 559 kr/72 hours, 779 kr/120 hours—sold at the TI and some hotels).

Alternative Sources of Tourist Information: As the TI's bottom line competes with its mission to help tourists, you may want to seek out other ways to inform yourself. The weekly English-language newspaper, *The Copenhagen Post*, has good articles about what's going on in town (often available free at TI or some hotels, or buy it at a newsstand, www.cphpost.dk). The witty alternative website, www.aok.dk, has several articles in English (and many more in Danish—readable and very insightful if you translate them online).

ARRIVAL IN COPENHAGEN

The **main train station** is linked by train to the airport (see page 222), to Frihavnen via Nordhavn Station (see page 223), and to Langelinie via Østerport Station (see page 223).

The main train station is a hive of travel-related activity (and 24-hour thievery). Locals call it Hovedbanegården (HOETH-bahn-gorn; look for *København H* on signs and schedules). Kiosks and fast-food eateries cluster in the middle of the main arrivals hall; other services include a ticket office, train information kiosk, baggage storage, pay WCs, a post office, and ATMs. The tracks at the back of the station (tracks 9-10 and 11-12) are for the suburban train (S-tog).

Just walk out the front door and you'll run into one of the entrances for Tivoli amusement park; if you go around its left side and up a couple of blocks, you'll be at Rådhuspladsen, where my "Copenhagen City Walk" begins.

HELPFUL HINTS

Pharmacy: Steno Apotek is across from the train station (open 24 hours, Vesterbrogade 6C—see map on page 224, tel. 33 14 82 66).

Blue Monday: As you plan, remember that most sights close on Monday, but these attractions remain open: Amalienborg Museum (closed Mon Nov-April), Christiansborg Palace (closed Mon Oct-April), City Hall, Museum of Copenhagen, Rosenborg Castle (closed Mon Nov-April), Round Tower, Royal Library, Our Savior's Church, Tivoli Gardens (generally closed late Sept-mid-April), and all of the various tours (canal, bus, walking, and bike). You can explore Christiania, but Monday is its rest day, so it's unusually quiet and some restaurants are closed.

Internet Access: Wi-Fi is easy to find in Copenhagen (available free at many cafés). If you need a terminal with Internet access, you can get online for free at the **Copenhagen Central Library** (Mon-Fri 10:00-19:00, Sat 10:00-14:00, closed Sun, midway between Nørreport and the Strøget at Krystalgade 15—see map on page 224) and **"Black Diamond" library** (see page 194). The **Telestation** call shop behind the train station offers pay Internet terminals (kitty-corner from TI, Mon-Fri 10:00-19:30, Sat 10:00-16:30, closed Sun, Banegårdspladsen 1, tel. 33 93 00 02).

Laundry: Pams Møntvask is a good coin-op laundry near Nørreport (wash-31 kr/load, soap-6 kr, dry-2 kr/minute, daily 6:00-21:00, 50 yards from Ibsens Hotel at 86 Nansensgade). **Tre Stjernet Møntvask** ("Three Star Laundry") is several blocks past the Meatpacking District (wash-27 kr/load, soap-5 kr, dry-1 kr/1.5 minutes, daily 6:00-21:00, Sønder Boulevard 97). For both locations, see the map on page 224. *Vaskel* is wash, *torring* is dry, and *sæbe* is soap.

Updates to This Book: For updates to this book, check www.ricksteves.com/update.

GETTING AROUND COPENHAGEN
By Public Transit

It's easy to navigate Copenhagen, with its fine buses, Metro, and S-tog (a suburban train system with stops in the city; rail passes valid on S-tog). For a helpful website that covers public-transport options (nationwide) in English, consult www.rejseplanen.dk.

The Story of Copenhagen

If you study your map carefully, you can read the history of Copenhagen in today's street plan. København (literally, "Merchants' Harbor") was born on the little island of Slotsholmen—today home of Christiansborg Palace—in 1167. What was Copenhagen's medieval moat is now a string of pleasant lakes and parks, including Tivoli Gardens. You can still make out some of the zigzag pattern of the moats and ramparts in the city's greenbelt.

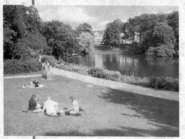

Many of these fortifications—and several other landmarks—were built by Denmark's most memorable king. You need to remember only one character in Copenhagen's history: Christian IV. Ruling from 1588 to 1648, he was Denmark's Renaissance king and a royal party animal (see the "King Christian IV" sidebar on page 197). The personal energy of this "Builder King" sparked a Golden Age when Copenhagen prospered and many of the city's grandest buildings were erected. In the 17th century, Christian IV extended the city fortifications to the north, doubling the size of the city, while adding a grid plan of streets and his Rosenborg Castle. This "new town" was the district around the Amalienborg Palace.

In 1850, Copenhagen's 140,000 residents all lived within this defensive system. Building in the no-man's-land outside the walls was only allowed with the understanding that in the event of an attack, you'd burn your dwellings to clear the way for a good defense.

Most of the city's historic buildings still in existence were built within the medieval walls, but conditions became too crowded, and outbreaks of disease forced Copenhagen to spread outside the walls. Ultimately those walls were torn down and replaced with "rampart streets" that define today's city center: Vestervoldgade (literally, "West Rampart Street"), Nørrevoldgade ("North"), and Østervoldgade ("East"). The fourth side is the harbor and the island of Slotsholmen, where København was born.

Tickets: The same tickets are used throughout the system. A 24-kr, **two-zone ticket** gets you an hour's travel within the center—pay as you board buses, or buy from station ticket offices, convenience stores, or vending machines for the Metro. (Ticket machines may not accept American credit cards, but I was able to use an American debit card with a PIN, and most machines also take Danish cash; if you want to use your credit card and the machine won't take it, find a cashier.) Assume you'll be within the

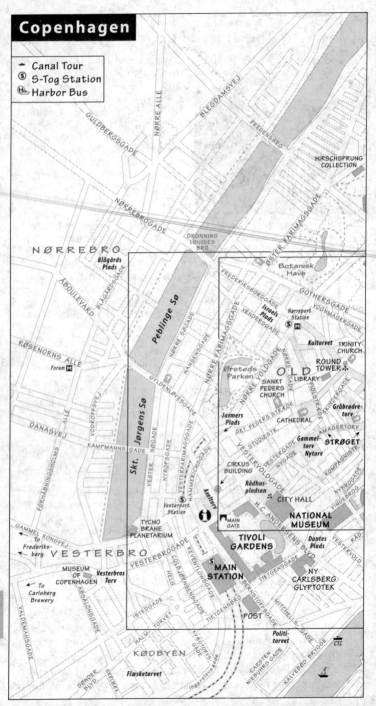

Copenhagen

- Canal Tour
- S-Tog Station
- Harbor Bus

NØRREBRO

VESTERBRO

KØDBYEN

COPENHAGEN

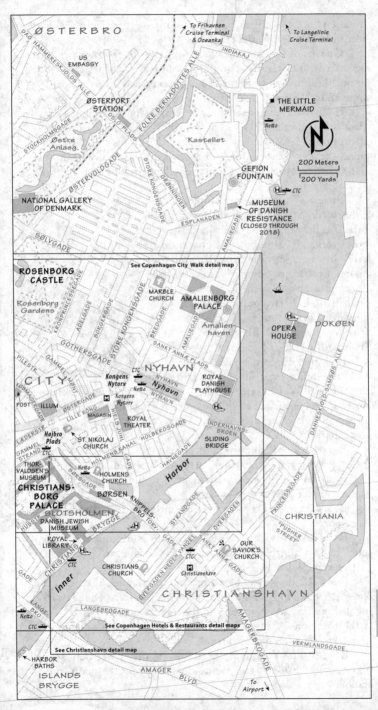

ØSTERBRO

DAG HAMMERESKJOLDS ALLE

US EMBASSY

ØSTERPORT STATION

Østre Anlaeg

STOCKHOLMSGADE

To Frihavnen Cruise Terminal & Oceankaj

To Langelinie Cruise Terminal

INDIAKAJ

OSLO PLADS

FOLKE BERNADOTTES ALLE

Kastellet

THE LITTLE MERMAID

Netto

200 Meters
200 Yards

ØSTERVOLDGADE

STORE KONGENSGADE

GRØNNINGEN

ESPLANADEN

GEFION FOUNTAIN

CTC

NATIONAL GALLERY OF DENMARK

SØLVGADE

AMALIEGADE

MUSEUM OF DANISH RESISTANCE (CLOSED THROUGH 2018)

See Copenhagen City Walk detail map

ROSENBORG CASTLE

Rosenborg Gardens

KRONPRINSESSEGADE

ADELGADE

BORGERGADE

STORE KONGENSGADE

GOTHERSGADE

PILESTR

GAMMEL MØNT

KØBMAGERGADE

MARBLE CHURCH

PPEGADE

AMALIEGADE

AMALIENBORG PALACE

Amalien-haven

SANKT ANNÆ PLADS

DOKØEN

OPERA HOUSE

CITY

Kongens Nytorv

NYHAVN

CTC

NYHAVN

Netto

Kongens Nytorv

Nyhavn

NYHAVN

ROYAL DANISH PLAYHOUSE

DANNESKJOLD-SAMSØS ALLE

POST

ILLUM

ØSTERGADE

NIELS JUELS

LILLE KONG

MAGASIN

ROYAL THEATER

HOLBERGSGADE

INDERHAVNS-BROEN

LÆDERSTR

Højbro Plads

CTC

ST. NIKOLAJ CHURCH

HOLMENS KANAL

Harbor

HAVNEGADE

SLIDING BRIDGE

GAMMEL STRAND

THOR-VALDSEN'S MUSEUM

Netto

BRGADE

HOLMENS CHURCH

CHRISTIANS-BORG PALACE

BØRSEN

KNIPPELS BRO TORV

STRANDGADE

OVERGADEN

PRINSESSEGADE

CHRISTIANIA

"PUSHER STREET"

SLOTSHOLMEN

HUSET

DANISH JEWISH MUSEUM

ROYAL LIBRARY

CHRISTIANS GADE

CTC

Inner

OVERGADEN NEDEN VANDET

SANKT ANNÆ GADE

CTC

OUR SAVIOR'S CHURCH

CHRISTIANS CHURCH

Christianehavn

CHRISTIANSHAVN

AMAGERBROGADE

LANGE BRO

Netto

CTC

LANGEBROGADE

See Copenhagen Hotels & Restaurants detail maps

See Christianhavn detail map

VERMLANDSGADE

HARBOR BATHS

ISLANDS BRYGGE

AMAGER BLVD.

To Airport

COPENHAGEN

middle two zones unless traveling to or from the airport, which requires a **three-zone ticket** (36 kr).

One handy option is the blue, two-zone *klippekort,* which can be shared—for example, two people can take five rides each (150 kr for 10 rides, insert it in the validation box each time you board a train and it'll snip off one of your rides).

If you're traveling exclusively in central Copenhagen, the **City Pass** is a good value (80 kr/24 hours, 200 kr/72 hours, covers travel within zones 1-4, including the airport). All passes are sold at stations, the TI, 7-Elevens, and other kiosks. Validate any all-day or multiday ticket by stamping it in the yellow machine on the bus or at the station.

Buses: While the train system is slick (Metro and S-tog, described later), its usefulness is limited for the typical tourist—but buses serve all of the major sights in town every five to eight minutes during daytime hours. If you're not riding a bike everywhere, get comfortable with the buses. Bus drivers are patient, have change, and speak English. City maps list bus routes. Locals are usually friendly and helpful. There's also a floating "Harbor Bus" (described next).

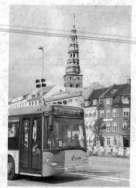

Bus lines that end with "A" (such as #1A) use quiet, eco-friendly, electric buses that are smaller than normal buses, allowing access into the narrower streets of the old town. Designed for tourists, these provide an easy overview to the city center. Among these, the following are particularly useful:

Bus **#1A** loops from the train station up to Kongens Nytorv (near Nyhavn) and then farther north, to Østerport.

Bus **#2A** goes from Christianshavn to the city center, then onward to points west.

Bus **#5A** connects the station more or less directly to Nørreport.

Bus **#6A** also connects the station to Nørreport, but on a much more roundabout route that twists through the central core (with several sightseeing-handy stops).

Bus **#11A** does a big loop from the train station through the core of town up to Nørreport, then down to Nyhavn before retracing its steps back via Nørreport to the train station.

Other non-"A" buses, which are bigger and tend to be more direct, can be faster for some trips:

Bus **#14** runs from Nørreport down to the city center, stopping near the Strøget, and eventually going near the main train station.

Bus **#26** runs a handy route right through the main tourist zone: train station/Tivoli to Slotsholmen Island to Kongens Nytorv (near Nyhavn) to the Amalienborg Palace/*Little Mermaid* area. It continues even farther north to the city's three main cruise ports, but the line splits, so check with the driver to make sure you're on the right bus (see sidebar on page 151 for details).

Bus **#66** goes from Nyhavn to Slotsholmen Island to Tivoli.

Metro: Copenhagen's Metro line, while simple, is super-futuristic and growing. For most tourists' purposes, only the airport and three consecutive stops within the city matter: Nørreport (connected every few minutes by the S-tog to the main train station), Kongens Nytorv (near Nyhavn and the Strøget's north end), and Christianshavn.

The city is busy at work on the new Cityringen (City Circle) Metro line. When it opens in 2018, the Metro will instantly become far handier for tourists—linking the train station, Rådhuspladsen, Gammel Strand (near Slotsholmen Island), and Kongens Nytorv (near Nyhavn). In the meantime, expect to see massive construction zones at each of those locations. Eventually the Metro will also extend to Ørestad, the industrial and business center created after the Øresund Bridge was built between Denmark and Sweden (for the latest on the Metro, see www.m.dk).

S-tog Train: The S-tog is basically a commuter line that links stations on the main train line through Copenhagen; for cruisers, the most important stops are the main train station, Nørreport (where it ties into the Metro system), Østerport (for Langelinie), and Nordhavn (for the Frihavnen port).

By Boat

The hop-on, hop-off "Harbor Bus" (Havnebus) boat stops at the "Black Diamond" library, Christianshavn (near Knippels Bridge), Nyhavn, the Opera House, and Nordre Toldbod, which is a short walk from *The Little Mermaid* site (and a slightly longer walk from the Langelinie cruise pier). The boat is part of the city bus system (lines #991 and #992) and is covered by the tickets described earlier. Taking a long ride on this boat—from the library to the end of the line—is the "poor man's cruise," without commentary, of course (runs 6:00-19:00). Or, for a true sightseeing trip, consider a guided harbor cruise (described later, under "Tours in Copenhagen").

By Taxi

Taxis are plentiful, easy to call or flag down, and pricey (35-kr pickup charge and then 15 kr/kilometer). For a short ride, four people spend about the same by taxi as by bus. Calling 35 35 35 35 will get you a taxi within minutes...with the meter already well on its way.

By Bike

Cyclists see more, save time and money, and really feel like locals. With a bike, you have Copenhagen at your command. I'd rather have a bike than a car and driver at my disposal. Virtually every street has a dedicated bike lane (complete with bike signal lights). Warning: Police routinely issue 500-kr tickets to anyone riding on sidewalks or through pedestrian zones. Note also that bikes can't be parked just anywhere. Observe others and park your bike among other bikes. The simple built-in lock that binds the back tire is adequate.

Renting a Bike: Consider one of these rental outfits in or near the city center (see map on page 158 for locations):

• **Københavns Cyklebørs,** near Nørreport Station, has a good selection of three-gear bikes (75 kr/1 day, 140 kr/2 days, 200 kr/3 days, 350 kr/week; Mon-Fri 9:00-17:30, Sat-Sun 10:00-14:00 & 18:00-20:00, closed Sat evening and all day Sun in off-season; Gothersgade 157, tel. 33 14 07 17, www.cykelborsen.dk).

• **Cykelbasen,** even closer to Nørreport, rents three- and seven-gear bikes (80 kr/day, 400 kr/week, includes lock; Mon-Fri 9:00-17:30, Sat 9:00-14:30, closed Sun; Gothersgade 137, tel. 22 18 06 42, www.cykel-basen.dk, click on "Info").

• **Copenhagen Bicycles,** at the entrance to Nyhavn by the Inderhavnsbroen pedestrian/bicycle bridge, rents basic three-gear bikes (70 kr/3 hours, 80 kr/6 hours, 110 kr/24 hours, includes lock, helmet–40 kr, daily 8:30-17:30, Nyhavn 44, tel. 33 93 04 04, www.copenhagenbicycles.dk). They also offer guided tours in English and Danish (100 kr, mid-April-Sept daily at 11:00, 2.5-3 hours).

Using City Bikes: The city's public bike-rental program, called **Bycyklen,** lets you ride shiny-white, three-gear "smart bikes" (with built-in GPS and an electric motor, should you need a boost) for 25 kr/hour. You'll find them parked in racks near

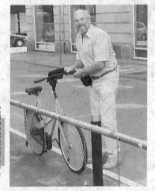

the train station, on either side of City Hall, and at many other locations around town. Use the touch-screen on the handlebars to create an account, enter your credit card info, and off you go (but be sure to return the bike to a Bycyklen docking station or face a 200-kr fine). At their website (http://bycyklen.dk), you can locate docking stations, reserve a bike at a specific station, and create an account in advance. I'd use the bikes for a one-way pedal here or there, but for more than a couple of hours, it's more cost-efficient to rent a regular bicycle.

Tours in Copenhagen

ON FOOT
Copenhagen is an ideal city to get to know by foot. You have several good options:

▲▲Hans Christian Andersen Tours by Richard Karpen
Once upon a time, American Richard Karpen visited Copenhagen and fell in love with the city. Now, 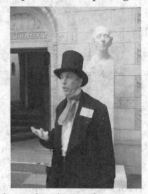 dressed as Hans Christian Andersen in a 19th-century top hat and long coat, he leads 1.5-hour tours that wander in and out of buildings, courtyards, back streets, and unusual parts of the old town. Along the one-mile route, he gives insightful and humorous background on the history, culture, and contemporary life of Denmark, Copenhagen, and the Danes (100 kr, kids under 12 free; departs from the TI, up the street from the main train station at Vesterbrogade 4A—at the corner with Bernstorffsgade; mid-May-mid-Sept Mon-Sat at 9:30, none on Sun; Richard departs promptly—if you miss him, try to catch up with the tour at the next stop on Rådhuspladsen).

Richard also gives excellent one-hour tours of **Rosenborg Castle,** playing the role of a dapper Renaissance "Sir Richard" (90 kr, doesn't include castle entry, mid-May-mid-Sept Mon and Thu at 12:00, meet outside castle ticket office). No reservations are needed for any of Richard's scheduled tours—just show up.

You can also hire Richard for private tours of the city or of Rosenborg Castle (1,000 kr/1.5 hours, June-Aug, mobile 91 61 95 02, www.copenhagenwalks.com, copenhagenwalks@yahoo.com).

▲Daily City Walks by Red Badge Guides
Five local female guides work together, giving two-hour English-language city tours. Their walks mix the city's highlights, back lanes, history, and contemporary social issues, and finish at Amalienborg Palace at noon for the changing of the guard (100 kr, daily mid-April-Sept at 10:00, departs from TI, just show up, pay direct, no minimum, tel. 20 92 23 87, www.redbadgeguides.dk, redbadgeguides@gmail.com). They also offer private guided tours upon request.

▲▲Copenhagen History Tours
Christian Donatzky, a charming young Dane with a master's degree in history, runs a walking tour on Saturday mornings.

Hans Christian Andersen (1805-1875)

The author of such classic fairy tales as *The Ugly Duckling* was an ugly duckling himself—a misfit who blossomed. Hans Christian

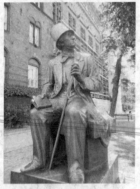

Andersen (called H. C., pronounced "hoe see" by the Danes) was born to a poor shoemaker in Odense. As a child he was gangly, high-strung, and effeminate. He avoided school because the kids laughed at him, so he spent his time in a fantasy world of books and plays. When his father died, the 11-year-old was on his own, forced into manual labor. He loved playing with a marionette theater that his father had made for him, sparking a lifelong love affair with the theater. In 1819, at the age of 14, he moved to Copenhagen to pursue an acting career and worked as a boy soprano for the Royal Theater. When his voice changed, the director encouraged him to return to school. He dutifully attended—a teenager among boys—and eventually went on to the university. As rejections piled up for his acting aspirations, Andersen began to shift his theatrical ambitions to playwriting.

After graduation, Andersen won a two-year scholarship to travel around Europe, the first of many trips he'd make and write about. His experiences abroad were highly formative, providing inspiration for many of his tales. Still in his 20s, he published an (obviously autobiographical) novel, *The Improvisatore*, about a poor young man who comes into his own while traveling in Italy. The novel launched his writing career, and soon he was hobnobbing with the international crowd—Charles Dickens, Victor Hugo, Franz Liszt, Richard Wagner, Henrik Ibsen, and Edvard Grieg.

In April and May, the theme is "Reformed Copenhagen" (covering the period from 1400 to 1600); in June and July, "King's Copenhagen" (1600-1800); and in August and September, "Hans Christian Andersen's Copenhagen" (1800-present). Those with a serious interest in Danish history will find these tours time well spent (80 kr, Sat at 10:00, approximately 1.5 hours, small groups of 5-15 people, tours depart from statue of Bishop Absalon on Højbro Plads between the Strøget and Christiansborg Palace, English only, no reservations necessary—just show up, tel. 28 49 44 35, www.historytours.dk, info@historytours.dk).

BY BOAT

For many, the best way to experience the city's canals and harbor is by canal boat. Two companies offer essentially the same live,

Despite his many famous friends, Andersen remained a lonely soul who never married. He had very close male friendships and journaled about unrequited love affairs with several women, including the famous opera star of the day, Jenny Lind, the "Swedish Nightingale." Without a family of his own, he became very close with the children of his friends—and, through his fairy tales, with a vast extended family of kids around the world.

Though he wrote novels, plays, and travel literature, it was his fairy tales, including *The Ugly Duckling, The Emperor's New Clothes, The Princess and the Pea, The Little Mermaid, The Snow Queen*, and *The Red Shoes*, that made him famous in Denmark and abroad. They made him Denmark's best-known author, the "Danish Charles Dickens." Some stories are based on earlier folk tales, and others came straight from his inventive mind, all written in an informal, conversational style that was considered unusual and even surprising at the time.

Andersen's compelling tales appeal to children and adults alike. They're full of magic and touch on strong, universal emotions—the pain of being different, the joy of self-discovery, and the struggle to fit in. The ugly duckling, for example, is teased by his fellow ducks before he finally discovers his true identity as a beautiful swan. In *The Emperor's New Clothes,* a boy is derided by everyone for speaking the simple, self-evident truth that the emperor is fooling himself. J. K. Rowling recently said, "The indelible characters he created are so deeply implanted in our subconscious that we sometimes forget that we were not born with the stories." (For more on Andersen's famous story *The Little Mermaid*—and what it might tell us about his life—see page 182.)

By the time of his death, the poor shoemaker's son was wealthy, cultured, and had been knighted. His rise through traditional class barriers mirrors the social progress of the 19th century.

three-language, one-hour cruises. Both boats leave at least twice an hour from Nyhavn and Christiansborg Palace, cruise around the palace and Christianshavn area, and then proceed into the wide-open harbor. Best on a sunny day, it's a relaxing way to see *The Little Mermaid* and munch on a lazy picnic during the slow-moving narration.

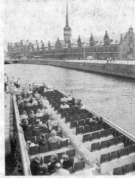

▲Netto-Bådene

These inexpensive cruises cost about half the price of their rival, Canal Tours Copenhagen. Go with Netto; there's no reason to pay nearly double (40 kr, mid-March-mid-Oct daily 10:00-17:00, runs later in summer, shorter hours in winter, sign at dock shows next departure, generally every 30 minutes, dress warmly—boats are open-top until Sept, tel. 32 54 41 02, www.havnerundfart.dk). Netto boats often make two stops where passengers can get off, then hop back on a later boat—at the bridge near *The Little Mermaid*, and at the Langebro bridge near Danhostel. Not every boat makes these stops; check the clock on the bridges for the next departure time.

Don't confuse the cheaper Netto and pricier Canal Tours Copenhagen boats: At Nyhavn, the Netto dock is midway down the canal (on the city side), while the Canal Tours Copenhagen dock is at the head of the canal. Near Christiansborg Palace, the Netto boats leave from Holmen's Bridge in front of the palace, while Canal Tours Copenhagen boats depart from Gammel Strand, 200 yards away. Boats leaving from Christiansborg are generally less crowded than those leaving from Nyhavn.

Canal Tours Copenhagen

This more expensive option does the same cruise as Netto for 75 kr (daily March-late Oct 9:30-18:00, runs later in summer, shorter hours in winter, no tours Jan-Feb, boats are sometimes covered if it's raining, tel. 32 96 30 00, www.stromma.dk).

In summer, Canal Tours Copenhagen also runs audioguided hop-on, hop-off **"water bus"** tours (95 kr/24 hours, daily late May-mid-Sept 9:30-19:00).

BY BUS
Hop-on, Hop-off Bus Tours

Several buses with recorded narration circle the city for a basic 1.25- to 1.5-hour orientation, allowing you to get on and off as you like at the following stops: Tivoli Gardens, Gammel Strand near Christiansborg Palace, *The Little Mermaid*, Rosenborg Castle, Nyhavn sailors' quarter, and more. Cruise passengers arriving at Langelinie can catch a hop-on, hop-off bus there; those arriving at other ports can take their cruise shuttle to *The Little Mermaid*, where you can pick up a hop-on, hop-off bus.

The same company runs **City Sightseeing**'s red buses and **Open Top Tours**' green buses. Both offer a Mermaid route for 175 kr and Carlsberg Brewery and Christiania routes for 195 kr (tickets good for 24 hours, pay driver, 2/hour, May-mid-Sept daily 9:30-18:00, shorter hours off-season, buses depart near the TI at the Radisson Blu Royal Hotel and at many other stops throughout city, tel. 25 55 66 88, www.city-sightseeing.dk). Open Top Tours also offers a 225-kr ticket that includes all tour routes and a cruise on their hop-on, hop-off canal boat.

Another operation—called **Red Blue Bus Tours**—does

a similar route but runs a little less frequently (every 45 minutes in summer, hourly in winter; 190 kr/1 day, 230 kr/2 days, www.sightseeing-cph.dk).

BY BIKE
▲Bike Copenhagen with Mike

Mike Sommerville offers three-hour guided bike tours of the city. A Copenhagen native, Mike enjoys showing off his city to visitors, offering both historic background and contemporary cultural insights along the way (April-Sept daily at 10:00, second departure Wed and Sat at 14:00; 300 kr includes bike rental, price same with or without a bike, 50-kr discount with this book—maximum 2 discounts per book and must have book with you, cash only). All tours are in English and depart from his bike shop at Sankt Peders Straede 47, in the Latin Quarter (see map on page 158). Mike also offers private tours; see the details at www.bikecopenhagenwithmike.dk.

Copenhagen City Walk

This self-guided walk takes about two hours. It starts at Rådhuspladsen (City Hall Square) and heads along the pedestrian street, the Strøget, through the old city, onto "Castle Island" (home of Christiansborg Palace), along the harbor promenade, and through Nyhavn, the sailors' quarter with the city's iconic canalfront houses. The walk officially ends at Kongens Nytorv ("King's New Square"), though you can continue another 10 minutes to Amalienborg Palace and then another 15 minutes beyond that to *The Little Mermaid*.

❶ Rådhuspladsen

Start from Rådhuspladsen (City Hall Square), the bustling heart of Copenhagen, dominated by the tower of the City Hall. Today

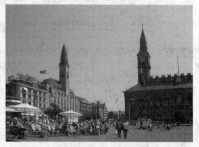

this square always seems to be hosting some lively community event, but it was once Copenhagen's fortified west end. For 700 years, Copenhagen was contained within its city walls. By the mid-1800s, 140,000 people were packed inside. The overcrowding led to hygiene problems. (A cholera outbreak killed 5,000.) It was clear: The walls needed to come down...and they did. Those formidable town walls survive today only in echoes—a circular series of roads and the

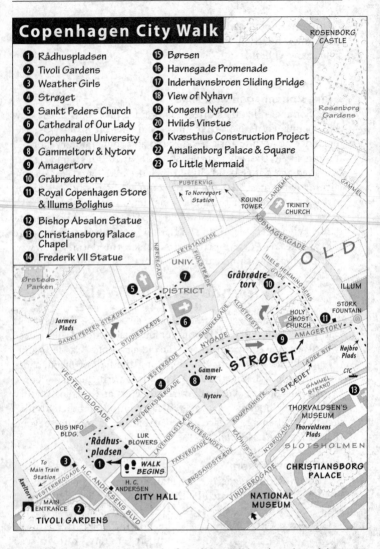

Copenhagen City Walk

1. Rådhuspladsen
2. Tivoli Gardens
3. Weather Girls
4. Strøget
5. Sankt Peders Church
6. Cathedral of Our Lady
7. Copenhagen University
8. Gammeltorv & Nytorv
9. Amagertorv
10. Gråbrødretorv
11. Royal Copenhagen Store & Illums Bolighus
12. Bishop Absalon Statue
13. Christiansborg Palace Chapel
14. Frederik VII Statue
15. Børsen
16. Havnegade Promenade
17. Inderhavnsbroen Sliding Bridge
18. View of Nyhavn
19. Kongens Nytorv
20. Hviids Vinstue
21. Kvæsthus Construction Project
22. Amalienborg Palace & Square
23. To Little Mermaid

remnants of moats, now people-friendly city lakes (see the sidebar on page 157).

• *Stand 50 yards in front of City Hall and turn clockwise for a...*

Rådhuspladsen Spin-Tour: The **City Hall**, or Rådhus, is worth a visit (described on page 185). Old **Hans Christian Andersen** sits to the right of City Hall, almost begging to be in another photo (as he used to in real life). Climb onto his well-worn knee. (While up there, you might take off your shirt for a racy photo, as many Danes enjoy doing.)

He's looking at **2 Tivoli Gardens** (across the street), which

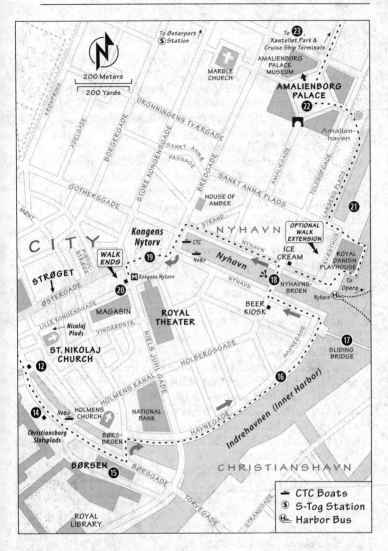

he loved and which inspired him when writing some of his stories. Tivoli Gardens was founded in 1843, when magazine publisher Georg Carstensen convinced the king to let him build a pleasure garden outside the walls of crowded Copenhagen. The king quickly agreed, knowing that happy people care less about fighting for democracy. Tivoli became Europe's first great public amusement park. When the train lines came, the station was placed just beyond Tivoli.

The big, glassy building with the *DI* sign is filled with the offices of Danish Industry—a collection of Danish companies whose logos you can see in the windows (plus the Irma grocery store at street level).

The big, broad boulevard is **Vesterbrogade** ("Western Way"), which led to the western gate of the medieval city (behind you, where the pedestrian boulevard begins). Here, in the traffic hub of this huge city, you'll notice...not many cars. Denmark's 180 percent tax on car purchases makes the bus, Metro, or bike a sweeter option. In fact, the construction messing up this square is part of a huge expansion of the Metro system.

Down Vesterbrogade towers the **Radisson Blu Royal Hotel** (formerly the SAS building), Copenhagen's only skyscraper. Locals say it seems so tall because the clouds hang so low. When it was built in 1960, Copenhageners took one look and decided—that's enough of a skyline. Notice there are no other buildings taller than the five-story limit in the old center.

The golden ❸ **weather girls** (on the corner, high above Vesterbrogade) indicate the weather: on a bike (fair weather) or with an umbrella. These two have been called the only women in Copenhagen you can trust, but for years they've been stuck in the almost-sunny mode...with the bike just peeking out. Notice that the red temperature dots max out at 28° Celsius (that's 82° Fahrenheit...a good memory aid: transpose 28 to get 82).

To the right, just down the street, is the Tiger Store (a popular local "dollar store"...nearly everything is under 50 kr). The next street (once the local Fleet Street, with the big newspapers) still has the offices for *Politiken* (the leading Danish newspaper) and the best bookstore in town, Boghallen.

As you spin farther right, three fast-food joints stand at the entry to the Strøget (STROY-et), Copenhagen's grand pedestrian boulevard—where we're heading next. Just beyond that and the Art Deco-style Palace Hotel (with a tower to serve as a sister to the City Hall) is the *Lur Blowers* **sculpture,** which honors the earliest warrior Danes. The *lur* is a curvy, trombone-sounding horn that was used to call soldiers to battle or to accompany pagan religious processions. The earliest bronze *lurs* date as far back as 3,500 years ago. Later, the Vikings used a wood version of the *lur*. The ancient originals, which still play, are displayed in the National Museum.

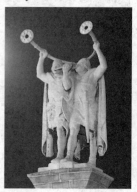

• *Now head down the pedestrian boulevard (pickpocket alert).*

❹ The Strøget

The American trio of Burger King, 7-Eleven, and KFC marks

the start of this otherwise charming pedestrian street. Finished in 1962, Copenhagen's experimental, tremendously successful, and much-copied pedestrian shopping mall is a string of lively (and individually named) streets and lovely squares that bunny-hop through the old town from City Hall to the Nyhavn quarter, a 20-minute stroll away. Though the Strøget has become hamburgerized, historic bits and attractive pieces of old Copenhagen are just off this commercial can-can.

As you wander down this street, remember that the commercial focus of a historic street like the Strøget drives up the land value, which generally trashes the charm and tears down the old buildings. Look above the modern window displays and street-level advertising to discover bits of 19th-century character that still survive. This end of the Strøget is young and cheap, while the far end has the high-end designer shops. Along the way, wonderfully quiet and laid-back areas are just a block or two away on either side.

After one block (at Kattesundet), make a side-trip three blocks left into Copenhagen's colorful **university district.** Formerly the old brothel neighborhood, later the heart of Copenhagen's hippie community in the 1960s, today this "Latin Quarter" is SoHo chic. Enjoy the colorful string of artsy shops and cafés. Because the old town was densely populated and built of wood, very little survived its many fires. After half-timbered and thatched buildings kept burning down, the city finally mandated that new construction be made of stone. But because stone was so expensive, many people built half-timbered structures, then disguised their facades with stucco, which made them look like stone. Exposed half-timbered structures are seen in courtyards and from the back sides. At Sankt Peders Stræde, turn right and walk to the end of the street. Notice the old guild signs (a baker, a key maker, and so on) identifying the original businesses here.

Along the way, look for large mansions that once circled expansive **courtyards.** As the population grew, the city walls constricted Copenhagen's physical size. The courtyards were gradually filled with higgledy-piggledy secondary buildings. Today, throughout the old center, you can step off a busy pedestrian mall and back in time in these characteristic, half-timbered, time-warp courtyards. Replace the parked car with a tired horse and the bikes with a line of outhouses, and you're in 19th-century Copenhagen. If you see an open courtyard door, you're welcome to discreetly wander in and look around.

You'll also pass funky shops and the big brick ❺ **Sankt Peders Church**—the old German merchant community's church, which still holds services in German. Its fine 17th-century brick grave chapel (filling a ground-floor building out back due to the boggy nature of the soil) is filled with fancy German tombs (25 kr to enter).

• *When Sankt Peders Stræde intersects with Nørregade, look right to find the big, Neoclassical...*

❻ Cathedral of Our Lady (Vor Frue Kirche)

The obelisk-like **Reformation Memorial** across the street from the cathedral celebrates Denmark's break from the Roman Catholic

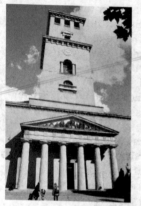

Church to become Lutheran in 1536. Walk around and study the reliefs of great Danish reformers protesting from their pulpits. The relief facing the church shows King Christian III presiding over the pivotal town council meeting when they decided to break away from Rome. As a young man, Prince Christian had traveled to Germany, where he was influenced by Martin Luther. He returned to take the Danish throne by force, despite Catholic opposition. Realizing the advantages of being the head of his own state church, Christian confiscated church property and established the state Lutheran Church. King Christian was crowned inside this cathedral. Because of the reforms of 1536, there's no Mary in the Cathedral of Our Lady. The other reliefs show the popular religious uprising, with people taking control of the word of God by translating the Bible from Latin into their own language.

Like much of this part of town, the church burned down in the British bombardment of 1807 and was rebuilt in the Neoclassical style. The cathedral's **facade** looks like a Greek temple. (Two blocks to the right, in the distance, notice more Neoclassicism—the law courts.) You can see why Golden Age Copenhagen (early 1800s) fancied itself a Nordic Athens. Old Testament figures (King David and Moses) flank the cathedral's entryway. Above, John the Baptist stands where you'd expect to see Greek gods. He invites you in...into the New Testament.

The **interior** is a world of Neoclassical serenity (free, open daily 8:00-17:00). It feels like a pagan temple that now houses Christianity. The nave is lined by the 12 apostles, clad in classical robes—masterpieces by the great Danish sculptor Bertel Thorvaldsen (see sidebar on page 193). Each strikes a meditative pose, carrying his identifying symbol: Peter with keys, Andrew with the X-shaped cross of his execution, Matthew and John writing their books, and so on. They lead to a statue of the *Risen Christ* (see photo), standing where the statue of Zeus would have

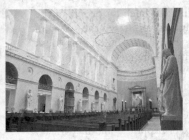

been: inside a temple-like niche, flanked by columns and topped with a pediment. Rather than wearing a royal robe, Jesus wears his burial shroud, opens his arms wide, and says, "Come to me." (Mormons will recognize this statue—a replica stands in the visitors' center at Salt Lake City's Temple Square and is often reproduced in church publications.) The marvelous acoustics are demonstrated in free organ concerts Saturdays in July and August at noon. Notice how, in good Protestant style, only the front half of the pews are "reversible," allowing the congregation to flip around and face the pulpit (in the middle of the church) to better hear the sermon.

• *Head back outside. If you face the church's facade and look to the left (across the square called Frue Plads), you'll see...*

❼ Copenhagen University

Now home to 30,000 students, this university was founded by the king in the 15th century to stop the Danish brain drain to Paris. Today tuition is free (but room, board, and beer are not). Locals

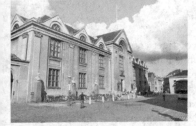

say it's easy to get in, but given the wonderful student lifestyle, very hard to get out.

Step up the middle steps of the university's big building; if the doors are open, enter a colorful lobby, starring Athena and Apollo. The frescoes celebrate high thinking, with themes such as the triumph of wisdom over barbarism. Notice how harmoniously the architecture, sculpture, and painting work together.

Outside, busts honor great minds from the faculty, including (at the end) Niels Bohr, a professor who won the 1922 Nobel Prize for theoretical physics. He evaded the clutches of the Nazi science labs by fleeing to America in 1943, where he helped develop the atomic bomb.

• *Rejoin the Strøget (one block downhill from the Reformation Memorial to the black-and-gold fountain) at the twin squares called...*

❽ Gammeltorv and Nytorv

This was the old town center. In Gammeltorv ("Old Square"), the Fountain of Charity (Caritas) is named for the figure of Charity on top. It has provided drinking water to locals since the early 1600s. Featuring a pregnant woman squirting water from her breasts next to a boy urinating, this was just too much for people of the Victorian Age. They corked both figures and raised the statue to what they hoped would be out of view. The exotic-looking kiosk was one of the city's first community telephone centers from the days before phones were privately owned. Look at the reliefs ringing its top: an airplane with bird wings (c. 1900) and two women talking on a newfangled telephonic device. (It was thought business would popularize the telephone, but actually it was women.)

While Gammeltorv was a place of happiness and merriment, Nytorv ("New Square") was a place of severity and judgment. Walk to the small raised area 20 yards in front of the old ancient-Greek-style former City Hall and courthouse. Do a 360. The square is Neoclassical (built mostly after the 1807 British bombardment). Read the old Danish on the City 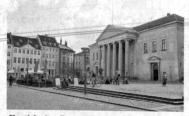 Hall facade: "With Law Shall Man Build the Land." Look down at the pavement and read the plaque: "Here stood the town's *Kag* (whipping post) until 1780."

• *Now walk down the next stretch of the Strøget—called Nygade—to reach...*

❾ Amagertorv

This is prime real estate for talented street entertainers. Walk to the stately brick Holy Ghost church (Helligåndskirken). The fine spire is typical of old Danish churches. Under the stepped gable was a medieval hospital run by monks (one of the oldest buildings in town, dating from the 12th century). Today the hospital is an antiques hall. In summer the pleasant courtyard is shared by a group of charities selling light bites and coffee.

Walk behind the church, down Valkendorfsgade—the street just before the church—and through a passage under the rust-colored building at #32 (if locked, loop back and go down Klosterstræde); here you'll find the leafy and beer-stained ❿ **Gråbrødretorv.** Surrounded by fine old buildings, this "Grey 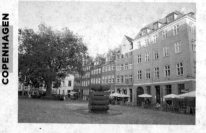 Friars' Square"—a monastic square until the Reformation made it a people's square—is a popular place for an outdoor meal or drink in the summer. At the end of the square, the street Niels Hemmingsens Gade returns to the Strøget.

Once back on busy Strøget, turn left and continue down Amagertorv, with its fine inlaid Italian granite stonework, to the next square with the "stork" fountain (actually three herons). The Victorian WCs here (free, steps down from fountain) are a delight.

This square, Amagertorv, is a highlight for shoppers, with the ⓫ **Royal Copenhagen store**—stacked with three floors of porcelain—and **Illums Bolighus**—a fine place to ogle modern Danish design (see "Shopping in Copenhagen," later). A block toward the canal—running parallel to the Strøget—starts Strædet, which is a "second Strøget" featuring cafés and antique shops.

North of Amagertorv, a broad pedestrian mall called **Købmagergade** leads past a fine modern bakery (Holm's Bager) to Christian IV's Round Tower and the Latin Quarter (university district). The recommended Café Norden overlooks the fountain—a good place for a meal or coffee with a view. The second floor offers the best vantage point.

• *Looking downhill from the fountain, about halfway to an imposing palace in the distance, you'll see a great man on a horse. Walk here to view this statue of Copenhagen's founder,* ⓬ *Bishop Absalon, shown in his Warrior Absalon get-up.*

From the bishop, you'll continue across a bridge toward the palace and the next statue—a king on a horse. As you cross the bridge, look right to see the City Hall tower, where this walk started. (A couple of the city's competing sightseeing boat tours depart from near here—see page 164.)

Christiansborg Palace and the Birthplace of Copenhagen

You're stepping onto the island of Slotsholmen (or Castle Island), the easy-to-defend birthplace of Copenhagen in the 12th century. It's dominated by the royal palace complex. Christiansborg Palace (with its "three crowns" spire)—the imposing former residence of kings—is now the Parliament building.

Ahead of you, the Neoclassical Lutheran church with the low dome is the ⓭ **Christiansborg Palace Chapel,** site of 350 years of royal weddings and funerals (free, only open Sun 10:00-17:00).

Walk to the next green copper equestrian statue. ⓮ **Frederik VII** was crowned in 1848, just months before Denmark got its constitution on June 5, 1849. (Constitution Day is celebrated with typical Danish understatement—stores are closed and workers get the day off.) Frederik, who then ruled as a constitutional monarch, stands in front of **Christiansborg Palace,** which Denmark's royal family now shares with its people's assembly (queen's wing on right, Parliament on left; for information on visiting the palace, see page 190). This palace, the seat of Danish government today, is considered the birthplace of Copenhagen. It stands upon the ruins

Copenhagen at a Glance

▲▲▲**Tivoli Gardens** Copenhagen's classic amusement park, with rides, music, food, and other fun. **Hours:** Mid-April-late Sept daily 11:00-23:00, Fri-Sat until 24:00, also open daily 11:00-22:00 for a week in mid-Oct and mid-Nov-New Year's Day. See page 183.

▲▲▲**National Museum** History of Danish civilization with tourable 19th-century Victorian Apartment. **Hours:** Museum—Tue-Sun 10:00-17:00, closed Mon; Victorian Apartment—English tours June-Sept Sat at 14:00, Danish tours Sat-Sun at 11:00, 12:00, and 13:00 year-round. See page 187.

▲▲▲**Rosenborg Castle and Treasury** Renaissance castle of larger-than-life "warrior king" Christian IV. **Hours:** June-Aug daily 10:00-17:00; May and Sept-Oct daily 10:00-16:00; Nov-Dec Tue-Sun 11:00-14:00 (treasury until 16:00), closed Mon; Jan-April Tue-Sun 11:00-16:00, closed Mon. See page 196.

▲▲▲**Christiania** Colorful counterculture squatters' colony. **Hours:** Always open; guided tours at 15:00 (daily late June-Aug, only Sat-Sun rest of year). See page 205.

▲▲**Christiansborg Palace** Royal reception rooms with dazzling tapestries. **Hours:** Reception rooms, castle ruins, and stables open daily except closed Mon in Oct-April. Hours vary by sight: Reception rooms 9:00-17:00, ruins 10:00-17:00, stables 13:30-16:00 except 10:00-17:00 in July. See page 190.

▲▲**Thorvaldsen's Museum** Works of the Danish Neoclassical sculptor. **Hours:** Tue-Sun 10:00-17:00, closed Mon. See page 191.

▲**City Hall** Copenhagen's landmark, packed with Danish history and symbolism and topped with a tower. **Hours:** Mon-Fri 8:30-16:00, some Sat 10:00-13:00, closed Sun. See page 185.

of Absalon's 12th-century castle (literally under your feet). The big stones between the statue and the street were put in for security after the 2011 terror attacks in Norway (in which 77 people were murdered, most of them teens and young adults). While Danes strive to keep government accessible, security measures like this are today's reality.

This is Denmark's power island, with the Parliament, Supreme Court, Ministry of Finance (to the left), and ⓯ **Børsen**—the historic stock exchange (farther to the left, with the fanciful dragon's tail spire; not open to tourists). The eye-catching red-brick stock exchange was inspired by the Dutch Renaissance, like much of 17th-century Copenhagen. Built to promote the mercantile

▲**Ny Carlsberg Glyptotek** Scandinavia's top art gallery, featuring Egyptians, Greeks, Etruscans, French, and Danes. **Hours:** Tue-Sun 11:00-17:00, closed Mon. See page 186.

▲**Museum of Copenhagen** The story of Copenhagen, displayed in an old house. **Hours:** Daily 10:00-17:00. See page 190.

▲**Danish Jewish Museum** Exhibit tracing the 400-year history of Danish Jews, in a unique building by American architect Daniel Libeskind. **Hours:** June-Aug Tue-Sun 10:00-17:00; Sept-May Tue-Fri 13:00-16:00, Sat-Sun 12:00-17:00; closed Mon year-round. See page 194.

▲**Amalienborg Museum** Quick and intimate look at Denmark's royal family. **Hours:** May-Oct daily 10:00-16:00; Nov-April Tue-Sun 11:00-16:00, closed Mon. See page 195.

▲**Rosenborg Gardens** Park surrounding Rosenborg Castle, filled with statues and statuesque Danes. **Hours:** Always open. See page 202.

▲**National Gallery of Denmark** Good Danish and Modernist collections. **Hours:** Tue-Sun 10:00-17:00, Wed until 20:00, closed Mon. See page 202.

▲**Our Savior's Church** Spiral-spired church with bright Baroque interior. **Hours:** Church—daily 11:00-15:30 but may close for special services; tower—July-mid-Sept Mon-Sat 10:00-19:00, Sun 10:30-19:00; April-June and mid-Sept-Nov daily until 16:00, closed Dec-March and in bad weather. See page 204.

ambitions of Denmark in the 1600s, it was the "World Trade Center" of Scandinavia. The facade reads, "For the profitable use of buyer and seller." The dragon-tail spire with three crowns represents the Danish aspiration to rule a united Scandinavia—or at least be its commercial capital.

Notice Copenhagen's distinctive green copper spires all around you. Beyond the old stock exchange lies the island of **Christianshavn,** with its own distinct spire. It tops the Church of Our Savior and features an external spiral staircase winding to the top for an amazing view. While political power resided here on Slotsholmen, commercial power was in the merchant's district, Christianshavn (neighborhood and church described later, under

"Sights in Copenhagen"). The Børsen symbolically connected Christianshavn with the rest of the city, in an age when trade was a very big deal.

• *Walk along the old stock exchange toward Christianshavn, but turn left at the crosswalk with the signal before you reach the end of the building. After crossing the street, go over the canal and turn right to walk along the harborfront promenade, enjoying views of Christianshavn across the water to your right.*

⑯ Havnegade Promenade

The Havnegade promenade to Nyhavn is a delightful people zone with trampolines, harborview benches (a good place to stop, look across the water, and ponder the trendy apartments and old-warehouses-turned-modern-office-blocks), and an ice-cream-licking ambience. Stroll several blocks from here toward the new **⑰ Inderhavnsbroen sliding bridge** for pedestrians and bikes. This "Kissing Bridge" (it's called that because the two sliding, or retractable, sections "kiss" when they come together) is designed to link the town center with Christianshavn and to make the new Opera House (ahead on the right, across the water) more accessible to downtown. Walk until you hit the Nyhavn canal.

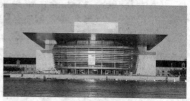

Across the way, at the end of Nyhavn canal, stands the glassy Royal Danish Theatre's Playhouse. While this walk finishes on Kongens Nytorv, the square at the head of this canal, you could extend it by continuing north along the harbor from the playhouse.

• *For now, turn left and walk to the center of the bridge over the canal for a...*

⑱ View of Nyhavn

Established in the 1670s along with Kongens Nytorv, Nyhavn ("New Harbor") is a recently gentrified sailors' quarter. (Hong Kong is the last of the nasty bars from the rough old days.) With its trendy cafés, jazz clubs, and tattoo shops (pop into Tattoo Ole at #17—fun photos, very traditional), Nyhavn is a wonderful place to hang out. The canal is filled with glamorous old sailboats of all sizes. Historic sloops are welcome to moor here in Copenhagen's ever-changing boat museum. Hans Christian Andersen lived and wrote his first stories here (in the red double-gabled building at #20).

From the bridge, take a few steps left to the cheap **beer kiosk** (on Holbergsgade, open daily until late). At this minimarket, let friendly manager Nagib give you a little lesson in Danish beer, and then buy a bottle or can. Choose from Carlsberg (standard

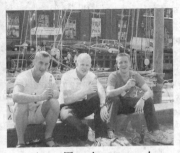

lager, 5 percent alcohol), Carlsberg Elephant (strong, 7.2 percent), Tuborg Grøn (standard lager, 4.6 percent), Tuborg Gold (stronger, 5.8 percent), and Tuborg Classic (dark beer, 4.6 percent). The cost? About 10-15 kr depending on the alcohol level. Take your beer out to the canal and feel like a local. A note about all the public beer-drinking here: There's no more beer consumption here than in the US; it's just out in public. Many young Danes can't afford to drink in a bar, so they "picnic drink" their beers in squares and along canals, at a quarter of the price for a bottle.

If you crave **ice cream** instead, cross the bridge, where you'll find a popular place with freshly made waffle cones facing the canal (Vaffelbageren).

Now wander the quay, enjoying the frat-party parade of tattoos (hotter weather reveals more tattoos). Celtic and Nordic mythological designs are in (as is bodybuilding, by the looks of things). The place thrives—with the cheap-beer drinkers dockside and the richer and older ones looking on from comfier cafés.

• *Make your way to the head of the canal, where you'll find a minuscule amber museum, above the House of Amber (see "Shopping in Copenhagen," page 210). Just beyond the head of Nyhavn canal sprawls the huge and stately King's New Square. Check it out.*

⑲ Kongens Nytorv

The "King's New Square" is home to the National Theater, French embassy, and venerable Hotel d'Angleterre, where VIPs and pop stars stay. In the mid-1600s the city expanded, pushing its wall farther east. The equestrian statue in the middle of the square celebrates Christian V, who made this square the city's geographical and cultural center. In 1676, King Christian rode off

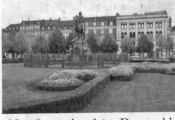

to reconquer the southern tip of Sweden and reclaim Denmark's dominance. He returned empty-handed and broke. Denmark became a second-rate power, but Copenhagen prospered. In the winter this square becomes a popular ice-skating rink.

Across the square on the left, small glass pyramids mark the Metro. The **Metro** that runs underground here features state-of-the-art technology (automated cars, no driver...sit in front to watch the tracks coming at you). As the cars come and go without drivers, compare this system to the public transit in your town.

Wander into ⓴ **Hviids Vinstue,** the town's oldest wine cellar (from 1723, just beyond the Metro station, at #19, under an Indian restaurant) to check out its characteristic interior and fascinating old Copenhagen photos. It's a colorful spot for an open-face sandwich and a beer (three sandwiches and a beer for 70 kr at lunchtime). Their wintertime *gløgg* (hot spiced wine) is legendary. Across the street, towering above the Metro station, is Magasin du Nord, the grandest old department store in town.

• *You've reached the end of this walk. But if you'd like to extend it by heading out to Amalienborg Palace and* The Little Mermaid, *retrace your steps to the far side of Nyhavn canal.*

Nyhavn to Amalienborg

Stroll along the canal to the Royal Danish Theatre's Playhouse and follow the harborfront promenade from there left through the big ㉑ **Kvæsthus construction project.** The Kvæsthus project's exhibition pavilion shows the vision for enhancing this waterfront area. You'll then stroll a delightful promenade to the modern fountain of Amaliehaven Park, immediately across the harbor from Copenhagen's slick Opera House. The Opera House is bigger than it looks—of its 14 floors, five are below sea level. Its striking design is controversial. Completed in 2005 by Henning Larsen, it was a $400 million gift to the nation from an oil-shipping magnate.

• *A block inland (behind the fountain) is the orderly...*

㉒ Amalienborg Palace and Square

Queen Margrethe II and her husband live in the mansion to your immediate left as you enter the square from the harborside. (If the flag's flying, she's home.) The mansion across the street (on the right as you enter) is where her son and heir to the throne, Crown Prince Frederik, lives with his wife, Australian busi-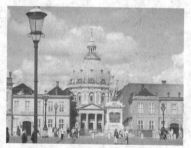nesswoman Mary Donaldson, and their four children. The royal guesthouse palace is on the far left. And the palace on the far right is the **Amalienborg Museum,** which offers an intimate look at royal living (described on page 195).

Though the guards change daily at noon, they do it with royal fanfare only when the queen is in residence (see page 195 for details). The royal guard often has a police escort when it marches through town on special occasions—leading locals to joke that theirs is "the only army in the world that needs police protection."

The equestrian statue of Frederik V is a reminder that this square was the centerpiece of a planned town he envisioned in 1750. It was named for him—Frederikstaden. During the 18th century, Denmark's population grew and the country thrived (as trade flourished and its neutrality kept it out of the costly wars impoverishing much of Europe). Frederikstaden, with its strong architectural harmony, was designed as a luxury neighborhood for the city's business elite. Nobility and other big shots moved in, but the king came here only after his other palace burned down in a 1794 fire.

Just inland, the striking Frederikskirke—better known as the **Marble Church**—was designed to fit this ritzy new quarter. If it's open, step inside to bask in its vast, serene, Pantheon-esque atmosphere (free, Mon-Thu 10:00-17:00, Fri-Sun 12:00-17:00).

• *From the square, Amaliegade leads two blocks north to...*

Kastellet Park

In this park, you'll find some worthwhile sightseeing. The 1908 **Gefion Fountain** illustrates the myth of the goddess who was

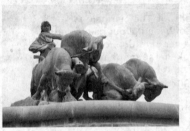

given one night to carve a hunk out of Sweden to make into Denmark's main island, Sjælland (or "Zealand" in English), which you're on. Gefion transformed her four sons into oxen to do the job, and the chunk she removed from Sweden is supposedly Vänern, Sweden's largest lake. If you look

at a map showing Sweden and Denmark, the island and the lake are, in fact, roughly the same shape. Next to the fountain is an Anglican church built of flint.

• *Climb up the stairs by the fountain and continue along the top of the rampart about five minutes to reach the harborfront site of the overrated, overfondled, and overphotographed symbol of Copenhagen,* Den Lille Havfrue, *or...*

㉓ *The Little Mermaid*

The Little Mermaid statue was a gift to the city of Copenhagen in 1909 from brewing magnate Carl Jacobsen (whose art collection forms the basis of the Ny Carlsberg Glyptotek). Inspired by a ballet performance of Andersen's story, Jacobsen hired the young sculptor Edvard Eriksen to immortalize the mermaid as a statue. Eriksen used his wife Eline as the model. The statue sat unappreciated for 40 years until Danny Kaye sang "Wonderful Copenhagen" in the movie *Hans Christian Andersen,* and the tourist board decided to use the mermaid as a marketing symbol for the

The Little Mermaid and Hans Christian Andersen

"Far out in the ocean, where the water is as blue as a corn-flower, as clear as crystal, and very, very deep..." there lived a young mermaid. So begins one of Hans Christian Andersen's best-known stories. The plot line starts much like the Disney movie, but it's spiced with poetic description and philosophical dialogue about the immortal soul.

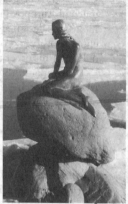

The mermaid's story goes like this: One day, a young mermaid spies a passing ship and falls in love with a handsome human prince. The ship is wrecked in a storm, and she saves the prince's life. To be with the prince, the mermaid asks a sea witch to give her human legs. In exchange, she agrees to give up her voice and the chance of ever returning to the sea. And, the witch tells her, if the prince doesn't marry her, she will immediately die heartbroken and without an immortal soul. The mermaid agrees, and her fish tail becomes a pair of beautiful but painful legs. She woos the prince—who loves her in return—but he eventually marries another. Heartbroken, the mermaid prepares to die. She's given one last chance to save herself: She must kill the prince on his wedding night. She sneaks into the bedchamber with a knife...but can't bear to kill the man she loves. The mermaid throws herself into the sea to die. Suddenly, she's miraculously carried up by the mermaids of the air, who give her an immortal soul as a reward for her long-suffering love.

The tale of unrequited love mirrors Andersen's own sad love life. He had two major crushes—one of them for the famous opera singer, Jenny Lind—but he was turned down both times, and he never married. He had plenty of interest in sex but likely died a virgin. He had close brotherly and motherly relations with women but stayed single, had time to travel and write, and maintained a child-like wonder about the world to his dying days.

city. For the non-Disneyfied *Little Mermaid* story—and insights into Hans Christian Andersen—see the sidebar. For more on his life, see page 164.

• *This is the end of our extended, wonderful "Copenhagen City Walk." From here you can get back downtown on foot, by taxi or on bus #1A from Store Kongensgade on the other side of Kastellet Park. You can also catch bus #26 (either downtown or back to your port) from farther north, along Folke Bernadottes Allé (confirm with driver that the bus you're getting on goes to your port; see page 151 for details). If your cruise ship is at Langelinie and you're ready to head back, you're just a short walk away.*

Sights in Copenhagen

NEAR THE TRAIN STATION

Copenhagen's great train station, the Hovedbanegården, is a fascinating mesh of Scandinavian culture and transportation efficiency. From the station, delightful sights fan out into the old city. The following attractions are listed roughly in order from the train station to Slotsholmen Island (except for the Museum of Copenhagen, which is several blocks from the station, in the opposite direction).

▲▲▲Tivoli Gardens

The world's grand old amusement park—since 1843—is 20 acres, 110,000 lanterns, and countless ice-cream cones of fun. You pay

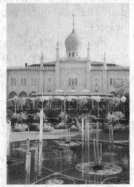

one admission price and find yourself lost in a Hans Christian Andersen wonderland of rides, restaurants, games, marching bands, roulette wheels, and funny mirrors. A roller coaster screams through the middle of a tranquil Asian food court, and the Small World-inspired Den Flyvende Kuffert ride floats through Hans Christian Andersen fairy tales. It's a children's fantasyland midday, but it becomes more adult-oriented later on. With or without kids, this place is a true magic kingdom. Tivoli doesn't try to be Disney. It's wonderfully and happily Danish. (Many locals appreciate the lovingly tended gardens.) I find it worth the admission just to see Danes—young and old—at play.

As you stroll the grounds, imagine the place in the mid-1800s, when it was new. Built on the site of the old town fortifications (today's lake was part of the old moat), Tivoli was an attempt to introduce provincial Danes to the world (for example, with the

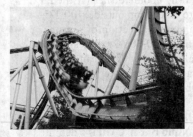

Asian Pavilion) and to bring people of all classes together.

Cost: 99 kr, free for kids under 8. To go on rides, you must buy ride tickets (from booth or machine, 25 kr/ticket, color-coded rides cost 1, 2, or 3 tickets apiece); or you can buy a multiride pass for 199 kr. If you'll be using at least eight tickets, buy the ride pass instead. To leave and come back later, you'll have to buy a 25-kr re-entry ticket before you exit. Tel. 33 15 10 01, www.tivoli.dk.

Hours: Mid-April-late Sept daily 11:00-23:00, Fri-Sat until 24:00. Dress warm for chilly evenings any time of year. There are lockers by each entrance.

Entertainment at Tivoli: If you're overnighting in Copenhagen before or after your cruise, Tivoli is a festive place to spend the evening. Upon arrival (through main entrance, on left in the service center), pick up a map and look for the events schedule. Take a moment to sit down and plan your entertainment for the evening. Events are generally spread between 15:00 and 23:00; the 19:30 concert in the concert hall can be as little as 50 kr or as much as 1,200 kr, depending on the performer (box office tel. 33 15 10 12). If the Tivoli Symphony is playing, it's worth paying for. The ticket box office is outside, just to the left of the main entrance (daily 10:00-20:00; if you buy a concert ticket you get into Tivoli for free).

Free concerts, pantomime theater, ballet, acrobats, puppets, and other shows pop up all over the park, and a well-organized visitor can enjoy an exciting evening of entertainment without spending a single krone beyond the entry fee. Friday evenings feature a (usually free) rock or pop show at 22:00. People gather around the lake 45 minutes before closing time for the "Tivoli Illuminations." Fireworks blast a few nights each summer. The park is particularly romantic at dusk, when the lights go on.

Eating at Tivoli: Inside the park, expect to pay amusement-park prices for amusement-park-quality food. Still, a meal here is part of the fun. **Søcafeen** serves only traditional open-face sandwiches in a fun beer garden with lakeside ambience. They allow picnics if you buy a drink (and will rent you plates and silverware for 10 kr/person). The *pølse* (sausage) stands are cheap, and a bagel sandwich place is in the amusements corner. **Færgekroen** offers a quiet, classy lakeside escape from the amusement-park intensity, with traditional dishes washed down by its own microbrew (200-300-kr hearty pub grub). **Wagamama,** a modern pan-Asian slurpathon from the UK, serves healthy noodle dishes (at the far back side of the park, also possible to enter from outside, 100-175-kr meals). **Nimb Terrasse** offers a simple selection of seasonal meat and fish dishes in a garden setting (200-300-kr dishes). **Café Georg,** to the left of the concert hall, has tasty 85-kr sandwiches and a lake view (also 100-kr salads and omelets). The kid-pleasing **Piratiriet** lets you dine on a pirate ship (150-180-kr main dishes).

For something more upscale, consider the complex of Nimb restaurants, in the big Taj Mahal-like pavilion near the entrance facing the train station. For dinner, **Nimb Bar 'n' Grill** is a definite splurge, with sophisticated 95-500-kr starters (such as veal tartare and caviar) and 220-600-kr meat dishes. **Nimb Brasserie,** sharing the same lobby, serves French classics (230-300-kr main dishes).

If it's chilly, you'll find plenty of **Mamma Mokka** coffee take-away stands. If you get a drink "to go," you'll pay an extra 5-kr deposit for the cup, which you can recoup by returning it to a machine (marked on maps).

▲City Hall (Rådhus)

This city landmark, between the train station/Tivoli and the Strøget, is free and open to the public (including a public WC). You can wander throughout the building and into the peaceful garden out back. It also offers private tours and trips up its 345-foot-tall tower.

Cost and Hours: Free to enter building, Mon-Fri 8:30-16:00; you can usually slip in Sat 10:00-13:00 when weddings are going on, or join the Sat tour; closed Sun. Guided English-language tours—30 kr, 45 minutes, gets you into more private, official rooms; Mon-Fri at 13:00, Sat at 10:00. Tower by escort only—20 kr, 300 steps for the best aerial view of Copenhagen, Mon-Fri at 11:00 and 14:00, Sat at 12:00, closed Sun. Tel. 33 66 33 66.

Visiting City Hall: It's draped, inside and out, in Danish

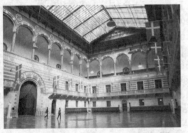

symbolism. The city's founder, Bishop Absalon, stands over the door. Absalon (c. 1128-1201)—bishop, soldier, and foreign-policy wonk—was King Valdemar I's right-hand man. In Copenhagen, he drove out pirates and built a fort to guard the harbor, turning a miserable fishing village into a humming Baltic seaport. The polar bears climbing on the rooftop symbolize the giant Danish protectorate of Greenland. Six night watchmen flank the city's gold-and-green seal under the Danish flag.

Step inside. The info desk (on the left as you enter) has racks of tourist information (city maps and other brochures). The building and its huge tower were inspired by the city hall in Siena, Italy (with the necessary bad-weather addition of a glass roof). Enormous functions fill this grand hall (the iron grate in the center of the floor is an elevator for bringing up 1,200 chairs), while the marble busts of four illustrious local boys—fairy-tale writer Hans Christian Andersen; sculptor Bertel Thorvaldsen; physicist Niels Bohr; and the building's architect, Martin Nyrop—look on. Underneath the floor are national archives dating back to 1275, popular with Danes researching their family roots.

As you leave, pop into the amazing clock opposite the info desk. Jens Olsen's World Clock, built from 1943 to 1955, was the mother of all astronomical clocks in precision and function. And it came with something new: tracking the exact time across the world's time zones. One of its gears does a complete rotation only every 25,753 years.

▲Ny Carlsberg Glyptotek

Scandinavia's top art gallery is an impressive example of what beer money can do. Brewer Carl Jacobsen (son of J. C. Jacobsen, who funded the Museum of National History at Frederiksborg Castle)

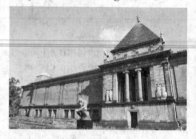

was an avid collector and patron of the arts. (Carl also donated *The Little Mermaid* statue to the city.) His namesake museum has intoxicating artifacts from the ancient world, along with some fine art from our own times. The next time you sip a Carlsberg beer, drink a toast to Carl Jacobsen and his marvelous collection. *Skål!*

Cost and Hours: 75 kr, free on Sun; open Tue-Sun 11:00-17:00, closed Mon; behind Tivoli at Dantes Plads 7, tel. 33 41 81 41, www.glyptoteket.com. It has a classy cafeteria under palms, as well as a rooftop terrace with snacks, drinks, and city views.

Visiting the Museum: Pick up a floor plan as you enter to help navigate the confusing layout. For a chronological swing, start with Egypt (mummy coffins and sarcophagi, a 5,000-year-old hippo statue), Greece (red-and-black painted vases, statues), the Etruscan world (Greek-looking vases), and Rome (grittily realistic statues and portrait busts).

The sober realism of 19th-century Danish Golden Age painting reflects the introspection of a once-powerful nation reduced to second-class status—and ultimately embracing what made them unique. The "French Wing" (just inside the front door) has Rodin statues. A heady, if small, exhibit of 19th-century French paintings (in a modern building within the back courtyard) shows how Realism morphed into Impressionism and Post-Impressionism, and includes a couple of canvases apiece by Géricault, Delacroix, Monet, Manet, Millet, Courbet, Degas, Pissarro, Cézanne, Van Gogh, Picasso, Renoir, and Toulouse-Lautrec. Look for art by Gauguin—from before Tahiti (when he lived in Copenhagen with his Danish wife and their five children) and after Tahiti. There's also a fine collection of modern (post-Thorvaldsen) Danish sculpture.

Linger with marble gods under the palm leaves and glass

dome of the very soothing winter garden. Designers, figuring Danes would be more interested in a lush garden than in classical art, used this wonderful space as leafy bait to cleverly introduce locals to a few Greek and Roman statues. (It works for tourists, too.) One of the original *Thinker* sculptures by Rodin (wondering how to scale the Tivoli fence?) is in the museum's backyard.

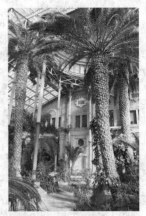

▲▲▲National Museum

Focus on this museum's excellent and curiously enjoyable Danish collection, which traces this civilization from its ancient beginnings. Its prehistoric collection is the best of its kind in Scandinavia. Exhibits are laid out chronologically and are eloquently described in English.

Cost and Hours: Free, Tue-Sun 10:00-17:00, closed Mon, mandatory lockers, enter at Ny Vestergade 10, tel. 33 13 44 11, www.natmus.dk. The café overlooking the entry hall serves coffee, pastries, and lunch (90-145 kr).

Visiting the Museum: Pick up the museum map as you enter, and head for the Danish history exhibit. It fills three floors, from the bottom up: prehistory, the Middle Ages and Renaissance, and modern times (1660-2000).

Danish Prehistory: Start before history did, in the Danish Prehistory exhibit (on the right side of the main entrance hall). Follow the room numbers in order, working counterclockwise around the courtyard and through the millennia.

In the Stone Age section, you'll see primitive tools and still-clothed skeletons of Scandinavia's reindeer hunters. The oak coffins were originally covered by burial mounds (called "barrows"). People put valuable items into the coffins with the dead, such as a folding chair (which, back then, was a real status symbol). In the farming section, ogle the ceremonial axes and amber necklaces.

The Bronze Age brought the sword (several are on display).

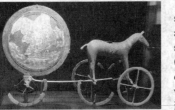

The "Chariot of the Sun"—a small statue of a horse pulling the sun across the sky—likely had religious significance for early Scandinavians (whose descendants continue to celebrate the solstice with fervor). In the same room are those iconic horned helmets. Contrary to popular belief (and countless tourist shops), these helmets were not worn by the Vikings, but by their predecessors—for ceremonial purposes, centuries earlier. In the next room are huge cases filled with still-playable *lur* horns (see page 170). Another room shows off a bitchin' collection of well-translated rune stones proclaiming heroic deeds.

This leads to the Iron Age and an object that's neither Iron nor Danish: the 2,000-year-old Gundestrup Cauldron of art-textbook fame. This 20-pound, soup-kitchen-size bowl made of silver was found in a Danish bog, but its symbolism suggests it was originally from Thrace (in northeast Greece) or Celtic Ireland. On the sides, hunters slay bulls, and gods cavort with stags, horses, dogs, and dragons. It's both mysterious and fascinating.

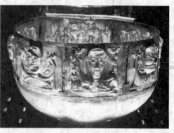

Prehistoric Danes were fascinated by bogs. To make iron, you need ore—and Denmark's many bogs provided that critical material in abundance, leading people to believe that the gods dwelled there. These Danes appeased the gods by sacrificing valuable items (and even people) into bogs. Fortunately for modern archaeologists, bogs happen to be an ideal environment for preserving fragile objects. One bog alone—the Nydam bog—has yielded thousands of items, including three whole ships.

No longer bogged down in prehistory, the people of Scandinavia came into contact with Roman civilization. At about this time, the Viking culture rose; you'll see the remains of an old warship. The Vikings, so feared in most of Europe, are still thought of fondly here in their homeland. You'll notice the descriptions straining to defend them: Sure, they'd pillage, rape, and plunder. But they also founded thriving, wealthy, and cultured trade towns. Love the Vikings or hate them, it's impossible to deny their massive reach—Norse Vikings even carved runes into the walls of the Hagia Sophia church (in today's Istanbul).

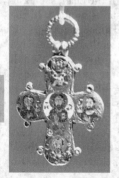

Middle Ages and Renaissance: Next, go upstairs and follow signs to Room 101 to start this section. You'll walk through the Middle Ages, where you'll find lots of bits and pieces of old churches, such as golden altars and *aquamaniles*, pitchers used for ritual hand-washing. The Dagmar Cross is the prototype for a popular form of crucifix worn by many Danes (Room 102, small glass display case—with colorful enamel paintings). Another cross in this case (the Roskilde Cross, studded with gemstones) was found inside the wooden head of Christ displayed high on the opposite wall. There are also exhibits on tools and trade, weapons, drinking horns, and fine, wood-carved winged altarpieces. Carry on to find a fascinating room on the Norse settlers of Greenland, material on the Reformation, and an exhibit on everyday town life in the 16th and 17th centuries.

Modern Times: The next floor takes you through the last few centuries, with historic toys and a slice-of-Danish-life (1660-

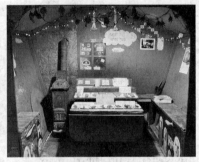

2000) gallery where you'll see everything from rifles and old bras to early jukeboxes. You'll learn that the Danish Golden Age (which dominates most art museums in Denmark) captured the everyday pastoral beauty of the countryside, celebrated Denmark's smallness and peace-loving nature, and mixed in some Nordic mythology. With industrialization came the labor movement and trade unions. After delving into the World Wars, Baby Boomers, creation of the postwar welfare state, and the "Depressed Decade" of the 1980s (when Denmark suffered high unemployment), the collection is capped off by a stall that, until recently, was used for selling marijuana in the squatters' community of Christiania.

The Rest of the Museum: If you're eager for more, there's plenty left to see. The National Museum also has exhibits on the history of this building (the Prince's Palace), a large ethnology collection, antiquities, coins and medallions, temporary exhibits, and a good children's museum. The floor plan will lead you to what you want to see.

▲National Museum's Victorian Apartment

The National Museum (listed above) inherited an incredible Victorian apartment just around the corner. The wealthy Christensen family managed to keep its plush living quarters a 19th-century time capsule until the granddaughters passed away in 1963. Since then, it's been part of the National Museum, with all but two of its rooms looking just as they did around 1890.

Cost and Hours: 50 kr, required one-hour tours leave from the National Museum reception desk (in Danish Sat-Sun at 11:00, 12:00, and 13:00 year-round; in English, June-Sept Sat only at 14:00).

▲Museum of Copenhagen (Københavns Museum)

This fine old house is filled with an entertaining and creative exhibit telling the story of Copenhagen. The ground floor covers the city's origins, the upper floor is dedicated to the 19th century, and the top floor includes a fun year-by-year walk through Copenhagen's 20th century, with lots of fun insights into contemporary culture.

Cost and Hours: 40 kr, daily 10:00-17:00, about 6 blocks past the train station at Vesterbrogade 59, tel. 33 21 07 72, www.copenhagen.dk.

ON SLOTSHOLMEN ISLAND

This island, where Copenhagen began in the 12th century, is a short walk from the train station and Tivoli, just across the bridge from the National Museum. It's dominated by Christiansborg Palace and several other royal and governmental buildings. Note that my "Copenhagen City Walk" (earlier) cuts right through Slotsholmen and covers other landmarks on the island (see page 175).

▲▲Christiansborg Palace

A complex of government buildings stands on the ruins of Copenhagen's original 12th-century fortress: the Parliament, Supreme Court, prime minister's office, royal reception rooms, royal library, several museums, and royal stables. Although the current palace dates only from 1928 and the royal family moved out 200 years ago, this building— the sixth to stand here in 800 years—is rich with tradition.

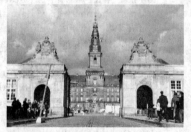

Three palace sights (the reception rooms, old castle ruins, and stables) are open to the public, giving us commoners a glimpse of the royal life.

Cost and Hours: Reception rooms-80 kr, castle ruins-40 kr, stables-40 kr, combo-ticket for all three-110 kr. All three sights are open daily (except in Oct-April, when they're closed on Mon) but have different hours: reception rooms 9:00-17:00 (may close at any time for royal events), ruins 10:00-17:00, stables and carriage museum 13:30-16:00 except July, when they're open 10:00-17:00. Tel. 33 92 64 92, www.christiansborg.dk.

Visiting the Palace: From the equestrian statue in front, go through the wooden door; the entrance to the ruins is in the corridor on the right, and the door to the reception rooms is out in the next courtyard, also on the right.

Royal Reception Rooms: While these don't rank among Europe's best palace rooms, they're worth a look. This is still the place where Queen Margrethe II impresses visiting dignitaries. The information-packed, hour-long English tours of the rooms are excellent (included in ticket, daily at 15:00). At other times, you'll wander the rooms on your own in a one-way route, reading the sparse English descriptions. As you slip-slide on protect-the-floor slippers through 22 rooms, you'll gain a good feel for Danish history, royalty, and politics. Here are a few highlights:

After the Queen's Library you'll soon enter the grand Great Hall, lined with boldly colorful (almost gaudy) tapestries. The palace highlight is this dazzling set of modern tapestries—Danish-designed but Gobelin-made in Paris. This gift, given to the queen on her 60th birthday in 2000, celebrates 1,000 years of Danish history, from the Viking age to our chaotic times...and into the future. Borrow the laminated descriptions for blow-by-blow explanations of the whole epic saga. The Velvet Room is where royals privately greet VIP guests before big functions.

In the corner room on the left, don't miss the family portrait of King Christian IX, which illustrates why he's called the "father-in-law of Europe"—his children eventually became, or married into, royalty in Denmark, Russia, Greece, Britain, France, Germany, and Norway.

In the Throne Room you'll see the balcony where new monarchs are proclaimed (most recently in 1972). And at the end, in the Hall of Giants (where you take off your booties among heroic figures supporting the building), you'll see a striking painting of Queen Margrethe II from 2010 on her 70th birthday. The three playful lions, made of Norwegian silver, once guarded the throne and symbolize absolute power—long gone since 1849, when Denmark embraced the notion of a constitutional monarch.

Castle Ruins: An exhibit in the scant remains of the first fortress built by Bishop Absalon, the 12th-century founder of Copenhagen, lies under the palace. A long passage connects to another set of ruins, from the 14th-century Copenhagen Castle. There's precious little to see, but it is, um, old and well-described. A video covers more recent palace history.

Royal Stables and Carriages Museum: This facility is still home to the horses that pull the queen's carriage on festive days, as well as a collection of historic carriages. While they're down from 250 horses to about a dozen, the royal stables are part of a strong tradition and, as the little video shows, will live on.

▲▲Thorvaldsen's Museum

This museum, which has some of the best swoon-worthy art you'll see anywhere, tells the story and shows the monumental work of

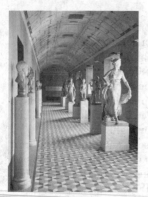

the great Danish Neoclassical sculptor Bertel Thorvaldsen (see sidebar). Considered Canova's equal among Neoclassical sculptors, Thorvaldsen spent 40 years in Rome. He was lured home to Copenhagen with the promise to showcase his work in a fine museum, which opened in the revolutionary year of 1848 as Denmark's first public art gallery. Of the 500 or so sculptures Thorvaldsen completed in his life—including 90 major statues—this museum has most of them, in one form or another (the plaster model used to make the original or a copy done in marble or bronze).

Cost and Hours: 40 kr, free on Wed, Tue-Sun 10:00-17:00, closed Mon, includes excellent English audioguide on request, located in Neoclassical building with colorful walls next to Christiansborg Palace, tel. 33 32 15 32, www.thorvaldsensmuseum.dk.

Visiting the Museum: The ground floor showcases his statues. After buying your ticket, go straight in and ask to borrow a free audioguide at the desk. This provides a wonderful statue-by-statue narration of the museum's key works.

Just before the audioguide desk, turn left into the Great Hall, which was the original entryway of the museum. It's filled with replicas of some of Thorvaldsen's biggest and grandest statues—national heroes who still stand in the prominent squares of their major cities (Munich, Warsaw, the Vatican, and others). Two great equestrian statues stare each other down from across the hall; while they both take the classic, self-assured pose of looking one way while pointing another (think Babe Ruth calling his home run), one of them (Jozef Poniatowski) is modeled after the ancient Roman general Marcus Aurelius, while the other (Bavaria's Maximilian I) wears modern garb.

Then take a spin through the smaller rooms that ring the central courtyard. Each of these is dominated by one big work—mostly classical subjects drawn from mythology. At the far end of the building stand the plaster models for the iconic *Risen Christ* and the 12 Apostles (the final marble versions stand in the Cathedral of Our Lady—see page 172). Peek into the central courtyard to see the planter box tomb of Thorvaldsen himself (who died in 1844).

Bertel Thorvaldsen (1770-1844)

Bertel Thorvaldsen was born, raised, educated, and buried in Copenhagen, but his most productive years were spent in Rome. There he soaked up the prevailing style of the time: Neoclassical. He studied ancient Greek and Roman statues, copying their balance, grace, and impassive beauty. The simple-but-noble style suited the patriotism of the era, and Thorvaldsen got rich off it. Public squares throughout Europe are dotted with his works, celebrating local rulers, patriots, and historical figures looking like Greek heroes or Roman conquerors.

In 1819, at the height of his fame and power, Thorvaldsen returned to Copenhagen. He was asked to decorate the most important parts of the recently bombed, newly rebuilt Cathedral of Our Lady: the main altar and nave. His *Risen Christ* on the altar (along with the 12 apostles lining the nave) became his most famous and reproduced work—without even realizing it, most people imagine the caring features of Thorvaldsen's Christ when picturing what Jesus looked like.

The prolific Thorvaldsen depicted a range of subjects. His grand statues of historical figures (Copernicus in Warsaw, Maximilian I in Munich) were intended for public squares. Portrait busts of his contemporaries were usually done in the style of Roman emperors. Thorvaldsen carved the Lion Monument, depicting a weeping lion, into a cliff in Luzern, Switzerland. He did religious statues, like the *Risen Christ*. Thorvaldsen's most accessible works are from Greek mythology—*The Three Graces*, naked *Jason with the Golden Fleece*, or Ganymede crouching down to feed the eagle Jupiter.

Though many of his statues are of gleaming white marble, Thorvaldsen was not a chiseler of stone. Like Rodin and Canova, Thorvaldsen left the grunt work to others. He fashioned a life-sized model in plaster, which could then be reproduced in marble or bronze by his assistants. Multiple copies were often made, even in his lifetime.

Thorvaldsen epitomized the Neoclassical style. His statues assume perfectly balanced poses—maybe even a bit stiff, say critics. They don't flail their arms dramatically or emote passionately. As you look into their faces, they seem lost in thought, as though contemplating deep spiritual truths.

In Copenhagen, catch Thorvaldsen's *Risen Christ* at the Cathedral of Our Lady, his portrait bust at City Hall, and the full range of his long career at the Thorvaldsen's Museum.

Continue into the next row of rooms: In the far corner room look for Thorvaldsen's (very flattering) self-portrait, leaning buffly against a partially finished sculpture.

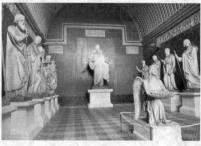

Downstairs you'll find a collection of plaster casts (mostly ancient Roman statues that inspired Thorvaldsen) and a video about his career.

Upstairs, get into the mind of the artist by perusing his personal possessions and the private collection of paintings from which he drew inspiration.

Royal Library

Copenhagen's "Black Diamond" (Den Sorte Diamant) library is a striking, supermodern building made of shiny black granite, leaning over the harbor at the edge of the palace complex. From the inviting lounge chairs, you can ponder this stretch of harborfront, which serves as a showcase for architects. Inside, wander through the old and new sections, catch the fine view from the "G" level, read a magazine, use the free computers (in the skyway lobby over the street nearest the harbor), and enjoy a classy—and pricey—lunch.

Cost and Hours: Free, special exhibits generally 30 kr; different parts of the library have varying hours but reading room generally open July-Aug Mon-Fri 8:00-19:00, Sat 10:00-16:00, longer hours rest of the year, closed Sun year-round; tel. 33 47 47 47, www.kb.dk.

▲Danish Jewish Museum (Dansk Jødisk Museum)

This museum, which opened in 2004 in a striking building by American architect Daniel Libeskind, offers a very small but well-exhibited display of 400 years of the life and impact of Jews in Denmark.

Cost and Hours: 50 kr; June-Aug Tue-Sun 10:00-17:00; Sept-May Tue-Fri 13:00-16:00, Sat-Sun 12:00-17:00; closed Mon year-round; behind "Black Diamond" library at Proviantpassagen 6—enter from the courtyard behind the red-brick, ivy-covered building; tel. 33 11 22 18, www.jewmus.dk.

NEAR THE STRØGET
Round Tower

Built in 1642 by Christian IV, the tower connects a church, library, and observatory (the oldest functioning observatory in Europe) with a ramp that spirals up to a fine view of Copenhagen (though the view from atop Our Savior's Church is far better—see page 204).

Cost and Hours: 25 kr, nothing to see inside but the ramp and the view; tower—daily mid-May-mid-Sept 10:00-20:00, off-season until 18:00; observatory—summer Sun 13:00-16:00, mid-Oct-mid-March Tue-Wed 19:00-22:00; just off the Strøget on Købmagergade.

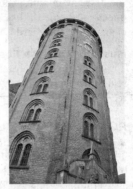

AMALIENBORG PALACE AND NEARBY

For more information on this palace and nearby attractions, including the famous *Little Mermaid* statue, see the end of my "Copenhagen City Walk" (page 181).

▲Amalienborg Museum (Amalienborgmuseet)

While Queen Margrethe II and her husband live quite privately in one of the four mansions that make up the palace complex, another mansion has been open to the public since 1994. It displays the private studies of four kings of the House of Glucksborg, who ruled from 1863 to 1972 (the immediate predecessors of today's queen). Your visit is short—six or eight rooms on one floor—but it affords an intimate and unique peek into Denmark's royal family. You'll see the private study of each of the last four kings of Denmark. They feel particularly lived-in—with cluttered pipe collections and bookcases jammed with family pictures—because they were. It's easy to imagine these blue-blooded folks just hanging out here, even today. The earliest study, Frederik VIII's (c. 1869), feels much older and more "royal"—with Renaissance gilded walls, heavy drapes, and a polar bear rug. With a little luck, the upstairs gala hall will be open during your visit.

Cost and Hours: 70 kr (90 kr on Sat), 130-kr combo-ticket also includes Rosenborg Palace; May-Oct daily 10:00-16:00; Nov-April Tue-Sun 11:00-16:00, closed Mon; with your back to the harbor, the entrance is at the far end of the square on the right; tel. 33 15 32 86, www.dkks.dk.

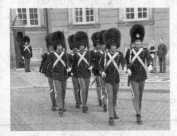

Amalienborg Palace Changing of the Guard

This noontime event is boring in the summer, when the queen is not in residence—the guards just change places. (This goes on for quite a long time—no need to rush here at the stroke of noon, or to crowd in during the first few minutes; you'll have plenty of good photo ops.) If the queen's at home (indicated by a flag flying above her home), the changing of the guard is accompanied by a military band.

Museum of Danish Resistance (Frihedsmuseet)

This museum, which tells the story of Denmark's heroic Nazi-resistance struggle (1940-1945), is closed through 2018 for reconstruction.

ROSENBORG CASTLE AND NEARBY
▲▲▲Rosenborg Castle (Rosenborg Slot) and Treasury

This finely furnished Dutch Renaissance-style castle was built by King Christian IV in the early 1600s as a summer residence. Rosenborg was his favorite residence and where he chose to die. Open to the public since 1838, it houses the Danish crown jewels and 500 years of royal knickknacks. While the old palace interior is a bit dark and not as immediately impressive as many of Europe's later Baroque masterpieces, it has a certain lived-in charm. It oozes the personality of the fascinating Christian IV and has one of the finest treasury collections in Europe. For more on Christian, read the sidebar on the next page.

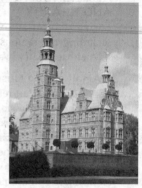

Cost and Hours: 90 kr, 130-kr ticket also includes Amalienborg Museum; June-Aug daily 10:00-17:00; May and Sept-Oct daily 10:00-16:00; Nov-Dec Tue-Sun 11:00-14:00 (treasury until 16:00), closed Mon; Jan-April Tue-Sun 11:00-16:00, closed Mon; mandatory lockers take 20-kr coin, which will be returned; Metro or S-tog: Nørreport, then 5-minute walk on Østervoldgade and through park; tel. 33 15 32 86, www.dkks.dk.

Tours: Richard Karpen leads fascinating one-hour tours in princely garb (90 kr plus entry fee, mid-May-mid-Sept Mon and Thu at 12:00, meet outside castle ticket office; see listing on page 163, under "Tours in Copenhagen"). Or take the following self-guided tour that I've woven together from the highlights of Richard's walk. You can also use your mobile device to take advantage of the palace's free Wi-Fi signal, which is intended to let you follow the "Konge Connect" step-by-step tour through the palace highlights (with audio/video/text explanations for your smartphone or tablet—bring earphones; instructional brochure at the ticket desk).

◉ Self-Guided Tour: Buy your ticket, then head back out and look for the *castle* sign. You'll tour the ground floor room by

King Christian IV:
A Lover and a Fighter

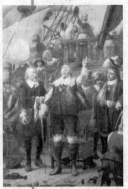

King Christian IV (1577-1648) inherited Denmark at the peak of its power, lived his life with the exuberance of the age, and went to his grave with the country in decline. His legacy is obvious to every tourist—Rosenborg Castle, Frederiksborg Palace, the Round Tower, Christianshavn, and on and on. Look for his logo adorning many buildings: the letter "C" with a "4" inside it and a crown on top. Thanks to both his place in history and his passionate personality, Danes today regard Christian IV as one of their greatest monarchs.

During his 50-year reign, Christian IV reformed the government, rebuilt the army, established a trading post in India, and tried to expand Denmark's territory. He took Kalmar from Sweden and captured strategic points in northern Germany. The king was a large man who also lived large. A skilled horseman and avid hunter, he could drink his companions under the table. He spoke several languages and gained a reputation as outgoing and humorous. His lavish banquets were legendary, and his romantic affairs were numerous.

But Christian's appetite for war proved destructive. In 1626, Denmark again attacked northern Germany, but was beaten back. In late 1643, Sweden launched a sneak attack, and despite Christian's personal bravery (he lost an eye), the war went badly. By the end of his life, Christian was tired and bitter, and Denmark was drained.

The heroics of Christian and his sailors live on in the Danish national anthem: "King Christian Stood by the Lofty Mast."

room, then climb to the third floor for the big throne room. After a quick sweep of the middle floor, finish in the basement (enter from outside) for the jewels.

• *Begin the tour on the palace's ground floor (turn right as you enter), in the Winter Room.*

Ground Floor: Here in the wood-paneled **Winter Room,** all eyes were on King Christian IV. Today, your eyes should be on him, too. Take a close look at his bust by the fireplace (if it's not here, look for it out in the corridor by the ticket taker). Check this guy out—fashionable braid, hard drinker, hard lover, energetic statesman, and warrior king. Christian IV was dynamism in the flesh, wearing a toga: a true Renaissance guy. During his reign, Copenhagen doubled in size. You're surrounded by Dutch paintings (the Dutch had a huge influence on 17th-century Denmark). Note the smaller statue of the 19-year-old king, showing him jousting jauntily on his coronation day. In another case, the golden astronomical clock—with musical works and moving figures—did everything you can imagine. Flanking the fireplace (opposite where you entered), beneath the windows, look for the panels in the tile floor that could be removed to let the music performed by the band in the basement waft in. (Who wants the actual musicians in the dining room?) The audio holes were also used to call servants.

The **study** (or "writing closet," nearest where you entered) was small (and easy to heat). Kings did a lot of corresponding. We know a lot about Christian because 3,000 of his handwritten letters survive. The painting on the right wall shows Christian at age eight. Three years later, his father died, and little Christian technically ascended the throne, though Denmark was actually ruled by a regency until Christian 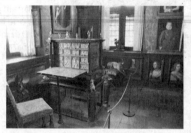 was 19. A portrait of his mother hangs above the boy, and opposite is a portrait of Christian in his prime—having just conquered Sweden—standing alongside the incredible coronation crown you'll see later.

Going back through the Winter Room, head for the door to Christian's **bedroom.** Before entering, notice the little peephole 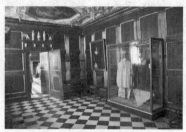 in the door (used by the king to spy on those in this room—well-camouflaged by the painting, and more easily seen from the other side), and the big cabinet doors for Christian's clothes and accessories, flanking the bedroom door (notice the hinges and keyholes). Heading into the bedroom, you'll see paintings showing the king as an old man...and as a dead man. (Christian died in this room.) In the case are the clothes he wore at his finest hour. During a naval battle against Sweden (1644), Christian stood directing the action when an explosion ripped across the deck, sending him sprawling and riddling him with shrapnel. Unfazed, the 67-year-old monarch bounced right back up and kept going, inspiring his men to carry on the fight. Christian's stubborn determination during this battle is commemorated in Denmark's national anthem. Shrapnel put out Christian's eye. No problem: The warrior king with a knack for heroic publicity stunts had the shrapnel bits removed from his eye and forehead and made into earrings as a gift for his mistress. The earrings hang in the case with his blood-stained clothes (easy to miss, right side). Christian lived to be 70 and fathered 25 children (with two wives and three mistresses). Before moving on, you can peek into Christian's private bathroom—elegantly tiled with Delft porcelain.

Proceed into the **Dark Room.** Here you'll see wax casts of royal figures. This was the way famous and important people were portrayed back then. The chair is a forerunner of the whoopee cushion. When you sat on it, metal cuffs pinned your arms down, allowing the prankster to pour water down the back of the chair (see hole)—making you "wet your pants." When you stood up, the chair made embarrassing tooting sounds.

The **Marble Room** has a particularly impressive inlaid marble floor. Imagine the king meeting emissaries here in the center, with the emblems of Norway (right), Denmark (center), and Sweden (left) behind him.

The end room, called the **King's Chamber,** was used by Christian's first mistress. Notice the ceiling painting, with an orchestra looking down on you as they play.

The long **stone passage** leading to the staircase exhibits an intriguing painting (by the door to the King's Chamber) showing

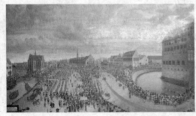

the crowds at the coronation of Christian's son, Frederik III. After Christian's death, a weakened Denmark was invaded, occupied, and humiliated by Sweden (Treaty of Roskilde, 1658). Copenhagen alone held out through the long winter of 1658-1659 (the Siege of Copenhagen), and Sweden eventually had to withdraw from the country. During the siege, Frederik III distinguished himself with his bravery. He seized upon the resulting surge of popularity as his chance to be anointed an absolute, divinely ordained monarch (1660). This painting marks that event—study it closely for slice-of-life details. Next, near the ticket taker, a sprawling family tree makes it perfectly clear that Christian IV comes from good stock. Notice the tree is labeled in German—the second language of the realm.

• *The queen had a hand-pulled elevator, but you'll need to hike up two flights of stairs to the throne room.*

Throne Room (Third Floor): The **Long Hall**—considered one of the best-preserved Baroque rooms in Europe—was great for banquets. The decor trumpets the accomplishments of Denmark's great kings. The four corners of the ceiling feature the four continents known at the time. (America—at the far-right end of the hall as you enter—was still considered pretty untamed; notice the decapitated head with the arrow sticking out of it.) In the center, of course, is the proud seal of the Danish Royal Family. The tapestries, designed for this room, are from 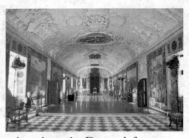 the late 1600s. Effective propaganda, they show the Danes defeating their Swedish rivals on land and at sea. The king's throne—still more propaganda for two centuries of "absolute" monarchs—was made of "unicorn horn" (actually narwhal tusk from Greenland). Believed to bring protection from evil and poison, the horn was the most precious material in its day. The queen's throne is of hammered silver. The 150-pound lions are 300 years old.

The small room to the left holds a delightful **royal porcelain** display with Chinese, French, German, and Danish examples of the "white gold." For five centuries, Europeans couldn't figure out how the Chinese made this stuff. The difficulty in just getting it back to Europe in one piece made it precious. The Danish pieces, called "Flora Danica" (on the left as you enter), are from a huge royal set showing off the herbs and vegetables of the realm.

• *Heading back down, pause at the middle floor, which is worth a look.*

Middle Floor: Circling counterclockwise, you'll see more fine clocks, fancy furniture, and royal portraits. The queen enjoyed her royal lathe (with candleholders for lighting and pedals to spin it hidden away below; in the Christian VI Room). The small mirror room (up the stairs from the main hall) was where the king played Hugh Hefner—using mirrors on the floor to see what was under those hoop skirts. In hidden cupboards, he had a fold-out bed and a handy escape staircase.

• *Back outside, turn right and find the stairs leading down to the...*

Royal Danish Treasury (Castle Basement): The palace was a royal residence for a century and has been the royal vault right up until today. As you enter, first head to the right, into the **wine cellar,** with thousand-liter barrels and some fine treasury items. The first room has a vast army of tiny golden soldiers, and a wall lined with fancy rifles. Heading into the next room, you'll see fine items of amber (petrified tree resin, 30-50 million years old) and ivory. Study the large box made of amber (in a freestanding case, just to the right as you enter)—the tiny figures show a healthy interest in sex.

Now head back past the ticket taker and into the main part of the treasury, where you can browse through exquisite royal knickknacks.

The diamond- and pearl-studded **saddles** were Christian IV's—the first for his coronation, the second for his son's wedding. When his kingdom was nearly bankrupt, Christian had these constructed lavishly—complete with solid-gold spurs—to impress visiting dignitaries and bolster Denmark's credit rating.

The next case displays **tankards.** Danes were always big drinkers, and to drink in the top style, a king had narwhal steins (#4030). Note the fancy Greenland Inuit (Eskimo) on the lid (#4023). The case is filled with exquisitely carved ivory. On the other side of that case, what's with the mooning snuffbox (#4063)? Also, check out the amorous whistle (#4064).

Drop by the case on the wall in the back-left of the room: The 17th century was the age of **brooches.** Many of these are made of freshwater pearls. Find the fancy combination toothpick and ear spoon (#4140). Look for #4146: A queen was caught having an affair after 22 years of royal marriage. Her king gave her a special present: a golden ring—showing the hand of his promiscuous queen shaking hands with a penis.

Step downstairs, away from all this silliness. Passing through the serious vault door, you come face-to-face with a big, jeweled **sword.** The tall, two-handed, 16th-century coronation sword was drawn by the new king, who cut crosses in the air in four directions, symbolically promising to defend the realm from all attacks. The cases surrounding the sword contain everyday items used by the king (all solid gold, of course). What looks like a trophy case of gold records is actually a collection of dinner plates with amber centers (#5032).

Go down the steps. In the center case is Christian IV's **coronation crown** (from 1596, seven pounds of gold and precious

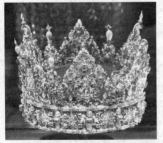

stones, #5124), which some consider to be the finest Renaissance crown in Europe. Its six tallest gables radiate symbolism. Find the symbols of justice (sword and scales), fortitude (a woman on a lion with a sword), and charity (a nursing woman—meaning the king will love God and his people as a mother loves her child). The pelican, which according to medieval legend pecks its own flesh to feed its young, symbolizes God sacrificing his son, just as the king would make great sacrifices for his people. Climb the footstool to look inside—it's as exquisite as the outside. The shields of various Danish provinces remind the king that he's surrounded by his realms.

Circling the cases along the wall (right to left), notice the fine enameled lady's goblet with traits of a good woman spelled out in

Latin (#5128) and above that, an exquisite prayer book (with hand-written favorite prayers, #5134). In the fifth window, the big solid-gold baptismal basin (#5262) hangs above tiny oval silver boxes that contained the royal children's umbilical cords (handy for protection later in life, #5272); two cases over are royal writing sets with wax, seals, pens, and ink (#5320).

Go down a few more steps into the lowest level of the treasury and last room. The two **crowns** in the center cases are more modern (from 1670), lighter, and more practical—just gold and diamonds without all the symbolism. The king's crown is only four pounds, the queen's a mere two.

The cases along the walls show off the **crown jewels.** These were made in 1840 of diamonds, emeralds, rubies, and pearls from earlier royal jewelry. The saber (#5540) shows emblems of the realm's 19 provinces. The sumptuous pendant features a 19-carat diamond cut (like its neighbors) in the 58-facet "brilliant" style for maximum reflection (far-left case, #5560). Imagine these on the dance floor. The painting shows the anointing of King Christian V at the Frederiksborg Castle Chapel in 1671. The crown jewels are still worn by the queen on special occasions several times a year.

▲Rosenborg Gardens

Rosenborg Castle is surrounded by the royal pleasure gardens and, on sunny days, a minefield of sunbathing Danish beauties and picnickers. While "ethnic Danes" grab the shade, the rest of the Danes worship the sun. When the royal family is in residence, there's a daily changing-of-the-guard mini parade from the Royal Guard's barracks adjoining Rosenborg Castle (at 11:30) to Amalienborg Palace (at 12:00). The Queen's Rose Garden (across the moat from the palace) is a royal place for a picnic. The fine statue of Hans Christian Andersen in the park—erected while he was still alive (and approved by him)—is meant to symbolize how his stories had a message even for adults.

▲National Gallery of Denmark (Statens Museum for Kunst)

This museum fills a stately building with Danish and European paintings from the 14th century through today. It's particularly worthwhile for the chance to be immersed in great art by the Danes, and to see its good collection of French Modernists, all well-described in English.

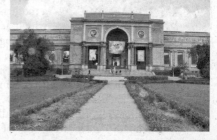

Cost and Hours: Permanent collection-free,

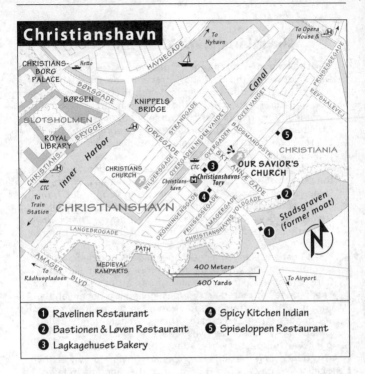

Christianshavn

To Nyhavn
To Opera House &

CHRISTIANS-BORG PALACE — Netto

BØRSEN

BØRSGADE

KNIPPELS BRIDGE

SLOTSHOLMEN

ROYAL LIBRARY

CHRISTIANS BRYGGE

Inner Harbor

CTC

To Train Station

HAVNEGADE

Canal

TORVEGADE

STRANDGADE

WILDERSGADE

OVERGADEN NEDEN VANDET

OVERGADEN OVEN VANDET

BÅDSMANDSSTR.

PRINSESSEGADE

REFSHALEVEJ

CHRISTIANS CHURCH

CTC

Christians-havn

Christianshavns Torv

OUR SAVIOR'S CHURCH

SKT. ANNÆ GADE

CHRISTIANIA

CHRISTIANSHAVN

DRONNINGENSGADE

PRINSESSEGADE

AMAGERGADE

CHRISTIANSHAVNS VOLDGADE

Stadsgraven (former moat)

LANGEBROGADE

PATH

MEDIEVAL RAMPARTS

AMAGER BLVD

To Rådhuspladsen

400 Meters

400 Yards

To Airport

1 Ravelinen Restaurant
2 Bastionen & Løven Restaurant
3 Lagkagehuset Bakery
4 Spicy Kitchen Indian
5 Spiseloppen Restaurant

---

special exhibits-110 kr, Tue-Sun 10:00-17:00, Wed until 20:00, closed Mon, Sølvgade 48, tel. 33 74 84 94, www.smk.dk.

CHRISTIANSHAVN

Across the harbor from the old town, Christianshavn—the former merchant's district—is one of the most delightful neighborhoods in town to explore. It offers pleasant canalside walks and trendy restaurants, along with two things to see: Our Savior's Church (with its fanciful tower) and Christiania, a colorful alternative-living community. Before visiting, make sure to read the background on Christianshavn, which helps explain what you'll see (see sidebar).

Your first look at the island will likely be its main square. Christianshavns Torv has a Metro stop, an early Copenhagen phone kiosk (from 1896), a fine baker across the street (Lagkagehuset), and three statues celebrating Greenland. A Danish protectorate since 1721, Greenland, with 56,000 people, is represented by two members in the Danish Parliament. The square has long been a hangout for Greenlanders, who appreciate the cheap beer and long hours of the big supermarket fronting the square.

Christianshavn: Then and Now

Christianshavn—Copenhagen's planned port—was vital to Danish power in the 17th and 18th centuries. Denmark had always been second to Sweden when it came to possession of natural resources, so the Danes tried to make up for it by acquiring resource-rich overseas colonies. They built Christianshavn (with Amsterdam's engineering help) to run the resulting trade business—giving this neighborhood a "little Amsterdam" vibe today.

Since Denmark's economy was so dependent on trade, the port town was the natural target of enemies. When the Danes didn't support Britain against Napoleon in 1807, the Brits bombarded Christianshavn. In this "blackest year in Danish history," Christianshavn burned down. That's why today there's hardly a building here that dates from before that time.

Christianshavn remained Copenhagen's commercial center until the 1920s, when a modern harbor was built. Suddenly, Christianshavn's economy collapsed and it became a slum. Cheap prices attracted artsy types, giving it a bohemian flavor. In 1971, squatters set up shop in an old military camp in Christianshavn and created their own community called Christiania, which still survives today.

Over the past few decades, Christianshavn has had a resurgence, and these days, prices are driven up by wealthy locals (who pay about 60 percent of their income in taxes) spending too much for apartments, renting them cheaply to their kids, and writing off the loss. Demand for property is huge. Today the neighborhood is inhabited mostly by rich students and young professionals, living in some of the priciest real estate in town.

▲Our Savior's Church (Vor Frelsers Kirke)

Following a recent restoration, the church gleams inside and out. Its bright Baroque interior (1696) is shaped like a giant cube. The magnificent pipe organ is supported by elephants (a royal symbol of the prestigious Order of the Elephant). Looking up to the ceiling, notice elephants also sculpted into the stucco of the dome, and a little one hanging from the main chandelier. Best of all, you can climb the unique spiral spire (with an outdoor staircase winding up to its top—398 stairs in all) for great views of the city and of the Christiania commune below.

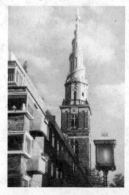

Cost and Hours: Church interior—free, open daily 11:00-15:30 but may close for special services; church tower—40 kr;

July-mid-Sept Mon-Sat 10:00-19:00, Sun 10:30-19:00; April-June and mid-Sept-Nov daily until 16:00; closed Dec-March and in bad weather; bus #2A, #19, or Metro: Christianshavn, Sankt Annægade 29, tel. 41 66 63 57, www.vorfrelserskirke.dk.

▲▲▲Christiania

In 1971, the original 700 Christianians established squatters' rights in an abandoned military barracks just a 10-minute walk from the Danish Parliament building. Two generations later, this "free city" still stands—an ultra-human mishmash of idealists, hippies, potheads, nonmaterialists, and happy children (600 adults, 200 kids, 200 cats, 200 dogs, 2 parrots, and 17 horses). There are even a handful of Willie Nelson-type seniors among the 180 remaining here from the original takeover. And an amazing thing has happened: The place has become the second-most-visited sight among tourists in Copenhagen, behind Tivoli Gardens. Move over, *Little Mermaid*.

"Pusher Street" (named for the sale of soft drugs here) is Christiania's main drag. Get beyond this touristy side of Christiania, and you'll find a fascinating, ramshackle world of moats and earthen ramparts, alternative housing, cozy tea houses, carpenter shops, hippie villas, children's playgrounds, peaceful lanes, and people who believe that "to be normal is to be in a straitjacket." A local slogan claims, *"Kun døde fisk flyder med strømmen"* ("Only dead fish swim with the current").

Hours and Tours: Christiania is open all the time but quiet (and some restaurants closed) on Mondays, which is its rest day (though "resting" from what, I'm not sure). Guided tours leave from the main entrance at 15:00 (just show up, 40 kr, 1.5 hours, daily late June-Aug, only Sat-Sun rest of year, in English and Danish, info tel. 32 95 65 07, www.rundvisergruppen.dk). You're welcome to snap photos, except on Pusher Street (but ask residents before you photograph them).

The Community: Christiania is broken into 14 administrative neighborhoods on a former military base. Most of the land, once owned by Denmark's Ministry of Defense, has been purchased by the Christiania community; the rest of it is leased from the state

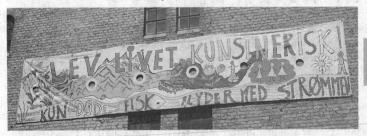

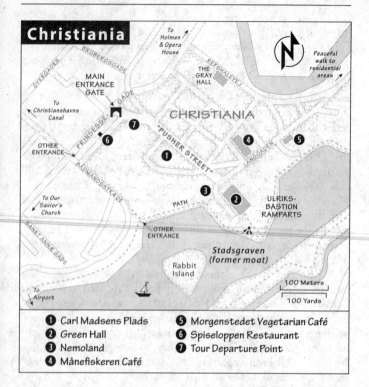

Christiania

To Holmen & Opera House

BRØBERGSGADE

OVERGADEN

MAIN ENTRANCE GATE

PRINSESSE-GADE

To Christianshavns Canal

OTHER ENTRANCE

BÅDMANDSSTRÆDE

SANKT ANNÆ GADE

To Our Savior's Church

To Airport

REFSHALEVEJ

THE GRAY HALL

CHRISTIANIA

"PUSHER STREET"

LANGGADEN

Peaceful walk to residential areas

PATH

ULRIKS-BASTION RAMPARTS

OTHER ENTRANCE

Stadsgraven (former moat)

Rabbit Island

100 Meters

100 Yards

❶ Carl Madsens Plads
❷ Green Hall
❸ Nemoland
❹ Månefiskeren Café
❺ Morgenstedet Vegetarian Café
❻ Spiseloppen Restaurant
❼ Tour Departure Point

(see the sidebar for details). Locals build their homes but don't own them—individuals can't buy or sell property. When someone moves out, the community decides who will be invited in to replace that person. A third of the adult population works on the outside, a third works on the inside, and a third doesn't work much at all.

There are nine rules: no cars, no hard drugs, no guns, no explosives, and so on. The Christiania flag is red and yellow because when the original hippies took over, they found a lot of red and yellow paint onsite. The three yellow dots in the flag are from the three "i"s in Christiania (or, some claim, the "o"s in "Love, Love, Love").

The community pays the city about $1 million a year for utilities and has about $1 million a year more to run its local affairs. A few "luxury hippies" have oil heat, but most use wood or gas. The ground here was poisoned by its days as a military base, so nothing is grown in Christiania. There's little industry within the commune (Christiania Cykler, which builds fine bikes, is an exception—www.pedersen-bike.dk). A phone chain provides a system of communal security (they have had bad experiences calling the police). Each September 26, the day the first squatters took over the barracks in 1971, Christiania has a big birthday bash.

Tourists are entirely welcome here, because they've become a major part of the economy. Visitors react in very different ways to the place. Some see dogs, dirt, and dazed people. Others see a haven of peace, freedom, and no taboos. Locals will remind judgmental Americans (whose country incarcerates more than a quarter of the world's prison inmates) that a society must make the choice: Allow for alternative lifestyles...or build more prisons.

Visiting Christiania: The main entrance is down Prinsessegade, behind the Our Savior's Church spiral tower. Passing under the gate, take Pusher Street directly into the community. The first square—a kind of market square (souvenirs and marijuana-related stuff)—is named Carl Madsens Plads, honoring the lawyer who took the squatters' case to the Danish supreme court in 1976 and won. Beyond that is Nemoland (a food circus, on the right). A huge warehouse called the Green Hall (Den Gronne Hal) is a recycling center and hardware store (where people get most of their building materials) that does double duty at night as a concert hall and as a place where children work on crafts. If you go up the stairs between Nemoland and the Green Hall, you'll climb up to the ramparts that overlook the canal. As you wander, be careful to distinguish between real Christianians and Christiania's motley guests—drunks (mostly from other countries) who hang out here in the summer for the freedom. Part of the original charter guaranteed that the community would stay open to the public.

On the left beyond the Green Hall, a lane leads to the Månefiskeren café, and beyond that, to the Morgenstedet vegetar-

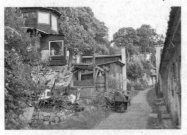

ian restaurant (the best place for a simple, friendly meal; see "Eating in Christiania," later). Beyond these recommended restaurants, you'll find yourself lost in the totally untouristy, truly local residential parts of Christiania, where kids play in the street and the old folks sit out on the front stoop—just like any other neighborhood. Just as St. Mark's Square isn't the "real Venice," the hippie-druggie scene on Pusher Street isn't the "real Christiania"—you can't say you've experienced Christiania until you've strolled these back streets.

A walk or bike ride through Christiania is a great way to see how this community lives. When you leave, look up—the sign above the gate says, "You are entering the EU."

Smoking Marijuana: Pusher Street was once lined with stalls selling marijuana, joints, and hash. Residents intentionally destroyed the stalls in 2004 to reduce the risk of Christiania

The Fight for Christiania

Ever since several hundred squatters took over an unused military camp in 1971, Christiania has been a political hot potato. No one in the Danish establishment wanted it. And no one had the nerve to mash it.

Part of Christiania's history has been ongoing government attempts to shut the place down. At first, city officials looked the other way because back then, no one cared about the land. But skyrocketing Christianshavn land values brought pressure to open Christiania to market forces. By the 1980s, the neighborhood had become gentrified, and both the city and developers were eyeing the land Christiania's hippies were squatting on. And when Denmark's conservative government took over in 2001, they vowed to "normalize" Christiania (with pressure from the US), with police regularly conducting raids on pot sellers.

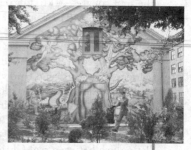

Things were looking grim for the Christianians until 2012, when the Danish government offered to sell most of the land to the residents at below the market rate, and offered guaranteed loans. In exchange, the Christianians had to promise to upgrade and maintain water, sewage, and electrical services, and preserve rights of way and "rural" areas. Accepting the offer, Christianians formed a foundation—Freetown Christiania—to purchase and control the property. The parts of Christiania that were not sold are leased to the residents and are still owned by the state.

For many Christianians, it's an ironic, capitalistic twist that they now own property, albeit collectively. They even sell

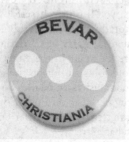

symbolic Christiania "shares" to help pay for the land. And, every adult over age 18 now owes a monthly rent that goes toward paying off the loans and to support services. But on the flip side, this is the greatest degree of security Christiania has ever experienced in its four-plus decades of existence. Even so, mistrust of the establishment is by no means dead, and there are still those who wonder what the government might be up to next.

being disbanded by the government. (One stall was spared and is on display at the National Museum.) Walking along Pusher Street today, you may witness policemen or deals being made—but never at the same time. You may also notice wafts of marijuana smoke and whispered offers of "hash" during your visit. And, in fact, on my last visit there was a small stretch of Pusher Street dubbed the "Green Light District," where pot was being openly sold (signs acknowledged that this activity was still illegal, and announced three rules here: 1. Have fun; 2. No photos; and 3. No running—"because it makes people nervous"). However, purchasing and smoking may buy you more time in Denmark than you'd planned—possession of marijuana is illegal.

About hard drugs: For the first few years, junkies were toler-

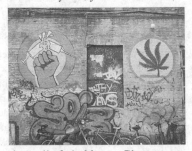

ated. But that led to violence and polluted the mellow ambience residents envisioned. In 1979, the junkies were expelled—an epic confrontation in the community's folk history now—and since then the symbol of a fist breaking a syringe is as prevalent as the leafy marijuana icon. Hard drugs are emphatically forbidden in Christiania.

Eating in Christiania: The people of Christiania appreciate good food and count on tourism as a big part of their economy. Consequently, there are plenty of decent eateries. Most of the restaurants are closed on Monday (the community's weekly holiday). **Pusher Street** has a few grungy but tasty falafel stands, as well as a popular burger bar. **Nemoland** is the hangout zone—a fun collection of stands peddling Thai food, burgers, *shawarma*, and other fast hippie food with great, tented outdoor seating (30-110-kr meals). Its stay-a-while atmosphere comes with backgammon, foosball, bakery goods, and fine views from the ramparts. **Månefiskeren** ("Moonfisher Bar") looks like a modern-day Brueghel painting, with billiards, chess, snacks, and drinks (Tue-Sun 10:00-23:00, closed Mon). **Morgenstedet** ("Morning Place") is a good, cheap vegetarian café with a mellow, woody interior and a rustic patio outside (50-100-kr meals, Tue-Sun 12:00-21:00, closed Mon, left after Pusher Street). **Spiseloppen** is *the* classy, good-enough-for-Republicans restaurant in the community (closed Mon, described on page 218).

COPENHAGEN

Shopping in Copenhagen

Shops are generally open Monday through Friday from 10:00 to 19:00 and Saturday from 9:00 to 16:00 (closed Sun). While big department stores dominate the scene, many locals favor the characteristic, small artisan shops and boutiques.

Uniquely Danish souvenirs to look for include intricate paper cuttings with idyllic motifs of swans, flowers, or Christmas themes; mobiles with everything from bicycles to Viking ships (look for the quality Flensted brand); and the colorful artwork of Danish artist Bo Bendixen (posters, postcards, T-shirts, and more). Jewelry lovers look for amber, known as the "gold of the North." Globs of this petrified sap wash up on the shores of all the Baltic countries.

WHERE TO SHOP

Consider the following stores, markets, and neighborhoods:

For a street's worth of shops selling **"Scantiques,"** wander down Ravnsborggade from Nørrebrogade.

Copenhagen's colorful **flea markets** are small but feisty and surprisingly cheap (May-Nov Sat 8:00-14:00 at Israels Plads; May-Sept Fri and Sat 8:00-17:00 along Gammel Strand and on Kongens Nytorv). For other street markets, ask at the TI.

The city's top **department stores** (Illum at Østergade 52, and Magasin du Nord at Kongens Nytorv 13) offer a good, if expensive, look at today's Denmark. Both are on the Strøget and have fine cafeterias on their top floors. The department stores and the Politiken Bookstore on Rådhuspladsen have a good selection of maps and English travel guides.

The section of the Strøget called **Amagertorv** is a highlight for shoppers. The **Royal Copenhagen** store here sells porcelain on three floors (Mon-Fri 10:00-19:00, Sat 10:00-18:00, Sun 12:00-17:00). The first floor up features figurines and collectibles. The second floor has a second-quality department for discounts, proving that "even the best painter can miss a stroke." Next door, **Illums Bolighus** shows off three floors of modern Danish design (Mon-Fri 10:00-19:00, Sat 10:00-18:00, Sun 11:00-18:00).

House of Amber, which has a shop and a tiny two-room museum with about 50 examples of prehistoric insects trapped in the amber (remember *Jurassic Park*?) under magnifying glasses. You'll also see remarkable items made of amber, from necklaces and chests to Viking ships and chess sets (25 kr, daily May-Aug 10:00-19:00, Sept-April 10:00-18:00, at the top of Nyhavn at Kongens Nytorv 2). If you're visiting Rosenborg Castle, you'll see the ultimate examples of amber craftsmanship in its treasury.

Eating in Copenhagen

While most of the restaurants listed here are lunch places, I've also included a few dinner options in case you spend a night here before or after your cruise.

CHEAP MEALS

For a quick lunch, try a *smørrebrød*, a *pølse*, or a picnic. Finish it off with a pastry.

Smørrebrød

Denmark's 300-year-old tradition of open-face sandwiches survives. Find a *smørrebrød* take-out shop and choose two or three that look good (about 25 kr each). You'll get them wrapped and ready for a park bench. Add a cold drink, and you have a fine, quick, and very Danish lunch. Tradition calls for three sandwich courses: herring first, then meat, and then cheese. Downtown, you'll find these handy local alternatives to Yankee fast-food chains. They range from splurges to quick stop-offs.

Between Copenhagen University and Rosenborg Castle

My three favorite *smørrebrød* places are particularly handy when connecting your sightseeing between the downtown Strøget core and Rosenborg Castle.

Restaurant Schønnemann is the foodies' choice—it has been written up in international magazines and frequently wins awards for "Best Lunch in Copenhagen." It's a cozy cellar restaurant crammed with small tables—according to the history on the menu, people "gather here in intense togetherness." The sand on the floor evokes a bygone era when passing traders would leave their horses out on the square while they lunched here. You'll need to reserve to get a table, and you'll pay a premium for their *smørrebrød* (70-170 kr, two lunch seatings Mon-Sat: 11:30-14:00 & 14:14-17:00, closed Sun, no dinner, Hauser Plads 16, tel. 33 12 07 85, www.restaurantschonnemann.dk).

Café Halvvejen is a small mom-and-pop place serving traditional lunches and open-face sandwiches in a woody and smoke-stained café, lined with portraits of Danish royalty. You can eat inside or at an outside table in good weather (50-70-kr *smørrebrød*, 80-110-kr main dishes, food served Mon-Sat 12:00-15:00, closed Sun, next to public library at Krystalgade 11, tel. 33 11 91 12).

Slagteren ved Kultorvet, a few blocks northwest of the university, is a small butcher shop with bowler-hatted clerks selling good, inexpensive sandwiches to go for about 35 kr. Choose from ham, beef, or pork (Mon-Thu 8:00-17:30, Fri 8:00-18:00,

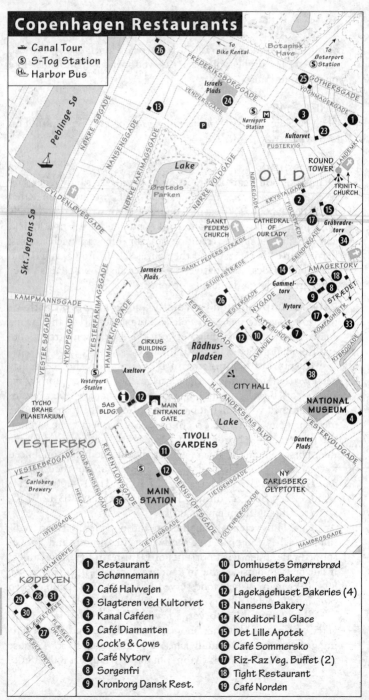

Copenhagen Restaurants

- Canal Tour
- S S-Tog Station
- Harbor Bus

1 Restaurant Schønnemann	10 Domhusets Smørrebrød
2 Café Halvvejen	11 Andersen Bakery
3 Slagteren ved Kultorvet	12 Lagekagehuset Bakeries (4)
4 Kanal Caféen	13 Nansens Bakery
5 Café Diamanten	14 Konditori La Glace
6 Cock's & Cows	15 Det Lille Apotek
7 Café Nytorv	16 Café Sommersko
8 Sorgenfri	17 Riz-Raz Veg. Buffet (2)
9 Kronborg Dansk Rest.	18 Tight Restaurant
	19 Café Norden

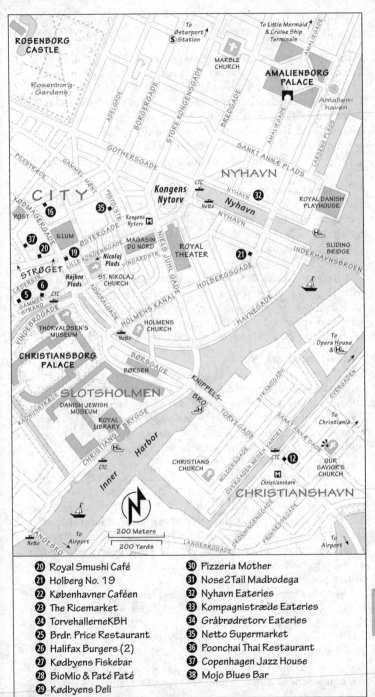

20 Royal Smushi Café
21 Holberg No. 19
22 Københavner Caféen
23 The Ricemarket
24 TorvehallerneKBH
25 Brdr. Price Restaurant
26 Halifax Burgers (2)
27 Kødbyens Fiskebar
28 BioMio & Paté Paté
29 Kødbyens Deli
30 Pizzeria Mother
31 Nose2Tail Madbodega
32 Nyhavn Eateries
33 Kompagnistræde Eateries
34 Gråbrødretorv Eateries
35 Netto Supermarket
36 Poonchai Thai Restaurant
37 Copenhagen Jazz House
38 Mojo Blues Bar

COPENHAGEN

Sat 8:00-15:00, closed Sun, just off Kultorvet square at #4 Frederiksborggade, look for gold bull's head hanging outside).

Near Christiansborg Palace

These eateries are good choices when sightseeing on Slotsholmen.

Kanal Caféen, on Frederiksholms Kanal across from Christiansborg Palace, serves lunch only and is a nice place for a traditional open-face sandwich. Inside, you'll rub elbows with locals in what feels like the cozy confines of a low-ceilinged, old sailing ship; outside you can dine right above the canal and watch the tour boats go by (60-90-kr sandwiches, Mon-Fri 11:30-17:00, Sat 11:30-15:00, closed Sun, Frederiksholms Kanal 18, tel. 33 11 57 70).

Café Diamanten serves open-face sandwiches, warm dishes, and salads—and pours microbrews from the tap. Take a seat inside the comfy café or under the parasols out front, with a view across the square to Thorvaldsen's Museum (65-95-kr sandwiches, Mon-Fri 10:00-20:30, Sat-Sun 10:00-19:00, Gammel Strand 50, tel. 33 93 55 45).

Burgers: **Cock's & Cows** is a trendy burger-and-cocktail bar with a happy, young vibe on an elegant street. Eat inside the brick-walled restaurant or in the courtyard out back (90-130-kr burgers—some piled almost ridiculously high, Sun-Thu 12:00-21:30, Fri-Sat 12:00-22:30, Gammel Strand 34, tel. 69 69 60 00).

Near Gammeltorv/Nytorv

Café Nytorv has pleasant outdoor seating on Nytorv (with cozy indoor tables available nearby) and a great deal on a *smørrebrød* sampler for about 200 kr—perfect for two people to share (if you smile, they'll serve it for dinner even though it's only on the lunch menu). This "Copenhagen City Plate" gives you a selection of the traditional sandwiches and extra bread on request (daily 9:00-22:00, Nytorv 15, tel. 33 11 77 06).

Sorgenfri offers a local experience in a dark, woody spot just off the Strøget (80-100 kr, Mon-Sat 11:00-20:45, Sun 12:00-18:00, Brolæggerstræde 8, tel. 33 11 58 80).

Or duck (literally) into **Kronborg Dansk Restaurant,** across the street from Sorgenfri, for finer-quality *smørrebrød* in a wood-beamed nautical setting (90-110-kr meat and fish sandwiches plus herring specialties, Mon-Sat 11:00-17:00, closed Sun, Brolæggerstræde 12, tel. 33 13 07 08).

Another option is **Domhusets Smørrebrød** (Mon-Fri 8:00-15:00, closed Sat-Sun, off the City Hall end of the Strøget at Kattesundet 18, tel. 33 15 98 98).

The Pølse

The famous Danish hot dog, sold in *pølsevogne* (sausage wagons) throughout the country, is another typically Danish institution that has resisted the onslaught of our global, prepackaged, fast-food culture. Study the photo menu for variations. These are fast, cheap, tasty, and, like their American cousins, almost worthless nutritionally. Even so, what the locals call the "dead man's finger" is the dog Danish kids love to bite.

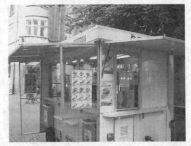

There's more to getting a *pølse* than simply ordering a "hot dog" (which in Copenhagen simply means a sausage with a bun on the side, generally the worst bread possible). The best is a *ristet* (or grilled) hot dog *med det hele* (with the works). Employ these other handy phrases: *rød* (red, the basic boiled weenie), *medister* (spicy, better quality), *knæk* (short, stubby, tastier than *rød*), *brød* (a bun, usually smaller than the sausage), *svøb* ("swaddled" in bacon), *Fransk* (French style, buried in a long skinny hole in the bun with sauce). *Sennep* is mustard and *ristet løg* are crispy, fried onions. Wash everything down with a *sodavand* (soda pop).

By hanging around a *pølsevogn,* you can study this institution. Denmark's "cold feet cafés" are a form of social care: People who have difficulty finding jobs are licensed to run these wiener-mobiles. As they gain seniority, they are promoted to work at more central locations. Danes like to gather here for munchies and *pølsesnak*—the local slang for empty chatter (literally, "sausage talk"). And traditionally, after getting drunk, guys stop here for a hot dog and chocolate milk on the way home—that's why the stands stay open until the wee hours.

For sausages a cut above (and from a storefront—not a cart), stop by the little grill restaurant **Andersen Bakery,** directly across the street from the train station (next to the Tivoli entrance). The menu is limited—either pork or veal/beef—but the ingredients are high-quality and the weenies are tasty (50-kr gourmet dogs, daily 7:00-19:00, Bernstorffsgade 5, tel. 33 75 07 35).

Picnics

Throughout Copenhagen, small delis *(viktualiehandler)* sell fresh bread, tasty pastries, juice, milk, cheese, and yogurt (drinkable, in tall liter boxes). Two of the largest supermarket chains are **Irma** (in the glassy DI—Danish Industry—building on Vesterbrogade next to Tivoli) and **Super Brugsen. Netto** is a cut-rate outfit with the cheapest prices and a good bakery section. And, of course, there's the ever-present **7-Eleven** chain, with branches seemingly on every corner; while you'll pay a bit more here, there's a reason they're called "convenience" stores—and they also serve pastries and hot dogs.

Pastry

The golden pretzel sign hanging over the door or windows is the Danes' age-old symbol for a bakery. Danish pastries, called *wienerbrød* ("Vienna bread") in Denmark, are named for the Viennese bakers who brought the art of pastry-making to Denmark, where the Danes say they perfected it. Try these bakeries: **Lagkagehuset** (multiple locations around town; the handiest options include one right in the train station, another nearby inside the TI, one along the Strøget at Frederiksborggade 21, and another on Torvegade just across from the Metro station in Christianshavn) and **Nansens** (on corner of Nansensgade and Ahlefeldtsgade, near Ibsens Hotel). **Emmerys**, a trendy, gluten-free, Starbucks-like organic bakery and café, has more than 20 branches around Copenhagen, and sells good pastries and sandwiches. For a genteel bit of high-class 1870s Copenhagen, pay a lot for a coffee and a fresh Danish at **Konditori La Glace,** just off the Strøget at Skoubogade 3.

RESTAURANTS

I've listed restaurants in four areas: the downtown core, the funky Christianshavn neighborhood across the harbor, near Nørreport, and in the trendy Meatpacking District behind the main train station.

In the Downtown Core

Det Lille Apotek ("The Little Pharmacy") is a reasonable, candlelit place. It's been popular with locals for 200 years, and today it's a hit with tourists. Their specialty is "Stone Beef," a big slab of tender, raw steak plopped down and cooked in front of you on a scalding-hot soapstone. Cut it into smaller pieces and it's cooked within minutes (traditional dinners for 125-190 kr, nightly from 17:30, just off the Strøget, between Frue Church and Round Tower at Store Kannikestræde 15, tel. 33 12 56 06).

Café Sommersko is a venerable eatery serving French-inspired Danish dishes in an elegant setting (125-165-kr lunches, 145-230-kr main courses, 300-kr three-course dinner, daily 11:00-22:30, Kronprinsensgade 6, tel. 33 14 81 89).

Riz-Raz Vegetarian Buffet has two locations in Copenhagen: around the corner from the canal boat rides at Kompagnistræde 20 (tel. 33 15 05 75) and across from Det Lille Apotek at Store Kannikestræde 19 (tel. 33 32 33 45). At both places, you'll find a healthy all-you-can-eat Middle Eastern/Mediterranean/vegetarian buffet lunch for 80 kr (cheese but no meat, great falafel, daily 11:30-16:00) and a bigger dinner buffet for 100 kr (16:00-24:00).

Use lots of plates and return to the buffet as many times as you like. Tap water is 11 kr per jug.

Tight resembles a trendy gastropub, serving an eclectic international array of food and drink (Canadian, Aussie, French, and burgers, with Danish microbrews) in a split-level maze of hip rooms that mix old timbers and brick with bright colors (150-200-kr main courses, 140-kr burgers, daily 17:00-22:00, just off the Strøget at Hyskenstræde 10, tel. 33 11 09 00).

Café Norden, very Danish with modern "world cuisine," good light meals, and fine pastries, is a big, venerable institution overlooking Amagertorv by the heron fountain. It's family-friendly, with good seats outside on the square, in the busy ground-floor interior, or with more space and better views upstairs (great people-watching from the window seats). Order at the bar—it's the same price upstairs or down. Consider their 185-kr Nordic tapa plate or their 170-kr "triple salad" (120-170-kr sandwiches and salads, 150-kr main courses, huge splittable portions, daily 9:00-24:00, Østergade 61, tel. 33 11 77 91).

Royal Smushi Café is a hit with dainty people who like the idea of small, gourmet, open-face sandwiches served on Royal Copenhagen porcelain. You can sit in their modern chandeliered interior or the quiet courtyard (3 little "smushi" sandwiches for 135 kr, Mon-Sat 10:00-19:00, Sun 10:00-18:00, next to Royal Copenhagen porcelain store at Amagertorv 6, tel. 33 12 11 22).

Holberg No. 19, a cozy American-run café with classic ambience, sits just a block off the tourist crush of the Nyhavn canal. With a loose, friendly, low-key vibe, it offers more personality and lower prices than the tourist traps along Nyhavn (no real kitchen but 65-95-kr salads and sandwiches, selection of wines and beers, order at the bar, Mon-Fri 8:00-22:00, Sat 10:00-20:00, Sun 10:00-18:00, Holberg 19, tel. 33 14 01 90).

Københavner Caféen, cozy and a bit tired, feels like a ship captain's dining room. The staff is enthusiastically traditional, serving local dishes and elegant open-face sandwiches for a good value. Lunch specials (80-100 kr) are served until 17:00, when the more expensive dinner menu kicks in (plates for 120-200 kr, daily, kitchen closes at 22:00, at Badstuestræde 10, tel. 33 32 80 81).

The Ricemarket, an unpretentious Asian fusion bistro, is buried in a modern cellar between the Strøget and Rosenborg Castle. It's a casual, more affordable side-eatery of a popular local restaurant, and offers a flavorful break from Danish food (65-95-kr small dishes, 115-185-kr big dishes, seven-dish family-style meal for 285 kr, daily 12:00-22:00, Hausergade 38 near Kultorvet, tel. 35 35 75 30).

Illum and **Magasin du Nord** department stores serve cheery, reasonable meals in their cafeterias. At Illum, eat outside at tables along the Strøget, or head to the elegant glass-domed top floor

(Østergade 52). Magasin du Nord (Kongens Nytorv 13) also has a great grocery and deli in the basement.

Also try **Café Nytorv** at Nytorv 15 or **Sorgenfri** at Brolægger-stræde 8 (both are described under *"Smørrebrød,"* earlier).

In Christianshavn

This neighborhood is a 10-minute walk across the bridge from the old center, or a 3-minute ride on the Metro. Choose one of my listings (for locations, see map on page 203), or simply wander the blocks between Christianshavns Torv, the main square, and the Christianshavn Canal—you'll find a number of lively neighborhood pubs and cafés.

Ravelinen Restaurant, on a tiny island on the big road 100 yards south of Christianshavn, serves traditional Danish food at reasonable prices to happy local crowds. Dine indoors or on the lovely lakeside terrace (which is tented and heated, so it's comfortable even on blustery evenings). This is like Tivoli without the kitsch and tourists. They offer a shareable "Cold Table" meal for 200 kr at lunch only (80-130-kr lunch dishes, 180-280-kr dinners, mid-April-late Dec daily 11:30-21:00, closed off-season, Torvegade 79, tel. 32 96 20 45).

Bastionen & Løven, at the little windmill (Lille Mølle), serves gourmet Danish nouveau cuisine with a French inspiration from a small but fresh menu, on a Renoir terrace or in its Rembrandt interior. The classiest, dressiest, and most gourmet of all my listings, this restaurant fills a classic old mansion. Reservations for indoor dining are required; they don't take reservations for outdoor seating, as weather is unpredictable (95-175-kr lunches, 200-kr dinners, 375-kr three-course meal; Tue-Sat 11:00-23:00, Sun 11:00-18:00, closed Mon; walk to end of Torvegade and follow ramparts up to restaurant, at south end of Christianshavn, Christianshavn Voldgade 50, tel. 31 34 09 40, www.bastionenloven.dk).

Lagkagehuset is everybody's favorite bakery in Christianshavn. With a big selection of pastries, sandwiches, excellent fresh-baked bread, and award-winning strawberry tarts, it's a great place for breakfast or picnic fixings (pastries for less than 20 kr, take-out coffee for 30 kr, daily 6:00-19:00, Torvegade 45). For other locations closer to the town center, see page 216 under "Pastry."

Ethnic Strip on Christianshavn's Main Drag: Torvegade, which is within a few minutes' walk of the Christianshavn Metro station, is lined with appealing and inexpensive ethnic eateries, including Italian, cheap kebabs, Thai, Chinese, and more. **Spicy Kitchen** serves cheap and good Indian food—tight and cozy, it's a hit with locals (80-kr plates, daily 17:00-23:00, Torvegade 56).

In Christiania: **Spiseloppen** ("The Flea Eats") is a wonderfully classy place in Christiania. It serves great 140-kr vegetarian meals and 175-250-kr meaty ones by candlelight. It's gourmet anarchy—a good fit for Christiania, the free city/squatter town (Tue-Sun 17:00-22:00, kitchen closes at 21:00, closed Mon, reservations often necessary Fri-Sat; 3 blocks behind spiral spire of Our Savior's Church, on top floor of old brick warehouse, turn right just inside Christiania's main gate, enter the wildly empty warehouse, and climb the graffiti-riddled stairs; tel. 32 57 95 58, http://spiseloppen.dk). Other, less-expensive Christiania eateries are listed on page 209.

Near Nørreport

TorvehallerneKBH is in a pair of modern, glassy market halls right on Israel Plads. Survey both halls and the stalls on the square before settling in. In addition to produce, fish, and meat stalls, it has several inviting food counters where you can sit to eat a meal, or grab something to go. I can't think of a more enjoyable place in Copenhagen to browse for a meal than this upscale food court (pricey but fun, with quality food; Tue-Thu 10:00-19:00, Fri 10:00-20:00, Sat 9:00-17:00, Sun 10:00-15:00, most places closed Mon; Frederiksborggade 21).

Brdr. Price Restaurant—an elegant, highly regarded bistro serving creative Danish and international meals just across from Rosenborg Castle—is good for a dressy splurge (150-250-kr main courses, daily 12:00-22:00, Rosenborggade 15, tel. 38 41 10 20, www.brdr-price.dk). They have a more formal, classic French-Danish restaurant downstairs.

Halifax, part of a small local chain, serves up "build-your-own" burgers, where you select a patty, a side dish, and a dipping sauce for your fries (120-135 kr, daily 12:00-22:00, Sun until 21:00, Frederiksborggade 35, tel. 33 32 77 11). They have another location just off the Strøget (at Larsbjørnsstræde 9).

In the Meatpacking District (Kødbyen)

Literally "Meat Town," Kødbyen is an old warehouse zone huddled up against the train tracks behind the main station. Danes raise about 25 million pigs a year (five per person), so there's long been lots of "meatpacking." Today, much of the meatpacking action is diners chowing down.

There are three color-coded sectors in the district—brown, gray, and white—and each one is a cluster of old industrial buildings. At the far end is the white zone (Den Hvide Kødby), which has been overtaken by some of the city's most trendy and enjoyable eateries, mingling with surviving offices and warehouses for the local meatpacking industry. All of the places I list here are within a few steps of each other (except for the Mother pizzeria, a block away).

COPENHAGEN

The curb appeal of this area is zilch (it looks like, well, a meatpacking district), but inside, these restaurants are bursting with life, creativity, and flavor. While youthful and trendy, this scene is also very accessible. Most of these eateries are in buildings with old white tile; this, combined with the considerable popularity of this area, can make the dining rooms quite loud. These places can fill up, especially on weekend evenings, when it's smart to reserve ahead.

It's a short stroll from the station: If you go south on the bridge called Tietgens Bro, which crosses the tracks just south of the station, and carry on for about 10 minutes, you'll run right into the area. Or you can ride the S-tog to the Dybbølsbro stop.

Kødbyens Fiskebar ("Fish Bar") is one of the first and still the most acclaimed restaurant in the Meatpacking District. Focusing on small, thoughtfully composed plates of modern Nordic seafood, the Fiskebar has a stripped-down white interior with a big fish tank and a long cocktail bar surrounded by smaller tables. It's extremely popular (reservations are essential), and feels a bit too trendy for its own good. While the prices are high, so is the quality; diners are paying for a taste of the "New Nordic" style of cooking that's so in vogue here (100-145-kr small plates, 200-245-kr main courses; open in summer daily from 18:00, in winter generally closed Sat-Sun; Flæsketorvet 100, tel. 32 15 56 56, http://fiskebaren.dk).

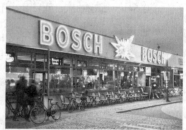

BioMio, in the old Bosch building, serves rustic Danish, vegan, and vegetarian dishes, plus meat and fish. It's 100-percent organic, and the young boss, Rune, actually serves diners (200-kr plates, daily 12:00-22:00, Halmtorvet 19, tel. 33 31 20 00, http://biomio.dk).

Paté Paté, next door to BioMio, is a tight, rollicking bistro in a former pâté factory. While a wine bar at heart—with a good selection of wines by the glass—it has a fun and accessible menu of creative modern dishes and a cozy atmosphere rare in the Meatpacking District. Ideally diners choose about three dishes per person and share (Mon-Sat from 17:30, closed Sun, Slagterboderne 1, tel. 39 69 55 57, www.patepate.dk).

Kødbyens Deli is this district's budget fast-food joint, serving chili, fish-and-chips, and burgers. You can take away or eat there on humble tables (70-kr plates, daily 17:00-21:00, facing Paté Paté at Slagterboderne 8, tel. 24 84 09 82).

Pizzeria Mother is named for the way the sourdough for their crust must be "fed" and cared for to flourish. You can taste that care in the pizza, which has a delicious tangy crust. Out front are comfortable picnic benches, while the interior curls around the busy pizza oven with chefs working globs of dough that will soon be the basis for your pizza (75-150-kr pizzas, daily 11:00-23:00, a block beyond the other restaurants listed here at Høkerboderne 9, tel. 22 27 58 98).

Nose2Tail Madbodega (*mad* means "food") prides itself on locally sourced, sustainable cooking, using the entire animal for your meal (hence the name). You'll climb down some stairs into an unpretentious white-tiled cellar (50-kr small plates, 70-180-kr large plates, Mon-Sat 18:00-24:00, closed Sun, Flæsketorvet 13A, tel. 33 93 50 45, http://nose2tail.dk).

Other Central Neighborhoods to Explore

To find a good restaurant, try simply window-shopping in one of these inviting districts.

Nyhavn's harbor canal is lined with a touristy strip of restaurants set alongside its classic sailboats. Here thriving crowds are served mediocre, overpriced food in a great setting. On any sunny day, if you want steak and fries (120 kr) and a 50-kr beer, this can be fun. On Friday and Saturday, the strip becomes the longest bar in the world.

Kompagnistræde is home to a changing cast of great little eateries. Running parallel to the Strøget, this street has fewer tourists and lower rent, and encourages places to compete creatively for the patronage of local diners.

Gråbrødretorv ("Grey Friars' Square") is perhaps the most popular square in the old center for a meal. It's like a food court, especially in good weather. Choose from Italian, French, or Danish. Two steakhouses are **Jensen's Bøfhus**, a kid-friendly chain (100-kr burgers, 120-220-kr main dishes), and the pricier but better **Bøf & Ost** (170-250-kr main dishes). **Skildpadden** ("The Turtle") is a student hit, with make-it-yourself sandwiches (70 kr, choose the type of bread, salami, and cheese you want) and a 60-kr salad bar, plus draft beer. It's in a cozy cellar with three little tables on the lively square (daily 10:00-20:00, Gråbrødretorv 9, tel. 33 13 05 06).

Istedgade and the surrounding streets behind the train station (just above the Meatpacking District) are home to an assortment of inexpensive ethnic restaurants. You will find numerous places serving kebabs, pizza, Chinese, and Thai (including tasty 65-130-kr meals at **Poonchai Thai Restaurant**—across the street from Hotel Nebo at Istedgade 1). The area can be a bit seedy, especially right behind the station, but walk a few blocks away to take your pick of inexpensive, ethnic eateries frequented by locals.

Starting or Ending Your Cruise in Copenhagen

If your cruise begins or ends in Copenhagen, you'll want some extra time here; for most travelers, at least a full day is a minimum for seeing the city's highlights. For a longer visit here, pick up my *Rick Steves Snapshot Copenhagen & the Best of Denmark* guidebook; for other nearby destinations, see my *Rick Steves Scandinavia* book.

Airport Connections

COPENHAGEN AIRPORT (KASTRUP)

Copenhagen's international airport is a traveler's dream, with a TI, baggage check, bank, ATMs, post office, shopping mall, grocery store, bakery, and more (airport code: CPH, airport info tel. 32 31 32 31, www.cph.dk). The three check-in terminals are within walking distance of each other (departures screens tell you which terminal to go to). On arrival, all flights feed into one big lobby in Terminal 3. When you pop out here, a TI kiosk is on your left, taxis are out the door on your right, trains are straight ahead, and shops and eateries fill the atrium above you. You can use dollars or euros at the airport, but you'll get change back in kroner.

Getting Between the Airport and Downtown

If you're spending the night in central Copenhagen before meeting your ship, your options for reaching your hotel include the Metro, trains, and taxis. There are also buses into town, but the train/Metro is generally better.

The **Metro** runs directly from the airport to Christianshavn, Kongens Nytorv (near Nyhavn), and Nørreport, making it the best choice for getting into town if you're staying in any of these areas (36-kr three-zone ticket, yellow M2 line, direction: Vanløse, 4-10/hour, 11 minutes to Christianshavn). The Metro station is located at the end of Terminal 3 and is covered by the roof of the terminal.

Convenient **trains** also connect the airport with downtown (36-kr three-zone ticket, covered by rail pass, 4/hour, 12 minutes). Buy your ticket from the ground-level ticket booth (look for *DSB: Tickets for Train, Metro & Bus* signs) before riding the escalator down to the tracks. Track 2 has trains going into the city (track 1 is for trains going east, to Sweden). Trains into town stop at the main train station (signed *København H;* handy if you're sleeping at my recommended hotels behind the train station), as well as the Nørreport and Østerport stations. At Nørreport, you can connect to the Metro for Kongens Nytorv (near Nyhavn) and Christianshavn.

With the train/Metro trip being so quick, frequent, and cheap, I see no reason to take a taxi. But if you do, **taxis** are fast, civil, accept credit cards, and charge about 250-300 kr for a ride to the town center.

Getting from Copenhagen Airport to Frihavnen or Oceankaj Ports

To reach either of these ports (where nearly all cruises that begin and end in Copenhagen dock), the easiest choice is to spring for a **taxi** (figure around 350-400 kr to either port).

It's much cheaper to take **public transportation,** though this option involves a train-to-bus transfer, making it less convenient for people with lots of luggage. From the airport, ride the train to Østerport Station, just one stop to the south (for details on taking the train from the airport, see "Getting Between the Airport and Downtown," earlier). After getting off at Østerport, hop on bus #26 to either cruise port (confirm with driver that the bus will stop at your port). To find the bus stop, exit the train station, turn left, and walk to the corner. The stop is across the busy street (for details on taking bus #26, see the sidebar on page 151).

Getting from Downtown to Frihavnen or Oceankaj Ports

If spending the night in Copenhagen before your trip, the easiest option for reaching either port is a **taxi** (200 kr or more from downtown).

Another option is to catch **bus #26** at various points downtown, including in front of the train station, near Rådhuspladsen (City Hall Square), and at Kongens Nytorv (near Nyhavn). Be aware that the bus splits into two different routes north of the city, so check with the driver that you're on a bus headed for your port. Also note that on weekends, you'll have to transfer at Østerport Station (for details on taking bus #26, see page 151).

If your ship is leaving from Frihavnen, you can take the **train** from either the main train station or the Nørreport Station (near some recommended hotels) to Nordhavn Station, then walk 10 minutes (a hassle if toting lots of luggage; for details, see page 153).

Hotels in Copenhagen

If you need a hotel in Copenhagen before or after your cruise, here are a few to consider. Note that big Copenhagen hotels have an exasperating pricing policy. Their high rack rates are actually charged only about 20 or 30 days a year—the rest of the time you'll probably pay less. Check hotel websites for deals. Prices include breakfast unless noted otherwise. All of these hotels are big and

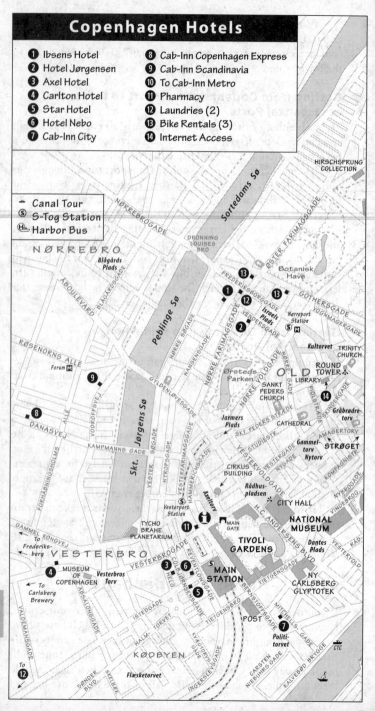

Copenhagen Hotels

1. Ibsens Hotel
2. Hotel Jørgensen
3. Axel Hotel
4. Carlton Hotel
5. Star Hotel
6. Hotel Nebo
7. Cab-Inn City
8. Cab-Inn Copenhagen Express
9. Cab-Inn Scandinavia
10. To Cab-Inn Metro
11. Pharmacy
12. Laundries (2)
13. Bike Rentals (3)
14. Internet Access

- Canal Tour
- S-Tog Station
- Harbor Bus

COPENHAGEN

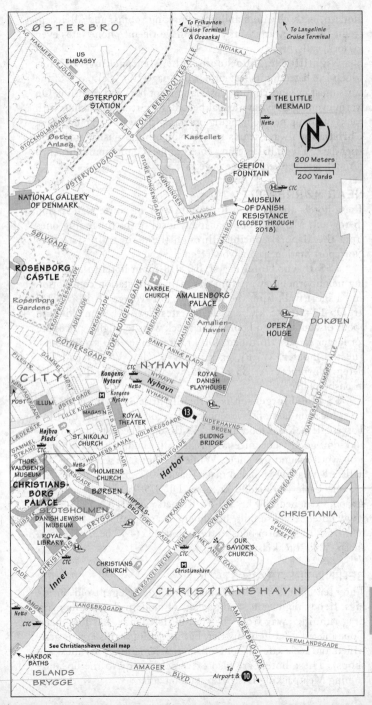

ØSTERBRO

To Frihavnen
Cruise Terminal
& Oceankaj

To Langelinie
Cruise Terminal

INDIAKAJ

DAG HAMMERSKJÖLDS ALLE

US
EMBASSY

ØSTERPORT
STATION

OSLO PLADS

FOLKE BERNADOTTES ALLE

THE LITTLE
MERMAID

STOCKHOLMSGADE

Østre
Anlaeg

Netto

Kastellet

N

200 Meters

ØSTERVOLDGADE

GRØNNINGEN

STORE KONGENSGADE

GEFION
FOUNTAIN

200 Yards

NATIONAL GALLERY
OF DENMARK

ESPLANADEN

CTC

AMALIEGADE

MUSEUM
OF DANISH
RESISTANCE
(CLOSED THROUGH
2018)

SØLVGADE

ROSENBORG
CASTLE

Rosenborg
Gardens

KRONPRINCESSEGADE

APELGADE

BORGERGADE

STORE KONGENSGADE

BREDGADE

MARBLE
CHURCH

AMALIEGADE

AMALIENBORG
PALACE

Amalien-
haven

OPERA
HOUSE

DOKØEN

PILESTR.

GOTHERSGADE

GAMMEL MØNT

SANKT ANNÆ PLADS

DANNESKIOLD-SAMSØS ALLE

CITY

Kongens
Nytorv

Netto

NYHAVN

CTC

NYHAVN

Nyhavn

NYHAVN

ROYAL
DANISH
PLAYHOUSE

KØBMAGERGADE

POST

ILLUM

ØSTERGADE

LILLE KONG.

NIELS JUEL

Kongens
Nytorv

MAGASIN

ROYAL
THEATER

HOLBERGSGADE

13

INDERHAVNS-
BROEN

LÆDERSTR.

Højbro
Plads

CTC

ST. NIKOLAJ
CHURCH

HOLMENS KANAL

GADE

HAVNEGADE

SLIDING
BRIDGE

THOR-
VALDSEN'S
MUSEUM

Gammel Strand

Netto

BØRSGADE

HOLMENS
CHURCH

Harbor

CHRISTIANS-
BORG
PALACE

DANISH JEWISH
MUSEUM

SLOTSHOLMEN

BØRSEN

KNIPPELS-
BRO-TORV.

STRANDGADE

PRINCESSEGADE

CHRISTIANIA

HAVGUS.

KNIPPELS-
BRO

GADE

OVERGADEN

PUSHER
STREET

ROYAL
LIBRARY

CTC

CHRISTIANS
CHURCH

OVERGADEN NEDEN VANDET

SANKT ANNÆ GADE

OUR
SAVIOR'S
CHURCH

CTC

CHRISTIAN

Inner

Christianshavn

CHRISTIANSHAVN

GADE

LANGE-
BRO

Netto

CTC

LANGEBROGADE

OVERGADEN OVEN VANDET

AMAGERBROGADE

VERMLANDSGADE

See Christianshavn detail map

HARBOR
BATHS

ISLANDS
BRYGGE

AMAGER BLVD.

To
Airport &

10

COPENHAGEN

modern, with elevators and non-smoking rooms, and all accept credit cards. Beware: Many hotels have rip-off phone rates even for local calls.

Nightlife Neighborhoods: The **Meatpacking District,** which I've listed for its restaurants (see page 219), is also one of the city's most up-and-coming destinations for bars and nightlife. On warm evenings, **Nyhavn** canal becomes a virtual nightclub, with packs of young people hanging out along the water, sipping beers. **Christiania** always seems to have something musical going on after dark. **Tivoli** has evening entertainment daily from mid-April through late September (see page 183).

NEAR NØRREPORT

These hotels are within a 10-minute walk of Nørreport Station (S-tog and Metro). Note that many local trains (including ones from the airport) continue through the main train station to Nørreport Station, saving you a transfer.

$$$ Ibsens Hotel is a stylish 118-room hotel in a charming neighborhood away from the main train station commotion and a short walk from the old center (on average Sb-1,145-1,245 kr, Db-1,145-1,445 kr, very slushy rates flex with demand—ask about discounts when booking or check website; higher prices are for larger rooms, third bed-400 kr, great bikes-150 kr/24 hours, guest computer, Wi-Fi, parking-185 kr/day, Vendersgade 23, S-tog: Nørreport, tel. 33 13 19 13, www.ibsenshotel.dk, hotel@ ibsenshotel.dk).

$$ Hotel Jørgensen is a friendly little 30-room hotel in a great location just off Nørreport, kitty-corner from the bustling TorvehallerneKBH food market. With some cheap, grungy rooms and some good-value, nicer rooms, it's a fine budget option, though a bit worn around the edges. While the lounge is welcoming, the halls are a narrow, tangled maze (basic S-475-525 kr, Sb-675-725 kr, very basic D-750-800 kr, nicer Db-875-950 kr, cheaper off-season, extra bed-200 kr, Wi-Fi, Rømersgade 11, tel. 33 13 81 86, www.hoteljoergensen.dk, hoteljoergensen@mail.dk). They also rent 175-200-kr dorm beds to those under 35 (4-12 beds per room, sheets-30 kr, breakfast-45 kr).

BEHIND THE TRAIN STATION

The area behind the train station mingles elegant old buildings, trendy nightspots, and pockets of modern sleaze. The main drag running away from the station, Istedgade, has long been Copenhagen's red-light district, but increasingly this area is gentrified and feels safe (in spite of the few remaining, harmless sex shops). These hotels are also extremely handy to the up-and-coming Meatpacking District restaurant zone.

COPENHAGEN

$$$ **Axel Hotel** and $$$ **Carlton Hotel,** operated by the Guldsmeden ("Dragonfly") company, have more character than most—a restful spa-like ambience decorated with imported Balinese furniture, and an emphasis on sustainability and organic materials. I've listed average prices, but rates can change dramatically, depending on when you book—check their website for the best deals (Axel: Sb-845-975 kr, Db-985-1,145 kr, breakfast-170 kr, 129 rooms, request a quieter back room overlooking the pleasant garden, guest computer, Wi-Fi, restful spa area with sauna and Jacuzzi-295 kr/person per stay, a block behind the train station at Helgolandsgade 7, tel. 33 31 32 66, booking@hotelguldsmeden. com; Carlton: a bit cheaper than Axel, 64 rooms, Vesterbrogade 66, tel. 33 22 15 00, carlton@hotelguldsmeden.com). They share a website: www.hotelguldsmeden.com.

$$ **Star Hotel** has 134 charmless, cookie-cutter rooms at reasonable prices. Rates vary with the season and online specials (Sb-700-1,300 kr, Db-875-1,555 kr but usually around 950-1,000 kr, some rates include breakfast—otherwise 85 kr, guest computer, Wi-Fi, nice courtyard out back, Colbjørnsensgade 13, tel. 33 22 11 00, www.copenhagenstar.dk, star@copenhagenstar.dk).

$$ **Hotel Nebo,** a secure-feeling refuge with a friendly welcome and 84 comfy rooms, is a half-block from the station (S-420 kr, Sb-620 kr, D-650-700 kr, Db-900-950 kr, most rates include breakfast—otherwise 65 kr, cheaper Oct-April, periodic online deals, extra bed-200 kr, guest computer, Wi-Fi, Istedgade 6, tel. 33 21 12 17, www.nebo.dk, nebo@nebo.dk).

A DANISH MOTEL 6

$$ **Cab-Inn** is a radical innovation and a great value, with several locations in Copenhagen: identical, mostly collapsible, tiny but comfy, cruise-ship-type staterooms, all bright, molded, and shiny, with TV, coffeepot, shower, and toilet. Each room has a single bed that expands into a twin-bedded room with one or two fold-down bunks on the walls. It's tough to argue with this kind of efficiency (general rates: teensy "economy" Sb-495 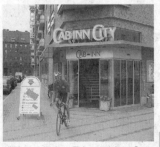 kr, Db-625 kr; still small "standard" Sb-545 kr, Db-675 kr, flip-down bunk Tb-805 kr; larger "commodore" Sb-645 kr, Db-775 kr; relatively gigantic "captain's" Sb-745 kr, Db-875; larger family rooms also available, breakfast-70 kr, easy parking-60 kr, guest computer, Wi-Fi, www.cabinn.com). The best of the bunch is **Cab-Inn City,** with 350 rooms and a great central location (a short

What If I Miss My Boat?

Remember that you can get help from the cruise line's port agent (listed on the destination information sheet distributed on the ship) or the local TI (see page 155). If the port agent suggests a costly solution (such as a private car with a driver), you may want to consider public transit.

To reach **Oslo,** you could hop on the night boat (DFDS, tel. 33 42 30 10, www.dfdsseaways.us). Otherwise, you can take the train; in addition to Oslo, trains run regularly to **Stockholm, Berlin** (a 3-hour connection to **Warnemünde**), **Amsterdam,** and **Brussels** (a 1.5-hour connection to **Zeebrugge**). For other points in **Norway,** connect through Oslo; for **Gdańsk,** you'll connect through Berlin. To look up specific connections, use www.bahn.com.

For some destinations, it may be best to take a **plane.** Copenhagen's airport, is easily reached by train from downtown (for airport details, see page 222).

Local **travel agents** in Copenhagen can help you sort through your options. For more advice on what to do if you miss the boat, see page 139.

walk south of the main train station and Tivoli at Mitchellsgade 14, tel. 33 46 16 16, city@cabinn.com). Two more, nearly identical Cab-Inns are a 15-minute walk northwest of the station: **Cab-Inn Copenhagen Express** (86 rooms, Danasvej 32, tel. 33 21 04 00, express@cabinn.com) and **Cab-Inn Scandinavia** (201 rooms, some quads, Vodroffsvej 55, tel. 35 36 11 11, scandinavia@cabinn.com). The newest and largest is **Cab-Inn Metro,** near the Ørestad Metro station (710 rooms, some quads, on the airport side of town at Arne Jakobsens Allé 2, tel. 32 46 57 00, metro@cabinn.com).

Danish Survival Phrases

The Danes tend to say words quickly and clipped. In fact, many short vowels end in a "glottal stop"—a very brief vocal break immediately following the vowel. While I haven't tried to indicate these in the phonetics, you can listen for them in Denmark...and (try to) imitate.

Three unique Danish vowels are æ (sounds like the *e* in "egg"), ø (sounds like the German *ö*—purse your lips and say "oh"), and *å* (sounds like the *o* in "bowl"). The letter *r* is not rolled—it's pronounced farther back in the throat, almost like a *w*. A *d* at the end of a word sounds almost like our *th*; for example, *mad* (food) sounds like "math." In the phonetics, ī sounds like the long *i* sound in "light," and bolded syllables are stressed.

English	Danish	Pronunciation
Hello. (formal)	Goddag.	goh-**day**
Hi. / Bye. (informal)	Hej. / Hej-hej.	hī / hī-hī
Do you speak English?	Taler du engelsk?	**tay**-lehr doo **eng**-elsk
Yes. / No.	Ja. / Nej.	yah / nī
Please. (May I?)*	Kan jeg?	kahn yī
Please. (Can you?)*	Kan du?	kahn doo
Please. (Would you?)*	Vil du?	veel doo
Thank you (very much).	(Tusind) tak.	(**too**-sin) tack
You're welcome.	Selv tak.	sehl tack
Can I help (you)?	Kan jeg hjælpe (dig)?	kahn yī **yehl**-peh (dī)
Excuse me. (to pass)	Undskyld mig.	**oon**-skewl mī
Excuse me. (Can you help me?)	Kan du hjælpe mig?	kahn doo **yehl**-peh mī
(Very) good.	(Meget) godt.	(**mī**-ehl) goht
Goodbye.	Farvel.	fah-**vehl**
one / two	en / to	een / toh
three / four	tre / fire	tray / feer
five / six	fem / seks	fehm / sehks
seven / eight	syv / otte	syew / **oh**-deh
nine / ten	ni / ti	nee / tee
hundred	hundred	**hoo**-nuh
thousand	tusind	**too**-sin
How much?	Hvor meget?	vor **mī**-ehl
local currency: (Danish) crown	(Danske) kroner	(**dahn**-skeh) **kroh**-nah
Where is...?	Hvor er...?	vor ehr
...the toilet	...toilettet	toy-**leh**-teht
men	herrer	**hehr**-ah
women	damer	**day**-mah
water / coffee	vand / kaffe	van / **kah**-feh
beer / wine	øl / vin	uhl / veen
Cheers!	Skål!	skohl
Can I have the bill?	Kan jeg få regningen?	kahn yī foh **rī**-ning-ehn

*Because Danish has no single word for "please," they approximate that sentiment by asking "May I?", "Can you?", or "Would you?", depending on the context.

STOCKHOLM
Sweden

Sweden Practicalities

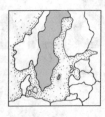

Scandinavia's heartland, Sweden (Sverige) is far bigger than Denmark and far flatter than Norway (174,000 square miles—just larger than California). This family-friendly land is home to Ikea, Volvo, ABBA, and long summer vacations at red-painted, white-trimmed summer cottages. Today's population numbers 9.7 million people. Once the capital of blond, Sweden is now home to a huge mix of immigrants. The majority of ethnic Swedes are nominally Lutheran. A mountain range and several islands separate Sweden's heavily forested landscape from Norway.

Money: 7 Swedish kroner (kr, officially SEK) = about $1. An ATM is called a *bankomat*. The local VAT (value-added sales tax) rate is 25 percent; the minimum purchase eligible for a VAT refund is 200 kr (for details on refunds, see page 134).

Language: The native language is Swedish. For useful phrases, see page 299.

Emergencies: Dial 112 for police, medical, or other emergencies. In case of theft or loss, see page 125.

Time Zone: Sweden is on Central European Time (the same as most of the Continent, and six/nine hours ahead of the East/West Coasts of the US). That puts Stockholm one hour behind Helsinki, Tallinn, and Rīga; and two hours behind St. Petersburg.

Embassies in Stockholm: The **US embassy** is at Dag Hammarskjölds Väg 31 (tel. 08/783-4375, http://stockholm.us embassy.gov). The **Canadian embassy** is at Klarabergsgatan 23 (tel. 08/453-3000, www.canadaemb.se). Call ahead for passport services.

Phoning: Sweden's country code is 46; to call from another country to Sweden, dial the international access code (011 from the US/Canada, 00 from Europe, or + from a mobile phone), then 46, followed by the area code (without initial zero) and the local number. For calls within Sweden, dial just the number if you are calling locally, and add the area code if calling long distance. To place an international call from Sweden, dial 00, the code of the country you're calling (1 for US and Canada), and the phone number. For more help, see page 1146.

Tipping: A gratuity is included in the price of sit-down meals, so you don't need to tip further. But for great service, round up your bill—no more than 10 percent. Tip a taxi driver by rounding up the fare a bit (pay 90 kr on an 85-kr fare). For more tips on tipping, see page 138.

Tourist Information: www.visitsweden.com

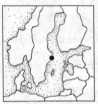

STOCKHOLM

One-third water, one-third parks, one-third city, on the sea, surrounded by woods, bubbling with energy and history, Sweden's stunning capital is green, clean, and underrated.

The city is built on an archipelago of islands connected by bridges. Its location midway along the Baltic Sea made it a natural port, vital to the economy and security of the Swedish peninsula. In the 1500s, Stockholm became a political center when Gustav Vasa established the monarchy (1523). A century later, the expansionist King Gustavus Adolphus made it an influential European capital. The Industrial Revolution brought factories and a flood of farmers from the countryside. In the 20th century, the fuming smokestacks were replaced with steel-and-glass Modernist buildings housing high-tech workers and an expanding service sector.

Today, with more than two million people in the greater metropolitan area (one in five Swedes), Stockholm is Sweden's largest city, as well as its cultural, educational, and media center. It's also the country's most ethnically diverse city. Despite its size, Stockholm is committed to limiting its environmental footprint. Development is strictly monitored, and pollution-belching cars must pay a toll to enter the city.

For the visitor, Stockholm offers both old and new. Explore Europe's best-preserved old warship and relax on a scenic harbor boat tour. Browse the cobbles and antique shops of the lantern-lit Old Town. Take a trip back in time at Skansen, Europe's first and best open-air folk museum. Marvel at Stockholm's glittering City Hall, slick shopping malls, and art museums.

While progressive and sleek, Stockholm respects its heritage. In summer, military bands parade daily through the heart of town

---

Excursions from Stockholm

Stockholm, a large and spread-out city, can be challenging to see in a hurry. If your sightseeing is focused, you can do it on your own—but a cruise-line excursion can help you get a good overview. Excursions within Stockholm may include bus or canal-boat trips in town; a walking tour of Gamla Stan (the Old Town); a panoramic visit to Fjällgatan (a scenic viewpoint in Södermalm, just above the cruise port); and/or tours of the Vasa Museum, City Hall, or Royal Palace. Less appealing are the visits to the Ice Bar (one of many such touristy ventures in Scandinavia) and the Ericsson Globe Arena (a gigantic, spherical sports arena with "SkyView" observation pods offering distant views of Stockholm). Jewish-themed tours of the city generally include stops in Gamla Stan, the Great Synagogue, and the Holocaust Monument. There's also a "rooftop walk" along the ridgeline of a building on the downtown island of Riddarholmen. Bike tours around Djurgården may entice you, but it's easy to rent your own bike, pick up a free map, and tour the island on your own.

Out of town, options include the grand **Drottningholm Palace** (impressive and described on page 278, but time-consuming to reach—Copenhagen has similar palaces that are easier to see), **Sigtuna** (a historic and touristy small town with traditional architecture), **Lake Mälaren** (the huge lake just west of Stockholm—less beautiful and far less convenient than the archipelago your cruise ship will sail through in the opposite direction), and **Haga Park** (another garden-and-palace ensemble, but second-rate after Drottningholm). While some of these—particularly Drottningholm—could be well worth your while on a longer visit, with a short day in port I'd stick to Stockholm proper.

---

to the Royal Palace, announcing the Changing of the Guard and turning even the most dignified tourist into a scampering kid.

PLANNING YOUR TIME

Stockholm is a spread-out city with a diverse array of sightseeing choices scattered across several islands. Because sailing all the way through the archipelago takes lots of time, most cruises leave Stockholm hours earlier than other ports of call. Your time here will be rushed compared to other ports. On a short, one-day cruise visit, you'll have to be selective. Here are your basic options:

• **Gamla Stan (Old Town):** Follow my self-guided stroll through the historic (if touristy) core of town, allowing about an hour. Add an hour to also tour the Nobel Museum, or 1-2 hours for the sights at the Royal Palace (depending on which sights you see, and how long you stay). If your timing is right, you can catch the Changing of the Guard—or even just the parade through town (begins summer Mon-Sat at 11:45, reaches palace at 12:15, one hour later on Sun; not every day off-season).

STOCKHOLM

• **Djurgården:** Stockholm's lush park island has three great sights that could easily gobble up a day: The Vasa Museum, Sweden's single most-visited sight, is tops for the chance to see an astonishingly well-preserved 17th-century warship (allow 1.5-2 hours). The Nordic Museum traces local history (allow 1-2 hours). And Skansen is Europe's original open-air folk museum (allow 2 hours). These time estimates are the minimum for a brief but meaningful visit; if you delve into details, any of these could consume hours. On a nice day, you could also rent a bike for a 1.5-hour spin around the island.

• **Modern City:** My self-guided walk leads you through the hardworking urban core of town in about 1.5 hours. It may not be particularly charming, but this is ground zero for shoppers.

• **City Hall:** Touring Stockholm's City Hall is worthwhile, but its location (on a different island beyond the train station, about a 15-minute walk from either the station or Gamla Stan) makes it tougher to squeeze into a tightly scheduled day in port. Once there, allow an hour for the required tour, plus another hour (including the walk up and down, plus possible waiting time) if you want to climb the tower.

• **Outlying Sights:** If you've already seen Stockholm's biggies or are in town for more than a short port visit (i.e., your cruise begins or ends here), you could visit Drottningholm Palace. You'll need to allow about an hour of travel time each way, plus an hour for the guided tour, and at least another hour to explore the grounds—a total of four hours minimum. Another option is the sculpture park at Millesgården (allow about 1.5 hours round-trip travel time, plus at least an hour to see the sculptures—a total of 2.5 hours minimum). Taking a boat trip through Stockholm's archipelago makes little sense, since you'll see much the same scenery as you sail into and/or out of the city.

The Best Plan: Choose either the Djurgården sights or Gamla Stan, or squeeze in a few items from each.

When planning your day, think carefully through your transportation options. Public transit is expensive, and taxis are even more so (especially if you get ripped off—for tips on avoiding this, see page 247). But there are several different ways to connect any two points: Consider the subway (T-bana), buses, trams, and the often-overlooked boats that shuttle passengers strategically between visit-worthy points (such as the one that connects Djurgården and Gamla Stan). The hop-on, hop-off harbor boat tours can also help you get around efficiently.

The Port of Stockholm

Arrival at a Glance: From **Stadsgården's** berth 167, the hop-on, hop-off boat is a handy way to reach both Djurgården and Gamla Stan; otherwise, you can walk to Gamla Stan in about 30 minutes; from Stadsgården's berth 160, it's an easy 15-minute walk to Slussen and across the bridge to Gamla Stan. From **Frihamnen,** the best plan is to take bus #76 to Djurgården or Gamla Stan.

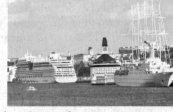

From either port, if your cruise line offers a shuttle bus, consider taking it downtown.

Port Overview

Stockholm has two main port areas: **Stadsgården** and **Frihamnen.** Stadsgården is used mainly for ships that are just stopping for the day, while cruises that begin or end in Stockholm typically use Frihamnen. A few small ships (or big ships dropping anchor and using tenders) may occasionally dock right along the embankment of **Gamla Stan;** as this is right in the center of the city (and arrivals here are both easy and rare), I haven't described it in detail.

Stadsgården: This embankment stretches along the northern edge of the island called Södermalm, which faces the city center across the water. It's dominated by the Viking Line Terminal, a hub for overnight boats to Helsinki. The cruise-ship berths (160 and 167) flank the terminal. Everything here is within walking distance of town. For more about Stadsgården, see page 239.

Frihamnen: This sprawling port is about three miles northeast of the city center. It's used by cruise ships as well as industrial ships and overnight ferries to Helsinki, Tallinn, St. Petersburg, Rīga, and other places. That means it's a large and potentially confusing area at first glance. Fortunately, most cruises use one section of the port, and bus connections into town are fairly straightforward. For more about Frihamnen, see page 241.

Tourist Information: TI kiosks (with bus tickets, city guides, and maps) open at both cruise ports when ships arrive, and remain open for about three hours.

GETTING INTO TOWN

First I'll cover the options that work from either Stadsgården or Frihamnen: cruise-line shuttle buses, tours, and taxis. Then I'll give directions for getting to town on foot and/or public transportation from each port.

By Cruise-Line Shuttle Bus

From both ports, many cruise lines offer shuttle buses into Stockholm. While these can be pricey (about 100 kr round-trip), they can be convenient. And, given the expense of public transit in Stockholm (even a basic one-way bus or subway ride costs about $5), the shuttle can be a good value.

Cruise-line shuttles generally drop off along the waterfront side of the Opera House, facing the Royal Palace and Gamla Stan across the harbor. From this point, here are your options:

• To reach **Gamla Stan,** simply cross the bridge, and you'll find yourself directly below the Royal Palace.

• To reach **Djurgården** (and the Vasa Museum), first walk up the big, long park (called Kungsträdgården) that runs alongside the Opera House. At the top end of the square, cross one lane of traffic behind the TGI Friday's to reach the tram stop. Take tram #7 going to the right (direction: Djurgården/Waldemarsudde), which takes you straight to Djurgården. Get off after crossing the bridge, at the Nordiska museet/Vasamuseet stop.

• My **"Stockholm Modern City"** self-guided walk begins from Kungsträdgården, the big park right around the corner from where the shuttle drops you off.

By Tour

At either cruise port, you'll be met by **hop-on, hop-off tour buses** that make a circuit around the city. From Stadsgården, you'll also see **hop-on, hop-off boats.** Both types of tours are operated by competing companies that offer similar trips (for details, see page 248).

For information on local tour options in Stockholm—including local guides for hire, walking tours, and bus tours—see "Tours in Stockholm" on page 248.

By Taxi

Taxis meet arriving cruise ships, but many overcharge. Taxis can charge whatever rates they want; one taxi can literally charge triple what the next one does. Before hopping in a cab, check the rates (posted in the back window) and read my advice on page 247 to be sure you get a fair fare. Here are the suggested one-way rates for likely journeys:

From **Stadsgården** (taxis wait in the big parking lot outside the Viking Line Terminal), here are approximate rates: to Gamla Stan—115 kr; to City Hall—150 kr; to the Vasa Museum (across the harbor, at Djurgården)—190 kr.

From **Frihamnen,** these are roughly the rates you should be charged: to the Vasa Museum (at Djurgården)—150 kr; and to Gamla Stan or City Hall—235 kr.

Other Options from Stadsgården to Town

Arriving at Stadsgården, everything is within walking distance of town. But if you dock at the more distant **berth 167** (on the far side of the Viking Line Terminal), it's a long 30-minute walk to Gamla Stan, making other transit options worth considering. The best plan depends on where you'd like to go in town. If you're heading for Djurgården (with the Vasa Museum), the hop-on, hop-off sightseeing boat may be your best option. But if you want to head for the modern city center (Kungsträdgården park), consider the cruise-line shuttle bus.

From **berth 160** (at the near side of the Viking Line Terminal), it's a short 15-minute walk to Gamla Stan, where you can start exploring or hop a harbor ferry to Djurgården (with the Vasa Museum). Hop-on, hop-off sightseeing boats also stop nearby.

For services available at the port, see the sidebar.

By Foot and/or Public Transportation

To get just about anywhere you'll want to go in the city, your first goal is Slussen, an underground hub for subway (T-bana) and bus lines, located at the west end of the Stadsgården embankment. Slussen will be a gloomy, huge, and messy construction site for the next few years, but will remain open. From Slussen, it's just a five-minute walk across the bridge to Gamla Stan. Once in Gamla Stan, many sights in downtown Stockholm are within walking distance. Boats leave from Gamla Stan for Djurgården (Vasa Museum, Nordic Museum, and Skansen).

Here are instructions for walking from either berth into town, and for reaching the bus stop:

From the Port to Slussen: As you exit **berth 167,** you'll see three color-coded lines painted on the pavement. The red and yellow lines lead left, to the dock for convenient **hop-on, hop-off sightseeing boats.** The blue line leads right, to the exit from the port area.

To head toward town, follow the blue line and exit the port gate, then continue along past the small **TI kiosk, taxi stands,** and the stops for the **hop-on, hop-off bus tours.** On your right is the huge Viking Line Terminal; a handy though infrequent shuttle runs to the train station from here (see posted schedule, 40 kr).

Continue past the terminal and up the slight incline. At the first traffic light, if you want to take a public bus, make a sharp left turn and walk along the viaduct (with the port area and parking garage just below you on the left) to reach the bus stop (see "Bus Options," later). Otherwise, continue straight through the traffic light, between the port and the busy road.

After a few minutes, you'll pass **berth 160.** (It's right next to the red-brick Fotografiska, a photography museum with excellent

Services at the Port of Stadsgården

A TI kiosk opens during ship arrivals near berth 167. The hub for other services is the Viking Line Terminal building, next to berth 167; inside you'll find WCs, an ATM, lockers, Internet access, and an automated pharmacy vending machine labeled *Mini Apotek*. For a real pharmacy, you'll have to head into the city (see "Medical Help" on page 244).

rotating exhibits, open daily, www.fotografiska.eu.) At the small boat dock just past the museum building, there's another stop for the **hop-on, hop-off sightseeing boat.** From this point, it's about another 10 minutes on foot—past the Birka Cruises terminal (serving a party cruise to Finland)—along the waterfront to Slussen.

Bus Options: A bus stop (called "Londonviadukten") connects Stadsgården to Slussen and points beyond, though it's inconveniently located on a busy road above the port area. But if you want to use it, here are your options (buy a ticket at the TI kiosk; you can't get one on the bus):

Any bus starting with #4 (such as #401) zips directly to the Slussen stop, under the bridge to Gamla Stan (just find the stairs up to Gamla Stan) and the Slussen subway/T-bana stop, with connections throughout the city.

Bus #53 (5-8/hour Mon-Fri, 3-4/hour Sat-Sun) loops up through the fun Södermalm area, then goes past Slussen and along the west side of Gamla Stan to the train station, and finally up to Odenplan.

Bus #71 (2/hour) begins the same way, then goes along the eastern edge of Gamla Stan and ends near Kungsträdgården (the starting point of my self-guided walk through the modern city).

From Slussen to Other Points in Stockholm: Slussen has a subway (T-bana) and bus station, with connections around the city (including the train station, T-Centralen).

Approaching Slussen on foot from the cruise ports, you'll see the T-bana and bus lines beneath the huge underpass. But due to heavy traffic, the easiest way to reach them is from above: First, bear right and uphill along the ramp to the bridge. Once at the bridge, turn left and walk up to the base of the big elevator; here you'll find stairs down to the T-bana and bus station. Or turn right on the bridge, to reach Gamla Stan and the embankment with ferries across the harbor to Djurgården.

By Hop-On, Hop-Off Sightseeing Boat

These boats (which stop near both berths at Stadsgården) are likely the easiest, most affordable, and all-around best solution for getting around town—particularly from berth 167. Departing right from the dock where you exit your cruise ship (follow yellow- and red-painted lines on the pavement), the boats make a handy circle to stops you'll likely want to visit: Slussen/Gamla Stan, the Royal Palace, Nybro harbor, the Vasa Museum, the modern art museum of Skeppsholmen Island, and Gröna Lund amusement park (on Djurgården). Competing companies run virtually the same one-hour route with tape-recorded narration (2-3 boats/hour, May-mid-Sept; see page 249 for details). This can be a great value if it connects the places you want to visit. For example, you could ride the boat from the cruise dock to Djurgården; then from Djurgården to Gamla Stan; then from Gamla Stan back to your awaiting ship.

Other Options from Frihamnen to Town

Frihamnen is a huge port just over a wooded hill from downtown Stockholm. Large and potentially confusing, it's used by cruise ships as well as industrial ships and overnight Baltic ferries. Fortunately, most cruise ships use one of three berths in one section of the port (indicated on the free welcome map for tourists): **berth 638,** at the end of a gigantic pier, is the main berth (and the only one with a dedicated termi-

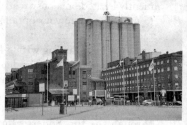

nal building); **berth 650,** on the pier across the water from berth 638; or **berth 634,** sharing the same pier as berth 638, but situated closer to land. For services available at the port, see the sidebar.

By Public Bus

Regardless of which Frihamnen berth you arrive at, you'll use the same stop for the public bus into town. It's along the road that skirts the port, near the red-and-white TI booth, which sells bus tickets—just follow the blue line painted on the ground. (See below for specific directions from each berth to the bus stop.)

Bus #76 is the most convenient, passing several major sights in town (4-7/hour Mon-Fri, 2-3/hour Sat, none Sun). Stops include Djurgårdsbron (at the bridge a short walk from the Vasa Museum and other Djurgården sights), Nybroplan, Kungsträdgården (near the Opera House and the start of my self-guided walk through the modern city), Slottsbacken (by the palace in Gamla Stan), Räntmästartrappan (at the southern end of Gamla Stan), Slussen, then through Södermalm and back the way it came. The only catch is the limited frequency on weekends—especially on Sunday—when you may be better off on bus #1.

Bus #1 is less convenient, cutting across the top of Östermalm

Services at the Port of Frihamnen

The cruise terminal building is at berth 638, marked **Stockholm Cruise Center** (a.k.a. Kryssningsterminal). Inside you'll find a user-friendly TI (with maps, Stockholm Cards, and bus tickets), WCs, and a gift shop, but no ATMs. They have free Wi-Fi, making it a popular place to hang out until last call (the password is posted on the wall). Otherwise, here are your options:

ATMs: The handiest one is inside the Frihamnsterminalen building, at the base of the pier. Just ride up the escalator.

Tourist Information: In addition to the TI inside the Stockholm Cruise Center, you'll find a TI window, dispensing maps and selling bus tickets, in the little red shed with white trim next to the bus stop.

Supermarket: While not particularly handy for the port, if you need to stock up on groceries, there's an **ICA Kvantum** supermarket a dreary 10-minute walk from the port entrance. To find it from the main pier and Frihamnsterminalen, go straight out and bear right with the road; continue as the road goes up and crosses an overpass; as you crest the hill, look over the parking lot on your right to see the supermarket (at Malmvägen 13).

and Norrmalm to the train station (every 5-8 minutes daily).

Bus Tickets: You can't buy tickets on board, so be sure to get them before you reach the stop. You can buy a ticket at the TI inside the terminal at berth 638 or at the booth near the bus stop. There's also a machine at the bus stop. It takes credit cards, but getting the correct ticket can be tricky: First, select English. Then choose "Purchase and Load Tickets," then "All Tickets." Now you'll have to arrow down (past several choices you don't want) to either "Zone A Ticket Full" (for a single ride, 36 kr) or "24 Hours Ticket Full" (for an all-day ticket covering buses, subway, and boats, 115 kr).

From Berth 638: To reach the bus stop, follow the blue line on the pavement for the 10-minute walk to the base of the pier; you'll pass (on the right) the Frihamnsterminalen—the terminal building for Tallink Silja and St. Peter Line ships. Inside and up the escalator, you'll find an ATM (labeled *Uttagsautomat*) and WCs. From this terminal building, cross the street and turn left to reach the TI window, and just beyond it, the bus stop; along this street, you'll also find stops for **hop-on, hop-off buses.**

From Berth 650: You'll exit the port gate at a red-and-white souvenir stand. Follow the blue line out of the parking lot, and turn right at the road. Ahead on the left, you'll pass the bus stop for buses #76 and #1, and just beyond it, a TI kiosk where you can buy a bus ticket. If you kept going on this road, you'd pass the Frihamnsterminalen (described on previous page; ATM upstairs) on the right.

From Berth 634: This one's simple: Just head straight down the pier, and you'll run right into the bus stop and TI, across the street.

RETURNING TO YOUR SHIP

Stadsgården: You can **walk** back here from Gamla Stan—you can see your ship in the distance—though leave yourself plenty of time for the relatively long distance (figure about 15 minutes to berth 160, and 30 minutes to berth 167).

If you ride back to berth 167 by **public bus,** get off at the stop called Londonviadukten. Buses serving this stop include #53 (from the train station, or from the embankment on the west side of Gamla Stan); and bus #71 (from the Opera House or Gamla Stan's eastern embankment). Both buses circle high above the port on Södermalm, then loop down to the Londonviadukten stop. From here, you'll walk along the busy road back toward town to reach the ramp leading down to the port area. (Note: Do not take buses starting with #4 from Slussen; while these work going *from* the port *to* Slussen, they go back along a different route.) There's no point taking a bus to return to berth 160, as the Londonviadukten bus stop is a 15-minute walk away—you're better off returning to Slussen and walking from there.

Frihamnen: From several points in town (see list of stops earlier), you can take **public bus** #76 or #1. Get off at the Frihamnen stop (closer to berth 650) or—if you're on bus #76—stay on one more stop to "Magasin 3," which drops you directly in front of the red-brick Frihamnsterminalen building. Then walk up the pier to the right of that building to reach berths 634 and 638, both on the right-hand side of the pier.

See page 291 for help if you miss your boat.

Stockholm

Greater Stockholm's two million residents live on 14 islands woven together by 54 bridges. Visitors need only concern themselves with these districts, most of which are islands:

Norrmalm is downtown, with many hotels and shopping areas, and the combined train and bus station. **Östermalm,** to the east, is more residential.

Kungsholmen, the mostly suburban island across from Norrmalm, is home to City Hall and inviting lakefront eateries.

Gamla Stan is the Old Town island of winding, lantern-lit

STOCKHOLM

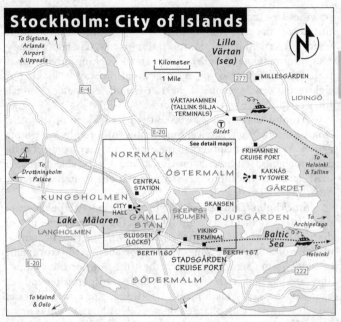

Stockholm: City of Islands

To Sigtuna, Arlanda Airport & Uppsala

Lilla Värtan (sea)

1 Kilometer

1 Mile

277 ■ MILLESGÅRDEN

LIDINGÖ

E-4

VÄRTAHAMNEN (TALLINK SILJA TERMINALS)

Ⓣ Gärdet

E-20

See detail maps

FRIHAMNEN CRUISE PORT

To Helsinki & Tallinn

NORRMALM

ÖSTERMALM

KAKNÄS TV TOWER

GÄRDET

To Drottningholm Palace

CENTRAL STATION

KUNGSHOLMEN

CITY HALL

SKEPPS-HOLMEN

SKANSEN

DJURGÅRDEN

Lake Mälaren

GAMLA STAN

To Archipelago

LÅNGHOLMEN

SLUSSEN (LOCKS)

VIKING TERMINAL

Baltic Sea

To Helsinki

BERTH 160

BERTH 167

E-20

STADSGÅRDEN CRUISE PORT

222

SÖDERMALM

To Malmö & Oslo

streets, antiques shops, and classy cafés clustered around the Royal Palace. The adjacent **Riddarholmen** is similarly atmospheric, but much sleepier. The locks between Lake Mälaren (to the west) and the Baltic Sea (to the east) are at a junction called **Slussen,** just south of Gamla Stan on the way to Södermalm.

Skeppsholmen is the small, central, traffic-free park/island with the Museum of Modern Art.

Djurgården is the park-island—Stockholm's wonderful green playground, with many of the city's top sights (bike rentals just over bridge as you enter island).

Södermalm, just south of the other districts, is sometimes called "Stockholm's Brooklyn"—young, creative, and trendy. Apart from its fine views and some good eateries, this residential island may be of less interest to those on a quick visit.

Orientation to Stockholm

TOURIST INFORMATION

Stockholm has two TI organizations, one far better than the other. The helpful city-run TI—called **Visit Stockholm**—has two branches. The main office is downtown in the Kulturhuset, facing Sergels Torg (Mon-Fri 9:00-19:00—until 18:00 off-season, Sat 9:00-16:00, Sun 10:00-16:00, Sergels Torg 3, T-bana: T-Centralen, tel. 08/5082-8508, www.visitstockholm.com). The efficient staff provides free city maps, the glossy *Stockholm Guide* booklet that introduces the city, the monthly *What's On* leaflet, Stockholm Cards (described later), transportation passes, day-trip and bus-tour information and tickets, and a room-booking service (small fee). Take a number as you enter, or avoid the wait by looking up sightseeing details on one of the user-friendly computer terminals (they can also give you the code for free Wi-Fi).

Around town, you'll also see the green *i* logo of the other "tourist information" service, **Stockholm Info,** run by a for-profit agency. While less helpful than the official TI, they hand out maps and brochures, sell Stockholm Cards, and may be able to answer basic questions (locations include train station's main hall, Gamla Stan, and Gallerian mall).

Stockholm Card: This 24-hour pass includes all public transit, entry to almost every sight (80 attractions), plus some free or discounted tours for 525 kr. An added bonus is the substantial pleasure of doing everything without considering the cost (many of Stockholm's sights are worth the time but not the money). The card pays for itself if you use public transportation and see Skansen, the Vasa Museum, and Drottningholm Palace. You can stretch it by entering Skansen on your 24th hour. A child's pass (age 7-17) costs about 60 percent less. The Stockholm Card also comes in 48-hour (675 kr), 72-hour (825 kr), and 120-hour (1,095 kr) versions. Cards are sold at the Visit Stockholm TIs, the unofficial Stockholm Info offices, many hotels and hostels, larger subway stations, and at www.visitstockholm.com.

HELPFUL HINTS

Theft Alert: Even in Stockholm, when there are crowds, there are pickpockets (such as at the Royal Palace during the Changing of the Guard). Too-young-to-arrest teens—many from other countries—are hard for local police to control.

Medical Help: For around-the-clock medical advice, call 1177. The **C. W. Scheele** 24-hour pharmacy is near the train station at Klarabergsgatan 64 (tel. 08/454-8130).

English Bookstore: The aptly named **English Bookshop,** in Gamla Stan, sells a variety of reading materials (including Swedish-interest books) in English (Mon-Fri 10:00-18:30, Sat 10:00-16:00, Sun 12:00-15:00, Lilla Nygatan 11, tel. 08/790-5510).

Laundry: Tvättomaten is a rare find—the only independent launderette in Stockholm (self-service-100 kr/load, open Mon-Fri 8:30-18:30—until 17:00 in July-mid-Aug, Sat 9:30-13:00, closed Sun; across from Gustav Vasa church, Västmannagatan 61 on Odenplan, T-bana: Odenplan, tel. 08/346-480, www.tvattomaten.com).

Updates to This Book: For updates to this book, check www. ricksteves.com/update.

GETTING AROUND STOCKHOLM
By Public Transit

Stockholm's fine but pricey public transport network (officially Storstockholms Lokaltrafik—but signed as *SL*) includes subway

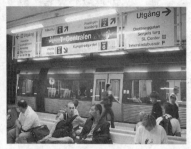

(Tunnelbana, called "T-bana") and bus systems, and a single handy tram from the commercial center to the sights at Djurgården. It's a sprawling city, so most visitors will need public transport at some point (transit info tel. 08/600-1000, press * for English, www.sl.se/english). The subway is easy to figure out, but

many sights are better served by bus. The main lines are listed on the back of the official city map. A more detailed system map is posted around town and available free from subway ticket windows and SL info desks in main stations. Check out the modern public art in the subway (such as at Kungsträdgården Station).

Tickets: A single ride for subway, tram, or bus costs 36 kr (up to 1.25 hours, including transfers); a 24-hour pass is 115 kr, while a 72-hour pass is 230 kr. Tickets are sold on the tram, but not on board buses—have one before you board.

You can choose whether to buy paper tickets or get an SL-Access fare card. **Paper tickets** are sold at the Pressbyrån newsstands scattered throughout the city, inside almost every T-bana station, and at some transit-ticket offices (all SL ticket-sellers are clearly marked with a blue flag with the *SL* logo); they are not available at self-service machines.

Locals and savvy tourists carry a blue **SL-Access card,** which you touch against the blue pad to enter the T-bana turnstile or when boarding a bus or tram. If planning to use public transit for more than a few rides, the card can save you money (200 kr for 8 rides, 20-kr deposit for card). You can top up your card at self-service machines (US credit cards work if you know your PIN).

By Harbor Shuttle Ferry

In summer, ferries let you make a fun, practical, and scenic shortcut across the harbor to Djurgården Island. Boats leave from Slussen (at the south end of Gamla Stan), docking near the Gröna Lund amusement park on Djurgården (45 kr, covered by public-transit passes, 3-4/hour, May-mid-Sept only, 10-minute trip, tel. 08/679-5830, www.waxholmsbolaget.se). On some runs, this ferry also

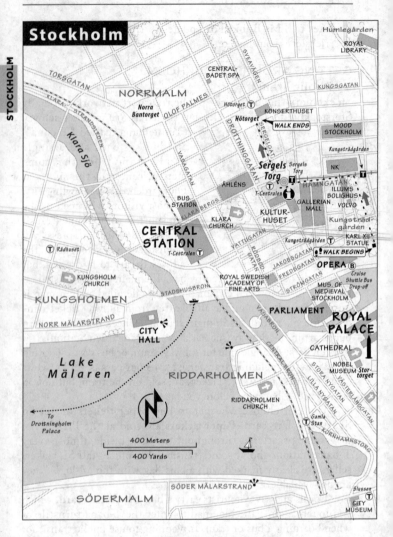

stops near the Museum of Modern Art on Skeppsholmen Island. The Nybro ferry makes the five-minute journey from Nybroplan to Djurgården, landing next to the Vasa Museum (55 kr, credit cards only, 1/hour, April-Sept daily 9:00-18:00, tel. 08/731-0025, www. ressel.se). While buses and trams run between the same points more frequently, the ferry option gets you out onto the water and can be faster—and certainly more scenic—than overland connections. The hop-on, hop-off boat tour (see page 249) also connects many of these stops.

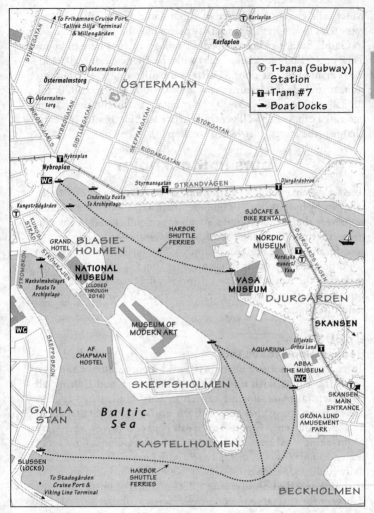

By Taxi

Stockholm is a good taxi town—provided you find a reputable cab that charges fair rates. Taxis are unregulated, so companies can charge whatever they like. Before hopping in a taxi, look carefully at the big yellow label in the back window, which lists various fares. On the left, you'll see the per-kilometer fares for weekdays, evenings and weekends, and holidays. The largest number, on the right, shows their "highest comparison price" *(högsta jämförpriset)* for a 10-kilometer ride that lasts 15 minutes; this number should be between 290 and 390—if it's higher, move on. (Legally, you're not obligated to take the first cab in line—feel free to compare fares.)

Most cabs charge a drop fee of about 45 kr. Taxis with inflated rates tend to congregate at touristy places like the Vasa Museum or in Gamla Stan. I've been ripped off enough by cabs here to know: Take only "Taxi Stockholm" cabs with the phone number (08/150-000) printed on the door. (Other companies that are reportedly honest include Taxi Kurir, tel. 08/300-000, and Taxi 020, tel. 08/850-400 or 020-20-20-20.) Your hotel, restaurant, or museum can call a cab, which will generally arrive within minutes (no extra charge—the meter starts when you hop in).

Tours in Stockholm

The sightseeing company **Strömma** has a lock on most city tours, whether by bus, by boat, or on foot. Their website (www.stromma. se) covers the entire program, much of which is listed below. For more information on their tours, call 08/1200-4000. Tours can be paid for in advance online, or simply as you board. The Stockholm Card provides discounts or even covers some of Strömma's tours, including the Royal Canal or Historic Canal boat trip (free), their orientation bus tour (half-price), and their hop-on, hop-off bus tour (discounted).

BY BUS
Hop-on, Hop-off Bus Tour

Three hop-on, hop-off buses make a 1.5-hour circuit of the city, orienting riders with a recorded commentary and linking all the essential places from Skansen to City Hall; when cruises are in town, they also stop at both cruise ports (Stadsgården and Frihamnen). **Open Top Tours'** green buses and **City Sightseeing's** red buses both cooperate with Strömma (260 kr/24 hours, 350 kr/72 hours, ticket covers both buses; May-Sept 2/hour daily 10:00-16:00, fewer off-season, none mid-Jan-mid-Feb, www. stromma.se). **Red Sightseeing** offers a similar hop-on, hop-off itinerary for the same price (3/hour, www.redbuses.se). All bus companies offer free Wi-Fi.

Quickie Orientation Bus Tour

Several different city bus tours leave from the Royal Opera House on Gustav Adolfs Torg. Strömma's Stockholm Panorama tour provides a good overview—but, as it's the same price as the 24-hour hop-on, hop-off ticket, I'd take this tour only if you want a quick and efficient loop with no unnecessary stops (260 kr, 4-6/day, fewer in Oct-May, 1.25 hours).

BY BOAT
▲City Boat Tours

For a good floating look at Stockholm and a pleasant break, consider a sightseeing cruise. I enjoy these various boat tours at the end of the

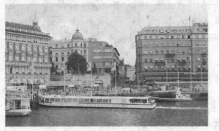

day, when the light is warm and the sights and museums are closed. The handiest are the Strömma/Stockholm Sightseeing boats, which leave from Strömkajen, in front of the Grand Hotel, and also stop at Nybroplan five minutes later.

Hop-On, Hop-Off Boat Tour

Stockholm is a city surrounded by water, making this boat option enjoyable and practical. Strömma and Royal Sightseeing offer the same small loop, stopping at key spots such as Djurgården (Skansen and Vasa Museum), Gamla Stan (near Slussen and again near Royal Palace), the Viking Line dock next to the cruise terminal at Stadsgården, and Nybroplan. Use the boat strictly as transport from Point A to Point B, or make the whole one-hour, eight-stop loop and enjoy the recorded commentary (Strömma-160 kr/24 hours, Royal Sightseeing-120 kr/24 hours, 2-3/hour May-mid-Sept, pick up map for schedule and locations of boat stops, www.stromma.se or www.royalsightseeing.com).

ON FOOT
Old Town Walk

Strömma offers a 1.25-hour Old Town walk (150 kr, 2/day July-Aug only, departs from obelisk next to Royal Palace on Gamla Stan, www.stromma.se).

Local Guides

Håkan Fränden is an excellent guide who brings Stockholm to life (mobile 070-531-3379, hakan.franden@hotmail.com). You can also hire a private guide through the Association of Qualified Tourist Guides of Stockholm (www.guidestockholm.com, info@guidestockholm.com). The standard rate is about 1,500 kr for up to three hours. **Marita Bergman** is a teacher and a licensed guide who enjoys showing visitors around during her school breaks (1,650 kr/half-day tour, mobile 073-511-9154, maritabergman@bredband.net).

BY BIKE

To tour Stockholm on two wheels, you can either use one of the city bikes or rent your own.

Using City Bikes: Stockholm's City Bikes program is a good option for seeing this bike-friendly town. While you'll find similar bike-sharing programs all over Europe, Stockholm's is the most usable and helpful for travelers. It's easy, the bikes are great, and the city lends itself to joy-riding.

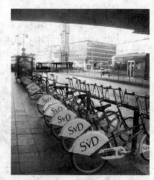

Purchase a 165-kr, three-day City Bike card at the TI, at the SL Center (Stockholm Transport) office at Sergels Torg, or at many hotels and hostels. The card allows you to grab a bike from one of the more than 90 City Bike racks around the city. You must return it within three hours (to any rack), but if you want to keep riding, just check out another bike. You can do this over and over for three days (available April-Oct only, www.citybikes.se).

The downside: Unless you have a lock, you can't park your bike as you sightsee. You'll need to return it to a station and get another when you're ready to go—which sounds easy enough, but in practice many stations are full (without an empty port in which to leave a bike) or have no bikes available. To overcome this problem, download the fun, easy, and free app from the website, which can help you find the nearest racks and bikes.

Renting a Bike: You can also rent bikes (and boats) at **Sjöcaféet,** next to Djurgårdsbron bridge near the Vasa Museum. It's ideally situated as a springboard for a pleasant bike ride around the park-like Djurgården island—use their free and excellent bike map/guide. For details, see page 270.

Stockholm Walks

This section includes two different self-guided walks to introduce you to Stockholm, both old (Gamla Stan) and new (the modern city).

▲▲OLD TOWN (GAMLA STAN) WALK

Stockholm's historic island core is charming, photogenic, and full of antiques shops, street lanterns, painted ceilings, and surprises. Until the 1600s, all of Stockholm fit in Gamla Stan. Stockholm traded with other northern ports such as Amsterdam, Lübeck, and Tallinn. German culture influenced art, building styles, and even the language, turning Old Norse into modern Swedish. With its narrow alleys and stairways, Gamla Stan mixes poorly with cars and modern economies. Today, it's been given over to the Royal Palace and to the tourists, who throng Gamla Stan's main drag,

STOCKHOLM

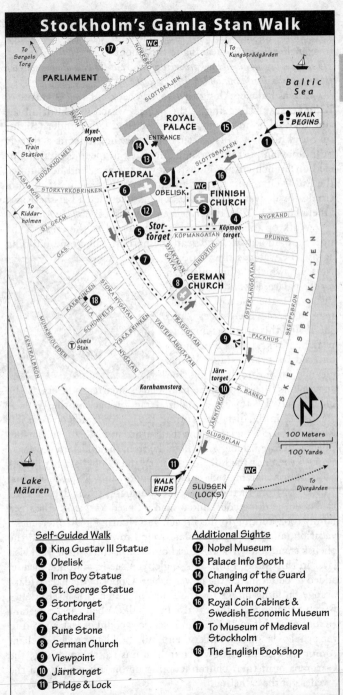

Stockholm's Gamla Stan Walk

To Sergels Torg

To 17

WC NORRBRO

To Kungsträdgården

PARLIAMENT

Baltic Sea

SLOTTSKAJEN

STALLBRON

RIDDARHOLMEN

To Train Station

Mynt-torget

ROYAL PALACE

15

WALK BEGINS

1

ENTRANCE

14

SLOTTSBACKEN

13

VASABRON

To Riddar-holmen

CATHEDRAL

STORKYRKOBRINKEN

6

2

OBELISK

16

WC

FINNISH CHURCH

NYGRAND.

3

BRUNNS.

4

Köpman-torget

ST. GERAN

12

Stor-torget

5

KÖPMANGATAN

GAS.

SVARTMAN GATAN

7

KINDSTUG

ÖSTERLANGGATAN

SKEPPSBRON

SKEPPSBROKAJEN

GERMAN CHURCH

8

KÄKBRINKEN

STORA NYGATAN

18

LILLA

SCHONFELTS

PRÄSTGATAN

VÄSTERLANGGATAN

MUNKBROLEDEN

TYSKA BRINKEN

9

PACKHUS

CENTRALBRON

NYGATAN

T Gamla Stan

Järn-torget

10

S. BANKO

Kornhamnstorg

JÄRNTORG

N

SLUSSPLAN

100 Meters

100 Yards

Lake Mälaren

11

WALK ENDS

SLUSSEN (LOCKS)

WC

To Djurgården

Self-Guided Walk

1 King Gustav III Statue
2 Obelisk
3 Iron Boy Statue
4 St. George Statue
5 Stortorget
6 Cathedral
7 Rune Stone
8 German Church
9 Viewpoint
10 Järntorget
11 Bridge & Lock

Additional Sights

12 Nobel Museum
13 Palace Info Booth
14 Changing of the Guard
15 Royal Armory
16 Royal Coin Cabinet & Swedish Economic Museum
17 To Museum of Medieval Stockholm
18 The English Bookshop

Västerlånggatan, seemingly unaware that most of Stockholm's best attractions are elsewhere. While you could just happily wander, this quick walk gives meaning to Stockholm's Old Town.

• *Our walk begins along the harborfront. Start at the base of Slottsbacken (the Palace Hill esplanade) leading up to the...*

Royal Palace: Along the water, check out the ❶ **statue of King Gustav III** gazing at the palace, which was built on the site of Stockholm's first castle (described later, under "Sights in Stockholm"). Gustav turned Stockholm from a dowdy Scandinavian port into a sophisticated European capital, modeled on French culture. Gustav loved the arts, and he founded the Royal Dramatic Theater and the Royal Opera in Stockholm. Ironically, he was assassinated at a masquerade ball at the Royal Opera House in 1792, inspiring Verdi's opera *Un Ballo in Maschera*.

Walk up the broad, cobbled boulevard to the crest of the hill. Stop, look back, and scan the harbor. The grand building across the water is the National Museum, which is often mistaken for the palace. Beyond that, in the distance, is the fine row of buildings on Strandvägen street. Until the 1850s, this area was home to peasant shacks, but as Stockholm entered its grand stage, it was cleaned up and replaced by fine

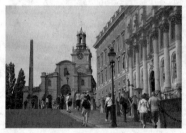

apartments, including some of the city's smartest addresses. The blocky gray TV tower—a major attraction back in the 1970s—stands tall in the distance. Turn to the palace facade on your left (finished in 1754, replacing one that burned in 1697). The niches are filled with Swedish bigwigs (literally) from the mid-18th century.

As you crest the hill, you're facing the ❷ **obelisk** that honors Stockholm's merchant class for its support in a 1788 war against Russia. In front of the obelisk are tour buses (their drivers worried about parking cops) and a sand pit used for *boules*. The royal family took a liking to the French game during a Mediterranean vacation, and it's quite popular around town today. Behind the obelisk stands Storkyrkan, Stockholm's cathedral (which we'll visit later in this walk). From this angle, you see its Baroque facade, added to better match the newer palace. Opposite the palace (dark orange building on left) is the Finnish church (Finska Kyrkan), which originated as the royal tennis hall. When the Protestant Reformation hit in 1527, church services could at last be said in the peoples' languages rather than Latin. Suddenly, each merchant community needed its own church. Finns worshiped here, the Germans built their church (coming up on this walk), and the Swedes got the cathedral.

Stroll up the lane to the right of the Finnish church into the shady churchyard where you'll find the fist-sized ❸ *Iron Boy,* the tiniest public statue (out of about 600 statues) in Stockholm. Swedish grannies knit caps for him in the winter. Local legend says the statue honors the orphans who had to transfer cargo from sea ships to lake ships before Stockholm's locks were built. Some people rub his head for good luck (which the orphans didn't have).

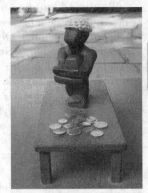

Others, likely needy when it comes to this gift, rub his head for wisdom. The artist says it's simply a self-portrait of himself as a child, sitting on his bed and gazing at the moon.

• *Continue through the yard, turn left onto Trädgårdsgatan, then bear right with the lane until you pop out at...*

Köpmangatan: Take a moment to explore this street from one end to the other. With its cobbles and traditional pastel facades, this is a quintessential Gamla Stan lane—and one of the oldest in town. The mellow yellow houses are predominantly from the 18th century; the red facades are mostly 17th century. Once merchants' homes, today these are popular with antique dealers. Back when there was comfort living within a city's walls, Gamla Stan streets like this were densely populated.

Head left, and you'll emerge on Köpmantorget square, with the breathtaking ❹ **statue of St. George** slaying the dragon. About 10 steps to the right of that is a maiden (representing Stockholm), looking on with thanks and admiration. At the other (top) end of the lane is old Stockholm's main square, our next stop.

❺ **Stortorget, Stockholm's Oldest Square:** Colorful old buildings topped with gables line this square, which was the heart of medieval Stockholm (pop. 6,000 in 1400). This was where the

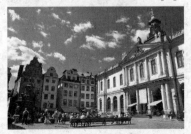

many tangled lanes intersected, becoming the natural center for shopping and the town well. Today Stortorget is home to lots of tourists—including a steady storm of cruise groups following the numbered Ping-Pong paddle of their guides on four-hour blitz tours of the city (300 ships call here between June and September each year). The square also hosts concerts, occasional demonstrators, and—in winter—Christmas shoppers at an outdoor market.

The grand building on the right is the **Stock Exchange.** It now houses the noble Nobel Museum (described later, under "Sights in Stockholm"). On the immediate left is the social-services agency **Stockholms Stadsmission** (offering the cheapest and best lunch around at the recommended Grillska Huset). If you peek into the adjacent bakery, you'll get a fine look at the richly decorated ceilings characteristic of Gamla Stan in the 17th century—the exotic flowers and animals implied that the people who lived or worked here were worldly. You'll also spy some tempting marzipan cakes (a local favorite) and *kanelbullar* (cinnamon buns). There's a cheap sandwich counter in the back and lots of picnic benches in the square.

The town well is still a popular meeting point. This square long held the town's pillory. Scan the fine old facades. The site of the **Stockholm Bloodbath** of 1520, this square has a notorious history. During a Danish power grab, many of Stockholm's movers and shakers who had challenged Danish rule—Swedish aristocracy, leading merchants, and priests—were rounded up, brought here, and beheaded. Rivers of blood were said to have flowed through the streets. Legend holds that the 80 or so white stones in the fine red facade across the square symbolize the victims. (One victim's son escaped, went into hiding, and resurfaced to lead a Swedish revolt against the Danish rulers. Three years later, the Swedes elected that rebel, Gustav Vasa, as their first king. He went on to usher in a great period in Swedish history—the Swedish Renaissance.)

• *At the far end of the square (under the finest gables), turn right and follow Trångsund toward the cathedral.*

❻ **Cathedral (Storkyrkan):** Just before the church, you'll see my personal phone booth (Rikstelefon) and the gate to the churchyard—guarded by statues of Caution and Hope. Enter the yellow-brick church—Stockholm's oldest, from the 13th century (40 kr; daily 9:00-16:00, open later Mon-Fri in summer—until 17:00 or 18:00). Signs explain events (busy with tours and services in summer).

When buying your ticket, pick up the free, worthwhile English-language flier. Exploring the cathedral's interior, you'll find many styles, ranging from medieval to modern. The front of the nave is paved with centuries-old **tombstones.** At one time, more than a thousand people were buried under the church. The tombstone of the Swedish reformer Olaus Petri is appropriately simple and appropriately located—under the finely carved and gilded pulpit. A witness to the Stockholm Bloodbath, Petri was nearly executed himself. He went on to befriend Gustav Vasa and guide him in Lutheranizing Sweden (and turning this cathedral from Catholic to Protestant). The fine 17th-century altar is made of silver and ebony. Above it, the silver Christ stands like a conquering general evoking the 1650s, an era of Swedish military might.

Opposite the pulpit, find the **bronze plaque** in the pillar. It recalls the 1925 Swedish-led ecumenical meeting of all Christian leaders—except the pope—that encouraged the Church to speak out against the type of evil that resulted in World War I's horrific death toll.

The **royal boxes** (carved wood, between the pulpit and the altar) date from 1684. In June of 2010, this church hosted a royal wedding (Crown Princess Victoria, heir to the throne, married Daniel Westling, her personal trainer). Imagine the pomp and circumstance as the nation's attention was drawn to this spot.

The remarkably detailed **statue** to the left of the altar, *Saint George and the Dragon* (1489)—a copy of which you saw outside a few minutes ago—is carved of oak and elk horn. To some, this symbolizes the Swedes' overcoming the evil Danes (commemorating a Swedish military victory in 1471). In a broader sense, it's an inspiration to take up the struggle against even non-Danish evil. Regardless, it must be the gnarliest dragon's head in all of Europe.

Return to the back of the church to find the exit. Before leaving, just to the left of the door, notice the **painting** that depicts Stockholm in the early 1500s, showing a walled city filling only today's Gamla Stan. It's a 1630 copy of the 1535 original. The church with its black spire dominated the town back then. The strange sun and sky predicted big changes in Sweden—and as a matter of fact, that's what happened. Gustav Vasa brought on huge reforms in religion and beyond. (The doors just to the left and right of the painting lead to a free WC.)

Heading outside, you'll emerge into the kid-friendly churchyard, which was once the cemetery.

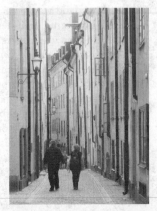

• *With your back to the church's front door, turn right and continue down Trångsund. At the next corner, turn left and go downhill on Storkyrkobrinken and take the first left on...*

Prästgatan: Enjoy a quiet wander down this peaceful, 15th-century "Priests' Lane." Västerlånggatan, the touristy drag, parallels this lane one block over.

(While we'll skip it now, you can walk back up it from the end point of this walk.) As you stroll Prästgatan, look for bits of its past: hoists poking out horizontally from gables (merchants used these to lift goods into their attics), tie bolts (iron bars necessary to bind the timber beams of tall buildings together), small coal or wood hatches (for fuel delivery back in the good old days), and flaming gold phoenixes under red-crown medallions (telling firefighters which houses paid insurance and could be saved in case of fire—for example, #46). Like other Scandinavian cities, Stockholm was plagued by fire until it was finally decreed that only stone, stucco, and brick construction (like you see here) would be allowed in the town center.

After a few blocks (at Kåkbrinken), a cannon barrel on the corner (look down) guards a Viking-age ❼ **rune stone.** In case you can't read the old Nordic script, it says: "Torsten and Frogun erected this stone in memory of their son."

• *Continue one block farther down Prästgatan to Tyska Brinken and turn left. You will see the powerful brick steeple of the German Church.*

❽ **German Church** (Tyska Kyrkan): The church's carillon has played four times a day since 1666. Think of the days when German merchants worked here. Today, Germans come to Sweden not to run the economy, but to enjoy its pristine nature (which is progressively harder to find in their own crowded homeland). Sweden formally became a Lutheran country even before the northern part of Germany—making this the very first German Lutheran church (free, Mon-Sat 11:00-15:00, Sun 12:30-17:00).

• *Wander through the churchyard (past a cute church café) and out the back. Exit right onto Svartmangatan and follow it to the right, ending at an iron railing overlooking Österlånggatan.*

❾ **Viewpoint:** From this perch, survey the street below to the left and right. Notice how it curves. This marks the old shoreline. In medieval times, piers stretched out like fingers into the harbor. Gradually, as land was reclaimed and developed, these piers were extended, becoming lanes leading to piers farther away. Behind you is a cute shop where elves can actually be seen making elves.

• *Walk right along Österlånggatan to...*

❿ **Järntorget:** A customs square in medieval times, this was the home of Sweden's first bank back in 1680 (the yellow building with the bars on the windows). The Co-op Nära supermarket on this square offers picnic fixings. From here, Västerlånggatan—the eating, shopping, and commercial pedestrian mall of Gamla Stan—leads back across the island. You'll be there in a minute, but first finish this walk.

• *Continue out of the square (opposite where you entered) down Järntorgsgatan, walk (carefully) out into the traffic hell, passing an equestrian statue of Jean-Baptiste Bernadotte—the French son of a lawyer invited to establish the current Swedish royal dynasty in the early 1800s. Continue ahead 50 yards until you reach a viewpoint overlooking a lock.*

⓫ Bridge Overlooking Slussen: This area is called Slussen, named for the locks between the salt water of the Baltic Sea (to your left) and the fresh water of the huge Lake Mälaren (to your right). In fact, Stockholm exists because this is where Lake Mälaren meets the sea. Traders would sail their goods from far inland to this point, where they'd meet merchants who would ship the goods south to Europe. In the 13th century, the new Kingdom of Sweden needed revenue, and began levying duty taxes on all the iron, copper, and furs shipped through here. From the bridge, you may notice a current in the water, indicating that the weir has been lowered and water is spilling from Lake Mälaren (about two feet above sea level) into the sea. Today, the locks are nicknamed "the divorce lock" because this is where captains and first mates learn to communicate under pressure and in the public eye.

Survey the view. Opposite Gamla Stan is the island of **Södermalm**—bohemian, youthful, artsy, and casual—with its popular Katarina viewing platform. Moored on the saltwater side are the cruise ships, which bring thousands of visitors into town each day during the season. Many of these boats are bound for Finland. The towering white syringe is the Gröna Lund amusement park's free-fall ride. The revolving *Djurgården Färjan* sign, along the embankment to your left, marks the ferry that zips from here directly to Gröna Lund and Djurgården.

You could catch bus #2, which heads back downtown (the stop is just beyond Bernadotte, next to the waterfront). But better yet, linger longer in Gamla Stan—day or night, it's a lively place to enjoy. Västerlånggatan, Gamla Stan's main commercial drag, is a touristy festival of distractions that keeps most visitors from seeing the historic charms of the Old Town—which you just did. Now you're free to window-shop and eat (see page 282).

• *For more sightseeing, consider the other sights in Gamla Stan or at the Royal Palace (all described later, under "Sights in Stockholm"). If you continue back up Västerlånggatan (always going straight), you'll reach the Parliament building and cross the water back over onto Norrmalm (where the street becomes Drottninggatan). This pedestrian street leads back into Stockholm's modern, vibrant new town.*

From here it's also a 10-minute walk to Kungsträdgården, the starting point of my Modern City self-guided walk (described next). You can either walk along the embankment and take the diagonal bridge directly across to the square, or you can walk back through the middle of Gamla Stan, taking the stately walkway past the Parliament, then turning right when you cross the bridge.

STOCKHOLM'S MODERN CITY WALK

On this walk, we'll use the park called Kungsträdgården as a springboard to explore the modern center of Stockholm—a commercial zone designed to put the focus not on old kings and mementos of superpower days, but on shopping. For the route, see the map on page 246.

• *Find the statue of King Karl XII, facing the waterfront at the harbor end of the park.*

Kungsträdgården: Centuries ago, this "King's Garden" was the private kitchen garden of the king, where he grew his cabbage salad. Today, this downtown people-watching center, worth ▲, is considered Stockholm's living room, symbolizing the Swedes' freedom-loving spirit. While the name implies that the garden is a private royal domain, the giant clump of elm trees just behind the statue reminds locals that it's the people who rule now. In the 1970s, demonstrators chained themselves to these trees to stop the building of an underground train station here. They prevailed, and today, locals enjoy the peaceful, breezy ambience of a teahouse instead. Watch the AstroTurf zone with "latte dads" and their kids, and enjoy a summer concert at the bandstand. There's always something going on. High above is a handy reference point—the revolving NK clock.

Kungsträdgården—surrounded by the harborfront and tour boats, the Royal Opera House, and shopping opportunities (including a welcoming Volvo showroom near the top left side of the square, showing off the latest in Swedish car design)—is *the* place to feel Stockholm's pulse (but always ask first: *"Kan jag kanna på din puls?"*).

Kungsträdgården also throws huge parties. The Taste of Stockholm festival runs for a week in early June, when restaurateurs show off and bands entertain all day. Beer flows liberally—a rare public spectacle in Sweden.

• *Stroll through Kungsträdgården, past the fountain and the Volvo store, and up to Hamngatan street. From here, we'll turn left and walk the length of the NK department store (across the street) as we wade through...*

Stockholm's Urban Shopping Zone (Hamngatan): In just a couple of blocks, we'll pass some major landmarks of Swedish consumerism. First, at the top of Kungsträdgården on the left, look for the gigantic **Illums Bolighus** design shop. (You can enter from the square and stroll all the way through it, popping out at Hamngatan on the far end.) This is a Danish institution, making its play for Swedish customers with this prime location. Across the street (on your right as you walk down Hamngatan), notice the giant gold *NK* marking the **Nordiska Kompaniet** department store (locals joke that the NK stands for "no kronor

Fika: **Sweden's Coffee Break**

Swedes drink more coffee per capita than just about any other country in the world. The Swedish coffee break—or *fika*—is a

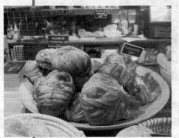

ritual. *Fika* is to Sweden what tea-time is to Britain. The typical *fika* is a morning or afternoon break in the workday, but can happen any time, any day. It's the perfect opportunity (and excuse) for tourists to take a break as well.

Fika fare is coffee with a snack—something sweet or savory. Your best bet is a *kanel-bulle,* a Swedish cinnamon bun,

although some prefer *pariserbulle,* a bun filled with vanilla cream. These can be found nearly everywhere coffee is sold, including just about any café or *konditori* (bakery) in Stockholm. A coffee and a cinnamon bun in a café will cost you about 40 kr. (Most cafés will give you a coffee refill for free.) But at Pressbyrån, the Swedish convenience stores found all over town, you can satisfy your *fika* fix for 25 kr by getting a coffee and bun to go. Grab a park bench or water-side perch, relax, and enjoy.

left"). It's located in an elegant early 20th-century building that dominates the top end of Kungsträdgården. If it feels like an old-time American department store, that's because its architect was inspired by grand stores he'd seen in the US (circa 1910).

Another block down, on the left, is the sleeker, more modern **Gallerian mall.** Among this two-story world of shops, upstairs you'll find a Clas Ohlson hardware and electronics shop (a men's favorite, as most Stockholmers have a cabin that's always in need of a little DIY repair). And there are plenty of affordable little lunch bars and classy cafés for your *fika* (Swedish coffee-and-bun break). You may notice that American influence (frozen yogurt and other trendy food chains) is challenging the entire notion of the traditional *fika*.

• *High-end shoppers should consider heading into the streets behind NK, with exclusive designer boutiques and the chichi Mood Stockholm mall (see page 281). Otherwise, just beyond the huge Gallerian mall, you'll emerge into Sergels Torg. Note that the handy tram #7 goes from here directly to Skansen and the other important sights on Djurgården (departures every few minutes; tickets sold on board).*

Sergels Torg and Kulturhuset: Sergels Torg square, worth ▲, dominates the heart of modern Stockholm with its stark 1960s-era functionalist architecture. The glassy tower in the middle of the fountain plaza is ugly in daylight but glows at night, symbolic of Sweden's haunting northern lights.

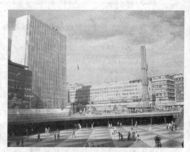

Kulturhuset, the hulking, low-slung, glassy building over-looking the square (on your left) is Stockholm's "culture center." Inside, just past the welcoming info desk, you'll find a big model of the city that locals use to check in on large infrastructure proj-ects. Push a few buttons and see what's happening. In this lively cultural zone, there's a space for kids, a library (with magazines and computer terminals), chessboards, fun shops, fine art cinema, art exhibits, and a venue for new bands (tel. 08/5083-1508, www. kulturhuset.stockholm.se).

I like to take the elevator to the top and explore each level by riding the escalator back down to the ground floor. On the roof-top, choose from one of two recommended eateries with terrific city views: Cafeteria Panorama has cheap meals and a salad bar while the Mat and Bar café is trendier and pricier (see page 290).

Back outside, stand in front of the Kulturhuset (across from the fountain) and survey the expansive square nicknamed "Plattan" (the platter). Everything around you dates from the 1960s and 1970s, when this formerly run-down area was reinvented as an urban "space of the future." In the 1970s, with no nearby resi-dences, the desolate Plattan became the domain of junkies. Now the city is actively revitalizing it, and the Plattan is becoming a people-friendly heart of the commercial town.

DesignTorget (enter from the lower level of Kulturhuset) is a place for independent Swedish designers to showcase and sell their clever products. (Local designers submit their creations, and the DesignTorget staff votes on and carries their favorites—per-haps you need a banana case?) Nearby are the major boutiques and department stores, including, across the way, H&M and Åhléns.

Sergelgatan, a thriving pedestrian and commercial street, leads past the five uniform white towers you see beyond the foun-tain. These office towers, so modern in the 1960s, have gone from seeming hopelessly out-of-date to being considered "retro," and are now quite popular with young professionals.

• *Walk up Sergelgatan past the towers, enjoying the public art and people-watching, to the market at Hötorget.*

Hötorget: "Hötorget" means "Hay Market," but today its stalls feed people rather than horses. The adjacent indoor market, Hötorgshallen, is fun and fragrant. It dates from 1914 when, for hygienic reasons, the city forbade selling fish and meat outdoors. Carl Milles' statue of *Orpheus Emerging from the Underworld* (with seven sad muses) stands in front of the city concert hall (which hosts the annual Nobel Prize award ceremony). The concert house, from 1926, is Swedish Art Deco (a.k.a. "Swedish Grace"). The lobby (open through much of the summer, 70-kr tours) still evokes Stockholm's Roaring Twenties. If the door's open, you're welcome to look in for free. Popping into the Hötorget T-bana station provides a fun glimpse at local urban design. Stockholm's subway system was inaugurated in the 1950s, and many stations are modern art installations in themselves.

• *Our walk ends here. For more shopping and an enjoyable pedestrian boulevard leading back into the Old Town, cut down a block to Drottninggatan and turn left. This busy drag leads straight out of the commercial district, passes the Parliament, then becomes the main street of Gamla Stan.*

Sights in Stockholm

GAMLA STAN (OLD TOWN)

The best of Gamla Stan is covered in my self-guided "Old Town Walk," earlier. But here are a few ways to extend your time in the Old Town.

On Stortorget
▲Nobel Museum (Nobelmuseet)

Opened in 2001 for the 100-year anniversary of the Nobel Prize, this wonderful little museum tells the story of the world's most prestigious prize. Pricey but high-tech and eloquent, it fills the grand old stock exchange building that dominates Gamla Stan's main square, Stortorget.

Cost and Hours: 100 kr, free Tue after 17:00; open June-Aug daily 10:00-20:00; Sept-May Tue 11:00-20:00, Wed-Sun 11:00-17:00, closed Mon; audioguide-20 kr, free 30-minute orientation tours in English: 6/day in summer, fewer off-season; on Stortorget in the center of Gamla Stan a block from the Royal Palace, tel. 08/5348-1800, www.nobelmuseum.se.

Background: Stockholm-born Alfred Nobel was a great inventor, with more than 300 patents. His most famous invention: dynamite. Living in the late 1800s, Nobel was a man of his age. It was a time of great optimism, wild ideas, and grand projects. His dynamite enabled entire nations to blast their way into the modern age with canals, railroads,

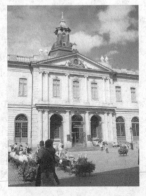

Stockholm at a Glance

▲▲▲**Skansen** Europe's first and best open-air folk museum, with more than 150 old homes, churches, shops, and schools. **Hours:** Park—daily May-late-June 10:00-19:00, late-June-Aug 10:00-22:00, Sept 10:00-18:00, Oct and March-April 10:00-16:00, Nov-Feb 10:00-15:00; historical buildings—generally 11:00-17:00, late June-Aug some until 19:00, most closed in winter. See page 271.

▲▲▲**Vasa Museum** Ill-fated 17th-century warship dredged from the sea floor, now the showpiece of an interesting museum. **Hours:** Daily June-Aug 8:30-18:00; Sept-May 10:00-17:00 except Wed until 20:00. See page 273.

▲▲**Military Parade and Changing of the Guard** Punchy pomp starting near Nybroplan and finishing at Royal Palace outer courtyard. **Hours:** Mid-May-mid-Sept daily, mid-Sept-April Wed and Sat-Sun only, start time varies with season but always at midday. See page 264.

▲▲**Royal Armory** A fine collection of ceremonial medieval royal armor, historic and modern royal garments, and carriages, in the Royal Palace. **Hours:** May-June daily 11:00-17:00; July-Aug daily 10:00-18:00; Sept-April Tue-Sun 11:00-17:00, Thu until 20:00, closed Mon. See page 265.

▲▲**City Hall** Gilt mosaic architectural jewel of Stockholm and site of Nobel Prize banquet, with tower offering the city's best views. **Hours:** Required tours daily generally June-Aug every 30 minutes 9:30-16:00, off-season hourly 10:00-15:00. See page 268.

▲▲**Nordic Museum** Danish Renaissance palace design and five fascinating centuries of traditional Swedish lifestyles. **Hours:** Daily 10:00-17:00, Wed until 20:00 Sept-May. See page 275.

and tunnels. It made warfare much more destructive. And it also made Alfred Nobel a very wealthy man. Wanting to leave a legacy that celebrated and supported people with great ideas, Alfred used his fortune to fund the Nobel Prize. Every year since 1901, laureates have been honored in the fields of physics, chemistry, medicine, literature, and peacemaking.

Visiting the Museum: Inside, portraits of all 700-plus prize-winners hang from the ceiling—shuffling around the room like shirts at the dry cleaner's (miss your favorite, and he or she will come around again in six hours). Behind the ticket desk are video screens honoring the six Nobel Prize categories, each running a

▲**Nobel Museum** Star-studded tribute to some of the world's most accomplished scientists, artists, economists, and politicians. **Hours:** June-Aug daily 10:00-20:00; Sept-May Tue 11:00-20:00, Wed-Sun 11:00-17:00; closed Mon. See page 261.

▲**Royal Palace Museums** Complex of Swedish royal museums, the two best of which are the Royal Apartments and Royal Treasury. **Hours:** Mid-May-mid-Sept daily 10:00-17:00; mid-Sept-mid-May Tue-Sun 12:00-16:00, closed Mon. See page 266.

▲**Royal Coin Cabinet and Swedish Economic Museum** Europe's best look at the history of money, with a sweep through the evolution of the Swedish economy to boot. **Hours:** Daily June-Aug 11:00-17:00, Sept-May 10:00-16:00. See page 266.

▲**Kungsträdgården** Stockholm's lively central square, with life-size chess games, concerts, and perpetual action. **Hours:** Always open. See page 258.

▲**Sergels Torg** Modern square with underground mall. **Hours:** Always open. See page 259.

▲**ABBA: The Museum** A super-commercial and wildly-popular-with-ABBA-fans experience. **Hours:** Daily 10:00-20:00, shorter hours off-season. See page 276.

▲**Thielska Galleriet** Enchanting waterside mansion with works of Scandinavian artists Larsson, Zorn, and Munch. **Hours:** Tue-Sun 12:00-17:00, closed Mon. See page 277.

▲**Millesgården** Dramatic cliffside museum and grounds featuring works of Sweden's greatest sculptor, Carl Milles. **Hours:** Daily 11:00-17:00 except closed Mon in Oct-April. See page 278.

clip about the most recent laureate in that category.

Flanking the main hall beyond that—where touchscreens organized by decade invite you to learn more about the laureates of your choice—two video rooms run a continuous montage of quick programs (three-minute bios of various winners in one program, five-minute films celebrating various intellectual environments—from Cambridge to Parisian cafés—in the other).

To the right of the ticket desk, find "The Gallery," with an endearingly eccentric collection of items that various laureates have cited as important to their creative process, from scientific equipment to inspirational knickknacks. The randomness of the items offers a fascinating and humanizing insight into the great minds of our time. Beyond that are a room dedicated to Alfred Nobel and a small children's area.

Royal Palace Complex (Kungliga Slottet)

Although the royal family beds down at Drottningholm, this complex in Gamla Stan is still the official royal residence. The palace, designed in Italian Baroque style, was completed in 1754 after a fire wiped out the previous palace—a much more characteristic medieval/Renaissance complex. This blocky Baroque replacement, which houses various museums, is big and (frankly) pretty dull. Note two of the sights—the Royal Armory and the Royal Coin Cabinet—are operated by different organizations, so they have separate entrances and tickets.

Planning Your Time: Visiting the several sights in and near the palace could fill a day, but Stockholm has far better attractions elsewhere. Prioritize. The Changing of the Guard and the awesome Royal Armory are the highlights.

The information booth in the semicircular courtyard (at the top, where the guard changes) gives out a list of the day's guided tours and an explanatory brochure/map that marks the entrances to the different sights. The main entrance to the Royal Palace (including the apartments, chapel, and treasury) faces the long, angled square and obelisk.

Tours: In peak season, the main Royal Palace offers a full slate of English tours covering the different sights (included in the admission)—allowing you to systematically cover nearly the entire complex. If you're paying the hefty price for a ticket, you might as well try to join at least one of the tours—otherwise, you'll struggle to appreciate the place. Some tours are infrequent, so be sure to confirm times when you purchase your admission (for more on tours, see the individual listings below).

Expect Changes: Since the palace is used for state functions, it is sometimes closed to tourists. And, as the exterior is undergoing a 20-year renovation, don't be surprised if parts are covered in scaffolding.

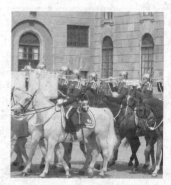

▲▲Military Parade and Changing of the Guard

Starting two blocks from Nybroplan (in front of the Army Museum at Riddargatan 13), Stockholm's daily military parade marches over Norrbro bridge, in front of the Parliament building, and up to the Royal Palace's outer courtyard, where the band plays and the guard changes. Smaller contingents of guards spiral in from other parts of the palace complex, eventually convening in the same place.

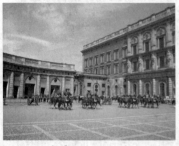

The performance is fresh and spirited, because the soldiers are visiting Stockholm just like you—and it's a chance for young soldiers from all over Sweden in every branch of the service to show their stuff in the big city. Pick your place at the palace courtyard, where the band arrives at about 12:15 (13:15 on Sun). The best spot to stand is along the wall in the inner courtyard, near the palace information and ticket office. There are columns with wide pedestals for easy perching, as well as benches that people stand on to view the ceremony (arrive early). Generally, after the barking and goose-stepping formalities, the band shows off for an impressive 30-minute marching concert. Though the royal family now lives out of town at Drottningholm, the palace guards are for real. If the guard by the cannon in the semicircular courtyard looks a little lax, try wandering discreetly behind him.

Cost and Hours: Free; mid-May-mid-Sept Mon-Sat parade begins at 11:45 (reaches palace at 12:15), Sun at 12:45 (palace at 13:15); April-mid-May and mid-Sept-Oct Wed and Sat at 11:45 (palace at 12:15), Sun at 12:45 (palace at 13:15); Nov-March starts at palace Wed and Sat at 12:15, Sun at 13:15. Royal appointments can disrupt the schedule; confirm times at TI. In summer, you might also catch the mounted guards (but they do not appear on a regular schedule).

▲▲Royal Armory (Livrustkammaren)

The oldest museum in Sweden is more than an armory and less than an armory. Rather than dusty piles of swords and muskets, it focuses on royal clothing: impressive ceremonial armor (never used in battle) and other fashion through the ages (including a room of kidswear), plus a fine collection of coaches. It's an engaging slice of royal life. Everything is displayed under sturdy brick vaults, beautifully lit, and well-described in English and by the museum's evocative audioguide.

Cost and Hours: 90 kr, half-price if you've already bought your Royal Palace ticket—so if you're touring both sights, buy your palace ticket before you come here; May-June daily 11:00-17:00; July-Aug daily 10:00-18:00; Sept-April Tue-Sun 11:00-17:00, Thu until 20:00, closed Mon; 20-kr audioguide is excellent—romantic couples can share it if they crank up the volume, information sheets in English available in most rooms; entrance at bottom of Slottsbacken at base of palace, tel. 08/402-3010, www. livrustkammaren.se.

▲Royal Palace

The Royal Palace consists of a chapel and four museums. Compared with many grand European palaces, it's underwhelming and flooded with cruise-excursion groups who don't realize that Stockholm's best sightseeing is elsewhere. It's worth a quick walk-through if you have a Stockholm Card (and, as a bonus, cardholders can go straight into each museum, bypassing the ticket office).

Cost and Hours: 150-kr combo-ticket covers all four museums and the chapel, includes guided tour; mid-May-mid-Sept daily 10:00-17:00; mid-Sept-mid-May Tue-Sun 12:00-16:00, closed Mon; tel. 08/402-6130, www.royalcourt.se.

Royal Apartments: The stately palace exterior encloses 608 rooms (one more than Britain's Buckingham Palace) of glittering 18th-century Baroque and Rococo decor. Guided 45-minute **tours** in English run twice daily.

Royal Treasury (Skattkammaren): Refreshingly compact compared to the sprawling apartments, the treasury gives you a good, up-close look at Sweden's crown jewels. It's particularly worthwhile with an English guided **tour** (daily at 13:00) or the included **audioguide** (which covers basically the same information).

Museum of Three Crowns (Museum Tre Kronor): This museum shows off bits of the palace from before a devastating 1697 fire. The models, illustrations, and artifacts are displayed in vaulted medieval cellars that are far more evocative than the run-of-the-mill interior of today's palace. But while the stroll through the cellars is atmospheric, it's basically just more old stuff, interesting only to real history buffs (guided tours in English offered on summer afternoons).

Chapel: If you don't want to spring for a ticket, but would like a little taste of palace opulence, climb the stairs inside the main entrance for a peek into the chapel—the only free sight at the palace. It's standard-issue royal Baroque: colorful ceiling painting, bubbly altars, and a giant organ.

Gustav III's Museum of Antiquities (Gustav III's Antikmuseum): In the 1700s, Gustav III traveled through Italy and brought home an impressive gallery of classical Roman statues. These are displayed exactly as they were in the 1790s. This was a huge deal for those who had never been out of Sweden (English tour at 16:00).

▲Royal Coin Cabinet (Kungliga Myntkabinettet)

More than your typical royal coin collection, this is the best money museum I've seen in Europe. A fine exhibit tells the story of money from crude wampum to credit cards, and traces the development of the modern Swedish economy. The mellow but informative included audioguide helps make sense of the collection (which has only some English descriptions).

Cost and Hours: 70 kr, free on Mon, open daily June-Aug 11:00-17:00, Sept-May 10:00-16:00, Slottsbacken 6, tel. 08/5195-5304, www.myntkabinettet.se.

More Gamla Stan Sights

These sights sit on the Gamla Stan islet of Helgeandsholmen (just north of the Royal Palace).

Parliament (Riksdag)

For a firsthand look at Sweden's government, tour the Parliament buildings. Guides enjoy a chance to teach a little Swedish poli-sci along the standard tour of the building and its art. It's also possible to watch the Parliament in session.

Cost and Hours: Free one-hour tours go in English late June-late Aug, usually 4/day Mon-Fri (when Parliament is not in session). The rest of the year tours run 1/day Sat-Sun only; you're also welcome to join Swedish citizens in the viewing gallery (free); enter at Riksgatan 3a, call 08/786-4862 between 9:00 and 11:00 to confirm tour times, www.riksdagen.se.

Museum of Medieval Stockholm (Medeltidsmuseet)

This modern, well-presented museum offers a look at medieval Stockholm. When the government was digging a parking garage near the Parliament building in the 1970s, workers uncovered a major archaeological find: parts of the town wall that King Gustav Vasa built in the 1530s, as well as a churchyard. This underground museum preserves these discoveries and explains how Stockholm grew from a medieval village to a major city, with a focus on its interactions with fellow Hanseatic League trading cities. Lots of artifacts, models, life-size dioramas, and sound and lighting effects—all displayed in a vast subterranean space—help bring the story to life.

Cost and Hours: 100 kr ticket normally includes Stockholm City Museum in Södermalm, but that's closed for restoration through 2017, so ticket price may change; Tue-Sun 12:00-17:00, Wed until 19:00, closed Mon; English audioguide-20 kr, enter museum from park in front of Parliament—down below as you cross the bridge, tel. 08/5083-1790, www.medeltidsmuseet. stockholm.se.

Nearby: The museum sits in **Strömparterren** park. With its café and Carl Milles statue of the *Sun Singer* greeting the day, it's a pleasant place for a sightseeing break (pay WC in park, free WC in museum).

DOWNTOWN STOCKHOLM

I've organized these sights and activities in the urban core of Stockholm by island and/or neighborhood.

On Kungsholmen, West of Norrmalm
▲▲City Hall (Stadshuset)

The Stadshuset is an impressive mix of eight million red bricks, 19 million chips of gilt mosaic, and lots of Stockholm pride. While

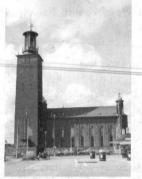

churches dominate cities in southern Europe, in Scandinavian capitals, city halls seem to be the most impressive buildings, celebrating humanism and the ideal of people working together in community. Built in 1923, this is still a functioning city hall. The members of the city council—101 people (mostly women) representing the 850,000 people of Stockholm—are hobby legislators with regular day jobs. That's why they meet in the evening. One of Europe's finest public buildings, the site of the annual Nobel Prize banquet, and a favorite spot for weddings (they do two per hour on Saturday afternoons, when some parts of the complex may be closed), City Hall is particularly enjoyable and worthwhile for its entertaining and required 50-minute tour.

Cost and Hours: 100 kr; English-only tours offered daily, generally June-Aug every 30 minutes 9:30-16:00, off-season hourly 10:00-15:00; schedule can change due to special events—call to confirm; 300 yards behind the central train station—about a 15-minute walk from either the station or Gamla Stan, bus #3 or #62, tel. 08/5082-9059, www.stockholm.se/cityhall. City Hall's cafeteria, which you enter from the courtyard, serves complete lunches for 95 kr (Mon-Fri 11:00-14:00, closed Sat-Sun).

Visiting City Hall: On the tour, you'll see the building's sumptuous National Romantic style interior (similar to Britain's

Arts and Crafts style), celebrating Swedish architecture and craftwork, and created almost entirely with Swedish materials. Highlights include the so-called Blue Hall (the Italian piazza-inspired, loggia-lined courtyard that was originally intended to be open air—hence the name—where

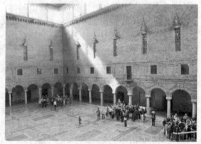

the 1,300-plate Nobel banquet takes place); the City Council Chamber (with a gorgeously painted wood-beamed ceiling that resembles a Viking longhouse—or maybe an overturned Viking boat); the Gallery of the Prince (lined with frescoes executed by Prince Eugene of Sweden); and the glittering, gilded, Neo-Byzantine-style (and aptly named) Golden Hall, where the Nobel recipients cut a rug after the banquet.

▲City Hall Tower

This 348-foot-tall tower rewards those who make the climb with the classic Stockholm view: The old church spires on the atmo-

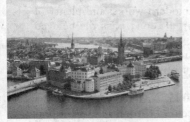

spheric islands of Gamla Stan pose together, with the rest of the green and watery city spread-eagle around them.

Cost and Hours: 40 kr, daily June-Aug 9:15-17:15, May and Sept 9:15-15:55, closed Oct-April.

Crowd-Beating Tips: Only 30 people at a time are allowed up into the tower, every 40 minutes throughout the day. To ascend, you'll need a timed-entry ticket, which you can only get in person at the tower ticket office on the same day (no phone or Internet orders). It can be a long wait for the next available time, and tickets can sell out by midafternoon. If you're touring City Hall, come to the tower ticket window first to see when space is available. Ideally an appointment will coincide with the end of your tour.

On Blasieholmen and Skeppsholmen

The peninsula of Blasieholmen pokes out from downtown Stockholm, and is tethered to the island of Skeppsholmen by a narrow bridge (with great views and adorned with glittering golden crowns). It is not connected to the city by T-bana or tram, but you can reach this area by bus #65 or the harbor shuttle ferry. Although Skeppsholmen is basically a "dead end" from a transportation perspective, it offers a peaceful break from the bustling city, with glorious views of Gamla Stan on one side and Djurgården on the other.

▲National Museum of Fine Arts (Nationalmuseum)

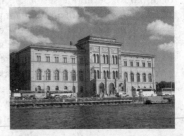

Stockholm's 200-year-old art museum, though mediocre by European standards, owns a few good pieces. Highlights include several canvases by Rembrandt and Rubens, a fine group of Impressionist works, and a sizeable collection of Russian icons. Seek out the exquisite paintings by the Swedish artists Anders Zorn and Carl Larsson.

Cost and Hours: The museum is closed for an extensive renovation (reopening in 2017); for the latest, see www. nationalmuseum.se.

Museum of Modern Art (Moderna Museet)

This bright, cheery gallery on Skeppsholmen island is as far out as can be. For serious art lovers, it warrants ▲▲. The impressive permanent collection includes modernist all-stars such as Picasso, Braque, Dalí, Matisse, Munch, Kokoschka, and Dix; lots of goofy Dada art (including a copy of Duchamp's urinal); Pollock, Twombly, Bacon, and other postmodern works; and plenty of excellent contemporary stuff as well (don't miss the beloved Rauschenberg *Goat with Tire*).

The building also houses the Architecture and Design Center, with changing exhibits on those topics (www.arkdes.se, covered by a separate ticket).

Cost and Hours: Museum-120 kr, Architecture and Design Center-80 kr, 180 kr for both, free on Fri from 18:00; Tue and Fri 10:00-20:00, Wed-Thu and Sat-Sun 10:00-18:00, closed Mon; free audioguide app, fine bookstore, harborview café, T-bana: Kungsträdgården plus 10-minute walk, or take bus #65, tel. 08/5202-3500, www.modernamuseet.se.

DJURGÅRDEN

Four hundred years ago, Djurgården was the king's hunting ground (the name means "Animal Garden"). You'll see the royal gate to the island immediately after the bridge that connects it to the mainland. Now this entire lush island is Stockholm's fun center, protected as a national park. It still has a smattering of animal life among its biking paths, picnicking families, art galleries, various amusements, and museums, which are some of the best in Scandinavia.

Orientation: Of the three great sights on the island, the Vasa and Nordic museums are neighbors, and Skansen is a 10-minute walk away (or hop on any bus or tram—they come every couple of minutes). Several lesser or special-interest attractions (from the ABBA museum to an amusement park) are also nearby.

To get around more easily, consider **renting a bike** as you enter the island. You can get one at Sjöcaféet, a café just over the Djurgårdsbron bridge; they also rent boats (bikes-80 kr/hour, 275 kr/day; canoes-150 kr/hour, kayaks-125 kr/hour; open May-Oct daily 9:00-21:00, closed off-season and in bad weather; handy city cycle maps, tel. 08/660-5757, www.sjocafeet.se).

In the concrete building upstairs from the café, you'll find a

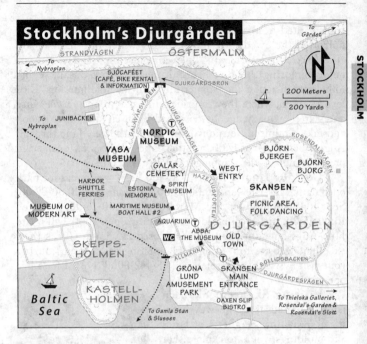

STOCKHOLM

Stockholm's Djurgården

ÖSTERMALM

STRANDVÄGEN

To Nybroplan

To Gärdet

SJÖCAFÉET (CAFÉ, BIKE RENTAL & INFORMATION)

DJURGÅRDSBRON

200 Meters
200 Yards

To JUNIBACKEN
Nybroplan

GALÄRVARVSVÄGEN

DJURGÅRDSVÄGEN

ROSENDALSVÄGEN

NORDIC MUSEUM

BJÖRN BJERGET

BJÖRN BJORG

VASA MUSEUM

GALÄR CEMETERY

SPIRIT MUSEUM

WEST ENTRY

HAZELIUSPORTEN

SKANSEN

HARBOR SHUTTLE FERRIES

ESTONIA MEMORIAL

PICNIC AREA, FOLK DANCING

MUSEUM OF MODERN ART

MARITIME MUSEUM BOAT HALL #2

AQUARIUM

DJURGÅRDEN

ABBA: THE MUSEUM

OLD TOWN

WC

SKEPPS-HOLMEN

ALLMÄNNA

SOLLIDSBACKEN

GRÖNA LUND AMUSEMENT PARK

SKANSEN MAIN ENTRANCE

DJURGÅRDSVÄGEN

Baltic Sea

KASTELL-HOLMEN

OAXEN SLIP BISTRO

To Thielska Galleriet, Rosendal's Garden & Rosendal's Slott

To Gamla Stan & Slussen

Djurgården visitors center, with free maps, island bike routes, brochures, and information about the day's events (you can also buy ABBA museum tickets here; center open daily in summer 8:00-20:00, shorter hours off-season).

Getting There: Take tram #7 from Sergels Torg (the stop is right under the highway overpass) or Nybroplan (in front of the gilded theater building) and get off at one of these stops: Nordic Museum (used also for Vasa Museum), Liljevalc Gröna Lund (for ABBA museum), or Skansen. In summer, you can take a ferry from Nybroplan or Slussen (see "Getting Around Stockholm," earlier). Walkers enjoy the harborside Strandvägen promenade, which leads from Nybroplan directly to the island.

Museums on Djurgården
▲▲▲Skansen

Founded in 1891, Skansen was the first in what became a Europe-wide movement to preserve traditional architecture in open-air museums. It's a huge park gathering more than 150 historic buildings (homes, churches, shops, and schoolhouses)

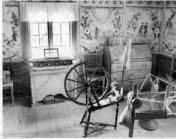

transplanted from all corners of Sweden. Other languages have borrowed the Swedish term "Skansen" (which originally meant "the Fort") to describe an "open-air museum." Today, tourists enjoy exploring this Swedish-culture-on-a-lazy-Susan, seeing folk crafts in action and wonderfully furnished old interiors. Kids love Skansen, where they can ride a life-size wooden *Dala*-horse and stare down a hedgehog, visit Lill-Skansen (a children's zoo), and take a minitrain or pony ride. While it's lively June through August before about 17:00, at other times of the year it can seem pretty dead; consider skipping it if you're here off-season.

Cost and Hours: 160 kr, kids-60 kr, less off-season; park open daily May-late-June 10:00-19:00, late-June-Aug 10:00-22:00, Sept 10:00-18:00, Oct and March-April 10:00-16:00, Nov-Feb 10:00-15:00; historical buildings generally open 11:00-17:00, late June-Aug some until 19:00, most closed in winter. Check their excellent website for "What's Happening at Skansen" during your visit (www.skansen.se) or call 08/442-8000 (press 1 for a live operator).

Visiting Skansen: Skansen isn't designed as a one-way loop; it's a sprawling spaghetti of lanes and buildings, yours to explore. For the full story, invest in the 75-kr museum guidebook. With the book, you'll understand each building you duck into and even learn about the Nordic animals awaiting you in the zoo. Check the live crafts schedule at the information stand by the main entrance to make a smart Skansen plan.

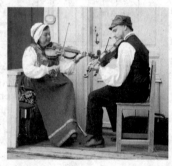

From the entrance, bear left to find the escalator, and ride it up to **"The Town Quarter"** (Stadskvarteren), where shoemakers, potters, and glassblowers are busy doing their traditional thing

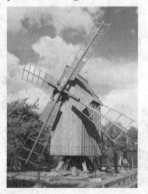

(daily 10:00-17:00) in a re-created Old World Stockholm. Continuing deeper into the park—past the bakery, spice shop/grocery, hardware store, and a cute little courtyard café—you'll reach the central square, **Bollnästorget** (signed as "Central Skansen" but labeled on English maps as "Market Street"), with handy food stands. The rest of Sweden spreads out from here. Northern Swedish culture and architecture is in the north (top of park map), and southern Sweden's in the south (bottom of map). Various home-steads—each one clustered protectively around an inner court-yard—are scattered around the complex.

Poke around. Follow signs—or your instincts. It's worth stepping into the old, red-wood Seglora Church (just past Bollnästorget), which aches with atmosphere under painted beams.

Eating at Skansen: The park has ample eating options to suit every budget. The most memorable—and affordable—meals are at the small folk food court on the main square, **Bollnästorget.** Here, among the duck-filled lakes, frolicking families, and peace-nik local toddlers who don't bump on the bumper cars, kiosks dish up "Sami slow food" (smoked reindeer), waffles, hot dogs, and more. There are lots of picnic benches—Skansen encourages **picnicking.** (A small grocery store is tucked away across the street and a bit to the left of the main entrance.)

▲▲▲Vasa Museum (Vasamuseet)

Stockholm turned a titanic flop into one of Europe's great sight-seeing attractions. The glamorous but unseaworthy warship *Vasa*—top-heavy with an extra cannon deck—sank 40 minutes into her 1628 maiden voyage when a breeze caught the sails and blew her over. After 333 years at the bottom of Stockholm's harbor, she rose again from the deep with the help of marine archaeologists. Rediscovered in 1956 and raised in 1961, this Edsel of the sea is today the best-preserved ship of its age anywhere—housed since 1990 in a brilliant museum. The masts perched atop the roof—best seen from a distance—show the actual height of the ship.

Cost and Hours: 130 kr, includes film and tour; daily June-Aug 8:30-18:00; Sept-May 10:00-17:00 except Wed until 20:00; WCs on level 3, good café, Galärvarvet, Djurgården, tel. 08/5195-4800, www.vasamuseet.se.

Getting There: The *Vasa* is on the waterfront immedi-ately behind the stately brick Nordic Museum (described later), a 10-minute walk from Skansen. Or you can take tram #7 from downtown. To get from the Nordic Museum to the Vasa Museum, face the Nordic Museum and walk around to the right (going left takes you into a big dead-end parking lot).

Crowd-Beating Tips: The museum can have very long lines, but they generally move quickly—you likely won't wait more than 15-20 minutes. If crowds are a concern, get here either right when it opens, or after about 16:00 (but note that the last tour starts at 16:30).

Tours: The free 25-minute **tour** is worthwhile. Because each guide is given license to cover whatever he or she likes, no two tours are alike—if you're fascinated by the place, consider taking two different tours to pick up new details. In summer, English tours run on the hour and half-hour (last tour at 16:30); off-season (Sept-May) tours go 3/day Mon-Fri, hourly Sat-Sun (last tour at 15:30). Listen for the loudspeaker announcement, or check at the info desk for the next tour. Alternatively, you can access the **audioguide** by logging onto the museum's Wi-Fi (www.vasamuseet.se/audioguide).

Film: The excellent 17-minute film digitally re-creates *Vasa*-era Stockholm (and the colorfully painted ship itself), dramatizes its sinking, and documents the modern-day excavation and preservation of the vessel. It generally runs three times per hour; virtually all showings are either in English or with English subtitles.

Visiting the Museum: For a thorough visit, plan on spending at least an hour and a half—watch the film, take a guided tour, and linger over the exhibits (this works in any order). After buying your ticket, head inside. Sort out your film and tour options at the information desk to your right.

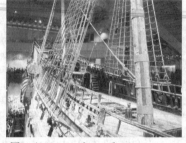

Upon entry, you're prow-to-prow with the great ship. The *Vasa*, while not quite the biggest ship in the world when launched in 1628, had the most firepower, with two fearsome decks of cannons. The 500 carved wooden statues draping the ship—once painted in bright colors—are all symbolic of the king's power. The 10-foot lion on the magnificent prow is a reminder that Europe considered the Swedish King Gustavus Adolphus the "Lion from the North." With this great ship, Sweden was preparing to establish its empire and become more engaged in European power politics. Specifically, the Swedes (who already controlled much of today's Finland and Estonia) wanted to push south to dominate the whole of the Baltic Sea, in order to challenge their powerful rival, Poland.

Designed by a Dutch shipbuilder, the *Vasa* had 72 guns of the same size and type (a rarity on mix-and-match warships of the age), allowing maximum efficiency in reloading—since there was no need to keep track of different ammunition. Unfortunately, the king's unbending demands to build it high (172 feet tall) but skinny made it extremely unstable; no amount of ballast could weigh the ship down enough to prevent it from tipping.

Now explore the **exhibits,** which are situated on six levels around the grand hall, circling the ship itself. All displays are well described in English. You'll learn about the ship's rules (bread can't be older than eight years), why it sank (heavy bread?), how it's preserved (the ship, not the bread), and so on. Best of all is the chance to do slow laps around the magnificent vessel at different levels.

Now painstakingly restored, 98 percent of the *Vasa*'s wood is original (modern bits are the brighter and smoother planks).

On **level 4** (the entrance level), right next to the ship, you'll see a 1:10 scale model of the *Vasa* in its prime—vividly painted and fully rigged with sails. Farther along, models show how the *Vasa* was salvaged; a colorful children's section re-creates the time period; and a 10-minute multimedia show explains why the *Vasa* sank (alternating between English and Swedish showings). Heading behind the ship, you'll enjoy a great view of the sculpture-slathered stern of the *Vasa*. The facing wall features full-size replicas of the carvings, demonstrating how the ship was originally colorfully painted.

Several engaging displays are on **level 5**. "Life On Board" lets you walk through the gun deck and study cutaway models of the hive of activity that hummed below decks (handy, since you can't enter the actual ship). Artifacts—including clothes actually worn by the sailors—were salvaged along with the ship. "Battle!" is a small exhibit of cannons and an explanation of naval warfare.

Level 6 features "The Sailing Ship," with models demonstrating how the *Vasa* and similar vessels actually sailed. You'll see the (very scant) remains of some of the *Vasa*'s actual riggings and sails. **Level 7** gives you even higher views over the ship.

Don't miss **level 2**—all the way at the bottom (ride the handy industrial-size elevator)—with some of the most interesting exhibits. "The Shipyard" explains how this massive and majestic vessel was brought into being using wood from tranquil Swedish forests. Tucked under the ship's prow is a laboratory where today's scientists continue with their preservation efforts. The "Objects" exhibit shows off actual items found in the shipwreck, while "Face to Face" introduces you to some of those who perished when the *Vasa* sank—with faces that were re-created from skeletal remains. Nearby, you'll see some of the skeletons found in the shipwreck.

▲▲Nordic Museum (Nordiska Museet)

Built to look like a Danish Renaissance palace, this museum offers a fascinating peek at 500 years of traditional Swedish lifestyles. The exhibits insightfully place everyday items into their social/historical context in ways that help you really grasp various chapters of Sweden's past. It's arguably more informative than Skansen. Take time to let the excellent, included audioguide enliven the exhibits.

Cost and Hours: 100 kr, free Wed after 17:00 Sept-May; daily 10:00-17:00, Wed until 20:00 Sept-May; Djurgårdsvägen 6-16, at Djurgårdsbron, tram #7 from downtown, tel. 08/5195-6000, www.nordiskamuseet.se.

Visiting the Museum: Entering the museum's main hall, you'll be face-to-face with Carl Milles' huge painted-wood statue of Gustav Vasa, father of modern Sweden. The rest of this floor is usually devoted to temporary exhibits. Highlights of the permanent collection are on the top two floors. Head up the stairs, or take the elevator just to the left of Gustav. Begin on floor 4 and work your way down.

On **floor 4,** four different exhibits ring the grand atrium. The "Homes and Interiors" section displays 400 years of home decor.

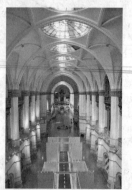

As you travel through time—from dark, heavily draped historical rooms to modern living rooms, and from rustic countryside cottages to aristocratic state bedrooms—you'll learn the subtle meaning behind everyday furniture that we take for granted. For example, the advent of television didn't just change entertainment—it gave people a reason to gather each evening in the living room, which, in turn, became a more-used (and less formal) part of people's homes. You'll learn about the Swedish designers who, in the 1930s, eschewed stiff-backed traditional chairs in favor of sleek perches that merged ergonomics and looks—giving birth to functionalism.

Also on this floor, the "Folk Art" section shows off colorfully painted furniture and wood carvings; vibrant traditional costumes; and rustic Bible-story illustrations that adorned the walls of peasants' homes. The "Sápmi" exhibit tells the fascinating and often overlooked story of the indigenous Sami people (formerly called "Lapps"), who lived in the northern reaches of Norway, Sweden, Finland, and Russia centuries before Europeans created those modern nations. On display are shoes, ceremonial knives, colorful hats and clothing, and other features of Sami culture.

Floor 3 has several smaller exhibits. The most interesting are "Table Settings" (with carefully set tables from the last century, representing different time periods, social classes, and occasions—from an elegant tea party to a rowdy pub) and "Traditions" (showing and describing each old-time celebration of the Swedish year—from Christmas to Midsummer—as well as funerals, confirmations, and other life events).

▲ABBA: The Museum

The Swedish pop group ABBA was, for a time, a bigger business than Volvo. After bursting on the scene in 1974 by winning the Eurovision Song Contest with "Waterloo," and increasing their fame by serenading Sweden's newly minted queen with "Dancing

Queen" in 1976, they've sold more than 380 million records, and the musical based on their many hits, *Mamma Mia!*, has been enjoyed by 50 million people. It was only a matter of time before Stockholm opened an ABBA museum, which is conveniently located just across the street from Skansen and next to Gröna Lund amusement park. Like everything ABBA, it is aggressively for-profit and slickly promoted, with the steepest ticket price in town (not covered by Stockholm Card). True to its subject, it's bombastic, glitzy, and highly interactive. If you like ABBA, it's lots of fun; if you love ABBA, it's ▲▲▲ nirvana.

Cost and Hours: 195 kr, 500-kr family ticket covers two adults and up to four kids, cash not accepted, daily 10:00-20:00, shorter hours off-season—likely until 18:00, Djurgårdsvägen 68, bus #44 or tram #7 to Liljevalc Gröna Lund stop, tel. 08/1213-2860, www.abbathemuseum.com.

Audioguide: ABBA aficionados will happily fork over 40 kr extra for the intimate audioguide, in which Agnetha, Benny, Björn, and Anni-Frid share their memories, in their own words.

Getting In: To control the crowds, only 75 people are let in every 15 minutes with timed-entry tickets. The museum strongly encourages getting tickets in advance from their website or at the TI. In fact, they'll charge you 20 kr extra per ticket to book one in person (but computer terminals are standing by if you want to "pre-book" on the spot). It can be crowded on summer weekends, in which case you may have to wait for a later time.

Other Djurgården Sights
Gröna Lund Amusement Park
Stockholm's venerable and lowbrow Tivoli-type amusement park still packs in the local families and teens on cheap dates. It's a busy venue for local pop concerts.

Cost and Hours: 110 kr, late April-late Sept daily 12:00-23:00, closed off-season, www.gronalund.com.

▲Thielska Galleriet
If you liked the Larsson and Zorn art in the National Gallery, and/or if you're a Munch fan, this charming mansion on the water at the far end of the Djurgården park is worth the trip.

Cost and Hours: 100 kr, Tue-Sun 12:00-17:00, closed Mon, bus #69 (not #69K) from downtown, tel. 08/662-5884, www.thielska-galleriet.se.

▲Biking the Garden Island
In all of Stockholm, Djurgården is *the* natural place to enjoy a bike ride. There's a good and reasonably priced bike-rental place just over the bridge as you enter the island (see page 270), and a world of park-like paths and lanes with harbor vistas to enjoy.

STOCKHOLM

Ask for a free map and route tips when you rent your bike. Figure about an hour to pedal around Djurgården's waterfront perimeter; it's mostly flat, but with some short steeper stretches that take you up and over the middle of the island. Those who venture beyond the Skansen park find themselves nearly all alone in the lush and evocative environs.

ON THE OUTSKIRTS
Two worthy sights sit on Stockholm's doorstep: the home and garden of Carl Milles, Sweden's greatest sculptor, and Drottningholm Palace, the summer residence of the Swedish royal family.

▲Millesgården
The villa and garden of Carl Milles is a veritable forest of statues by Sweden's greatest sculptor. Millesgården is dramatically situated on a bluff overlooking the harbor in
Stockholm's upper-class suburb of Lidingö. While the art is engaging and enjoyable, even the curators have little to say about it from an interpretive point of view—so your visit is basically without guidance. But in Milles' house, which dates from the 1920s, you can see his north-lit studio and get a sense of his creative genius.

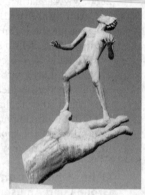

Cost and Hours: 100 kr; daily 11:00-17:00 except closed Mon in Oct-April; English booklet explains the art, restaurant and café, tel. 08/446-7590, www.millesgarden.se.

Getting There: Catch the T-bana to Ropsten, then take bus #207 to within a five-minute walk of the museum; several other #200-series buses also get you close enough to walk (allow about 45 minutes total each way).

▲▲Drottningholm Palace (Drottningholms Slott)
The queen's 17th-century summer castle and current royal residence has been called "Sweden's Versailles." Touring the palace, you'll see art that makes the point that Sweden's royalty is divine and belongs with the gods. You can walk the two floors on your own, but with no explanations or audioguides, it makes sense to take the included guided tour.

Cost and Hours: 120 kr, May-Aug daily 10:00-16:30, Sept daily 11:00-15:30, Oct and April Fri-Sun only 11:00-15:30, Nov-Dec and mid-Jan-March Sat-Sun only 12:00-15:30, closed last two weeks of Dec; free-with-admission palace tours in English are offered 4/day June-Aug, fewer off-season; tel. 08/402-6280, www.royalcourt.se.

Services: The gift shop/café at the entrance to the grounds (near the boat dock and bus stop) acts as a visitors center; Drottningholm's only WCs are in the adjacent building.

Getting There: The castle is an easy boat or subway-plus-bus ride from downtown Stockholm. Consider approaching by water (as the royals traditionally did) and then returning by bus and subway (as a commoner).

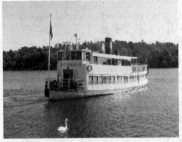

Boats depart regularly from near City Hall for the relaxing hour-long trip (145 kr one-way, 195 kr round-trip, discount with Stockholm Card, departs from Stadshusbron across from City Hall on the hour through the day, likely additional departures at :30 past the hour on weekends or any day in July-Aug, fewer departures Sept-April, tel. 08/1200-4000, www.stromma.se).

It can be faster (30-45 minutes total) to take **public transit:** Ride the T-bana about 20 minutes to Brommaplan, where you can catch any #300-series bus for the five-minute ride to Drottningholm (as you leave the Brommaplan Station, check monitors to see which bus is leaving next—usually from platform A, E, or F; 54 kr one-way).

Visiting the Palace: While not the finest palace interior in Europe (or even in Scandinavia), Drottningholm offers a chance to stroll through a place where a monarch still lives. You'll see two floors of lavish rooms, where Sweden's royalty did their best to live in the style of Europe's divine monarchs.

Ascend the grand staircase (decorated with faux marble and relief-illusion paintings) and buy your ticket on the first floor. Entering the state rooms on the **first floor,** admire the craftsmanship of the walls, with gold leaf shimmering on expertly tooled leather. Then pass through the Green Cabinet and hook right into Hedvig Eleonora's State Bed Chambers. The richly colored Baroque decor here, with gold embellishments, is representative of what the entire interior once looked like.

This room was also the residence of a later monarch, Gustav III. That's why it looks like (and was) more of a theater than a place for sleeping. In the style of the French monarchs, this is where the ceremonial tucking-in and dressing of the king would take place.

Backtrack into the golden room, then continue down the other hallway. You'll pass through a room of royal portraits with very consistent characteristics: pale skin with red cheeks; a high forehead with gray hair (suggesting wisdom); and big eyes (windows to the soul). At the end of the hall is a grand library, which once held some 7,000 books. The small adjoining room is filled by a large model of a temple in Pompeii; Gustav III—who ordered this built—was fascinated by archaeology, and still today, there's a museum of antiquities named for him at the Royal Palace in Stockholm.

On the **second floor,** as you enter the first room, notice the faux doors, painted on the walls to create symmetry, and the hidden doors for servants (who would scurry—unseen and unheard—through the walls to service the royal family). In the Blue Drawing Room is a bust of the then-king's cousin, Catherine the Great. This Russian monarch gave him—in the next room, the Chinese Drawing Room—the (made-in-Russia) faux "Chinese" stove. This dates from a time when exotic imports from China (tea, silk, ivory, Kung Pao chicken) were exciting and new. (Around the same time, in the mid-18th century, the royals built the Chinese Pavilion on Drottningholm's grounds.) The Gobelins tapestries in this room were also a gift, from France's King Louis XVI. In the next room, the darker Oskar Room, are more tapestries—these a gift from England's King Charles I. (Sensing a trend?) You'll pass through Karl XI's Gallery (overlooking the grand staircase)—which is still used for royal functions—and into the largest room on this floor, the Hall of State. The site of royal weddings and receptions, this room boasts life-size paintings of very important Swedes in golden frames and a bombastically painted ceiling.

Drottningholm Court Theater: This 18th-century theater (Drottningholms Slottsteater) has miraculously survived the ages—complete with its instruments; hand-operated sound-effects machines for wind, thunder, and clouds; and original stage sets. Visit it on a 40-minute guided tour, which some find more enjoyable than the palace tour.

Cost and Hours: 100 kr for guided tour, English tours about hourly May-Aug 11:00-16:30, Sept 12:00-15:30—these are first and last tour times, shop open before and after, may be limited tours on weekends in April and Oct-Dec, no tours Jan-March, tel. 08/759-0406, www.dtm.se.

Shopping in Stockholm

Sweden offers a world of shopping temptations. Smaller stores are open weekdays 10:00-18:00, Saturdays until 17:00, and Sundays 11:00-16:00. Some of the bigger stores (such as NK, H&M, and Åhléns) are open later on Saturdays and Sundays.

Fun Chain Stores

DesignTorget, dedicated to contemporary Swedish design, receives a commission for selling the unique works of local designers (generally Mon-Fri 10:00-19:00, Sat 10:00-18:00, Sun 11:00-17:00, big branch underneath Sergels Torg—enter from basement level of Kulturhuset, other branches are at Nybrogatan 23 and at the airport, www.designtorget.se).

Systembolaget is Sweden's state-run liquor store chain. A sample of each bottle of wine or liquor sits in a display case. A card in front explains how it tastes and suggests menu pairings. Look for the item number and order at the counter. Branches are in Hötorget underneath the movie theater complex, in Norrmalm at Vasagatan 21, and just up from Östermalmstorgat Nybrogatan 47 (Mon-Wed 10:00-18:00, Thu-Fri 10:00-19:00, Sat 10:00-15:00, closed Sun, www.systembolaget.se).

Hamngatan

The main shopping zone between Kungsträdgården and Sergels Torg (described in "Stockholm's Modern City Walk" on page 258) has plenty of huge department stores. At the top of Kungsträdgården, Illums Bolighus is a Danish design shop. Across the street, Nordiska Kompaniet (NK) is elegant and stately; the Swedish design (downstairs) and kitchenware sections are particularly impressive. The classy Gallerian mall is just up the street from NK and stretches seductively nearly to Sergels Torg. The Åhléns store, kitty-corner across Sergels Torg, is less expensive than NK and has two cafeterias and a supermarket. Affordable clothing chain H&M has a store right across the street.

Mood Stockholm

The city's most exclusive mall is a downtown block filled with big-name Swedish and international designers, plus a pricey food court and restaurants. The preciously upscale decor and mellow music give it a Beverly Hills vibe (Mon-Fri 10:00-20:00, Sat 10:00-18:00, Sun 11:00-17:00, Regeringsgatan 48). This mall anchors a ritzy, pedestrianized shopping zone; for additional trendy and exclusive shops, browse the nearby streets Jakobsbergsgatan and Biblioteksgatan.

Södermalm

When Swedes want the latest items by local designers, they skip the downtown malls and head for funky Södermalm. Götgatan, the main drag that leads from Slussen up to this neighborhood, is a particularly good choice, with shop after shop of mostly Swedish designers. Boutiques along here—some of them one-offs, others belonging to Swedish chains—include Weekday (jeans and dressed-up casual), Filippa K (smart casual and business attire), and Tiogruppen (bold bags and fabrics).

Nybrogatan

This short and pleasant traffic-free street, which connects Östermalmstorg with the Nybroplan waterfront, is lined with small branches of interesting design shops, including Nordiska Galleriet (eye-catching modern furniture, at #11), DesignTorget (described earlier, at #16), and Hemslöjden (Swedish handicrafts, at #23). It also has shoe and handbag stores, and an enticing cheese shop and bakery.

Flea Markets

For a *smörgåsbord* of Scanjunk, visit the **Loppmarknaden,** northern Europe's biggest flea market, at Vårberg Center (free entry weekdays and Sat-Sun after 15:00, 15 kr on weekends—when it's busiest; open Mon-Fri 11:00-18:00, Sat 10:00-16:00, Sun 11:00-16:00; T-bana: Vårberg, tel. 08/710-0060, www.loppmarknaden.se). Hötorget, the produce market, also hosts a Sunday flea market in summer (see page 260).

Eating in Stockholm

At lunch, cafés and restaurants have 95-kr daily special plates called *dagens rätt* (generally Mon-Fri only). Most museums have handy cafés (with lots of turnover and therefore fresh food, 100-kr lunch deals, and often with fine views). Convenience stores serve gas station-style food (and often have seats). As anywhere, department stores and malls are eager to feed shoppers and can be a good, efficient choice. If you want culturally appropriate fast food, stop by a local hot dog stand. Picnics are a great option. There are plenty of park-like, harborside spots to give your cheap picnic some class.

For the location of restaurants in Gamla Stan, see the map on page 284. For other neighborhoods, see page 294.

IN GAMLA STAN

Most restaurants in Gamla Stan serve the 95-kr weekday lunch special mentioned above, which comes with a main dish, small salad, bread, and tap water. Choose from Swedish, Asian, or Italian cuisine. Several popular places are right on the main square (Stortorget) and near the cathedral. Järntorget, at the far end, is another fun tables-in-the-square scene. Touristy places line Västerlånggatan. You'll find more romantic spots hiding on side lanes. I've listed my favorites here (for

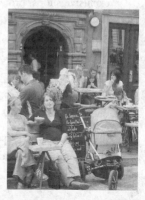

Swedish Cuisine

Most people don't travel to Sweden for the food. Though potatoes and heavy sauces are a focus of the country's cuisine, its variety of meat and fish dishes can be surprisingly satisfying. If you don't think you'll like Swedish or Scandinavian food, be sure to splurge at a good-quality place before you pass final judgment.

Every region of Sweden serves different specialties, but you'll always find *svenska köttbullar* on the menu (Swedish meatballs made from beef and pork in a creamy sauce). This Swedish favorite is topped with lingonberry jam, which is served with many meat dishes across Scandinavia. Potatoes, seemingly the only vegetable known to Sweden, make for hearty *kroppkakor* dumplings filled with onions and minced meat. The northern variation, *pitepalt,* is filled with pork. Southern Sweden takes credit for *pytt i panna,* a medley of leftover meat and diced potatoes that's fried and served with an egg yolk on top. And it seems that virtually every meal you'll eat here includes a side of boiled, small new potatoes.

Though your meals will never be short on starch, be sure to try Sweden's most popular baked good, *kanelbulle,* for a not-so-light snack during the day. This pastry resembles a cinnamon roll, but it's made with cardamom and topped with pearl sugar. Enjoy one during *fika,* the daily Swedish coffee break so institutionalized that many locals use the term as a verb (see page 259).

Like those of its Nordic neighbors, Sweden's extensive coastline produces some of the best seafood in the world. A light, tasty appetizer is *gravad lax,* a dill-cured salmon on brown bread or crackers. You'll also likely encounter *Toast Skagen.* This appetizer-spread is made from shrimp, dill, mayonnaise, and Dijon mustard, and is eaten on buttered toast.

For a main course, the most popular seafood dish is crayfish. Though only eaten by the aristocracy in the 16th century, these shellfish have since become a nationwide delicacy; they're cooked in brine with dill and eaten cold as a finger food. Traditional crayfish parties take place outdoors on summer evenings, particularly in August. Friends and family gather around to indulge in this specialty with rye bread and a strong cheese. The Swedes also love Baltic herring; try *stekt strömming,* a specialty of the east coast, which is herring fried with butter and parsley. As usual, it's served with potatoes and lingonberry jam. Adventurous diners can have their herring pickled or fermented—or order more unusual dishes like reindeer.

As for beer, the Swedes classify theirs by alcohol content. The higher the number, the higher the alcohol content—and the price. *Klass 1* is light beer—very low-alcohol. *Klass 2* is stronger, but still mild. And *Klass 3* has the most body, the most alcohol, and the highest price.

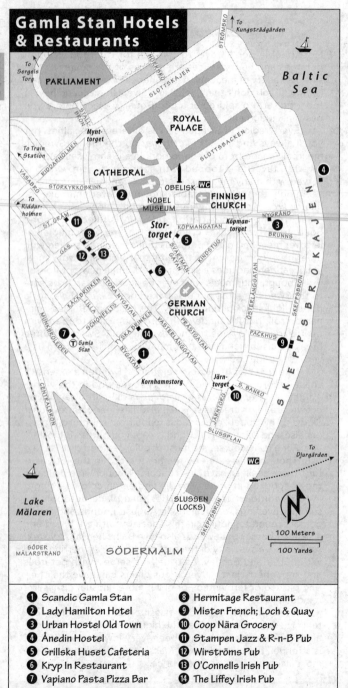

Gamla Stan Hotels & Restaurants

1. Scandic Gamla Stan
2. Lady Hamilton Hotel
3. Urban Hostel Old Town
4. Ånedin Hostel
5. Grillska Huset Cafeteria
6. Kryp In Restaurant
7. Vapiano Pasta Pizza Bar
8. Hermitage Restaurant
9. Mister French; Loch & Quay
10. Coop Nära Grocery
11. Stampen Jazz & R-n-B Pub
12. Wirströms Pub
13. O'Connells Irish Pub
14. The Liffey Irish Pub

locations, see the map on page 284).

Grillska Huset is a cheap and handy cafeteria run by Stockholms Stadsmission, a charitable organization helping the poor. It's grandly situated right on the old square, with indoor and outdoor seating (tranquil garden up the stairs and out back), fine daily specials, a hearty salad bar, and a staff committed to helping others. You can feed the hungry (that's you) and help house the homeless at the same time. The 95-kr daily special gets you a hot plate, salad, and coffee, or choose the 90-kr salad bar—both available Mon-Fri 11:00-14:00 (also 100-kr meals, café serves sandwiches and salads daily 10:00-18:00, Stortorget 3, tel. 08/787-8605). They also have a fine little bakery *(brödbutik)* with lots of tempting cakes and pastries (30-40-kr premade sandwiches, closed Sun).

Kryp In, a small, cozy restaurant (the name means "hide away") tucked into a peaceful lane, has a stylish hardwood and candlelit interior, great sidewalk seating, and an open kitchen letting you in on Vladimir's artistry. If you dine well in Stockholm once (or twice), I'd do it here. It's gourmet without pretense. They serve delicious, modern Swedish cuisine with a 475-kr three-course dinner. In the good-weather months, they serve weekend lunches, with specials starting at 120 kr. Reserve ahead for dinner (200-290-kr plates, daily 17:00-23:00, May-Oct Sat-Sun from 12:30, a block off Stortorget at Prästgatan 17, tel. 08/208-841, www.restaurangkrypin.se).

Vapiano Pasta Pizza Bar, a bright, high-energy, family-oriented eatery, issues you an electronic card as you enter. Circulate to the different stations, ordering up whatever you like as they swipe your card (80-150-kr pastas, pizzas, and salads). Portions are huge and easily splittable. As you leave, your card indicates the bill. Season things by picking a leaf of basil or rosemary from the potted plant on your table. Because tables are often shared, this is a great place for solo travelers (daily 11:00-24:00, right next to entrance to Gamla Stan T-bana station, Munkbrogatan 8, tel. 08/222-940). They also have locations on Östermalm (facing Humlegården park at Sturegatan 12) and Norrmalm (between the train station and Kungsholmen at Kungsbron 15)—for these locations, see the map on page 295.

Hermitage Restaurant is a friendly, faded, hippie-feeling joint that serves a tasty vegetarian buffet in a warm communal dining setting (120 kr gets you a meal, Mon-Fri 11:00-21:00, Sat-Sun 12:00-21:00, Stora Nygatan 11, tel. 08/411-9500).

Picnic Supplies in Gamla Stan: The handy and affordable **Coop Nära** mini supermarket is strategically located on Järntorget, at the Slussen end of Gamla Stan; the **Munkbrohallen** supermarket downstairs in the Gamla Stan T-bana station is also very picnic-friendly (both open daily 7:00-22:00).

DINING ON THE WATER

In Gamla Stan: The harbor embankment of Gamla Stan, facing a gorgeous Stockholm panorama, is lined with swanky quayside eateries and al fresco tables. While prices are high, the setting is memorably romantic—sophisticated, yet waterfront-casual. The listings below are open daily 11:30-24:00 in good weather, when it's smart to call ahead to reserve a view table.

Mister French is the classiest option, with French and American cuisine and a sleek black-and-white color scheme. Choose between the bar (200-kr simple bar food) or the full restaurant (200-300-kr main courses, cheaper half-portions available). They serve a 150-kr lunch special. While the brasserie interior is classy, I'd eat here only for the outdoor views (Tullhus 2, tel. 08/202-095, www.mrfrench.se).

Loch & Quay, next door, is a simpler "summer pub" with lower prices (160-220-kr pub grub, 120-150-kr lunches available until 14:30, Tullhus 2, tel. 08/225-755).

In Kungsholmen, Behind City Hall: On a balmy summer's eve, **Mälarpaviljongen** is a dreamy spot with hundreds of locals enjoying the perfect lakefront scene, as twinkling glasses of rosé shine like convivial lanterns. From City Hall, walk 15 minutes along Lake Mälaren (a treat in itself) and you'll find a hundred casual outdoor tables on a floating restaurant and among the trees on shore. Line up at the cafeteria to order a drink, snack, or complete meal. When it's cool, they have heaters and blankets. The walk along the lake back into town caps the experience beautifully (60-kr beer, 130-kr cocktails, 110-kr lunch plates, 180-240-kr evening meals, open in good weather April-Sept daily 11:00-late, easy lakeside walk or T-bana to Fridhemsplan plus a 5-minute walk to Nörr Mälarstrand 63, no reservations, tel. 08/650-8701).

In Djurgården: **Sjöcaféet,** beautifully situated and greedily soaking up the afternoon sun, fills a woody terrace stretching along the harbor just over the Djurgårdsbron bridge. In summer, this is a fine place for a meal or just a drink before or after your Skansen or *Vasa* visit. They have affordable lunch plates (105 kr, Mon-Fri 11:00-13:00 only); after 14:00, you'll pay 130-180 kr per plate (also 12-kr pizzas, order at the bar, daily 8:00-20:00, often later in summer, closed off-season, tel. 08/661-4488). For the location, see the map on page 271.

Oaxen Slip Bistro, a trendy harborfront place 200 yards below the main Skansen gate, serves creative Nordic cuisine with sturdy local ingredients in a sleek interior or on its delightfully woody terrace. Overlooking a canal in what feels like an old shipyard, and filled with in-the-know locals, this place is a real treat. Reservations are smart (200-kr plates, game and seafood, daily

12:00-14:00 & 17:00-21:30, Beckholmsvägen 26, tel. 08/5515-3105, www.oaxen.com). For location, see the map on page 271.

SÖDERMALM STREETS AND EATS

This quickly gentrifying, working-class district, just south of Gamla Stan (steeply uphill from Slussen), has some of Stockholm's most enticing food options—especially for beer lovers. It's also a bit less swanky, and therefore more affordable, than many of the city's more touristy neighborhoods.

Götgatan and Medborgarplatsen

The neighborhood's liveliest street is the artery called Götgatan, which leads from Slussen (where Södermalm meets Gamla Stan) steeply up into the heart of Södermalm. Here, mixed between the boutiques, you'll find cafés tempting you to join the Swedish coffee break called *fika*, plus plenty of other eateries. Even if you don't dine in Södermalm, it's worth a stroll here just for the window-shopping fun.

At the top of the street, you'll pop out into the big square called Medborgarplatsen. This neighborhood hang-out is a great scene, with almost no tourists and lots of options—especially for Swedish fast food. (My favorite, Melanders Fisk, is listed next.) Outdoor restaurant and café tables fill the square, which is fronted by a big food hall. (There's also a T-bana stop here.) The recommended Kvarnen beer hall (see later) is just around the corner to the left.

Melanders Fisk, facing the square, has only outside tables (and is therefore an option only in warm weather). You order at the bar and join locals in this classic scene. *Skagenröra*, shrimp with mayo on toast or filling a baked potato, is the signature dish—and dear to the Swedish heart (115 kr; also 90-kr lunch plates daily, 130-150-kr fish plates served daily, Medborgarplatsen 3, tel. 08/644-4040).

Skånegatan and Nytorget

A bit farther south, these cross-streets make another good spot to browse among fun and enticing restaurants, particularly for ethnic cuisine.

Nytorget Urban Deli is the epitome of Södermalm's trendy-hipster vibe and an amazing scene. It's half fancy artisanal delicatessen—with all manner of ingredients—and half white-subway-tile-trendy eatery, with indoor and outdoor tables filled with Stockholm yuppies eating well. If it's busy—as it often is—they'll scrawl your name at the bottom of the long butcher-paper waiting list (no reservations). If it's full, you can grab a place at the bar and eat there (international and Swedish modern dishes, 100-190-kr light meals, 190-225-kr bigger meals, daily 8:00-23:00, at the far end of Skånegatan at Nytorget 4, tel. 08/5990-9180).

Nytorget Urban Deli Picnic: The upscale grocery store attached to the deli seems designed for picnickers, with lots of creative boxed meals and salads to go (same address and hours—see listing above). The park across the street has lots of benches and picnic tables.

Kohphangan, with almost a laughably over-the-top island atmosphere that belies its surprisingly good Thai food, has been a hit for 20 years. (Thailand is to Sweden what Mexico is to Americans—the sunny "south of the border" playground.) The ambience? Mix a shipwreck, Bob Marley, and a Christmas tree, and you've got it (160-220-kr dishes, daily 12:00-24:00, Skånegatan 57, tel. 08/642-5040).

Gossip is a mellow, unpretentious hole-in-the-wall serving Bangladeshi street food (120-160-kr dishes, Mon-Fri 11:00-23:00, Sat-Sun 13:00-23:00, Skånegatan 71, tel. 08/640-6901).

Classic Swedish Beer Halls: Three different but equally traditional Södermalm beer halls serve well-executed, hearty Swedish grub in big, high-ceilinged, orange-tiled spaces with rustic wooden tables.

Kvarnen ("The Mill") is a reliable choice with a 1908 ambience. As it's a football-club base, it can be rough. Pick a classic Swedish dish from their fun and easy menu (100-130-kr starters, 140-200-kr main courses, daily 17:00-24:00, Tjärhovsgatan 4, tel. 08/643-0380). **Pelikan,** an old-school beer hall, is less sloppy and has nicer food. It's a bit deeper into Södermalm (120-230-kr starters, 190-270-kr main courses, Mon-Thu 16:00-23:00, Fri-Sun 13:00-23:00, Blekingegatan 40, tel. 08/5560-9290). **Akkurat** has a staggering variety of microbrews—both Swedish and international (on tap and bottled)—as well as whisky. It's great if you wish you were in England with a bunch of Swedes (short menu of 190-240-kr pub grub, Mon-Fri 11:00-24:00, Sat 15:00-24:00, Sun 18:00-24:00, Hornsgatan 18, tel. 08/644-0015).

IN NORRMALM
At or near the Grand Hotel

Royal Smörgåsbord: To stuff yourself with all the traditional Swedish specialties (a dozen kinds of herring, salmon, reindeer, meatballs, lingonberries, and shrimp, followed by a fine table of cheeses and desserts) with a super harbor view, consider splurging at the Grand Hotel's dressy **Veranda Restaurant.** While very touristy, this is considered the finest *smörgåsbord* in town. The Grand Hotel, where royal guests and Nobel Prize winners stay, faces the harbor across from the palace. Pick up their English flier for a good explanation of the proper way to enjoy this grand buffet. Reservations are often necessary (485 kr in evening, 445 kr for lunch, drinks extra, open nightly 18:00-22:00, also open for lunch Sat-Sun 13:00-16:00 year-round and Mon-Fri 12:00-15:00 in May-Sept, no shorts after 18:00, Södra Blasieholmshamnen 8, tel. 08/679-3586, www.grandhotel.se).

Restaurang B.A.R. has a fun energy, with diners surveying the meat and fish at the ice-filled counter, talking things over with the chef, and then choosing a slab. Prices are on the board, and everything's grilled (250-300-kr meals, open daily except closed Sun-Mon in July, behind the Grand Hotel at Blasieholmsgatan 4, tel. 08/611-5335).

At the Royal Opera House
The Operakällaren, one of Stockholm's most exclusive restaurants, runs a little "hip pocket" restaurant called **Bakfickan** on the side, specializing in traditional Swedish quality cooking at reasonable prices. It's ideal for someone eating out alone, or for anyone wanting an early dinner. Choose from two different daily specials or pay 180-280 kr for main dishes from their regular menu (160-180-kr specials served daily from 12:00 until they run out—which can be early or as late as 20:00, no specials in July). Sit inside—at tiny private side tables or at the big counter with the locals—or, in good weather, grab a table on the sidewalk, facing a cheery red church (Mon-Sat 12:00-22:00, closed Sun, on the inland side of Royal Opera House, tel. 08/676-5809).

At or near Hötorget
Hötorget ("Hay Market"), a vibrant outdoor produce market just two blocks from Sergels Torg, is a fun place to picnic-shop. The outdoor market closes at 18:00, and many merchants put their unsold produce on the push list (earlier closing and more desperate merchants on Sat).

Hötorgshallen, next to Hötorget (in the basement under the modern cinema complex), is a colorful indoor food market with an old-fashioned bustle, plenty of exotic and ethnic edibles, and—in the tradition of food markets all over Europe—some great little eateries (Mon-Fri 10:00-18:00, Sat 10:00-15:00, closed Sun). The best is **Kajsas Fisk,** hiding behind the fish stalls. They serve delicious fish soup to little Olivers who can hardly believe they're getting...more. For 95 kr, you get a big bowl of hearty soup, a simple salad, bread and crackers—plus one soup refill. Their *stekt strömming* (traditional fried herring and potato dish) is a favorite (90-150-kr daily fish specials, Mon-Fri 11:00-18:00, Sat 11:00-16:00, closed Sun, Hötorgshallen 3, tel. 08/207-262). There's a great kebab and falafel place a few stalls away.

Kungshallen, an 800-seat indoor food court across the square from Hötorget, has more than a dozen eateries. The main floor is a bit more upscale, with sit-down places and higher prices, while the basement is a shopping-mall-style array of fast-food counters, including Chinese, sushi, pizza, Greek, and Mexican. This is a handy place to comparison-shop for a meal at lower prices (Mon-Fri 9:00-22:00, Sat-Sun 12:00-22:00).

Near Sergels Torg

Kulturhuset Rooftop Eateries: Two places (one cheap and the other trendy) are handy for simple meals with great city views. **Cafeteria Panorama,** offering cheap eats and a salad bar, has both inside and outside seating with jaw-dropping vistas (90-kr lunch specials with salad bar, Sat-Mon 11:00-18:00, Tue-Fri 11:00-20:00). The more stylish **Mat and Bar café** has a pleasant garden setting with pricier food (daily until 21:00).

The many modern shopping malls and department stores around Sergels Torg all have appealing, if pricey, eateries catering to the needs of hungry local shoppers. **Åhléns** department store has a Hemköp supermarket in the basement (daily until 21:00) and two restaurants upstairs with 80-110-kr daily lunch specials (Mon-Fri 11:00-19:30, Sat 11:00-18:30, Sun 11:00-17:30).

IN ÖSTERMALM

Saluhall, on Östermalmstorg (near recommended Hotel Wellington), is a great old-time indoor market with top-quality artisanal producers and a variety of sit-down and take-out eateries. While it's nowhere near "cheap," it's one of the most pleasant market halls I've seen, oozing with upscale yet traditional Swedish class. Inside you'll find Middle Eastern fare, sushi, classic Scandinavian open-face sandwiches, sea- 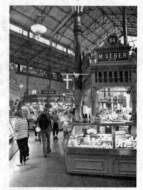 food salads, healthy wraps, cheese counters, designer chocolates, gourmet coffee stands, and a pair of classic old sit-down eater- ies (Elmqvist and Tystamare). This is your chance to pull up a stool at a lunch counter next to well-heeled Swedish yuppies (Mon-Thu 9:30-18:00, Fri until 19:00, Sat until 16:00, closed Sun).

Örtagården, upstairs from the Saluhall, is primarily a veg-etarian restaurant and serves a 145-kr buffet weekdays until 17:00 and a larger 155-kr buffet evenings and weekends (Mon-Fri 11:00-22:00, Sat-Sun 11:00-21:00, entrance on side of market building at Nybrogatan 31, tel. 08/662-1728).

What If I Miss My Boat?

Remember that you can get help from the cruise line's port agent (listed on the destination information sheet distributed on the ship) and the local TI (see page 243).

Many cruise port cities are accessible by train from Stockholm, including **Oslo** and **Copenhagen** (via Malmö; buses also connect to Oslo and Copenhagen); for points south (such as **Warnemünde/Berlin, Amsterdam,** and **Gdańsk**), you'll probably have to go via Copenhagen. For points in Norway (such as **Bergen, Stavanger,** or **Flåm**), you'll take the train to Oslo and connect from there.

Stockholm is a hub for overnight boats on the Baltic. From here, you can sail overnight to **Helsinki** (two companies: Viking Line, tel. 08/452-4000, www.vikingline.fi; or Tallink Silja, tel. 08/222-140, www.tallinksilja.com), to **Tallinn** (Tallink Silja), to **Rīga** (Tallink Silja), and—in two nights—to **St. Petersburg** (St. Peter Line, www.stpeterline.com). It's faster to reach St. Petersburg by taking the night boat first to Helsinki, then hopping on the express train (www.vr.fi). But you'll need a visa to enter Russia (arranged well in advance of your trip, not possible at the last minute); if you don't have one, you'll likely need to meet your ship at a later port of call.

You may find it's faster to **fly** to many places. Stockholm's Arlanda Airport is an easy train ride from downtown; for more on the airport, see "Starting or Ending Your Cruise in Stockholm" on page 292.

For more advice on what to do if you miss the boat, see page 139.

Restaurang Volt is a destination restaurant for foodies looking to splurge on "New Nordic" cooking: fresh, locally sourced ingredients fused into bold new recipes with fundamentally Swedish flavors. Owners Fredrik Johnsson and Peter Andersson fill their minimalist black dining room with just 31 seats, so reservations are essential (550 kr/four courses, 700 kr/six courses, no à la carte, Tue-Sat 18:00-24:00, closed Sun-Mon, Kommendörsgatan 16, tel. 08/662-3400, www.restaurangvolt.se).

Riche, a Parisian-style brasserie just a few steps off Nybroplan at Östermalm's waterfront, is a high-energy environment with a youthful sophistication. They serve up pricey but elegantly executed Swedish and international dishes in their winter garden, bright dining room, and white-tile-and-wine-glass-chandeliered bar (140-230-kr starters, 200-340-kr main courses, 175-kr plat du jour, Mon-Fri 7:30-24:00, Sat-Sun 12:00-24:00, Birger Jarlsgatan 4, tel. 08/5450-3560).

STOCKHOLM

Starting or Ending Your Cruise in Stockholm

If your cruise begins and/or ends in Stockholm, you'll want some extra time here. While you can squeeze the city into a day, two days will let you see more. For a longer visit, pick up my *Rick Steves Snapshot Stockholm* or *Rick Steves Scandinavia* guidebooks.

Airport Connections

ARLANDA AIRPORT

Stockholm's Arlanda Airport is 28 miles north of town (airport code: ARN, tel. 08/797-6000, www.arlanda.se). The airport TI (in Terminal 5, where most international flights arrive, long hours daily) can advise you on getting into Stockholm and on your sightseeing plans.

Getting Downtown from Arlanda Airport

The **airport train,** the Arlanda Express, is the fastest way to zip between the airport and the central train station. Traveling most of the way at 125 mph, it gets you downtown in just 20 minutes—but it's not cheap (260 kr one-way, 490 kr round-trip, free for kids under age 17 with adult, covered by rail pass; generally 4/hour—departing at :05, :20, :35, and :50 past the hour in each direction; toll-free tel. 020-222-224, www.arlandaexpress.com). Buy your ticket either at the window near the track or from a ticket-vending machine, or pay an extra 100 kr to buy it on board. In summer and on weekends, a special fare lets two people travel for nearly half-price (two for 280 kr one-way, available daily mid-June-Aug, Thu-Sun year-round).

Airport shuttle buses (Flygbussarna) run between the airport and Stockholm's train/bus stations (119 kr, 6/hour, 40 minutes, may take longer at rush hour, buy tickets from station kiosks or at airport TI, www.flygbussarna.se).

Taxis between the airport and the city center take 30-40 minutes (about 520 kr, depends on company, look for price printed on side of cab). Establish the price first. Reputable taxis accept credit cards.

The **cheapest airport connection** is to take bus #583 from the airport to Märsta, then switch to the *pendeltåg* (suburban train, 4/hour), which goes to Stockholm's central train station (72 kr, 1 hour total journey time, covered by Stockholm Card).

GETTING TO FRIHAMNEN CRUISE PORT

When meeting your cruise at this sprawling port, it helps to know which berth your ship leaves from—berth 650, 634, or 638.

The easiest but most expensive way to reach your cruise ship is by **taxi**—figure about 520 kr from the airport to Frihamnen, or around 200-250 kr from downtown.

Public transportation is workable (and often cheaper), but there's no direct connection from the airport. First make your way downtown using one of the methods outlined above; then catch the bus to the port: Ride bus #1 from the train station, or bus #76 from various points downtown. On weekends (when bus #76 runs infrequently or not at all), you'll likely need to take bus #1. For more on these buses, see page 240.

Arriving at Frihamnen: Near the cruise terminals, there are two stops: Both buses stop at "Frihamnen" (near berth 650), while bus #76 continues one more stop to "Magasin 3" (closer to berths 634 and 638). A blue line painted on the sidewalk leads to each of the three berths.

If getting off at the "Frihamnen" stop, continue straight ahead along the street to the first intersection, where you'll bear right to reach berth 650 and left to reach berth 634 or 638.

If you get off the bus at "Magasin 3," proceed straight until you reach the Frihamnsterminalen; turn right just before it and head out the long, wide pier—first passing berth 634, then berth 638. (Berth 638 and the cruise terminal are near warehouse, or *magasin*, #6 and #8.)

ALTERNATE AIRPORT

Some discount airlines use Skavsta Airport, about 60 miles south of Stockholm (airport code: NYO, www.skavsta.se). Flygbussarna shuttle buses connect to the city (159 kr, cheaper if you buy online in advance, about 1-2/hour—generally timed to meet arriving flights, 80 minutes, www.flygbussarna.se).

Hotels in Stockholm

If you need a hotel in Stockholm before or after your cruise, here are a few to consider (see the maps on pages 284 and 295 for locations).

Between business travelers and the tourist trade, demand for Stockholm's hotels is healthy but unpredictable, and most hotels' rates vary from day to day. For each hotel (for comparison's sake), I've listed the average price for a standard double room in high season (mid-June-mid-Aug)—but your rate will almost certainly be higher or lower, depending on the timing of your visit.

STOCKHOLM

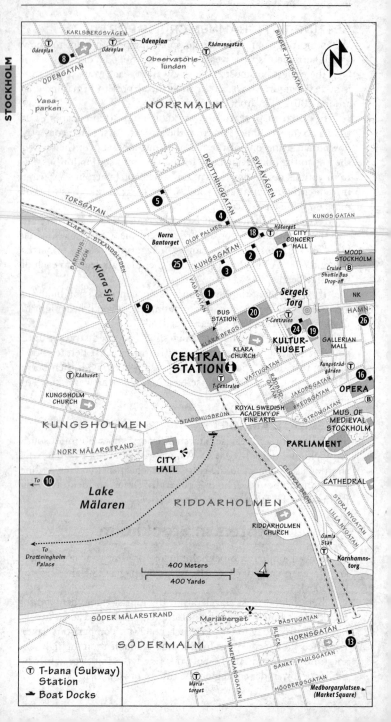

KARLSBERGSVÄGEN

Odenplan

←Odenplan

Rådmansgatan

8

ODENGATAN

Observatorie-
lunden

Vasa-
parken

NORRMALM

BIRGER JARLSGATAN

DROTTNINGGATAN

SVEAVÄGEN

TORSGATAN

5

KUNGS GATAN

KLARA

STRANDSLEDEN

BARNHUS-
BRON

Klara
Sjö

4

OLOF PALMES

18

Hötorget

T

CITY
CONCERT
HALL

MOOD
STOCKHOLM

Norra
Bantorget

25

KUNGSGATAN

2

17

B

Cruise
Shuttle Bus
Drop-off

NK

VASAGATAN

3

1

Sergels
Torg

HAMN-

9

BUS
STATION

20

T-Centralen

24

19

26

KLARABERGS

Klara
Church

T-Centralen

KULTUR-
HUSET

GALLERIAN
MALL

Rådhuset

CENTRAL
STATION

Kungsträd-
gården

16

VATTUGATAN

T

KUNGSHOLMEN

KUNGSHOLM
CHURCH

T-Centralen

RÖDBO-
GATAN

JAKOBSGATAN

BREDGATAN

STRÖMGATAN

Opera

B

NORR MÄLARSTRAND

STADSHUSBRON

ROYAL SWEDISH
ACADEMY OF
FINE ARTS

MUS. OF
MEDIEVAL
STOCKHOLM

PARLIAMENT

CATHEDRAL

To 10

CITY
HALL

Lake
Mälaren

RIDDARHOLMEN

CENTRALBRON

STORA NYGATAN

LILLA NYGATAN

To
Drottningholm
Palace

RIDDARHOLMEN
CHURCH

Gamla
Stan

T

Kornhamns-
torg

400 Meters

400 Yards

SÖDER MÄLARSTRAND

Mariaberget

BÄSTUGATAN

BLEK

HORNSGATAN

13

SÖDERMALM

TIMMERMANSGATAN

SANKT PAULSGATAN

Maria-
torget

T

HÖGBERGSGATAN

Medborgarplatsen
(Market Square)→

Ⓣ T-bana (Subway)
Station
⬌ Boat Docks

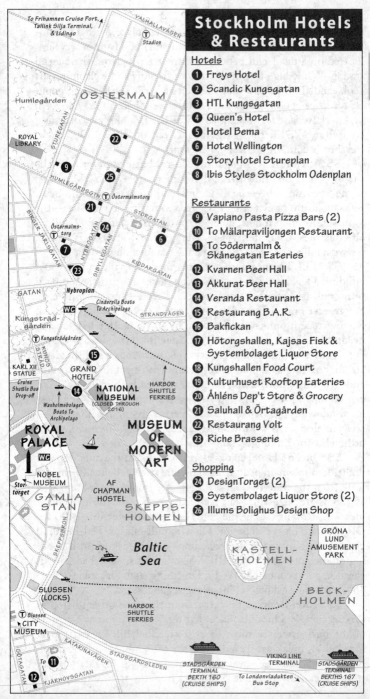

STOCKHOLM

Stockholm Hotels & Restaurants

Hotels

1. Freys Hotel
2. Scandic Kungsgatan
3. HTL Kungsgatan
4. Queen's Hotel
5. Hotel Bema
6. Hotel Wellington
7. Story Hotel Stureplan
8. Ibis Styles Stockholm Odenplan

Restaurants

9. Vapiano Pasta Pizza Bars (2)
10. To Mälarpaviljongen Restaurant
11. To Södermalm & Skånegatan Eateries
12. Kvarnen Beer Hall
13. Akkurat Beer Hall
14. Veranda Restaurant
15. Restaurang B.A.R.
16. Bakfickan
17. Hötorgshallen, Kajsas Fisk & Systembolaget Liquor Store
18. Kungshallen Food Court
19. Kulturhuset Rooftop Eateries
20. Åhléns Dep't Store & Grocery
21. Saluhall & Örtagården
22. Restaurang Volt
23. Riche Brasserie

Shopping

24. DesignTorget (2)
25. Systembolaget Liquor Store (2)
26. Illums Bolighus Design Shop

NEAR THE TRAIN STATION

$$$ Freys Hotel is a Scan-mod, four-star place, with 127 compact, smartly designed rooms. It's well-situated for train travelers, located on a dead-end pedestrian street across from the central station. While big, it works hard to be friendly and welcoming. Its cool, candlelit breakfast room becomes a bar in the evening, popular for its selection of Belgian microbrews (Sb-1,750 kr, Db-2,470 kr, check website for specials as low as Db-1,750 kr, air-con, guest computer, Wi-Fi, Bryggargatan 12, tel. 08/5062-1300, www.freyshotels.com, freys@freyshotels.com).

$$$ Scandic Kungsgatan, central but characterless, fills the top floors of a downsized department store with 270 rooms. If the Starship *Enterprise* had a low-end hotel, this would be it. Save about 100 kr by taking a "cabin" room with no windows—the same size as other rooms, quiet, and well-ventilated (Db-2,000 kr, air-con, guest computer, Wi-Fi, Kungsgatan 47, tel. 08/723-7220, www.scandichotels.com, kungsgatan@scandichotels.com).

$$ HTL Kungsgatan, jamming modernity into a classic old building a few blocks from the station, takes a futuristic approach to providing just what travelers really need—and nothing else. You reserve online, then check in at a self-service kiosk on arrival. Roving receptionists are standing by in the coffee bar for any needs. The 274 rooms are small and functional (no desk or chairs) but trendy and comfortable. Everything surrounds a stylish, glassy atrium boasting a hip lounge/restaurant with a youthful party vibe and live music until 24:00 on most weekends (Sb/Db-1,700 kr, can be much lower—around 700 kr—in slow times, 100 kr less for windowless but well-ventilated "sleeper" room, breakfast-75 kr, air-con, elevator, Wi-Fi, Kungsgatan 53, tel. 08/4108-4150, www.htlhotels.com, htlkungsgatan@htlhotels.com).

$$ Queen's Hotel enjoys a great location at the quiet top end of Stockholm's main pedestrian shopping street (about a 10-minute walk from the train station, or 15 minutes from Gamla Stan). The 59 rooms are well worn, but reasonably priced for the convenient location. Rooms facing the courtyard are quieter (Sb-1,100 kr, Db-1,300 kr, bigger "superior" Db with pull-out sofa bed-1,900, 10 percent discount for readers who book direct—ask for it; if booking online enter rate code "RICKS" in all caps, extra bed-250 kr, elevator, guest computer, Wi-Fi, Drottninggatan 71A, tel. 08/249-460, www.queenshotel.se, info@queenshotel.se).

$$ Hotel Bema, a bit farther out than the others listed in this section, is a humble place that rents 12 fine rooms for some of the best prices in town (S-900 kr, Db-1,100 kr, extra person-250 kr, breakfast served at nearby café, bus #65 from station to Upplandsgatan 13—near the top of the Drottninggatan pedestrian street, or walk about 15 minutes from the train station—exit toward *Vasagatan* and head straight up that street, tel. 08/232-675, www.hotelbema.se, info@hotelbema.se).

IN QUIETER RESIDENTIAL AREAS

$$$ Hotel Wellington, two blocks off Östermalmstorg, is in a less handy but charming part of town. It's modern and bright, with hardwood floors, 60 rooms, and a friendly welcome. While it may seem pricey, it's a cut above in comfort, and its great amenities—such as a very generous buffet breakfast, free coffee all day long, and free buffet dinner in the evening—add up to a good value (prices range widely, but in summer generally Db-1,820 kr, smaller Db for 200 kr less, mention this book when you book direct for a 10 percent discount, guest computer, Wi-Fi, free sauna, old-fashioned English bar, garden terrace bar, T-bana: Östermalmstorg, exit to Storgatan and walk past big church to Storgatan 6; tel. 08/667-0910, www.wellington.se, cc.wellington@choice.se).

$$$ Story Hotel Stureplan is a colorful boutique hotel with a creative hipster vibe. Conveniently located near a trendy dining zone between Östermalmstorg and the Nybroplan waterfront, it has 83 rooms above a sprawling, cleverly decorated, affordably priced restaurant. You'll book online, check yourself in at the kiosk, and receive a text message with your door key code (tight bunk-bed Db-1,700 kr, standard Db-2,000 kr, more for bigger rooms, elevator, free minibar drinks, Wi-Fi, Riddargatan 6, tel. 08/5450-3940, www.storyhotels.com).

$$$ Ibis Styles Stockholm Odenplan rents 76 cookie-cutter rooms on several floors of a late-19th-century apartment building (Db-1,950 kr, about 300 kr cheaper with nonrefundable "advance saver" rate, Wi-Fi, T-bana: Odenplan, Västmannagatan 61, reservation tel. 08/1209-0000, reception tel. 08/1209-0300, www.ibisstyles.se, odenplan@uniquehotels.se).

IN GAMLA STAN

$$$ Scandic Gamla Stan offers Old World elegance in the heart of Gamla Stan (a 5-minute walk from Gamla Stan T-bana station). Its 52 small rooms are filled with chandeliers and hardwood floors (Sb-1,400 kr, Db-2,000 kr, 200 kr extra for larger room, elevator, Wi-Fi, Lilla Nygatan 25, tel. 08/723-7250, www.scandichotels.com, gamlastan@scandichotels.com).

$$$ Lady Hamilton Hotel, classic and romantic, is shoe-horned into Gamla Stan on a quiet street a block below the cathedral and Royal Palace. The centuries-old building has 34 small but plush and colorfully decorated rooms. Each one is named for a Swedish flower and is filled with antiques (Db-2,200 kr, a few hundred kronor more for a bigger "corner" room with a better view, elevator, guest computer, Wi-Fi, Storkyrkobrinken 5, tel.

08/5064-0100, www.ladyhamiltonhotel.se, info@ladyhamilton hotel.se).

$$ Urban Hostel Old Town is a sane and modern hostel conveniently located in an untrampled part of Gamla Stan, just a few steps off the harbor. Conscientiously run, with 135 beds in small but tidy, modern rooms, it's not a party hostel—grown-ups will feel comfortable here (bunk in 16-bed dorm-295 kr, S-695 kr, D-900 kr, Db-1,500 kr, T-1,100 kr, Q-1,400 kr, Qb-2,200 kr, breakfast-75 kr, air-con, elevator, Wi-Fi, Nygränd 5, tel. 08/1214-0444, www.urbanhostels.se, info@urbanhostels.se).

$$ Ånedin Hostel is a floating hotel, moored near the foot of the Royal Palace. Once a cruise boat, the classic liner *MS Birger Jarl* has 130 cabins, varying from small simple rooms to superior cabins with private baths (Db-600 kr, Qb-900 kr, prices vary by size of room and berth configuration, breakfast-90 kr, Wi-Fi in public spaces, Skeppsbron Tullhus 1, tel. 08/6841-0130, www. anedinhostel.com, info@anedinhostel.com).

Nightlife in Stockholm

The easiest choices are the bars and other live-music venues in Gamla Stan. The street called Stora Nygatan, with several lively bars, has perhaps the most accessible and reliable place for good jazz in town—**Stampen Jazz & Rhythm n' Blues Pub.** It has two venues: a stone-vaulted cellar below and a fun-loving saloon-like bar upstairs (check out the old instruments and antiques hanging from the ceiling). From Monday through Thursday, there's live music only in the saloon. On Friday and Saturday, bands alternate sets in both the saloon and the cellar (160-kr cover Fri-Sat only, open Mon-Thu 17:00-late, Fri-Sun 20:00-late, Stora Nygatan 5, tel. 08/205-793, www.stampen.se). For the location, see the map on page 284.

Several other lively spots are within a couple of blocks of Stampen on Stora Nygatan. Your options include **Wirströms Pub** (live blues bands play in crowded cellar Tue-Sat 21:00-24:00, no cover, 62-kr beers, open daily 11:00-late, Stora Nygatan 13, www. wirstromspub.se); **O'Connells Irish Pub** (a lively expat sports bar with music—usually Tue-Sat at 21:00, open daily 12:00-late, Stora Nygatan 21, www.oconnells.se); and **The Liffey** (classic Irish pub with 150-180-kr pub grub, live music Wed and Fri-Sun at 21:30, open daily 11:00-late, Stora Nygatan 40-42, www.theliffey.se).

Swedish Survival Phrases

Swedish pronunciation (especially the vowel sounds) can be tricky for Americans to say, and there's quite a bit of variation across the country; listen closely to locals and imitate, or ask for help. The most difficult Swedish sound is *sj,* which sounds roughly like a guttural "*h*w" (made in your throat); however, like many sounds, this is pronounced differently in various regions—for example, Stockholmers might say it more like "shw."

English	Swedish	Pronunciation
Hello. (formal)	*Goddag!*	goh-**dah**
Hi. / Bye. (informal)	*Hej. / Hej då.*	hey / hey doh
Do you speak English?	*Talar du engelska?*	**tah**-lar doo **eng**-ehl-skah
Yes. / No.	*Ja. / Nej.*	yaw / nay
Please.	*Snälla: / Tack.**	**snehl**-lah / tack
Thank you (very much).	*Tack (så mycket).*	tack (soh **mee**-keh)
You're welcome.	*Ingen orsak.*	**eeng**-ehn **oor**-sahk
Can I help you?	*Kan jag hjälpa dig?*	kahn yaw **jehl**-pah day
Excuse me.	*Ursäkta.*	**oor**-sehk-tah
(Very) good.	*(Mycket) bra.*	(**mee**-keh) brah
Goodbye.	*Adjö.*	ah-**yew**
one / two	*en / två*	ehn / tvoh
three / four	*tre / fyra*	treh / **fee**-rah
five / six	*fem / sex*	fehm / sehks
seven / eight	*sju / åtta*	*h*woo / **oh**-tah
nine / ten	*nio / tio*	**nee**-oh / **tee**-oh
hundred	*hundra*	**hoon**-drah
thousand	*tusen*	**too**-sehn
How much?	*Hur mycket?*	hewr **mee**-keh
local currency: (Swedish) kronor	*(Svenske) kronor*	(svehn-**skeh**) **kroh**-nor
Where is...?	*Var finns...?*	var feens
...the toilet	*...toaletten*	toh-ah-**leh**-tehn
men	*man*	mahn
women	*kvinna*	**kvee**-nah
water / coffee	*vatten / kaffe*	**vah**-tehn / **kah**-feh
beer / wine	*öl / vin*	url / veen
Cheers!	*Skål!*	skohl
The bill, please.	*Kan jag få notan, tack.*	kahn yaw foh **noh**-tahn tack

*Swedish has various ways to say "please," depending on the context. The simplest is *snälla,* but Swedes sometimes use the word *tack* (thank you) the way we use "please."

HELSINKI
Finland

Finland Practicalities

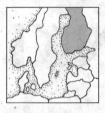

We think of Finland (Suomi) as Scandinavian, but it's better to call it Nordic (along with Iceland and Estonia). Finland is bordered by Russia to the east, Sweden and Norway to the north, the Baltic Sea to the west, and Estonia (across the Gulf of Finland) to the south. After gaining independence from Russia in 1917, Finland resisted invasion during World War II—and a low-key but pervasive Finnish pride has percolated here ever since. A mostly flat, forested, lake-filled country of 130,500 square miles (almost twice the size of Washington state), Finland is home to 5.3 million people. Finland's population is more than 79 percent Lutheran, and the vast majority (93.4 percent) is of Finnish descent.

Money: €1 (euro) = about $1.40. An ATM is called a *pankkiautomaatti;* these are often marked *Otto.* The local VAT (value-added sales tax) rate is 24 percent; the minimum purchase eligible for a VAT refund is €40 (for details on refunds, see page 134).

Language: The native language is Finnish. For useful phrases, see page 346.

Emergencies: Dial 112 for police, medical, or other emergencies. In case of theft or loss, see page 125.

Time Zone: Finland is one hour ahead of Central European Time (seven/ten hours ahead of the East/West Coasts of the US). That puts Helsinki in the same time zone as Tallinn and Rīga; one hour ahead of Stockholm, the rest of Scandinavia, and most other continental cruise ports (including Gdańsk and Warnemünde); and one hour behind St. Petersburg.

Embassies in Helsinki: The **US embassy** is at Itäinen Puistotie 14B (tel. 40/140-5957, emergency tel. 09/616-250, http://finland.usembassy.gov). The **Canadian embassy** is at Pohjoisesplanadi 25B (tel. 09/228-530, www.canada.fi). Call ahead for passport services.

Phoning: Finland's country code is 358; to call from another country to Finland, dial the international access code (011 from the US/Canada, 00 from Europe, or + from a mobile phone), then 358, followed by the area code (without initial zero) and the local number. For calls within Finland, dial just the number if you are calling locally, and add the area code if calling long distance. To place an international call from Finland, dial 00, the code of the country you're calling (1 for US and Canada), and the phone number. For more help, see page 1146.

Tipping: The bill for a sit-down meal already includes gratuity, so you don't need to add more, though it's nice to round up about 5-10 percent for good service. Round up taxi fares a bit (pay €3 on an €2.85 fare). For more tips on tipping, see page 138.

Tourist Information: www.visitfinland.com

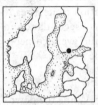

HELSINKI

Helsinki is the only European capital with no medieval past. Although it was founded in the 16th century by the Swedes in hopes of countering Tallinn as a strategic Baltic port, it never amounted to more than a village until the 18th century. Then, in 1746, Sweden built a huge fortress on an island outside Helsinki's harbor, and the village boomed as it supplied the fortress. After taking over Finland in 1809, the Russians decided to move Finland's capital and university closer to St. Petersburg—from Turku to Helsinki. They hired a young German architect, Carl Ludvig Engel, to design new public buildings for Helsinki and told him to use St. Petersburg as a model. This is why the oldest parts of Helsinki (around Market Square and Senate Square) feel so Russian—stone buildings in yellow and blue pastels with white trim and columns. Hollywood used Helsinki for the films *Gorky Park* and *Dr. Zhivago*, because filming in Russia was not possible during the Cold War.

Though the city was part of the Russian Empire in the 19th century, most of its residents still spoke Swedish, which was the language of business and culture. In the mid-1800s, Finland began to industrialize. The Swedish upper class in Helsinki expanded the city, bringing in the railroad and surrounding the old Russian-inspired core with neighborhoods of four- and five-story apartment buildings, including some Art Nouveau masterpieces. Meanwhile, Finns moved from the countryside to Helsinki to take jobs as industrial laborers. The Finnish language slowly acquired equal status with Swedish, and eventually Finnish speakers became the majority in Helsinki (though Swedish remains a co-official language).

Since downtown Helsinki didn't exist until the 1800s, it was more conscientiously designed and laid out than other European capitals. With its many architectural overleafs and fine Neoclassical and Art Nouveau buildings, Helsinki often turns guests into students of urban design and planning. Good neighborhoods for architecture buffs to explore are Katajanokka, Kruununhaka, and Eira. If you're intrigued by what you see, look for the English-language guide to Helsinki architecture (by Arvi Ilonen) in bookstores.

All of this makes Helsinki sound like a very dry place. It's not. Despite its sometimes severe cityscape and chilly northern latitude, the city bursts with vibrant street life and a joyful creative spirit. In 2012, Helsinki celebrated its stint as a "World Design Capital" and spiffed up the city with exciting new projects—including the Helsinki Music Centre concert hall, an extensive underground bike tunnel that cuts efficiently beneath congested downtown streets, and an all-around rededication to its already impressive design. While parts of the city may seem dark and drab, splashes of creativity and color hide around every corner—but you'll only discover them if you take the time to look.

PLANNING YOUR TIME

Helsinki will keep you busy on your day in port. While the downtown core, with most of the big sights, is compact and walkable, several worth-a-detour attractions require a longer walk or bus/tram/taxi ride. Below I've listed the most important sights in town, starting from Market Square and moving outward; while this order makes sense for those arriving at the South Harbor, if you're arriving at the West Harbor, it may be more logical to link these sights differently. To best manage your time, start at the farthest-flung sights, then work your way back toward the town center (and your ship).

• **Market Square:** This delightful harborfront zone is worth at least a 30-minute browse—more if you shop or grab lunch here.

• **Helsinki Walk:** Starting at Market Square, you can take this two-part self-guided walk (allow about two hours without stops) for an introduction to the city's sightseeing spine.

• **Senate Square and Churches:** Near Market Square and the start of my self-guided walk, be sure to stroll through Senate Square, visit the **Lutheran Cathedral** (allow 30 minutes or less), and tour the **Uspenski Orthodox Cathedral** (figure on 30 minutes). This part of town won't take you much more than an hour.

• **Orientation Bus Tour:** Early in your visit, consider a 1.75-hour bus tour (or one of the one-hour hop-on, hop-off loops) to conveniently link the outlying areas of Helsinki (including the **Sibelius Monument**—which is worth seeing, but not worth the long trip to see on your own).

• **National Museum:** For those curious about Finland's story, this pleasant museum tells it well; allow at least an hour (likely more). The landmark Finlandia Hall is across the street and also worth a peek (10 minutes).

• **Temppeliaukio:** The dramatic "Church in the Rock" is one of Helsinki's best sights—but also one of its least convenient, burrowed into a residential zone a 10-minute walk behind the National Museum. Allow 30 minutes (plus the time it takes to get there).

• **Out of Town:** Two out-of-town sights are worth the trek for those with a special interest, but either one will eat up the better part of your time in port. **Suomenlinna Fortress,** the fortified island defending Helsinki's harbor, is reached by a 15-minute boat trip; once there, you'll want at least an hour to explore, plus 30 minutes for the museum and 25 minutes for the entertaining "multivision" show. **Seurasaari Open-Air Folk Museum** requires a 30-minute bus ride each way from downtown, plus at least 1.5 hours to see the dozens of historic structures.

If you move fast on a longish day in port, you can probably squeeze in all the in-town sights; if you're tight on time, skip the National Museum.

The Port of Helsinki

Arrival at a Glance: If arriving at the West Harbor, your best bet for getting downtown is public transportation (bus #14 from Hernesaari terminal, tram #9 from West/Länsi terminal). From the South Harbor (Katajanokan and Olympia terminals), you can walk into town in about 15 minutes (or hop on a tram—#4T from Katajanokan, #2 from Olympia).

Port Overview

Cruises arrive at several ports in Helsinki. These circle two large harbors: West Harbor (most big ships) or South Harbor (often for the smaller ships). Each individual cruise berth is designated by a two- or three-letter code (noted below, along with each terminal's name in Finnish and Swedish). The setup can be confusing—but you need to pay attention only to the port you're arriving at. For a detailed map, see www.portofhelsinki.fi.

Most of the port areas lack services (though a few have terminal buildings with ATMs or Internet access, and the tiny TI at the Hernesaari terminal is helpful). For most services, you'll do best if you wait to get into downtown Helsinki, where ATMs—usually marked *Otto*—are abundant, especially along the Esplanade.

West Harbor (Länsistama/Västra Hamnen): This ugly industrial port is about 1.5 miles west of downtown and has two cruise ports:

• **Hernesaari Terminaali** (Ärtholmen in Swedish), the primary cruise port for Helsinki, sits on the eastern side of West Harbor. It has two berths (Quay B, code: LHB; and Quay C, code: LHC), a handy TI kiosk, and a nearby stop for public bus #14, which heads into town.

• **West Terminal** (Länsiterminaali/Västra Terminalen), on the western side of West Harbor, has a cruise berth at Melkki Quay (code: LMA), a 10-minute walk from tram #9 into town.

South Harbor (Eteläsatama/Södra Hamnen): This conveniently and scenically located port is within walking distance of downtown. Ringing this harbor are several terminals for both cruises and overnight ferries; two of these are most commonly used by cruise ships:

• **Katajanokan Terminaali** (Skatudden in Swedish), along the harbor's northern embankment, is near two cruise berths (codes: ERA and ERB). A third berth (code: EKL), used more by overnight ferries than cruise ships, is closer to town. From any of these, it's an easy walk or quick ride on tram #4T into town.

• **Olympiaterminaali** (code: EO), along the southern embankment, is used mostly by smaller cruise ships, and is also an easy walking distance into town (or hop on tram #2).

• The South Harbor berths that are closest to downtown (**Kanavaterminaali** and **Makasiiniterminaali**) are used mostly by overnight ferries, though occasionally overflow cruise ships may end up here.

Tourist Information: Among the cruise ports, the only one with a dedicated TI is the Hernesaari terminal. Otherwise, head into town and visit the helpful TI right on Market Square.

GETTING INTO TOWN

Below, I cover arrival details for each of Helsinki's four ports. From any harbor, your cruise line may offer a **shuttle bus,** dropping you off near Stockmann department store downtown—so I've also included arrival instructions for that option. In addition, I've listed some **tour** options.

West Harbor

You can walk downtown from the West Harbor (about 2 miles/40-50 minutes). While long, it can be nice. Start by following the green line. You can walk along the seaside or down the trendy, shop-filled Bulevardi (passing the red-brick Hietalahti Market Hall and its popular outdoor flea market, described later).

Helsinki Excursions

Helsinki itself has plenty to fill a day, but many of its sights—including its architectural highlights, the remarkable Church in the Rock, and the Sibelius Monument—are spread far and wide. This, plus the fact that Helsinki is unusually car-friendly (and less pedestrian-oriented), makes an orientation **bus tour** a good way to get your bearings. While your cruise line likely offers an excursion for this, you'll have a similar experience and pay far less if you join a local bus tour when you arrive (see options on page 315). The short, basic Helsinki bus tours generally make three stops: at the Church in the Rock (45 minutes, plus a four-block hike from where the bus parks), the Sibelius Monument (10 minutes), and Senate Square/Market Square (30 minutes). But you'll likely get more information from this chapter than on one of these excursions. Various cruise lines also offer **walking tours** of downtown Helsinki, including Senate Square and the Esplanade, but you'll do just as well following my self-guided Helsinki Walk (see page 317). Finally, you might combine either a bus ride or a walking tour with a Helsinki **harbor tour,** offering a closer look at the Suomenlinna islands (described on page 316) or, far beyond that, the Archipelago Sea (studded with thousands of little islands, but less scenic than the Stockholm Archipelago).

While gimmicky "ice bar" experiences in other cities are skippable, excursions to Helsinki's **"Winter World"** facility offers something extra—a complete, snowy indoor world where you can ride a sled, toss a snowball, and hike on a snowy hill. While undoubtedly a tourist trap, this may be worth it on a hot day if you have a limited appetite for Helsinki and prefer snowballs and vodka to sightseeing.

Out-of-town excursions can include the excellent **Seurasaari Open-Air Museum,** offering a look at traditional Finnish culture (and described on page 336); **Porvoo,** the second-oldest town in Finland, with fine wooden architecture; **Sipoo,** a very old and traditional farming area with the stone St. Sigfrid's Church; and **Hvitträsk,** a landmark of Finnish architecture in a pleasant forests-and-lake countryside setting. While any of these might be interesting on a longer visit, with just one day I'd rather explore Helsinki proper (or, if you have a special interest, choose an excursion combining one of these outlying sights with places in town).

Arriving at Hernesaari Terminaali

Leaving your ship, you'll run right into a small souvenir store (with free Wi-Fi), waiting excursion buses, and, hiding in a nondescript kiosk 50 yards away, a TI (which is open only in the morning when ships are in). This is a good place to pick up a map, get questions answered, and buy an all-day transit pass (credit cards only). There is no ATM here, but the TI (like other vendors here) accepts credit cards. Just beyond the TI is a parking lot with cruise shuttle buses, taxis (figure €15-20 to downtown), and hop-on, hop-off tour buses (for details, see later). A big port construction plan in the works will bring (in coming years) a typical Finnish sauna in this area—a nice way to relax, Helsinki-style, if you have time to kill before re-boarding your ship.

If riding **public bus #14** into town, buy an €8 all-day transit pass at the TI kiosk (credit card only, no individual tickets sold), or wait to buy a €3 single-ride ticket from the driver (cash only). The bus stop is about a five-minute walk: From the port gate and TI, follow the green line through the parking lot (passing all the buses) to the far end. When you reach the street, turn left and follow it for a short block; the bus stop on the right (marked *Pajamäki/ Smedjebacka*). From here, bus #14 takes you downtown (runs every 10-20 minutes). Two stops are most useful: First, after about 10 minutes, the bus stops at Kamppi (a 10-minute walk from the train station area, Stockmann department store, and the Esplanade); and second, the stop called Kauppakorkeakoulut/Handelshögskolorna (for the Church in the Rock). Stepping off the bus here, continue straight ahead one block (in the direction the bus was headed) and turn right up Luthernikatu to reach the back of the church; circle around the right side to find the entrance.

In summer, a **ferry** goes from Hernesaari to Market Square (€7 one-way, €10 all day, only 3/day starting at 9:30, late June-early Aug daily, early-late June and early-late Aug Sat-Sun only, 30 min-utes, mobile 040-736-2329, www.seahelsinki.fi).

Arriving at West Terminal(Länsiterminaali)

If you arrive here, your ship puts in at the most desolate part of the port. Exiting, you'll pass through the deserted-feeling **Ristelly Terminal** building, with a few souvenir shops and no real services. Once outside, you'll see taxis (figure about €15-20 downtown) and bus stops for cruise excursions. To head into town on your own, proceed straight out the port gate, then follow the green line on the pavement for about 10 minutes, through dull shipyards to the **Länsiterminaali** building (which is used primarily by Tallink and St. Peter Line boats). Inside the terminal are ATMs, WCs, lockers, a newsstand, and a rack of TI brochures. A taxi stand is just outside the terminal's side door. Across the wide street is the big Verkkokauppa.com shopping complex; its lobby (open 24/7) has free Internet terminals, and upstairs is a sprawling Best Buy-like electronics store (Mon-Fri 9:00-21:00, Sat 9:00-18:00, Sun 12:00-18:00).

Directly in front of the Länsiterminaali building is the stop for **tram #9,** which takes you downtown. You can buy tickets at the newsstand inside the terminal, or at the automated machine by the tram stop (cash or credit card, €2.50 for a single ticket, €8 for an all-day ticket). This is the start of the line, so you can't go in the wrong direction—just hop on any tram that shows up (runs every 10 minutes). Get off at the train station (Rautatieasema/ Järnvägsstationen stop), right in the middle of my self-guided Helsinki Walk, and an easy walking distance to many top sights.

South Harbor

From any of the South Harbor berths, you can see the green dome marking the Lutheran Cathedral and Helsinki's city center. If the weather's nice and you're up for a walk, just stroll toward the dome. I've noted your other options below. (If you happen to arrive at **Kanavaterminaali** or **Makasiiniterminaali**—which few cruises do—walking is certainly the easiest option, as both are within a five-minute walk of Market Square.)

While it makes little sense to hire a taxi for the short ride into town, figure about €10-15 for a trip from any of these terminals to any sights in the downtown area.

Arriving at Katajanokan Terminaali

As you exit the port area, turn left and walk until you see the Viking Line terminal building. Inside, you'll find an ATM, WCs, lockers, and a newsstand; out front are hop-on, hop-off buses and (at 10:30) Helsinki Expert's orientation tour buses ("Helsinki Panorama" tours, see page 315). Directly across the street from the terminal building is the start-of-the-line stop for **tram #4T.** You can ride it straight into town (4-8/hour): the fourth stop, Ritarihuone/ Riddarhuset, is the City Hall (near Market Square and TI); the next stop is Senate Square (Senaatintori/Senatstorget); and from there, the tram continues along Aleksanterinkatu, parallel to the Esplanade, to the train station area (Lasipalatsi/Glaspalatset stop), then the National Museum (Kansallismuseo/Nationalmuseet stop).

Alternatively, you can **walk** into town in about 15 minutes: simply proceed past the Viking Line terminal and continue straight ahead (with the harbor on your left, passing a gas station, then several brick warehouses) to Market Square.

Arriving at Olympiaterminaali

Ships put in near the Olympiaterminaali building (used primarily by Tallink Silja overnight boats to Stockholm), which has ATMs, WCs, lockers, and a newsstand. Out front are hop-on, hop-off buses and (at 10:30) Helsinki Expert's orientation tour buses. It's an easy 15-minute **walk** around the harbor to Market Square (just walk toward the green dome). To shave some time off the trip, hop on **tram #2,** which departs from the street in front of the terminal and zips you into town (ride it to the right, direction: Eläintarha).

The third stop is Senate Square (Senaatintori/Senatstorget); the sixth stop is the train station (Rautatieasema/Järnvägsstationen); and the tenth stop (Sammonkatu) is near Temppeliaukio, the Church in the Rock.

By Cruise-Line Shuttle Bus

Regardless of which port they use, many cruise lines offer a shuttle bus into downtown (price varies, but usually around €8 one-way, €12 round-trip). This is especially worth considering if you're arriving at the far-flung ports of the West Harbor (Hernesaari terminal or West/Länsi terminal).

Arrival in Downtown Helsinki: Most cruise shuttles drop off across the street from Stockmann department store (near the corner of Mannerheimintie and Lönnrotinkatu). While this is a handy entry point that lets you walk to many sights, it can be hard to get your bearings in this bustling shopping zone. From the bus stop, cross the busy boulevard with the tram tracks and proceed straight down the street between the huge, red-brick Stockmann and the white, round Swedish Theater (Svenska Teatern). This is the start of the Esplanade, which leads regally down to Market Square and the beginning of my self-guided Helsinki Walk.

By Tour

Bus tours can be an excellent way to get your bearings in this somewhat spread-out city; after getting oriented, you can choose where to spend the rest of your time.

You have two options: **orientation bus tours** that do a 1.75-hour circuit around the big sights; or **hop-on, hop-off bus tours** that allow you to get off wherever you like and catch another bus later. Neither type of tour serves all of the cruise ports (though hop-on, hop-off buses do meet arriving cruisers at the primary Hernesaari terminal, and orientation tours leave from near the Katajanokan and Olympia terminals in the morning after the overnight boats from Stockholm arrive); in most cases, you'll need to make your way downtown to catch the bus. If considering the hop-on, hop-off tour, carefully note the frequency of buses (which can be sparse), and make sure you understand the schedule and departure point for the bus back to your port.

Other tour options in Helsinki include harbor boat tours, a "pub tram," an architectural walk, and local guides for hire.

For more on all of these, see "Tours in Helsinki" on page 315.

RETURNING TO YOUR SHIP
By Shuttle Bus
If your cruise line offers a shuttle bus, you'll likely find it across the street from the Stockmann department store, along the busy and wide Mannerheimintie boulevard. The easiest way to get there from Market Square is to head straight up the Esplanade, curl around the right side of the big, white Swedish Theater, then cross the busy street straight ahead.

On Your Own
West Harbor: If returning to West Harbor terminals, leave plenty of time for public transportation. To get to **Hernesaari,** hop on bus #14 (direction: Hernesaaren laituri) and get off at the last stop (you'll see your ship). The only catch is finding a handy bus stop for the #14 downtown; the most convenient is probably Kamppi, a 10-minute walk down Salomonkatu from the train station/Finlandia Hall area. To get to the **West/Länsi** terminal, ride tram #9 (direction: Länsiterminaali); the easiest place to catch it downtown is in front of the train station. Remember to leave yourself at least 10 minutes for the walk from the tram stop to your ship.

   South Harbor: Returning to South Harbor ports, it's probably easiest just to walk—you should be able to see your ship from Market Square, and it won't take longer than 15 minutes. (If you have time to kill before heading back, it's a delight to spend it on Market Square or the adjacent Senate Square.) But if you want to get there faster—or are coming from another part of town—you can take the tram: To reach the **Katajanokan** terminal, catch tram #4T (not #4) from various points in town—including the National Museum, Lasipalatsi (near the train station), Senate Square, and the Ritarihuone stop by City Hall—and ride it to its end point at the Katajanokan terminaali stop. To reach the **Olympia** terminal, take tram #2 from various points in town—including Sammonkatu (near Temppeliaukio), the train station, Senate Square, and City Hall—to its end station, Olympialaituri.

   See page 344 for help if you miss your boat.

Helsinki

Helsinki (pop. 604,000) has a compact core. The city's natural gateway is its main harbor, where ships from Stockholm and Tallinn dock. At the top of the harbor is Market Square (Kauppatori), an outdoor food and souvenir bazaar. Nearby are two towering, can't-miss-them landmarks: the white Lutheran Cathedral and the red-brick Orthodox Cathedral.

Helsinki's grand pedestrian boulevard, the Esplanade, begins right at Market Square, heads up past the TI, and ends after a 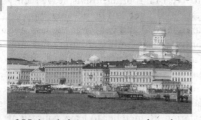 few blocks in the central shopping district. At the top end of the Esplanade, the broad, traffic-filled Mannerheimintie avenue veers north through town past the train and bus stations on its way to many of Helsinki's museums and architectural landmarks. For a do-it-yourself orientation to town along this route, follow my self-guided Helsinki Walk on page 317.

Linguistic Orientation: Finnish is completely different from the Scandinavian languages of Norwegian, Danish, and Swedish. That can make navigating a bit tricky. Place names ending in *-katu* are streets, *-tie* is "road" or "way," and *-tori* or *-aukio* means "square." Finland's bilingual status means that most street names, tram stops, and map labels appear in both Finnish and Swedish. In any event, I've rarely met a Finn who doesn't speak excellent English.

Orientation to Helsinki

TOURIST INFORMATION

The friendly, energetic **main TI,** just off the harbor, offers great service, and its brochure racks are fun to graze through. It's located a half-block inland from Market Square, on the right just past the fountain, at the corner of the Esplanade and Unioninkatu (May-Sept Mon-Fri 9:00-20:00, Sat-Sun 9:00-18:00, Oct-April closes two hours earlier, free Wi-Fi, guest computer, tel. 09/3101-3300, www.visithelsinki.fi). Pick up a city map, a public-transit map, and the free *Helsinki This Week* magazine (nicely illustrated, with articles on what to do in town as well as lists of sights, hours, concerts, and events). If interested in design, ask for publications about the local design culture; if music's your thing, ask about concerts—popular venues are Kallio Church and the Lutheran Cathedral.

The tiny **train station TI,** which consists of a one-person desk inside the Helsinki Expert office, provides many of the same services and publications.

Helsinki Expert: This private service, owned by Strömma/Sightseeing Helsinki, sells the Helsinki Card (described next), ferry tickets (€8 booking fee), and sightseeing tours by bus and boat. They have one branch in the train station hall, another occupying the front desks in the main TI on Market Square, and small, summer-only sightseeing kiosks on the Esplanade and by the harbor (all branches open Mon-Fri 9:00-15:00, Sat 10:00-14:00, closed Sun, tel. 09/2288-1600, www.stromma.fi).

Helsinki Card: If you're planning to visit a lot of museums in Helsinki, this card can be a good deal. The card includes free entry to over 50 museums, fortresses, and other major sights; free use of buses, trams, and the ferry to Suomenlinna; a free city bus tour or harbor cruise (your choice—plus a discount on the other, plus a discount on the hop-on, hop-off bus); and a 72-page booklet (€44/24 hours, €54/48 hours, €64/72 hours, €3 less if bought online and picked up on arrival at the main TI's Helsinki Expert desk; sold at all Helsinki Expert locations and both Viking Line and Tallink Silja ferry terminals, www.helsinkicard.com).

For a cheaper alternative, you could buy a public-transit day ticket (see "Getting Around Helsinki," later), take my self-guided walk, visit the free churches (Temppeliaukio Church, Lutheran Cathedral, Uspenski Orthodox Cathedral, and Kamppi Chapel of Silence), and stop by the free Helsinki City Museum.

HELPFUL HINTS

Internet Access: For the tourist, Helsinki is one of Europe's handiest cities for free Wi-Fi; along the Esplanade and throughout the city center, look for the "Helsinki City Open" network. Most hotels, cafés, and museums also have hot spots. The **City Hall,** facing Market Square and the harbor, has six free, fast terminals and speedy Wi-Fi in its inviting lobby (get code for terminal from desk, Mon-Fri 9:00-19:00, Sat-Sun 10:00-16:00).

Pharmacy: A **24-hour pharmacy**—*apteekki*—is located at Mannerheimintie 96 (at Kansaneläkelaitos stop for tram #2, #4/4T, or #10, tel. 020-320-200).

Laundry: PesuNet, primarily a dry-cleaning shop, welcomes travelers to use its half-dozen self-service machines. It's around the corner from the Iso Roobertinkatu stop for tram #3. Multitaskers can browse the nearby Design District to pass waiting time (€10/load, not coin-op—pay staff who will help, Mon-Thu 8:00-19:00, Fri 8:00-18:00, Sat 10:00-15:00, closed Sun, Punavuorenkatu 3, tel. 09/622-1146).

Bike Rental: Try **Greenbike** (one-speed bike-€5/hour or €20/ all day; three-speed bike-€30/all day; May-Aug daily 10:00-18:00, shorter hours and closed Sun-Mon off-season, Bulevardi 32—but entrance is just around the corner on Albertinkatu, mobile 050-550-1020, www.greenbike.fi). Another option is at the locksmith shop just inside the Metro station facing the **Kamppi plaza**—but they have higher prices and less helpful service (€24/4 hours, €30/all day, €35/24 hours, Mon-Fri 7:00-21:00, Sat 9:00-18:00, Sun 12:00-18:00, tel. 09/739-010); Greenbike sometimes has a temporary location set up on this plaza, as well.

Best View: The **Torni Tower's Ateljee Bar** offers a free panorama view. Ride the elevator from the lobby of the venerable Torni Hotel (built in 1931) to the 12th floor, where you can browse around the perch or sit down for a pricey drink (€5 coffee, €8-10 alcohol, Sun-Thu 14:00-24:00, Fri-Sat 12:00-24:00, Yrjönkatu 26, tel. 020-123-4604).

What's With the Slot Machines? Finns have a love affair with lotteries and petty gambling. You'll see coin-operated games of chance everywhere, including restaurants, supermarkets, and the train station.

Updates to This Book: For updates to this book, check www. ricksteves.com/update.

GETTING AROUND HELSINKI

In compact Helsinki, you won't need to use public transportation as much as in big cities like Stockholm.

By Bus and Tram: With the public-transit route map (available at the TI, also viewable on the Helsinki Region Transport website—www.hsl.fi) and a little mental elbow grease, the buses and trams are easy, giving you Helsinki by the tail. The single Metro line is also part of the system, but it isn't useful for short-term visitors.

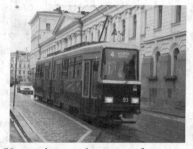

Single tickets are good for an hour of travel (€3 from driver, €2.50 at ticket machines at a few larger bus and tram stops). A day ticket (€8/24 hours of unlimited travel, issued on a plastic card you'll touch against the card reader when entering the bus or tram) pays for itself if you take four or more rides; longer versions are also available (€4 per extra 24 hours, 7-day maximum). Day tickets can be bought at the ubiquitous yellow-and-blue R-Kiosks (convenience stores), as well as at TIs, the train station, Metro stations, and ticket machines at a

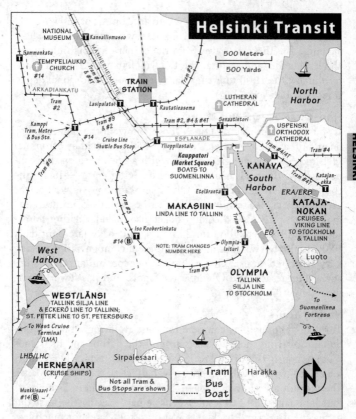

handful of stops, but not from drivers. The Helsinki Card also covers public transportation. All of these tickets and cards are valid only within the city of Helsinki, not the suburbs.

Tours in Helsinki

As in Stockholm, the big company Strömma (also called Sightseeing Helsinki and Helsinki Expert) has a near monopoly on city tours, whether by bus, boat, or foot.

▲▲▲Orientation Bus Tours

These 1.75-hour "Helsinki Panorama" bus tours give an ideal city overview with a look at all of the important buildings, from the remodeled Olympic Stadium to Embassy Row. You stay on the bus the entire time, except for a 10-minute stop or two (when possible, they try to stop at the Sibelius Monument and/or Temppeliaukio Church). You'll learn strange facts, such as how Finns took down the highest steeple in town during World War II so that Soviet bombers flying in from Estonia couldn't see their target. Tours get booked up, so it's wise to reserve in advance online or call 09/2288-1600 (€31, free with Helsinki Card, www.stromma.fi, sales@stromma.fi). The tour leaves from the corner of Fabianinkatu and the Esplanade (and stops at the Katajanokan and Olympia cruise terminals); the 11:00 tour runs daily year-round (additional departures possible April-Aug).

Hop-On, Hop-Off Bus Tours

If you'd enjoy the tour described above, but want the chance to hop on and off at will, consider **Open Top Tours** (owned by Strömma/Helsinki Sightseeing, green buses), with a 1.5-hour loop that connects downtown Helsinki, several outlying sights—including the Sibelius Monument and Olympic Stadium—as well as the Hernesaari cruise terminal. Buses run every 30-45 minutes and make 13 stops (€27, €39 combo-ticket also includes harbor tour—see next, all tickets good for 24 hours, mid-May-late Sept daily 10:00-16:00, www.stromma.fi). A different company, **Sightseeing City Tour** (red buses), offers a similar route for similar prices, stops at the Hernesaari and Olympia terminals, and has fewer departures (www.citytour.fi).

Harbor Tours

Three boat companies compete for your attention along Market Square, offering snoozy cruises around the harbor and its islands roughly hourly from 10:00 to 18:00 in summer (typically 1.5 hours for €17-24; www.royalline.net, www.ihalines.fi, www.stromma.fi). The narration is slow-moving—often recorded and in as many as four languages. I'd call it an expensive nap. Taking the ferry out to Suomenlinna and back gets you onto the water for much less money (€5 round-trip, covered by day ticket or Helsinki Card). If you do take a harbor cruise, here's how the competing companies differ: **Helsinki Sightseeing/Strömma** (yellow-and-white boats) offers the best and priciest route, going through a narrow channel in the east to reach sights that the other cruises miss. The other companies focus on the harbor itself and Suomenlinna fortress; of these, **Royal Line** (green-and-white boats) has the best food service on board, while **IHA** (blue-and-white boats) is more likely to have a live guide (half their boats have live guides, the others have recorded commentary).

Pub Tram

In summer, this antique red tram makes a 50-minute loop through the city while its passengers get looped on the beer for sale on board (€9 to ride, €6 beer, mid-May-Aug Tue-Sat 14:00-20:00, no trams Sun-Mon, leaves at the top of each hour from in front of the Fennia building, Mikonkatu 17, across from train-station tower, www.koff.net).

Local Guides

Helsinki Expert can arrange a private guide (book at least three days in advance, €204/2 hours, tel. 09/2288-1222, sales@stromma. fi). **Christina Snellman** is a good licensed guide (mobile 050-527-4741, chrisder@pp.inet.fi). **Archtour** offers local guides who specialize in Helsinki's architecture (tel. 09/477-7300, www.archtours. com).

Helsinki Walk

This self-guided walk—worth ▲▲▲—offers a convenient spine for your Helsinki sightseeing. I've divided the walk into two parts: On a quick visit, focus on Part 1 (which takes about an hour). To dig deeper into the city's architectural landmarks—and reach some of its museums—continue with Part 2 (which adds about another 45 minutes). Note that several points of interest on this walk are described in more detail later, under "Sights in Helsinki."

PART 1: THE HARBORFRONT, SENATE SQUARE, AND ESPLANADE

• *Start at the obelisk in the center of the harborfront market.*

❶ Market Square

At the heart of the square is the **Czarina's Stone,** with its double-headed eagle of imperial Russia. It was the first public monument in Helsinki, designed by Carl Ludvig Engel and erected in 1835 to celebrate the visit by Czar Nicholas I and Czarina Alexandra. Step over the chain and climb to the top step for a clockwise spin-tour:

Begin by facing the **harbor.** The big, red Viking ship and white Silja ship are each floating hotels for those making the

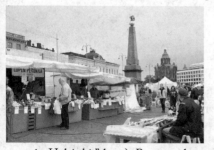

40-hour Stockholm-Helsinki round-trip. Now pan to the right. The brick-and-tan building along the harborfront is the Old Market Hall, with some enticing, more upscale options than the basic grub at the outdoor market (for a rundown on both options, see "Eating in Helsinki," later). Between here and there, a number of harbor cruise boats vie for your business. Farther to the right, the trees mark the beginning of Helsinki's grand promenade, the Esplanade (where we're heading). Hiding in the leaves is the venerable iron-and-glass Café Kappeli. The yellow building across from the trees is the TI. From there, a string of Neoclassical buildings face the

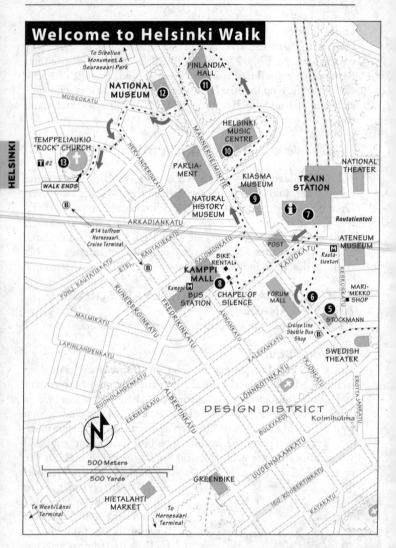

Welcome to Helsinki Walk

To Sibelius Monument & Seurasaari Park

FINLANDIA HALL **11**

NATIONAL MUSEUM **12**

MUSEOKATU

HELSINKI MUSIC CENTRE **10**

MANNERHEIMINTIE

TEMPPELIAUKIO "ROCK" CHURCH **13**

T #2

WALK ENDS

PARLIA-MENT

NEVANLINNANKATU

NATIONAL THEATER

KIASMA MUSEUM **9**

TRAIN STATION

NATURAL HISTORY MUSEUM

B

#14 to/from Hernesaari Cruise Terminal

ARKADIANKATU

Rautatientori

B

RAUTATIEKATU

SALOMONKATU

POST

ATENEUM MUSEUM

Rauta-tientori

KAIVOKATU

KESKUSKATU

POHJ. RAUTATIEKATU

ETELÄ

RUNEBERGINKATU

BIKE RENTAL

KAMPPI MALL **8**

Kamppi

BUS STATION

CHAPEL OF SILENCE

FORUM MALL

6

5

MARI-MEKKO SHOP

STOCKMANN

FREDRIKINKATU

MALMIKATU

LAPINLAHDENKATU

ANNANKATU

Cruise Line Shuttle Bus Stop

B

SWEDISH THEATER

RUOHOLAHDENKATU

EERIKINKATU

ALBERTINKATU

KALEVANKATU

LÖNNROTINKATU

YRJÖNKATU

DESIGN DISTRICT

Kolmihulma

EROTTAJANKATU

BULEVARDI

UUDENMAANKATU

N

500 Meters

500 Yards

GREENBIKE

ISO ROOBERTINKATU

To West/Länsi Terminal

HIETALAHTI MARKET

To Hernesaari Terminal

KATAKATU

---

harbor. The blue-and-white City Hall building was designed by Engel in 1833 as the town's first hotel, built to house the czar and czarina. The Lutheran Cathedral is hidden from view behind this building (we'll go there soon). Next, after the short peach-colored building, is the Swedish Embassy (flying the blue-and-yellow Swedish flag and designed to look like Stockholm's Royal Palace). Then comes the Supreme Court and, tucked back in the far corner, Finland's Presidential Palace. Finally, standing proud, and reminding Helsinki of the Russian behemoth to its east, is the Uspenski Orthodox Cathedral.

HELSINKI

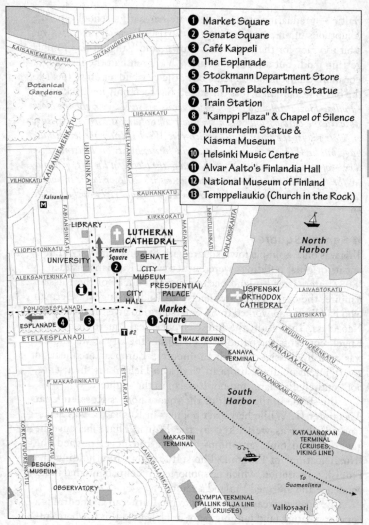

1. Market Square
2. Senate Square
3. Café Kappeli
4. The Esplanade
5. Stockmann Department Store
6. The Three Blacksmiths Statue
7. Train Station
8. "Kamppi Plaza" & Chapel of Silence
9. Mannerheim Statue & Kiasma Museum
10. Helsinki Music Centre
11. Alvar Aalto's Finlandia Hall
12. National Museum of Finland
13. Temppeliaukio (Church in the Rock)

Explore the colorful **outdoor market**—part souvenirs and crafts, part fruit and veggies, part fish and snacks. Sniff the stacks of trivets, made from cross-sections of juniper twigs—an ideal, fragrant, easy-to-pack gift for the folks back home (they smell even nicer when you set something hot on them).

Done exploring? With your back to the water, walk left to the end of Market Square and cross the street (tiptoeing over tram tracks) to reach the *Havis Amanda* fountain. Designed by Ville Vallgren and unveiled here in 1908, the fountain has become the symbol of Helsinki, the city known as the "Daughter of the

Baltic"—graduating students decorate her with a school cap. The voluptuous figure, modeled after the artist's Parisian mistress, was a bit too racy for the conservative town, and Vallgren had trouble getting paid. But as artists often do, Vallgren had the last laugh: For more than a hundred years now, the city budget office (next to the Sasso restaurant across the street) has seen only her backside.

• *Follow Havis Amanda's right cheek across the street, go right one block (toward the harborfront), then turn left up Sofiankatu street (passing, on your right, the City Hall—with free Wi-Fi, Internet terminals, huge public WCs in the basement, and free exhibits on Helsinki history—often photography). Near the end of the block, on the left, you may see the free* **Helsinki City Museum** *(unless it's 2016 or later, in which case it will have moved one block east). You'll pop out right in the middle of...*

❷ Senate Square

This was once a simple town square with a church and City Hall—but its original buildings were burned when Russians invaded in 1808. Later, after Finland became a grand duchy of the Russian Empire, the czar sent in architect Carl Ludvig Engel (a German who had lived and worked in St. Petersburg) to give the place some Neo-class. The result: the finest Neoclassical square in Europe. Engel represents the paradox of Helsinki: The city as we know it was built by Russia, but with an imported European architect, in a very intentionally "European" style. So Helsinki is, in a sense, both entirely Russian...and not Russian in the slightest.

The statue in the center of the square honors **Russian Czar Alexander II.** While he wasn't popular in Russia (he was assassinated), he was well-liked by the Finns. That's because he gave Finland more autonomy in 1863 and never pushed the "Russification" of Finland. The statue shows him holding the Finnish constitution, which he supported. It defined internal independence and affirmed Finland's autonomy.

The huge **staircase** leading up to the **Lutheran Cathedral** is a popular meeting (and tanning) spot in Helsinki. This is where students from the nearby university gather...and romances are born.

Head up those stairs and survey Senate Square from the top. Scan the square from left to right. First, 90 degrees to your left is the **Senate building** (now the prime minister's office). The small, blue, stone building with the slanted mansard roof in the far-left corner, from 1757, is one of just two pre-Russian-conquest buildings remaining in Helsinki. **Café Engel** (opposite the cathedral at Aleksanterinkatu 26) is a fine place for a light lunch or cake and coffee. The café's winter lighting seems especially designed to boost the spirits of glum, daylight-deprived Northerners.

Continue looking right. Facing the Senate directly across

the square is its twin, the **University of Helsinki's** main building (36,000 students, 60 percent female). Symbolically (and physically), the university and government buildings are connected via the cathedral, and both use it as a starting point for grand ceremonies.

Farther to the right, and tucked alongside the cathedral, the line of once-grand Russian administration buildings now house the **National Library.** In czarist times, the National Library received a copy of every book printed in the Russian Empire. With all the chaos Russia suffered throughout the 20th century, a good percentage of its Slavic texts were destroyed. But Helsinki, which enjoyed relative stability, claims to have the finest collection of Slavic books in the world. This fine, purpose-built Neoclassical building is generally open to the public and worth a look (though it may be closed for renovation through late 2015).

If you'd like to visit the **cathedral interior,** now's your chance; the entrance is tucked around the left side as you face the towering dome (see page 330 for a description).

• *When you're ready, head back down the stairs and angle right through the square, continuing straight down Unioninkatu.*

Along **Unioninkatu,** do a little window-shopping; this is the first of many streets we'll see lined with made-in-Finland shops (though these are more touristy than the norm). In addition to the jewelry shops and clothes boutiques, look for the Schröder sporting goods store (on the left, at #23), which shows off its famous selection of popular Finnish-made Rapala fishing lures—ideal for the fisher folk on your gift list. At the end of this street (on the right), you'll spot the TI, with a Helsinki Expert desk inside (handy for booking bus tours and other activities).

• *Facing Havis Amanda's backside once more, turn right and head into the grassy median, with the delightful...*

❸ Café Kappeli

If you've got some time, dip into this old-fashioned, gazebo-like oasis of coffee, pastry, and relaxation (get what you like at the bar inside and sit anywhere). In the 19th century, this was a popular hangout for local intellectuals and artists. Today the café offers romantic tourists waiting for their ship a great €3-cup-of-coffee memory (daily 9:00-24:00). The bandstand in front hosts nearly daily music and dance performances in summer.

• *Beyond Café Kappeli stretches...*

❹ The Esplanade

Helsinki's top shopping boulevard sandwiches a park in the middle (another Engel design from the 1830s). The grandiose street names Esplanadi and Bulevardi, while fitting today, must have been bombastic and almost comical in rustic little 1830s Helsinki. To help you imagine this elegant promenade in the 19th century, informative signs (in English) explain Esplanade Park's background and its many statues.

The north side (on the right, with the TI) is interesting for window-shopping, people-watching, and sun-worshipping. In fact, after the first block, browsers may want to leave the park and cross over to that side of the street. In just a few steps, you'll pass flagship stores for several household-name Finnish designers.

First up, at #25B, **Ittala** displays dishes and other glassware, both decorative and functional. Popping into the shop, you'll see Alvar Aalto's signature wavy-mouthed vases, which haven't gone out of fashion since they arrived in 1936; Oiva Toikka's iconic "dew drop"-patterned chalices and pedestal bowls, from 1964, as well as his bird sculptures; and a minimuseum of glass art in the back (Art & Design Studio).

Back on the Esplanade, a few doors down at #27C, **Kalevala Jewelry** sells quality made-in-Finland jewelry. Some pieces look modern, while others are inspired by old Scandinavian, Finnish, and Sami themes. Next door (also at #27C), **Aarikka** is more affordable and casual, with costume jewelry, accessories, and home decor made mostly from big, colorful spheres of wood.

In the next block, the hulking, ornately decorated **Hotel Kämp** (#29) is a city landmark. **Galleria Esplanad** (entrance at #31) is a super-exclusive mall with big-name Finnish and international fashion stores. Then, after the recommended **Strindberg Café** (one of many fine spots along the Esplanade to nurse a drink), at the corner, is perhaps Finland's most famous export: **Marimekko,** whose mostly floral patterns adorn everything from purses to shower curtains to iPhone cases (two more Marimekko branches—specializing in clothes and in kids' stuff—are within a block of here).

Directly across the Esplanade's park median from Marimekko is another landmark of world design, **Artek.** Founded by designers Alvar and Elissa Aalto, this shop showcases expensive, high-end housewares in the modern, practical style that Ikea commercialized successfully for the mass market.

In the block after Marimekko, at #39, is the huge **Academic Bookstore** (Akateeminen Kirjakauppa), designed by Alvar Aalto, with an extensive map and travel section, periodicals, English books, and Café Aalto.

At the very top of the Esplanade, the park dead-ends at the **Swedish Theater.** Built under Russian rule to cater to Swedish residents of a Finnish city, this building encapsulates Helsinki's complex cultural mix. (The theater's recommended Teatterin Grilli is handy for a drink or meal out in the park.) The Finnish National

Theater—catering to the other segment of the city's bilingual population—is nearby, close to the train station.

• *At the end of the Esplanade, on the right, you'll reach...*

❺ Stockmann Department Store

This prestigious local institution is Finland's answer to Harrods or Macy's. Stockmann is the biggest, best, and oldest department store in town, with a great gourmet supermarket in the basement. Just beyond is Helsinki's main intersection, where Esplanade and Mannerheimintie meet.

• *Turn right on Mannerheimintie. At the far side of Stockmann, you'll see a landmark statue, the...*

❻ Three Blacksmiths

While there's no universally accepted meaning for this statue (from 1932), most say it celebrates human labor and cooperation and

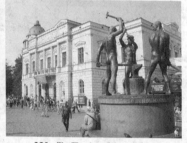

shows the solid character of the Finnish people. On the base, note the rare, surviving bullet damage from World War II. The Soviet Union used that war as an opportunity to invade Finland—which it had lost just 20 years prior—to try to reclaim their buffer zone. In a two-part war (the "Winter War," then the "Continuation War"), Finland held fast and emerged with its freedom—and relatively little war damage.

Stockmann's entrance on Aleksanterinkatu, facing the *Three Blacksmiths,* is one of the city's most popular meeting points. Everyone in Finland knows exactly what it means when you say: "Let's meet under the Stockmann's clock." Across the street from the clock, the Old Student Hall is decorated with mythic Finnish heroes.

• *For a shortcut to our next stop, duck through the passage (marked* City-Käytävä*) directly across the street from Stockmann's clock. This will take you through a bustling commercial zone. You'll enter—and continue straight through—the City Center shopping mall. Emerging on the far side, you're face-to-face with the harsh (but serene) architecture of the...*

❼ Train Station

This Helsinki landmark was designed by Eliel Saarinen (see sidebar). The four people on the facade symbolize peasant farmers with lamps coming into the Finnish capital. Duck into the main hall and the Eliel Restaurant inside to catch the building's ambience.

Exiting, with your back to the train station, look to the left;

Two Men Who Remade Helsinki

Eliel Saarinen (1873-1950)

At the turn of the 20th century, architect Eliel Saarinen burst on the scene by pioneering the Finnish National Romantic style. Inspired by peasant and medieval architectural traditions, his work was fundamental in creating a distinct—and modern—Finnish identity. The château-esque National Museum of Finland, designed by Saarinen and his two partners after winning a 1902 architectural competition, was his first major success (see page 332). Two years later, Saarinen won the contract to construct the Helsinki train station (completed in 1919). Its design marks a transition into 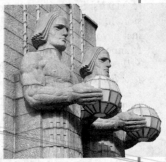 the Art Nouveau style of the early 1900s. The landmark station—characterized by massive male sculptures flanking its entrance, ornate glass and metalwork, and a soaring clock tower—presently welcomes over 300,000 travelers each day.

In the early 1920s, Saarinen and his family emigrated to the US, where his son, Eero, would become the architect of such iconic projects as the Gateway Arch in St. Louis and the main terminal at Dulles International Airport near Washington, DC.

Alvar Aalto (1898-1976)

Alvar Aalto was a celebrated Finnish architect and designer working in the Modernist tradition; his buildings used abstract 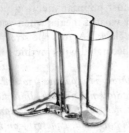 forms and innovative materials without sacrificing functionality. Finlandia Hall in Helsinki is undoubtedly Aalto's most famous structure, but that's just the beginning. A Finnish Frank Lloyd Wright, Aalto concerned himself with nearly every aspect of design, from furniture to light fixtures. Perhaps most notable of these creations was his sinuous Savoy Vase, a masterpiece of simplicity and sophistication that is emblematic of the Aalto style. His designs became so popular that in 1935 he and his wife opened Artek, a company that manufactures and sells his furniture, lamps, and textiles to this day (see page 322).

diagonally across the square is Finland's National Gallery, the **Ateneum** (with works by obscure but talented Finns, as well as better-known international artists). Directly across the square (and not visible from here), it faces the **Finnish National Theater**—the counterpoint to the Swedish Theater we saw earlier.

• *We've worked our way through the central part of town. Now, if you're ready to explore some interesting buildings and monuments, continue with...*

PART 2: MANNERHEIMINTIE AND HELSINKI'S ICONIC ARCHITECTURE

The rest of this walk follows the boulevard called Mannerheimintie, which serves as a showcase for much of Helsinki's iconic architecture; this walk also helps you reach some of the city's farther-flung sights. (Details on many of these appear later, under "Sights in Helsinki.")

• *With your back to the station, turn right and follow the tram tracks (along Kaivokatu street) back out to the busy boulevard called Mannerheimintie. Cross the street and the tram tracks, and continue straight ahead, toward what looks like a giant wood block. You'll pop out of the bustling plaza in front of the Kamppi shopping mall, called...*

❽ "Kamppi Plaza" (Narinkkatori) and the Chapel of Silence

This is a hub of Helsinki—both for transportation (with a Metro stop and bus station nearby) and for shopping (with the towering Kamppi Center shopping mall). Turn your attention to the round, wooden structure at the corner of the plaza nearest the Esplanade. This is one of Helsinki's newest and most surprising bits of architecture: the Kamppi **Chapel of Silence.** Enter through the doorway in the black building just to the right, and enjoy a moment or three of total serenity. (For more on the chapel, see page 331.)

• *Leaving the chapel, cut through the middle of the big plaza, with the shopping mall on your left and the low-lying yellow building on your right. Through the gap at the end of the square, you'll see an equestrian statue. Go meet him.*

❾ Carl Gustaf Mannerheim and the Kiasma Museum

The busy street's namesake was a Finnish war hero who frustrated the Soviets both in Finland's "Civil War" for independence, and again later, in World War II. Mannerheim and his fellow Finns put up a fierce resistance, and the Soviets finally gave up and redirected their efforts to the race to Berlin. While the Baltic States—across the Gulf of Finland—were "liberated" by the Red Army, dooming them to decades under the Soviet system, the Finns managed to refuse this assistance. Mannerheim became Finland's first postwar president, and thanks to his efforts (and those of countless others), Finland was allowed to chart its own democratic, capitalist course after the war. (Even so, Finland remained officially neutral through the Cold War, providing both East and West a political buffer zone.)

Mannerheim is standing in front of the glassy home of the **Kiasma Museum,** with changing exhibits of contemporary art. A bit farther along and across the street from Kiasma, with its stoic row of Neoclassical columns, stands the Finnish **Parliament.**

From Mannerheim and Kiasma, head down into the grassy, sloping park. At the lowest point, watch out—you're crossing a busy **bicycle highway** that cuts right through the middle of the city center. Look left under the tunnel to see how they turned a disused old rail line into a subterranean pedalers' paradise.

• *The glassy building dominating the end of the park is the...*

⑩ Helsinki Music Centre (Musiikkitalo)

Built in 2011, this structure is even bigger than it looks: two-thirds of it is underground, and the entire complex houses seven separate venues. It's decorated, inside and out, with bold art (such as the gigantic pike on tiptoes that stands in the middle of the park). As you approach the bottom of the building, step into the atrium (Mon-Fri 8:00-22:00, Sat 10:00-22:00, Sun 10:00-20:00) and look up to ogle the shimmering silver sculpture. Upstairs is a music store. The interior features a lot of pine and birch accents, which warm up the space and improve the (Japanese-designed) acoustics. It didn't take long for the Music Centre to become an integral part of the city's cultural life; in the first season of performances alone, some 400,000 people attended events here. They also offer English tours of the facility (see "Sights in Helsinki," later).

Back outside, circle around the back side of the Music Centre. Follow the straight, flat promenade that runs alongside a grassy park used for special events, and a former industrial zone that's slated for further redevelopment; the train tracks are just beyond.

• *Crossing the street, you'll see (on the left) perhaps the most important work of Finnish architecture...*

⑪ Alvar Aalto's Finlandia Hall

While famous, this big, white building can be a bit difficult for nonarchitects to appreciate. Walk through the long parking lot all the way to the far end, and look back for a more dramatic view. The building—entirely designed by Aalto, inside and out—opened in 1971 and immediately became a national icon. Notice how Aalto employs geometric shapes and sweeping lines to create a striking concert hall, seating up to 1,700 guests. Aalto designed the inclined roof to try to maximize the hall's acoustics—imitating the echo chamber of an old-fashioned church tower—with marginal success.

Turn to face shimmering **Töölönlahti Bay** (not a lake, but an inlet of the Baltic Sea)—ringed by a popular walking and jogging track. From here, you can see more Helsinki landmarks: across the lake and a bit to the left, the white tower marks the Olympic Stadium that hosted the world in 1952. And to the right are the rides of Helsinki's old-time amusement park, Lenininpuisto.

• *If you'd like to extend this walk with a leisurely stroll, join the natives on the waterfront path (offering even better views of Finlandia Hall). Otherwise, consider...*

More Helsinki Sights

To reach two more major sights, go up the stairs immediately to the right of Finlandia Hall, then continue all the way up to the main road. Directly across the street stands what looks like a château with a steeple. This building houses the fine ❶ **National Museum of Finland,** which tells this country's story with lots of artifacts.

There's one more great architectural treasure in Helsinki, about a 10-minute walk behind the National Museum: the sit-and-wipe-a-tear beautiful Church in the Rock, ❸ **Temppeliaukio.** Once inside, sit. Enjoy the music. It's a wonderful place to end this walk.

To continue on to the **Sibelius Monument,** located in a lovely park setting, take bus #24 (direction: Seurasaari) from nearby Arkadiankatu street. The same ticket is good for your return trip (within one hour), or ride it to the end of the line for the bridge to Seurasaari Island and Finland's open-air folk museum. From there, bus #24 returns to the top of the Esplanade.

All three of these sights are explained in more detail next, under "Sights in Helsinki."

Sights in Helsinki

NEAR THE SOUTH HARBOR
▲▲Uspenski Orthodox Cathedral

This house of worship was built for the Russian military in 1868 (at a time when Finland belonged to Russia). *Uspenski* is Russian for the Assumption of Mary. It hovers above Market Square and faces the Lutheran Cathedral, just as Russian culture faces Europe.

Cost and Hours: Free; Tue-Fri 9:30-20:00, Sat 10:00-15:00, Sun 12:00-15:00, closed Mon, Kanavakatu 1 (about a 5-minute walk beyond the harborfront market).

Visiting the Cathedral: Before heading inside, view the exterior. The uppermost "onion dome" represents the "sacred heart of

Helsinki at a Glance

▲▲▲**Temppeliaukio Church** Awe-inspiring, copper-topped 1969 Church in the Rock. **Hours:** June-Sept Mon-Sat 10:00-17:45, Sun 11:45-17:45; closes one hour earlier off-season. See page 332.

▲▲**Uspenski Orthodox Cathedral** Orthodoxy's most prodigious display outside of Eastern Europe. **Hours:** Tue-Fri 9:30-20:00, Sat 10:00-15:00, Sun 12:00-15:00, closed Mon. See page 327.

▲▲**Lutheran Cathedral** Green-domed, 19th-century Neo-classical masterpiece. **Hours:** June-Aug Mon-Sat 9:00-24:00, Sun 12:00-24:00; Sept-May Mon-Sat 9:00-18:00, Sun 12:00-18:00. See page 329.

▲▲**Suomenlinna Fortress** Helsinki's harbor island, sprinkled with picnic spots, museums, and military history. **Hours:** Museum daily May-Sept 10:00-18:00; Oct-April 10:30-16:30. See page 334.

▲▲**Seurasaari Open-Air Folk Museum** Island museum with 100 historic buildings from Finland's farthest corners. **Hours:** June-Aug daily 11:00-17:00; late May and early Sept Mon-Fri 9:00-15:00, Sat-Sun 11:00-17:00, buildings closed mid-Sept-mid-May. See page 336.

▲**Senate Square** Consummate Neoclassical square, with Lutheran Cathedral. **Hours:** Always open. See page 320.

Jesus," while the smaller ones represent the hearts of the 12 apostles.

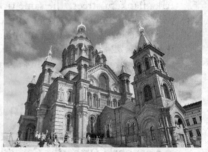

The cathedral's interior is a potentially emotional icon experience. Its rich images are a stark contrast to the sober Lutheran Cathedral. While commonly called the "Russian church," the cathedral is actually Finnish Orthodox, answering to the patriarch in Constantinople (Istanbul). Much of eastern Finland (parts of the Karelia region) is Finnish Orthodox.

The cathedral's Orthodox Mass is beautiful, with a standing congregation, candles, incense, icons in action, priests behind the iconostasis (screen), and timeless music (human voices only—no instruments). In the front left corner, find the icon featuring the Madonna and child, surrounded by rings and jewelry (under glass), given in thanks for prayers answered. Across from the icon is a

▲**Helsinki City Museum** Tells the city's history well and in English. **Hours:** Mon-Fri 9:00-17:00, Thu until 19:00, Sat-Sun 11:00-17:00. See page 330.

▲**Ateneum, The National Gallery of Finland** Largest collection of art in Finland, including local favorites plus works by Cézanne, Chagall, Gauguin, and Van Gogh. **Hours:** Tue and Fri 10:00-18:00, Wed-Thu 9:00-20:00, Sat-Sun 10:00-17:00, closed Mon. See page 330.

▲**National Museum of Finland** The scoop on Finland, featuring folk costumes, an armory, czars, and thrones; the prehistory and 20th-century exhibits are best. **Hours:** Tue-Sun 11:00-18:00, closed Mon. See page 332.

▲**Sibelius Monument** Stainless-steel sculptural tribute to Finland's greatest composer. **Hours:** Always open. See page 333.

▲**Design Museum** A chronological look at Finland's impressive design pedigree, plus cutting-edge temporary exhibits. **Hours:** June-Aug daily 11:00-18:00; Sept-May Tue 11:00-20:00, Wed-Sun 11:00-18:00, closed Mon. See page 333.

white marble table with candle holes and a dish of wheat seeds, representing recent deaths. Wheat seeds symbolize that death is not the end, but just a change.

Though the cathedral is worthwhile, the one in Tallinn is more richly decorated; skip this one if you're visiting both cities and are short on time.

▲▲Lutheran Cathedral

With its prominent green dome, gleaming white facade, and the 12 apostles overlooking the city and harbor, this church is Carl Ludvig Engel's masterpiece.

Cost and Hours: Free; June-Aug Mon-Sat 9:00-24:00, Sun 12:00-24:00; Sept-May Mon-Sat 9:00-18:00, Sun 12:00-18:00; sometimes closes for events; on Senate Square, www.helsingin seurakunnat.fi. In summer, free

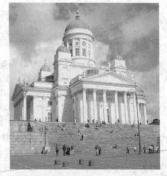

organ concerts are held on Sundays at 20:00.

Visiting the Cathedral: Enter the building around the left side. Finished in 1852, the interior is pure architectural truth. Open a pew gate and sit, surrounded by the saints of Protestantism, to savor Neoclassical nirvana. Physically, this church is perfectly Protestant—austere and unadorned—with the emphasis on preaching (prominent pulpit) and music (huge organ). Statuary is limited to the local Reformation big shots: Martin Luther, Philipp Melanchthon (Luther's Reformation sidekick), and the leading Finnish reformer, Mikael Agricola. A follower of Luther at Wittenberg, Agricola brought the Reformation to Finland. He also translated the Bible into Finnish and is considered the father of the modern Finnish language. Agricola's Bible is to Finland what the Luther Bible is to Germany and the King James Bible is to the English-speaking world.

▲Helsinki City Museum

This interesting museum, a few steps off of Senate Square, gives an excellent, accessible overview of the city's history in English. At the beginning of 2016, they are scheduled to move one block east, to Katariinankatu. But until then, they'll be showing off the enjoyable "Mad About Helsinki" exhibit. The ground floor is a sentimental look at some of the people of Helsinki's favorite places: seafront gardens, the cathedral steps, amusement park attractions, and home sweet home (with a mock-up of a typical Helsinki kitchen). The upstairs exhibit traces the history of the city from the 1550s, taking the novel approach of zooming in on individual, everyday people—from different historical periods and social classes—to better understand why each of them chose to call Helsinki home.

Cost and Hours: Free, Mon-Fri 9:00-17:00, Thu until 19:00, Sat-Sun 11:00-17:00, Sofiankatu 4—or one block east on Katariinankatu beginning in 2016, www.helsinkicitymuseum.fi.

BEYOND THE ESPLANADE

These sights are scattered in the zone west of the Esplanade, listed roughly in the order you'll reach them from the city center (and in the order they appear on my self-guided walk, earlier).

▲Ateneum, The National Gallery of Finland

This museum showcases Finnish artists (mid-18th to 20th century) and has a fine international collection, including works by Cézanne, Chagall, Gauguin, and Van Gogh. They also have good temporary exhibits. However, as the building is being renovated through late 2015, many of their star canvases are out on loan, and the "greatest hits" of their Finnish collection has been condensed on the ground floor. Before buying your ticket, be clear on what's on view today. Either way, the collection is hard to appreciate without the €3 audioguide (though the laminated English information sheets in a few rooms are helpful).

Cost and Hours: €12, Tue and Fri 10:00-18:00, Wed-Thu 9:00-20:00, Sat-Sun 10:00-17:00, closed Mon, near train station at Kaivokatu 2, tel. 0294-500-401, www.ateneum.fi.

▲Kamppi Chapel of Silence (Kampin Kappeli)

Sitting unassumingly on the busy, commercialism-crazy plaza in front of the Kamppi shopping mall/bus-station complex, this restful space was opened by the city of Helsinki in 2012 to give residents and visitors a place to escape the modern world. The teacup-shaped wooden structure, clad in spruce and with an oval footprint, encloses a 38-foot-tall cylinder of silence. Indirect light seeps in around the edges of the ceiling, bathing the clean, curved, alder-wood paneling in warmth and tranquility. Does it resemble Noah's Ark? The inside of an egg? The architects left it intentionally vague. Although it's a church, there are no services; the goal is to keep it open for anyone needing a reflective pause. Along with the Church in the Rock, it's one more example of a poignant and peaceful spot where secular modern architecture and spiritual sentiment converge beautifully.

Cost and Hours: Free, Mon-Fri 7:00-20:00, Sat-Sun 10:00-18:00, Simonkatu 7, enter through adjacent low-profile black building.

Helsinki Music Centre (Musiikkitalo)

This modern facility provides a home for the arts in Helsinki, but its biggest draw may be the park that surrounds it—decorated with wildly creative contemporary art. You can stop in to look around the building any time it's open, and architecture fans may want to take an English tour.

Cost and Hours: Building open Mon-Fri 8:00-22:00, Sat 10:00-22:00, Sun 10:00-20:00; English tours offered most days in summer for €12, check website for schedule; Mannerheimintie 13A, tel. 020-707-0400, www.musiikkitalo.fi.

Finlandia Hall (Finlandia-Talo)

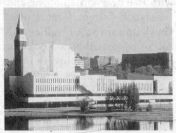

Alvar Aalto's most famous building in his native Finland means little to the nonarchitect without a tour. To see the building from its best angle, view it from the seaside parking lot, not the street—where nearly everyone who looks at the building thinks, "So what?" (For the answer to that question, see page 326 of my self-guided walk, earlier.)

Cost and Hours: €12.50 for a tour, call ahead or visit website to check times; hall information shop open Mon-Fri 9:00-19:00, closed Sat-Sun; Mannerheimintie 13e, tel. 09/40241, www.finlandiatalo.fi.

▲National Museum of Finland (Kansallismuseo)

This pleasant, easy-to-handle collection is in a grand building designed by three of this country's greatest architects—including Eliel Saarinen—in the early 1900s. Divided into four sections, the exhibit chronologically traces the land of the Finns from prehistory to the 20th century. The Neoclassical furniture, folk costumes, armory, and other artifacts are interesting, but the highlights are Finland's largest permanent archaeological collection (covering the prehistory of the country) and the 20th-century exhibit, which brings Finland's story up to the modern day. While the collection is impressive and well-described in English, those descriptions are quite dry, and the museum is a bit hard to appreciate. The interactive top-floor workshop is worth a look for its creative teaching.

Cost and Hours: €8, free on Fri 16:00-18:00; open Tue-Sun 11:00-18:00, closed Mon; Mannerheimintie 34, tel. 09/4050-9552, www.nba.fi. The museum café, with a tranquil outdoor courtyard, has light meals and Finnish treats such as lingonberry juice and reindeer quiche (open until 17:00). It's just a five-minute walk from Temppeliaukio Church.

▲▲▲Temppeliaukio Church

A more modern example of great church architecture (from 1969), this Church in the Rock was blasted out of solid granite. It was

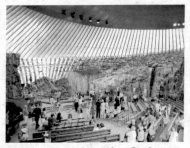

designed by architect brothers Timo and Tuomo Suomalainen, and built within a year's time. Barren of decor except for a couple of simple crosses, the church is capped with a copper-and-skylight dome; it's normally filled with live or recorded music and awestruck visitors. Grab a pew. Gawk upward at a 13-mile-long coil of copper ribbon. Look at the bull's-eye and ponder God. Forget your camera. Just sit in the middle, ignore the crowds, and be thankful for peace...under your feet is a bomb shelter that can accommodate 6,000 people.

Cost and Hours: Free, June-Sept Mon-Sat 10:00-17:45, Sun 11:45-17:45, closes one hour earlier off-season and for special events and concerts, Lutherinkatu 3, tel. 09/2340-6320, www. helsinginseurakunnat.fi.

Getting There: The church is at the top of a gentle hill in a residential neighborhood, about a 15-minute walk north of the bus station or a 10-minute walk behind the National Museum (or take tram #2 to Sammonkatu stop).

▲Sibelius Monument

Six hundred stainless-steel pipes called "Love of Music"—built on solid rock, as is so much of Finland—shimmer in a park to honor

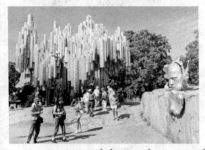

Finland's greatest composer, Jean Sibelius. It's a forest of pipe-organ pipes in a forest of trees. The artist, Eila Hiltunen, was forced to add a bust of the composer's face to silence critics of her otherwise abstract work. City orientation bus tours stop here for 10 minutes—long enough. Bus #24 stops here (30 minutes until the next bus, or catch a quick glimpse on the left from the bus) on its way to the Seurasaari Open-Air Folk Museum. The #2 tram, which runs more frequently, stops a few blocks away.

THE DESIGN DISTRICT

Exploring Helsinki's Design District—described in detail under "Shopping in Helsinki," later—can be a sightseeing highlight for many visitors. A good starting point is the Design Museum a few blocks south of the Esplanade.

▲Design Museum

Design is integral to contemporary Finnish culture, and this fine museum—with a small but insightful permanent collection tracing the evolution of domestic design from the 1870s, plus well-presented temporary exhibits—offers a good overview. Worth ▲▲▲ to those who came to Finland just for the design, it's interesting to anybody.

Cost and Hours: €10; June-Aug daily 11:00-18:00; Sept-May Tue 11:00-20:00, Wed-Sun 11:00-18:00, closed Mon; Korkeavuorenkatu 23, www.designmuseum.fi.

OUTER HELSINKI

A weeklong car trip up through the Finnish lakes and forests to Mikkeli and Savonlinna would be relaxing, but you can actually enjoy Finland's green-trees-and-blue-water scenery without leaving Helsinki. Here are two great ways to get out and go for a walk on a sunny summer day.

▲▲Suomenlinna Fortress

The island guarding Helsinki's harbor served as a strategic fortress for three countries: Finland, Sweden, and Russia. It's now a popular park, with delightful paths, fine views, and a visitors center. On a sunny day, it's a simply delightful place to stroll among hulking buildings with recreating Finns. The free Suomenlinna guidebooklet (stocked at the Helsinki TI, ferry terminal, and the visitors center)

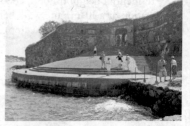

covers the island thoroughly. The island has one good museum (the Suomenlinna Museum, at Suomenlinna Centre—described later) and several skippable smaller museums, including a toy museum and several military museums (€3-4 each, open summer only).

Getting There: Catch a ferry to Suomenlinna from Market Square. Walk past the high-priced excursion boats to the public HKL ferry (€5 round-trip, covered by day ticket and Helsinki Card, 15-minute trip, May-Aug 2-3/hour—generally at :00, :20, and :40 past the hour, but pick up schedule to confirm; Sept-April every 40-60 minutes). If you'll be taking at least two tram rides within 24 hours of visiting Suomenlinna, it pays to get a day ticket instead of a round-trip ticket. A private ferry, JT Line, also runs a "water bus" to Suomenlinna from Market Square in summer (€7 round-trip, May-Sept 2/hour, tel. 09/534-806, www.jt-line.fi). As it costs a bit more and runs less frequently, the JT Line is only worthwhile if you're in a rush to get to the Suomenlinna Centre and museum (since the water bus uses a dock here instead of the northern port used by the public ferry).

Tours: The one-hour English-language island tour departs from the Suomenlinna Centre (€10, free with Helsinki Card; June-Aug daily at 11:00, 12:30, and 14:30; Sept-May 1/day Sat-Sun only). The tour is fine if you're a military history buff, but it kind of misses the point of what's now essentially a giant playground for all ages.

Background: The fortress was built by the Swedes with French financial support in the mid-1700s to counter Russia's rise to power. (Russian Czar Peter the Great had built his new capital, St. Petersburg, on the Baltic and was eyeing the West.) Named Sveaborg ("Fortress of Sweden"), the fortress was Sweden's military pride and joy. With five miles of walls and hundreds of cannons, it was the second strongest fort of its kind in Europe after Gibraltar. Helsinki, a small community of 1,500 people before 1750, soon became a boomtown supporting this grand "Gibraltar of the North."

The fort, built by more than 10,000 workers, was a huge investment and stimulated lots of innovation. In the 1760s, it had the world's biggest and most modern dry dock. It served as a key naval base during a brief Russo-Swedish war in 1788-1790. But in 1808, the Russians took the "invincible" fort without a fight—by siege—as a huge and cheap military gift.

Today, Suomenlinna has 1,000 permanent residents, is home to Finland's Naval Academy, and is most appreciated by locals for its fine scenic strolls. The island is large—actually, it's six islands connected by bridges—and you and your imagination get free run of the fortifications and dungeon-like chambers. When it's time to eat, you'll find a half-dozen cafés and plenty of picnic opportunities.

Visiting Suomenlinna: Across from the public ferry landing are the Jetty Barracks, housing a small information desk (a good place to pick up the free island map/booklet, if you haven't already), convenient WC, free modern art exhibit, and the pricey Panimo brewpub/restaurant. From here, start your stroll of the island. You'll wander on cobbles past dilapidated shiplap cottages that evoke a more robust time for this once-strategic, now-leisurely island. The garrison church on your left, which was Orthodox until its 20th-century conversion to Lutheranism, doubled as a lighthouse.

A five-minute walk from the ferry brings you to the **Suomenlinna Centre,** which houses the worthwhile Suomenlinna Museum. Inside the (free) lobby, you'll find an information desk, gift shop, café, and giant model of all six islands that make up Suomenlinna—handy for orientation. The exhibits themselves are well-presented but dryly explained: fragments of old walls, cannons, period clothing, model ships, and so on; the upstairs focuses on the site's transition from a fortress to a park. The main attraction is the fascinating 25-minute "multivision" show, presenting the island's complete history, which runs twice hourly and has a headphone soundtrack in English (€6.50 for museum and film, daily May-Sept 10:00-18:00, Oct-April 10:30-16:30, tel. 09/684-1850, www.suomenlinna.fi).

From the Suomenlinna Centre, cross the bridge—noticing the giant, rusted seaplane hall on the right, housing the Regatta Club, with a fun sailboat photo exhibition and shop. On the far side of the hall, peer into the gigantic dry dock.

Back on the main trail, climb five minutes uphill to the right into **Piper Park** (Piperin Puisto). Hike up past its elegant 19th-century café (with rocky view tables), and continue up and over the ramparts to a surreal swimming area. From here, follow the waterline—and the ramparts—to the south. You'll walk above bunkers burrowed underground, like gigantic molehills (or maybe Hobbit houses). Periodic ladders let you scramble down onto the rocks. Imposing cannons, now used as playsets and photo-op props for kids, are still aimed ominously at the Gulf of Finland—in case, I imagine, of Russian invasion...or if they just get fed up with all of those cruise ships. Reaching the southern tip of the island, called King's Gate, peek out through the cannon holes. Then make your walk a loop by circling back to the Suomenlinna Centre and, beyond that, the ferry dock for the ride home.

▲▲Seurasaari Open-Air Folk Museum

Inspired by Stockholm's Skansen, also on a lovely island on the edge of town, this is a collection of 100 historic buildings from every corner of Finland. It's 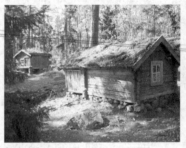 wonderfully furnished and gives rushed visitors an opportunity to sample the far reaches of Finland without leaving the capital city. If you're not taking a tour, get the €1.20 map or the helpful €6 guidebook. You're welcome to bring a picnic, or you can have a light lunch (snacks and cakes) in the Antti farmstead at the center of the park.

Cost and Hours: Free park entry, €8 to enter buildings; June-Aug daily 11:00-17:00; late May and early Sept Mon-Fri 9:00-15:00, Sat-Sun 11:00-17:00; buildings closed mid-Sept-mid-May; tel. 09/4050-9660, www.seurasaari.fi.

Tours: English tours are free with €8 entry ticket, offered mid-June-mid-Aug generally at 15:00, and take one hour (confirm times on their website).

Getting There: To reach the museum, ride bus #24 (from the top of the Esplanade, 2/hour) to the end (note departure times for your return) and walk across the quaint footbridge.

Shopping in Helsinki

Helsinki may be the top shopping town in the Nordic countries. Even in this region that prides itself on its creative design culture, Helsinki is a trendsetter; many Finnish designers are household names worldwide. The easiest place to get a taste of Finnish design is along the Esplanade, but with even a little more time, it's worth delving into the nearby Design District.

Opening Times: Most shops are open all day long Mondays through Fridays (generally 10:00 until 17:00 or 18:00), often have shorter hours on Saturday (likely opening at 10:00 or 12:00 and closing around 16:00), and most are closed on Sundays. Larger shops have longer hours, including brief opening hours on Sundays. While specific hours are not listed for each shop below, I have noted those that seriously buck these trends (and you can find complete hours for any shop online).

ALONG THE ESPLANADE

Helsinki's elegant main drag, the Esplanade, is a coffee-sipper's and window-shopper's delight. Practically every big name in Finnish design (and there are lots of them) has a flagship store along this people-pleasing strip. These tend to be open a bit longer than the hours noted above; most are open until 19:00 (or even 20:00) on weekdays, until 17:00 on Saturdays, and even on Sundays (typically 12:00-16:00 or 17:00).

On my self-guided walk, earlier, I pointed out several Esplanade shops worth dipping into: Consider the purses, scarves, clothes, and fabrics from **Marimekko,** the well-known Finnish fashion company famous for floral designs (at #33A, www.marimekko.com). (Two more Marimekko branches are a short walk away: one specializing in children's items halfway up the cross-street, Mikonkatu, at #2D; and another specializing in clothing one block farther up the Esplanade, then right up Keskuskatu to the intersection with Aleksanterinkatu.) **Aarikka** (#27C, www.aarikka.com) and **Iittala** (#25B, www.iittala.com) have Finnish housewares and ceramics, while **Kalevala** (at #27C, along with Aarikka) sells finely crafted, handmade jewelry (www.kalevalakoru.com).

Across the street, on the south side of the Esplanade, are more shops: **Artek,** Alvar and Elissa Aalto's flagship store (#18, www.artek.fi); **Finlayson** is a more affordable option for Finnish home decor and design (one block closer to the harbor at #14, www.finlayson.fi).

The Esplanade is capped by the enormous, eight-floor **Stockmann** department store, arguably the Nordic region's most impressive (Mon-Fri 9:00-21:00, Sat 9:00-18:00, Sun 12:00-18:00, great basement supermarket, Aleksanterinkatu 52B, www.stockmann.fi). Bookworms enjoy the impressive **Academic Bookstore** just downhill from Stockmann (#39, same hours as Stockmann).

Fans of Tove Jansson's Moomin children's stories will enjoy the **Moomin Shop,** on the second floor of the Forum shopping mall at Mannerheimintie 20, across the busy tram-lined street from Stockmann (Mon-Fri 9:00-21:00, Sat 9:00-18:00, Sun 12:00-18:00, www.moomin.fi).

THE DESIGN DISTRICT

Helsinki's Design District is a several-block cluster of streets that are lined with a dizzying array of one-off boutiques, galleries, and other shops highlighting local designers. From high fashion to comfy everyday clothes, and from lovingly handcrafted jewelry to clever kitchen doodads, this is an engaging zone to explore. For a handy orientation to the options in this ever-changing area, visit www.designdistrict.fi, and get tips at the TI—they often hand out maps or brochures illustrating your options.

While the Design District sprawls—roughly southwest of the Esplanade nearly all the way to the waterfront—the following sub-areas are most worthy of exploration.

Kolmikulma Park and Nearby

Just a block south of the Esplanade's top end (down Erottajankatu), the park called Kolmikulma (literally "Triangular," also called Diana Park for its spear-throwing statue centerpiece) is a handy epicenter of Design District liveliness. From here, streets fan out to the west. A few choices ring the park itself, while several more line the streets that stretch southwest.

Uudenmaankatu has the highest concentration of shops, especially fashion boutiques of local designers. **Nounou** (on the left, at #2) has very colorful glass pieces (open only Tue, Thu, and Sat); the recommended **Café Bar No. 9,** across the street, is a popular place to grab a filling meal. Farther along, **Astra Taivas** (on the right, at #13) is a hole-in-the-wall crammed with precarious shelves of secondhand glassware—causing even the most cautious visitor to feel like the proverbial bull in a china shop. At the end of the block, **Ivana Helsinki** (at #15, on the right) has pattered casual dresses. A detour to the right up the next street (Annankatu) takes you to **Momono,** a tight and endearing shop highlighting Finnish design (on the left at Annankatu 12).

Back on Uudenmaankatu, it's just one more (less interesting) block to Fredrikinkatu, with a lot more choices (described later).

Meanwhile, a block south, pedestrianized **Iso Roobertinkatu** has a few more less interesting choices, and also has lots of cheap eateries. **Formverk,** at the corner with Annankatu, has fun home decor and kitchenware (Annankatu 5).

Fredrikinkatu

This street, which crosses Uudenmaankatu two blocks west of the park, is one of the most engaging streets in town. (For a sneak peek of the many shops lining this street—only a few of which are noted here—see www.fredashops.fi.)

At the corner with Uudenmaankatu, **C. Hagelstam** is an antiquariat with cool vintage prints and antique books, while across the street, **Peroba** (at Uudenmaankatu 33) displays bold Scan design. From here, head north along Fredrikinkatu, which is lined with mostly fashion designers, plus **Kauniste** (on the left at #24, uniquely patterned fabrics and prints) and, at the end of the block on the left, **Chez Marius** (#26, a world of fun kitchen gadgets and cooking gear). This shop also marks the pleasant intersection with the tree- and tram-lined Bulevardi. **Day,** kitty-corner from the Chez Marius, has funky, quirky home decor and gifts (Bulevardi 11).

Continuing north across Bulevardi and along Fredrikinkatu, the next block has several home-decor shops, including **Casuarina** (on the left at #30, with a spare, rustic, reclaimed aesthetic) and **Primavera Interiors** (across the street at #41, with a more artistic and funky style).

Browse your way two more blocks up Fredrikinkatu to the cross-street, **Eerikinkatu,** which also has lots of inviting little galleries and boutiques; two are at the same address, just around the corner to the left (at Eerikinkatu 18): **DesiPeli,** with a variety of home decor, including some very cool, Marimekko-type fabrics (closed Sun-Mon); and **Napa & Paja,** a collective gallery of three jewelry designers, showcasing their beautiful, unique, delicate designs. They also stock casual handbags and books about Finland.

OTHER SHOPPING OPTIONS

Market Square: This harborfront square is packed not only with fishmongers and producers, but also with stands selling Finnish

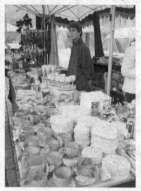

souvenirs and more refined crafts (roughly Mon-Fri 6:30-17:00—or until 18:00 in summer, Sat 6:30-16:00, only tourist stalls open on Sun 10:00-16:00).

Modern Shopping Mall: For less glamorous shopping needs, the **Kamppi** mall above and around the bus station is good.

Flea Market: If you brake for garage sales, Finland's biggest flea market, the outdoor **Hietalahti Market,** is worth the 15-minute walk from the harbor or a short ride on tram #6 from Mannerheimintie to the Hietalahdentori stop (June-Aug Mon-Fri 9:00-19:00, Sat 8:00-16:00, Sun 10:00-16:00; less action, shorter hours, and closed Sun off-season). The adjacent red-brick indoor Hietalahti Market Hall houses food stands (described later, under "Eating in Helsinki").

Eating in Helsinki

Helsinki's many restaurants are smoke-free and a good value for lunch on weekdays. Finnish companies get a tax break if they distribute lunch coupons (worth €9) to their employees. It's no surprise that most downtown Helsinki restaurants offer weekday

HELSINKI

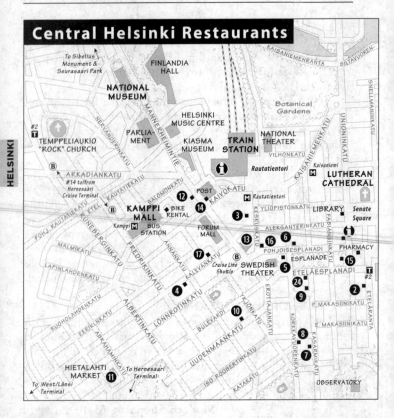

Central Helsinki Restaurants

lunch specials that cost exactly the value of the coupon. These low prices evaporate on Saturday and Sunday, when picnics and Middle Eastern kebab restaurants are the only budget options.

FUN HARBORFRONT EATERIES

Stalls on Market Square: Helsinki's delightful and vibrant square is magnetic any time of day...but especially at lunchtime. This really is the most memorable, casual, quick-and-cheap lunch place in town. A half-dozen orange tents (erected to shield diners from bird bombs) serve fun food on paper plates until 18:00. It's not unusual for the Finnish president to stop by here with visiting dignitaries. There's a crêpe place, and at the far end—my favorites—several salmon grills (€10-13 for a good meal). The only real harborside dining in this part of town is picnicking. While these places provide picnic tables, you can also have your food foil-wrapped to go and grab benches right on the water down near Uspenski Orthodox Cathedral.

   Old Market Hall (Vanha Kauppahalli): Just beyond the harborside market is a cute, red-brick, indoor market hall. It's

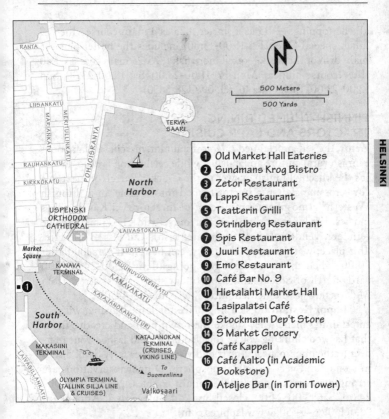

1. Old Market Hall Eateries
2. Sundmans Krog Bistro
3. Zetor Restaurant
4. Lappi Restaurant
5. Teatterin Grilli
6. Strindberg Restaurant
7. Spis Restaurant
8. Juuri Restaurant
9. Emo Restaurant
10. Café Bar No. 9
11. Hietalahti Market Hall
12. Lasipalatsi Café
13. Stockmann Dep't Store
14. S Market Grocery
15. Café Kappeli
16. Café Aalto (in Academic Bookstore)
17. Ateljee Bar (in Torni Tower)

HELSINKI

beautifully renovated with upscale-feeling woodwork, and quite tight inside (Mon-Sat 8:00-18:00, closed Sun). Today, along with produce stalls, it's a hit for its fun, inexpensive eateries. You'll find lots of enticing coffee shops with tempting pastries; various grilled, smoked, or pickled fish options (you'll smell it before you see it); mounds of bright-yellow paella; deli counters with delectable open-face sandwiches; a handy chance to sample reindeer meat; and an array of ethnic eats, from Middle Eastern and Lebanese meals to Vietnamese banh mi sandwiches. In the market hall, **Soppakeittiö** ("Soup Kitchen") serves big bowls of filling, tasty seafood soup for €9.50, including bread and water (Mon-Fri 11:00-16:00, Sat 11:00-15:00—except closed Sat in summer, closed Sun year-round).

Sundmans Krog Bistro is sedate and Old World but not folkloric, filling an old merchant's mansion facing the harbor. As it's the less fussy and more affordable (yet still super-romantic) little sister of an adjacent, posh, Michelin-rated restaurant, quality is assured. A rare and memorable extra is their Baltic fish buffet—featuring salmon, Baltic sprat, and herring with potatoes and all the toppings—€15 as a starter, €25 as a main course. The €19 lunch special (Mon-Fri 11:00-15:00) includes the buffet plus the main dish of the week—often more fish (€23-25 main courses, €40 three-course dinners, Mon-Fri 11:00-23:00, Sat 12:00-23:00, Sun 13:00-23:00, Eteläranta 16, tel. 09/6128-5450).

FINNISH-THEMED DINING: TRACTORS AND LAPP CUISINE

Zetor, the self-proclaimed *traktor* restaurant, mercilessly lampoons Finnish rural culture and cuisine (while celebrating it deep down). It's the kitschy Finnish answer to the Cracker Barrel. Sit next to a cow-crossing sign at a tractor-turned-into-a-table, in a "Finnish Western" atmosphere reminiscent of director Aki Kaurismäki's movies. For lunch or dinner, main courses run €17-23 and include reindeer, vendace (small freshwater fish), and less exotic fare. This place, while touristy and tacky, can be fun. It gets loud after 20:00, when the dance floor gets going (daily 12:00-24:00, 200 yards north of Stockmann department store, across street from McDonald's at Mannerheimintie 3, tel. 010-766-4450).

Lappi Restaurant is a fine place for Lapp cuisine, with an entertaining menu (they smoke their own fish) and creative decor that has you thinking you've traveled north and lashed your reindeer to the hitchin' post. The friendly staff serves tasty Sami dishes in a snug and very woody atmosphere. Dinner reservations are strongly recommended (€24-39 main courses, Mon-Fri 16:00-24:00, Sat 13:00-24:00, closed Sun, off Bulevardi at Annankatu 22, tel. 09/645-550, www.lappires.com).

VENERABLE ESPLANADE CAFÉS

Highly competitive restaurants line the sunny north side of the Esplanade—offering creative lunch salads and light meals in their cafés (with fine sidewalk seating), plush sofas for cocktails in their bars, and fancy restaurant dining upstairs.

Teatterin Grilli, attached to the landmark Swedish Theater, has several interconnected eateries inside and fine, park-side seating indoors and out. Order a salad from the café counter in the "Wine & Deli & Juice" bar, facing the Academic Bookstore (€10 with bread, choose two meats or extras to add to crispy base, Caesar salad option). The long cocktail bar is popular with office workers yet comfortable for baby-boomer tourists. Whether you order a meal or a drink, you're welcome to find a seat out on the leafy Esplanade terrace (café counter open Mon-Fri 9:00-20:30, Sat 11:00-20:30, Sun 12:00-20:30 except closed Sun in winter, at the top of the Esplanade, Pohjoisesplanadi 2, tel. 09/6128-5000). There's also a fancy restaurant.

Strindberg, near the corner of the Esplanade and Mikonkatu, has several parts—each one oozing atmosphere and class. Down-stairs is an elegant café with outdoor and indoor tables great for people-watching (€8-15 sandwiches and salads). The upstairs cock-tail lounge—with big sofas and bookshelves giving it a den-like coziness—attracts the after-work office crowd. Also upstairs, the inviting restaurant has huge main dishes for €20-30, with fish, meat, pasta, and vegetarian options; reserve in advance to try to get a window seat overlooking the Esplanade (restaurant open Mon 11:00-23:00, Tue-Sat 11:00-24:00, closed Sun; café open Mon 9:00-23:00, Tue-Sat 9:00-24:00, Sun 10:00-22:00, Pohjoisesplanadi 33, tel. 09/681-2030).

TRENDY EATERIES IN AND NEAR THE DESIGN DISTRICT

Predictably, several creative eateries cluster in the Design District, a short stroll south and west of the Esplanade. While these aren't for budget diners, they do offer a fresh and updated take on the cuisine of Finland. Many of these restaurants highlight the excit-ing "New Nordic" school of cooking, featuring fresh, seasonal ingredients—often foraged or locally sourced—and modern, inventive presentations.

Spis is your best Helsinki bet for splurging on Finnish New Nordic. Reserve ahead for one of the prized tables in its tiny, peeling-plaster, rustic-chic dining room (tasting menus only: €57/4 courses, €77/6 courses, Tue-Sat from 17:30, last seating at 20:30, closed Sun-Mon, Kasarmikatu 26, mobile 045-305-1211, www.spis.fi).

Juuri has a trendy, casual interior and serves a variety of "sapas" (Suomi tapas)—small plates highlighting Finland's culi-nary bounty. It's lunch-only on weekdays (€5 small plates, €28 main courses, Mon-Fri 11:00-14:30 only, Sat 12:00-22:00, Sun 16:00-22:00, Korkeavuorenkatu 27, tel. 09/635-732).

Emo Restaurant is a pleasantly unpretentious, blue-jeans wine bar in a sleepy zone just a block off of the Esplanade. They serve up €10 small plates; most patrons share several (lunch Tue-Thu 11:30-14:30; dinner Mon-Sat 17:00-24:00, closed Sun; Kasarmikatu 44, mobile 010-505-0900, www.emo-ravintola.fi).

Pub Grub: **Café Bar No. 9** is a simpler, cheaper choice right in the heart of the Design District. Tucked between design shops, its borderline-divey bar vibe attracts a loyal local following, who enjoy digging into plates of unpretentious pub food (€10-16 meals, Uudenmaakatu 9, tel. 09-621-4059).

Market Hall: Hiding in a nondescript neighborhood at the edge of the Design District, the **Hietalahti Market Hall** (at Lönnrotinkatu 34, just north of the Bulevardi) is a fun place to browse for a meal. It's similar to the Old Market Hall along the

What If I Miss My Boat?

Remember that you can get help from the cruise line's port agent (listed on the destination information sheet distributed on the ship) and the local TI (see page 312). If the port agent suggests a costly solution (such as a private car with a driver), you may want to consider public transit.

Two fine and fiercely competitive lines—Viking Line (tel. 0600-15700, www.vikingline.fi) and Tallink Silja (tel. 0600-41577, www.tallinksilja.com)—connect Helsinki to **Stockholm.** Several companies run fast boats to **Tallinn,** including Tallink Silja, Viking Line, Linda Line (www.lindaline.ee), and Eckerö Line (www.eckeroline.fi). To reach points farther west, you could take the night boat to Stockholm, then the train from there to **Copenhagen** or **Oslo** (or take the overnight boat from Stockholm to **Rīga**). To research train schedules, see www.bahn.com. But for many of these places, you're probably better off flying.

St. Petersburg is well connected to Helsinki, but your options depend on whether you have a Russian visa (impossible to get last-minute if you don't already have one). With a visa, you can take a speedy train (www.vr.fi) or a slower bus. But if you don't have a visa, you're likely better off waiting and meeting your ship at the next stop.

If you need to catch a **plane** to your next destination, you can take a bus to Helsinki's airport, about 10 miles north of the city (www.helsinki-vantaa.fi).

Local **travel agents** in Helsinki can help you; I'd check first with the user-friendly Helsinki Expert desk inside the main TI (see page 312). For more advice on what to do if you miss the boat, see page 139.

South Harbor, but far less touristy. The elegantly renovated old food hall is filled with an enticing array of vendors, and delightful seating upstairs (Mon-Fri 8:00-18:00, Sat 8:00-17:00, closed Sun).

FUNCTIONAL EATING

Lasipalatsi, the renovated, rejuvenated 1930s Glass Palace, is on Mannerheimintie between the train and bus stations. The café (with a youthful terrace on the square out back) offers a self-service buffet (€10 weekday lunch before 15:00, €17 weekend brunch, €13 dinner after 15:00 any day); there are always €5 sandwiches and cakes (Mon-Fri 7:30-22:00, Sat 9:00-23:00, Sun 11:00-22:00, more expensive restaurant upstairs—closed Sun, across from post office at Mannerheimintie 22, tel. 09/612-6700).

PICNICS

In supermarkets, buy the semi-flat bread (available dark or light) that Finns love—every slice is a heel. Finnish liquid yogurt is also a treat (sold in liter cartons). Karelian pasties, filled with rice or mashed potatoes, make a good snack. A beautiful, upscale supermarket is in the basement of the **Stockmann** department store—follow the *Delikatessen* signs downstairs (Mon-Fri 9:00-21:00, Sat 9:00-18:00, open most Sun 12:00-18:00, Aleksanterinkatu 52B). Two blocks north, a more workaday, inexpensive supermarket is **S Market,** under the Sokos department store next to the train station (Mon-Sat 7:00-22:00, Sun 10:00-22:00).

Finnish Survival Phrases

In Finnish, the emphasis always goes on the first syllable. Double vowels
(e.g., *ää* or *ii*) sound similar to single vowels, but are held a bit longer.
The letter *y* sounds like the German *ü* (purse your lips and say "oh").
In the phonetics, ī sounds like the long *i* in "light," and bolded syllables
are stressed.

English	Finnish	Pronunciation
Good morning. (formal)	*Hyvää huomenta.*	**hew**-vaah **hwoh**-mehn-tah
Good day. (formal)	*Hyvää päivää.*	**hew**-vaah **pī**-vaah
Good evening. (formal)	*Hyvää iltaa.*	**hew**-vaah **eel**-taah
Hi. / Bye. (informal)	*Hei. / Hei-hei.*	hey / hey-hey
Do you speak English?	*Puhutko englantia?*	**poo**-hoot-koh **ehn**-glahn-tee-yah
Yes. / No.	*Kyllä. / Ei.*	**kewl**-lah / ay
Please.	*Ole hyvä.*	**oh**-leh **hew**-vah
Thank you (very much).	*Kiitos (paljon).*	**kee**-tohs (**pahl**-yohn)
You're welcome.	*Kiitos. / Ei kestä.*	**kee**-tohs / ay **kehs**-tah
Can I help you?	*Voinko auttaa?*	**voin**-koh **owt**-taah
Excuse me.	*Anteeksi.*	**ahn**-teek-see
(Very) good.	*(Oikein) hyvä.*	(**oy**-kayn) **hew**-vah
Goodbye.	*Näkemiin.*	**nah**-keh-meen
one / two	*yksi / kaksi*	**ewk**-see / **kahk**-see
three / four	*kolme / neljä*	**kohl**-meh / **nehl**-yah
five / six	*viisi / kuusi*	**vee**-see / **koo**-see
seven / eight	*seitsemän / kahdeksan*	**sayt**-seh-mahn / **kah**-dehk-sahn
nine / ten	*yhdeksän / kymmenen*	**ew**-dehk-sahn / **kewm**-meh-nehn
hundred	*sata*	**sah**-tah
thousand	*tuhat*	**too**-haht
How much?	*Paljonko?*	**pahl**-yohn-koh
local currency: euro	*euro*	**ay**-oo-roh
Where is...?	*Missä on...?*	**mee**-sah ohn
...the toilet	*...WC*	**vay**-say
men	*miehet*	**mee**-ay-heht
women	*naiset*	**nī**-seht
water / coffee	*vesi / kahvi*	**veh**-see / **kah**-vee
beer / wine	*olut / viini*	**oh**-luht / **vee**-nee
Cheers!	*Kippis!*	**kip**-pis
The bill, please.	*Saisinko laskun, kiitos.*	**sī**-seen-koh **lahs**-kuhn **kee**-tohs

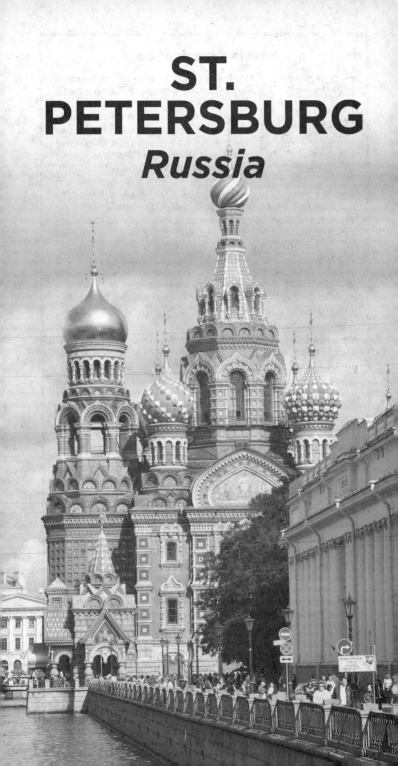

ST.
PETERSBURG
Russia

Russia Practicalities

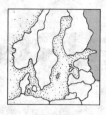

Russia (Россия) is a vast, multiethnic country of more than 142 million people. The world's biggest country by area (6.6 million square miles), it is nearly double the size of the US. Though no longer the great military and political power that it was during the Cold War, Russia remains a country of substantial natural resources, including oil. St. Petersburg—Russia's "window on the West"—is the country's northwestern outpost, peering across the Baltic Sea to Europe.

Money: The currency has been in flux recently, so check the latest rates. As of this writing (in early 2015), 65 Russian rubles (R, official RUB) = about $1. An ATM is called a bankomat (банкомат). The local value-added sales tax (called ндс/NDS) is 18 percent; the minimum purchase eligible for a VAT refund is 10,000 R (for details on refunds, see page 134). At some sights, you'll see higher "foreigner prices" for non-Russians.

Language: The native language is Russian, which uses the Cyrillic alphabet (see page 363).

Emergencies: Dial 112 for police or other emergencies. Pickpockets and petty theft are a problem in St. Petersburg; for tips, see page 362. In case of theft or loss, see page 125.

Time Zone: St. Petersburg is on Moscow Time (one hour ahead of Helsinki, Tallinn, and Rīga; two hours ahead of Scandinavia and most of the Continent, including Stockholm and Copenhagen; and eight/eleven hours ahead of the East/West Coasts of the US).

Consulate in St. Petersburg: The **US consulate** is at Furshtadtskaya 15 (tel. 331-2600, http://stpetersburg.usconsulate.gov). There is no **Canadian embassy** in St. Petersburg; instead, contact the Moscow branch (23 Starokonyushenny Pereulok, tel. 495/925-6000, www.russia.gc.ca). Call ahead for passport services.

Phoning: Russia's country code is 7, and St. Petersburg's area code is 812. To call from another country to Russia, dial the international access code (011 from the US/Canada, 00 from Europe, or + from a mobile phone), then 7, followed by the area code and local number. For calls within Russia, dial just the number if you are calling locally; if you're calling long distance, dial 8, then the area code and the number. To call the US or Canada from Russia, dial 8, then dial 10, then 1, then your area code and phone number. For more tips, see page 1146.

Tipping: As service is included at sit-down meals, you don't need to tip further. Tip a taxi driver by rounding up the fare a bit (pay 300 R on an 280-R fare). For more tips on tipping, see page 138.

Tourist Information: www.visit-petersburg.ru

ST. PETERSBURG

Санкт-Петербург

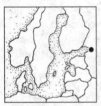

Once a swamp, then an imperial capital, and now a showpiece of vanished aristocratic opulence shot through with the dingy ruins of communism, St. Petersburg is Russia's most accessible and most tourist-worthy city. During the Soviet era, it was called Leningrad, but in 1991 St. Petersburg reverted to its more fitting historic name. Designed by imported French, Dutch, and Italian architects, this is, arguably, European Russia's least "Russian" city.

Palaces, gardens, statues, and arched bridges over graceful waterways bring back the time of the czars. Neighborhood markets bustle with gregarious honey maids offering samples, and brim with exotic fishes and meats, pickled goodies, and fresh produce. Stirring monuments—still adorned with hammers, sickles, and red stars—tower over the masses, evoking Soviet times. Jammed with reverent worshippers, glorious Orthodox churches are heavy with incense, shimmer with icons, and filled with hauntingly beautiful music. Topping things off are two of the world's premier art museums—the Hermitage and the Russian Museum—and one of its most opulent royal houses, the Catherine Palace.

St. Petersburg can challenge its visitors, most of whom have to jump through hoops to get a visa—and then struggle with not enough time, limited English, and an idiosyncratic (and not quite Western) approach to "service" and predictability. But most visitors leave St. Petersburg with vivid memories of a magnificent city, one that lives according to its own rules. While this place can be exasperating, it is worth grappling with. Beyond its brick-and-mortar sights, St. Petersburg gives first-timers a perfect peek into the enigmatic Russian culture.

Save time on a sunny day just to walk. Keep your head up: The upper facades are sun-warmed and untouched by street grime. While Nevsky Prospekt—the city's famous main boulevard— encapsulates all that's wonderful and discouraging about this quixotic burg, get beyond that axis. Explore the back streets along the canals. Stroll through the Summer Garden. Shop for a picnic at a local market hall. Go for a canal boat cruise. Step into a neighborhood church to watch people get intimate with an icon. Take a Metro ride anywhere, just for the experience. Climb St. Isaac's Cathedral for the view. When the Baltic Sea brings clouds and drizzle, plunge into the Hermitage or the Russian Museum.

PLANNING YOUR TIME

St. Petersburg is fantastic and gigantic, with much to see. With two days here, your priorities should include the following (see later for a specific hour-by-hour plan).

• **Hermitage:** One of the world's finest palaces, housing one of the world's best art collections. Four hours is just enough for a quick taste (one hour for the staterooms, one hour for Old Masters art, one hour for Modern Masters, and an extra hour just to move around the huge and crowded complex).

• **Russian Museum:** Excellent, manageable, and relatively uncrowded collection of Russian art. Allow two hours.

• **Nevsky Prospekt:** St. Petersburg's bustling main drag, explained by my self-guided walk from Palace Square (behind the Hermitage) to the Fontanka River, and passing several of the biggies listed here. Allow two hours for the walk, not counting sightseeing stops.

• **Fabergé Museum:** One of the world's best collections of Fabergé eggs fills a mansion near the end of my self-guided Nevsky Prospekt walk. An hour gives you a speedy look; you're required to join a tour until 18:00, after which you can visit on your own.

• **Kazan Cathedral, Church on Spilled Blood, and St. Isaac's:** St. Petersburg's three best Orthodox churches—each very different (so they're complementary). Allow about 30 minutes apiece for a quick visit, plus another 30 minutes to climb to the viewpoint atop St. Isaac's.

• **Peter and Paul Fortress:** The city's fortified-island birthplace, with stout ramparts, the burial cathedral of the czars, and a smattering of mildly interesting museums. For a targeted visit (cathedral and quick stroll around the grounds), allow about an hour; an additional hour lets you dip into some of the museums. Either way, budget about 30 minutes each way to get here from the city center (by foot over the Neva, or by Metro from Nevsky Prospekt).

• **Other Museums:** These include the Russian Museum of

Ethnography, Kunstkamera (international ethnography and oddities), and Museum of Russian Political History. Allow 30-60 minutes for each one—potentially much more if you're especially interested in their subjects.

• **Out-of-Town Sights:** Those who love opulent palaces can make a pilgrimage to two over-the-top Romanov residences on the city outskirts: **Peterhof** (with gorgeous gardens) or **Tsarskoye Selo** (with the Catherine Palace and its sumptuous Amber Room). Given the relative complexity of reaching either palace, most cruisers skip these to focus on the abundant sights in the city center, or opt for a cruise-run excursion. On your own, either place can be seen in a half-day targeted tour by taxi or with a hired driver; otherwise, allow a full day.

BEST TWO- OR THREE-DAY PLAN

Most cruises stop in St. Petersburg for two days. I've also provided suggestions for a third day, in case you have it. To maximize your daytime sightseeing, see if your cruise line offers an evening visit to the Hermitage (see page 356).

Day 1

9:00	Follow my self-guided walk along Nevsky Prospekt to acquaint yourself with the city.
11:00	Visit the Kazan Cathedral and Church on Spilled Blood, and grab a quick lunch.
13:00	Tour the Russian Museum.
15:00	Take a canal boat cruise.
16:30	Visit St. Isaac's Cathedral.
18:30	Dinner.
Evening	Ballet, a concert, or the circus—or possibly an evening Hermitage visit (through your cruise line).

Day 2

10:30	Plunge into the Hermitage.
13:30	Grab a quick lunch, then walk across the Neva River to the Strelka viewpoint, continuing to Peter and Paul Fortress.
15:30	Tour the Kunstkamera and/or the Museum of Russian Political History; for a break, stroll through the Summer Garden.
18:00	Visit the Fabergé Museum.
19:30	Return to the city center for dinner (if your ship's departure time allows it).

Day 3

With more time, do days 1 and 2 at a more relaxed tempo, with more time in the Hermitage or the Russian Museum—letting

To Visa or Not to Visa?

Note: The following information was accurate as of early 2015, but Russian visa regulations are notoriously changeable. Confirm everything stated here before you make your plans. For the latest requirements, see www.ricksteves.com/russianvisa.

To enter Russia, residents of most countries, including the US and Canada, are required to obtain a visa in advance. The only exception is for travelers arriving by sea (on a cruise ship or passenger ferry), who can be in the country for up to 72 hours without a visa.

However, there's a catch: Once you leave your ship, you are required to remain with your guide or escort the entire time—which means you'll have virtually no free time to explore. (A loophole in St. Petersburg allows some tour operators to provide a downtown "shuttle service" to passengers arriving on the St. Peter Line ferries, but this service isn't extended to those arriving on a cruise ship.)

Cruisers in St. Petersburg have three options: 1) **Obtain a visa** to explore the city on your own; 2) **hire a private guide** to handle the red tape and accompany you on shore; or 3) see the city with a **cruise-line excursion.**

Obtaining a visa is the most hassle, but it gives you the most freedom—and even with the fees, it's the most affordable choice. Hiring a guide is more expensive than going it alone, but you'll have a nice combination of structure and independence—although technically you have to stay with your guide, which effectively rules out a relaxing dinner or ballet in the evening (for more on private guides, including hiring one for a no-visa visit, see page 371). An excursion is likely about half the cost of a private guide, but you'll do everything as part of a large group (for

what you don't get to spill over to today. Other choices are to visit other museums that interest you; ride the Metro to less-touristed parts of the city (such as the back streets of Vasilyevsky Island; see page 383); or go to Peterhof or Tsarskoye Selo for the day. WWII history buffs should consider a visit to Piskaryovskoye Memorial Cemetery.

One-Day Plan

A few cruises are in town for only one day. In this case, devout art lovers should tour the Hermitage, then follow my self-guided Nevsky Prospekt walk. For a wider-ranging experience, skip the Hermitage and follow this ambitious plan (if you're not up for it all, omit the Russian Museum):

more on the excursion option, see the sidebar on page 356).

How to Get a Visa: Before applying for a visa, you must first get an official document called a "visa invitation" (*priglashenie*; sometimes called a "letter of invitation," "visa sponsor," or "visa support letter") from a Russian organization recognized by the Russian Foreign Ministry. Visa invitations are typically issued either by a hotel or by a tour operator. If you're arriving by cruise, you'll need to arrange an invitation through a third-party agency. These agencies specialize in steering your visa application through the process. They can also help you arrange visa invitations and navigate the confusing application. I've had a good experience with Passport Visa Express.com (www.passportvisas express.com).

In addition to the $160 visa price, visa agencies charge a service fee of about $80-110 (including the invitation fee). To ship your passport securely to and from the visa agency costs another $50 or so. Figure at least $350 total per person.

Entering Russia with a Visa: When you enter the country, the immigration officer will ask you to fill out a migration card in duplicate, listing your name, passport number, and other details. The officer will stamp both parts of the card and keep one. Don't lose the other half—it must be presented when you leave the country. (A digital version of this card is being phased in, but you'll still need to carry the hard copy.)

While in Russia, you are required to carry your original passport (not just a copy) with you at all times. Police in Russia can stop you at any time and ask to see your documents, though this seldom happens to tourists.

9:00   Follow my self-guided Nevsky Prospekt walk (about 2 hours), stopping in the Kazan Cathedral (30 minutes), Church on Spilled Blood (30 minutes), and Russian Museum (2 hours). Along the way, grab a quick lunch (30 minutes) and take some time to shop and linger (30 minutes).

15:00 Take a canal boat cruise.

16:00 Ride the Metro to the Peter and Paul Fortress, and tour the Romanov tombs at Sts. Peter and Paul Cathedral.

18:00 Walk back across the Neva, pausing at Strelka for a panoramic view. Consider an early-evening visit to the Fabergé Museum (back on Nevsky Prospekt).

19:00 Dinner, ballet, or...return to your ship.

The Port of St. Petersburg

Arrival at a Glance: From the **Marine Facade port,** either take a taxi or brave the fun and very cheap bus-plus-Metro option to reach Nevsky Prospekt. If your ship docks along the river in the city, at the **Lieutenant Schmidt** or **English embankments,** it's a longish walk or quick taxi ride to major sights.

Port Overview

St. Petersburg's enormous, U-shaped cruise port is called the **Marine (Morskoy) Facade.** Built on reclaimed land at the western tip of Vasilyevsky Island (facing the Gulf of Finland), it can accommodate a staggering seven big ships at once, feeding into four separate terminal buildings (each with roughly the same services; for port information, see www.ppspbmf.ru). If you sail in during muggy weather, keep your veranda door closed; St. Petersburg was built on a swamp, and bugs can still swarm here.

A lucky few ships—generally smaller, luxury vessels—dock along the Neva River embankment (either the **Lieutenant Schmidt embankment** or the **English embankment**) close to the city center, a long but scenic walk from the Hermitage and other sights.

Tourist Information: There are small TI kiosks at the Marine Facade terminals, but they're not particularly helpful (and often closed). If you happen to see an open one, pick up a map. Otherwise, make your way downtown to find the TI on Palace Square (see page 362).

GETTING INTO TOWN FROM MARINE FACADE

Leaving your ship, you'll go through the **immigration** checkpoint (regardless of whether you have a visa or are with a private guide or excursion, you'll go through the same process).

After the immigration checkpoint, you'll enter a sleek terminal building with a crowd of prearranged drivers and tour guides (holding signs with the names of their clients), an **ATM** dispensing rubles, a desk for booking a taxi, and several souvenir stands perfectly positioned to help departing cruisers burn through whatever rubles remain in their pockets.

Given the size of the port, before heading out, be sure you know both your ship's terminal building number and the docking berth number.

By Taxi

Taxis line up in front of the terminal, charging 600-800 R for a ride downtown (figure 1,400 R one-way to Peterhof, or 1,200 R to Tsarskoye Selo). If no taxis are standing by, look for someone with a *TAXI* clipboard (they may be at a small desk inside the terminal).

By Public Transportation

It's easy, cheap, and very local to ride public transportation from the Marine Facade into downtown. The basic plan: Ride a bus to the nearest Metro station, then either whoosh under the city by subway all the way downtown, or get off at the first stop and walk through interesting neighborhoods the rest of the way into the city.

At the curb in front of the terminal, look for the stop for **bus #158** (2/hour, stops at each terminal, 25 R—pay the conduc-

tor). You'll get off at the **Primorskaya Metro** station: After leaving the port and driving past apartment blocks, the bus turns left onto a big boulevard with tram tracks, with several shops on the right. This is where you hop off (if you're not sure, ask fellow passen-

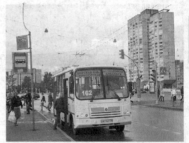

gers: "Metro?"). Exiting the bus, walk straight ahead, and proceed alongside the big shopping center. Look for the Metro sign—an "M" that's bulging on the sides.

Head into the Metro station, turn right to find the ticket window, and buy a token (31 R). Use the token to pass through the turnstile, and head down the long escalator. This is the terminus of the green line, so trains run only in the direction of downtown (toward Rybatskoye). For more on St. Petersburg's Metro system, see page 368.

Option 1: Metro to Downtown

The easiest plan on a tight schedule is to ride the Metro two stops to the **Gostiny Dvor** station. This pops you out onto the city's main avenue, Nevsky Prospekt. From here, it's a 10-minute walk to several major sights, including the Russian Museum, Church on Spilled Blood, and Kazan Cathedral. If you want to reach the start of Nevsky Prospekt (near Palace Square, behind the Hermitage), ride bus #3, #7, #24, or #191; or take trolley bus #1, #5, #7, #10, #11, or #22. Of these, trolley buses #5 and #22 continue to St. Isaac's Cathedral. Alternatively, to get to Peter and Paul Fortress, ride the Metro to Gostiny Dvor, then switch to the other Metro line (blue, Nevsky Prospekt stop); ride this line in the direction of Parnas, and get off at the first stop, Gorkovskaya—about a 10-minute walk from the fortress (see directions on page 358).

Excursions from St. Petersburg

The majority of cruisers in St. Petersburg don't want to go through the hassle of getting a visa (see page 352), so they see the city exclusively with excursions. But remember that you'll likely be in town for two full days and, without a visa, you can leave the ship *only* with an excursion (or with a private guide you've arranged in advance; for more on this option, see page 371).

And excursion costs can add up. For example, on a mid-range cruise line, a two-day itinerary that includes a once-over-lightly bus-and-walking tour, a guided Hermitage tour, and trip to one of the countryside palaces the next day, costs about $500 per person. Evening activities (such as ballet, folk shows, or a nighttime Hermitage visit) are extra. A small cabal of tour operators controls all the cruise tourism business in St. Petersburg. They employ their own stable of guides (whose quality varies widely), and generally take you only to shops and restaurants that they own. (This means that virtually none of the money you spend "in St. Petersburg" supports the broader community.)

While I prefer getting my own visa, or hiring a guide to sort through the red tape for me, the reality is that the majority of cruisers landing in St. Petersburg will opt for the simplicity of cruise-line excursions. Here's a rundown of the typical choices:

The basic St. Petersburg visit includes a narrated **bus ride** around town, with brief photo-op stops at major landmarks. Many also include a shopping stop and a meal. To add more substance, you can book a tour that includes in-depth tours of individual sights. The most popular choice is the **Hermitage/Winter Palace.** Excursions usually consist of a surgical strike of the main historical rooms and a few select masterpieces from the art collection. Don't expect "free time" to linger at your favorites or to explore rooms not on the tour. (For example, lovers of Impressionism should be sure to book a tour that explicitly includes this collection—some don't.) If your cruise line offers an after-hours **evening visit of** the Hermitage (which may include a

Option 2: Back-Street and Riverfront Walk to Downtown

If you're interested in exploring some back streets where few tourists venture, here's another option: Ride the Metro one stop to Vasileostrovskaya, where you can start my "Back-Streets Walk on Vasilyevsky Island" (described on page 383). This walk takes you to the riverfront, the Strelka viewpoint, and ends either at the Peter and Paul Fortress or the Hermitage and Nevsky Prospekt.

GETTING INTO TOWN FROM THE NEVA EMBANKMENT

Smaller ships sometimes put in along either embankment of the Neva River, closer to the city center. Consider yourself lucky if

concert in one of the grand halls), it's worth considering simply because it spares you from the crowds and saves valuable daylight time for other priorities.

Other popular stops are the two sprawling countryside palaces outside town: **Peterhof** (sometimes called the **Summer Palace**) to the west; and **Tsarskoye Selo** (usually billed as the **Catherine Palace** for its grandest structure, sometimes called by its village name, Pushkin), to the south. On a short visit, seeing both is overkill—choose just one. Peterhof has more impressive grounds, while Tsarskoye Selo has more opulent interiors. Some tours to the Catherine Palace tack on a quick stop at yet another nearby palace, **Pavlovsk.**

You may also see excursions that include a **river cruise,** which is well worthwhile for the excellent orientation it provides. Other excursions specialize either in **cathedrals and churches** (of which St. Petersburg has many fascinating and lavish examples) or the **Grand Choral Synagogue** (worthwhile only if you have a special interest). Some excursions include a ride on the **Metro,** just for kicks—an enlightening and local-feeling peek at an impressive people-mover.

Evening entertainment includes **folklore shows** and **ballet.** While ballet is a Russian forte, note that great venues such as the Mariinsky and Mikhailovsky Theaters are on hiatus between mid-July and mid-September; carefully read the fine print of any ballet excursion you're offered. Often, it's a crowd-pleasing, made-for-tourists show put on by lower-tier performers in a tired old ballroom.

And, believe it or not, some cruise lines offer one-day excursions all the way to **Moscow** (round-trip by plane).

Unfortunately, cruise-line excursions rarely go to a few excellent sights—including the outstanding Russian Museum, the powerful WWII-era Piskaryovskoye Memorial Cemetery, or Peter the Great's quirky Kunstkamera; to see those, you'll need a visa or a private guide.

your ship docks here, as it's within (fairly long) walking distance of the big sights.

Lieutenant Schmidt Embankment (North Bank): Named for a naval officer executed for his role in a failed 1905 revolution, the Lieutenant Schmidt (Leytenanta Shmidta) embankment is a scenic 30-minute walk (1.5 miles) from the heart of town. It's right in front of the beautiful, golden-domed Optina Pustyn church (described on page 386—be sure to drop in for a peek). Because there is no ATM at or near the terminal, consider changing some cash on board before you arrive, or be ready to walk into town to find an ATM.

To **walk** into town, simply stroll with the river on your

right. Cross at the second bridge, Dvortsovy Most, to reach the Hermitage, Palace Square, and Nevsky Prospekt; or turn left just after that bridge to find the Strelka viewpoint and the bridge to Peter and Paul Fortress.

To reach handy **buses, trolley buses, and trams** from the north embankment, walk to the Optina Pustyn church and turn up the street called "Ulitsa 14-ya Liniya/Ulitsa 15-ya Liniya" (улица 14-я Линия/улица 15-я Линия). After one long block, you'll hit a main thoroughfare, Bolshoy Prospekt. Turn left and walk a half-block to the stop for trolley bus #10 or #11 or bus #7, all of which cross Dvortsovy Most to reach Palace Square, then continue up Nevsky Prospekt to Uprising Square.

If you're heading to Peter and Paul Fortress, walk one very long block beyond the busy Bolshoy Prospekt to Sredny Prospekt; once there, turn right a half-block to the stop for tram #6 or #40. Ride this going to the right; you'll hop out at the first stop after crossing the river—at Zverinskaya street; you can also stay on for three more stops and get off right next to the Gorkovskaya Metro station (it looks like a flying saucer), and walk through the park to the fortress. For either option, once you've boarded the tram, wait for the conductor to come to you to pay the fare (28 R).

English Embankment (South Bank): The nearest berth to the town center, the English (Angliyskaya) embankment is a 20-minute walk from the Hermitage (about a mile away)—head out with the river on your left until you reach the second bridge (Dvortsovy Most). There's no easy, direct public-transit connection.

RETURNING TO YOUR SHIP

Marine Facade: To return to the Marine Facade from the Gostiny Dvor area downtown (on Nevsky Prospekt), hop on the green Metro line and ride two stops to the end of the line, Primorskaya. Head out front and find bus #158. (From where you got off the bus, cross the busy street and tram tracks to find the "A" stop.) The bus runs about every 30 minutes back to the Marine Facade.

Neva Embankment: Both embankment terminals are walkable (and visible) from the city center. If you get turned around, just make your way to the Neva and look downriver for your ship. But leave yourself plenty of time to walk back—it's farther than it looks, and may take as long as 30 minutes from the Hermitage to either terminal. Or consider the tram, bus, and trolley bus connections noted above.

St. Petersburg

St. Petersburg is gigantic and decentralized; you'll want to carefully plan your time to minimize backtracking. Most of the sights (and the dense urban core) are on the south bank of the Neva River; to the north are the historic Peter and Paul Fortress and the tidy, grid-planned residential zone of Vasilyevsky Island (with the cruise port at its western tip). The city—built over a swamp—is a horizontal one. Foundations for skyscrapers are too challenging.

Orientation to St. Petersburg

Don't go looking for a cutesy, cobbled "old town"; the entire city was carefully planned to fit within its three concentric waterways: first the Moyka (Мойка) River, then the Griboyedov Canal (Канал Грибоедова), and finally the Fontanka (Фонтанка) River.

The geographical center of the city is the Admiralty building, with a slender, golden spire that shines like a beacon (next to the river, Hermitage, and Palace Square). From here, bustling avenues (called *prospekty*) radiate out to the distant suburbs. The busiest and most interesting thoroughfare is Nevsky Prospekt (Невский Проспект). Almost everything you'll want to see is either along Nevsky or a few blocks to either side of it. Uprising Square (Ploshchad Vosstaniya, Площадь Восстания)—home to a tall obelisk and the Moskovsky train station—marks the end of the usual tourist zone.

Maps make St. Petersburg appear smaller than it is. What looks like "just a few blocks" can easily translate into a half-hour walk. The two-mile walk along Nevsky from the Admiralty to Uprising Square takes about an hour at a brisk pace. Make things easier on yourself by getting comfortable with the city's cheap and generally well-coordinated public transit. The Metro boasts frequent trains that zip effortlessly beneath clogged streets. A well-planned network of buses, trolley buses, and shared minibuses called *marshrutki* help you bridge the (sometimes long) gaps between sights and Metro stops; while a bit less user-friendly to the uninitiated, these can save tons of time when mastered.

A few terms you'll see on maps: *ulitsa* is "street," *ploshchad* is "square," *prospekt* is "avenue," and *most* is "bridge." Many street signs are conveniently bilingual. They usually list the house number of the building they're on, as well as the numbers of the buildings to either side (this is convenient, as buildings can be very large).

You may see free maps around town, but if you'll be navigating

ST. PETERSBURG

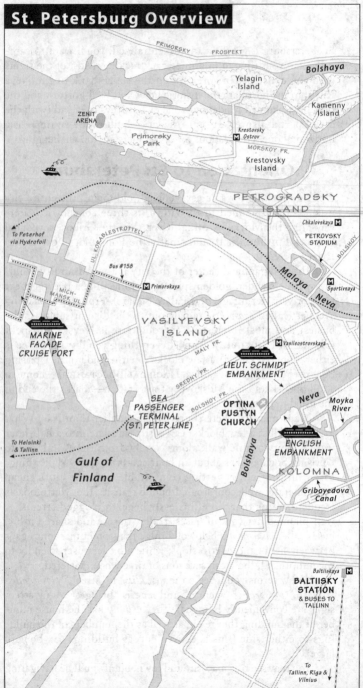

St. Petersburg Overview

PRIMORSKY PROSPEKT

Bolshaya

Yelagin Island

Kamenny Island

ZENIT ARENA

Primorsky Park

Krestovsky Ostrov Ⓜ

MORSKOY PR.

Krestovsky Island

PETROGRADSKY ISLAND

To Peterhof via Hydrofoil

UL. KORABLESTROITELY

Chkalovskaya Ⓜ

PETROVSKY STADIUM

BOLSHOY

Bus #158

Ⓜ Primorskaya

Malaya Neva

Ⓜ Sportivnaya

MICH-MANSK. UL.

MARINE FACADE CRUISE PORT

VASILYEVSKY ISLAND

MALY PR.

LIEUT. SCHMIDT EMBANKMENT

Ⓜ Vasileostrovskaya

SREDNY PR.

Neva

Moyka River

SEA PASSENGER TERMINAL (ST. PETER LINE)

BOLSHOY PR.

OPTINA PUSTYN CHURCH

ENGLISH EMBANKMENT

To Helsinki & Tallinn

Bolshaya

KOLOMNA

Gulf of Finland

Griboyedova Canal

Baltiiskaya Ⓜ

BALTIISKY STATION
& BUSES TO TALLINN

To Tallinn, Riga & Vilnius

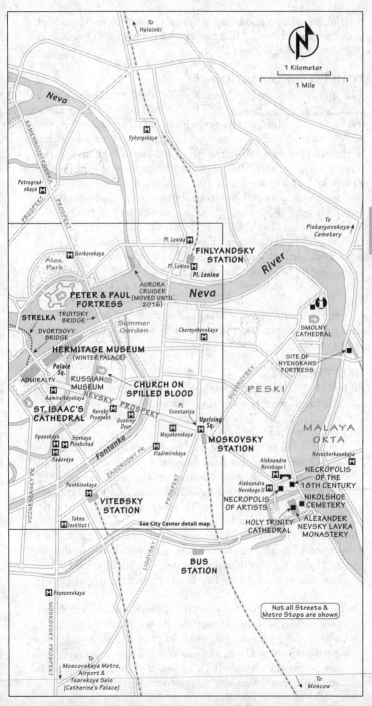

on your own, buy a good map at one of the bookstores listed later, under "Helpful Hints." I like the "city tourist map" by Discus, with labels in both English and Cyrillic.

TOURIST INFORMATION

The city TI has several branches. While they aren't as well-organized as many European TIs, the staff tries hard, speaks at least a bit of English, and may be willing to call around to help you with a question they can't answer. The most convenient branch is in the glass pavilion just to the left of the **Hermitage** (as you face it from Palace Square); the main branch is a few steps off **Nevsky Prospekt** (at Sadovaya 14, across from Gostiny Dvor—watch for the low-profile door and go up one flight of stairs; Mon-Fri 10:00-19:00, closed Sat-Sun, tel. 310-2231, www.visit-petersburg.ru or www.ispb.info). You'll also see TI kiosks in high-tourist areas such as St. Isaac's Cathedral, Peter and Paul Fortress, on Uprising Square (Ploshchad Vosstaniya) near Moskovsky train station, and at the airport (all generally open daily 9:00-19:00, but hours and services are unpredictable). The city also runs a 24-hour "Tourist Help Line," with English operators, at tel. 303-0555.

The bimonthly *St. Petersburg In Your Pocket* guidebook is good; look for free copies around town or browse it online at www.inyourpocket.com.

HELPFUL HINTS

Sightseeing Schedules: Opening times for St. Petersburg's museums and churches are very changeable—particularly the closed days, and days when sights are open late. When planning your visit, confirm hours online.

Take note of closed days: The Hermitage, Kunstkamera, and Peterhof are closed on Mondays, the Russian Museum and Tsarskoye Selo on Tuesdays, many religious sites (St. Isaac's, Church on Spilled Blood) on Wednesdays, the Museum of Russian Political History on Thursdays, and the Fabergé Museum on Fridays.

Don't Drink the Water: While new water treatment plants have improved quality in recent years, and most locals wash fruit and brush their teeth with tap water, they still don't drink it—and neither should you. Buy bottled water cheaply in grocery stores.

Theft Alert: Russia has hardworking, often unusually aggressive pickpockets who target tourists. Be particularly aware anywhere along Nevsky Prospekt, in crowded shopping areas (such as Gostiny Dvor), and on public transport. Assume that any scuffle is a distraction by a team of thieves, and that anyone who approaches you on the street is trying to pull off a

Learning the Cyrillic Alphabet

If you're going to Russia—even if just for a couple of days on a cruise—you'll have a much richer, smoother experience if you take the time to learn the Cyrillic alphabet. Once you know the basics, you can (slowly) sound out signs around town, and some of those very long, confusing words will become familiar. It's actually a fun pastime to try to figure out signs while you're walking down the street, waiting for a bus, or riding a long Metro escalator.

The table shows the Cyrillic alphabet (both capital and lowercase), and in the second column, the Roman equivalent. Notice that the letters fall—very roughly—into four categories: Some letters are basically the same sound as in English, such as A, E, K, M, O, and T. Others are easy if you know the Greek alphabet: Γ—gamma (g), Д—delta (d), Π—pi (p), and Φ—phi (f). Some are unique to Russian; most of these are "fricative" sounds, like *ts, sh, ch,* or *kh* (Ж, З, Ц, Ч, Ш, Щ, Х). And the fourth category seem designed to trip you up: "false friends" that have a different sound than the Roman letter they resemble, such as В, С, Н, Р, Х, and У. It can be helpful to remember that the "backwards" Roman consonants are actually vowels (И, Й, Я).

The letter Ы, which sounds somewhat similar to the *i* in English "ill," looks like two letters but is treated as one. The "hard sign" and "soft sign" are silent letters that affect the pronunciation of the preceding consonant in ways you need not worry about.

Two important words which you'll often see are easy to confuse: вход means entrance, but выход is an exit. For more Russian words and phrases, see page 440.

Cyrillic	Roman
Аа	a
Бб	b
Вв	v
Гг	g
Дд	d
Ее	ye, e
Ёё	yō
Жж	zh
Зз	z
Ии	i
Йй	y
Кк	k
Лл	l
Мм	m
Нн	n
Оо	o
Пп	p
Рр	r
Сс	s
Тт	t
Уу	u
Фф	f
Хх	kh
Цц	ts
Чч	ch
Шш	sh
Щщ	shch
Ъъ	hard sign
Ыы	y
Ьь	soft sign
Ээ	e
Юю	yu
Яя	ya

scam. Some thieves are well-dressed and even carry guidebooks to fool you. Thieves can be rough—they've even been known to detach and steal big camera lenses in one smooth motion. Keep anything precious close (wear a money belt for your passport, credit cards, and other valuables, leave the fancy jewelry at home, and don't be careless with cameras, smartphones, and tablets).

Pedestrian Safety: Russian drivers are shockingly forceful, zipping between lanes and around any obstructions. They drive fast, even on small downtown streets. Don't jaywalk: *Always* use crosswalks and look both ways before crossing—especially along Nevsky Prospekt, with its eight lanes of traffic moving at terrifying speeds.

Online Translation Tip: If a website you want is available only in Russian, try using the Chrome browser (www.google.com/chrome), which can (roughly) translate the page for you.

Business Hours: Most shops, restaurants, and services are open the same hours seven days a week (the legacy of communism, which tried to do away with weekends). You'll see a surprising number of shops and restaurants open 24/7 (look for *24* Часа).

"Sightseeing Tax" for Foreigners: You may notice that the admission price for Russians to various sights can be cheaper than the cost for foreigners. I've listed only the "foreigner" price, but if you happen to have a Russian passport, insist on the lower price.

Dress Code: In Orthodox churches, modest dress is expected (no shorts or bare shoulders; women are encouraged to cover their heads with a scarf).

Pharmacy: Look for the chain called **36.6**—as in the normal Celsius body temperature. The most central location is at Gorokhovaya 16, near the Admiralteyskaya Metro stop (open long hours daily).

Medical/Dental Services: The (entirely Russian-staffed) **American Medical Clinic** is near St. Isaac's Cathedral on the Moyka embankment (Naberezhnaya reki Moyki 78, tel. 740-2090, www.amclinic.com, info@amclinic.ru).

Internet Access: Many cafés and restaurants, and even some museums, have free Wi-Fi hotspots. If you need a computer, you can get online at the Internet café at the back of the Subway restaurant at Nevsky Prospekt 11 (enter on side street and take stairs to second floor; Skype installed, open 24 hours, tel. 314-6705).

Bookstore: The city's best-known bookstore, **Dom Knigi** ("House of Books," Дом Книги), is in the old Singer sewing machine building at Nevsky Prospekt 28 (by the Griboyedov Canal, across from Kazan Cathedral). It sells English novels and locally produced guidebooks and has a pretty second-floor café with a view over the Kazan Cathedral (daily 9:00-24:00). **Anglia Bookshop** (Англия), just off Nevsky Prospekt facing the Fontanka River (next to the horse statues on the Anichkov Bridge, at the end of my self-guided Nevsky Prospekt walk), has a fine selection of English-language books by Russian authors and about Russian history (Mon-Sat 11:00-20:00, Sun 12:00-20:00, Fontanka 38, tel. 579-8284). You'll also see the **Bukvoyed** (Буквоед) bookstore chain around town, with several handy branches along Nevsky Prospekt (generally daily 9:00-22:00).

Currency Fluctuation: The ruble is on a roller-coaster ride—mostly going down. Depending on economic conditions when you travel, you may find higher prices (in rubles) than those quoted here. Because of the currency instability, in some listings I've given prices in US dollars, especially for personal services and smaller vendors (walking tours, private guides, etc.). For current exchange rates, check www.oanda.com.

ATMs: The word for ATM is банкомат *(bankomat)*. They are most commonly inside banks, hotels, restaurants, and other establishments, though you will find a few out on the street. Locals advise using machines inside bank lobbies when possible.

Telephones: There are no pay phones in St. Petersburg. For international calls, your best bet is to use Skype or another computer-based service from an Internet café.

Mail: Mailboxes are blue with "Почта России" in white lettering. The central post office, open 24 hours, is in a historic building a couple of blocks beyond St. Isaac's Cathedral at Pochtamtskaya Ulitsa 9 (look for the archway that crosses the street). The Russian mail service has a reputation for delivering things extremely slowly, if at all, but just for postcards—well, you can take the risk.

Convenience Stores: There are small stores in every neighborhood (often down a few steps from street level and open late or even 24 hours) where you can pick up basic necessities. Look for signs saying Продукты ("foodstuffs") or Универсам (Universam, meaning "self-service store"). In the very center, the 24-hour *universam* at Bolshaya Konyushennaya Ulitsa 4 (at the corner of Shvedsky Pereulok) is convenient and decent-sized.

What's With All the Weddings? It's a Russian tradition for bride and groom to visit about 10 different parks and monuments around town on their wedding day and have their photo taken.

Timeline of Russian History

800s — Spurred by Viking trade along Russia's rivers, states form around the cities of Novgorod and Kiev. ("Russia" comes from a Viking word.)

988 — Kiev converts to Christianity and becomes part of the Eastern Orthodox world.

1224-1242 — Tatar (Mongol) hordes conquer Russia and exact tribute. But Russia succeeds where the Baltics fail: keeping the Germans out.

1465-1557 — The Russian czars consolidate power in Moscow, drive away the Tatars, and form a unified Russian state.

1613 — Foundation of the Romanov dynasty, which lasts until 1917. (For a full rundown of the Romanovs, see "Romanovs 101" on page 430.)

1703 — Czar Peter the Great founds St. Petersburg as Russia's forward-looking capital and "window on the West." Russia expands southward and eastward under Peter and his successor, Catherine.

1812 — Napoleon invades Russia and burns Moscow, but loses an army on the way home.

1855-1861 — Russia loses Crimean War and decides to modernize, including freeing the serfs.

1905 — Russia loses a war with the Japanese, contributing to a failed revolution later glorified by the communists as a manifestation of the workers' consciousness.

1917 — In March, the Romanov czar is ousted by a provisional government led by Alexander Kerensky; in the October Revolution, the provisional government is ousted by the Bolsheviks (communists), led by Vladimir Lenin. A few months later, the entire Romanov family is executed.

1924 — Lenin dies on January 26, and in his honor St. Petersburg is renamed Leningrad (it reverted to St. Petersburg again in 1991).

1924-1939 — Josef Stalin purges the government and the army. Forced collectivization causes famine and tens of millions of deaths in Ukraine.

1939-1945 — In World War II, Russia loses 20 million people to the Germans (including as many as a million in the Siege of Leningrad), but winds up with control over a sizable chunk of Eastern and Central Europe.

1945-1962	At the peak of the Cold War, Russia acquires the atom bomb, and launches the first satellite and the first manned space mission.
1970s	During a time of stagnation under Leonid Brezhnev, the communist system slowly fails.
1985	Mikhail Gorbachev comes to power and declares the beginning of *glasnost* (openness) and *perestroika* (restructuring) in the Soviet system.
1991	Reactionaries try to topple Gorbachev. They fail to keep power, but so does Gorbachev. Boris Yeltsin takes control of the government and starts reforms.
1993	Reactionaries fail to topple Yeltsin. Weakened, Yeltsin manages to hang on to power until 1999, despite grumbling from the ultra-nationalist right and the communist left.
1999	On New Year's Eve, Yeltsin suddenly and inexplicably resigns, handing the country over to former KGB officer Vladimir Putin.
2000-2008	Putin serves as president.
2008-2012	The term-limited Putin becomes prime minister, keeping a close watch on the presidency of his handpicked successor, Dmitry Medvedev. (Cynical onlookers dub the arrangement a "tandemocracy.")
2012	Surprise! A conveniently timed change in the law allows Putin to return as president, while Medvedev swaps roles to become prime minister. Russian protesters and international observers grumble about "reforms" that shore up Putin's power.
2014	The Russian city of Sochi, on the Black Sea, hosts the Winter Olympics, amid controversy over Putin's laws against "gay propaganda." Soon after the Olympics, Ukraine's Crimea region (a highly strategic, traditionally Russian Black Sea peninsula) falls under Russian control, and warfare rages in eastern Ukraine between pro-Russian and pro-Ukrainian factions. US- and EU-driven sanctions, coupled with declining oil prices, cause the ruble to plummet on the international market.
2016	Russia hosts the World Cup.

GETTING AROUND ST. PETERSBURG

The best available English-language **journey planner** for St. Petersburg's public transportation is www.spb.rusavtobus.ru/en. Though not very user-friendly, it covers both the Metro and surface transport. The official Metro website (www.metro.spb.ru) is in Russian only.

By Metro: Compared to systems in many other European metropolises, St. Petersburg's Metro has fewer stations and lines. This means it's a longer walk between stations—but beneath the city you'll move at a shockingly fast pace. The system is clean, efficient, very cheap, and—with a little practice—easy to use (everything is clearly labeled in English). You'll marvel at one of the most impressive people-movers on the planet—at rush hour, it's astonishing to simply stand on the platform and watch the hundreds upon hundreds of commuters pile in and out of each train. It's worth taking at least once just for the experience.

You enter with a metal token (*zheton*, жетон), which you can buy for 31 R—either at the ticket windows, or from machines in station entrances (in Russian and English, easy to figure out: push button labeled Купить жетоны—"buy tokens," select the number of tokens you want, then insert money). A 10-journey pass is sold at ticket windows only (295 R, valid 7 days, cannot be shared). There are no day passes.

Signs in the Metro are fully bilingual, and maps of the system are posted widely. Each of the five lines is numbered and color-coded. It helps to know the end station in the direction you're traveling. Unlike most European subway systems, transfer stations (where two lines meet) have two names, one for each line. Some stations in the center have flood doors along the boarding area that open only when trains arrive. Trains run from about 6:00 in the morning to a little after midnight.

Pickpocket Alert: Metro stations, especially at rush hour, are particularly high-risk for pickpocketing. While any line near a touristy sight is targeted, the busy green line—connecting the cruise port to the city center (Gostiny Dvor)—is particularly plagued. A common strategy: A team of thieves spot a tourist. Then, as everyone loads into the train, the thief in front stumbles, your arms go out, the guy behind you grabs his target, the door closes...and it's just you without your wallet, zipping across town on the train.

By Bus and Trolley Bus: Buses and trolley buses (with overhead wires) are very quick, cheap, and convenient for getting around the center of town. They're useful for connecting locations not served by the Metro, and let you see the city instead of burying you underground (especially nice when zipping along Nevsky Prospekt). The system takes a little patience to figure out (it helps if you can sound out Cyrillic to decipher posted schedules); ideally, ask a knowledgeable local which bus number to look for.

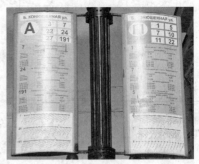

Along the street, stops are marked by an **A** (for buses), a flat-topped **M** for trolley buses, and a **K** for *marshrutki* minibuses (explained later). Signs at bus stops—in Russian only—list the route number, frequency, and sometimes the names of the stops en route. (Tram lines, marked by a T, run only in the city's outer districts.)

All surface transport costs 28 R per ride; pay the conductor, who wears a reflective vest and will give you a thin paper-slip ticket. There are no transfers, so you pay again if you switch buses.

The buses and trolley buses that run along Nevsky Prospekt (between its start, at Malaya Morskaya Ulitsa, and Uprising Square/Ploshchad Vosstaniya) are useful: buses #3, #7, #24, and #191, and trolley buses #1, #5, #7, #10, #11, and #22. Don't be afraid to make mistakes; if you take the wrong bus and it turns off Nevsky, just hop out at the next stop. Trolley buses #5 and #22 conveniently veer off from the lower end of Nevsky down Malaya Morskaya Ulitsa to St. Isaac's Cathedral and the Mariinsky Theater.

***Marshrutki* (Minibuses):** These "share taxis"—operated by private companies—travel along set, numbered routes, prefixed with the letter K. You can wave them down anywhere along the way and ask to be dropped off at any point along the route. They're designed more for residents than for tourists, but can be useful for going to Peterhof, Tsarskoye Selo, or the airport.

By Taxi: Locals tend to avoid cabs, and you should use them only with caution. You won't see taxi stands in St. Petersburg, and you should walk away from cabbies who hail *you* down ("Taxi?"). But you can always call and order an **official taxi** by phone (you'll probably need a Russian speaker to help, as few dispatchers or cabbies speak English). Official taxis are a little more expensive and safer than those hailed on the street. Pay the fare on the meter, rounding up a little. Beware that congested city traffic can make a taxi ride slow. Official taxis typically have a set minimum fare—typically 350-400 R—which covers most trips within the city center.

Two reliable companies are **068** (tel. 068, www.taxi068.ru) and **Novoye Zhyoltoye** (New Yellow Taxis, Новое Жёлтое; tel.

600-8888, www.peterburg.nyt.ru/en). You can send in a form from the English-language section of either website to order a taxi, but you'll need to give a local phone number. The **Ladybird** taxi service (tel. 900-0504, www.ladybird-taxi.ru) has only women drivers and provides car seats for kids.

Tours in St. Petersburg

Walking Tours

Peterswalk has been doing excellent, English-language walking tours of the city since 1996. I like this tour because rather than visiting the crowded, famous sights, you'll simply walk through the city and learn about contemporary life and culture ($22/person, 4 hours, mobile +7-921-943-1229, www.peterswalk.com, info@peterswalk.com). From April through October, the tour begins every day at 10:30 at Hostel Life, around the corner from Nevsky Prospekt 47 (near the Fontanka River—ring the bell at Vladimirsky Prospekt 1 and go up to the fourth floor; tour may run sporadically off-season—check website). Peterswalk also does bike tours, private guided tours, and visa-free tours for cruise travelers (see below).

Bike Tours

Peterswalk offers 3.5-hour weekend and late-night bike tours (mid-May-Sept Sat-Sun at 11:00, also mid-May-Aug Tue and Thu at 22:30, $40/person, starts at SkatProkat bike shop at Goncharnaya Ulitsa 7, near Moskovsky train station and Ploschad Vosstaniya).

Boat Tours in English

St. Petersburg is a delight to see from the water. Low-slung canal boats ply their way through the city, offering a handy orientation to major landmarks. After curling through narrow, urban waterways, your boat pops out onto the wide Neva River and a grand panorama of the Hermitage, Admiralty, and Peter and Paul Fortress. Various companies advertise at touristy points near canals 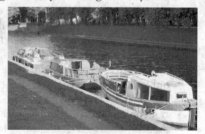 and offer essentially the same one-hour cruise, most with recorded or live narration in Russian. It's worth asking the various hawkers around town whether they have an English option. One that does is **Neptun** (Нептун), near the Hermitage (600 R one-hour cruise, 3/hour; recorded narration in English typically available at 13:00, 15:00, and 17:00; on Moyka embankment at #26, near recommended Troitsky Most restaurant—see map on page 360, tel. 924-4452, www.neptun-boat.ru).

Hop-on Hop-off Bus Tours

CityTour runs red, double-decker, hop-on, hop-off buses that make a circuit of major sights in the center, with recorded commentary. Buses start at Ostrovsky Square (near the statue of Catherine the Great, along Nevsky Prospekt) about every 30 minutes from 9:00 to 19:00; the full circle takes two hours (600 R all-day ticket, buy on board, tel. 718-4769, mobile +7-961-800-0755, www.citytourspb.ru).

Private Guides for Travelers with Visas

Each of the following guide organizations is smart, small, reliable, and committed to helping visitors enjoy and understand their city. I work with them when my tour groups are in town, and they are consistently excellent. If you have a visa, you can hire them privately for walking or car tours (generally $40/hour for up to 8 people on foot, 4-hour minimum). If you're coming on a cruise without a visa, see the next section.

Natalya German-Tsarkova: Natalya and her team of guides make touring the city easy and meaningful ($40/hour, $300/4 hours, $450/8 hours with car, up to 6 people; mobile +7-921-391-1894, www.original-tours.com, natalya.german@gmail.com).

Timofey Kruglikov's "Tailored Tours of St. Petersburg": Tim and his team of guides are passionate about art and history, and they're all Russian scholars ($40/hour, $70/hour with car, 4-hour minimum, www.tour-petersburg.com, info@tour-petersburg.com).

Peterswalk Private Guides: The most entrepreneurial and "Back Door" of these guide groups, Peterswalk offers daily public walks and bike tours (explained above) as well as private tours. Their passion is to be out and about in town, connecting with today's reality ($40/hour for up to 8 people, 4-hour minimum, mobile +7-921-943-1229, www.peterswalk.com, info@peterswalk.com).

Private Guides for Cruise Travelers Without Visas

The three outfits recommended above can also work with cruise passengers who don't have visas. For many cruisers, this is the ideal way to experience St. Petersburg: It's less hassle than getting a visa and offers more freedom than a typical cruise-line excursion.

You'll have to book well in advance to allow time for your guide to handle all the red tape (expect to provide your passport details). For two full eight-hour days of sightseeing with a guide and car, a couple can expect to pay around $550 per person. Larger groups are cheaper per person ($350/person for 4, $270/person for 6). The price typically includes admission fees. Your guide can pick you up at your cruise terminal, and bring you back there at the end of each day.

St. Petersburg Walks

Two self-guided walks take you through two sides of St. Petersburg: "A Stroll on Nevsky Prospekt" cuts through the bustling historical center of town, while my "Back-Streets Walk on Vasilyevsky Island" (see page 383) reveals a local neighborhood and an aspect of the city that most tourists never see.

A STROLL ON NEVSKY PROSPEKT

Taking about two hours (not counting sightseeing stops), this walk, worth ▲▲▲, offers a fascinating glimpse into the heart of the city.

Nevsky Prospekt (Невский Проспект)—St. Petersburg's famous main thorough-fare—represents the best and the worst of this beguiling metropolis. Along its two-mile length from the Neva River to Uprising Square (Ploshchad Vosstaniya, Площадь Восстания), this superlative boulevard passes some of the city's most opu- 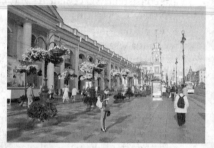 lent palaces (the Hermitage), top museums (the Hermitage and Russian Museum), most important churches (Kazan Cathedral, Church on Spilled Blood), finest urban architecture, liveliest shopping zones, lushest parks, and slice upon slice of Russian life.

This walk also gives you a taste of the smog, congestion, and general chaos with which the city perennially grapples. Pickpockets are brazen here (blurring the line between petty theft and mugging), as are drivers—it's essential to be watchful, remain calm, and cross the street only at designated crosswalks (and even then, use caution). If it's crowded and you're getting stressed, duck into a serene shopping gallery or café for a break.

As Nevsky Prospekt cuts diagonally through town from the Admiralty building (the bull's eye of this city's urban layout), it crosses three waterways. We'll focus on the first mile-and-a-quarter stretch to the Fontanka River—though you could carry on all the way to Uprising Square and beyond.

• *Begin your walk on the vast square facing the Hermitage.*

Palace Square to the Admiralty

The impressively monumental **Palace Square** (Dvortsovaya Ploshchad)—with the arcing, Neoclassical General Staff Building facing the bubbly, Baroque Hermitage—lets you know you're in an imperial capital. It oozes blue-blood class.

Take a moment just to let the grand scale of this space sink in. Like all of St. Petersburg, it was custom-built to impress—and intimidate—visiting dignitaries. If your trip also takes you to

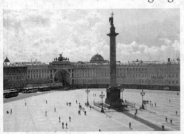

Estonia, ponder this: The entire Old Town of Tallinn could fit comfortably inside the footprint of this square and palace.

The **Alexander Column** honors Czar Alexander I and celebrates Russia's military victory over Napoleon in 1812. Along with Moscow's Red Square, this is the stage upon which much of early modern Russian history played out. On January 22, 1905, the czar's imperial guard opened fire on peaceful protesters here, massacring hundreds (or possibly thousands). By 1917, the czar was ousted. The provisional government that replaced him was in turn dislodged by the Bolsheviks' October Revolution—kicking off 75 years of communist rule.

• *As you face the Hermitage, exit the square over your left shoulder, toward the glittering dome. When you reach the corner, before continuing, look across the busy street.*

The **Alexander Garden** (Alexandrovsky Sad), with benches and jungle gyms, are a favorite place for families. It's the backyard of the **Admiralty** building—the stately structure with the golden spire. When Peter the Great was laying out his new capital in the early 18th century, he made the Admiralty its centerpiece—indicating the importance he placed on his imperial navy. From here, three great avenues fan out through the city; of these, Nevsky Prospekt is *the* main drag.

Before we head up the street, notice that **St. Isaac's Cathedral**—with that shimmering dome—is a 10-minute walk away (to the right, with your back to the Admiralty, at the far end of this park; for more on this church, see page 418).

• *Standing at the corner across from the garden, you're already at the start of Nevsky Prospekt. Use the crosswalk to reach the right side of the street and the first part of this walk.*

Admiralty to the Moyka River

A few steps down this first block, watch on the right for the shop marked КОФЕ ХАУЗ. Visitors are intimidated by the Cyrillic alphabet, but with a little practice (and the alphabet tips on page 363), you can decode signs easily—often surprising yourself when they turn out to be familiar words. In this case, Кофе Хауз is Kofe Haus...coffeehouse. This Moscow-based Starbucks clone is popular, but very expensive. Russia's deeply stratified society has an enormous lower class, a tiny upper class, and virtually no

ST. PETERSBURG

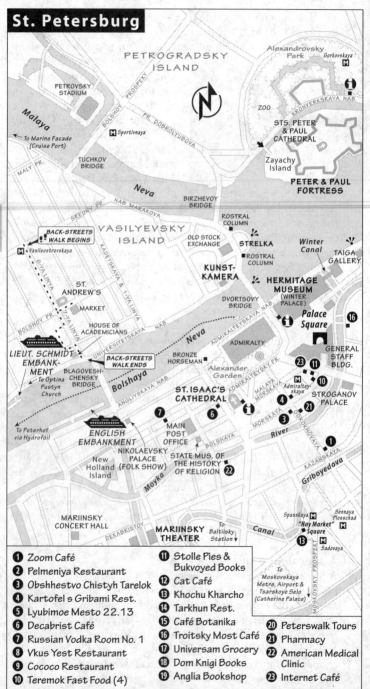

St. Petersburg

PETROGRADSKY ISLAND

PETROVSKY STADIUM

Alexandrovsky Park

Gorkovskaya

ZOO

STS. PETER & PAUL CATHEDRAL

Malaya

BOLSHOY PROSPEKT

PR. DOBROLYUBOVA

Sportivnaya

KRONVERKSKAYA NAB.

TUCHKOV BRIDGE

MALY PR.

Zayachy Island

PETER & PAUL FORTRESS

To Marine Facade (Cruise Port)

Neva

BIRZHEVOY BRIDGE

NAB MARAKOVA

SREDNY PR.

ROSTRAL COLUMN

BACK-STREETS WALK BEGINS

Vasileostrovskaya

VASILYEVSKY ISLAND

OLD STOCK EXCHANGE

STRELKA

ROSTRAL COLUMN

Winter Canal

TAIGA GALLERY

6-YA LINIYA

KADETSKAYA & 1-YA LINIYA

ST. ANDREW'S

KUNST-KAMERA

HERMITAGE MUSEUM (WINTER PALACE)

Palace Square

16

MARKET

DVORTSOVY BRIDGE

BOLSHOY PR.

HOUSE OF ACADEMICIANS

UNIVERSITETSKAYA NAB.

ADMIRALTEYSKAYA NAB.

ADMIRALTY

GENERAL STAFF BLDG.

LIEUT. SCHMIDT EMBANK-MENT

BACK-STREETS WALK ENDS

Neva

23

11

To Optina Pustyn Church

BLAGOVESH-CHENSKY BRIDGE

Bolshaya

BRONZE HORSEMAN

Alexander Garden

ADMIRALTEYSKY PR.

Admiralteyskaya

10

STROGANOV PALACE

ANGLIYSKAYA NAB.

ST. ISAAC'S CATHEDRAL

MALAYA MORSKAYA

4

21

7

6

3

MORSKAYA

River

To Peterhof via Hydrofoil

ENGLISH EMBANKMENT

MAIN POST OFFICE

GOROKHOVAYA

New Holland Island

NIKOLAEVSKY PALACE (FOLK SHOW)

STATE MUS. OF THE HISTORY OF RELIGION

BOLSHAYA

1

KAZANSKAYA

Moyka

22

Griboyedova

MARIINSKY CONCERT HALL

DEKABRISTOV

MARIINSKY THEATER

To Baltiisky Station

Canal

Spasskaya

Sennaya Ploschad

"Hay Market" Square

13

Sadovaya

To Moskovskaya Metro, Airport & Tsarskoye Selo (Catherine Palace)

MOSKOVSKY PROSPEKT

1 Zoom Café
2 Pelmeniya Restaurant
3 Obshhestvo Chistyh Tarelok
4 Kartofel s Gribami Rest.
5 Lyubimoe Mesto 22.13
6 Decabrist Café
7 Russian Vodka Room No. 1
8 Vkus Yest Restaurant
9 Cococo Restaurant
10 Teremok Fast Food (4)

11 Stolle Pies & Bukvoyed Books
12 Cat Café
13 Khochu Kharcho
14 Tarkhun Rest.
15 Café Botanika
16 Troitsky Most Café
17 Universam Grocery
18 Dom Knigi Books
19 Anglia Bookshop

20 Peterswalk Tours
21 Pharmacy
22 American Medical Clinic
23 Internet Café

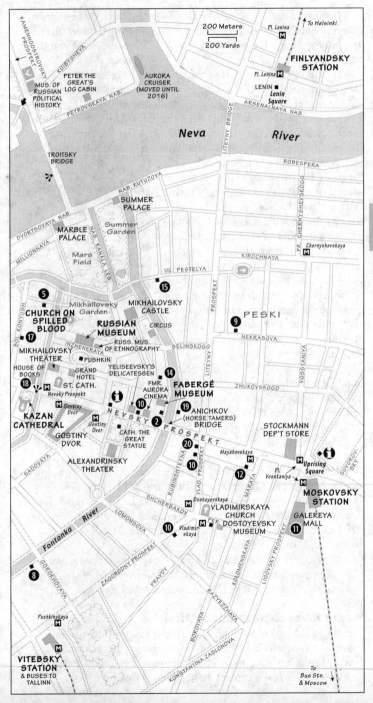

middle class. Trendy shops like this (where a latte costs double your hometown Starbucks) are filled with upwardly mobile urbanites, but the poorer locals around you could never dream of affording a drink here.

In the next block, halfway down on the right, the recommended **Stolle** (Штолле) is a chain restaurant good for a snack or light lunch. They specialize in savory and sweet pies.

Look directly across the street at the building with *1939* above the door. On the pillar just to the right of the door, notice the small length of barbed wire and blue plaque. This is a monument to the **Siege of Leningrad,** as the city was named during the Soviet era. During World War II, Nazi forces encircled the city and bombarded it for 872 days (from September 1941 through January 1944). At the outset, the city's population, swollen with refugees, was at 3 million—but by the siege's end, a million or more people were dead, mostly civilians who succumbed to starvation. The

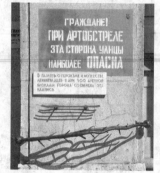

assault claimed more lives than any other siege in world history. St. Petersburg's buildings were ravaged, but not the spirit of those who refused to surrender.

Here, the north side of the street was in the direct line of fire from Nazi shells, lobbed in from German positions southwest of the city. The blue sign reads, roughly, "Citizens: During artillery bombardment, this side is more dangerous."

About 30 yards down, on the right, the Буквоед sign marks an outlet of the **Bukvoyed** bookstore chain—a handy place to pick up a St. Petersburg map if you need one. At the next intersection, look left down Bolshaya Morskaya street to see the magnificent **yellow arch** of the General Staff Building. The archway opens to Palace Square—where we started this walk. To the right, the street leads to a handy branch of the **Teremok** (Теремок) Russian fast-food chain (see page 436) and, beyond that, to the square in front of St. Isaac's Cathedral.

• *Continuing one more block on Nevsky Prospekt brings you to the first of St. Petersburg's concentric waterways, the Moyka River. As you proceed straight across the bridge, stick to the right side of the street.*

Moyka River to Kazan Cathedral

Crossing the Moyka, you'll likely see many touts selling tickets for **canal boat tours.** While this is an excellent way to get your bearings in St. Petersburg, most offer commentary only in Russian. Confirm the language before you hop aboard (see page 370).

The river is lined with fine 19th-century architecture. The pink building with white columns (on your right as you cross the water) is the **Stroganov**

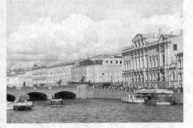

Palace. The aristocratic family that resided here left their mark all over Russia—commissioning opulent churches, financing the czars' military agenda, and fostering the arts—but their lasting legacy is the beef dish, likely named for them, that has made "Stroganoff" a household name around the world.

Continue another long block, and watch across the street (on the left) for another chance to practice your Russian—though the distinctive logo may give it away: САББЭЙ ("SABVAY" = Subway).

Just beyond Subway, looking left (across the street), notice the pretty, park-like street (Bolshaya Konyushennaya) flanked by beautiful buildings. On the

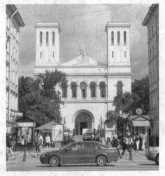

left side is a sort of community center for **Dutch** transplants, while the building on the right is for **Germans.** Catherine the Great (r. 1762-1796), who—like Peter the Great—loved to promote the multiethnic nature of her empire, encouraged various cultural enclaves to settle in community buildings like these. Each enclave consisted of several apartment houses clustered around a church. You'll see another example as you proceed up Nevsky Prospekt, where the German **Lutheran Church of St. Peter and St. Paul** is set back between two yellow buildings (on the left). The church is a reminder that much of St. Petersburg was built by Lutherans: Dutch, Germans, Swedes, and so on. This is only one of the many houses of worship built along this avenue under the auspices of the czars. Later, the aggressively atheistic communist regime repurposed churches all over the city; in this case, the church was turned into a swimming pool.

• *Coming up on the right is the Kazan Cathedral, with its stately semi-circular colonnade and grand dome.*

Kazan Cathedral to Griboyedov Canal

Built in the early 1800s and named for a revered Russian icon, **Kazan Cathedral** was later converted into a "Museum of

Atheism" under the communists. It's since been restored to its former glory and is free to enter. To find the main entrance, go down Kazanskaya street (perpendicular to Nevsky, just before the church). Go in through what looks like a "side" door, and soak in the mystical Orthodox ambience. Inside you'll find a dim interior, a much-venerated replica of the icon of Our Lady of Kazan, a monument to the commander who fended off Napoleon's 1812 invasion, and lots of candles and solemn worshippers (for more on the cathedral's interior, see the listing on page 414). You'll exit through the left transept, which pops you out into a delightful little **grassy park** facing Nevsky Prospekt. This is a good spot to sit, relax, and maybe buy a drink from a vendor.

It's appropriate that Nevsky Prospekt is lined with so many important churches. The street leads to the monastery that holds relics of Alexander Nevsky (1220-1263), an esteemed Russian saint who, as an influential prince, fought off encroaching German and Swedish foes—including in a pivotal 1240 battle on the Neva River, near what would later become St. Petersburg.

• *Leaving the park, head to the intersection and cross over Nevsky Prospekt.*

Scrutinize the distinctive oxidized-copper tower of the Art Nouveau building on the corner (at #28).

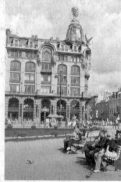

At the base of the globe-topped turret is an unlikely symbol—an American bald eagle, wings spread wide, grasping a laurel wreath in its talon and wearing a stars-and-stripes shield on its breast. Architecture fans know this building as the Singer House (yes, the Russian headquarters of the American sewing machine company—the globe at the top proclaims Singer's worldwide reach). Today it's home to **Dom Knigi** ("House of Books"). Up close, take a minute to examine the building's fine decorative details. Inside, the inviting bookshop has a delightfully atmospheric—if pricey—turn-of-the-century café on the second floor (daily 9:00-23:00).

• *The Singer building sits next to the Griboyedov Canal. Walk to the midsection of the intersection/bridge over the water (watch out for pickpockets in this highly concentrated tourist zone—they work in groups and can get physical all along Nevsky Prospekt).*

Griboyedov Canal to Gostiny Dvor

Looking down the length of the river, you can't miss one of Russia's most distinctive buildings: the **Church on Spilled Blood.** Dramatically scenic from here, it gets even prettier as you get closer. To snap some classic photos, work your way to the small bridge partway down the river. If you plan to visit this church, now's a good time; the **Russian Museum** is also nearby (the yellow building fronting the canal just before the church is a side-wing of that museum; we'll reach the museum's main entrance later on this walk). The church and museum are both described in more detail later, under "Sights in St. Petersburg." If you want to do some souvenir shopping, see if the handy (if touristy and overpriced) **crafts market** just behind the church is open. I'll wait right here.

Back already? Let's continue down Nevsky Prospekt (for now, stay on the left side). Just after the river is the **Small Philharmonic (Малый филармония)**—one of the "big four" cultural institutions in St. Petersburg (the others are the Great Philharmonic, the Mariinsky Theater, and the Mikhailovsky Theater). Consider taking in a performance while you're in town; on a short visit, the ballet is a popular choice (for details, see "Entertainment in St. Petersburg," later).

A half-block farther along, tucked between buildings on the left, you'll see the pale yellow facade of the Roman Catholic **St.**

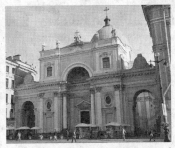

Catherine's Church. This is one of several "St. Catherines" that line Nevsky Prospekt—many congregations named their churches for the empress who encouraged their construction. This one has an endearing starving artists' market out front.

At the next corner, on the left, is the **Grand Hotel Europe**—an ultra-fancy (if dated) five-star hotel that opened in 1875. Its opulence attracted the likes of Tchaikovsky, Stravinsky, Debussy, and H. G. Wells as guests.

The hotel sits at the corner of Mikhailovskaya street. If you detour one long block down this street, you'll find the main entrance of the **Russian Museum,** with a fantastic collection of works by exclusively Russian artists. (While the Hermitage's art collection is world-class, there's nothing "local" or Russian about it.) For a self-guided tour of the highlights of the Russian Museum, see page 404. Presiding over the park in front of the museum (Ploshchad Iskusstv, "Square of the Arts") is a statue of **Alexander Pushkin** (1799-1837)— Russia's leading poet, considered by many to have raised modern Russian literature to an art form.

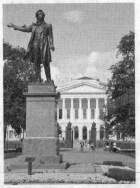

Back on Nevsky, capping the red tower across the boulevard from the hotel, notice the black metal skeletal **spire**—like a naked Christmas tree. This was part of an early 19th-century optical telegraph system that stretched more than 800 miles from here to Warsaw (which was then part of the Russian Empire). Each tower in this line-of-sight chain across the empire winked Morse code signals at the next with mirrors.

· *Continue along Nevsky to the middle of the next block.*

In a gap in the buildings on the left, you'll see yet another church—the beautiful robin-egg-blue home of the local Armenian community. **St. Catherine's Gregorian Church** belongs to the Armenian Apostolic faith, one of the oldest branches of Christianity—founded in A.D. 301, when St. Gregory the Illuminator baptized the Armenian king. Approaching the front door, look for the little shop window on the

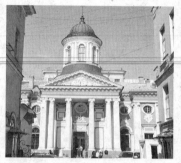

right, which sells breads, jams, and honey imported from Armenia to comfort homesick transplants here.

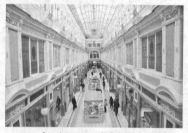

Now face across the street to confront the gigantic, yellow Gostiny Dvor shopping complex. We'll cross over later to take a look, but for now, continue past the church. Keep an eye out on the left for #48 (look for the Пассажъ sign above the door; it's before the ramp leading to a pedestrian underpass). Step inside and climb the stairs into the gorgeously restored, glass-roofed **"Passazh" arcade,** an elite haven for high-class shoppers since 1846 (daily 10:00-21:00), making it one of the first shopping malls in the world. The communists converted the Passazh into a supermarket and, later, into a "model store," intended to leave foreigners with a (misleadingly) positive impression of the availability of goods in the USSR. These days it sells perfume, jewels, and decorative glass, giving off a genteel air as mellow music plays in the background.

· *At the end of the block, use the pedestrian underpass (which also leads to a pair of convenient downtown Metro stops—Nevsky Prospekt on the blue line, and Gostiny Dvor on the green line) to cross beneath Nevsky Prospekt: Take the ramp down, turn right, then turn right again up the next ramp.*

Gostiny Dvor to Fontanka River

You'll pop out of the underpass at **Gostiny Dvor** (which means, basically, "merchants' courtyard"—like a Turkish caravanserai). Built in the 1760s, this marketplace is a giant but hollow structure,

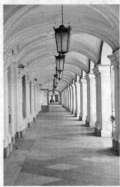

with two stories of shops (more than 100 in all) wrapping around a central courtyard. To see an undiscovered corner of Nevsky that most tourists miss, head upstairs: At the corner of the building nearest the underpass, go through the door and up the stairs, then find your way back outside to reach the tranquil, beautifully symmetrical arcades. Standing at the corner, the arches seem to recede in both directions nearly as far as the eye can see.

Looking out, take note of the open plaza in front of Gostiny Dvor. This is a popular place for **political protests**—which, in Putin's Russia, are barely tolerated. Article 31 of the Russian constitution guarantees the freedom of assembly—a right that seems always to be in question, especially since any protest must be officially registered. To push the boundaries, on the 31st of every month, peaceful demonstrators routinely seek government permission to stage a protest here, are denied, then stage the protest anyway—only to be dutifully arrested by riot-gear-clad cops. This "Strategy-31" movement tries to keep the issue of free speech alive in the consciousness of a Russia that seems willing to let that freedom lapse.

• *Go back into the underpass, and this time, stay on the right side of Nevsky Prospekt for one more block.*

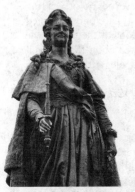

You'll soon reach **Ostrovsky Square** (Ploshchad Ostrovskogo), a fine park anchored by a statue of **Catherine the Great.** While Peter the Great gets founding credit for this city, Catherine arguably made it great. A Prussian blue-blood (born in today's Poland), Catherine married Russia's Czar Peter III, then quickly overthrew him in a palace coup. Throughout her 34-year reign, Catherine never remarried, but she is believed to have cleverly parlayed sexual politics to consolidate her power.

On the pillar below and to the right of Catherine is **Prince Grigory Potemkin,** one of the statesmen and military leaders with whom Catherine collaborated and consorted. Potemkin is the namesake of a fascinating story about how even a great ruler can be fooled. After Potemkin conquered the Crimean peninsula during the Russo-Turkish War, Catherine visited to survey her new domain. To convince her that "Russification" of the Crimea had been a success, Potemkin supposedly created artificially perfect villages, with stage-set houses peopled by "Russian villagers" custom-ordered from Centralsky Casting. To this day the term "Potemkin village" describes something artificial used to hoodwink a gullible target—a term as applicable to modern Russian and American politics as it was to Catherine's nation-building. In 1972, when President Nixon visited this city, Nevsky Prospekt itself was similarly spruced up to disguise the USSR's economic hardships. (Because Nixon viewed the street from a limo, the authorities only fixed up the bottom two floors of each facade.)

• From the square, use the crosswalk to head back over Nevsky Prospekt.

Just across from the park is the pleasantly pedestrianized street called Malaya Sadovaya. On the corner, **Yeliseevsky's delicatessen** occupies a sumptuously decorated Art Nouveau building (at #56). Once the purveyor of fine food to the Russian aristocracy (like Dallmayr's in Munich), Yeliseevsky's was bumped down several pegs when the communists symbolically turned it into "Grocery Store #1." Now, in another sign of the times, it's been remodeled into an almost laughably over-the-top boutique deli with a small, expensive café—drop in to browse the selection of cheese and chocolates (daily 10:00-23:00, photography strictly prohibited).

A few steps beyond Yeliseevsky's, find the passage (at #60, just past the Teremok fast-food joint) leading to the Zara department store. The store fills a space once occupied by the historic **Aurora (Аврора) Cinema**—one of the first movie houses in St. Petersburg. Entering, you'll step upon the original tiles and head up the grand staircase to the elegantly decorated main hall (daily 10:00-22:00).

• Continue along Nevsky Prospekt for another block and a half, until you hit the Fontanka River.

Fontanka River to Uprising Square

Of St. Petersburg's many beautiful and interesting bridges, the **Anichkov Bridge** is one of the finest. On pillars anchoring each end are statues of a man with a horse. The ensemble, sculpted in 1841 and known collectively as *The Horse Tamers*, expresses humanity's ongoing desire to corral nature. Watch the relationship between horse and man evolve: In one view, it's a struggle, with the man overwhelmed by the wild beast's power; in another, it's a cooperative arrangement, with the man leading the bridled and saddled horse. Looking over the Fontanka River, it's easy to take this as a metaphor for St. Petersburg's relationship to the water. To survive and prosper, the city had to tame the inhospitable, swampy delta on which it is built.

• *You've walked the most interesting stretch of Nevsky Prospekt, but if you'd like to see more of the city center, continue by foot or by bus down Nevsky for a half-mile until you reach* **Uprising Square** *(this intimidatingly huge transit hub is a showcase of Russia's bigger-is-better city-planning aesthetic, with some surviving Soviet touches; for bus numbers, see page 369).*

Otherwise, you have several options. Just to the left along the Fontanka embankment is the exquisite **Fabergé Museum** *(see page 412). To sightsee at the* **Russian Museum, Church on Spilled Blood, Kazan Cathedral,** *or* **Hermitage,** *walk back along Nevsky the way you came, or hop on a bus (see page 369 for buses that make the trip; note that a few trolley buses veer off from the end of Nevsky for* **St. Isaac's Cathedral,** *saving an extra 10-minute walk).*

To easily reach the **Peter and Paul Fortress,** *take the Metro: Backtrack to the underpass in front of Gostiny Dvor, find the Nevsky Prospekt station on the blue line, and ride one stop to Gorkovskaya—a short walk from the fortress.*

Or, from the same Metro station, locate the Gostiny Dvor station on the green line, which you can ride one stop to the Vasileostrovskaya stop to begin my **"Back-Streets Walk,"** *described next.*

BACK-STREETS WALK ON VASILYEVSKY ISLAND

Tourists in St. Petersburg typically visit just a handful of famous sights and walk the grand Nevsky Prospekt. That's exciting, but if that's all you do, you'll miss the workaday city. This self-guided walk, worth ▲▲, is the remedy.

To start, ride the subway to the Vasileostrovskaya station (green line, first westbound stop after Gostiny Dvor). From this stop, you'll walk 15 minutes (passing a local market) to the riverfront, another 15 scenic minutes along the riverfront to the Strelka viewpoint, and 15 more minutes to either the Peter and Paul Fortress or the Hermitage and Nevsky Prospekt (in opposite directions).

This walk works great for cruisers who arrive at the Marine Facade terminal complex; simply follow my instructions for taking the public bus to the Metro (see page 355), then ride one stop to Vasileostrovskaya.

• *Exiting the Metro station, you'll be kitty-corner from a palatial McDonald's. Turn right, then right again, and pause in the middle of the pedestrian street. You're smack-dab in...*

The Heart of the Island

This street, called Ulitsa 7-ya Liniya/Ulitsa 6-ya Liniya (улица 7-я Линия/улица 6-я Линия), is in the center of an upscale residential zone that stretches from the city center all the way to the massive Marine Facade cruise port. Carefully planned Vasilyevsky Island has 30 numbered north/west streets (called "lines") that cross its three big east/west thoroughfares (named "big"/*bolshoy*, "medium"/*sredny*, and "small"/*maly*). Each side of the street has a different number—in this case, 6 on the left, 7 on the right.

You're standing upon what was a canal—part of the planned town that was laid out in the 1720s, during Peter the Great's lifetime. Directly in front of the Metro station, just before the park-like center strip, notice the statue of a horse-driven tram. In the 19th century (after the canal was filled in), trams like this shuttled from river to river. The lowest buildings (on the left) date from the original 18th-century town.

Head to the center strip and stroll under the larch trees down this lively, colorful, traffic-free street—one of the oldest in the city. Gurgling fountains punctuate the walk. Look for food trucks parked on the sidewalk, selling cheap, tasty pastries. You'll pass several chain stores: mobile phones (Мегафон— that's "Megafon"); fast-food joints both Russian (Теремок) and American (Subway); and American-sounding chains that are actually Russian (Coffeeshop Company). Imagine this street under communism: less colorful...less tacky.

• *After one very long block, on the left you'll see a pink church.*

St. Andrew's Cathedral

While a church was first built here in the 1720s as part of the original street plan, the present building dates from the 1760s. Today this is a neighborhood church, where ordinary people stop by on the way home (visitors are welcome—no photos; women can borrow a scarf to cover their heads). Step inside for a totally untouristy Russian Orthodox experience (for more on the faith and the features of its churches, see page 416). Like most of St. Petersburg, this church echoes European styles—its Baroque exterior would be at home in Bavaria. But the interior is filled with Orthodox icons. Its iconostasis, or altar screen, survived communism. Discreetly notice the ritual: Women cover their heads, while sullen teens just flip up the hoods of their windbreakers. Upon leaving, worshippers turn back, face the church, and cross themselves. The reverence of these acts illustrates how faith has been reincorporated into Russian life in a huge way since the end of the atheistic communist era.

• *Continuing past the church, you'll reach a big intersection (Bolshoy Prospekt, "Big Avenue"). Cross the street, then detour a block to the left (cutting through the little park) to reach the yellow building with a big green* Рынок *sign over the gate. This is the neighborhood's...*

Farmer's Market

Poke through the gateway into the inner courtyard to find some open-air stalls, including a tasty tandoor bakery from Uzbekistan, the former Soviet republic in Central Asia (on the left as you enter the courtyard). Inside the market, wade through the clothing stalls to find the food—just follow your nose.

Backtrack to the street you were on (Ulitsa 6-ya Liniya), cross to the right side, and continue in the direction you were headed. After about 50 yards, pop into the historic, brick-and-stone **pharmacy** (on your right, Аптека). While open for business, it's like a little museum taking you back to 1908 (Mon-Fri 9:00-21:00).

• *Detour around the pharmacy (leaving the building, take three left turns) for a quick look at some...*

Back Streets

While these are a bit sterile, you can imagine how they originally served as a mews (stables). Throughout the town, formal parade entries to grand buildings face the front, while the rough "back entries" are for servants and the poor. With the 1917 Revolution, larger buildings were divided up to house many families—Doctor Zhivago-style. Partitions were put into staircases, and bathrooms were retrofitted into kitchens. Vast blocks were divided into a series of courtyards, with apartments becoming cheaper the deeper they were buried. Walking around town, you can see how fine 19th-century features survive on some buildings, and other buildings—shelled in World War II—were rebuilt more simply in the 1950s and 1960s. Continue walking around the old pharmacy block—exploring the unpolished back sides of 18th- and 19th-century buildings, and peeking into courtyards and playgrounds—then turn left again to return to the main street.

• *Turn right, and notice the yellow building with sculpted heads over the windows, just before the river. This is the...*

House of Academicians

This was where big brains lived in the 18th century, and in Soviet times it functioned as a residential think tank. Each of the black plaques between the windows honors a great Russian scientist. The blue plaque by the door identifies the former apartment of Ivan Pavlov. If that name rings a bell, it's because he famously studied conditioned responses (and was the first Russian to win a Nobel Prize).

• *Continuing along, you'll pop out at the...*

Neva Riverbank

You're separated from the nicely pedestrianized embankment by a busy highway. (The nearest crosswalk is one very long block to your right, as you face the river.)

To your left, the **Annunciation (Blagoveshchensky) Bridge,** from 1850, was the first permanent bridge over the Neva.

Just to your right, notice the many **cargo ships** stacked up along the embankment. St. Petersburg is at the mouth of the Neva River, but its 342 bridges impede the progress of ships wanting to head upstream. The solution: Each night, from about 1:30 to 5:00 in the morning, drawbridges throughout the city center open, allowing cargo boats to proceed. Boats arriving during the day tie up here to wait their turn. From here, ships can go upstream and reach either the Arctic Sea (far to the north) or the Black Sea (far to the south) via a series of industrial canals built in Soviet times to connect the Neva with the great rivers of Russia's interior.

• *From here, you have two choices: Head right, to the Schmidt embankment and Optina Pustyn Church (described next), or walk left to the Strelka viewpoint, from where you can circle around to either the Peter and Paul Fortress or the Hermitage (described later, under "Sights in St. Petersburg").*

Schmidt Embankment

Turning right, the fine riverside promenade is lined with muscular Russian-made ships (note their ports of registry painted on their sterns). A stroll along here leads to the Schmidt embankment, where smaller luxury cruise ships tie up. St. Petersburg is Russia's leading port, and looking downstream, you can see the huge cranes that are part of its big shipbuilding and shipping industry. Although marine shipping is still important to St. Petersburg, imagine when the town was newly founded in the early 18th century, and the only real access was by sea.

• *Across from the Schmidt embankment is a dazzling gold-domed church.*

Optina Pustyn

This is one of the many branch churches of the Eastern Orthodox Optina monastery. Step inside to enjoy one of St. Petersburg's most beautiful church interiors—with splendid frescoes, ornate icons, and shimmering gold (daily 8:00-20:00; tourists welcome but be discreet). Repurposed by the communists, this house of worship spent time as a hockey rink. Restorers even found a hard-hit puck still embedded in one wall. Now the building has reclaimed its sacred purpose, and its male choir is one of Russia's most beloved. Its café and bookshop face the busy embankment road.

Sights in St. Petersburg

Most of St. Petersburg's major sights and landmarks are in the central zone that radiates out from the south bank of the Neva River, starting with the city's most famous sight—the Hermitage museum.

▲▲▲THE HERMITAGE (ЭРМИТАЖ)

Built by Peter the Great's daughter, Elizabeth, the Hermitage was later filled with the art collection of Catherine the Great.

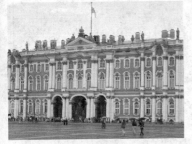

The Hermitage's vast collections of just about everything—but especially its European masterworks—make it one of the world's top art museums, ranking with the Louvre and the Prado. Housed in the Romanovs' Winter Palace, the Hermitage (EHR-mee-tazh, officially the State Hermitage, Государственный Эрмитаж), is actually two top-notch sightseeing experiences in one: an art gallery of European works and an imperial residence. Enjoy the Leonardos, Rembrandts, and Matisses while imagining the ostentatious lifestyles of the czars who collected them. Between the canvases, you glide through some of the most opulent ballrooms and throne rooms ever built. *Warning:* Dense crowds tarnish the Hermitage experience, and visiting early or late makes only a minimal difference. If you're particularly bugged by crowds, consider skipping the visit.

Cost and Hours: 400 R (students free), Tue-Sun 10:30-18:00, Wed until 21:00, closed Mon.

Information: Tel. 710-9625 (recorded info) or 710-9079, www.hermitagemuseum.org.

Ticket-Buying Tips: Handy **machines** in the main courtyard sell tickets without a line (available 10:00-16:00 only, clearly explained in English). It's also possible to buy a ticket in advance **online** for a slightly inflated price ($18/1 day, $26/2 days—bring email confirmation to exchange for ticket on-site, www.hermitageshop.org). You're not tied to a particular entry time. If you buy a ticket online or from one of the machines and want to add extras (such as a guided tour), go to the ticket windows inside, with typically shorter lines.

Getting In: Individual visitors enter through the courtyard that faces the grand Palace Square with the Alexander Column. From the column and square, you'll go through a passageway—if you bought tickets online, exchange your voucher for tickets at the

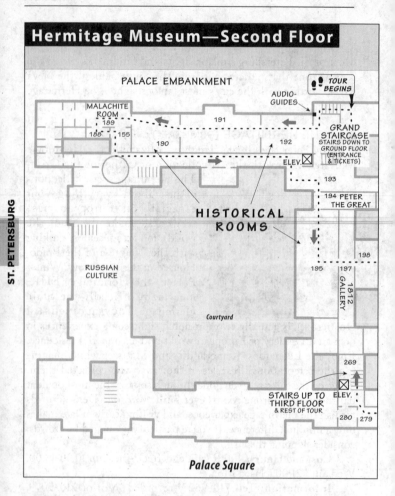

Hermitage Museum—Second Floor

kiosk here. Next you'll emerge into a large courtyard with **ticket machines** scattered around—use one of these if you didn't book ahead. You'll see a long **ticket line** at the far end of the courtyard, by the entrance door, but that's primarily for Russians (who qualify for a discounted price unavailable at the machines). With tickets in hand, skip the line and head right into the entry hall. There, line up at the security checkpoint to scan your ticket at the turnstile and enter the museum.

Tours: Immediately beyond the security checkpoint is a desk where you can rent an English **audioguide** (350 R, leave ID as deposit; less-crowded audioguide stand at top of main stairway). The audioguide has handy, digestible descriptions of the palace's historical rooms and of major paintings, but isn't worth the high price for a single traveler on a short visit. It's possible to customize

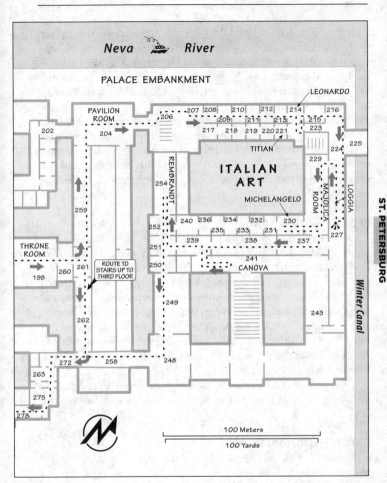

your own tour with the museum's **audioguide app** (see the website). **Guided tours** are offered in the entry hall (300 R, times posted in courtyard).

Services: Pick up a free **map** at the information desk. Down the stairs from the entry hall is an **ATM,** a **cloakroom** (remember which of the 14 sections you use), a tiny **bookstore** (there are better ones later, inside the museum), and a crowded **WC** (there are more later). In the hall to the right, before you reach the stairway, are more **WCs,** a mediocre and crowded **café,** several gift shops, and a large **bookstore.**

Photography: You'll technically need a photo permit (200 R, sold in entry hall or at the machines)—but this rule is only loosely enforced.

Expect Changes to Modern Collection: The General Staff

Building (the yellow building with the arch, across the square from the Hermitage) has been renovated into a gleaming exhibition space, and over time much of the Hermitage's modern art collection will relocate here. If Impressionist and Post-Impressionist art is your priority, confirm which building these works are in before buying your ticket.

Cruise-Line Evening Visits: If you're visiting St. Petersburg on a cruise, consider taking the evening Hermitage excursion-tour that's offered by many cruise lines. It's a more peaceful museum experience, saves your daylight hours for other activities, and is a good option if you don't mind a short and limited look at the collection's highlights.

❂ Self-Guided Tour

This tour will take you quickly through the Hermitage's highlights, divided into three parts: 1) historical rooms; 2) Old Masters (Leonardo, Raphael, Rembrandt, etc.); and 3) Modern Masters (Matisse, Chagall, Picasso, etc.). Very roughly, the first (ground) floor, where you enter, shows ancient art; the second floor has the historical rooms plus galleries covering the medieval, Renaissance, and Baroque eras (Old Masters); and the third floor is devoted to the 19th and 20th centuries (Modern Masters). Room numbers are posted over the doors to each room, but they're easy to miss in these opulent surroundings.

Length of This Tour: It should take about four hours—including one full hour just to fight the crowds and connect the dots.

Part 1: Historical Rooms

• *At the end of the entry area (the hall with the metal detectors and audioguide stand), head up the...*

Ambassador's Stairs: You are in the Winter Palace, the czar's official city residence, built by Italian architects (notably Francesco Bartolomeo Rastrelli) between 1754 and 1762 in the style called Elizabethan Baroque—named for the czarina who popularized it. At this time, all of St. Petersburg—like this staircase—drew on the talents of artists and artisans imported from Western Europe. The palace is designed 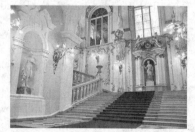 to impress, astonish, and humble visitors with the power of the Romanov dynasty. The stairway gives you a good feeling for the building's architecture, with its gilded ceiling showing the Greek gods relaxing in the clouds. A serious fire damaged the palace in

1837, but it was quickly restored. The museum occupies the Winter Palace plus two connected buildings, the Small Hermitage and the Large Hermitage, which were built in the late 18th century. The museum takes its name from these buildings, where the royal art collections were originally housed.

• *At the top of the stairs, go through the door and pass through a series of large rooms—192, 191 (imagine grand balls of the czar in this room, with inlaid floors and three crystal chandeliers; today it generally hosts temporary exhibits), and 190 (with the tomb of Alexander Nevsky, adorned with two tons of silver)—to reach Room 189.*

The Malachite Room: This drawing room, which dates from just after the 1837 fire, is decorated with malachite, a green cop-per-based mineral found in Russia's Ural Mountains. After the first stage of the Russian Revolution in spring 1917, in which the czar was ousted, a provisional government led by Alexander Kerensky declared Russia a republic. This government took over the Winter Palace and met in the Malachite Room, over-looking the Neva River. Their last meeting was on November 7, 1917. That evening, communist forces, loyal to Vladimir Lenin and the Bolshevik Party, seized power of the city in a largely bloodless coup. (Although the Bolsheviks took over in November, back then Russia still used the old Julian calendar—so technically it was an "October" Revolution.)

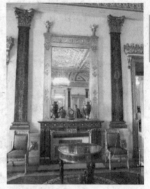

• *At the end of the Malachite Room, turn left into Room 188, then Room 155, and find the long series of smaller rooms filled with Romanov por-traits (Rooms 153 and 151), which returns you parallel to the way you came. At the end of the hall, turn right, directly into Room 193.*

Field Marshals' Hall: This hall was for portraits of Russia's military generals—perhaps so that the ruling family could keep names and faces straight. After 1917, the paintings were taken down and moved to other museums. But in recent years, the original portraits, dating from 1814 to the 1830s (and evoking the Russian victory over Napoleon and the French), have been returned to their places here.

• *The next, very red room (194) is the...*

Memorial Hall of Peter the Great: This hall pays homage to Peter the Great, who founded this city a generation before the Winter Palace's construction. You see his portrait (with Minerva, the goddess of wisdom) and a copy of his throne. Above, on the wall to either side, are paintings commemorating his decisive victories over Sweden—at Lesnaya in 1708 and Poltava in 1709. (For more on the dynamic Peter, see the sidebar on page 426.)

• *Continue into the **Armorial Hall** (Room 195), a banquet hall with golden columns and sculptures of knights with spears in each corner, and take a left into the long, skinny Room 197, known as the...*

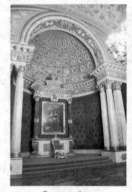

War Gallery of 1812: Opened in 1826, this hall displays over 300 portraits of the generals who helped to expel Napoleon from Russia in 1812 and chase him back to France. The Russian and French armies fought to a draw at the battle of Borodino, just west of Moscow, in September. The French troops were lured into Moscow, but the city was deliberately burned, Russian forces refused to submit to French control, and after some days, Napoleon's troops realized they were overextended and began to retreat through the deepening winter cold. Napoleon had entered Russia with 400,000 men, but only a tenth would make it back out. This crushing reversal ended his plans for European dominance.

The large portraits show the most important figures in Napoleon's defeat—practice your Cyrillic by reading the names. At the far-left end of the hall, the largest of all is an equestrian portrait of Czar Alexander I (the czar who pushed out the French). To either side of him are the Austrian emperor Franz I (Франц I) and the Prussian emperor Friedrich Wilhelm III (Фридрих-Вильхельм III). Next comes Grand Duke Konstantin Pavlovich (Константин Павлович), the czar's unruly brother and heir to the throne; across from him is Field Marshal Mikhail Golenishchev-Kutuzov (Голенищев-Кутузов), the strategist of the battle of Borodino. To the other side of the doors are Britain's Duke of Wellington (Веллингтон) and Michael Barclay de Tolly (Барклай де Толли), a Russian general of Baltic German and Scottish descent. (A few generals weren't available for sittings, so they're remembered by squares of green cloth.)

At the end opposite Alexander, one painting depicts the battle of Borodino, while the other (Peter von Hess's *Crossing the Berezina*) shows Napoleon's troops retreating through the snow in rags and disarray, crossing a bridgeless river.

• *Back in the middle of this long hallway, proceed into Room 198.*

Throne Room: This grand hall, created in the early 1840s, was of great importance as the setting for official ceremonies and receptions in czarist times. The magnificent parquet floor, made from 16 types of wood, is original. The Soviets added to the grandeur by installing a huge map of the USSR inlaid with semiprecious stones (now gone).

• *From Room 198, pass through the smaller room beyond it (260) into Room 261; here, hang a left and pass through the looong Room 259 and little Room 203 before stepping into Room 204, the...*

Pavilion Room: You've left the Winter Palace and entered the original Small Hermitage (founded by Catherine the Great).

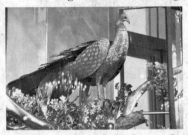

Consisting of two long and parallel galleries, this was where Catherine hung her original art collection in 1762. Admire the fine view of the interior courtyard. Decorated in the 1850s in French Renaissance style, the room contains the fun Peacock Clock, a timepiece made by British goldsmith James Cox and purchased by Catherine the Great. (The controls are in the large mushroom—a video shows it in action.) Across the hall, scrutinize the remarkably detailed inlaid floor.

• *You've seen the most important historical rooms in the Hermitage. At this point, it's best to focus on one or two artistic periods from among the Hermitage's vast collections. The basic options are to proceed directly into the **Old Masters** collection in the adjoining rooms (described next, in "Part 2" of this tour); or to skip forward several centuries and head upstairs to the fine **Modern Masters** collection (described later, in "Part 3").*

To find the modern section, head through the long and skinny Rooms 259 and 262, then turn right and loop through smaller Rooms 272-280 to find the stairs up to the third floor—watch on the right for Room 280. Once there, turn to "Part 3" of this tour. (Before following these directions, confirm that the modern collection is still in the building—it may be relocated to the General Staff Building, across Palace Square, by the time you visit.)

Part 2: Old Masters

• *The Italian Renaissance works we'll see are on the same floor as the historic rooms. Just beyond the Pavilion Room and the Peacock Clock, proceed straight, cross the bridge between the hermitages, and then pass the top of the stairwell (with the huge, green malachite-and-bronze vase) to enter a long hallway. Here begins the Old Hermitage's collection of Italian art. While there's a lot to see, for now pass through Rooms*

ST. PETERSBURG

207–213 (but pause in Room 209, at the Fra Angelico fresco of Mary and Baby Jesus, and in Room 210, with some fine Della Robbia ceramic works)—until you emerge in the exquisite Room 214.

Leonardo da Vinci

Considering that there are only about 20 paintings in existence by the great Renaissance genius, the two humble Madonnas in the Hermitage are world-class treasures. Leonardo da Vinci (1452-1519) reinvented the art of painting and influenced generations of artists, and these two small works were landmarks in technique, composition, and the portrayal of natural human emotion.

Paintings of mother Mary with Baby Jesus had always been popular in Renaissance Italy. But before Leonardo, large altarpieces typically showed the Madonna and Child seated formally on a throne, surrounded by saints, angels, elaborate architecture, and complex symbolism. Leonardo reinvented the theme in intimate, small-scale works for private worship. He deleted extraneous characters and focused on the heart of the story—a mother and her child alone in a dark room, sharing a private moment.

• *First up, on the wooden panel straight ahead as you enter the room is the...*

Benois Madonna (1475-1478): A youthful Mary shows Jesus a flower. Jesus (with his Casper-the-Friendly-Ghost-like head)

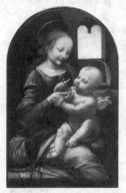

inspects this wondrous thing with a curiosity and concentration that's wise beyond his years. Mary practically giggles with delight. It's a tender, intimate moment, but with a serious psychological undertow. The mustard flower—with four petals—symbolizes the cross of Jesus' eventual Crucifixion. Jesus and Mary play with it innocently, oblivious to the baby's tragic destiny.

This is one of Leonardo's earliest known works. In fact, it may be the first painting he did after quitting the workshop of his teacher, Verrocchio, to strike out on his own. The painting, which was often copied (including by Raphael), was revolutionary. The painstaking detail astonished Leonardo's contemporaries—the folds in Mary's clothes, Jesus' dimpled flesh, the tiniest wisps of haloes, Mary's brooch. How did he do it? The secret was a new technological advance—oil-based paints. Unlike the more common tempera (egg-based) paint, oils could be made nearly transparent. This allowed Leonardo to apply layer after layer to make the subtlest transitions of color, mimicking real life.

• *Farther along the room is another panel, with the...*

Litta Madonna (1490-1491): Mary nurses Baby Jesus, gazing down proudly. Jesus stays locked onto Mary's breast but turns his eyes outward absentmindedly—dreamy-eyed with milk—to face the viewer, drawing us into the scene. The high-light of the painting is clearly Mary's radiant face, gracefully tilted down and beaming with tenderness.

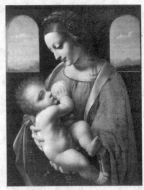

Compare the *Litta Madonna* and *Benois Madonna*—each is a slight variation on a popular theme. Both are set in dark interiors lit by windows looking out on a dis-tant landscape (though the *Benois* landscape remains unfinished). Subconsciously, this accentuates the intimacy and tranquility of the setting. Both paintings were originally done on wood panel before being transferred to canvas (and retouched) a century ago. Both paintings are named for the family that at one point owned them. One difference is in the style. The *Litta Madonna* has crisper outlines—either because it was done in (less subtle) tempera or by a (less subtle) apprentice.

What they have in common is realistic emotion, and this sets all of Leonardo's Madonnas apart from those of his contempo-raries. With a tilt of the head, a shining face, a downturned mouth, the interplay of touching hands and gazes, Leonardo captured an intimacy never before seen in painting. He draws aside a curtain to reveal an unguarded moment, showing mother and child interact-ing as only they can. These holy people don't need haloes (or only the wispiest) to show that sacred bond.

Before leaving this room, notice the palace architecture itself. The doors are inlaid with ebony, bronze, and tortoiseshell. The scenes decorating the fireplaces are delightful micro-mosaics.

• *The door across from the* Benois Madonna *leads to Room 221, where we'll find...*

Titian

Danae (1553-1554): One of art history's most blatantly sexual paint-ings, this nude has fascinated people for centuries—both for its subject matter and for Titian's bravura technique. The Hermitage's canvas is the second (or third) of five nearly identical paintings Titian painted of the popular legend.

It shows Danae from Greek mythology, lying naked in her bedchamber. Her father has locked her up to prevent a dreadful prophecy from coming true—that Danae will bear a son who will grow up to kill him. As Danae daydreams, suddenly a storm cloud

gathers overhead. In the light-
ning, a divine face emerges—it's
Zeus. He transforms himself
into a shower of gold coins.
Danae tilts her head and gazes
up, transfixed. She goes weak-
kneed with desire, and her left
leg flops outward. Zeus rains
down between Danae's legs,

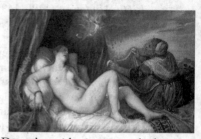

impregnating her. Meanwhile, Danae's maid tries to catch the
divine spurt with her apron.

This legend has been depicted since ancient times.
Symbolically, it represented how money can buy sexual favors. In
medieval times, Danae was portrayed as being as money-hungry
as the maid. But Titian clearly wants to contrast Danae and the
maid. He divides the canvas, with Danae's warm, golden body
on one side and the frigid-gray old maid on the other. Zeus rains
straight down, enriching them both, and uniting the composition.
Danae is a celebration of giving yourself to love.

• *Backtrack through the Leonardo room (214), continue through Rooms
215 and 216 (at the corner, with a love scene by Giulio Romano from
Catherine's private erotica collection), and bear right. Pass straight
through Room 224 to reach Room 227 and an homage to...*

Raphael

Loggia: This long, narrow hallway—more than 200 feet long,
only 13 feet wide, and decorated with colorful paintings—is a replica of one of the painter Raphael's crowning
achievements, the Vatican Loggia in Rome.
(The original loggia, in the Vatican Palace,
was designed by the architect Bramante—who
also authored St. Peter's Basilica in Rome;
Raphael and his assistants completed the loggia's fresco decorations in 1518-1519.)

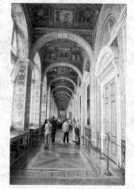

In the 1780s, after admiring color engrav-
ings of the Vatican Loggia, Catherine the
Great had this exact replica built of Raphael's
famous hallway. It's virtually identical to
the original, though the paintings here are
tempera on canvas. They were copied from
the frescoes in Rome (under the direction of Austrian painter
Christoph Unterberger) and sent to St. Petersburg along with a
scale model of the entire ensemble.

The Loggia exudes the spirit of the Renaissance, melding the
Christian world (52 biblical scenes on the ceiling) and the Classical
world (fanciful designs on the walls and arches). The ceiling tells

Christian history chronologically, starting with the Creation and the expulsion of Adam and Eve and ending with Christ's Last Supper. For the walls, Raphael used the ancient "grotesque" style found in archaeological sites (or "grottos"): lacy designs, garlands, flowers, vases, and mythological animals. Raphael resurrected these motifs, which became extremely popular with European nobility. The complex symbolism, mixing the Christian and pagan, also intrigued the educated elite, and the Loggia has come to be called "Raphael's Bible."

• *When you're done in the Loggia, go back to the start of the hallway (Room 226) and turn left into Room 229, the* **Majolica Room.** *Here you'll find two authentic masterpieces by Raphael.*

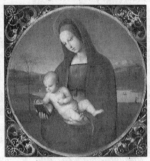

Conestabile Madonna (c. 1504): The dinner-plate-size painting in the gilded frame just opposite the entrance is one of Raphael's first known works, painted when he was still a teenager. Mother Mary multitasks, cradling Baby Jesus while trying to read. Precocious Jesus seems to be reading, too. Though realistic enough, the work shows a geometrically perfect world: Mary's oval face, Jesus' round head, and the perfect oval frame. The influence of Leonardo is clear: in the tilt of Mary's head and position of Jesus' pudgy legs (similar to the *Litta Madonna*) and in the child's beyond-his-years focus on an object (from the *Benois Madonna*). The picture is remarkable for its color harmonies and its perfected forms—characteristics that Raphael would beautifully develop in his later works.

While you're in this room, look also for Raphael's somber **Holy Family** (c. 1507), another rare early work. It's also known as *Madonna with Beardless Joseph,* for obvious reasons.

• *At the far end of the Raphael room, hook right into Room 230. In the center of this gallery is a sculpture by…*

Michelangelo

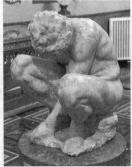

Crouching Boy (c. 1530): The nude figure crouches down within the tight "frame" of the block of marble he came from. The statue was likely intended to pose forlornly at the base of a tomb in the Medici Chapel in Florence, possibly to symbolize the vanquished spirit of the deceased's grieving relatives. Though the project (and this statue) were never fully finished, the work possesses Michelangelo's trademark pent-up energy.

• *We'll leave the Italian Renaissance now. Go back one room, turn immediately right, then right again at the blue vase. Head down the skylighted Rooms 247, 238, and 239 (with grand vases). At the last of these rooms (239), watch for the door on the left for the long, pastel-hazy, light-filled Room 241. Slow your pace and stroll through this gorgeous array of Neoclassical sculpture. Just after the doors, look for...*

Canova

The Three Graces (1813-1816): The great Venetian sculptor shows the three mythological ladies who entertained the Greek gods at

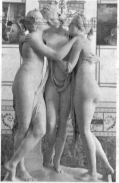

dinnertime. They huddle up, hugging and exchanging glances, their heads leaning together. Each pose is different, and the statue is interesting from every angle. But the group is united by their common origin—carved from a single block of marble—and by the sash that joins them. The ladies' velvety soft skin is Canova's signature element. Antonio Canova (1757-1822) combines the cool, minimal lines of Neoclassicism with the warm sentiment of Romanticism.

• *Go back into Room 239, then turn left into the smaller Room 251. Turn right and go through Room 252 and into the green-hued Room 254, with the best collection of Rembrandts outside the Netherlands.*

Rembrandt

The great Dutch painter is beautifully represented at the Hermitage. We'll tune into two works in particular.

• *As you enter the room, look to the left to find...*

Danae (1636): Compare this large-scale nude of the Greek demi-goddess to Titian's version, which we saw earlier. The scene is similar—a nude woman reclines diagonally on a cano-pied bed, awaiting her lover (the randy god Zeus), accompanied by her maid (in the dim background). But Rembrandt depicts a more practical, less ecstatic tryst. Where Titian's Danae was helpless with rapture, Rembrandt's is more in control. She's propped upright and focused, and her legs aren't splayed open. Danae motions to her offstage lover—either welcoming him into her boudoir or

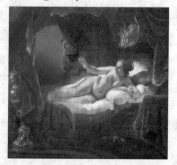

warning him to be cautious. Historians note that Danae has the body of Rembrandt's first wife (the original model) and the face of his mistress (painted over a decade later).

Catherine the Great—herself no stranger to bedroom visitors—bought this painting in 1772 as one of the works that grew into the Hermitage collection.

· *At the far end of the room, look for...*

The Prodigal Son (c. 1669): In the Bible, Jesus tells this story of the young man who wastes his inheritance on wine, women, and song. He returns home, drops to his knees before his father, and begs forgiveness. Rembrandt recounts the whole story—past, present, and future—in this single moment, frozen in time. The Prodigal Son's tattered clothes and missing shoe hint at the past—how he was once rich and wearing fine clothes, but ended up penniless, alone, bald, and living in a pigsty. His older brother (standing to the right) is the present:

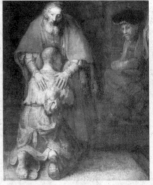

He looks down in judgment, ready to remind their dad what a bad son the Prodigal is. But the father's face and gestures foretell the story's outcome, as he bends down to embrace his son with a tenderness that says all will be forgiven. The father's bright-red cloak wraps around the poor Prodigal like loving arms.

The Prodigal Son is one of Rembrandt's last paintings. Some read Rembrandt's own life story into the painting: Rembrandt had been a young prodigy whose God-given talent brought him wealth, fame, and the love of a beautiful woman. Then he lost it all, and was even forced to sell off his possessions to pay his debts. His last years were spent in relative poverty and obscurity.

· *It's a long haul from here up to the modern collection on the third floor. Follow these directions carefully: From Rembrandt, go back through Room 252 into Room 251, and continue straight ahead through Room 250, then the long Room 249. Emerging into Room 248, turn right and use the corridor (Room 258) to cut back across the three hermitages (crossing the bridge, then passing the garden). Carry on straight into Room 272, hook left, and do a loop through Rooms 272–280 to find the stairs (on the right, in Room 280).*

Part 3: Modern Masters

The Hermitage has an impressive collection of paintings by Impressionist and Post-Impressionist masters. It's perfect for seeing how these artists—living in France in the late 19th century—influenced one another. The museum's core collection benefited greatly during the 1917 Russian Revolution. Many wealthy aristocrats with the taste and budget for these paintings fled the country. With not a hint of apology, the Soviet Union nationalized the collections you'll enjoy next so the proletariat could enjoy them. Remember: Some or all of this art may be relocated to the General Staff Building, across Palace Square. And in general, the art in these rooms is often shuffled around. Expect some changes to these descriptions.

Overview: So many canvases are crammed into these small rooms, it's hard to keep track of who's who. Here's a primer on just a few of the many famous names represented here: **Edouard Manet** (1832-1883) bucked the strict academic system to paint realistic scenes of everyday life, rather than prettified goddesses. Manet inspired his friend **Edgar Degas** (1834-1917) to sketch candid snapshots of the modern Parisian lifestyle—café scenes, workers, and well-dressed families bustling through Parisian streets. **Claude Monet** (1840-1926) and his close friend **Auguste Renoir** (1841-1919) took things another step, setting their canvases up outdoors and painting quickly to capture shimmering landscapes using a mosaic of bright colors. **Vincent van Gogh** (1853-1890), a moody Dutchman, learned this Impressionist technique from the bohemians in Paris, but infused his landscapes with swirling brushwork and an emotional expressiveness. Van Gogh's Post-Impressionist style was adopted by his painting partner, **Paul Gauguin** (1848-1903), who used bright patches of colors and simplified forms to re-create the primitive look of tribal art. **Henri Matisse** (1869-1954) went further, creating the art of "wild beasts" (Fauves), using even brighter colors and simpler forms than Gauguin. Gauguin had greatly admired a brilliant-but-struggling artist named **Paul Cézanne** (1839-1906), who also rejected traditional three-dimensionality to compose paintings as geometrical blocks of color. As the 20th century dawned, **Pablo Picasso** (1881-1973) broke Cezanne's blocks of colors into shards and "cubes" of color, all jumbled up, anticipating purely abstract art.

• *This floor's rooms are smaller—and more crowded. Sharpen your elbows and, from the top of the stairs, turn left into Room 314, turn left again, and do a loop through Rooms 332, 331, 330, and 323, and then right into Room 322. Finally, turn right into Room 321, where you'll find...*

Renoir

Later in life, Renoir—who, along with Monet, was one of the founding fathers of Impressionism—changed his style. He veered from the Impressionist credo of creating objective studies in color and light to begin painting things that were unabashedly "pretty."

He populated his canvases with rosy-cheeked, middle-class girls performing happy domestic activities, rendered in a warm, inviting style. As Renoir himself said, "There are enough ugly things in life."

• *Now head into Room 320 and continue into Room 319, dominated by* **Monet**. *Next up, Room 318 features lots of* **Cézanne** *(including* Lady in Blue*). And Room 317 is packed with works by...*

Vincent van Gogh

A self-taught phenom who absorbed the Impressionist technique before developing his own unique style, Vincent van Gogh struck out on his own in Arles, in the south of France, in 1888. For the next two years of his brief life, he cranked out a canvas nearly every other day. He loved painting the rural landscape and the colorful life of the locals.

• *On your left as you enter is...*

Arena at Arles (1888): Like a spontaneous photograph, this painting captures the bustle of spectators at the town's bullfighting ring. The scene is slightly off-kilter, focusing on the crowds rather than action in the ring. Van Gogh typically painted in a rush, and you can see it in the hurried lines and sketchy faces.

Memory of the Garden at Etten (*Ladies of Arles*, 1888): In the fall of 1888, Gauguin came to visit Van Gogh. The two friends

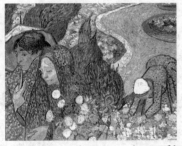

roomed together and painted side by side. It was Gauguin who suggested that Vincent change things up and paint something besides Impressionist scenes of everyday life. The result was this startling canvas, in which Vincent portrayed a garden he remembered from his childhood. The vivid colors had special meaning to him, representing the personalities of his mother and sister. The style shows the influence of Gauguin—big swaths of bright colors, divided by thick black outlines.

• *On the facing wall are two more notable paintings.*

The Lilac Bush (1889): On December 23, 1888, a drunk and angry Van Gogh turned on Gauguin, threatening him with a knife. Then he cut off a piece of his own ear and sent it to a prostitute. Judged insane, Van Gogh checked into a mental hospital for treatment. There he painted this simple subject that bristles with life, a forest of thick brushstrokes charged with Van Gogh's strong emotions.

The Cottages (1890): Van Gogh moved north of Paris in 1890 to be under a doctor's care. The wavy brushstrokes and surreal colors of this work suggest an uncertain frame of mind. This was one of Vincent's last paintings. A few weeks later, he wandered into a field near these homes and shot himself, having spent his life in poverty and artistic obscurity. No sooner had he died than his work took wings.

• *The next room (316) has a wonderful collection of works by...*

Paul Gauguin

The Hermitage typically displays about a dozen paintings of the French Post-Impressionist Paul Gauguin, who famously left his stockbroker job and family to paint full-time. Eventually he fulfilled his lifelong dream to live and work in the South Seas, especially Tahiti. He spent much of his later life there, painting island life in all its bright color and simplicity.

• *Just to the left as you enter the room is...*

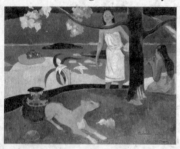

   Tahitian Pastorals (*Pastorales Tahitiennes*, 1892): This work, from Gauguin's first stay in Tahiti, captures the paradise Gauguin had always envisioned. He paints an island-dotted landscape peopled by exotic women doing simple tasks and making music. A lounging dog dominates the foreground. The style is intentionally "primitive," collapsing 3-D landscapes into a two-dimensional pattern of bright colors. In ***Woman Holding a Fruit*** (1893)—on the facing wall—a native girl enjoys the simple pleasures of life in all her naked innocence.

• *Continue straight across the bridge, peering down into a pastel-blue hall decorated with a whipped-cream can and Alexander's Wedgwood portrait at the end of the hall. Don't miss the wonderful view over Palace Square from the windows on your left. You'll head straight through Rooms 343–344 and into Room 345; the largest, most famous, and most important canvas here is by...*

Matisse

The Dance (1909-1910): Five dancers strip naked, join hands, and go ring-around-the-rosy, creating an infectious air of abandon. This large, joyous work was one of Matisse's personal favorites. It features his Fauvist colors—bright red dancers on a blue-and-green background.

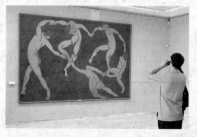

Meanwhile, the undulating lines that join the dancers create a pleasing design that anticipates modern, abstract art.

Other Matisse works in this room (and the previous one) trace his evolution from a realistic painter of still lifes to Impressionism to bright Fauvist colors to his semi-abstract works that pioneer modern abstract art.

• *Pass through Rooms 346–347 to reach Rooms 348 and 349, focusing on the works of...*

Pablo Picasso

In the year 1900, the 19-year-old Spaniard Pablo Picasso arrived in Paris, the world art capital. A relentless experimenter, Picasso would soon liberate himself from academic art traditions as he laid the basis for the new modern style. Besides groundbreaking examples of early Cubism and painted masterpieces from his Blue Period, the collection includes his playful ceramics. Be sure to enjoy these three paintings (all in Room 348):

• *On the left wall as you enter, between the windows, is...*

The Absinthe Drinker (1901): A woman sits alone in a grimy café, contemplating her fate, soothed by a glass of that highly potent and destructive form of alcohol. She leans on a table, deep in thought, with her distorted right arm wrapped around her protectively. All of the lines of sight—her unnaturally vertical forearm and the lines on the wall behind her—converge on her face, boxing her into a corner. The painting shows Picasso's facile mastery of the earlier generation of Impressionist and Post-Impressionists. It's a snapshot café scene like Degas, with the flat two-dimensional feel of Gauguin and the emotional expressiveness of Van Gogh.

• *Just to the left of the door you came in is...*

Two Sisters (1902): From Picasso's Blue Period, painted with a gloomy palette, this canvas looks sympathetically at people who, like Picasso, felt sad and alienated. The painting started with a sketch Picasso had made of two sisters—one a prostitute and one a nun. From that specific source, he developed a work of universal character.

• *On the facing wall is...*

Three Women (1908): This work (and the studies near it) shows how Picasso was rethinking how artists look at the world. He shattered reality into shards and cubes of color, then reassembled the pieces like a collage on canvas—the style called Cubism.

• *While there's much more to be seen, our tour is finished. If you're still craving more, the private apartments of Maria Alexandronovna (wife of Czar Alexander II; Rooms 289 and 304–307) are impressive, especially Room 304—the Empress' Drawing Room from the 1850s, with Catherine the Great's collection of gems and cameos. She claimed to be addicted to gems.*

Otherwise, make your way back down to the ground floor and plot your escape. Just follow signs with your new favorite word in the Russian language: ВЫХОД..."*exit.*" *If you're looking for extra credit, you can head across the Palace Square for the special exhibits shown in the...*

General Staff Building

Designed in Russian Empire style as a headquarters for the Russian military, this building is now a palatial art gallery. It's currently being used for special shows of big-name modern artists and themed exhibits, but in time some or all of the Hermitage's 19th- and 20th-century painting collection will be relocated here. If and when that happens, these galleries, like those of its big sister across the square, will be worth ▲▲▲—and best of all, the art will become much easier to appreciate than in the cramped Hermitage attic. While things are in flux, your best source for what's where is the Hermitage website.

Most likely, you'll enter below the big yellow arch directly across from the Hermitage entrance (door on the left as you go under the arch). After the ticket desk, you'll find a lower level with a cloakroom, WCs, and other services, and—above that—a cavernous atrium with a wide, modern marble staircase leading up to the exhibition halls (200 R for special exhibits, Tue-Sun 10:00-18:00, Wed until 21:00, closed Mon).

MUSEUMS AND GARDENS NEAR NEVSKY PROSPEKT

Two adjacent, related museums—the Russian Museum, with a fine-art collection, and the Russian Museum of Ethnography—sit just beyond the Griboyedov Canal. Behind them is a pair of historic gardens, the Mikhailovsky and Summer Gardens. Farther down Nevsky, near the Fontanka River, is the dazzling Fabergé Museum.

▲▲▲Russian Museum (Русский Музей)

Here's a fascinating collection of Russian art, particularly 18th-and 19th-century painting and portraiture. People who are disappointed that the Hermitage is mostly Western European art love the Russian Museum, since the artists shown here are largely unknown in the West. Much of the work reveals Russians exploring their own culture and landscape: marshes, birch stands,

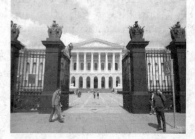

muddy village streets, the conquest of Siberia, fire-lit scenes in family huts, and Repin's portrait of Tolstoy standing barefoot in the woods.

This comparatively uncrowded museum adds depth to the experience you have as a visitor to St. Petersburg—the artists represented here saw the same rooftops, churches, and street scenes as you do. Their art brings you in touch with the country's turbulent political history and captures the small-town wooden architecture and forest landscapes that you won't see on a visit to this big city.

The museum occupies the Mikhailovsky Palace, built in the 1820s for Grand Duke Mikhail Pavlovich (a grandson of Catherine the Great). Though the interiors aren't as impressive as those at the Hermitage, original decorations in a few rooms give you a taste of how the Russian nobility lived.

Cost and Hours: 350 R, Wed and Fri-Mon 10:00-18:00, Thu 13:00-21:00, closed Tue, last entry 30 minutes before closing, photo permit-250 R, English audioguide-250 R.

Information: The museum is at Inzhenernaya Ulitsa 4, two blocks north of Nevsky Prospekt along Griboyedov Canal, near the Church on Spilled Blood. Tel. 595-4248, www.rusmuseum.ru.

Entering the Museum: The entrance is at the basement (servants') level, in the right-hand corner as you enter the main courtyard. Purchase your tickets, pick up a map (listing room numbers), and go through the security checkpoint. On the basement level, you'll find cloakrooms, a bookstore, a post office (handy if you need stamps), WCs, and a small café. For later, notice the back exit, which gives you the option of leaving through the gardens on the north side of the museum (from where you can bear left through the park to reach the Church on Spilled Blood). To reach the exhibits, take the stairs up one flight and show your ticket. Here, at the base of the grand staircase, you can rent the good audioguide, which interprets 300 of the museum's best works (or, for a quick visit, just use the self-guided tour, below).

Layout: The museum has 109 numbered rooms (find numbers over doorways), which lend themselves to a route in more or less chronological order.

❷ Self-Guided Tour

The museum's most exciting works cover the period from roughly 1870 to 1940. Russia was in ferment during these years—first with the end of serfdom and agitation for social change and equality; later with World War I, industrialization, and the beginnings of communism; and throughout with artistic currents such as Impressionism, Art Nouveau, and Modernism that came in from the West. I suggest a chronological tour through the collection, but pace yourself to spend the majority of your time with the most important works, near the end. Here are things to look for as you enjoy a sweep through Russian history via its art.

• *Head up the grand staircase and turn left into Room 1. We'll do a quick counterclockwise spin around this floor.*

Early Russian Art

Rooms 1-4: These rooms house Russian icons, the earliest dating back to the 1100s. Icons are a key part of Orthodox traditions of worship, and have roots in medieval Greece and Byzantium ("icon" means image or likeness in Greek). Just as it's best to see animals in the wild rather than in a zoo, icons are best seen in the context of the churches for which they were designed. These depictions of sacred people or events gave the illiterate faithful a way to "see" and communicate with the holy. You can follow the evolution of icon style from the 12th to the 16th century, finishing in Room 4, where some of the most recent icons are tainted by a European realism that kills the mysticism.

18th- and Early 19th-Century Russian Painting

Rooms 5-12: The grandest architecture in the museum is seen in these rooms, which overlook the gardens out back and display mostly 18th-century portraits. Notice the cultural revolution portrayed here: Following Peter the Great's reforms, the upper crust of Russia is clean-shaven, speaks French, and wears European clothes. There's a new outlook, and portraits mirror a society where people are showing off their individuality. You'll also see a few rare 18th-century Russian-made tapestries.

In Room 6, on the left wall, Ivan Nikitin's *Portrait of the Field Hetman* (1720s), with red-rimmed eyes, conveys an unusual degree of real personality. Peter the Great's court painter succeeded in showing this battle-worn officer ("hetman" means captain) not as a stuffed suit, but as a man proudly doing his duty for Russia despite being worn down by the horrors of war.

In the gaudy Room 10, Dmitry Levitzky's big portrait of Catherine the Great (*The Legislatress at the Temple of Justice,* flanked by smaller portraits of the leading figures in her court) is filled with symbolism and captures her cult of personality. Catherine gestures toward a pedestal with smoldering poppies—indicating that she was always alert, sacrificing repose for the betterment of her nation. Her orange-and-black sash indicates that Catherine established Russia's highest military honor, the Order of St. George. At her feet, an eagle perches on a stack of books, representing her respect for the word of law. And out the window on the left, see the wind-filled sails of a ship, suggesting Catherine's connection to the world and the expansion of the Russian realm. A similar, sculptural version of Catherine stands in the same room.

Room 11 is a great example of the Russian Empire style of

Carlo Rossi, the architect who designed this building. Rossi's amped-up Neoclassicism, popularized by Catherine the Great's successor, Alexander I, pervades the city. Here you see the style at its cohesive zenith—from inlaid floor to furniture to architecture.

Rooms 13-17: These rooms cover the Romantic era of the early 19th century. Room 14 is dominated by Karl Brullov's *The Last Day of Pompeii* (1833), a painting every Russian student knows well. It and paintings nearby (such as the dramatic shipwreck scenes) show the Romanticism of the age: They're emotional and theatrical, a reaction to the formal Neoclassicism of Catherine the Great. These Russian artists paint with confidence, no longer parroting European styles. Although inspired by European trends, they're confidently Russian now.

At the far end of Room 15 is Alexander Ivanov's *Appearance of Christ to the People* (completed before 1855), a variant of his masterwork of the same name (in Moscow's Tretyakov Gallery). The entire wall is filled with studies for this, his magnum opus, to which the artist dedicated 20 years of his career.

• *Continue back to the landing, head down the grand staircase, and turn left into Room 18.*

Late 19th- and Early 20th-Century Painting

Rooms 18-22: Paintings in Room 18, from the 1860s, show artists capturing real life. As across Europe, class awareness and social consciousness was growing, and artists began to use their work to question social inequalities. You can see an example of this "critical realism" in Vasily Perov's *Monastery Refectory* (1865-76), which shows fat monks scraping their plates clean while ignoring the hungry beggars at their feet.

Room 19 draws attention to Russian history in realistic paintings such as Nikolai Ghe's *Peter I Interrogating the Czarevich Alexei at Peterhof.* Without excessive pathos, we see the czar bluntly questioning his son—before putting in motion the inquisition that would condemn Alexei to death.

Rooms 20 and 22 focus on Romantic landscapes from the 1860s and 1870s that celebrate Russia's tranquil forests and seaside. In this period countries all across Europe experienced a resurgence of nationalism, and it showed in their art. Room 21 focuses on classical themes: the death of Nero, Christian martyrs in the Colosseum, and so on.

• *Now we'll jump forward to the museum's highlights. Proceed to Room 33 (if some rooms are closed, you may have to backtrack through later rooms to reach 33). But don't rush—there are some powerful canvases in the intervening halls that set the tone for what's to come.*

Rooms 33-34 and 54: Ilya Repin (1844-1930), who came from a modest background, often explored the rural lives of common people—he could be called an early Socialist Realist. His painting met approval during the Soviet period for its focus on the working class. He specialized in brilliant portraits that combined landscape settings with psychological insight and historical realism. A prime example is in Room 33—Repin famously painted Leo Tolstoy in peasant clothing, standing barefoot in the woods (1901).

In Room 34, find the painting that makes you want to sing the Volga Boat Song. With *Barge Haulers on the Volga* (1870-1873), Repin polished his local celebrity and gained renown in the West. Eleven wretched workers (called *burlaks*)—bodies groaning and with pain etched on their faces—are yoked like

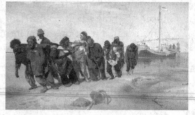

livestock for the Sisyphean task of pulling a ship against the current. The youngest *burlak* in the center, with inexplicable optimism, strikes a classically heroic pose. A steamship on the horizon emphasizes how cruelly outdated this form of labor is in the modern age. It's no wonder the Soviets embraced this painting as a perfect metaphor for the timeless struggle of the working class.

Also in Room 34, find *Seeing Off a Recruit* (1879), in which a young man hugs his mother as he prepares to let the army take him far away (25 years was a standard term of duty)—showing the sacrifice of military service in human terms that are still relevant today.

Rooms 36-37: One of Russia's foremost historical painters, Vasily Surikov (1848-1916) grew up in Siberia but later moved to European Russia. He excelled at creating dynamic battle scenes designed to spur Russian patriotism. In Room 36, his gigantic *Ermak's Conquest of Siberia* (1895) is a reminder that Russia has an uneasy relationship with its native peoples. Here, Caucasian-featured soldiers armed with guns cross a river by boat, meeting Siberian forces on the other shore armed with bow and arrow. In Room 37, Surikov's gigantic *Stepan Razin* (with the rowboat) commemorates the Cossack who led an uprising against the czar in 1670.

Room 38: Viktor Vasnetsov's *Knight at the Crossroads* (1882) evokes Russia's answer to Arthurian legend. A Russian knight on horseback, depicted in a natural landscape setting, ponders a stone with an inscription suggesting that any route he takes will present pitfalls. The skull and bones littering the grass and the ominous raven overhead drive home the somber message.

• *From here, backtrack to Room 35, and look for the door on the left that leads down into...*

Room 39: Vasily Vereshchagin (1842-1904) specialized in

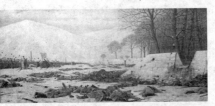

photorealistic paintings emphasizing two subjects: military scenes and exotic views of Eastern cultures (which he explored in his travels to the Balkans, Central Asia, and British India). Traveling with the military, he painted the reality of war vividly, but got too close and became a casualty himself in the Russo-Japanese War in 1904. Because he took a warts-and-all approach to combat, many of Vereshchagin's warfare paintings were deemed too graphic or unsettling to be exhibited during his lifetime. *Shipka-Sheynovo* shows Russia's 1877 victory over the Ottoman Empire at the battle of Shipka Pass, in what's now Bulgaria. The victorious Russian general rides past cheering troops, but the composition is dominated by the grotesque corpses of soldiers scattered in the snow. Vereshchagin's evocatively detailed *At the Entrance to the Mosque* makes evident the artist's fascination with the Eastern cultures whose decline is documented on his other canvases.

• *As you pass through Rooms 40–43, notice how the sun-dappled canvases of the Russian Impressionists were clearly influenced by the French Impressionists.*

Room 45: *Seventeenth-Century Moscow Street on a Public Holiday* (1895), by **Andrei Ryabushkin,** is a semiromanticized view of premodern Russian life: wooden houses, unpaved streets, women in headscarves and men in long beards, beggars, and the colorful, onion-domed St. Basil's Cathedral in the background.

Room 48: Here, in the small folk-art wing, you can get a glimpse of small-town Russia. It's worth perusal if only for its collection of village woodcarving. In addition, you'll see lace, lacquer boxes, pewter jewels, and folk dress (all described in English).

• *Now head back out to Room 48, turn left, and go down the corridor to reach a flight of stairs. Take this up to the top floor of the museum's Benois Wing (English descriptions in this wing for each room), housing most of the museum's 20th-century art. You'll begin in Room 66.*

More 20th-Century Art

Room 66: Mikhail Vrubel's *Bogatyr* (1898) was painted on the cusp of the new century. A massive, ogre-like knight errant sits on a fantastically fat horse. The decorative style borrows from the Art Nouveau movement, the theme echoes Russian myths and stories, and the surrealistic presentation anticipates expressionist painting. Vrubel (1856-1910) had a thing for demons and paintings beyond reality.

Rooms 69-70: Valentin Serov (1865-1911) made his name as the best Russian portrait painter of his day. Many Russian celebrities and aristocrats sat for him, eager for one of his freely brushed, technically adept portraits. It was said that his likenesses were so insightful that subjects could learn about themselves by viewing their Serov portrait.

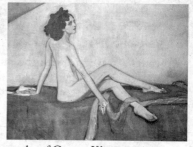

Serov departed from his usual approach for his 1910 nude portrait of Ida Rubinstein, a famous Russian ballerina (in Room 70). Daring in its simplicity and starkness, the painting has the flatness and sharp outlines of Art Nouveau—evoking the works of Gustav Klimt.

Room 71: Although his bread and butter was book illustration, Boris Kustodiev (1878-1927) was also known for colorful paintings such as *Shrovetide* (1916). Here you see the inescapably recurrent theme in Russian paintings of winter: sleigh rides, snow-covered roofs, festivals, and fairy-tale churches, all under an achingly beautiful winter sky of swirling pink-and-blue pastels. The artist appreciated plump models (as evidenced by *Merchant's Wife* and *Merchant's Wife at Tea*). Just as we say a woman's figure is Rubenesque, Russians say someone is Kustodievesque.

Russian Abstraction, the Avant-Garde, and Socialist Realism

Rooms 72 to 85 take us further into Russia's tumultuous 20th century. With the chaos and unprecedented destruction of World War I and the Bolshevik Revolution that followed, Russia was changing radically—as you'll see in the art displayed in these rooms. Zip through the first few rooms, seeing the Russian take on several modern European styles—Post-Impressionism, Cubism, Expressionism, Abstract Expressionism, and so on.

Rooms 78-80: Here you sense the 1920s. There was a feeling that a new world had been created; art and politics were parallel and complementary forces. But in 1928, with the strengthening of the idealistic communist movement under Stalin, there was a big change, as art became a servant of political ideology.

Rooms 80-83: The partition in the middle of Room 80 marks a major shift. Art from the early Soviet period glorified workers and the "dictatorship of the proletariat." Dubbed Socialist Realism, this government-sanctioned style had to be realistic and its content had to be socialist. Because the abstract cannot be controlled—it's open to free interpretation—it was not allowed. From 1928 on, art was acceptable only if it actively promoted socialist ideology. This was true for visual arts, literature, and even (as far as possible) for music.

In Room 80, Alexander Samokhvalov's *Militarized Komsomol* (1932-1933) conveys the Socialist Realist aesthetic: "realistically" showing everyday people who are, in an idealized way, eagerly participating in the socialist society. In this case, we see scouts learning how to scout—and potentially more than that, should the need arise.

In Room 81, you can see how art was used to build heroes, both in war and in the culture of sport.

The post-WWII canvases in Room 82 depict idyllic natural and peasant scenes, extolling the simple life held central in the Soviet worldview. These paintings make you want to sign up for a Russian-countryside summer vacation.

In Room 83, the Khrushchev-era art of the 1960s comes with a hint of spring—and a sense of the thawing that the summer of love (in 1967) blew across the Iron Curtain.

Rooms 84-85: It's subtle, but here you can feel change in the air. Rather than idealizing everyday Russian life, these works—

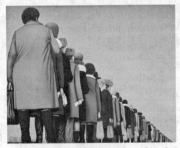

from the later Soviet years—are clearly critical of it. In Room 85, Alexei Sundukov's *Queue* (1986) is a perhaps too-on-the-nose depiction of the trials of a communist consumer. In the center of this room, Dmitry Kaminker's *The Oarsman* (1987), sculpted under perestroika, communicates the hopeless feeling of the last years of communism. This is dissident art, filled with political allegory, created not for the public but for an underground exhibition.

Then, in the late 1980s—just before the USSR fell apart—the Soviet leader Mikhail Gorbachev allowed a free art exhibit. This marked the end of Socialist Realism—and the end of real dissident art, because there was no longer any danger in showing it. The artistic spirit of the Russian people survived communism and came out of the closet.

▲Russian Museum of Ethnography
(Российский Этнографический Музей)

This branch of the Russian Museum offers an extensive, if dry, introduction to the various peoples of the former Soviet Union, reaching from Vilnius to Vladivostok. Fans of folk culture find it worthwhile, and anyone will be impressed by the diversity of one of the planet's biggest and most varied countries. The good, included audioguide (use the free Wi-Fi to download it) tells you more about each culture.

Cost and Hours: 350 R, Tue-Sun 10:00-18:00, closed Mon and last Fri of month, at Inzhenernaya 4—directly to the right as you face the main entrance of the Russian Museum, www.ethnomuseum.ru.

Summer Garden (Летний сад)

The zone behind the Russian Museum is filled with delightful parks and gardens. Directly behind the building, the inviting, tree-filled Mikhailovsky Garden (Михайловский сад) leads (across the canal) into the geometrically regimented Field of Mars (Марсово поле) park, designed to showcase military parades.

But best of all (just to the east, across another canal) is the Summer Garden (Летний сад), one of St. Petersburg's most enjoyable public spaces. The oldest garden in the city, it was laid out in 1710 under Peter the Great himself, right where the Fontanka River meets the Neva. It's laced with walking trails, studded with fountains and statues, and generously tree-shaded. Along the Fontanka is Peter's own **Summer Palace** (Летний дворец).

Cost and Hours: Free entry, garden open in summer daily 10:00-22:00; off-season Wed-Mon 10:00-19:30, closed Tue; fountains run Wed-Mon May-Sept only; audioguide-300 R.

▲▲Fabergé Museum (Музей Фаберже)

This sumptuous museum fills the beautifully restored Shuvalov Palace with the world's biggest collection of works by Carl Fabergé, jeweler to the czars. Opened in 2013, the museum is built around the collection assembled by the American publisher Malcolm Forbes (and later purchased by one of Russia's wealthy oligarchs). The undisputed highlight: 14 exquisite Fabergé eggs, including nine imperial Easter eggs. These jeweled fantasies—impossibly lavish, individually created "surprise"-loaded gifts given by the czars to their relatives and friends—represent the pinnacle of Romanov excess. Even those bored by treasury collections are wowed by the chance to get an up-close, 360-degree view of 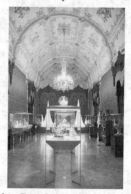 these incredible creations. The sight is a two-fer: Besides ogling the breathtaking treasury of priceless objects, you get to explore the halls of a grand canalside mansion, fueling fantasies of how the czars' aristocratic pals used to live.

Cost and Hours: 300 R, ticket office sells same-day admissions only—advance sales are online; Sat-Thu 9:30-20:45, closed Fri; dry audioguide-150 R; Fontanka 21, tel. 333-2655, www.fabergemuseum.ru.

Getting In: At this relatively new museum, logistics for your visit may be in flux (check their website for the latest). But as of this writing, you can visit with a **guided tour** before 18:00 (English tours generally run 2/day—otherwise you can join a Russian tour and pay for the audioguide; buy tickets online to be sure you'll get in, or call or email ahead to find out today's schedule—tel. 333-2655 or 3332655@fsv.ru). After 18:00, it's possible to visit **on your own** (with the help of the audioguide). On-your-own evening visit tickets go on sale at 17:45 (last ticket sold 1.5 hours before closing time).

Visiting the Museum: Ascend the grand staircase, under a gloriously stuccoed dome, and circle the collection counterclockwise. Each room is more amazing than the last.

From the **Knights' Hall**—filled with precious wine goblets, drinking horns, silver vessels, and military memorabilia—turn left into the **Red Room,** with silk walls and dark-stained walnut woodwork. Here you can get a close look at even more fine gold and silver work, from elaborate tankards to precious metals made to resemble wicker and cloth.

In the **Blue Room** are those 14 magnificent Fabergé eggs. They are displayed in chronological order, illustrating the evolution of their craftsmanship, inventiveness, and extravagance. Painstakingly crafted by court jeweler Peter Carl Fabergé (1846-1920), no two are alike. The variety of eggs and the surprises they hold is stunning: The first egg (commissioned by Czar Alexander III in 1885) held a golden yolk, which enclosed a golden hen concealing a diamond miniature of the royal crown and a ruby egg. Later eggs contain increasingly complex mechanisms: A miniature Jesus emerges from a tomb made of agates; a rose-colored egg contains a "bud," whose petals spring open with the press of a button to reveal a diamond crown. The coronation of Nicholas II (the last czar) is celebrated by an egg that reveals an astonishingly detailed miniature coronation carriage—complete with working wheels and suspension.

There's much more to see: snuff boxes, watches, belt buckles, paintings, and icons. If the door's open, peek into the spectacular **Concert Hall,** with a musicians' gallery up above. The **Gold Room** displays dozens of "cabinet gifts"—many of them *objets d'fantasie* (impossibly expensive knickknacks)—presented by people who curried favor with the Romanovs. In this room, also look for striking photos of the ramshackle palace before its long restoration. The **Gothic Room** is filled with exquisite icons, some dating back to the 1600s; the **Upper Dining Room** boasts a pristine collection of late 19th- and 20th-century paintings (including Renoir's *Place de la Trinité*); and the **White and Blue Room** shows off shimmering enamel, silverwork, filigree, and porcelain.

CHURCHES

Russian Orthodoxy has revived since the end of communism.
Duck into any neighborhood church, full of incense, candles, and

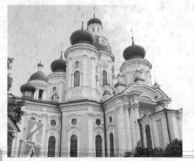

liturgical chants. It's usually OK to visit discreetly during services, when the priest opens the doors of the iconostasis, faces the altar, and leads the standing congregation in chant. Smaller churches are usually free to enter (though you can leave a small donation, or buy and light a candle) and full

of Russians morning, noon, and night, and will give you more of
a feeling for Russian religion than will church-museums such as
St. Isaac's or the Church on Spilled Blood. For more on Russian
Orthodoxy, see the sidebar on page 416.

▲▲Kazan Cathedral (Казанский Собор)

This huge, functioning house of worship, right along Nevsky
Prospekt next to the Griboyedov Canal, offers an accessible

Orthodox experience,
although its interior is not
very typical. Reopened as
a church after years as a
"Museum of Atheism," the
building has a sweeping
exterior portico patterned
after St. Peter's in Rome.

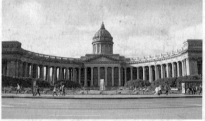

Cost and Hours: Free,
daily 9:00-20:00, services generally at 10:00 and 18:00, Kazanskaya
2, www.kazansky-spb.ru.

Visiting the Church: Although the church faces Nevsky
Prospekt, you'll enter through the west-facing main door, which is
down a side street (Ulitsa Kazanskaya).

Entering, let your eyes adjust to the low light. Built from
1799 to 1812 and now brilliantly restored, the cathedral seems to
rival its model, St. Peter's—typical of this city so determined to
be Western...only bigger and better. When Russia tunes in to TV
for Easter and Christmas services, the broadcast comes from this
church. It's often packed with Orthodox visitors from throughout
the country.

Straight ahead as you enter, appreciate the brilliant silver-
arched iconostasis. Worshippers wait in a long line to kiss the
church's namesake, the **Icon of Our Lady of Kazan** (left side of

the iconostasis). Considered the single most important icon of the Russian Orthodox faith, the original icon was discovered by a young girl (directed by a vision of the Virgin Mary) in a tunnel beneath the city of Kazan in 1579. A monastery was erected on that site, and replicas of the icon were sent to other Russian cities—including St. Petersburg—to be venerated by the faithful. The original icon was stolen from Kazan in 1904 and went missing for nearly 100 years (it resurfaced in the Vatican and was returned to Kazan in 2005, although its authenticity has been questioned). Either way, this is a replica, but still considered holy.

The icon is important partly because it was invoked in many successful military campaigns, including the successful defense of Russia during Napoleon's 1812 invasion. (The painting above shows the icon in action as Russian soldiers liberate Moscow from a brief Polish occupation in 1612.)

In the left transept, find the statue and tomb of **Field Marshal Mikhail Kutuzov** (1745-1813), who led Russian troops during the Napoleonic conflict. On the pillars flanking the tomb up above, notice the original Napoleonic banners seized in the invasion, and the keys to the cities that Kutuzov's forces retook from Napoleon as they pushed him back to Paris.

▲▲▲Church on Spilled Blood (Спас на Крови)

This exuberantly decorative church, with its gilded carrot top of onion domes, is a must-see photo op just a short walk off Nevsky

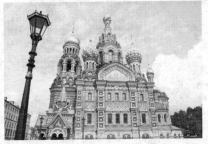

Prospekt. It's built on the place where a suicide bomber assassinated Czar Alexander II in 1881—explaining both the evocative name and the structure's out-of-kilter relationship to the surrounding street plan. Ticket windows are on the north side of the church, facing away from Nevsky Prospekt. Go inside to appreciate the mysteriously dim interior, slathered with vivid mosaics.

Cost and Hours: 250 R, Thu-Tue 10:30-18:00, closed Wed; may be open later May-Sept (likely until 22:30) for 350 R; last entry 30 minutes before closing, audioguide-100 R, Kanal Griboyedova 2b, tel. 315-1636, http://eng.cathedral.ru.

Background: Begun just after Alexander's assassination but not finished until 1907, the church is built in a neo-Russian, Historicist style. That means that its designers created a building that was a romantic, self-conscious, fairy-tale image of their own national history and traditions—similar to Neuschwanstein Castle

The Russian Orthodox Church

The Russian Orthodox Faith

In the 11th century, the Great Schism split the Christian faith into two branches: Roman Catholicism in the west (based in Rome), and Eastern or Byzantine Orthodoxy in the east (based in Constantinople—today's Istanbul).

The Eastern Orthodox Church stayed true to the earliest traditions of the Christian faith, rejecting some theological issues accepted in the West (infallibility of the pope, and the doctrines of Purgatory and the Immaculate Conception, among others). *Orthos* is Greek for "right belief"—and if you believe you've already got it right, you're resistant to change.

The Eastern Orthodox Church is divided into about a dozen branches that are administratively independent even as they share many of the same rituals. Each branch is ruled by a patriarch (similar to a pope). The largest of these—with about half of the world's 300 million Orthodox Christians—is the Russian Orthodox Church.

Under communism, the state religion—atheism—trumped the faith professed by the majority of Russians. The Russian Orthodox Church survived, but many church buildings were seized by the government and repurposed (as museums, municipal buildings, sports facilities, and so on). Many more were destroyed. Soviet citizens who openly belonged to the Church sacrificed any hope of advancement within the communist system. But since the fall of communism, Russians have flocked back to their faith. (Even President Vladimir Putin, a former KGB agent and avowed atheist, revealed that he had secretly been an Orthodox Christian all along.) These days, new churches are being built and destroyed ones are being rebuilt or renovated... and all of them, it seems, are filled with worshippers. Today, three out of every four Russian citizens follow this faith.

Visiting an Orthodox Church

The doctrines of Catholic and Orthodox churches remain similar, but many of the rituals and customs are different. These become apparent when you step inside an Orthodox church.

Before entering an active church, women should cover their heads; women and men both must have their knees covered. (Churches that are tourist attractions may be more flexible.)

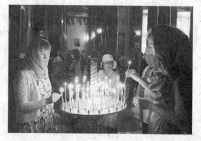

Watch worshippers arrive and go through the standard routine: Drop a coin in the wooden box, pick up a candle, say a prayer, light the candle, and place it in the candelabra. Make the sign of the cross and kiss the icon. You're welcome to join in.

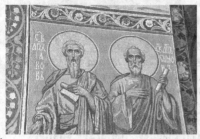

Most Orthodox church decorations consist of icons: paintings of saints, packed with intricate symbolism and cast against a shimmering golden background. These are not intended to be lifelike, but to remind viewers of the metaphysical nature of Jesus and the saints. You'll almost never see statues, which, to Orthodox people, feel a little too close to the forbidden worship of graven images.

Most Eastern Orthodox churches have at least one mosaic or painting of Christ in a standard pose—as *Pantocrator,* a Greek word meaning "Ruler of All." The image shows Christ as King of the Universe, facing directly out, with penetrating eyes and a halo-cross behind his head.

While the sanctuary is visible in Catholic churches, it's hidden in Orthodox ones. Instead, you'll see an iconostasis: an altar screen covered with curtains and icons. The standard design of the iconostasis calls for four icons flanking the central door. On the right are Jesus and John the Baptist, and on the left are Mary and the Baby Jesus (together in the first panel), and then an icon featuring the saint or event that the church is dedicated to.

The iconostasis divides the lay community from the priests— the material world from the spiritual one. The spiritual heavy lifting takes place behind the iconostasis, where the priests symbolically turn bread and wine into the body and blood of Christ. Then they open the doors or curtains and serve the Eucharist to their faithful flock.

Notice that there are few (if any) pews. Worshippers stand through the service as a sign of respect (though some older parishioners sit on the seats along the walls). Traditionally, women stand on the left side, and men on the right, equally distant from the altar (because all are equal before God). The Orthodox faith tends to use a Greek cross, with four equal arms (like a plus sign, sometimes inside a circle), which focuses on God's perfection. Many Orthodox churches have Greek-cross floor plans rather than the elongated nave-and-transept designs that are common in Western Europe.

Orthodox services generally involve chanting (a dialogue that goes back and forth between the priest and the congregation), and the church is filled with the evocative aroma of incense, heightening the experience for the worshippers.

ST. PETERSBURG

in Bavaria. Psychologically, it seems fitting that the Romanovs, as they fought a rising tide of people power and modernity, would build a church as old school and traditionally Russian as their policies and approach to governance.

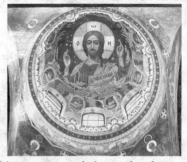

Alexander II, called "the Great Reformer," freed the serfs in 1861. He gave them land—but expected them to pay for it. The dumbfounded peasants responded by rioting, and the seeds of proletariat discontent were planted. (Alexander's liberal reforms unwittingly gave rise to the movements that would ultimately decapitate the dynasty.) Memorial plaques around the church exterior (translated in English) list Alexander's many reforms.

Jaw-droppingly beautiful as it was, the church had a short life as a place of worship. The very theme of the church—honoring an assassinated czar—was against what the Bolsheviks stood for, so it was looted with gusto during the 1917 Russian Revolution. To add insult to injury, during the communist era, the church was used for storing potatoes, and the streets around it were named for Alexander's assassins. (Out of about 300 churches in the city, only four continued to function during Soviet times.) The Church on Spilled Blood was damaged in World War II, when its crypt did duty as a morgue. Restored in the 1990s, today it serves mostly as a museum.

Visiting the Church: Enter the church and look up; Christ gazes down at you from the top of the dome, bathed in light from the windows and ringed by the gold balcony railing. The walls are covered with exquisite mosaics (nothing is painted) that show how Orthodoxy continues the artistic traditions of early Christianity. Walk up to the iconostasis (the partition at mid-church). Typically made of wood, this one is of marble, with inlaid doors. In the back of the church, the canopy shows an exposed bit of the cobbled street, marking the spot where Czar Alexander II was mortally wounded—where the czar's blood was spilled. Glass cases to the left show the painstaking restoration work.

▲▲St. Isaac's Cathedral (Исаакиевский Собор)

The gold dome of St. Isaac's glitters at the end of Malaya Morskaya Ulitsa, not far from the Admiralty. St. Isaac's was built between 1818 and 1858, and its Neoclassical exterior reminds Americans of the US Capitol building. Although the patriarch resides in Moscow, this is considered the leading church in the Russian Orthodox world.

Cost and Hours: Interior/"museum"—250 R, Thu-Tue 10:30-18:00, May-Sept may be open later (likely until 22:30) for 350 R, closed Wed year-round; roof ("colonnade")—150 R, daily 10:30-18:00, May-Oct may be open until 22:30—or even later during "White Nights"; last entry 30 minutes before closing, Isaakievskaya pl. 4, tel. 315-9732, http://eng.cathedral.ru.

Getting Tickets: Bypass the line at the ticket window by using the machines (in English, bills only—no coins). When the main ticket window takes breaks, you can buy tickets at the group window around the corner, or at the machines.

Visiting the Church: Before entering, take a minute to 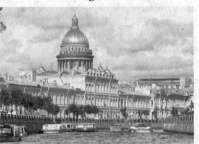 appreciate the facade. The granite steps and one-piece granite columns were shipped here from a Finnish quarry 150 miles away. (Massive stonework like this, the grand embankments, and promenades throughout the city date from Catherine the Great's rule.) The enormous building sits upon swampy land, which challenged the French architect and required a huge stone foundation.

The **interior** has a few exhibits, but ultimately it's all about the grand space. Find the case in the nave showing models of the three churches that stood here before this one. 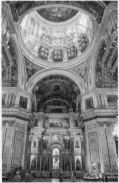 Then simply appreciate the massive scale of this church—by some measures, the fourth-largest in Christendom. Notice the grand iconostasis, with its malachite veneer columns. Because the brutal winter weather is tough on paintings, most of what looks like paintings in the church are actually mosaics, which date from the first half of the 19th century. The large mosaic panels at ground level, while made to replace canvas versions on the walls and in the dome, remain parked on the floor.

A photo display shows how, during the "Great Patriotic War" (World War II), this church's crypt protected many of the Hermitage treasures. Today, aside from a small side chapel that was reconsecrated in 1994 (at the left end of the iconostasis), this building is not a functioning house of worship—it's technically a museum.

ST. PETERSBURG

It's worthwhile to climb the colonnade stairway to the **roof** (262 steps) for the view. Every tenth step (heading up and down) is numbered in a countdown to your goal.

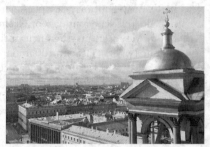

Nearby Sights: Between St. Isaac's Cathedral and the river stands one of the most evocative monuments in the city: the **Bronze Horseman.** This huge statue of a horseback Peter the Great stands atop a massive and symbolic rock inscribed, simply, "From Catherine II to Peter I, 1782."

SIGHTS NORTH OF THE NEVA RIVER

From the waterfront side of the Hermitage, you can spot several sights across the river that are worth visiting. But you'll have to allow plenty of time; while these places appear close, it takes a while to reach them by foot.

▲▲Strelka Spin-Tour

To reach the Peter and Paul Fortress from the Hermitage, you'll cross the Dvortsovy Bridge and then pass a strategic viewpoint, called Strelka. For a sweeping 360-degree view of St. Petersburg's core, head down to the park that fills the knob of land at water level (between the two pink columns).

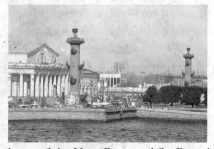

You're standing on a corner of the large **Vasilyevsky Island**—one of the many islands that make up St. Petersburg. (A nickname for the town is "City on 101 Islands," although an official count is elusive.)

Literally meaning "Little Arrow," **Strelka** sticks out into the very heart of the Neva River and St. Petersburg. The park filling the point is one of the sites around town where newlyweds are practically obligated to come for wedding pictures. They toast with champagne, then break their glasses against the big granite ball (watch your step).

To begin your spin-tour, face the can't-miss-it **Hermitage,** just across the Neva—the Winter Palace of the czars and today a world-class art museum. The sprawling complex has several wings: the main green-and-white structure, as well as the yellow and mint-green sections beyond it. No wonder it could take days to fully see the place.

Now begin spinning to the left. The Art Nouveau **Trinity Bridge** (Troitsky Most)—one of St. Petersburg's longest and most beautiful—was built in 1903, its design having beat out a submission by Gustav Eiffel. Before the 1850s, no permanent bridges spanned the Neva; one crossed only on pontoon bridges (in the summer) or a frozen river (in winter). It wasn't unusual for St. Petersburgers to get stranded while waiting for a deep freeze or a thaw. Just beyond the bridge (on its right end), you can faintly see the trees marking the delightful **Summer Garden**—the private garden for Peter the Great's cute little Summer Palace, and now a public park and a wonderful place for a warm-weather stroll (for details, see page 412).

On the left side of the river, you'll see the stoutly walled **Peter and Paul Fortress,** with its slender golden spire (for details, see page 422). St. Petersburg was born here in 1703, when Peter the Great began building this fortress to secure territory he had won in battle with the Swedes. Are there any sunbathers on the sandy beach out front?

Scanning the waterfront, think for a moment about how strategic this location is, at the mouth of the Neva River. Although very short (only 42 miles), the Neva is an essential link in a vital series of shipping waterways. It connects the Gulf of Finland to Lake Lagoda, which feeds (via a network of canals) into Russia's "mother river," the Volga—Europe's longest river, which cuts north-to-south through the Russian heartland all the way to the Caspian Sea. A series of Soviet-era shipping canals connects the Volga to the Moskva River, the Black Sea, and the Danube. That makes the Neva the outlet for all Russian waterways to all of Europe and beyond. In other words, you could sail from Iran to Volgograd to Istanbul to Budapest to Moscow to Lisbon—but you would have to go through St. Petersburg.

Turning farther left, you'll spot the first of the two giant, pink **rostral columns** that flank the Strelka viewpoint. Inspired by similar towers built by ancient Greeks and Romans to celebrate naval victories, these columns are decorated with anchors and studded with the symbolic prows of ships defeated in battle. Once topped by gaslights (now electric), the pillars trumpet St. Petersburg's nautical heritage. (A similar column stands in the middle of New York City's Columbus Circle.) Facing Strelka is the white-columned **Old Stock Exchange,** bordered by yellow warehouses.

Just to the left, the turreted pastel-blue building is Peter the Great's **Kunstkamera,** a sort of ethnographical museum built around the czar's original collection (described next). "Kunstkamera" and "Hermitage" are both European words and concepts that Peter the Great imported to class up his new, European-style capital.

Circle a bit farther to the left. The yellow buildings at the end of the bridge (just right of the Hermitage) are the **Admiralty,** the geographical center of St. Petersburg and the headquarters of Peter the Great's imperial navy.

▲Kunstkamera (Кунсткамера)

Peter the Great, who fancied himself a scientist, founded this—the first state public museum in Russia—in 1714. He filled it with

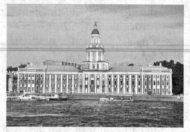

his personal collections, consisting of "fish, reptiles, and insects in bottles," scientific instruments, and books from his library. In the 19th century, Russian travelers returning from the Americas added a rich array of artifacts—and, amazingly, those original collections remain in this same building. The anthropological and ethnographic collections include the best exhibit on northern Native Americans that you'll find on this side of the Atlantic. While many tourists dismiss the Kunstkamera as a "museum of curiosities," locals are proud of its scientific tradition and its impressive collections. There's ample English information.

Cost and Hours: 250 R; Tue-Sun 11:00-19:00, closed Mon and last Tue of month, last entry at 18:00; Universitetskaya Naberezhnaya 3, enter around the left side as you face the steeple from the riverfront; tel. 328-1412, www.kunstkamera.ru.

▲▲Peter and Paul Fortress (Петропавловская Крепость)

Founded by Peter the Great in 1703 during the Great Northern War with Sweden, this fortress on an island in the Neva was the birthplace of St. Petersburg. Its gold steeple catches the sunlight,

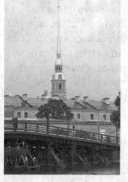

and its blank walls face the Winter Palace across the river. While it's a large complex, the most important parts are easy to see quickly: Wander the grounds, dip into the cathedral to visit the tombs of the Romanovs, and maybe do a little sunbathing on the beach. For those wanting to delve into history, the grounds also have museums about city history, space exploration, and the famous-to-Russians former prison.

Cost: It's free to enter and explore the grounds. The sights inside are covered by individual tickets (cathedral-250 R, prison-150 R, St. Petersburg history museum-100 R, fortress history museum-100 R, space/rocketry museum-50 R) and a variety of combo-tickets (cathedral and prison-350 R, everything-370 R). There are two ticket offices: one in the low, yellow pavilion just to the left of the cathedral, and another just inside the main gate.

Hours: Grounds open daily 6:00-22:00; cathedral and prison daily 10:00-19:00, last entry 30 minutes before closing; smaller museums Thu-Mon 11:00-19:00, Tue 11:00-18:00, closed Wed.

Tours and Information: The 250-R audioguide provides more information (www.spbmuseum.ru). You'll find pay WCs scattered around the grounds.

Getting There: Footbridges at either end of the fortress's island (Hare Island/Zayachy Ostrov) connect it to the rest of St. Petersburg. Getting there is easy: Just set your sights on the skinny golden spire. The main entrance is through the park from the Gorkovskaya Metro station. The other entrance is at the west end—a scenic, 20-minute walk from Palace Square and the Hermitage. Cross the bridge (Dvortsovy Most) by the Hermitage, angle right past the Strelka viewpoint (worth a quick stop to enjoy the view—described earlier), then cross the next bridge (Birzhevoy Most), turn right, and follow the waterline to a footbridge leading to the fortress' side entrance.

Background: There's been a fortress here as long as there's been a St. Petersburg. When he founded the city, in 1703, this was the first thing Peter the Great built to defend this strategic meeting point of the waterways of Russia and the Baltic. Originally the center of town was just east of here (near the preserved log cabin where Peter the Great briefly resided).

⊙ Self-Guided Tour: Pick up a map when you buy your ticket to navigate the sprawling complex. Begin at the cathedral, marked by the golden spire.

Sts. Peter and Paul Cathedral: The centerpiece of the fortress and—until modern times—the tallest building in the city, this church is the final resting place of the Romanov czars, who ruled Russia from 1613 through 1917.

The cathedral was designed by a Swiss-Italian architect who, like so many others, was imported by Peter the Great to introduce European culture to Russia. With the Bolshevik Revolution in 1917, mobs of workers and sailors ransacked the place—taking out their anger against the Romanov dynasty, desecrating the tombs, and looting everything they could. It's been a museum since 1922, and was extensively renovated in the last decade. Today, people are understandably caught up in the allure of the glamorous Romanov dynasty: White-marble monuments mark the graves of czars and czarinas, who are buried 10 feet below floor level.

ST. PETERSBURG

Entering the church, pick up a floor plan identifying each member of the dynasty. I'll cover just a few highlights.

Start by facing the main altar, with its glittering **iconostasis** and its traditional Orthodox imagery painted in the Russian Baroque style. From here we'll circle clockwise to visit the most important tombs. The tombs to the right (as you face the altar) include perhaps the two greatest czars. On the right, in front, is **Peter the Great** (1672-1725). Marked by his bronze bust, the founder of the city was the first czar to be buried here. He's surrounded by other 18th-century rulers, including **Catherine II "the Great"** (1729-1796, back left).

Now turn 180 degrees and walk straight back to the opposite end of the church. To the left of the entry door is a small chapel containing the tombs of the much-romanticized family of the final Romanov czar: **Nicholas II** (1868-1918), his wife, Alexandra, and their four daughters and one son. The czar abdicated in March 1917, and was imprisoned with the rest of his family. The Bolsheviks murdered them all on the night of July 16, 1918. The family was shot at point-blank range with handguns. Because the daughters had diamonds sewn into their dresses, some of the bullets deflected at crazy angles—to be sure they were dead, the assassins bayoneted them. Originally buried in an unmarked grave, the remains of most of the family members were only rediscovered in 1991, and reburied here in 1998.

Persistent legends surround the fate of the Romanov daughter **Anastasia,** who was rumored to have escaped the execution. In the decades since the massacre, different women emerged claiming to be the long-lost Anastasia—most famously Anna Anderson, who turned up in Berlin in the 1920s. But very recent DNA testing has positively identified the remains of the real Anastasia (found only in 2007 and now interred here), while similar tests disproved Anderson's claim.

In the middle of the church, about a third of the way from the main door to the iconostasis, on the left, is **Maria Fedorovna** (1847-1928). This popular Danish princess (known as Dagmar in her native land) moved from Copenhagen to St. Petersburg, married the second-to-the-last czar (Alexander III, next white tomb), gave birth to the last czar (Nicholas II), and fled the October Revolution to live in exile in Denmark. After her death, she was buried with her fellow Danish royals at Roskilde Cathedral; in 2006, her remains were brought back here with great fanfare to join her adopted clan. Hers is one of the most popular graves in the church.

History Exhibit: Exit through the gift shop (to the left of the main altar), but before leaving, turn right from the shop into a hall with a visual and well-described history of the church and the

Romanov dynasty, complete with a family tree and portraits. At the end of this corridor is a collection of tombs of other Romanovs including late 20th-century family members—grand dukes and grand duchesses—reminding us that many Romanov cousins long outlived their ancestors.

Tower Climb: To climb the spire for a grand view, find the stairs and buy a special 150-R ticket just inside the cathedral entry.

The Grounds: Strolling the grounds, you'll get an up-close look at the stout brick wall surrounding the island. From the cathedral, head out through the gateway for a peek at the river. You can also circle around the fortress exterior to find the delightful sandy beach huddled alongside the wall—an understandably popular place for St. Petersburgers to sunbathe on balmy days, and for newlyweds to snap wedding portraits.

There are two ways to **climb up onto the wall** encircling the fortress. The "Neva Curtain Wall" (facing away from the river) is included in the comprehensive combo-ticket; the more scenic "Neva Panorama" (on the river side) has a separate 250-R ticket.

▲Museum of Russian Political History
(Музея политической истории России)

This is the city's best exhibit about Russia's communist period. Across the moat from the Peter and Paul Fortress, it's partly housed in a mansion where Lenin had an office, and sprawls through several attached buildings. The eclectic collection is best appreciated by someone with a cursory understanding of modern Russian history. The core exhibit—"Man and Power in Russia, 19th-21st Centuries"—is modern and freshly presented, employing historical artifacts, photography, archival footage, sound clips, and touchscreens. Some English information is posted, and you can borrow descriptions in most exhibits, but it's worth investing in one of the audioguides (each with a different focus—ask about your options).

Cost and Hours: 150 R, Fri-Tue 10:00-18:00, Wed 10:00-20:00, closed Thu and last Mon of month, last entry one hour before closing, audioguides-200 R each, Kuybysheva 2-4 but enter around the corner facing the park at Kronverkskiy Prospekt 1, tel. 233-7052, www.polithistory.ru.

▲Peter the Great's Log Cabin

The oldest surviving building in St. Petersburg is the log cabin that served as Peter's first "palace" when he arrived to oversee the building of his great city in 1703. (He was only Peter I then, not becoming "Great" until 1721.) Peter was fighting Sweden (then a major European power), and with the foundation of St. Petersburg here, on former Swedish soil, he was making it clear: This was Russia...and Russia now had a gateway to the Baltic Sea, and

ST. PETERSBURG

Peter the Great

Every so often, an individual comes along who revolutionizes an entire people. While Russia has had more than its share of those figures, perhaps the most dynamic and influential was Peter the Great.

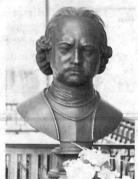

During the four decades he ruled Russia (1682-1725), Czar Peter I transformed his country into a major European power. Even more self-assured than your average monarch, Peter gave himself the nickname "Peter the Great"—and it stuck. He stood well over six feet tall, and he ruled Russia with a towering power and determination. Full of confidence and charm, Peter mixed easily with all classes of people and at times even dressed cheaply and spoke crudely.

Peter grew up at court in Moscow. In a formative episode, the newly crowned, 10-year-old Peter witnessed a bloody palace coup that sidelined him in a co-rulership for years. But Peter's exile put him in proximity to Moscow's German community, a source of bold new ideas that jolted his worldview. He was particularly taken with the Protestant work ethic, and was fascinated by the idea that humans could conquer nature. He saw this mindset as a refreshing antidote for the fatalistic Russian Orthodox outlook.

Peter came into his own as sole ruler in 1689, and quickly began making up for lost time. He became the first czar in a century to travel to Europe in peacetime, making an epic journey to

thus to Europe. All the buildings in the original settlement in the swamp were made of wood. This one (actually a log cabin contained within a bigger, modern brick structure, in a tidy riverfront park) is just six sparsely, yet evocatively, furnished rooms with an attached exhibit on the birth of St. Petersburg.

Cost and Hours: 200 R, Wed and Fri-Mon 10:00-18:00, Thu 13:00-21:00, closed Tue, Petrovskaya Naberezhnaya 6, tel. 232-4576.

▲Cruiser Aurora

The Soviet Union created a thrilling and inspirational mythology about the revolution that created it. According to popular history, that uprising kicked off with a shot from the battleship *Aurora*, a signal to revolutionaries to storm the Winter Palace. (Usually positioned on the Petrogradskaya embankment, the *Aurora* is currently under renovation elsewhere in the city until sometime in 2016.) State-of-the-art when built about 1900, the *Aurora* fought in the Russo-Japanese War (1904-1905). Later, its guns defended

Holland and England, great maritime powers from whom Peter wanted to learn everything he could about shipbuilding, technology, navigation, and seamanship. He even went undercover for a stint in an Amsterdam shipyard, sleeping in a humble cupboard bed.

Upon his return, Peter began implementing reforms to give Russia a fresh start. To encourage his subjects to be more enterprising, he created a 14-level "table of ranks," designed to reward hard work rather than simply heredity. He did away with symbols of the old world, such as long beards, literally shaving the beards right off of his advisors' faces.

Internationally, Peter the Great refashioned Russia's army to resemble Western models, and he founded the Russian navy. He started the Great Northern War with Sweden to ensure that Russia would have access to the Baltic Sea for trade and strategic purposes. He built an entirely new capital in St. Petersburg and established a shipbuilding industry there. He reorganized the government and introduced new taxes to support his foreign policy.

Although Peter is revered by many Russians today, his reign was not without scandal. A heavy drinker with a short temper, Peter was known to lash out against even his closest advisors. He had his own son killed and exiled his first wife to a convent.

Despite his cruelties, Peter left a positive imprint on Russian history. When Peter took the throne, Russia was a backwater, stuck in the Middle Ages. By the time he died, his country had become a European powerhouse.

Leningrad during the Nazi siege in World War II; when it looked like the Germans might take the city, the Soviets sunk the *Aurora* rather than let this relic of the Revolution fall into their hands. After the war, the much-adored ship was salvaged and substantially rebuilt. It's remained a symbol of the Revolution with an almost religious significance for pilgrims from throughout Russia. This is a first stop for many Russians touring St. Petersburg, and it's fun to make the scene here with them. The gun on the bow with the brass plaque tells the story. When it returns to the Petrogradskaya embankment, the cruiser will likely open for tours once again (for details, see www.aurora.org.ru).

OUTER ST. PETERSBURG
▲▲Peterhof (Петергоф)

Peter the Great's lavish palace at Peterhof (sometimes still called by its communist name, Petrodvorets/Петродворец) sits along the Gulf of Finland west of the city. With glorious gardens, this is Russia's Versailles and the target of many tour groups and travel poster photographers. Promenade along the grand canal, which runs through landscaped grounds from the boat dock up to the terraced fountains in front of the palace. You can visit the museum inside the palace if you want, but it's more fun to stay outdoors. Children love to run past the trick fountains—sometimes they splash you, sometimes they don't.

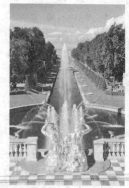

Cost and Hours: Park—500 R, open daily in summer 9:00-20:00, last entry 17:45; Grand Palace museum—550 R, Tue-Sun 10:30-18:00, until 19:00 in summer, closed Mon, May-mid-Oct open longer hours on Sat (10:00-21:00, last entry at 19:45); audioguide-500 R, www.peterhofmuseum.ru. Consider investing in the good 100-R guide-booklet that helps you locate each fountain.

Getting There: In summer, "Meteor" **hydrofoils,** run by competing companies, leave for Peterhof from docks to either side of the busy bridge by the Hermitage (first boat leaves around 10:00 and every 30 minutes thereafter, last boat returns from Peterhof at 18:00—or at 18:30 or 19:00 in summer, ask before you buy your ticket); 30-40-minute trip, 650-700 R one way, 1,100-1,200 R roundtrip, plus 500 R entry to the palace grounds; hydrofoils stop running in even mildly strong winds). Of the hydrofoil companies, only one has a good English website (www.peterhof-express.com, tel. 647-0017).

If it's windy, or to save money, you can take **public transportation:** Ride the Metro to the lavishly decorated Avtovo station, cross the street to the right, and find a gang of *marshrutka* minibuses with signs for *Peterhof.* For variety, consider riding the minibus to the top end of the gardens, enjoy the half-mile stroll downhill through the grounds, and return via hydrofoil.

▲▲▲Tsarskoye Selo (Царское Село)

About 15 miles south of St. Petersburg is the charming small town of Pushkin. Back when Peter the Great started construction of a summer palace here, it was called Tsarskoye Selo—literally "Czars' Village." The site features a spectacular cluster of over-the-top-opulent Romanov palaces, pavilions, and gardens, built by Peter and his heirs (mostly in the 18th century).

The main attraction is the **Catherine Palace,** famous for its breathtaking Amber Room. Arguably Russia's single most enjoyable palace to tour (and that's saying something), the Catherine Palace lacks the staggering scale and world-class paintings of the

Hermitage, but gives you much more insight into the dynamic czars and czarinas who ruled Russia. (For more on the Romanov family tree, see the sidebar on page 430.)

Peter the Great and his wife, Catherine I, built the original palace at Tsarskoye Selo starting in 1717—when St. Petersburg itself was still in its infancy. In the following decades, the palace was rebuilt and expanded many times, most notably by Peter and Catherine's daughter, Elizabeth, who wanted to make it Russia's answer to Versailles. Most of what you see today was designed by the Italian architect Francesco Bartolomeo Rastrelli in Elizabethan Baroque style. Later, Catherine the Great left her own mark on the palace, expanding and renovating in the more restrained Neoclassical style (with the help of Scottish architect Charles Cameron).

Because the palace had been turned into a museum (and carefully documented) after the Bolshevik Revolution, conservators could authentically restore it from the damage it suffered in World War II. The highlight of their restoration work (and of your visit) is the **Amber Room,** a

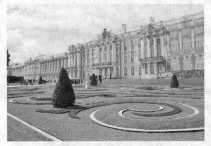

painstakingly accurate replica of the lavish original, whose decorative wall panels were a gift to the Romanovs from Frederick the Great, but looted and lost in the war. Outside, you could spend hours—or days—exploring the sprawling grounds of the **Catherine Park** that surrounds the palace. While it's possible to enter some of the garden's landmark attractions, it's perfectly enjoyable to simply go for a walk in the park.

Cost and Hours: Palace—400 R, 550 R if purchased in advance online; open Wed-Mon 10:00-18:00 (during May-Sept, individuals can enter only 12:00-16:00—see below), closed Tue year-round; off-season also closed last Mon of month; audioguide-150 R, tel. 466-6669, http://eng.tzar.ru. Park—120-R admission fee collected May-Sept 9:00-17:00, free at other times; open daily 7:00-21:00.

Getting There: Tsarskoye Selo is most easily reached with a **guide,** who can provide door-to-door service and an efficient, highly focused tour of just the highlights (for private guide services, see page 371).

Crowd-Beating Tips: In peak season (May-Sept), individuals may enter the Catherine Palace only from 12:00 until 16:00, and tickets can sell out. To be sure you'll get in, reserve a ticket online (550 R, up to 4 tickets per order, includes entry to Catherine

Romanovs 101

As you tour the many imperial sights in and near St. Petersburg, this cheat sheet will keep you oriented to the Romanov czars and czarinas who built this city and ruled it until the Bolshevik Revolution in the early 20th century. The Romanov dynasty began in 1613 with Mikhail Romanov—but I'll start with his more famous descendant...

Peter I "the Great" (1689-1725): Dynamic and reform-minded, Peter was the founder of modern Russia. He famously moved the capital city from Moscow to St. Petersburg. (For more on Peter, see the sidebar on page 426.) When Peter died, his wife Catherine (1684-1727) became empress; at her death, the throne passed to Peter's grandson from a prior marriage...

Peter II (1715-1730): He ruled only two years before dying of an illness. Because the teenaged Peter II lacked an heir, the throne reverted to Peter the Great's half-brother's daughter...

Anna (1693-1740): After a decade as czarina, Anna died of kidney disease. Her infant nephew, Ivan VI, was quickly deposed in a palace coup to install Anna's cousin...

Elizabeth (1709-1762): The overindulged daughter of Peter the Great and Catherine I, Elizabeth was raised in the lap of luxury at the Catherine Palace (which she later bathed in the frilly Elizabethan Baroque style). She never married, so the throne passed to her cousin Anna's son...

Peter III (1728-1762): He ruled just six months before being assassinated in a palace coup to install his wife...

Catherine II "the Great" (1729-1796): A German aristocrat who had married into the Romanov clan, Catherine enjoyed a very successful 34-year reign. She never remarried, but maintained (suspiciously) close relations with a trusted circle of mostly male advisors. The practical Catherine eschewed Baroque excess and popularized a more restrained Neoclassicism. Catherine wasn't fond of her only son, whom she was unable to prevent from succeeding her.

Paul I (1754-1801): Catherine's son ruled only five years before a palace coup assassinated him to install his son...

Park); you'll receive an email voucher that you'll exchange for a ticket at the booth near the Palace Church gate (look for onion domes, open Wed-Mon 12:00-16:00; must show ID).

▲Piskaryovskoye Memorial Cemetery
(Пискарёвское Мемориальное Кладбище)

This is a memorial to the hundreds of thousands who died in the city during the Nazi Siege of Leningrad in World War II. The cemetery, with its eternal flame, acres of mass grave bunkers (marked only with the year of death), moving statue of Mother Russia, and many pilgrims bringing flowers to remember lost

Alexander I (1777-1825): Alexander's grandmother Catherine aspired to make him the czar that she believed her son, Paul, could never be. Alexander enjoyed a long (nearly 25-year) but melancholy reign, while pursuing a more dynamic version of his grandma's Neoclassicism, called the Russian Empire style. When Alexander fell ill and died, he made way for his much younger brother...

Nicholas I (1796-1855): During his 30-year reign, Russia had high points (territorial expansion) and low points (the loss of the Crimean War). Upon his death, the throne passed to his son...

Alexander II (1818-1881): Alexander "the Liberator," who was czar for a quarter-century, boldly freed the serfs in 1861—but also instituted a convoluted land-redemption process that caused peasant uprisings (foreshadowing the eventual fall of the czarist regime). A left-wing terrorist group assassinated Alexander II in St. Petersburg (at the site of the Church on Spilled Blood). The throne passed to his son...

Alexander III (1881-1894): During his uneventful 15 years as czar, Alexander reversed some of his father's reforms and continued the Romanov trends of the 19th century: exuberant imperial decadence coupled with crippling societal ills. The empire was in decline, leaving a mess for Alexander III's son...

Nicholas II (1868-1918): This czar and his family have been much romanticized for their lavish lifestyle and tragic end. Seduced by the trappings of imperial life, and unwilling to grapple with the realities of a changing world, they retreated to Alexander's Place (in Tsarskoye Selo) and sought solace in the advice of the charismatic and enigmatic mystic, Rasputin. Nicholas oversaw Russia's failed foray into World War I (resulting in millions of Russian deaths) and was ultimately deposed by the February Revolution in 1917, setting the stage for the rise of Vladimir Lenin's Bolsheviks.

On July 17, 1918, Nicholas and his family (including his larger-than-life daughter, Anastasia) were executed by a firing squad—ending more than three centuries of Romanov rule from St. Petersburg.

loved ones, is an awe-inspiring experience even for an American tourist to whom the Siege of Leningrad is just another page from the history books.

Cost and Hours: Free, daily 9:00-21:00, until 18:00 in winter, www.pmemorial.ru.

Getting There: The memorial is northeast of the city at Nepokorennykh Prospekt 72. From downtown, take the red Metro line (catch it at Uprising Square, near the end of Nevsky Prospekt) and ride it toward Devyatkino, getting off at the Ploshchad Muzhestva stop. Exit to the street, cross to the eastbound bus stop, and take bus #123 to the sixth stop—you'll see the cemetery buildings on your left.

Shopping in St. Petersburg

With vivid cultural artifacts for sale at reasonable prices, St. Petersburg is an obvious shopping stop for many tourists.

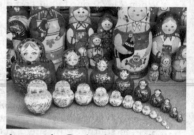

The famous Russian **nesting dolls** called *matryoshka* are one of the most popular items. The classic design shows a ruby-cheeked Russian peasant woman, wearing a babushka and traditional dress, but don't miss the entertaining modern interpretations. You'll see Russian heads of state (Peter the Great inside Lenin inside Stalin inside Gorbachev inside Putin), as well as every American professional and college sports team you can imagine—each individual player wearing his actual number. Other popular gifts include **amber** pieces and delicately painted **wooden eggs.**

High-quality **porcelain** is sold at numerous outlets of the Imperial Porcelain Factory (Императорский Фарфоровый Завод, sometimes referred to by its Soviet-era name, Lomonosov), which made fine tableware for the czars (there's one at Nevsky Prospekt 60, www.imp.ru).

You'll find colorful Russian **shawls** and **scarves** as well as tablecloths and **linens** at Pavloposadskie Platki (Павлопосадские платки, at Nevsky Prospekt 87 and elsewhere around town, www.platki.ru)—including entertaining themed patterns that memorialize events from Russian history and the lives of favorite saints.

St. Petersburg's major sights have excellent **museum gift shops,** such as those in the Hermitage and at the Russian Museum.

Big, glitzy **souvenir shops** (like the one facing the Moyka, just off Palace Square) offer a wide variety of items, but the prices are inflated to cover a 30 percent kickback for tour guides—even if you're on your own. Other, similar shops are typically located near major sights—consider popping in to Galeria Naslediye (Галерея Наследие) to check out the selection of *matryoshka*, imitation Fabergé eggs, and amber (between the Hermitage and the Church on Spilled Blood on the Moyka embankment at Naberezhnaya reki Moyki 37, www.souvenirboutique.com).

Entertainment in St. Petersburg

▲▲Ballet

St. Petersburg is synonymous with classical ballet. Durable masterpieces like "Swan Lake" were first staged at the city's Mariinsky Theater, and many of the world's star dancers, past and present (Anna Pavlova, Rudolf Nureyev, Mikhail Baryshnikov), have trained and performed here.

The best venues in St. Petersburg for ballet are the Mariinsky Theater and the Mikhailovsky Theater. Ballet season at both theaters runs from mid-September to mid-July. Both theaters have storied histories, classic opera-house interiors (the Mariinsky's is a bit more opulent), and well-designed websites that allow you to buy tickets online in advance, in English (you may first have to create a registration account). Same-day tickets are often available (though not for the most popular ballets).

Although the historic Mariinsky (formerly Kirov) company is the most famous, there are other ballet troupes in town. Some companies stage summer performances especially for tourists (but usually not with their "A-list" dancers).

The **Mikhailovsky Theater** is conveniently located, at Ploshchad Isskustv 1, by the Russian Museum, a block off Nevsky (box office open daily 10:00-21:00, tel. 595-4305, www.mikhailovsky.ru).

The **Mariinsky Theater** (formerly the Kirov Theater) has grown into a complex of buildings southwest of St. Isaac's Cathedral, at Teatralnaya Ploshchad. Two separate but associated buildings face each other across a canal near "Theater Square": the original, traditional Mariinsky Theater; and the brand-new, sleek, and state-of-the-art Mariinsky II opera house. A couple of long blocks to the west, on Pisareva street, is the modern, lower-profile Concert Hall. Be clear on which venue you're attending (box office open 11:00-19:00, tel. 326-4141, www.mariinsky.ru). Buses take you right to Theater Square. Alternatively, you can take the Metro to Sadovaya and walk about 20 minutes.

Opera and Classical Music

Besides ballet, the Mariinsky and Mikhailovsky theaters host world-class opera and musical performances. Your best bet is to peruse their websites to see what's on; unfortunately, the theaters go dark in August.

Folk Music and Dancing

Every night, a hardworking troupe puts on a touristy, crowd-pleasing Russian folklore show at the Nikolaevsky Palace (near the Neva embankment, southwest of St. Isaac's Cathedral). The show kicks off with a men's a cappella quartet, followed by two different dance groups. The experience includes some light snacks and drinks. Popular with big bus groups, it's a rollicking introduction to Russian folk clichés. As seating is first-come, first-served, be sure to arrive early (nightly shows at 19:00, box office open daily 11:00-21:00, Ploshchad Truda 4, tel. 312-5500, or reserve by email at office@folkshow.ru or online at www.folkshow.ru).

▲Circus

The St. Petersburg circus is a revelation: Performed in one intimate ring, it has the typical tigers and lions but also a zany assortment of other irresistible animal acts (ostriches, poodles) as well as aerial acrobats (no nets), impossibly silly clowns, and more. Its performers have been staging their shows since 1877 in the stone "big top" on the edge of the Fontanka River. It's just east of the Russian Museum; some maps label it "Ciniselli Circus" after the Italian circus family that first built the place. Like many other entertainment options in town, the circus shuts down in summer—the season typically runs from September through May (tickets 500-2,000 R, box office open daily 11:00-19:00, tel. 570-5390 or 570-5411, www.circus.spb.ru).

Eating in St. Petersburg

St. Petersburg has a huge selection of eating options. It's easy to find attractive cafés and restaurants, but hard to find value-priced ones. While Nevsky Prospekt is lined with inviting eateries, you'll eat better for less if you explore even a block off the main touristy drag. The listings below are all well-located or good values, and all have English-language menus.

Many cafés offer speedy, convenient light meals (sandwiches, light meals, salads, and crêpes—*bliny*). Столовая (Stolovaya, "diner") is a good word to look for if you're in need of a quick and easy meal. Russians are big on soups and appetizers, and it's perfectly reasonable to order two or three of these at a meal and skip the main dishes. Some restaurants have "business lunch" specials, served until 15:30 or 16:00.

RUSSIAN FOOD

Cosmopolitan St. Petersburg has international tastes, so truly "traditional" Russian restaurants are scarce (and mostly aimed at either at tourists or a fine-dining crowd). More commonly, you'll see restaurants with eclectic international menus (Mediterranean, Thai, burgers, etc.) and a few, token Russian classics.

Russians love soup—popular kinds are beet borscht, fish *ukha*, cabbage *shchi*, and meat *solyanka*. Russian cuisine is heavy on small dishes that we might think of as appetizers or sides, such as *pelmeni* and *vareniki* (types of dumplings), *kasha* (buckwheat groats) prepared in various ways, *bliny,* and high-calorie salads. Bread is often served as an automatic side order in restaurants.

In recent years, both local and Western franchise restaurants have sprouted up all over Russia. You'll see Subway, Pizza Hut, KFC, McDonald's, and more. Popular Russian chains such as Teremok and Chainaya Lozhka serve authentic food and can be convenient time-savers during a day of sightseeing.

Russian beer is good. It goes without saying that there are many vodkas to choose from. Russians like to drink inexpensive sparkling wine that's still called *Sovyetskoye shampanskoye* (Soviet champagne). Try *kvas,* a fizzy, fairly sweet, grain-based beverage that is marketed as non-alcoholic (but often has a negligible alcohol content) and *mors* (berry juice). In Russia, always drink bottled water, which is available widely in shops.

SIT-DOWN RESTAURANTS

All of these youthful places (except the Russian Vodka Room No. 1) offer a peek at Russian hipster culture and diverse menus with international and Russian dishes.

Zoom Café (Zoom Кафе) has a lively atmosphere and a fresh menu. Popular and a good value, it's in a pleasant basement-level dining room just off Griboyedov Canal, a bit south of Nevsky Prospekt (160-240-R soups, 240-480-R main courses, by the corner of Gorokhovaya and Kazanskaya at Gorokhovaya Ulitsa 22, Mon-Fri 9:00-24:00, Sat 11:00-24:00, Sun 13:00-24:00, food served until 22:30, tel. 612-1329).

Pelmeniya (Пельмения) is a great place to sample the food for which it's named: delicious filled dumplings. Besides Russian *pelmeni,* choices include *khinkali* (from Georgia, with a thick dough "handle"), *varenyky* (from Ukraine, like Polish pierogi), *manti* (from Turkey and the Caucasus), *gyoza* (from Asia), and even ravioli. The modern interior overlooks the Fontanka River next to the Anichkov Bridge (140-240-R small portion, 250-400-R large portion, well-described English menu, daily 11:00-23:00, Fontanka 25, tel. 571-8082).

Obshhestvo Chistyh Tarelok (Общество Чистых Тарелок/"Clean Plates Society") has a great energy, powered by loud music and a lively thirtysomething clientele. The mismatched-lumber bar and oversized Ikea chandeliers hint at the varied international fare, from burgers to curry to some Russian standbys (200-270-R soups, 300-500-R meals, daily 12:00-late, Gorokhovaya 13, tel. 934-9764, www.cleanplates.ru).

Kartofel s Gribami (Картофель с Грибами/"Potatoes with Mushrooms") is a fun, jazzy, and central hangout serving unpretentious but thoughtfully crafted Russian "street food"—such as *kapsalon* (a traditional casserole, available with various fillings) and the stuffed-pita sandwich called *shaverma* (300-400-R dishes, daily 12:00-24:00, Gorokhovaya 12, tel. 994-0983).

Lyubimoe Mesto 22.13 (Любимое Место/"Favorite Place 22.13") is a bombastic, multilevel, colorful restaurant just around the corner from the Church on Spilled Blood. Its trendy interior is crammed under old vaults, and the pricey but crowd-pleasing menu offers something for everyone (300-500-R starters, soups, and pizzas, 400-600-R main courses and big salads, Konyushennaya Ploshchad 2, tel. 647-8050).

Decabrist Café (Декабрист Кафе), casual and lively, has a rustic but modern interior in a handy location near St. Isaac's Cathedral. They have light meals and soups (200-350 R), burgers and traditional Russian dishes (300-400 R), and a 250-R three-course weekday lunch deal (daily 8:00-22:00, Yakubovicha 2, tel. 912-1891, www.decabrist.net).

Stuffy, Traditional Russian Cuisine: **Russian Vodka Room No. 1,** connected with St. Petersburg's vodka museum, is a fancier, more expensive restaurant with classy food and service (and yes, 200 types of vodka) that caters to tourists. You can choose between the elegant, old-time interior or the sidewalk seating, facing the busy boulevard. It's a little beyond St. Isaac's Cathedral—trolleybuses #5 and #22 stop conveniently on the same street. The huge building has multiple restaurants—look for the Vodka Room between entrances (подъезд) 5 and 6 (500-1,000-R main courses, daily 12:00-24:00, Konnogvardeisky Bulvar 4, tel. 570-6420).

"New Russian" Farm-to-Table Eateries: For something a notch above the places listed earlier, foodies dig into these two. **Vkus Yest** (Вкус Есть, "Taste Eat"), with a spare, bare-brick-walls dining room, faces the Bolshoi Drama Theater across the Fontanka River, and there's jazz on the soundtrack. Brief, constantly changing, and adventurous, the menu is fun to explore. The name is a pun: Есть means both "to eat" and "there is" (200-350-R soups and pastas, 350-600-R main courses, daily 12:00-23:00, Fontanka 23, tel. 983-3376, www.ofwgroup.ru). **Cococo** (Кококо) fills its laid-back, mellow cellar with rustic tables and decor that's a mix of old and new. The fun-to-read placemat menu includes old dishes done a new way, as well as some more innovative alternatives. Compared to Vkus Yest, it's pricier, the portions are smaller, and it's a bit hit-or-miss—but it's still well worth trying (350-450-R soups, 450-800-R main courses, open daily 12:00-late, Nekrasova 8, tel. 579-0016, www.kokoko.spb.ru).

Speedy Chain Restaurants

Teremok (Теремок) is a chain with branches literally all over town. It's quick and convenient for those who don't speak Russian,

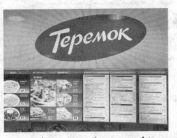

handy for families, and lets you share and try lots of different dishes. Though sometimes derided as "Russian fast food," it actually serves a perfectly healthy array of Russian standards at very affordable prices. Choose borscht, *ukha* (fish soup), *pelmeni* (dumplings), sweet or savory *bliny* (crepes), or *kasha* (buckwheat groats) prepared in various ways. *Kvas* and *mors* (berry juice) are on the drinks menu. It's the setting that is fast-foody, complete with orange uniforms for the staff, plastic trays filled at the sales counter, and trash bins for your paper plates and napkins. Expect somewhat brisk service, and if you don't see the English menu brochure, ask for it—or just point to the photos on the posted menu (100-200-R main courses; Bolshaya Morskaya Ulitsa 11, Nevsky Prospekt 60, and Vladimirsky Prospekt 3 are three of many locations; all open daily at least 10:00-23:00).

Stolle (Штолле), another chain, specializes in crispy pies, both savory and sweet. Their handiest location, near the start of Nevsky Prospekt (at #11), combines order-at-the-counter, point-to-what-you-want efficiency with a refined drawing-room atmosphere. This makes it popular with local tour guides...and with pickpockets. Ask for their English menu. They tend to sell out of many flavors later in the day (pies sold by size—figure about 200 R for a large portion, daily 9:00-22:00).

GEORGIAN FOOD

Although any Georgian will tell you it is not "Russian," Georgian cuisine is a much appreciated, flavorful alternative that's popular with Russians and visitors alike. Some of the classic Georgian dishes are *khachapuri* (хачапури)—hot bread filled with cheese, somewhat like a calzone; *khinkali* (хинкали)—a hearty filled dumpling gathered into a thick, doughy "handle" and dipped into sauces; *pkhali* (пхали)—chopped greens; chicken *satsivi* (сациви)—diced chicken in a spicy yellow sauce; *baklazhan* (баклажан)—eggplant; *lobio* (лобио)—beans, served hot or cold; and plenty of *lavash* (лаваш)—bread. If you want soup, try *kharcho* (харчо), a spicy broth with lots of meat and onions. Main dishes (often grilled meat) are less special.

Cat Café (КЭт Кафе)—an institution for expats in St. Petersburg since the end of communism—has a cozy, traditional interior with only eight tables and a friendly vibe (300-500-R *khachapuri*, 250-375-R soups, 300-500-R main courses, reservations recommended, Stremyannaya Ulitsa 22, daily 12:00-23:00, tel. 571-3377, www.cafe-cat.ru).

What If I Miss My Boat?

Remember that you can get help from the cruise line's port agent (listed on the destination information sheet distributed on the ship) and the local TI (see page 362). If the port agent suggests a costly solution (such as a private car with a driver), you may want to consider public transit.

Your biggest concern is a visa. If you've entered St. Petersburg with an excursion (meaning without a visa), chances are your ship won't leave without you, since they are responsible for your presence in Russia. On the off chance that you're left behind, head for the US embassy to navigate the red tape—your lack of a visa will make leaving the country next to impossible without soliciting help.

If do you have a visa and missed your ship, you can reach **Helsinki** on the fast train (trains leave from Finland Station/Finlyandsky Vokzal/Финляндский Вокзал, Metro: Ploshchad Lenina; train info: www.vr.fi) or a much slower bus. To **Tallinn,** ride the slow bus or the occasional St. Peter Line overnight boat (www.stpeterline.com). To reach **Stockholm** or **Rīga,** you'll probably do best to connect through Tallinn.

If you need to catch a **plane** to your next destination, St. Petersburg's Pulkovo airport is reachable by a Metro-plus-bus combination (via the Moskovskaya Metro stop; www.pulkovoairport.ru).

Local **travel agents** in St. Petersburg can help you. For more advice on what to do if you miss the boat, see page 139.

Khochu Kharcho (Хочу Харчо, literally "I want Georgian soup") is a big, boisterous, industrial-strength restaurant facing the busy Sennaya square (where three Metro lines converge). This sprawling mash-up of modern and traditional comes with several seating areas, a busy open kitchen with a wood-fired grill and tandoor oven, and an enticing photo menu that makes ordering easy. While aimed squarely at Russian tourists (think of it as the local answer to the Hard Rock Café), it offers a lively and accessible—if pricey—sample of Georgian fare (350-500-R soups, 400-550-R *khachapuri,* 450-800-R main dishes, open daily 24 hours, Sadovaya 39—next to the small footbridge at the southwest corner of the square, tel. 640-1616).

Tarkhun (Таркун, "Tarragon"), a block off the Fontanka River between the Fabergé Museum and the circus, is a more upscale place to try Georgian fare (300-400-R soups, 350-600-R main dishes, daily 12:00-23:30, Karavannaya 14, tel. 377-6525).

VEGETARIAN FARE

Café Botanika (Кафе Ботаника) is a few blocks beyond the Russian Museum, past the Summer Garden and just over the

Fontanka River. It's fresh and attractive, with seating both indoors and streetside. The menu includes Russian, Indian, Italian, and Japanese dishes (200-250-R soups, 300-500-R main courses, daily 11:00-24:00, Ulitsa Pestelya 7, tel. 272-7091).

Troitsky Most (Троицкий Мост) is a tiny, inexpensive vegetarian café just north of Nevsky along the Moyka River. Order at the counter and then find a seat—a board, partly translated into English, lists the day's specials (130-150-R main courses, daily 9:00-23:00, Naberezhnaya Reki Moyki 30).

Russian Survival Phrases

Russia comes with a more substantial language barrier than most of Europe. In general, young Russians know at least a little halting schoolroom English; hoteliers and museum clerks may speak only a few words; and older people speak none at all.

For help with decoding the Cyrillic alphabet, see the sidebar on page 363.

English	Russian / Transliteration	Pronunciation
Hello. (formal)	Здравствуйте. / Zdravstvuyte.	**zdrah**-stvee-tyeh
Hi. (informal)	Привет. / Privyet.	pree-**vyeht**
Goodbye.	До свидания. / Do svidaniya.	dah svee-**dahn**-yah
Do you speak English?	Вы говорите по-английски? / Vy govoritye po angliyski?	vih gah-vah-**ree**-tyeh pah ahn-**glee**-skee
I (don't) understand.	Я (не) понимаю. / Ya (nye) ponimaui.	yah (nyeh) poh-nee-**mah**-yoo
Yes.	Да. / Da.	dah
No.	Нет. / Nyet.	nyeht
Please.	Пожалуйста. / Pozhaluysta.	pah-**zhahl**-stah
Thank you.	Спасибо. / Spasibo.	spah-**see**-bah
Excuse me.	Извините. / Izvinitye.	eez-vee-**nee**-tyeh
(Very) good.	(Очень) хорошо. / (Ochen) khorosho	(**oh**-cheen) kha-**roh**-show
How much?	Сколько стоит? / Skolko stoit?	**skohl**-kah **stoh**-yeet
one, two	один, два / odin, dva	ah-deen, dvah
three, four	три, четыре / tri, chetyre	tree, cheh-**teer**-yeh
five, six	пять, шесть / pyat, shest	pyaht, shyest
seven, eight	семь, восемь / sem, vosem	syehm, **vwoh**-sehm
nine, ten	девять, десять / devyat, desyat	**dyeh**-veht, **dyeh**-seht
Where is...?	Где...? / Gdye...?	guh-**dyeh**
...the toilet	...туалет / tualet	too-ahl-**yeht**
men	мужчины / muzhchiny	moo-**shee**-neh
women	женщины / zhenshchiny	zhen-**shee**-neh
(to the) right	(на) право / (na) pravo	(nah) **prah**-vah
(to the) left	(на) лево / (na) levo	(nah) **leh**-vah
beer	пиво / pivo	**pee**-vah
vodka	водка / vodka	**vohd**-kah
water	вода / voda	vah-**dah**
coffee	кофе / kofe	**koh**-fyeh
Cheers! (To your health)	На здоровья! / Na zdorovya!	nah zdah-**roh**-veh

TALLINN
Estonia

Estonia Practicalities

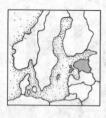

Wedged between Latvia and Russia, Estonia borders the Baltic Sea and Gulf of Finland (at 17,500 square miles, it's roughly the size of New Hampshire and Vermont combined). The country also encompasses more than 1,500 islands and islets. Like Finland, Estonia struggled against Swedish and Russian domination throughout its history. After World War I, Estonia achieved independence, but with the next world war, it fell victim to a 50-year communist twilight, from which it's still emerging. Joining the European Union in 2004 has helped bring the country forward. Estonia is home to 1.3 million people, a quarter of whom are of Russian descent. Even two decades after independence, tension still simmers between the ethnic Estonian population and its ethnic Russian population.

Money: €1 (euro) = about $1.40. An ATM is called a *pangaautomaat*, and is sometimes marked *Otto*. The local VAT (value-added sales tax) rate is 20 percent; the minimum purchase eligible for a VAT refund is €38 (for details on refunds, see page 134).

Language: The native language is Estonian. For useful phrases, see page 485.

Emergencies: In case of emergency, dial 112. For police, dial 110. In case of theft or loss, see page 125.

Time Zone: Estonia is one hour ahead of Central European Time (seven/ten hours ahead of the East/West Coasts of the US). That puts Tallinn in the same time zone as Helsinki and Rīga; one hour ahead of Stockholm, the rest of Scandinavia, and most other continental cruise ports (including Gdańsk and Warnemünde); and one hour behind St. Petersburg.

Embassies in Tallinn: The **US embassy** is at Kentmanni 20 (tel. 668-8128, emergency tel. 509-2129, http://estonia.us embassy.gov). The **Canadian embassy** is at Toomkooli 13 (tel. 627-3311, www.canada.ee). Call ahead for passport services.

Phoning: Estonia's country code is 372; to call from another country to Estonia, dial the international access code (011 from the US/Canada, 00 from Europe, or + from a mobile phone), then 372, followed by the local number. For local calls within Estonia, just dial the number as it appears in this book—whether you're calling from across the street or across the country. To place an international call from Estonia, dial 00, the code of the country you're calling (1 for US and Canada), and the phone number. For more tips, see page 1146.

Tipping: The bill for a sit-down meal includes gratuity, so you don't need to tip further, though it's nice to round up about 5-10 percent for good service. For taxis, round up the fare a bit (pay €5 on an €4.50 fare) For more tips on tipping, see page 138.

Tourist Information: www.visitestonia.com

TALLINN

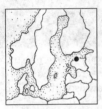

Tallinn is a rising star in the tourism world, thanks to its strategic location (an easy boat ride from Stockholm, Helsinki, and St. Petersburg); its perfectly preserved, atmospheric Old Town, bursting with quaint sightseeing options; and its remarkable economic boom since throwing off Soviet shackles just over two decades ago. Easily the most accessible part of the former USSR, Estonia was only the third post-communist country to adopt the euro (in 2011) and has weathered recent Europe-wide economic crises like a champ. While the city still struggles to more effectively incorporate its large Russian minority, Tallinn feels ages away from its Soviet past—having eagerly reclaimed its unique Nordic identity. Estonian pride is in the air...and it's catching.

Among Nordic medieval cities, there's none nearly as well-preserved as Tallinn. Its mostly intact city wall includes 26 watchtowers, each topped by a pointy red roof. Baroque and choral music ring out from its old Lutheran churches. I'd guess that Tallinn (with 400,000 people) has more restaurants, cafés, and surprises per capita and square inch than any city in this book—and the fun is comparatively cheap.

Though it's connected by boat to Helsinki and Stockholm, Tallinn is very different from those cities. Yes, Tallinn's Nordic Lutheran culture and language connect it with Scandinavia, but two centuries of tsarist Russian rule and 45 years as part of the Soviet Union have blended in a distinctly Russian flavor.

As a member of the Hanseatic League, the city was a medieval stronghold of the Baltic trading world. In the 19th and early 20th centuries, Tallinn industrialized and expanded beyond its walls. Architects encircled the Old Town, putting up broad streets of public buildings, low Scandinavian-style apartment buildings, and single-family wooden houses. After 1945, Soviet planners ringed the city with stands of now-crumbling concrete high-rises where many of Tallinn's Russian immigrants settled. Like Prague and Kraków, Tallinn has westernized at an astounding rate since the fall of the Soviet Union in 1991. Yet the Old World ambience within its walled town center has been beautifully preserved.

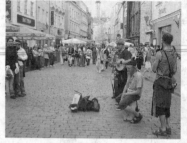

Tallinn is still busy cleaning up the mess left by the communist experiment. New shops, restaurants, and hotels are bursting out of old buildings. The city changes so fast, even locals can't keep up. The Old Town is getting a lot of tourist traffic now, so smart shopping is wise. You'll eat better for half the price by seeking out places that cater to locals.

Tallinn's Old Town is a fascinating package of pleasing towers, ramparts, facades, *striptiis* bars, churches, shops, and people-watching. It's a rewarding detour for those who want to spice their Scandinavian travels with a Baltic twist.

PLANNING YOUR TIME

Tallinn is a snap for cruisers: The port is within walking distance of the Old Town, which contains most of what you'll want to see. On a busy day in port, I'd do the following, in this order:

• To hit the ground running, walk 15 minutes to the Fat Margaret Tower and launch into my **self-guided Tallinn Walk**, which leads you past virtually all of the best sights (allow 2-3 hours, more if you want to linger).

• Spend the afternoon shopping and browsing—or, to get out of the cruiser rut, tram or taxi to **Kadriorg Park** for a stroll through the palace gardens and to tour the delightful Estonian art collection at Kumu (allow about an hour, including transit time, to see the park, and add another hour for Kumu).

• With more time, you could visit the Song Festival Grounds (beyond Kadriorg Park; allow at least an extra hour for a quick visit) or the Estonian Open-Air Museum (allow 30 minutes each way to get there, plus a couple of hours to tour the grounds).

While Tallinn's Old Town is understandably popular, sometimes it feels *too* popular; when several cruises are in town, the cobbles can be uncomfortably crammed. If crowds bother you, consider keeping your Old Town visit brief and instead focus on the sights just out of town, such as Kadriorg Park. You'll see a side

Excursions from Tallinn

Tallinn is so walkable, and its Old Town sights so easy to appreciate, that there's no reason to take an excursion here. Most cruise lines offer a walking tour through the **Old Town** with a few brief sightseeing stops (often including quick visits to Town Hall Square, Palace Square, the Russian Orthodox Cathedral, Dome Church, and various viewpoints)—but the self-guided walk in this chapter covers the same ground at your own pace. Other excursions may include a bus tour around the city, sometimes with stops at outlying sights such as the manicured, palatial **Kadriorg Park** and the stirring **Song Festival Grounds**—but these are also doable on your own (and even affordable by taxi).

A few places farther out of town are a bit more challenging to reach on your own on a short port visit. These include the **Estonian Open-Air Museum** at Rocca al Mare (described on page 477); the communist-planned apartment district of **Lasnamäe** (sometimes billed as "Pirita"); the town of **Rakvere**, about 60 miles east (with its 13th-century castle and "town citizen's museum" of 19th-century life); and the beaches and forests of the **Kakumäe** district, on the western edge of Tallinn. But Tallinn itself is so appealing that these excursions don't merit consideration on a brief visit. Just stick around the city and enjoy the Old World ambience.

TALLINN

of Tallinn that most cruisers miss entirely.

Remember to bring a jacket—Tallinn can be chilly even on sunny summer days. And, given that locals call their cobbled streets "a free foot massage," sturdy shoes are smart, too.

The Port of Tallinn

Arrival at a Glance: It's a quick 15-minute walk from Tallinn's cruise port into town; the fair taxi rate is less than €5.

Port Overview

All cruises come into Tallinn's Old Town Port, which is less than a mile northeast of the Old Town. Within this sprawling area, the primary cruise dock consists of a long, skinny pier at the northern edge; overflow cruise ships might dock near one of the port area's other terminals (which are mainly used for ferries and catamarans to Helsinki, Stockholm, and St. Petersburg). In this case, you'll arrive near A-Terminal/B-Terminal/C-Terminal (all three are clustered in the same area, between the main cruise port and the sailboat marina), D-Terminal (south of the marina), or

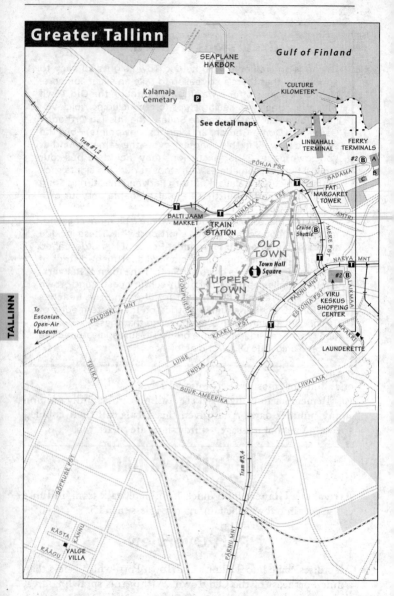

Greater Tallinn

Gulf of Finland

SEAPLANE HARBOR

Kalamaja Cemetery

"CULTURE KILOMETER"

See detail maps

LINNAHALL TERMINAL

FERRY TERMINALS

#2 B A

C B

Tram #1,2

PÕHJA PST

SADAMA

FAT MARGARET TOWER

AHTRI

BALTI JAAM MARKET

RAUNAMÄE TEE

TRAIN STATION

Cruise Shuttle B

MERE PST

OLD TOWN

Town Hall Square

NARVA MNT

T

UPPER TOWN

#2 B

VIRU KESKUS SHOPPING CENTER

To Estonian Open-Air Museum

TOOMPUESTE

PALDISKI MNT

PÄRNU MNT

ESTONIA PST

LAIKMAA

LAUNDERETTE

WAAKRI

KAARLI PST

TULIKA

LUISE

ENDLA

SUUR-AMEERIKA

LIIVALAIA

SÕPRUSE PST

Tram #3,4

PÄRNU MNT

RÄSTA

KANNU

RÄÄGU

VALGE VILLA

occasionally at the Linnahall terminal (west of the cruise port). Regardless of where you arrive, it's easy to walk into town.

Tourist Information: There's no TI at the port, though the main cruise terminal does have a privately run desk that hands out town maps, answers basic questions, and rents a 16-stop town audioguide (skip it—my self-guided walk in this chapter is better). The public terminal buildings (at A-Terminal and D-Terminal)

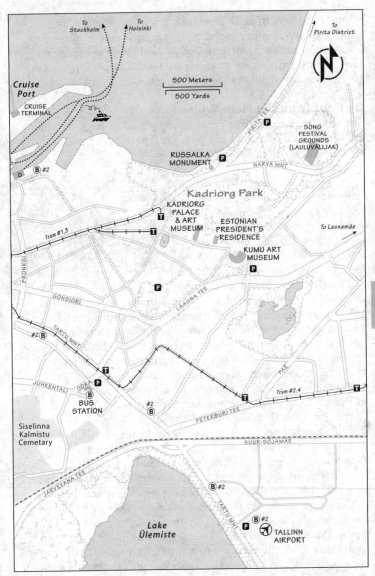

have racks of basic tourist brochures. Otherwise, head into the Old Town Square and visit the TI (see "Orientation to Tallinn," later).

GETTING INTO TOWN

Walking is the obvious way to reach the Old Town. If you arrive at the main cruise port (or the Linnahall terminal), figure about a 15-minute walk. If you arrive at A-/B-/C-Terminal, it's a few minutes shorter; from D-Terminal, it's a few minutes longer. Unless you have limited mobility, there's little reason to pay for a taxi or cruise-line shuttle bus, or to hassle with the local bus. Hop-on, hop-off bus tours stop near the port but are best if you are planning to visit sights outside the Old Town.

By Foot from the Main Cruise Port

The straightforward cruise port can accommodate large ships on either side. Walking down the pier, you'll pass the jagged breakwater and be met by a row of taxis and buses.

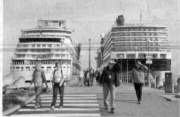

The small, metallic **main cruise terminal** building (on your right as you step off the pier) is a shopping mall in disguise, but inside you will find a nonofficial info desk. The terminal building also has several shops, a café, and a currency exchange booth (though there are no ATMs—the nearest is in the A-Terminal building, a 5-minute walk away). Free Wi-Fi is available in the area near the cruise terminal building; you can sit and get online at the tented picnic-table area out back.

Exit the terminal building at the far end. From here, you'll go through a gauntlet of shops to reach the port gate area. Overpriced taxis meet cruisers here, as do representatives selling all-day tickets for hop-on, hop-off bus tours (both explained later). Bypass all of this, find the blue line painted on the pavement, and follow it to the port gate. (If you'd rather first visit the Seaplane Harbor, described on page 474, look for a red-gravel path—straight ahead as you leave the cruise port, marked *Kultuurikilomeeter*—which takes you there on a long, scenic, mostly seaside stroll.)

After exiting the port gate, proceed across the street, then turn left with the crosswalks. At the next big cross street, Sadama, you can turn left to get to the A-Terminal building (ATM and local bus stop, described next), or turn right to reach the Old Town: Walk a couple of long blocks on Sadama (passing the erotic nudes that mark the entrance to a surely classy hotel). Then, at the gas station, you'll approach a confusing intersection; turn left across two lanes, then right, and head straight toward the pointy steeple. Soon after, angle right across the street, then straight, and climb the steps to the stout, round, stone Fat Margaret Tower; on the way up, you'll pass the ferry memorial mentioned at the start of my self-guided walk.

By Foot from the Other Terminals

If you arrive at any of the other terminals, look for a blue line painted on the pavement; this leads you out of the port area. The best strategy is to walk toward the tallest pointy tower and the round, fat stone gate at its base (visible from most of the port area), which mark the start of my self-guided walk.

From the pier beyond **D-Terminal,** walk five minutes (follow the blue line) to the D-Terminal building. Inside is an ATM, WCs, lockers, and stands with sparse tourist brochures. From the D-Terminal, you can see the spire marking the Old Town, about a 15-minute walk away.

If you arrive near **A-/B-/C-Terminals,** walk to the **A-Terminal building.** While primarily for ferry passengers, it has various services also useful to cruisers. Just outside the door are two ATMs, and inside are WCs, lockers, a café, and a newsstand selling bus tickets. The parking lot in front of the terminal is a good place to look for a taxi that charges fair rates. Public bus #2 leaves from the shelter at the edge of the parking lot in front of A-Terminal (for details on buses, see "Getting into Town," later). To reach the Old Town on foot, walk straight out of A-Terminal, following the walking instructions up Sadama street outlined earlier.

By Taxi

Taxis meet arriving cruise ships near the main cruise port, happy to overcharge arriving passengers for the laughably brief ride into town. A legitimate taxi using the meter should charge €5 or less to anywhere in the Old Town—though when I asked cabbies at the port, they shamelessly told me, "€10 to lower town, €15 to upper town." It can be worth the walk to the area in front of A-Terminal, where you may find a taxi with more reasonable posted rates. Before choosing a taxi, read my tips on page 454.

By Cruise-Line Shuttle Bus or Local Bus

Some cruise lines offer **shuttles** into town. Unless it's free, it's often not worth it: The bus takes you to a point at the edge of the Old Town that's only slightly more convenient than the port itself. Cruise shuttles drop off along the busy ring road, at the pleasant park next to the Russian Cultural Center (Vene Kultuurikeskus). Get off here, walk straight ahead in the same direction (with the busy street on your left), and pass the charming local-style Viru Turg market to reach Viru street (with a big taxi stand, flower vendors, and an archway from the old city wall). Walk straight up Viru street into town.

The **local bus #2** is affordable, but by the time you walk to the bus stop (in front of either A-Terminal or D-Terminal), wait for a bus, and walk into town from the stop, you could have walked all the way to town (2/hour, €1.60 on board; if you'll be taking more

Services near the Port

You'll find a few services at the port areas; for others, wait until you're downtown.

ATMs: There's no ATM at the cruise port itself, but there are two just outside the front door of the nearby A-Terminal building. There's also an ATM inside D-Terminal (useful only if your ship arrives there). Once in the Old Town, ATMs are easy to find.

Internet Access: The area near the main cruise terminal has free Wi-Fi. For Internet access in the city center, see "Helpful Hints," later.

Pharmacy: The best (and most memorable) choice is in the Old Town—the historic (and still-functioning) pharmacy on Old Town Square (described on page 461).

than three rides in a day, buy a Ühiskaart smartcard from R-Kiosk shops in terminals). It goes directly to a stop handy to the Old Town: Hop off at A. Laikmaa, and walk into town through the Viru Gate. For more on buses and the Ühiskaart, see page 453.

By Tour

Two fiercely competitive companies (Tallinn City Tour and CitySightseeing Tallinn) run different **hop-on, hop-off bus tour routes** and meet each arriving ship to drum up business (sometimes offering discounts). Aside from a stop near Toompea Castle, the routes are entirely outside the Old Town, and the frequency is low, which could leave you stranded if you want to hop on again soon. And realistically, on a short day in port, you'll likely spend most or all of your day in the walkable Old Town—making a bus trip unnecessary. However, if you're planning to get to outlying sights, these can be a good way to do it.

Tallinn City Tour offers three different one-hour bus tours—you can take all three on the same day for one price (€19/24 hours, free with Tallinn Card, tel. 627-9080, www.citytour.ee). **CitySightseeing Tallinn** runs three similar routes, with a similarly sparse frequency (€18 for all three lines, €15 for just one line, www.citysightseeing.ee).

For information on other local tour options in Tallinn—including local guides for hire, good Tallinn Traveller Tours offered by a youthful walking-tour company, bike tours, and more—see "Tours in Tallinn" on page 455.

RETURNING TO YOUR SHIP

The easiest choice is to simply walk back; it takes about 15 minutes to reach the main cruise terminal from the Old Town (a bit less to the A-/B-/C-Terminals, a bit longer to D-Terminal). Walk through town on Pikk street, popping out at Fat Margaret Tower; look right, and you'll see the ships.

If you catch a taxi, insist on the meter. It should be no more than €5 from the Old Town area (possibly a euro more from Kadriorg Park). From Old Town Square, walk down Viru street (see the last section of my self-guided walk) and go through Viru Gate, where you'll usually find several reputable taxis.

See page 484 for help if you miss your boat.

Tallinn

Tallinn's walled Old Town is an easy 15-minute walk from the ferry and cruise terminals, where most visitors land. The Old Town is divided into two parts (historically, two separate towns): the upper town (Toompea) and the lower town (with Town Hall Square). A remarkably intact medieval wall surrounds the two towns, which are themselves separated by another wall.

Town Hall Square (Raekoja Plats) marks the heart of the medieval lower town. The main TI is nearby, as are many sights and eateries. Pickpockets are a problem in the more touristy parts of the Old Town, so keep valuables carefully stowed. The area around the Viru Keskus mall and Hotel Viru, just east of the Old Town, is useful for everyday shopping (bookstores and supermarkets), practical services (laundry), and public transport.

Orientation to Tallinn

TOURIST INFORMATION
The hardworking TI has maps, concert listings, and free brochures (May-Aug Mon-Fri 9:00-19:00—until 20:00 mid-June-Aug, Sat-Sun 9:00-17:00—until 18:00 mid-June-Aug; Sept-April Mon-Fri 9:00-18:00, Sat-Sun 9:00-15:00; a block off Town Hall Square at Kullassepa 4, tel. 645-7777, www.tourism.tallinn.ee, visit@tallinn.ee). Look for the helpful *Tallinn in Your Pocket*, a booklet with restaurant, hotel, and sight listings (€2.50 at the TI and elsewhere around town, but you may find free copies at a hotel, and you can download it for free at www.inyourpocket.com).

Tallinn Card: This card—sold at the TIs, airport, train station, travel agencies, ferry ports, and big hotels—gives you free use of public transport and entry to more than 40 museums and major sights (€24/24 hours, €32/48 hours, €40/72 hours, comes with good info booklet, www.tallinncard.ee). It includes one tour of your choice (orientation walk or one of two hop-on, hop-off

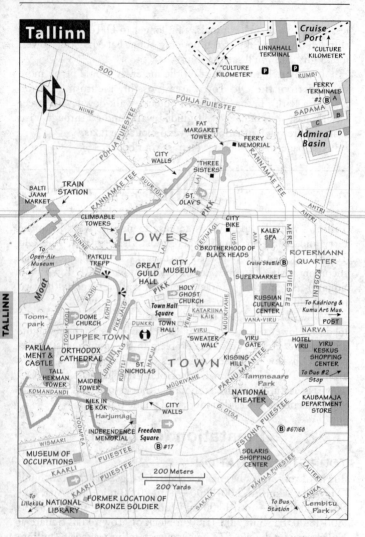

Tallinn

bus routes), plus a 50 percent discount on any others (see "Tours in Tallinn," later, for specifics). If you're planning to take one of these tours and to visit several sights, this card will likely save you money—do the math.

HELPFUL HINTS

Internet Access: Public Wi-Fi is easy to find around Tallinn; look for the free "Tallinn WiFi" network. The **main TI** has one terminal where you can briefly check your email for free.

Travel Agency: Estravel, at the corner of Suur-Karja and Müürivähe, is handy and sells boat tickets for no extra fee

(Mon-Fri 9:00-18:00, closed Sat-Sun, Suur-Karja 15, tel. 626-6233).

Bike Rental: Head for **City Bike,** at the north end of the Old Town near the ferry terminals (€10/6 hours, €13/24 hours; electric bikes—€5/hour, €20/6 hours, €25/24 hours; daily May-Sept 9:00-19:00, Oct-April 9:00-17:00, Uus 33, mobile 511-1819, www.citybike.ee). They also do bike tours (see "Tours in Tallinn," later).

GETTING AROUND TALLINN

By Public Transportation: The Old Town and surrounding areas can be explored on foot, but use public transit to reach outlying sights (such as Kadriorg Park, Kumu Art Museum, or the Estonian Open-Air Museum). Tallinn has buses, trams, and trolley buses (buses connected to overhead wires)—avoid mistakes by noting that they reuse the same numbers (bus #2, tram #2, and trolley bus #2 are totally different lines). Maps and schedules are posted at stops, or visit http://soiduplaan.tallinn.ee (for an overview of transit stops useful to visitors, see the "Greater Tallinn" map on page 446). As you approach a station, you'll hear the name of the impending stop, followed by the name of the next stop—don't get confused and hop off one stop too early.

You can buy a **single ticket** from the driver for €1.60 (exact change appreciated). If you'll be taking more than three rides in a day, invest in an **Ühiskaart smartcard.** You can buy one for €2 at any yellow-and-blue R-Kiosk convenience store (found all over town), and then load it up with credit, which is deducted as you travel (€1.10 for any ride up to 1 hour, €3/24 hours, €5/72 hours, €6/120 hours). The card is shareable by multiple people for single rides, but you'll need separate cards for the multiride options.

Bus #2 (Moigu-Reisisadam) is helpful on arrival and departure, running every 20-30 minutes between the port's A-Terminal and the airport. En route it stops at D-Terminal; at "A. Laikmaa," next to the Viru Keskus mall (a short walk south of the Old Town); and at the long-distance bus station.

By Taxi: Taxis in Tallinn are handy, but it's easy to get ripped off. The safest way to catch a cab is to order one by phone (or ask a trusted local to call for you)—this is what Estonians usually do.

Tulika is the largest company, with predictable, fair prices (€3.35 drop charge plus €0.69/kilometer, €0.80/kilometer from 23:00-6:00, tel. 612-0001 or 1200, check latest prices at www.tulika.ee). **Tallink Takso** is another reputable option with similar fares (tel. 640-8921 or 1921). Cabbies are required to use the meter and give you a meter-printed receipt. If you don't get a receipt, it's safe to assume you're being ripped off and legally don't need to pay. The trip from the cruise port to anywhere in the town center

Tallinn at a Glance

Central Tallinn

▲▲▲**Tallinn's Old Town** Well-preserved medieval center with cobblestoned lanes, gabled houses, historic churches, and turreted city walls. **Hours:** Always open. See page 456.

▲▲**Russian Orthodox Cathedral** Accessible look at the Russian Orthodox faith, with a lavish interior. **Hours:** Daily 8:00-19:00, icon art in gift shop. See page 463.

▲**Museum of Estonian History** High-tech exhibits explain Estonia's engaging national narrative. **Hours:** May-Aug daily 10:00-18:00, same hours off-season except closed Wed. See page 467.

▲**Museum of Occupations** Estonia's tumultuous, sometimes secret history under Soviet and Nazi occupiers from 1940 to 1991. **Hours:** June-Aug Tue-Sun 10:00-18:00, Sept-May Tue-Sun 11:00-18:00, closed Mon year-round. See page 469.

St. Nicholas Church Art museum displaying Gothic art in a restored old church. **Hours:** Wed-Sun 10:00-17:00, closed Mon-Tue. See page 461.

Town Hall and Tower Gothic building with history museum and climbable tower on the Old Town's main square. **Hours:** Museum—July-Aug Mon-Sat 10:00-16:00, closed Sun and rest of

should be no more than €5; longer rides around the city (e.g., from the Old Town to the Estonian Open-Air Museum) should run around €8-10.

If you must catch a taxi off the street, go to a busy taxi stand where lots of cabs are lined up. Before you get in, take a close look at the yellow price list on the rear passenger-side door; the base fare should be €3-4 and the per-kilometer charge under €1. If it's not, keep looking. Glance inside—a photo ID license should be attached to the middle of the dashboard. Don't negotiate or ask for a price estimate; let the driver use the meter. Rates must be posted by law, but are not capped or regulated, so the most common scam—unfortunately widespread, and legal—is to list an inflated price on the yellow price sticker (as much as €3/kilometer), and simply wait for a tourist to hop in without noticing. Singleton cabs lurking in tourist areas are usually fishing for suckers, as are cabbies who flag you down ("Taxi?")—give them a miss. It's fun to play spot-the-scam as you walk around town.

year; tower—May-mid-Sept daily 11:00-18:00, closed rest of year. See page 468.

Outside the Core

▲▲**Kumu Art Museum** The best of contemporary Estonian art displayed in a strikingly modern building. **Hours:** May-Sept Tue-Sun 11:00-18:00, Wed until 20:00, closed Mon; same hours off-season except closed Mon-Tue. See page 472.

▲▲**Seaplane Harbor** Impressive museum of boats and planes—including a WWII-era submarine—displayed in a cavernous old hangar along the waterfront. **Hours:** May-Sept daily 10:00-19:00; same hours off-season except closed Mon. See page 474.

▲**Kadriorg Park** Vast, strollable oasis with the palace gardens, Kumu Art Museum, and a palace built by Czar Peter the Great. **Hours:** Park always open. See page 471.

▲**Song Festival Grounds** National monument and open-air theater where Estonians sang for freedom. **Hours:** Open long hours daily. See page 475.

▲**Estonian Open-Air Museum** Authentic farm and village buildings preserved in a forested parkland. **Hours:** Late April-Sept—park open daily 10:00-20:00, buildings open until 18:00; Oct-late April—park open daily 10:00-17:00 but many buildings closed. See page 477.

Tours in Tallinn

Bus and Walking Tour

This enjoyable, narrated 2.5-hour tour of Tallinn comes in two parts: first by bus for an overview of sights outside the Old Town, such as the Song Festival Grounds and Kadriorg Park, then on foot to sights within the Old Town (€20, pay driver, covered by Tallinn Card, in English; daily morning and early afternoon departures from A-Terminal, D-Terminal, and major hotels in city center; tel. 610-8616, www.traveltoestonia.com).

Local Guides

Mati Rumessen is a top-notch guide, especially for car tours inside or outside town (€35/hour driving or walking tours, price may vary with group size, mobile 509-4661, www.tourservice.ee, matirumessen@gmail.com). Other fine guides are **Antonio Villacis** (mobile 5662-9306, antonio.villacis@gmail.com) and **Miina Puusepp** (€20/hour, mobile 551-7028, miinap@hot.ee).

TALLINN

Tallinn Traveller Tours

These student-run tours show you the real city without the political and corporate correctness of official tourist agencies. Check www.traveller.ee to confirm details for their ever-changing lineup, and to reserve (or call mobile 5837-4800). The **City Introductory Walking Tour** is free, but tips are encouraged (around €5/person if you enjoy yourself, daily at 12:00, 2 hours). They also typically offer a two-hour **Old Town Walking Tour** (€15, daily at 10:00, similar to the free tour but generally a much smaller group), and can also arrange private tours. They have a variety of **bike tours,** including a 2.5-hour "Welcome to Tallinn" overview (€16, daily at 11:00). All tours start from in front of the main TI.

City Bike Tours

City Bike offers a two-hour, nine-mile **Welcome to Tallinn** bike tour that takes you outside the city walls to Tallinn's more distant sights: Kadriorg Park, Song Festival Grounds, a beach at Pirita, and more (€16, 50 percent discount with Tallinn Card, daily at 11:00 year-round, departs from their office at Uus 33 in the Old Town, mobile 511-1819, www.citybike.ee).

Tallinn Walk

This self-guided walk, worth ▲▲▲, explores the "two towns" of Tallinn. The city once consisted of two feuding medieval towns separated by a wall. The upper town—on the hill, called Toompea—was the seat of government ruling Estonia. The lower town was an autonomous Hanseatic trading center filled with German, Danish, and Swedish merchants who hired Estonians to do their menial labor. Many of the Old Town's buildings are truly old, dating from the boom times of the 15th and 16th centuries. Decrepit before the 1991 fall of the Soviet Union, the Old Town has been slowly revitalized, though there's still plenty of work to be done.

Two steep, narrow streets—the "Long Leg" and the "Short Leg"—connect the upper town (Toompea) and the lower town. This two-part walk—"Part 1" focusing on the lower town, and "Part 2" climbing up to the upper town—goes up the short leg and down the long leg. Allow about two hours for the entire walk (not counting time to enter museums along the way).

PART 1: THE LOWER TOWN

• *The walk starts at the port—where cruise ships and ferries from Helsinki arrive. If you're coming from elsewhere in Tallinn, take tram #1 or #2 to the Linnahall stop, or just walk out to the Fat Margaret Tower from anywhere in the Old Town.*

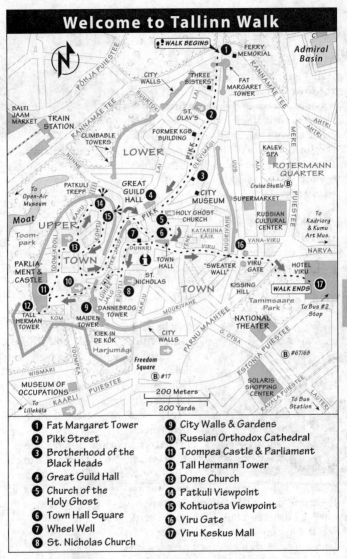

Welcome to Tallinn Walk

1 Fat Margaret Tower
2 Pikk Street
3 Brotherhood of the Black Heads
4 Great Guild Hall
5 Church of the Holy Ghost
6 Town Hall Square
7 Wheel Well
8 St. Nicholas Church
9 City Walls & Gardens
10 Russian Orthodox Cathedral
11 Toompea Castle & Parliament
12 Tall Hermann Tower
13 Dome Church
14 Patkuli Viewpoint
15 Kohtuotsa Viewpoint
16 Viru Gate
17 Viru Keskus Mall

❶ To Fat Margaret Tower and Start of Walk

From the port, hike toward the tall tapering spire, go through a small park, and enter the Old Town through the archway by the squat Fat Margaret Tower.

Just outside the tower, on a bluff overlooking the harbor, is half of a **black arch.** (The other half of the arch sits in the park just below the hill.) This is a memorial to 852 people who perished in September of 1994 when the *Estonia* passenger-and-car ferry sank in stormy conditions during its Tallinn-Stockholm run.

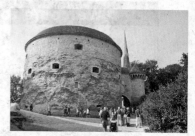

Fat Margaret Tower (Paks Margareeta, so called for its thick walls) guarded the entry gate of the town in medieval times (the sea once came much closer to this point than it does today). The relief above the gate dates from the 16th century, during Hanseatic times, when Sweden took Estonia from Germany. The Estonian Maritime Museum in the tower is paltry—skip it.

• *Once through the gate, head up Tallinn's main drag...*

❷ Pikk Street

Literally "Long Street," the medieval merchants' main drag—leading from the harbor up into town—is lined with interesting buildings. Many were warehouses, complete with cranes on the gables. Strolling here, you'll feel the economic power of those early German trading days.

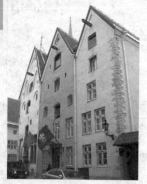

One short block up the street on the right, the buildings nicknamed **"Three Sisters"** (now a hotel) are textbook examples of a merchant home/warehouse/office from the 15th-century Hanseatic Golden Age. The charmingly carved door near the corner evokes the wealth of Tallinn's merchant class.

After another, longer block, you'll pass **St. Olav's Church** (Oleviste Kirik, a Baptist church today), notable for what was once the tallest spire in the land. If the name didn't tip you off that this was once a Lutheran church, then the stark, whitewashed interior guarantees it. Climbing 234 stairs up the tower rewards you with a great view. You can enter both the church and the tower around the back side (church—free entry, daily 10:00-18:00, July-Aug until 20:00; tower—€2, open April-Oct only; www.oleviste.ee).

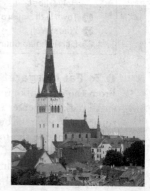

The once-handsome building at **Pikk #59** (the second house after the church, on the right) was, before 1991, the sinister local headquarters of the KGB. "Creative interrogation methods" were used here. Locals well knew that the road of suffering started here, as Tallinn's troublemakers were sent to Siberian gulags.

• *A few short blocks farther up Pikk (after the small park), on the left at #26, is the extremely ornate doorway of the...*

❸ Brotherhood of the Black Heads

Built in 1440, this house was used as a German merchants' club for nearly 500 years (until Hitler invited Estonian Germans back

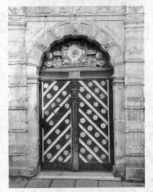

to their historical fatherland in the 1930s). Before the 19th century, many Estonians lived as serfs on the rural estates of the German nobles who dominated the economy. In Tallinn, the German big shots were part of the Great Guild (which we'll see farther up the street), while the German little shots had to make do with the Brotherhood of the Black Heads. This guild, or business fraternity, was limited to single German men. In Hanseatic towns, when a fire or battle had to be fought, single men were deployed first, because they had no family. Because single men were considered unattached to the community, they had no opportunity for power in the Hanseatic social structure. When a Black Head member married a local woman, he automatically gained a vested interest in the town's economy and well-being. He could then join the more prestigious Great Guild, and with that status, a promising economic and political future often opened up.

Today the hall is a concert venue (and, while you can pay to tour its interior, I'd skip it—it's basically an empty shell).

Keep going along Pikk street. Architecture fans enjoy several **fanciful facades** along here, including the boldly Art Nouveau #18 (on the left, reminiscent of the architectural bounty of fellow Baltic capital Rīga; appropriately enough, today this building houses one of Tallinn's leading cutting-edge architecture firms) and the colorful, eclectic building across the street (with the pointy gable).

On the left, at #16 (look for *Kalev* awnings), the famous and recommended **Maiasmokk** ("Sweet Tooth") coffee shop, in business since 1864, remains a fine spot for a cheap coffee-and-pastry break.

• *Just ahead, pause at the big yellow building on the right (at #17).*

❹ Great Guild Hall (Suurgildi Hoone)

With its wide (and therefore highly taxed) front, the Great Guild Hall was the epitome of wealth. Remember, this was the home of the most prestigious of Tallinn's Hanseatic-era guilds. Today it houses the worthwhile **Museum of Estonian History,** offering a concise, engaging, well-presented survey of this country's story (for details, see "Sights in Tallinn," later).

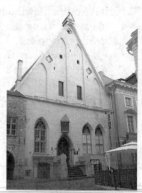

• *Across Pikk street from the Great Guild Hall is the...*

❺ Church of the Holy Ghost (Pühavaimu Kirik)

Sporting an outdoor clock from 1633, this pretty medieval church is worth a visit. (The plaque on the wall just behind the ticket desk is in Estonian and Russian, but not English; this dates from before 1991, when things were designed for "inner tourism"—within the USSR.) The church retains its 14th-century design. Flying from the back pillar, the old flag of Tallinn—the same as today's red-and-white Danish flag—recalls 13th-century Danish rule. (The name "Tallinn" means "Danish Town.") The Danes sold Tallinn to the German Teutonic Knights, who lost it to the Swedes, who lost it to the Russians. The windows are mostly from the 1990s (€1, Mon-Sat 9:00-18:00, closes earlier in winter, closed most of Sun to non-worshippers, Pühavaimu 2, tel. 646-4430, www.eelk.ee). The church hosts English-language Lutheran services Sundays at 15:00 (maybe earlier in summer).

• *If you were to go down the street to the left as you face the church, it's a three-minute walk to the **Tallinn City Museum** (described later, under "Sights in Tallinn").*

Leading alongside the church, tiny Saiakang lane (meaning "White Bread"—bread, cakes, and pies have been sold here since medieval times) takes you to...

❻ Town Hall Square (Raekoja Plats)

A marketplace through the centuries, with a cancan of fine old buildings, this is the focal point of the Old Town. The square was

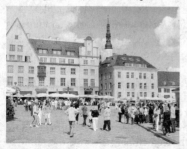

the center of the autonomous lower town, a merchant city of Hanseatic traders. Once, it held criminals chained to pillories for public humiliation and knights showing off in chivalrous tournaments; today it's full of Scandinavians and Russians savoring cheap beer, children singing on the bandstand, and cruise-ship groups following the numbered paddles carried high by their well-scrubbed local guides.

The 15th-century **Town Hall** (Raekoda) dominates the square; it's now a museum, and climbing its tower earns you a commanding view (see photo; for details, see page 468).

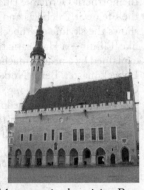

On the opposite side of the square, across from #12 in the corner, the **pharmacy** (Raeapteek) dates from 1422 and claims—as do many—to be Europe's oldest. With decor that goes back to medieval times, the still-operating pharmacy welcomes visitors with its painted ceiling beams, English descriptions, and long-expired aspirin. Past the functioning counter is a room of display cases with historical exhibits (free entry, Tue-Sat 10:00-18:00, closed Sun-Mon).

Town Hall Square is ringed by inviting but touristy eateries, a few of which are still affordable, such as Troika and the Kehrwieder cafés. The TI is a block away (behind Town Hall).

• *Facing the Town Hall, head right up Dunkri street—lined with several more eateries—one long block to the* ❼ ***wheel well***, *named for the "high-tech" wheel, a marvel that made fetching water easier.*

Turn left on Rataskaevu street (which soon becomes Rüütli) and walk two short blocks to...

❽ St. Nicholas Church (Niguliste Kirik)

This 13th-century Gothic church-turned-art-museum served the German merchants and knights who lived in this neighborhood 500 years ago. On March 9, 1944, while Tallinn was in German hands, Soviet forces bombed the city, and the church and surrounding area—once a charming district, dense with medieval buildings—were burned out; only the church was rebuilt.

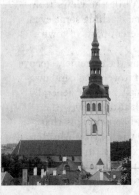

The church's interior houses a fine collection of mostly Gothic-era ecclesiastical art (€3.50, Wed-Sun 10:00-17:00, last entry 30 minutes before closing, closed Mon-Tue; organ concerts Sat and Sun at 16:00 included in admission).

You'll enter the church through the modern cellar, where you can see photos of the WWII destruction of the building (with its toppled steeple). Then make your way into the vast, open church interior.

Front and center is the collection's highlight: a retable (framed altarpiece) from 1481, by Herman Rode—an exquisite example of the northern Germanic late-Gothic style. Along with scenes from the life of St. Nicholas and an array of other saints, the altarpiece shows the skyline of Lübeck, Germany (Rode's hometown, and—like Tallinn—a Hanseatic trading city). The intricate symbolism is explained by a nearby touchscreen. Also look for another work by a Lübeck master, Bernt Notke's *Danse Macabre* ("Dance of Death"). Once nearly 100 feet long, the surviving fragment shows sinister skeletons approaching people from all walks of life. This common medieval theme reminds the viewer that life is fleeting, and no matter who we are, we'll all wind up in the same place.

• *As you face the church, if you were to turn left and walk downhill on Rüütli street, you'd soon pass near* **Freedom Square**—*for a taste of modern Tallinn (described on page 469).*

But for now, let's continue our walk into the upper town.

PART 2: THE UPPER TOWN (TOOMPEA)

• *At the corner opposite the church, climb uphill along the steep, cobbled, Lühike Jalg ("Short Leg Lane"), home to a few quality craft shops. At the top of the lane, pause at the giant stone tower, noticing the original oak door—one of two gates through the wall separating the two cities. This passage is still the ritual meeting point of the mayor and prime minister whenever there is an important agreement between town and country.*

Facing that tower and door, turn left and go through the café courtyard to its far end. You'll emerge into a beautiful view terrace in front of the...

❾ City Walls and Gardens

The imposing city wall once had 46 towers, of which 26 still stand. The gravel-and-grass strip that runs in front of the wall offers a fun stroll and fine views. If you have interest and energy, you can also climb some of the towers and ramparts. (While the views from the towers are nice, keep in mind that we'll be reaching some even more dramatic viewpoints—overlooking different parts of town—later on this walk.)

The easiest option is to simply scramble up the extremely steep and tight steps of the **Dannebrog restaurant tower;** you can buy a drink or a cheap meal here (€5 soups, €7 pastas), but they generally don't charge those who just want a quick look at the view.

To reach a higher vantage point—or if Dannebrog is charging admission—you can pay €3 to enter the nearby **Maiden Tower** (Neitsitorn). It has a few skippable exhibits, an overpriced café, and great views—particularly from the top floor, where a full glass wall reveals panoramic town views (tower and café open daily 10:30-22:00, exhibits open until 19:00, shorter hours Oct-April).

With more time, add a visit to the **Kiek in de Kök**—the stout, round tower that sits farther along the wall (with extremely tight, twisty, steep stone staircases inside). While fun to say, the name is Low German for "Peek in the Kitchen"— so called because it's situated to allow guards to literally peek into townspeople's homes. This tower is bigger than the Maiden Tower, with more impressive exhibits—not a lot of real artifacts, but plenty of cannons, mannequins, model ships, movies, and models of the castle to give you a taste of Tallinn's medieval hey-day. The €7 combo-ticket with the Maiden Tower lets you walk along the scenic rampart between the two towers (find the door marked *Väljapääs* on the second floor of the Maiden Tower, and open it with your wristband ticket; also possible to enter just Kiek in de Kök with €4.50 ticket; extra for tour of tunnels below the tower).

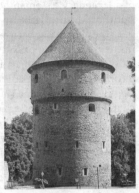

• *When you're finished with the towers and ramparts, go through the hole in the wall, and head uphill into the upper town.*

Circle around the left side of the big, onion-domed church; as you stroll, on your left is the so-called **"Danish King's Garden."** Tallinn is famous among Danes as the birthplace of their flag. According to legend, the Danes were losing a battle here. Suddenly, a white cross fell from heaven and landed in a pool of blood. The Danes were inspired and went on to win. To this day, their flag is a white cross on a red background.

• *Complete your circle around to the far side of the church (facing the pink palace) to enjoy a great view of the cathedral, and to find the entrance.*

❿ Russian Orthodox Cathedral

The Alexander Nevsky Cathedral—worth ▲▲—is a gorgeous

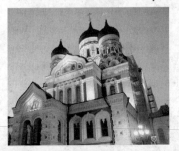

building. But ever since the day it was built (in 1900), it has been a jab in the eye for Estonians. The church went up near the end of the two cen-turies when Estonia was part of the Russian Empire. And, as through-out Europe in the late 19th century, Tallinn's oppressed ethnic groups— the Estonians and the Germans— were caught up in national revival movements, celebrating their own culture, language, and history rather than their Russian overlords'. So the Russians flexed their cultural muscle by building this church in this location, facing the traditional Estonian seat of power, and over the supposed grave of a legendary Estonian hero, Kalevipoeg. They also tore down a statue of Martin Luther to make room.

The church has been exquisitely renovated inside and out. Step inside for a sample of Russian Orthodoxy (church free and open daily 8:00-19:00, icon art in gift shop). It's OK to visit discreetly during services (daily at 9:00 and 18:00), when you'll hear priests singing the liturgy in a side chapel. Typical of Russian Orthodox churches, it has glittering icons (the highest concentration fills the big screen—called an iconostasis—that shields the altar from the congregation), no pews (worshippers stand through the service), and air that's heavy with incense. All of these features combine to create a mystical, otherworldly worship experience. Notice the many candles, representing prayers; if there's a request or a thank-you in your heart, you're welcome to buy one at the desk by the door. Exploring this space, keep in mind that about 40 percent of Tallinn's population is ethnic Russian.

• *Across the street is the...*

⓫ Toompea Castle (Toompea Loss)

The pink palace is an 18th-century Russian addition onto the medieval Toompea Castle. Today, it's the Estonian Parliament (Riigigoku) building, flying the Estonian flag—the flag of both the first (1918-1940) and second (1991-present) Estonian republics. Notice the Estonian seal: three lions for three great battles in Estonian history, and oak leaves for strength and stubbornness. Ancient pagan Estonians, who believed spirits lived in oak trees, would walk through forests of oak to toughen up. (To this day, Estonian cemeteries are in forests. Keeping some of their pagan sensibilities, they believe the spirits of the departed live on in the trees.)

• *Facing the palace, go left through the gate into the park to see the...*

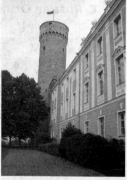

⓬ Tall Hermann Tower (Pikk Hermann)

This tallest tower of the castle wall is a powerful symbol here. For 50 years, while Estonian flags were hidden in cellars, the Soviet flag flew from Tall Hermann. As the USSR was unraveling, Estonians proudly and defiantly replaced the red Soviet flag here with their own black, white, and blue flag.

• *Backtrack and go uphill, passing the Russian church on your right. Climb Toom-Kooli street to the...*

⓭ Dome Church (Toomkirik)

Estonia is ostensibly Lutheran, but few Tallinners go to church. A recent Gallup Poll showed Estonia to be the least religious coun-

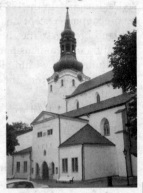

try in the European Union—only 14 percent of respondents identified religion as an important part of their daily lives. Most churches double as concert venues or museums, but this one is still used for worship. Officially St. Mary's Church—but popularly called the Dome Church—it's a perfect example of simple Northern European Gothic, built in the 13th century during Danish rule, then rebuilt after a 1684 fire. Once the church of Tallinn's wealthy German-speaking aristocracy, it's littered with more than a hundred coats of arms, carved by local masters as memorials to the deceased and inscribed with German tributes. The earliest dates from the 1600s, the latest from around 1900. For €5, you can climb 140 steps up the tower to enjoy the view (church entry free, daily 9:00-18:00, www.eelk.ee/tallinna.toom).

• *Leaving the church, turn left and hook around the back of the building. You'll pass a slanted tree, then the big, green, former noblemen's club-house on your right (at #1, vacated when many Germans left Estonia in the 1930s). Head down cobbled Rahukohtu lane (to the right of the yellow, pyramid-shaped house). Strolling the street, notice the embassy signs: Government offices and embassies have moved into these build-ings and spruced up the neighborhood. Continue straight under the arch and belly up to the grand...*

⓮ Patkuli Viewpoint

Survey the scene. On the far left, the Neoclassical facade of the executive branch of Estonia's government enjoys the view. Below

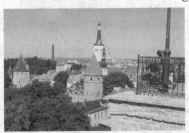

you, a bit of the old moat remains. The *Group* sign marks Tallinn's tiny train station, and the clutter of stalls behind that is the rustic market. Out on the water, ferries shuttle to and from Helsinki (just 50 miles away). Beyond the lower town's medi-eval wall and towers stands the green spire of St. Olav's Church, once 98 feet taller and, locals claim, the world's tallest tower in 1492. Far in the distance is the 1,000-foot-tall TV tower, the site of a standoff between Soviet paratroopers and Estonian patriots in 1991.

During Soviet domination, Finnish TV was even more important, as it gave Estonians their only look at Western lifestyles. Imagine: In the 1980s, many locals had never seen a banana or pineapple—except on TV. People still talk of the day that Finland broadcast the soft-porn movie *Emmanuelle*. A historic migration of Estonians purportedly flocked from the countryside to Tallinn to get within rabbit-ear's distance of Helsinki and see all that flesh onscreen. The TV tower was recently refurbished and opened to visitors.

• *Go back through the arch, turn immediately left down the narrow lane, turn right (onto Toom-Rüütli), take the first left, and pass through the trees to the...*

⓯ Kohtuotsa Viewpoint

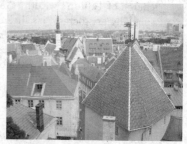

Scan the view from left to right. On the far left is St. Olav's Church, then the busy cruise port and the skinny white spire of the Church of the Holy Ghost. The narrow gray spire farther to the right is the 16th-century Town Hall tower. On the far right is the tower of St. Nicholas Church. Below you, visually trace Pikk street, Tallinn's historic main drag, which winds through the Old Town, leading from Toompea Castle down the hill (from right to left), through the gate tower, past the Church of the Holy Ghost, behind St. Olav's, and out to the harbor. Less picturesque is the clutter of Soviet-era apartment blocks on the distant hori-

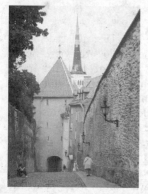

zon. The nearest skyscraper (white) is Hotel Viru, in Soviet times the biggest hotel in the Baltics, and infamous as a clunky, dingy slumbermill. Locals joke that Hotel Viru was built from a new Soviet wonder material called "micro-concrete" (60 percent concrete, 40 percent microphones). Underneath the hotel is the modern Viru Keskus, a huge shopping mall and local transit center, where this walk will end. To the left of Hotel Viru, between it and the ferry terminals, is the Rotermann Quarter, where old industrial buildings are being revamped into a new commercial zone.

• *From the viewpoint, descend to the lower town. Go out and left down Kohtu, past the Finnish Embassy (on your left). Back at the Dome Church, the slanted tree points the way, left down Piiskopi ("Bishop's Street"). At the onion domes, turn left again and follow the old wall down Pikk Jalg ("Long Leg Lane") into the lower town. Go under the tower, then straight on Pikk street, and after two doors turn right on Voorimehe, which leads into Town Hall Square.*

⑯ Through Viru Gate

Cross through the square (left of the Town Hall's tower) and go downhill (passing the kitschy medieval Olde Hansa Restaurant, with its bonneted waitresses and merry men). Continue straight down Viru street toward Hotel Viru, the blocky white skyscraper in the distance. Viru street is old Tallinn's busiest and kitschiest shopping street. Just past the strange and modern wood/glass/stone mall, Müürivahe street leads left along the old wall, called the "Sweater Wall." This is a colorful and tempting gauntlet of women selling knitwear (anything with images and bright colors is likely machine-made). Katariina Käik, a lane with glassblowing shops, leads left, beyond the sweaters. Back on Viru street, pass the golden arches and walk through the medieval arches—Viru Gate—that mark the end of old Tallinn. Outside the gates, opposite Viru 23, above the flower stalls, is a small park on a piece of old bastion known as the Kissing Hill (come up here after dark and you'll find out why).

• *Use the crosswalk to your right to reach the...*

⑰ Viru Keskus Mall

Here, behind Hotel Viru, at the end of this walk, you'll find the real world: basement supermarket, ticket service, bookstore, and many bus and tram stops. If you still have energy, you can cross the busy street by the complex and explore the nearby Rotermann Quarter (see page 470).

Sights in Tallinn

IN OR NEAR THE OLD TOWN

Central Tallinn has dozens of small museums, most suitable only for specialized tastes. The following sights are the ones I'd visit first.

▲Museum of Estonian History (Eesti Ajaloomuuseum)

The Great Guild Hall on Pikk street (described on my self-guided walk, earlier) houses this modern, well-presented-in-English exhibit. The museum's "Estonia 101" approach—combining lots of actual artifacts (from prehistory to today) and high-tech interactive exhibits—is geared toward educating first-time visitors about this obscure but endearing little country.

Cost and Hours: €5, May-Aug daily 10:00-18:00, same hours off-season except closed Wed, tel. 696-8690, www.ajaloomuuseum.ee.

Visiting the Museum: As you enter, download the free smartphone audioguide to navigate the collection. Pondering the question of what it means to be an Estonian, you'll view a coin collection of past currencies (including the Soviet ruble and the pre-euro krooni), then head into the whitewashed vaulted hall to see the "Spirit of Survival" exhibit, which traces 11,000 years of Estonian history. Steep steps lead down into the cellar, with an armory, ethnographic collection, items owned by historical figures, an exhibit about the Great Guild Hall itself, and a fun "time capsule" that lets you insert your face into videos illustrating episodes in local history.

Town Hall (Raekoda) and Tower

This museum facing Town Hall Square is open to the general public only in the summer. It has exhibits on the town's administration and history, along with an interesting bit on the story of limestone. The tower, the place to see all of Tallinn, rewards those who climb its 155 steps with a wonderful city view.

Cost and Hours: Museum—€5, entrance through cellar, July-Aug Mon-Sat 10:00-16:00, closed Sun and Sept-June; audioguide-€4.75; tower—€3, May-mid-Sept daily 11:00-18:00, closed rest of year; tel. 645-7900, www.tallinn.ee/raekoda.

Tallinn City Museum (Tallinna Linnamuuseum)

This humble museum, filling a 14th-century townhouse, features Tallinn history from 1200 to the 1950s. It displays everyday items through history. Even though there are basic English explanations, it's not enough; the museum is a loose collection of artifacts that offers a few intimate peeks at local lifestyles.

Cost and Hours: €3.20, March-Oct Wed-Mon 10:30-18:00, Nov-Feb Wed-Mon 10:00-17:30, closed Tue year-round, last entry 30 minutes before closing, Vene 17, at corner of Pühavaimu, tel. 615-5183, www.linnamuuseum.ee.

Visiting the Museum: You'll begin on the ground floor, at a model of circa-1825 Tallinn—looking much like it does today. Then you'll head up through three more floors, exploring exhibits on the port (with model ships), guilds (tools and products), advertising in the 1920s and 30s (chronicling the rise of modern local industries in pre-Soviet times), Tallinn's Estonian identity (with recreated rooms from the early 20th century), and the Soviet period (displaying propaganda, including children's art that celebrated the regime).

Freedom Square (Vabaduse Väljak)

Once a USSR-era parking lot at the southern tip of the Old Town, this fine public zone was recently revamped: The cars were moved underground, and now a glassy new plaza invites locals (and very few tourists) to linger. The recommended **Wabadus café,** with tables out on the square, is a popular hangout. The space, designed to host special events, feels a bit stern and at odds with the cutesy cobbles just a few steps away. But it's an easy opportunity to glimpse a contrast to the tourists' Tallinn.

The towering **cross** monument facing the square (marked *Eesti Vabadussõda 1918-1920*) honors the Estonian War of Independence. Shortly after the Bolshevik Revolution set a new course for Russia, the Estonians took advantage of the post-WWI reshuffling of Europe to rise up and create—for the first time ever—an independent Estonian state. The "cross of liberty" on top of the pillar represents a military decoration

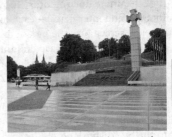

from that war (and every war since). The hill behind the cross has more monuments, and fragments of past fortifications.

Across the busy street from the square, the hulking, red-brick building houses the **office of Tallinn's mayor.** Edgar Savisaar, a former prime minister, has been mayor of this city twice (most recently since 2007). Criticized by some for his authoritarian approach and his coziness with Russia, Savisaar is adored by others for his aggressive legislation. For example, in 2013, he made all public transit completely free to anyone living within the city limits—a move designed to cut commuting costs (and carbon emissions) and to lure suburbanites to move into the town center. Younger locals grumble about what they jokingly term *"Homo soveticus"*—a different species of Estonian who was raised in Soviet times and is accustomed to a system where everything is free. To this day, governmental giveaways are the easiest way to boost approval ratings.

If you're interested in Estonia's 20th- and 21st-century history, it's an easy five-minute walk from this square to the next sight.

▲Museum of Occupations (Okupatsioonide Muuseum)

Locals insist that Estonia didn't formally lose its independence from 1939 to 1991, but was just "occupied"—first by the Soviets (for

TALLINN

one year), then by the Nazis (for three years), and then again by the USSR (for nearly 50 years). Built with funding from a wealthy Estonian-American, this compact museum tells the history of Estonia during its occupations.

Cost and Hours: €5, June-Aug Tue-Sun 10:00-18:00, Sept-May Tue-Sun 11:00-18:00, closed Mon year-round, skip the amateurish €4 audioguide, Toompea 8, at corner of Kaarli Puiestee, tel. 668-0250, www.okupatsioon.ee.

Visiting the Museum: Entering, you'll walk past a poignant monument made of giant suitcases—a reminder of people who fled the country. After buying your ticket, pick up the English descriptions and explore. (The ticket desk also sells a well-chosen range of English-language books on the occupation years.)

The exhibit is organized around seven TV monitors screening 30-minute **documentary films** (with dry commentary, archival footage, and interviews)—each focusing on a different time period. At each screen, use the mouse to select English. Surrounding each monitor is a display case crammed with artifacts of the era. The footage of the Singing Revolution is particularly stirring.

Before settling into the film loop, take a quick clockwise spin from the ticket desk to see the larger **exhibits,** which illustrate how the Soviets kept the Estonians in line. First you'll see a rustic boat that a desperate defector actually rowed across the Baltic Sea to the Swedish island of Gotland. Look for the unsettling surveillance peephole, which will make you want to carefully examine your stateroom tonight. Surrounded by a lot more of those symbolic suitcases, the large monument with a swastika and a red star is a reminder that Estonia was occupied by not one, but two different regimes in the 20th century. You'll also see vintage cars, phone boxes, and radios that give a flavor of that era. Near the center of the exhibit, somber prison doors evoke the countless lives lost to detention and deportation.

Near those prison doors, take the red-velvet staircase down to the **basement.** There, near the WCs, is a collection of Soviet-era statues of communist leaders—once they lorded over the people, now they're in the cellar guarding the toilets.

▲Rotermann Quarter (Rotermanni Kvartal)

Sprawling between Hotel Viru and the port, just east of the Old Town, this 19th-century industrial zone is being redeveloped into shopping, office, and living space. Characteristic old brick shells are being topped with visually striking glass-and-steel additions. For those interested in the gentrification of an aging city—and, quite possibly, even for those who aren't—it's worth a quick stroll to see the cutting edge of old-meets-new Nordic architecture. While construction is ongoing, and the area still feels a bit

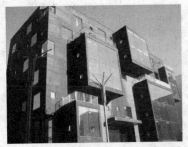

soulless (only a few shops and restaurants are open), developers are setting the stage for the creation of a vital new downtown district. I've recommended two good restaurants that give you an excuse to walk five minutes across the street from the Old Town to take a look around; see "Eating in Tallinn," later. To see the first completed section, start at Hotel Viru, cross busy Narva Maantee and walk down Roseni street. At #7 you'll find the hard-to-resist Kalev chocolate shop, selling Estonia's best-known sweets (Mon-Sat 10:00-20:00, Sun 11:00-18:00).

KADRIORG PARK AND THE KUMU MUSEUM
▲Kadriorg Park

This expansive seaside park, home to a summer royal residence and the Kumu Art Museum, is just a five-minute tram ride or a 25-minute walk from Hotel Viru. After Russia took over Tallinn in 1710, Peter the Great built the cute, pint-sized Kadriorg Palace for Czarina Catherine (the palace's name means "Catherine's Valley"). Stately, peaceful, and crisscrossed by leafy paths, the park has a rose garden, duck-filled pond, playground and benches, and old czarist guardhouses harkening back to the days of Russian rule. It's a delightful place for a stroll or a picnic. If it's rainy, duck

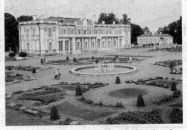

into one of the cafés in the park's art museums (described below).

Getting There: Reach the park on tram #1 or #3 (direction: Kadriorg; catch at any tram stop around the Old Town). Get off at the Kadriorg stop (the end of the line, where trams turn and head back into town), and walk 200 yards straight ahead and up Weizenbergi, the park's main avenue. Peter's summer palace is on the left; behind it, visit the formal garden (free). At the end of the avenue is the Kumu Art Museum, the park's most important sight. A taxi from Hotel Viru to this area should cost €5 or less. If you're returning from here directly to the port to catch your cruise ship, use tram #1—it stops at the Linnahall stop near the main cruise port and Terminals A, B, and C (a bit father from Terminal D).

Visiting Kadriorg Park: The palace's manicured **gardens** (free to enter) are a pure delight; on weekends, you'll likely see a steady parade of brides and grooms here, posing for wedding pictures. The summer palace itself is home to the **Kadriorg Art Museum** (Kadrioru Kunstimuuseum), with very modest Russian and Western European galleries (€4.80; May-Sept Tue-Sun 10:00-17:00, Wed until 20:00, closed Mon; same hours off-season except closed Mon-Tue; Weizenbergi 37, tel. 606-6400, www.kadriorumuuseum.ee).

The fenced-off yard directly behind the garden is where you'll spot the local "White House" (although it's pink)—home of **Estonia's president.** Walk around to the far side to find its main entrance, with the seal of Estonia above the door, flagpoles flying both the Estonian and the EU flags, and stone-faced guards.

A five-minute walk beyond the presidential palace takes you to the Kumu Art Museum, described next. For a longer walk from here, the rugged park rolls down toward the sea.

▲▲Kumu Art Museum (Kumu Kunstimuuseum)

This main branch of the Art Museum of Estonia brings the nation's best art together in a striking modern building designed by an international (well, at least Finnish) architect, Pekka Vapaavuori. The entire collection is accessible, well-presented, and engaging, with a particularly thought-provoking section on art from the Soviet period. The museum is well worth the trip for art lovers, or for anyone intrigued by the unique spirit of this tiny nation—particularly when combined with a stroll through the nearby palace gardens (described earlier) on a sunny day.

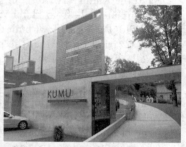

Cost and Hours: €5.50, or €4.20 for just the permanent collection; May-Sept Tue-Sun 11:00-18:00, Wed until 20:00, closed Mon; same hours off-season except closed Mon-Tue; audioguide-€3.20; trendy café, tel. 602-6000, www.kumu.ee.

Getting There: To reach the museum, follow the instructions for Kadriorg Park, explained earlier; Kumu is at the far end of the park. To get from the Old Town to Kumu directly without walking through the park, take bus #67 or #68 (each runs every 10-15 minutes, #68 does not run on Sun); both leave from Teatri Väljak, on the far side of the pastel yellow theater, across from the Solaris shopping mall. Get off at the Kumu stop, then walk up the stairs and across the bridge.

Visiting the Museum: Just off the ticket lobby (on the second floor), the **great hall** has temporary exhibits; however, the permanent collection on the third and fourth floors is Kumu's main draw. While you can rent an audioguide, I found the free laminated sheets in most rooms enough to enjoy the collection. The maze-like layout on each floor presents the art chronologically.

The **third floor** displays a concise "Treasury of Estonian Art" through the mid-20th century. It starts with 18th-century portraits of local aristocrats, then moves through 19th-century Romanticism (including some nice views of Tallinn, scenes of Estonian nature, and idealized images of Estonian peasant women in folk costumes). Eduard von Gebhardt's engaging *Sermon on the Mount* (1904) includes a wide variety of Estonian portraits—some attentive, others distracted—listening to Jesus' most famous address. You'll see the Estonian version of several Modernist styles: Pointillism (linger over the lyrical landscapes of Konrad Mägi and the recently rediscovered works of Herbert Lukk), Cubism, and Expressionism. In the 1930s, the Pallas School provided a more traditional, back-to-nature response to the wild artistic trends of the time. By the dawn of World War II, you can see the art growing even more conservative, and the final canvases, from the war years, convey an unmistakable melancholy.

The **fourth-floor exhibit,** called "Difficult Choices," is a fascinating survey of Estonian art from the end of World War II until "re-independence" in 1991. Some of the works are mainstream (read: Soviet-style), while others are by dissident artists.

Estonian art parted ways with Western Europe with the Soviet takeover in 1945. The Soviets insisted that artworks actively promote the communist struggle, and to that end, Estonian artists were forced to adopt the Stalinist formula, making paintings that were done in the traditional national style but that were socialist in content—in the style now called **Socialist Realism.**

Socialist Realism had its roots in the early 20th-century Realist movement, whose artists wanted to depict the actual conditions of life rather than just glamour and wealth—in America, think of John Steinbeck's novels or Walker Evans' photographs of the rural poor. In the Soviet Union, this artistic curiosity about the working class was perverted into an ideology: Art was supposed to glorify labor and the state's role in distributing its fruits. In a system where there was ultimately little incentive to work hard, art was seen as a tool to motivate the masses, and to support the Communist Party's hold on power.

In the collection's first room, called "A Tale of Happiness," you'll see syrupy images of what Soviet leadership imagined to be the ideal of communist Estonia. In *Agitator Amongst the Voters* (1952), a stern portrait of Stalin in the hazy background keeps an eye on a young hotshot articulating some questionable ideas; his listeners' reactions range from shudders of horror to smirks of superiority. *The Young Aviators* (1951) shows an eager youngster wearing a bright-red neckerchief (indicating his membership in the Pioneers, the propaganda-laden communist version of Scouts) telling his enraptured schoolmates stories about a model airplane.

The next room shows canvases of miners, protesters, speech-ifiers, metalworkers, tractor drivers, and more all doing their utmost for the communist society. You'll also see paintings of industrial achievements (like bridges) and party meetings. Because mining was integral to the Estonian economy, miners were portrayed as local heroes, marching like soldiers to their glorious labor. Women were depicted toiling side by side with men, as equal partners.

While supposedly a reflection of "real" life, Socialist Realism art was formulaic and showed little creative spirit. Though some Estonian artists flirted with social commentary and the avant-garde, a few ended up in Siberia as a result.

Later, in the Brezhnev years, Estonian artists managed to slip Surrealist, Pop, and Photorealist themes into their work (for example, Rein Tammik's large painting *1945-1975*, which juxtaposes an old tractor with the flower children of the Swingin' Sixties). Estonia was the only part of the USSR that recognized Pop Art. As the Soviets would eventually learn, change was unstoppable.

The rest of the museum is devoted to temporary exhibits, with contemporary art always on the **fifth floor** (where there's a nice view back to the Old Town from the far gallery).

ALONG THE HARBORFRONT
▲▲Seaplane Harbor (Lennusadam)

One of Tallinn's newest and most ambitious sights, this nautical, aviation, and military museum fills a gigantic old hangar along the

waterfront north of downtown. It has loads of hands-on activities for kids, and thrills anyone interested in transportation, while others find it off-puttingly militaris-tic. (The many Russian tour-ists who enjoy posing with its machine-gun simulators don't help matters.)

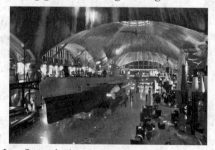

Cost and Hours: €10; May-Sept daily 10:00-19:00; same hours off-season except closed Mon; last entry one hour before closing, Vesilennuki 6, tel. 620-0550, www.seaplaneharbour.com.

Getting There: It's along the waterfront, about a mile north of the Old Town. It's a long but doable **walk,** made more enjoyable if you follow the red-gravel "Culture Kilometer" (Kultuurikilomeeter) seaside path from near the cruise terminals. While there's no handy tram or bus to the museum, a one-way **taxi**

from the town center shouldn't cost much more than €5. The **hop-on, hop-off buses** also stop here.

Visiting the Museum: When you buy your ticket, you'll be issued an electronic card, which you can use at terminals posted throughout the exhibit to email yourself articles on topics that interest you. The entire collection is enlivened by lots of interactive screens, giant movies, and simulators (such as huge-scale shoot-em-up video games with life-sized artillery). Touchscreens explain everything in three languages: Estonian, Russian, and English...in that order.

The cavernous old **seaplane hangar** cleverly displays exhibits on three levels: the ground floor features items from beneath the sea (such as a salvaged 16th-century shipwreck, plus a cinema that shows films subtitled in English); catwalks halfway up connect exhibits dealing with the sea surface (the impressive boat collection—from buoys to sailboats to the massive *Lembit* sub); and airplanes are suspended overhead. Touchscreens provide more information in English; just take your time exploring the collection. The star of the show is the 195-foot-long *Lembit* submarine from 1937: Estonian-commissioned and British-built, this vessel saw fighting in World War II and later spent several decades in the service of the USSR's Red Fleet. You can climb down below decks to see how the sailors lived, peek through the periscope, and even stare down the torpedo tubes. A cool café on the top level (above the entrance) overlooks the entire space, which feels endless.

Outside, filling the old harbor, is the maritime museum's collection of **historic ships,** from old-fashioned tall ships to modern-day military boats. The highlight is the steam-powered icebreaker *Suur Tõll*, from 1914. Sometimes you can pay to go out on a brief trip on one of the sailboats (ask at the ticket desk when you enter).

OUTER TALLINN
▲Song Festival Grounds (Lauluväljak)

At this open-air theater, built in 1959 and resembling an oversized Hollywood Bowl, the Estonian nation gathers to sing. Every five years, these grounds host a huge national song festival with 25,000 singers and 100,000 spectators. During the festival, the singers rehearse from Monday through Thursday, and then, on Friday morning, dress up in their traditional outfits and march out to the Song Festival Grounds from Freedom Square. While it hosts big pop-music acts, too, it's a national monument for the compelling role it played in Estonia's fight for independence.

Since 1988, when locals sang patriotic songs here in defiance of Soviet rule, these grounds have taken on a symbolic importance to the nation. Locals vividly recall putting on folk costumes knitted by their grandmothers (some of whom later died in Siberia)

Estonia's Singing Revolution

When you are a humble nation of just a million people lodged between Russia and Germany (and tyrants such as Stalin and Hitler), simply surviving is a challenge. Estonia was free from 1920 to 1939. Then they had a 50-year Nazi/Soviet nightmare. Estonians say, "We were so few in numbers that we had to emphasize that we exist. We had no weapons. Being together and singing together was our power." Singing has long been a national form of expression in this country; the first Estonian Song Festival occurred in 1869, and has been held every five years since then.

Estonian culture was under siege during the Soviet era. Moscow wouldn't allow locals to wave their flag or sing patriotic songs. Russians and Ukrainians were moved in, and Estonians were shipped out in an attempt to dilute the country's identity. But as cracks began to appear in the USSR, the Estonians mobilized—by singing.

In 1988, 300,000 Estonians—imagine...a third of the population—gathered at the Song Festival Grounds outside Tallinn to sing patriotic songs. On August 23, 1989—the 50th anniversary of a notorious pact between Hitler and Stalin—the people of Latvia, Lithuania, and Estonia held hands to make "the Baltic Chain," a human chain that stretched 360 miles from Tallinn to Vilnius in Lithuania. Some feared a Tiananmen Square-type bloodbath, but Estonians kept singing.

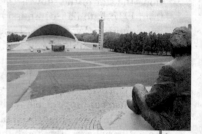

In February of 1990, the first free parliamentary elections took place in all three Baltic states, and pro-independence candidates won majorities. In 1991, hardline communists staged a coup against Soviet leader Mikhail Gorbachev, and Estonians feared a violent crackdown. The makeshift Estonian Parliament declared independence. Then, the coup in Moscow failed. Suddenly, the USSR was gone, and Estonia was free.

Watch the documentary film *The Singing Revolution* before your visit (www.singingrevolution.com) to tune into this stirring bit of modern history and to draw inspiration from Estonia's valiant struggle for freedom.

and coming here with masses of Estonians to sing. Overlooking the grounds from the cheap seats is a statue of Gustav Ernesaks, who directed the Estonian National Male Choir for 50 years through the darkest times of Soviet rule. He was a power in the drive for independence, and lived to see it happen.

Cost and Hours: Free, open long hours, bus #1A, #5, #8, #34A, or #38 to Lauluväljak stop.

▲Estonian Open-Air Museum (Vabaõhumuuseum)

Influenced by their ties with Nordic countries, Estonians are enthusiastic advocates of open-air museums. For this one, they salvaged farm buildings, windmills, and an old church from rural areas and transported them to a park-like setting just outside town (4 miles west of the Old Town). The goal: to both save and share their heritage. Attendants 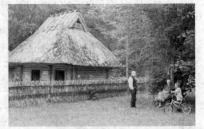 are posted in many houses, but to really visualize life in the old houses, rent the audioguide (€7/3 hours). The park's Kolu Tavern serves traditional dishes. You can rent a bike (€3/hour) for a breezy roll to quiet, faraway spaces in the park.

Cost and Hours: Late April-Sept: €7, park open daily 10:00-20:00, historic buildings until 18:00; Oct-late April: €5, park open daily 10:00-17:00 but many buildings closed; tel. 654-9100, www.evm.ee.

Getting There: Take bus #21 or #21B from the train station to the Rocca al Mare stop. Because buses back to Tallinn run infrequently, check the departure schedule as soon as you arrive, or ask staff how to find the Zoo stop, with more frequent service, a 15-minute walk away.

Shopping in Tallinn

With so many cruisers inundating Tallinn, the Old Town is full of trinkets, but it is possible to find good-quality stuff. Wooden goods, like butter knives and juniper-wood trivets, are a good value. Marvel at the variety on sale in Tallinn's liquor stores, popular with visiting Scandinavians. Tucked into the Old Town are many craft and artisan shops where prices are lower than in Nordic countries.

The **"Sweater Wall"** is a fun place to browse sweaters and woolens, though few are hand-knitted by grandmothers these 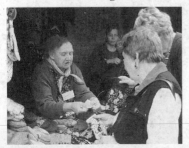 days. Find the stalls under the wall on Müürivahe street (daily 10:00-17:00, near the corner of Viru street, described on page 467). From there, explore **Katariina Käik,** a small alley between Müürivahe and Vene streets, which has several handicraft stores and workshops selling pieces that make nice souvenirs.

TALLINN

The cheery **Navitrolla Gallerii** is filled with work by the well-known Estonian artist who goes just by the name Navitrolla. His whimsical, animal-themed prints are vaguely reminiscent of *Where the Wild Things Are* (Mon-Fri 10:00-18:00, Sat 10:00-17:00, Sun 10:00-16:00, Sulevimägi 1, tel. 631-3716, www.navitrolla.ee).

The **Rahva Raamat** bookstore in the Viru Keskus mall (floors 3-4, high up in the glass atrium) has English-language literature on the main floor, and a huge wall of travel books upstairs (daily 9:00-21:00).

Balti Jaam Market, Tallinn's bustling traditional market, is behind the train station and has little of touristic interest besides

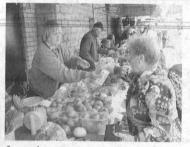

wonderful photo ops. That's why I like it. It's a great time-warp scene, fragrant with dill, berries, onions, and mushrooms. You'll hear lots of Russian. The indoor sections sell meat, clothing, and gadgets. You could also assemble a very rustic picnic here. To find the market from the train station, just walk across the head of the train platforms (following *Jaama Turg* signs) and keep going (Mon-Fri 8:00-18:00, Sat-Sun 8:00-17:00, better early).

For something tamer, the **Viru Turg outdoor market,** a block outside the Old Town's Viru Gate, has a lively, tourist-oriented collection of stalls selling mostly clothing, textiles, and flowers (daily May-Sept 9:00-17:00, Oct-April 10:00-16:00, north of Viru street at Mere Puiestee 1).

Eating in Tallinn

Tallinn's Old Town has a wide selection of largely interchangeable, mostly tourist-oriented eateries. Don't expect bargains here—you'll pay near-Scandinavian prices (average main dishes can cost €15-20). For a better value, roam at least a block or two off the

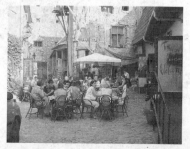

main drags, where you can find great food at what seems like fire-sale prices. At most of my listings, you can assemble a three-course meal for around €20. Some restaurants have good-value lunch specials on weekdays (look for the words *päeva praad*). As a mark of quality, watch for restaurants with an *Astu Sisse!* label in the window;

this Estonian equivalent of a Michelin star is awarded to just 50 restaurants each year. Tipping is not required, but if you like the service, round your bill up by 5-10 percent when paying.

A few years ago it was hard to find authentic local cuisine, but now Estonian food is trendy—a hearty Northern mixture of meat, potatoes, root vegetables, mushrooms, dill, garlic, bread, and soup. Pea soup is a local specialty. You usually get a few slices of bread as a free, automatic side dish. A typical pub snack is Estonian garlic bread *(küüslauguleivad)*—deep-fried strips of dark rye bread smothered in garlic and served with a dipping sauce. Estonia's Saku beer is good, cheap, and on tap at most eateries. Try the nutty, full-bodied Tume variety.

ESTONIAN CUISINE IN THE OLD TOWN

Restorant Aed is an elegant, almost gourmet, health-food eatery calling itself "the embassy of pure food." While not vegetarian, it is passionate about serving organic, seasonal, modern Estonian cuisine in a woody, romantic setting. Take your pick from four dining options: under old beams, in the cellar, out front on the sidewalk, or out back on the garden terrace (€10-15 main dishes, daily 12:00-23:00, Rataskaevu 8, tel. 626-9088, www.vonkrahl.ee/aed).

Vanaema Juures ("Grandma's Place"), an eight-table cellar restaurant, serves homey, traditional Estonian meals, such as pork roast with sauerkraut and horseradish. This is a fine bet for local cuisine. No tacky medieval stuff here—just good food at fair prices in a pleasant ambience, where you expect your waitress to show up with her hair in a bun and wearing granny glasses (€8-17 main dishes, daily 12:00-22:00, Rataskaevu 10/12, tel. 626-9080, www.vonkrahl.ee/vanaemajuures).

At **Leib** ("Back Bread"), just outside the walls at the seaside end of the Old Town, you enter up steps into a fun garden under the medieval ramparts, and can sit indoors or out. Peruse the classy and engaging menu, which changes with the seasons—their food has Estonian roots, but with international influences (€10-16 main courses, daily 12:00-15:00 & 18:00-23:00, Uus 31, tel. 611-9026, www.leibresto.ee/en).

Mekk is a small, fresh, upscale place whose name stands for "modern Estonian cuisine." While their à la carte prices are a bit higher than at my other listings, they offer artful weekday lunch specials for just €7 (not available July-Aug), and a €35 four-course fixed-price meal for serious eaters. Young, elegant locals take their lunch breaks here (€12-25 main dishes, Mon-Sat 12:00-23:00, closed Sun, Suur-Karja 17/19, tel. 680-6688, www.mekk.ee).

Modern Cuisine on Freedom Square: **Wabadus,** facing the vast and modern square, turns its back on old Tallinn. This sleek, urbane café/restaurant—which has been the town meeting

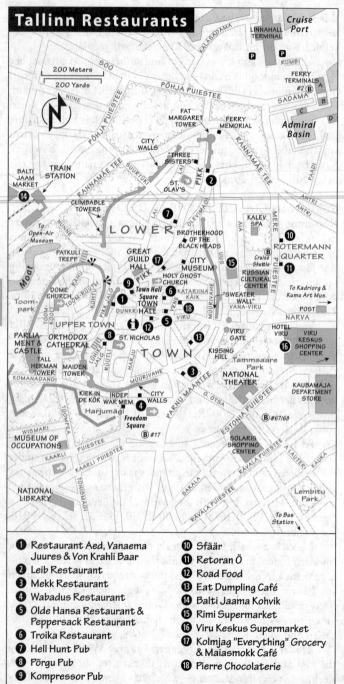

Tallinn Restaurants

1 Restaurant Aed, Vanaema Juures & Von Krahli Baar
2 Leib Restaurant
3 Mekk Restaurant
4 Wabadus Restaurant
5 Olde Hansa Restaurant & Peppersack Restaurant
6 Troika Restaurant
7 Hell Hunt Pub
8 Põrgu Pub
9 Kompressor Pub
10 Sfäär
11 Retoran Ö
12 Road Food
13 Eat Dumpling Café
14 Balti Jaama Kohvik
15 Rimi Supermarket
16 Viru Keskus Supermarket
17 Kolmjag "Everything" Grocery & Maiasmokk Café
18 Pierre Chocolaterie

place since 1937—serves coffee, cocktails, and international fare. To escape the cobbles and crowds of the Old Town, walk a few minutes to enjoy a moment of peace—ideally at one of the terrace tables on the square, if the weather's good (€5 weekday lunch specials, €7-10 salads, €7-18 main courses, Mon-Tue 11:00-19:00, Wed-Thu 11:00-21:00, Fri-Sat 11:00-24:00, closed Sun, Vabaduse Väljak 10, tel. 601-6461, www.wabadus.ee).

TOURIST TRAPS ON AND NEAR TOWN HALL SQUARE

Tallinn's central square is a whirlpool of tacky tourism, where aggressive restaurant touts (some dressed as medieval wenches or giant matryoshka dolls) accost passersby to lure them in for a drink or meal. While a bit off-putting, some of these restaurants have surprisingly good (if expensive) food. Of the many options ringing the square and surrounding streets, these are the ones most worth considering.

"Medieval" Estonian Cuisine: Two well-run restaurants just below Town Hall Square specialize in re-creating medieval food (from the days before the arrival of the potato and tomato from the New World). Each is grotesquely touristy, complete with gift shops where you can buy your souvenir goblet. Both have street seating, but you'll get all the tourists and none of the atmosphere.

Olde Hansa, filling three creaky old floors and outdoor tables with tourists, candle wax, and scurrying medieval waitresses, can be quite expensive. And yet, the local consensus is that the food here is far better than it has any right to be (€14-30 main dishes, daily 10:00-24:00, musicians circulate Tue-Sun after 18:00, a belch below Town Hall Square at Vana Turg 1, reserve in advance, tel. 627-9020, www.oldehansa.ee).

Peppersack, across the street, tries to compete in the same price range, and feels marginally less circus-like (Vana Turg 6, tel. 646-6800).

Russian Food: As more than a third of the local population is enthusiastically Russian, there are plenty of places serving Russian cuisine (see also "Budget Eateries," described later). **Troika** is my choice for Russian food. Right on Town Hall Square, with a folkloric-costumed waitstaff, they serve €7-11 *bliny* (pancakes) and *pelmeni* (dumplings), and €11-20 main dishes. Sit out on the square; in the more casual, Russian-village-themed tavern; or under a fine vault in the trendy, atmospheric cellar (which has slightly cheaper prices) (open daily 10:00-23:00, Raekoja Plats 15, tel. 627-6245, www.troika.ee).

TALLINN

PUBS IN THE OLD TOWN

Young Estonians eat well and affordably at pubs. In some pubs, you go to the bar to look at the menu, order, and pay. Then find a table, and they'll bring your food out when it's ready.

Hell Hunt Pub ("The Gentle Wolf") was the first Western-style pub to open after 1991, and it's still going strong, attracting a mixed expat and local crowd with its tasty food. Five of their own microbrews are on tap. Consider making a meal from the great pub snacks (€3-6) plus a salad (€5-6). Choose a table in its convivial, rustic-industrial interior or on the garden terrace across the street (€6 pastas, €10 main dishes, daily 12:00-24:00, Pikk 39, tel. 681-8333).

Von Krahli Baar serves cheap, substantial Estonian grub—such as potato pancakes *(torud)* stuffed with mushrooms or shrimp—in a big, dark space that doubles as a center for Estonia's alternative theater scene; there's also seating in the tiny courtyard where you enter. It started as the bar of the theater upstairs, then expanded to become a restaurant, so it has a young, avant-garde vibe. You'll feel like you're eating backstage with the stagehands (€6-7 main dishes, Mon-Sat 12:00-24:00, Sun 12:00-15:00, Rataskaevu 10/12, a block uphill from Town Hall Square, near Wheel Well, tel. 626-9090).

Põrgu is particularly serious about its beer, with a wide variety of international and Estonian brews on tap—including some microbrews. Its simple, uncluttered cellar feels like less of a tourist trap than the others listed here (€3-7 bar snacks and salads, €8-13 main dishes, Mon-Sat 12:00-24:00, closed Sun, Rüütli 4, tel. 644-0232).

Kompressor, a big, open-feeling beer hall, is in all the guidebooks for its cheap, huge, and filling €5 pancakes—savory or sweet (daily 11:00-24:00, Rataskaevu 3, tel. 646-4210).

IN THE ROTERMANN QUARTER

This modern, up-and-coming district (described on page 470), just across the busy road from Tallinn's Old Town, is well worth exploring for a jolt of cutting-edge architecture and hipster edginess. It's an antidote to the central area's ye-olde aura. As more and more buildings in this zone are being renovated, this is a fast-changing scene. But these two choices, in a long brick building facing the Old Town, are well-established and a good starting point.

Sfäär (Sphere), which combines an unpretentious bistro with a design shop, is a killing-two-birds look at the Rotermann Quarter. In this lively, cheery place, tables are tucked between locally designed clothes and home decor. The menu is bold but accessible and affordable, featuring Estonian and international fare with a hint of molecular flair (€6-10 starters and pastas, €12-16 main dishes, Mon-Wed 8:00-22:00, Thu-Fri 8:00-24:00, Sat 10:00-24:00, Sun 10:00-22:00, shop open daily 12:00-21:00, Mere Puiestee 6E, mobile 5699-2200, www.sfaar.ee).

Retoran Ö (Swedish for "Island"), just a few doors down in the same building, is your Rotermann Quarter splurge. The dressy, trendy, retrofitted-warehouse interior feels a sophisticated world away from the Old Town's tourist traps. The cuisine tries to highlight an Estonian approach to "New Nordic" cooking—small dishes carefully constructed with seasonal, local ingredients. Reservations are smart (€19-24 main courses, €70 tasting *menu*, Mon-Sat 18:00-23:00, closed Sun, Mere Puiestee 6E—enter from the parking lot around back, tel. 661-6150, www.restoran-o.ee).

BUDGET EATERIES

Road Food, tucked on a tiny lane immediately behind the Town Hall Tower, has some of the best cheap eats in the city. A branch of the Olde Hansa food empire, this sandwich shop serves up an excellent, quick taste of Estonia, stuffing its €4-5 sandwiches with local meats and sauces. It's attached to a well-stocked beer and wine shop, making it easy to browse for the perfect drink to wash things down (daily 11:00-24:00, shorter hours off-season, Vanaturo kael 8).

Eat, a laid-back, cellar-level student hangout with a big foos-ball table and a book exchange, serves the best-value lunch in town. Its menu is very simple: three varieties of *pelmeenid* (dumplings), plus sauces, beet salad, and pickles. You dish up what you like and pay by weight (€2-3/big bowl). Ask for an education in the various dumplings and sauces and then go for the complete experience. Enjoy with abandon—you can't spend much money here, and you'll feel good stoking their business (Mon-Sat 11:00-21:00, closed Sun, Sauna 2, tel. 644-0029).

At the Outdoor Market: **Balti Jaama Kohvik,** at the end of the train station near the Balti Jaam Market, is an unimpressive-looking 24-hour diner with no real sign (look for a faded red awning and *Kohvik avatud 24 tundi*—"café open 24 hours"—on the door; it's actually built into the train-station building). The bustling stainless-steel kitchen cranks out traditional Russian/Estonian dishes—the cheapest hot food in town. While you won't see or hear a word of English here, the glass case displays the various offerings and prices (€3 meals, €1.60 soups, dirt-cheap-yet-wonderful savory pancakes for less than €1, and tasty *beljaš*—a kind of pierogi). Unfortunately, the area feels sketchy after dark.

Supermarkets: For picnic supplies, try the **Rimi** supermarket just outside the Old Town at Aia 7, near the Viru Gate (daily 8:00-22:00). A larger, more upscale supermarket in the basement of the

What If I Miss My Boat?

Remember that you can get help from the cruise line's port agent (listed on the destination information sheet distributed on the ship) and the local TI (see page 451). If the port agent suggests a costly solution (such as a private car with a driver), you may want to consider public transit.

Frequent fast boats connect Tallinn to **Helsinki;** these are operated by Tallink Silja (tel. 640-9808, www.tallinksilja. com), Linda Line (tel. 699-9333, www.lindaline.ee), Eckerö Line (tel. 664-6006, www.eckeroline.fi), and Viking Line (tel. 666-3966, www.vikingline.fi). Tallink Silja boats also go to **Stockholm** overnight. St. Peter Line boats connect to **St. Petersburg,** but you can do this only if you've arranged a visa long in advance (www.stpeterline.com). To reach **Rīga,** the bus is easy. For many other destinations—such as **Copenhagen** or **Oslo**—you can take an overnight boat to Stockholm, then connect by train. (To research train schedules, see www.bahn.com.) But for these and other destinations, it may be even better to fly.

If you need to catch a **plane,** you can ride the bus to the convenient Tallinn airport (Tallinna Lennujaam), just three miles southeast of downtown (www.tallinn-airport.ee).

Local **travel agents** in Tallinn, such as Estravel, can help you (see page 452). For more advice on what to do if you miss the boat, see page 139.

Viru Keskus mall (directly behind Hotel Viru) has convenient, inexpensive take-away meals (daily 9:00-21:00). The handy little **Kolmjag "Everything"** grocery is a block off Town Hall Square (daily 24 hours, Pikk 11, tel. 631-1511).

PASTRIES

The **Maiasmokk** ("Sweet Tooth") café and pastry shop, founded in 1864, is the grande dame of Tallinn cafés—ideal for dessert. Even through the Soviet days, this was *the* place for a good pastry or a glass of herby Tallinn schnapps ("Vana Tallinn"). Point to what you want from the selection of classic local pastries at the counter, and sit down for coffee on the other side of the shop. Everything's reasonable (Mon-Fri 8:00-21:00, Sat 9:00-21:00, Sun 9:00-20:00, Pikk 16, across from church with old clock, tel. 646-4079). They also have a marzipan shop (separate entrance).

Pierre Chocolaterie at Vene 6 has scrumptious fresh pralines, sandwiches, and coffee in a courtyard filled with craft shops (also €5-8 light meals, daily 8:30-late, tel. 641-8061).

Estonian Survival Phrases

Estonian has a few unusual vowel sounds. The letter *ä* is pronounced "ah" as in "hat," but *a* without the umlaut sounds more like "aw" as in "hot." To make the sound *ö*, purse your lips and say "oh"; the letter *õ* is similar, but with the lips less pursed. Listen to locals and imitate. In the phonetics, ī sounds like the long *i* in "light," and bolded syllables are stressed.

English	Estonian	Pronunciation
Hello. (formal)	Tervist.	**tehr**-veest
Hi. / Bye. (informal)	Tere. / Nägemist.	**teh**-reh / **nah**-geh-meest
Do you speak English?	Kas te räägite inglise keelt?	kahs teh **raah**-gee-teh **een**-glee-seh kehlt
Yes. / No.	Jah. / Ei.	yah / ay
Please. / You're welcome.	Palun.	**pah**-luhn
Thank you (very much).	Tänan (väga).	**tah**-nahn (**vah**-gaw)
Can I help you?	Saan ma teid aidata?	saahn mah tayd ī-dah-tah
Excuse me.	Vabandust.	**vaw**-bahn-doost
(Very) good.	(Väga) hea.	(**vah**-gaw) **hey**-ah
Goodbye.	Hüvasti.	**hew**-vaw-stee
one / two	üks / kaks	ewks / kawks
three / four	kolm / neli	kohlm / **nay**-lee
five / six	viis / kuus	vees / koos
seven / eight	seitse / kaheksa	**sayt**-seh / **kaw**-hehk-sah
nine / ten	üheksa / kümme	**ew**-hehk-sah / **kew**-meh
hundred	sada	**saw**-daw
thousand	tuhat	**too**-hawt
How much?	Kui palju?	kwee **pawl**-yoo
local currency: (Estonian) crown	(Eesti) krooni	(**eh**-stee) **kroo**-nee
Where is...?	Kus asub...?	koos ah-**soob**
...the toilet	...tualett	**too**-ah-leht
men	mees	mehs
women	naine	**nī**-neh
water / coffee	vesi / kohvi	**vay**-see / **koh**-vee
beer / wine	õlu / vein	**oh**-loo / vayn
Cheers!	Terviseks!	**tehr**-vee-sehks
The bill, please.	Arve, palun.	**ahr**-veh **pah**-luhn

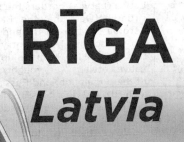

RĪGA
Latvia

Latvia Practicalities

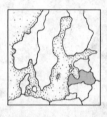

Latvia (Latvija) borders the Baltic Sea, sitting between the other Baltic states: Estonia (to the north) and Lithuania (to the south). The country's population (2.2 million) is made up largely of native Latvians (very roughly two-thirds of the population) and Russians (about a third). Latvia's terrain of generally low plains covers 25,000 square miles, about the size of West Virginia. Latvia's major city and capital is Rīga (at 700,000 residents, the Baltic states' largest city). Roughly half the jobs in Latvia are located in the city. Like its Baltic neighbors, Latvia spent most of its history occupied by foreign powers—Sweden, Russia, Germany, the USSR—but became independent in 1991 (following the breakup of the Soviet Union) and joined both NATO and the European Union in the spring of 2004.

Money: €1 (euro) = about $1.40. An ATM is called a *bankomāti*. The local VAT (value-added sales tax) rate is 21 percent; the minimum purchase eligible for a VAT refund is €44 (for details on refunds, see page 134).

Language: The native language is Latvian.

Emergencies: Dial 112 for police, medical, or other emergencies. (You can also dial 02 for police and 03 for an ambulance.) In case of theft or loss, see page 125.

Time Zone: Latvia is one hour ahead of Central European Time (seven/ten hours ahead of the East/ West Coasts of the US). That puts Rīga in the same time zone as Helsinki and Tallinn; one hour ahead of Stockholm, the rest of Scandinavia, and most other continental cruise ports (including Gdańsk and Warnemünde); and one hour behind St. Petersburg.

Embassies in Rīga: The **US embassy** is at 1 Samnera Velsa Iela (tel. 6710-7000, http://riga.usembassy.gov/). The **Canadian embassy** is at 20/22 Baznicas Iela (tel. 6781-3945, www.canada.ee). Call ahead for passport services.

Phoning: Latvia's country code is 371; to call from another country to Latvia, dial the international access code (011 from the US/Canada, 00 from Europe, or + from a mobile phone), then 371, followed by the local number. For local calls within Latvia, just dial the number as it appears in this book—whether you're calling from across the street or across the country. To place an international call from Latvia, dial 00, the code of the country you're calling (1 for US and Canada), and the phone number. For more help, see page 1146.

Tipping: If a gratuity is included in the price of your sit-down meal, you don't need to tip further; otherwise, a tip of roughly 10 percent is customary. Tip a taxi driver by rounding up the fare a bit (pay €3 on an €2.85 fare). For more tips on tipping, see page 138.

Tourist Information: www.latvia.travel

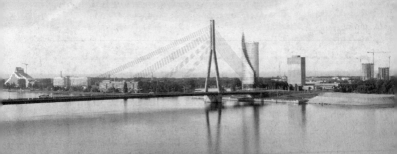

RĪGA

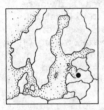

The biggest city of the Baltics is an under-rated gem, with a charming but not cutesy Old Town, a sprawling real-world market, a smattering of good museums, the finest collection of fanciful Art Nouveau buildings in Europe, a palpable civic pride expressed in its luscious parks and stately facades, and fewer cruise passengers clogging its cobbles than most other towns in this book. From a cruiser's perspective, Rīga (pronounced REE-gah) is the sleepy antidote to its Baltic rival, the tourist-crazed Tallinn. Rīga has a bit less Scandinavian-mod style and sugary Old World charm, but it enjoys more big-city realness. And, while Tallinn's ties to the former USSR feel like ancient history, Rīga's Russian connection is more palpable, giving visitors a glimpse into a "half-Russian" society without plunging into the full monty of St. Petersburg.

Centuries before it was Russian (or even Latvian), Rīga was a prominent trading city. Bishop Albert of Bremen, German merchants, and the Teutonic Knights made it the center of Baltic Christianization, commercialization, and colonization when they founded the city in the early 1200s. Rīga came under Polish control for a while during the 16th century; later, in the 17th century, the czars made it the Russian Empire's busiest commercial port. Latvia gained its independence for the first time following World War I in 1918, but that lasted just over two decades; with World War II, it was folded into the USSR's holdings.

Under Soviet rule, Rīga became first an important military center and later, because of its high standard of living, one of the favored places for high-ranking military officers to retire to (to keep them at arm's length from power, they were given a choice of

Excursions from Rīga

Rīga can easily be enjoyed without an excursion. Getting into town is simple, the sights are pleasant but don't require a lot of explanation to enjoy, and the basics are covered in this chapter. Even the outlying sights (such as the Central Market, and the Art Nouveau quarter and museum) are an easy and pleasant walk from downtown. And joining a tour or hiring your own guide in Rīga is easy and affordable (see "Tours in Rīga," later).

Most cruise lines offer walking tours of Rīga's **Old Town,** or a bus-plus-walking-tour option. You can't really see the Old Town core by bus, so if you'd like to get all the stories and legends, a walking tour is best. If you're interested in Rīga's **Art Nouveau** facades, choose a tour that includes some walking, not just a bus ride. A bus tour zips you past several fine examples, but doesn't allow you to linger over the stunning details.

Those with an interest in **Jewish history** may find worthwhile a tour that includes several sites related to Rīga's difficult Holocaust experience: the memorial at the site of the Grand Choral Synagogue (burned down by Nazis), the site of the Old Jewish Cemetery (defiled by Nazis), the monument at Rumbula (the site of a mass execution in a forest), and the memorial at Salaspils (the largest Nazi concentration camp in the Baltics).

Cruise lines offer a wide range of excursions to outlying attractions. These include **Jurmala** (Rīga's seaside resort, sometimes combined with a spa visit); **"Middle Ages Rīga"** (including the Gauja River northeast of town, the evocative ruins of Sigulda Medieval Castle, the reconstructed Turaida Castle and nearby church, and the legend-packed Gutmanis cave); and the **Latvian Open-Air Ethnographic Museum** (with 118 traditional buildings relocated here from around the country). Again, as Rīga itself is so easy to enjoy in a relaxed day, I'd skip all of these options.

RĪGA

anywhere in the USSR *except* Moscow, Kiev, and St. Petersburg). The Soviets encouraged Russian immigration, and by the time the USSR fell, Latvians were in the minority in their own capital city. Perceptive travelers will notice that Russian is still widely spoken here. Though Russian-Estonian tensions in neighboring Estonia grab more headlines, Latvia has its own tricky mix to negotiate.

But for visitors, Rīga is a purely enjoyable city, regardless of what language is spoken by the people you'll meet. Stroll the Old Town, browsing the shops and dipping into a museum or two; the excellent Museum of the Occupation of Latvia is tops for those intrigued by the Baltics' tumultuous 20th century. For a revealing look at an extremely local-feeling market, linger in the Central Market, which trudges on seemingly oblivious to the cruise passengers just over the berm. (As one of the cheapest destinations in this book, Rīga is a fine place to do a little shopping.) Save some time to stroll through some of Rīga's delightful parks, following the meandering river (once a moat) that runs right in front of the towering Freedom Monument. And make a pilgrimage to some of the city's gorgeous Art Nouveau facades, which scream out with fanciful, entertaining details. Making things even better, Rīga enjoyed a stint as a European Capital of Culture in 2014; several long-neglected buildings and museums received facelifts for the occasion.

PLANNING YOUR TIME

Get your bearings with a stroll through the Old Town. Mid-morning, walk to the Central Market for some people-watching and to harvest ingredients for a picnic lunch or snack. Then head back to town to see the Museum of the Occupation of Latvia (opens at 11:00) and/or the Art Museum Rīga Bourse. For a good picnic alternative, consider lunch at one of the many al fresco cafés downtown. In early afternoon, wander out of the Old Town core to see the Freedom Monument, Orthodox Cathedral, and (a few blocks north) the best of Rīga's many Art Nouveau facades, plus the wonderful little Art Nouveau Museum. From the Art Nouveau sights, it's a fairly short walk (mostly through parklands) to the cruise dock.

RĪGA

The Port of Rīga

Arrival at a Glance: It's an easy 10- to 20-minute stroll into town—no taxis or buses needed.

Port Overview

One of the simplest, most manageable cruise ports in northern Europe, Rīga is made-to-order for cruise passengers. Ships dock along a river embankment just a 10-minute walk from the edge of the Old Town, or a 20-minute walk from the very heart of town.

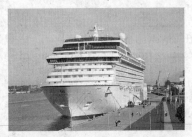

To reach Rīga, your ship will pick up a pilot for the journey up the Daugava River. The sailing from the Baltic up the river gives you a revealing glimpse of the grimy, hardworking industry that makes Rīga the Baltics' no-nonsense muscleman. Don't fret—the core of town (where

Services near the Port

Because the cruise port is so close to town, there's little need for services at the port itself. Stepping off the ship, turn left to find Rīga's passenger port terminal building (marked *Rīga Pasazieru Osta*), with **ATMs,** lockers, WCs, a newsstand, and a café. But you might as well turn right and walk into the Old Town, where ATMs abound. The Old Town also has several **pharmacies.**

you'll be spending time) is far more pleasant.

Tourist Information: There's no tourist information whatsoever at the port; just walk into town to find TIs on Town Hall Square and just to the north (see "Tourist Information," later).

GETTING INTO TOWN

To **walk** into town, just step off the ship, turn right, and head toward the spires. Here are the details: After turning right to walk along the embankment (with the river on your right), proceed straight and pass under the bridge. At the first crosswalk, turn left and cross the busy highway. Once across, continue straight up Poļu Gāte, alongside the pastel-blue church. At the intersection, turn right onto Pils Iela, which takes you directly to Cathedral Square in the heart of town. If you'd like to visit the TI, you can continue straight all the way to the far end of Cathedral Square (past all the al fresco tables), and turn right down the narrow, café-lined Tirgoņu Iela. The next small square has even more café tables, plus a fun outdoor souvenir market. As you walk through it, watch on your right for a big gap leading to an ugly modern building—this is the Museum of the Occupation of Latvia, which shares Town Hall Square with the TI (in the ornate building in the foreground).

Taxis may meet arriving ships, attempting to drastically overcharge cruisers €4-8 (or even more) for the laughably short ride into town. (The fair, metered rate would be closer to €3-4.) As you'll have trouble getting a fair price, you'll do better taking the easy walk into town.

RETURNING TO YOUR SHIP

Just head north along the river (with the river on your left); you'll run right into your ship. If you're coming from the Art Nouveau district, use a map to navigate your way diagonally through the big Kronvalda Park. When you pop out at the other end, you're just a quick walk from the dock. To cross the highway, it's easiest and safest to use the busy bridge that crosses over both the highway and the river (you can find steps up to the bridge level near the

RĪGA

Statoil gas station). Cross partway over, but before reaching the river, look for the stairs down (on your right) to the port gate area.

See page 505 for help if you miss your boat.

Rīga

With about 700,000 people, Rīga is the biggest city in the Baltics. But the town core feels small and manageable, and even just a few hours are enough to get a satisfying taste.

Orientation to Riga

Rīga's Old Town (called Vecrīga) is on the right bank of the wide Daugava River. The cruise port is next to the northernmost of Rīga's bridges. From the river, the main drag—Kaļķu Iela—leads through the Old Town to the Freedom Monument, where it becomes Brīvības Bulvāris and continues out of town. You'll find plenty to keep you busy within the Old Town or a short walk from it.

The Old Town is hemmed in on the east side by a chain of relaxing parks, with the once-genteel urban residential zone stretching beyond. One of Rīga's most worthwhile areas is the cluster of Art Nouveau facades about a 20-minute walk (or €3-4 taxi ride) northeast of the city center. There's no reason to cross the river.

A couple of terms you'll see around town: *Iela* is "street," and *Bulvāris* is "boulevard."

TOURIST INFORMATION
The tourist office is in the ornate brick building attached to the House of Blackheads, right on Town Hall Square (daily May-Sept 9:00-19:00, Oct-April 10:00-18:00, Rātslaukums 6, tel. 6703-7900, www.liveriga.com). A second branch is just a few short blocks away along the main drag, Kaļķu Iela (at #16, tel. 6722-7444).

Tours in Rīga

Since Rīga is best seen by foot, a **walking tour** is probably your best bet. Various local companies offer these, but the main operation is Smile Line, which has a kiosk by the statue of St. Roland in the middle of Town Hall Square, right in front of the TI. Their 1.5-hour introductory walk departs daily at 10:30 (€12), but for a bit more you can hire one of their guides to personally lead you through town (one person-€20, groups of 2 or more-€15/person). They also have a two-hour departure daily at 13:00 for €15. You

RĪGA

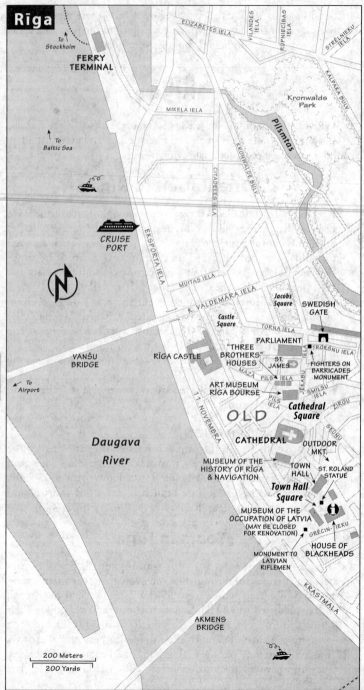

Rīga

To Stockholm

FERRY TERMINAL

To Baltic Sea

CRUISE PORT

ELIZABETES IELA

VILANDES IELA

RUPNIECIBAS IELA

STRELNIEKU IELA

Kronwalds Park

Pilsmtas

KALPAKA BULV.

MIKELA IELA

KRONVALDE BULV.

CITADELES IELA

EKSPORTA IELA

MUITAS IELA

K. VALDEMARA IELA

Jacobs Square

SWEDISH GATE

Castle Square

TORNA IELA

TROKSNU IELA

PARLIAMENT

"THREE BROTHERS" HOUSES

RĪGA CASTLE

ST. JAMES

MAZA PILS IELA

JEKABU IELA

FIGHTERS ON BARRICADES MONUMENT

ART MUSEUM RĪGA BOURSE

PILS IELA

SMILSU IELA

Cathedral Square

ZIRGU IELA

VANŠU BRIDGE

To Airport

OLD

11. NOVEMBRA

CATHEDRAL

SKUNU IELA

OUTDOOR MKT.

Daugava River

MUSEUM OF THE HISTORY OF RĪGA & NAVIGATION

TOWN HALL

ST. ROLAND STATUE

Town Hall Square

MUSEUM OF THE OCCUPATION OF LATVIA (MAY BE CLOSED FOR RENOVATION)

GRECIN-IEKU

HOUSE OF BLACKHEADS

MONUMENT TO LATVIAN RIFLEMEN

KRASTMALA

AKMENS BRIDGE

200 Meters
200 Yards

RĪGA

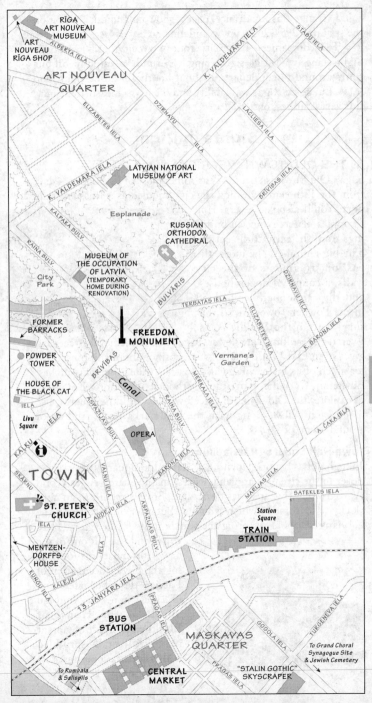

RĪGA

could arrange this in advance, or just show up and ask about it on the spot (tel. 2954-2626, www.smileline.lv).

Two companies—Rīga City Tour (www.citytour.lv) and Rīga Sightseeing (www.riga-sightseeing.lv)—run **hop-on, hop-off bus tours** around town, departing about hourly for a one-hour loop (€15). But given Rīga's walkability and the tours' measly frequency, this isn't your best option.

Sights in Rīga

IN THE OLD TOWN (VECRĪGA)

Rīga's Old Town isn't as "old" as some; most of its buildings date from the 18th century, when the city boomed as a Russian trade port. You'll also see several fine
examples of Art Nouveau build-
ings from the early 20th century.

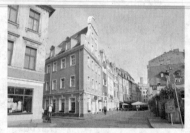

The big churches, the moat, the
bastion, fragments of the city
walls, a couple of dozen houses,
and the cannonballs embedded
in the Powder Tower are all that
survive from the Middle Ages.
Even if the buildings are newer, Rīga's twisty medieval street plan gives it an Old World charm. As a cosmopolitan shipping town for much of its history, Rīga also boasts a wide range of churches: Lutheran, Catholic, Anglican, Orthodox, and more. Enjoyable to explore, the Old Town is graced with several fine squares; I've listed each below, along with the landmarks you'll find on or around them.

Town Hall Square (Rātslaukums)

Though not as big or as inviting as Cathedral Square, this space—closer to the river—is arguably Rīga's "main square." After World War II, when this area was devastated, Soviets rebuilt in an ugly, blocky style (some of which remains). But after independence, the Latvians set about restoring the square to its former glory. Here

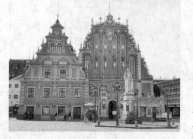

you'll find the TI, one of the city's top museums (outlining the Soviet occupation of Latvia—described later), and its finest non-Art Nouveau building: the **House of Blackheads.** Made of vibrant red brick liberally sprinkled with gilded decorations, this was originally the guildhall

RĪGA

of a merchant society that chose as its patron St. Mauritius, a third-century North African. The nickname came from the guild seal with disembodied black heads. (Racial sensitivity was clearly not a medieval forte—and, judging by the fact that the guild seal is still here, it's not quite a priority these days, either.) See the dates at the top: Although the guildhall was originally built in 1334, it was destroyed in World War II and only rebuilt in 1999. The left half of the building (containing the TI) looks as if it's part of the House of Blackheads, but was built centuries later.

Facing the House of Blackheads is Rīga's stately Town Hall. On the square between them stands a statue of **St. Roland,** Rīga's patron saint. Back then, the tip of Roland's sword was considered the geographical center of the city—the point from which all distances were measured.

A block above Town Hall Square is the towering, almost-onion steeple of **St. Peter's Church** (Petera Baznica), with an austere Lutheran interior and an elevator to an observation deck (€7, closed Mon).

Along the bottom of Town Hall Square is the Soviet-era building that now (with a flourish of poetic justice) houses the Museum of the Occupation of Latvia (described next). Around the far side of the building, facing the river, stands the proud **Monument to the Latvian Riflemen.** These soldiers fought on the side of the czar during World War I, but then defected to join Lenin's Bolshevik Revolution. During communist times, the Soviets strategically chose local heroes to venerate in each of its satellites (the heroes conveniently also echoed Soviet ideals).

▲Museum of the Occupation of Latvia (Latvijas Okupācijas Muzejs)

This spunky, thorough exhibit tells Latvia's story during the tumultuous five decades between 1940 and 1991. Located next to the House of Blackheads, it fills the large upstairs hall of the dreary, communist-style, corroded-copper building that mars the otherwise architecturally quaint Town Hall Square. The ragtag exhibits are undergoing a much-needed overhaul. During the 2015-2016 cruise season, you'll find the exhibit at either the main building or at its temporary home in the former US embassy, just outside the Old Town at Raiņa Bulvāris 7 (double-check with the TI for the current location).

The new collection promises to keep the focus on the periods of Nazi and Soviet oppression—particularly the deportations of Latvians to Siberia. (You can step into a replica of a gulag barrack and see prisoners' letters home written on strips of birch bark.) To get the full story, try to time your visit to join one of the guided tours.

Cost and Hours: Note that these details may change due to

RĪGA

ongoing renovations. Free, but donations suggested, €3 to take photos, May-Sept daily 11:00-18:00, Oct-April Tue-Sun 11:00-17:00, closed Mon, Strelnieku Laukums 1 or Raiņa Bulvāris 7 (temporary location), tel. 6721-2715, www.occupationmuseum.lv.

Tours: Guided tours are generally offered in English at 12:00 and 16:00, but confirm times; €3 per person with a €10 minimum.

▲▲Cathedral Square (Doma Laukums)

In old Rīga's biggest square, three things jockey for attention: The enormous cathedral, the Art Nouveau facade of the old stock

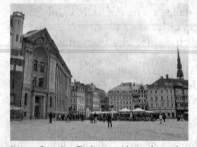

exchange museum (now an art museum—described next), and café tables spilling out over the cobbles in every direction.

The **cathedral** (Doma Baznica), with its distinctive copper roof, dates from 1211. Dwarfing everything around it, it's positively huge for the Baltics, where big churches are rare. With additions built over the generations, it's a hodgepodge of architectural styles. During Soviet times, the altars and other religious decorations were taken out and the cathedral was converted into a concert hall. Inside, the inscriptions recall Latvia's German Lutheran heritage, and the crypt holds what's left of Bishop Albert of Bremen, who started it all. It also has a particularly fine and gigantic organ (with more than 6,700 pipes), which is played for brief noontime concerts during the tourist season (generally Mon-Sat at 12:00, www.doms.lv).

Facing the cathedral from across the square is the ornately decorated former stock exchange building, or **Bourse,** which houses the Art Museum Rīga Bourse (described next). The second-story grille hides a carillon, which sweetly chimes the hour.

The far end of the square is the terrain of outdoor café and restaurant tables—a tempting place to sit, nurse a coffee or Latvian beer, and watch the parade of tourists and locals.

From here, you can tour the art museum, wander a couple of streets with fine Art Nouveau houses, or walk along Pils Iela to Rīga Castle (all described later).

Art Museum Rīga Bourse

Rīga's stately old stock exchange building has been meticulously restored to its original diarrhea-brown color, which glistens in the sun. Its interior (also gorgeously restored, and also diarrhea brown) houses temporary exhibits and a modest collection of "foreign art." While the changing collections are generally good, the permanent exhibits (fourth floor—Western European art and painting gallery, third floor—Asian art) take a backseat to the finely restored rooms that house them. The highlights are the airy atrium with beautiful tile floors (viewable for free) and the fourth floor, with gilded chandeliers and other details whose sumptuousness outshines the art.

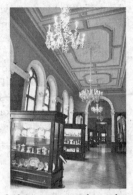

Cost and Hours: permanent exhibit-€2.85, extra for temporary exhibits or €6.40 combo-ticket for all; Tue-Sun 10:00-18:00, Fri until 20:00, closed Mon, Doma Laukums 6, tel. 6722-3434, www.rigasbirza.lv.

Rīga Castle

Leave Cathedral Square and walk down Pils Iela to this relatively unimpressive, blocky fortress (a "palace" it ain't) that was the no-nonsense headquarters of the Teutonic Knights who ruled Rīga. Built in the 14th century, the castle stoutly anchored the northern tip of the Old Town as it kept careful watch downriver for potential invaders. The door on the landward side of the castle, with a guard out front, is the office of the Latvian president; nearby is the entrance to the skippable Latvian National History Museum. During Soviet times, the castle was converted into the "Children's Palace"—many older Latvians recall visiting here as youngsters.

RĪGA

Walk to Swedish Gate and Former Barracks

From Rīga Castle, take a stroll through the most historic quarter of the Old Town. With your back to the big, round tower, walk

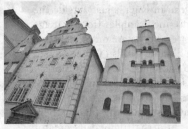

straight ahead up Mazā Pils Iela a block and a half to find (on the right) the **"Three Brothers"**—a trio of the oldest surviving houses in Rīga. The oldest, white house (#17) has minuscule windows—dating from the 15th century, when taxation was based on window size. Yellow #19 is newer, from 1646, while green and narrow #21 is the baby of the bunch, from the turn of the 18th century.

Continue past the Brothers and turn left up Jēkaba Iela. On the left, you'll pass the corner of Latvia's **parliament.** This is the building where—back when it was the seat of the Latvian Supreme Soviet—independence from the USSR was declared on May 4, 1990. On the nearby corner, look for the little pyramid-shaped monument to the **Fighters on the Barricades,** a brave group of about 15,000 Latvians who, at great personal risk, protected strategic Latvian areas when skirmishes with pro-Soviet forces broke out in January of 1991; seven were killed. The Latvians were unsure of whether Soviet leader Mikhail Gorbachev would send the full force of the Red Army to reclaim the Baltics. Although that never happened, Latvians still honor those who were willing to make the ultimate sacrifice for sovereignty.

Near the top of Jēkaba Iela, turn right down the tiny, rocky lane called **Trokšņu Iela.** Watch your step on this ankle-twisting

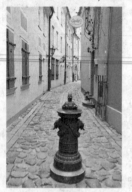

alley, paved with rocks originally carried as ballast on big ships. After a block on this street, you'll pop out at the so-called **Swedish Gate** (built in the 17th century by Swedish soldiers stationed here). Going through it, you'll discover a long row of yellow **barracks** filled with shops and cafés, facing a reconstructed stretch of the former town wall (along Torņa Iela). At the far end is the **Powder Tower,** which once housed the town's supply of gunpowder. The tower defended that cache well over the centuries, as nine Russian cannonballs (from the 17th and 18th centuries) are supposedly embedded in the walls. The Museum of War inside is skippable.

From the Powder Tower, you could turn right and head down Smilšu, for some fun Art Nouveau facades on the way back down to Cathedral Square.

Old Town Art Nouveau

While arguably the best Art Nouveau in Rīga is just outside the historic core (described later), several fine examples from that age line the Old Town streets. The best examples are on or near two streets leading off from Cathedral Square: Smilšu (especially #2 and #8), to the east; and Šķūņu, to the south. Just off of Smilšu, at Meistaru 10, is the famous **House of the Black Cat;** while the building itself is relatively tame, its corner turret is topped with a cat with its back arched defiantly, supposedly placed there as an offensive gesture toward a guild that denied its creator membership.

Other Museums

Rīga's Old Town is packed with small, modest museums that are worth perusing if you have a special interest or a rainy day. The **Museum of the History of Rīga and Navigation** (Rīgas Vestures un Kugniecibas Muzejs) gives a fairly good idea of Rīga's early history as a center on the Baltic-Black Sea trade route, explains the

Old Town's street plan in terms of a now-silted-up river that used to flow through the center, and shows you everything you wanted to see on interwar Rīga (May-Sept daily 10:00-17:00, Oct-April Wed-Sun 11:00-17:00, behind the cathedral at Palasta Iela 4, www.rigamuz.lv). The **Mentzendorffs House** is a meticulously restored 17th-century aristocrat's townhouse (May-Sept daily 10:00-17:00, Oct-April Wed-Sun 11:00-17:00, Grēcinieku Iela 18, enter on Kungu Iela, www.mencendorfanams.com).

OUTSIDE THE OLD TOWN

While many cruisers stick to the cobbles, some of Rīga's most appealing (and certainly its most local-feeling) attractions are just a short walk beyond the former city walls. The Central Market, mentioned first, is just south of the Old Town, while the other places noted here are to the east. I've listed these roughly in order, from nearest to farthest from the Old Town.

▲▲Central Market (Centralais Tirgus)

What do you do when you have five perfectly good zeppelin airship hangars left behind by the Germans after World War I? Latvia's

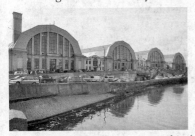

answer: Move them to the center of the capital city and turn them into extremely spacious market halls. Just beyond the southern edge of the Old Town—only a 15-minute walk from the quaint cobbled squares—is this vast, sprawling market that feels like the outskirts of Moscow. This is not a touristy souvenir market (though you may find a stall or two), but a real, thriving market where locals buy whatever they need at reasonable prices. If you've been cruising through Scandinavia's more expensive cities, you'll find basic foodstuffs here to be almost scandalously cheap. It's open and bustling every day, though some sections close on certain Mondays (www.centraltirgus.lv).

To get to the market, walk to the south end of the Old Town, cross the tram tracks, and find the underpass that runs beneath the big berm. Then explore to your heart's content, wishing you had a full kitchen in your stateroom to cook up all the tempting ingredients. Just past the one hangar that runs sideways, find the colorful and fragrant flower market. Then poke through all five of the zeppelin hangars, each one with a different variety of meats, cheeses, bakery items, dry goods, and (in the final, smelly hall) fish. While nothing here is exactly gourmet—this is not an artisan, organic market—it makes it easy to imagine life for an everyday Rīgan. The old brick warehouses just toward the river from the market zone have recently been refurbished and now house finer shops.

The Central Market also marks the Maskavas, or **"Little Moscow,"** neighborhood, which contains a huge Russian population. While all of the Baltic states have large Russian populations, Rīga became especially Russified during the Soviet period, leaving an awkward tension between its Latvian and Russian groups. As if to mark this territory, looming overhead is a classic "Stalin Gothic" tower (virtually identical in style to similar towers in Warsaw, Moscow, and elsewhere). Originally designed to be a hotel and conference center for collective farmers (who had little use for either hotels or a conference center), it later became, and remains, the Academy of Science.

▲▲Freedom Monument (Brivibas Piemniekelis)

Dedicated in 1935, located on a traffic island in the middle of Brīvības Bulvāris, this monument features Lady Liberty (here

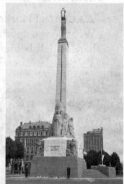

nicknamed "Milda") holding high three stars representing the three regions of Latvia. At the base of the tower, strong and defiant Latvians break free from their chains and march to the future. The Soviets must have decided that removing the monument was either too difficult or too likely to spur protests among Latvians, because they left it standing—but reassigned its major characters: The woman became Mother Russia, and the three stars, the Baltic states. (KGB agents apprehended anyone who tried to come near it.) Now it is again the symbol of independent Latvia, and locals lay flowers between the two soldiers who stand stoically at the monument's base. The grand building nearby is the Opera House. The bridge near the monument offers beautiful views over Rīga's great parks.

Parks

Rīga's Old Town is hemmed in on its eastern edge by delightful, manicured parks that line up along a picturesque stream that was once the fortified city's moat.

Russian Orthodox Cathedral

Just past the Freedom Monument on Rīga's main drag (Brīvības Bulvāris), sitting at the edge of a park, this striking house of worship dates from the 19th century. During the Soviet period, when the atheistic regime notoriously repurposed houses of worship, the building was used as a planetarium and "house of knowledge." While the interior is far from original—it was gutted by the Soviets—it's serene and otherworldly. Especially if you won't be visiting the Orthodox churches in Tallinn or St. Petersburg, it's worth the short walk out of the Old Town to take a peek.

Latvian National Museum of Art (Latvijas Valsts Makslas Muzejs)

Housed in a stately old building in the parklands just east of the town center, this fine museum collects works by Latvian and Russian artists. The collection, almost entirely from 1910 to 1940, concentrates all the artistic and political influences that stirred Latvia then: French Impressionism, German design, and Russian propaganda-poster style on the one hand; European internationalism, Latvian nationalism, rural romanticism, and Communism on the other. The Russian art section is particularly worthwhile if you won't be going to St. Petersburg's superb Russian Museum. The museum was recently extensively renovated; confirm its current hours at the TI before venturing out to the park.

Cost and Hours: €4.30, Wed-Mon 11:00-18:00, Fri until 20:00, closed Tue, Kr. Valdemara Iela 10, www.lnmm.lv.

▲▲Art Nouveau Rīga

Worth ▲▲▲ for architecture fans, but interesting even to those who don't know Art Nouveau from Art Garfunkel, Rīga's more

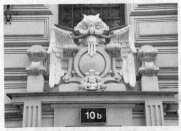

than 800 exuberantly decorated facades from the late 19th and early 20th centuries make it Europe's single best city for the distinctive, eye-pleasing style of Art Nouveau. These are not the flowing, organic curves of Barcelona's Modernista style, but geometrically precise patterns adorned with fanciful details, including an army of highly expressive, gargoyle-like heads.

Art Nouveau Walk: While easy-to-love facades are scattered throughout the city center (including some wonderful examples in the Old Town—see page 500), it's worth the 20-minute walk northeast of the center to find a particularly impressive batch. It's a pleasant stroll—you can follow the parks most of the way there, and you can tie in visits to the Orthodox Church and (if it's open) the Latvian National Museum of Art.

For the best short stretch of houses, begin at the corner of the park nearest Elizabets Iela, Strēlnieku Iela, and Kaplaka Bulvāris. Head up **Strēlnieku**; on the right, at #4, is a magnificent blue-and-white facade almost *too* cluttered with adornments: stripes, rings, slinky women holding wreaths of victory, and stylized helmeted heads over the windows. (This, like most buildings in this area, was decorated by Mikhail Eisenstein—whose director son

Sergei earned a place in every "Intro to Film" college class with his seminal 1925 film, *Battleship Potemkin*.) At the corner, you'll see the yellow turreted building that houses the Art Nouveau Museum, and the fine shop across the street (both described later). If you turn right just before this house, on **Alberta Iela,** you'll find several more grandiose examples: #13 (pale pink, on right; notice the moaning heads at the bases of the turrets), #8 (blue and white, on the left; tree-trunk supports grow and leaf into a lion's head), #4 (beige, on the left; with griffins flanking the ornately framed doorway, three Medusa heads up top, and lions guarding the towers), and (shabby but still impressive, the next two on the left) #2 and #2a. At the end of Alberta, jog right for a block, then head left down **Elizabets Iela** to find a couple more examples at #10a and #10b (blue and gray, with hoot-owls over the doors). All of these glorious buildings were turned into communal apartments under the communist regime.

Rīga Art Nouveau Museum: When you're done ogling the facades, head back the way you came, to the corner of Alberta and Strēlnieku. Head a few steps up Strēlnieku (to the right) to find the excellent little Rīga Art Nouveau Museum, in the bottom of the yellow castle-like building with the pointy red turret (€5, Tue-Sun 10:00-18:00, closed Mon, audioguide-€2.50, guided tour-€14.50/group—call or email ahead to arrange, Alberta 12, enter on Strēlnieku, tel. 6718-1465, www.jugendstils.riga.lv, jugendstils@riga.lv).

This museum shows what life was like behind those slinky facades back in the early 20th century. Buzz the doorbell to get inside, then peer up the stairwell. Inside the museum, you're greeted by docents dressed in period costumes, who invite you to don a fancy, feathery hat for your stroll through a finely decorated, circa-1903 apartment, with furniture, clothes, decorative items, rugs, and lots of other details dating from the age.

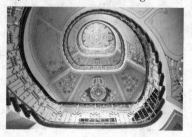

This was the personal apartment of architect Konstantīns Pēkšēns, whose photo you'll see in the first room. You'll go through several rooms, including a dining room, bedroom, kitchen (with tiny maid's chamber on the side), bathroom (the apartment had hot water and even central heating—cutting-edge at the time), and more. Take your time and savor all the details—the gently seductive curve of the plant stand, the ribbons delicately tied to flower vases on the dining table, the old-school icebox and coffee grinder in the kitchen, and the natural motifs painted high on the

What If I Miss My Boat?

Remember that you can get help from the cruise line's port agent (listed on the destination information sheet distributed on the ship) and the local TI (see page 493). If the port agent suggests a costly solution (such as a private car with a driver), you may want to consider public transit.

Buses connect Rīga to **Tallinn** (about hourly, 4.5 hours). For **Stockholm,** Tallink Silja offers overnight ferry trips (www.tallinksilja.com). To get to **St. Petersburg** or **Helsinki,** it's probably easier to go to Tallinn or Stockholm and connect from there (but remember that you'll need a visa—arranged weeks in advance—to enter Russia). **Gdańsk** requires a long overland journey; because the route from Latvia to Poland is flanked by Kaliningrad (part of Russia) and Belarus, both of which require transit visas, you'll need to determine a route via the relatively short Lithuanian-Polish border instead—ask the TI for help.

If you need to catch a **plane** to your next destination, you can ride a public bus to Rīga's international airport (www.riga-airport.com).

Local **travel agents** in Rīga can help you. For more advice on what to do if you miss the boat, see page 139.

walls in each room (based on items found in the Latvian countryside). Very few barriers or cordons separate you from the world of a century ago, making this a particularly appealing and immersive little museum.

Nearby: If you'd like to take some of this Art Nouveau home with you, directly across the street from the museum is the **Art Nouveau Rīga shop,** with piles of souvenirs inspired by this distinctive style (daily 10:00-19:00, Strēlnieku 9, tel. 6733-3030, www.artnouveauriga.lv).

More Art Nouveau: The tiny area described above is just the beginning of Rīga's Art Nouveau neighborhood. A couple of blocks to the west, just north of the parklands, **Vīlandes Iela** and the parallel **Rūpniecības Iela** have several fine facades. The area just south and east of the Brīvības Bulvāris main drag (such as **Tērbatas Iela** and **A.Čaka Iela**) also has several examples.

Shopping in Rīga

The souvenirs you'll see most often here are linens (tablecloths, placemats, and scarves) and carved-wood items (such as spoons and trivets). There are a few sparse souvenir stands at the **Central Market,** but that's really designed more for the natives. Souvenir shops are peppered through the Old Town, and an entertaining open-air **souvenir market** pops up in summer in the small square just north of Town Hall Square.

If you're turned on by Rīga's Art Nouveau bounty, another good option is "faux Nouveau"—replica items such as tiles, cards, textiles, jewelry, and so on. The best choices are at the **Art Nouveau Rīga shop,** across the street from the Art Nouveau Museum (described earlier).

Eating in Rīga

Central Rīga—particularly the area between Cathedral Square and Town Hall Square—is full of tempting open-air cafés and restaurants. Rather than seek out a particular place, I'd simply window-shop to find an appealing cuisine and people-watching vantage point.

GDAŃSK
Poland

Poland Practicalities

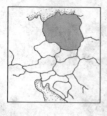

Poland (Polska), arguably Europe's most devoutly Catholic country, is sandwiched between Protestant Germany and Eastern Orthodox Russia. Nearly all of the 38.5 million people living in Poland are ethnic Poles. The country is 121,000 square miles (the same as New Mexico) and extremely flat, making it the chosen path of least resistance for many invading countries since its infancy. Poland was dominated by foreigners for the majority of the last two centuries, finally gaining true independence (from the Soviet Union) in 1989. While parts of the country are still cleaning up the industrial mess left by the Soviets, Poland also has some breathtaking medieval cities—such as Gdańsk—that show off its kind-hearted people, dynamic history, and unique cultural fabric.

Money: 1 złoty (zł, or PLN) = 100 groszy (gr) = about 30 cents; 3 zł = about $1. An ATM is called a *bankomat*. The local VAT (value-added sales tax) rate is 23 percent; the minimum purchase eligible for a VAT refund is 200 zł (for details on refunds, see page 134).

Language: The native language is Polish. For useful phrases, see page 558.

Emergencies: Dial 112 for police, medical, or other emergencies. In case of theft or loss, see page 125.

Time Zone: Poland is on Central European Time (the same as most of the Continent, one hour ahead of Great Britain, and six/nine hours ahead of the East/West Coasts of the US). That puts Gdańsk one hour behind Rīga, Tallinn, and Helsinki, and two hours behind St. Petersburg.

Embassies in Warsaw: The **US embassy** is at Ulica Piękna 12; appointments are required for routine services (tel. 022-504-2784, Document14http://poland.usembassy.gov). The **Canadian embassy** is at Ulica Jana Matejki 1-5 (tel. 022-584-3100, www.poland.gc.ca). Call ahead for passport services.

Phoning: Poland's country code is 48; to call from another country to Poland, dial the international access code (011 from the US/Canada, 00 from Europe, or + from a mobile phone), then 48, followed by the local number. For local calls within Poland, just dial the number as it appears in this book—whether you're calling from across the street or across the country. To place an international call from Poland, dial 00, the code of the country you're calling (1 for US and Canada), and the phone number. For more tips, see page 1146.

Tipping: A gratuity is included at sit-down meals, so you don't need to tip further, though it's nice to round up your bill about 5-10 percent for great service. Tip a taxi driver by rounding up the fare a bit (pay 30 zł on an 27-zł fare). For more tips on tipping, see page 138.

Tourist Information: www.poland.travel

GDAŃSK
and the PORT of GDYNIA

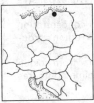

Gdańsk (guh-DAYNSK) is a true find on the Baltic Coast of Poland. You may associate Gdańsk with dreary images of striking dockworkers from the nightly news in the 1980s—but there's so much more to this city than shipyards, Solidarity, and smog. It's surprisingly easy to look past the urban sprawl to find one of northern Europe's most historic and picturesque cities. Gdańsk is second only to Kraków as Poland's most appealing destination.

Exploring Gdańsk is a delight. The gem of a Main Town boasts block after block of red-brick churches and narrow, colorful, ornately decorated Hanseatic burghers' mansions. The riverfront embankment, with its trademark medieval crane, oozes salty maritime charm. Gdańsk's history is also fascinating—from its 17th-century Golden Age to the headlines of our own generation, big things happen here. You might even see portly old Lech Wałęsa still wandering the streets. And yet, Gdańsk is also looking to its future, steadily repairing some of its WWII damage after a long communist hibernation. Over the past decade, whole swaths of the city have been remade with a bold new modernity... but always with a respect for the past.

Gdańsk is the anchor of the three cities that make up the metropolitan region known as the Tri-City (Trójmiasto). The other two parts are as different as night and day: a once-swanky resort town (Sopot) and a practical, nose-to-the-grindstone business center and cruise port (Gdynia). Although your ship arrives at Gdynia (guh-DIN-yah), don't waste your time there—make a beeline to the main attraction, Gdańsk (and with extra time, consider a quick visit to Sopot).

Excursions from Gdynia

Gdańsk is clearly the best choice. Most cruise-line excursions include a walking tour through the Main Town; some may include guided visits to the giant, red-brick **St. Mary's Cathedral** or the **European Solidarity Center** museum at the Solidarity shipyard. You'll want to explore the town after your tour, so look for an itinerary that includes some free time—or skip the return bus ride to your ship and head back later on your own (by train, using this book's instructions).

I'd prefer to spend a full day in Gdańsk, but excursions often tack on visits to other locations outside town. These may include (in order of worthiness):

Sopot: A relaxing beach resort, this town's location halfway between Gdynia and Gdańsk makes it an easy add-on.

Malbork Castle: The fearsome Teutonic Knights built this sprawling castle as their headquarters. Though impressive, it's farther from town than other sights, and the expansive complex takes time to fully see.

Stutthof Concentration Camp: This Nazi concentration camp memorial offers a poignant look at this region's troubled 20th century.

Oliwa Cathedral: This red-brick church is far from unique in this region, but its impressive organ (with animated figures that move when it plays) is a crowd-pleaser.

PLANNING YOUR TIME

Minimize your time in Gdynia and max out in Gdańsk. The best plan is to spend the morning in Gdańsk's Main Town and along the embankment, and the afternoon at the Solidarity shipyard. (From the shipyard, it's easy to get to the train station; for efficiency, wrap up your Main Town activities before heading to Solidarity.)

• **Gdańsk Main Town:** Follow Part 1 of my Gdańsk Walk, a self-guided walking tour of the picturesque old core and embankment (allow one hour, including a visit to St. Mary's Church interior, but if you can, take more time to linger and enjoy).

• **Main Town Sights:** Peruse this book's listings and choose the sights that appeal to you most; these include St. Mary's Church, Amber Museum, Uphagen House, Main Town Hall, Artus Court, and the National Maritime Museum (allow about 30 minutes apiece for a quick stop, more for an in-depth visit).

• **Walking to the Solidarity Shipyard:** Follow Part 2 of my self-guided Gdańsk Walk to bring meaning to this 30-minute stroll.

• **Visiting the Solidarity Shipyard and European Solidarity Center:** Allow about 2.5 hours for this entire area.

In addition to the sights in Gdańsk, if you have time to kill on your way back to Gdynia, you could hop off the train in Sopot and stroll down the manicured main drag to the pleasure pier and beach. Allow at least 15 minutes to walk between Sopot's station and its beachfront, plus up to 15 minutes waiting for the train to Gdynia, plus however much time you want to linger at the beach.

When planning your day, be sure to allow plenty of time to make it from your ship in Gdynia to your point of interest in Gdańsk. For example: 5-10 minutes for the shuttle from your ship into Gdynia, then 15 minutes walking to the Gdynia train station, then 35 minutes for the train ride into Gdańsk (plus whatever time you need to wait for your train—up to 15 minutes), then 15-20 minutes walking from Gdańsk's main train station to the Main Town. Rounding up, plan roughly 1.5 hours each way.

The Port of Gdynia

Arrival at a Glance: Ride the shuttle bus into Gdynia's town center (to avoid the dreary walk through industrial ports), then walk 15 minutes to the train station for the 35-minute ride into Gdańsk; from Gdańsk's train station, it's about a 15-minute walk into the heart of the Main Town.

Port Overview

Because Gdańsk's port is relatively shallow, the biggest cruise ships must put in at Gdynia...leaving confused tourists to poke around town looking for some medieval quaintness, before coming to their senses and heading for Gdańsk.

Gdynia is less historic (and less attractive) than Gdańsk or Sopot, as it was mostly built in the 1920s to be Poland's main harbor after Gdańsk became a "free city" (see "Gdańsk History" sidebar, later). Today, Gdynia is a major business center, and—thanks to its youthful, progressive city government—has edged ahead of the rest of Poland in transitioning from communism.

Like a Soviet Bloc bodybuilder, Gdynia's port area is muscular and hairy. Cruise ships are shuffled among hardworking industrial piers that make the area feel uninviting. Among northern European cruise ports, Gdynia is the least user-friendly for arriving passengers, with few amenities (such as ATMs) available in the immediate port area. Each of the sprawling port's many piers is named for a country or region. Three are used for cruises: **Nabrzeże Francuskie** (French Quay), where most large ships dock; **Nabrzeże Stanów Zjednoczonych** (United States Quay), farther out, a secondary option for large ships; and convenient **Nabrzeże Pomorskie** (Pomeranian Quay, part of the Southern

GDAŃSK

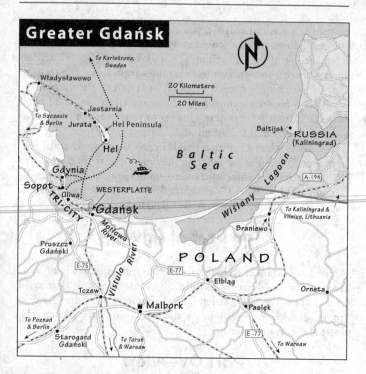

Greater Gdańsk

Pier), used by small ships and located alongside Gdynia's one "fun" pier, with museums and pleasure craft. Port information: www. port.gdynia.pl.

Money Matters: Gdynia has the only cruise port area I've seen with no ATMs or money-exchange options at or near the cruise-ship berths. If your ship offers on-board currency conversion, consider it. But if you're riding the shuttle or a taxi into downtown Gdynia (the easiest option), you'll find that ATMs are plentiful there, so you might as well wait. Taxi drivers generally take euros, though their off-the-cuff exchange rate may not be favorable.

The best place to find an **ATM** is along Skwer Kościuski, where the shuttle drops you off. Several banks line this square.

Tourist Information: There's no TI directly at the port, but TI representatives meet arriving cruise ships to hand out maps and answer questions. In Gdynia, the TI is on the main drag between the shuttle-bus drop-off and the train station (Mon-Fri 9:00-18:00, Sat-Sun 9:00-16:00, closes one hour earlier and closed Sun off-season, on the right at 24 ulica 10 Lutego, tel. 58-622-3766). In Gdańsk, the TI has handy offices at the train station and in the Main Town (see page 519).

Sights in Gdynia: Most of the city's sightseeing is along its waterfront. Directly toward the water from the shuttle-bus drop-off (through the park) is the **Southern Pier** (Molo Południowe). This concrete slab—nowhere near as charming as Sopot's wooden-boardwalk version—features a modern shopping mall and a smattering of sights, including an aquarium and a pair of permanently moored museum boats. If you have time to kill in Gdynia before returning to your ship, spend it here. Plans are afoot to convert the big warehouse at the base of the Nabrzeże Francuskie pier into an **emigration museum,** possibly as early as 2015; if and when this opens, it will offer a handy sightseeing opportunity for cruisers arriving here (for the latest, see www.muzeumemigracji.pl).

Alternate Port Near Gdańsk: A few small ships may dock at **Nabrzeże Oliwskie** (Oliwa Quay) at Gdańsk's New Port (Nowy Port), about four miles north of downtown. Used infrequently, this port has few services for cruisers, although TI representatives do meet arriving ships. Trams and buses connect this port to downtown Gdańsk, but because the port area has no ATM, these do you little good. If your cruise line offers a shuttle bus, take it; from the drop-off point, just walk over the two bridges to reach the center of the Main Town. An honest taxi should charge about 40-50 zł for the ride into town.

GETTING TO GDAŃSK

These instructions assume that you're arriving in Gdynia and plan to head directly to Gdańsk (which you should). While taxis are fast, they're pricey, and the public-transportation option is cheap and doable.

By Taxi

Taxi drivers line up to meet arriving cruise ships. While I've listed the legitimate fare estimates below, many cabbies try to charge far more. Try asking several drivers until you get a quote that resembles my figures, and be sure they use the meter. Remember, taxi drivers generally accept (and give quotes in) euros—though if you have Polish złotys, they'll take those, too.

To Gdynia's train station (*Dworzec*, DVOH-zhets): 20 zł (about €5)

To Gdańsk's Main Town: 125 zł (about €30)

To Sopot (beach resort between Gdynia and Gdańsk): 60-80 zł (about €15-20)

Many of the taxis that line up at the ship are looking for the long fare into Gdańsk and may not be willing to take you on the shorter trip to the Gdynia train station. If that's the case, walk out the port gate and look for a taxi there—but be warned that the outside-the-port cabbies are probably unregulated and more likely to overcharge.

By Public Transportation

The basic plan: From the **Nabrzeże Francuskie** or **Nabrzeże Stanów Zjednoczonych** piers, ride the shuttle bus (or walk) into downtown Gdynia, walk up to the train station, ride the train to Gdańsk, then walk into Gdańsk's historic Main Town. The step-by-step details are outlined below (it sounds more complicated than it is).

If you're fortunate enough to arrive at the **Nabrzeże Pomorskie** pier, you can simply walk straight up (away from the waterfront) about 10 minutes to reach Skwer Kościuski, then skip to step 2.

From anywhere in town, you can take a **taxi** to Gdynia's main train station (Dworzec Główna), and skip to step 3.

Step 1: From the Port to Downtown Gdynia (Skwer Kościuski)

The easiest option is to take your cruise line's **shuttle bus** into downtown (5-minute trip). The shuttle drops you off at Skwer Kościuski, in the heart of downtown Gdynia. (From here, look toward the waterfront, at the far end of the long park. You'll see a broad pier lined with museums and other attractions, with a beach next to it—a handy place to kill a little time on the way back to your ship.)

The very long, dull **walk**—though not advisable—is possible in a pinch. From the nearer Nabrzeże Francuskie, it takes about 20-30 minutes at a fast pace: Walk straight out of the port gate, bear left (past the bus stop), and continue with the industrial cranes on your right (following sporadic *City* arrow signs). At the roundabout, turn right and work your way straight into town; the road passes through industrial zones, wooded areas, residential neighborhoods, and over train tracks. (When the main road veers to the left to climb onto an overpass, continue straight on the low road.) You'll suddenly pop out in a downtown-feeling area on the street called Portowa; after a few blocks, this becomes Świętojańska, the city's main drag. Soon you'll hit the tree-lined boulevard called Skwer Kościuski (near the cruise-line shuttle bus stop—see next); turn right and head up ulica 10 Lutego to the train station, as described in step 2.

If you arrive at the even more distant Nabrzeże Stanów Zjednoczonych pier, the walk downtown will take up to 45 minutes. From the port gate, walk straight ahead to the roundabout, and continue straight along the same road as it bends left along the train tracks. Continue to the next big roundabout, where you'll cross the street, bear left, and walk along the road with the train tracks on your right. This will take you (after a long walk) to the roundabout described above. Turn right and continue into town to reach Skwer Kościuski.

Step 2: From Skwer Kościuski to Gdynia Main Train Station

From the shuttle-bus stop at Skwer Kościuski, it's about a 10-minute **walk** to the train station: Head up the broad, parklike boulevard, going away from the water (if you need cash, you'll spot several ATMs in this part of town). At the top of the square, the street becomes ulica 10 Lutego and continues straight (very gradually uphill)—follow it. A few short blocks later, watch for the Gdynia TI on the right (see "Tourist Information" on page 512). Just beyond that, the street curves to the right; once you're around the corner, use the crosswalk to reach the train station (marked *Dworzec Podmiejski*).

Step 3: From Gdynia Main Train Station to Gdańsk Main Train Station

Gdynia's main train station (Gdynia Główna) has an ATM just outside the station's front door; inside are lockers, WCs, and snack stands.

The station is best connected to Gdańsk, Sopot, and other towns by yellow-and-blue regional commuter trains (*kolejka*, operated by SKM). These **SKM trains** go in each direction about every 10-15 minutes (less often after 19:30), and make several stops en route to Gdańsk (35 minutes, 5.70 zł), including the resort town of Sopot (15 minutes, 3.80 zł).

As you enter the Gdynia train station, look to the right to see the **ticket office** *(kasa biletowa)*, where you can buy a ticket for Gdańsk. These tickets must be stamped in the easy-to-miss yellow slots at the bottom of the stairs leading up to the tracks (you're likely to be fined if you don't validate your ticket). You can also buy tickets at the **automated ticket machine** marked *SKM Bilety* (near the head of platform 4, with English instructions); these tickets do not need to be validated. Climb the stairs to platform 1; Gdańsk-bound trains leave from the side of the platform facing away from the city center and sea (labeled *tor 502;* look for *Gdańsk* on the list of stops).

Know Your Stop: Each city has multiple stops. In Gdańsk, you'll most likely hop off at the Gdańsk Główny stop (the main station). However, they're planning to add a new station, called Gdańsk Śródmieście, which is just beyond the Gdańsk Główny stop and even closer to the sights; if you can confirm that this station is open, use it. To visit Sopot, use the stop called simply Sopot (only one word). When returning to Gdynia, your stop is Gdynia Główna (the main station).

PKP Trains: Gdynia's main train station is also served by long-distance PKP trains, operated by the national railway. These are faster but less frequent than SKM commuter trains—unless one is leaving at a convenient time, stick with the easy SKM trains. Tickets for one system can't be used on the other. Trains for the two systems chug along on the same tracks, but use different (but nearby) platforms/stations (at Gdańsk's main train station, national PKP trains use platforms 1-3, while regional SKM trains use platforms 3-5; in Sopot, the SKM station is a few hundred feet before the PKP station).

Step 4: From Gdańsk Main Train Station to the Main Town

Gdańsk's main train station (Gdańsk Główny) is a pretty brick palace on the western edge of the old center. SKM trains arriving from Gdynia use the shorter tracks 3-5. Inside the terminal building, you'll find lockers, ATMs, and ticket windows.

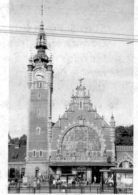

To reach the heart of the Main Town, it's an easy 15-miute walk: Find the pedestrian underpass (with a TI) near the McDonald's, and take it all the way under the busy highway. Emerging on the other side, bear right, circle around the right side of Cinema City, and follow the busy road until you reach the LOT airlines office, then head left toward the brick towers. (You could take a taxi or tram to shave a few minutes off the walk, but it's not necessary.)

Note: If the new Gdańsk Śródmieście station is open, this is the best place to get off. From here, it's easy to reach the entrance to the historic center: Just head outside and cross the busy highway.

Once in town, follow Part 1 of my self-guided Gdańsk Walk (on page 521).

By Tour

Few good tour options exist in Gdynia. I'd hightail it into Gdańsk, where you'll find the options described under "Tours in Gdańsk," page 520.

RETURNING TO YOUR SHIP

Taxis run passengers back to the ship for similar rates as those listed on page 520.

To take the train back to Gdynia, return to the Gdańsk main train station (figure about 15-20 minutes from the Main Town, or a little less from the shipyard area). Before boarding the train, buy tickets at any ticket window or automated machine marked *SKM*. If you buy the ticket from a kiosk (rather than a machine), be sure to stamp it in the yellow box for validation. Then take any blue-and-yellow SKM train heading for Gdynia. If you have lots

GDAŃSK

of time to spare before your ship leaves, consider hopping out at Sopot for a stroll down to the waterfront. In Gdynia, get off at the stop called **Gdynia Główna** (the main station). Exiting the station, simply head down toward the water on ulica 10 Lutego, and find your cruise shuttle-bus stop in the middle of Skwer Kościuski.

See page 557 for help if you miss your boat.

Gdańsk

Gdańsk, with 460,000 residents, is part of the larger urban area known as the Tri-City (Trójmiasto, total population of 1 million).

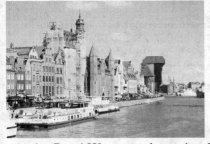

But the tourist's Gdańsk is compact, welcoming, and walkable—virtually anything you'll want to see is within a 20-minute stroll of everything else.

Focus on the Main Town (Główne Miasto), home to most of the sights described, including the spectacular Royal Way main drag: ulica Długa. The Old Town (Stare Miasto) has a handful of old brick buildings and faded, tall, skinny houses—but the area is mostly drab and residential, and not worth much time. Just beyond the northern end of the Old Town (about a 30-minute walk from the heart of the Main Town) is the entrance to the Gdańsk Shipyard, with the excellent European Solidarity Center and its top-notch museum. From here, shipyards sprawl for miles.

The second language in this part of Poland is German, not English. As this was a predominantly German city until the end of World War II, German tourists flock here in droves. But you'll win no Polish friends if you call the city by its more familiar German name, Danzig. You'll also find that Gdańsk is becoming an increasingly popular cruise destination, with about 100 ships calling here each year. During summer daytime hours, the town is filled with little tour groups.

Orientation to Gdańsk

TOURIST INFORMATION

Confusingly, Gdańsk has three different TI organizations. The regional TI occupies the **Upland Gate,** facing the busy road that hems in the Main Town, at the start of my self-guided walk

Gdańsk at a Gdlance

▲▲▲**Royal Way/Ulica Długa** Gdańsk's colorful showpiece main drag, cutting a picturesque swath through the heart of the wealthy burghers' neighborhood. **Hours:** Always open. See page 524.

▲▲▲**Solidarity Sights and Gdańsk Shipyard** Home to the beginning of the end of Eastern European communism, housing a towering monument and an excellent museum, the European Solidarity Center. **Hours:** Memorial and shipyard gate—always open. Solidarity Center—daily 10:00-18:00, Sat-Sun until 20:00 May-Sept. See page 542.

▲▲**Main Town Hall** Ornately decorated meeting rooms, town artifacts, and climbable tower with sweeping views. **Hours:** Mid-June-mid-Sept Mon-Thu 9:00-16:00, Fri-Sat 10:00-18:00, Sun 10:00-16:00; mid-Sept-mid-June Tue 10:00-13:00, Wed-Sat 10:00-16:00, Thu until 18:00, Sun 11:00-16:00, closed Mon. See page 540.

▲▲**Artus Court** Grand meeting hall for guilds of Golden Age Gdańsk, boasting an over-the-top tiled stove. **Hours:** Same as Main Town Hall, above. See page 540.

▲▲**St. Mary's Church** Giant red-brick church crammed full of Gdańsk history. **Hours:** June-Sept Mon-Sat 9:00-18:30, Sun 13:00-18:30; closes progressively earlier off-season. See page 532.

(May-Sept Mon-Fri 9:00-20:00, Sat-Sun 9:00-18:00; Oct-April daily 9:00-18:00; tel. 58-732-7041). The city TI has three branches: one conveniently located at the bottom (river) end of the main drag, at **Długi Targ 28** (just to the left as you face the gate; July-Aug daily 9:00-19:00; Sept-June Mon-Sat 9:00-17:00, Sun 9:00-16:00; tel. 58-301-4355, www.gdansk4u.pl). Satellite TIs are at the **main train station** (in the underpass, same hours, tel. 58-721-3277) and at the **airport** (open 24/7, tel. 58-348-1368). Skip the other TI, which has a prominent location (in the red, high-gabled building across ulica Długa from the Town Hall) but is sloppily run by the national government.

Sightseeing Card: Busy sightseers should consider the **Tourist Card,** which includes entry to 24 sights in Gdańsk, Gdynia, and Sopot, and discounts at others. Check the list of what's covered (most of the biggies in town are free with the card, while the European Solidarity Center is 50 percent off), and do the arithmetic. If you'll be seeing several included museums, this card could save you some money (sightseeing-only card: 38 zł/24

▲**Amber Museum** High-tech exhibit of valuable golden globs of petrified tree sap. **Hours:** Same as Main Town Hall, above. See page 539.

▲**Uphagen House** Tourable 18th-century interior, typical of the pretty houses that line ulica Długa. **Hours:** Same as Main Town Hall. See page 540.

▲**National Maritime Museum** Sprawling exhibit on all aspects of the nautical life, housed in several venues (including the landmark medieval Crane and a permanently moored steamship) connected by a ferry boat. **Hours:** July-Aug daily 10:00-18:00; Sept-Oct and March-June Tue-Sun 10:00-16:00, closed Mon; Nov-Feb Tue-Sun 10:00-15:00, closed Mon. See page 542.

Historical Zone of the Free City of Gdańsk Tiny museum examining Gdańsk's unique status as a "free city" between the World Wars. **Hours:** Tue-Sun 12:00-17:00, until 18:00 May-Aug, closed Mon year-round. See page 541.

Archaeological Museum Decent collection of artifacts from this region's past. **Hours:** July-Aug Tue-Fri 9:00-17:00, Sat-Sun 10:00-17:00; Sept-June Tue and Thu-Fri 8:00-16:00, Wed 9:00-17:00, Sat-Sun 10:00-16:00; closed Mon year-round. See page 541.

hours, 48 zł/72 hours; "max" card also includes local public transit: 58 zł/24 hours, 88 zł/72 hours; sold only at TIs).

HELPFUL HINTS

Blue Monday: Off-season, most of Gdańsk's museums are closed Monday. In the busy summertime, the Gdańsk Historical Museum branches are open—and free—for limited hours on Monday.

Internet Access: You'll find several free Wi-Fi hot spots in major tourist zones around central Gdańsk.

St. Dominic's Fair: Each summer for three weeks around St. Dominic's Day (last week in July through first half of August), Gdańsk is packed with visitors for its venerable St. Dominic's Fair. You'll find otherwise stately streets jammed with stalls selling crafts and edibles, concert stages (there's a lot of free music), and people from all over Poland milling about. While this is a huge draw, the fair has surprisingly little impact on sights or restaurants.

GDAŃSK

GETTING AROUND GDAŃSK

Most of the recommended sights are within easy walking distance. Public transportation is generally unnecessary for sightseers spending their time in town.

By Public Transportation: Gdańsk's trams and buses work on the same tickets: Choose between a single-ride ticket (3 zł), one-hour ticket (3.60 zł), and 24-hour ticket (12 zł). Major stops have handy ticket machines, which take coins, small bills, and credit cards. Otherwise, buy tickets *(bilety)* at kiosks marked *RUCH* or *Bilety ZKM*, or pay a little more to buy tickets on board. In the city center, the stops worth knowing about are Plac Solidarnośći (near the shipyards and European Solidarity Center), Gdańsk Główny (in front of the main train station), and Brama Wyżynna (near the Upland Gate and the new Gdańsk Śródmieście train station). When buying tickets, don't confuse *ZKM* (the company that runs Gdańsk city transit) with *SKM* (the company that runs commuter trains to outlying destinations).

One public bus worth knowing about is Gdańsk's **bus #100.** Every 20 minutes, this made-for-tourists minibus (designed to navigate the twisty streets of the town center) makes a loop through the Old Town and Main Town, with strategic stops near Mariacka street, just south of the Royal Way, at the main train station, and near Solidarity Square. As this is a relatively new service, confirm that it's running and get details at the TI (covered by regular transit ticket, may run in summer only).

By Taxi: Taxis cost about 8 zł to start, then 2-3 zł per kilometer (a bit more at night). Find a taxi stand, or call a cab (try Neptun, tel. 19686; or Dejan, tel. 58-19628).

Tours in Gdańsk

Private Guide

Hiring your own local guide is an exceptional value. **Agnieszka Syroka**—youthful, bubbly, and personable—is a wonderful guide (400 zł for up to 4 hours, more for all day, mobile 502-554-584, www.tourguidegdansk.com, asyroka@interia.pl or syroka. agnieszka@gmail.com). **Jacek "Jake" Podhorski,** who teaches economics at the local university, guides in the summer. He has fascinating personal memories of the communist days (400 zł/3 hours, 100 zł extra with his car, mobile 603-170-761, ekojpp@univ.gda.pl).

Gdańsk Walk

In the 16th and 17th centuries, Gdańsk was Poland's wealthiest city, with gorgeous architecture (much of it in the Flemish Mannerist style) rivaling that in the two historic capitals, Kraków and Warsaw. During this Golden Age, Polish kings would visit this city of well-to-do Hanseatic League merchants, and gawk along the same route trod by tourists today.

The following self-guided walk (rated ▲▲▲) introduces you to the best of Gdańsk. It bridges the two historic centers (the Main Town and the Old Town), dips into St. Mary's Church (the city's most important church), and ends at the famous shipyards and Solidarity Square (where Poland began what ultimately brought down the USSR). I've divided the walk into two parts (making it easier to split up, if you like): The first half focuses on a loop through the Main Town (with most of the high-profile sights), while the second part carries on northward, through the less touristy Old Town to the shipyards.

PART 1: THE MAIN TOWN

• *Begin at the west end of the Main Town, just beyond the last gate at the edge of the busy road (at a road sign that says* Sztokholm...*a reminder that the car ferry to Sweden leaves from near here).*

Upland Gate (Brama Wyżynna)

The Main Town's fortifications were expanded with a Renaissance wall bound by the Upland Gate (built in 1588). "Upland" refers to the hills you see beyond—considered high country in this flat region. Standing with your back to the busy arterial (which traces the old moat), study the gate. Find its three coats of arms (the black eagle for Royal Prussia, the crowned white eagle for Poland, and the two crosses for Gdańsk). Recall that this city has, for almost the entirety of its history before the mid-20th century, been (at least) bicultural—German and Polish, coexisting more or less peacefully. Also notice the little wheels that once hoisted a drawbridge.

• *It's a straight line from here to the river. Walk through the arch (which houses a TI) to the next arch, just a few steps ahead.*

Torture Chamber (Katownia) and Prison Tower (Wieża Więzienna)

The tall, Gothic brick gate before you was part of an earlier protective wall made useless after the Renaissance walls were built in 1588. While today these structures house the Amber Museum (described later), it's free to walk through the evocative passage (except on Mon, when the passage is closed). Inside, find gargoyles (on the left, a town specialty) and the shackles from which prisoners were hung (on the right). Look up at the inside of the high gable to the headless man, identifying this as the torture chamber. This old jail—with its 15-foot-thick walls—was used as a prison even in modern times, under Nazi occupation.

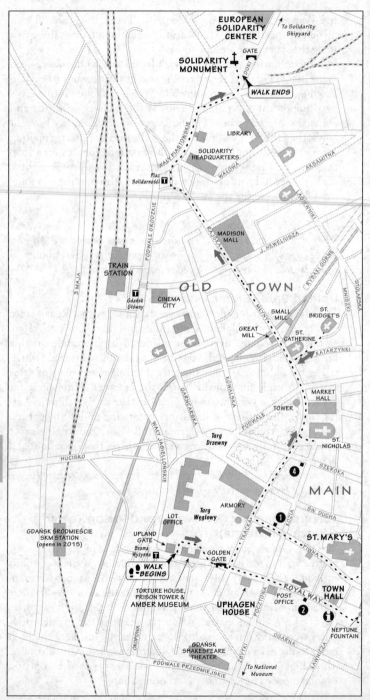

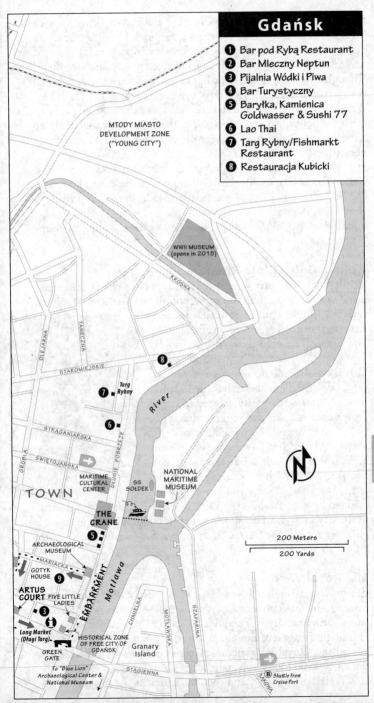

Gdańsk

1. Bar pod Rybą Restaurant
2. Bar Mleczny Neptun
3. Pijalnia Wódki i Piwa
4. Bar Turystyczny
5. Baryłka, Kamienica Goldwasser & Sushi 77
6. Lao Thai
7. Targ Rybny/Fishmarkt Restaurant
8. Restauracja Kubicki

MTODY MIASTO DEVELOPMENT ZONE ("YOUNG CITY")

WWII MUSEUM (opens in 2015)

KROSNA

River

STAROMIEJSKIE

Targ Rybny

STRAGANIARSKA

OLEJARNA

TANECZNA

ŚWIĘTOJAŃSKA

GROBLA

MARITIME CULTURAL CENTER

SS SOŁDEK

NATIONAL MARITIME MUSEUM

T O W N

THE CRANE

DŁUGIE POBRZEŻE

ARCHAEOLOGICAL MUSEUM

MARIACKA

GOTYK HOUSE

ARTUS COURT

FIVE LITTLE LADIES

EMBANKMENT

Motława

Long Market (Długi Targ)

GREEN GATE

To "Blue Lion" Archaeological Center & National Museum

HISTORICAL ZONE OF FREE CITY OF GDAŃSK

Granary Island

SCHMIELNA

MOTŁAWSKA

SZAFARNIA

STAGIEWNA

ŁĄKOWA

B Shuttle from Cruise Port

200 Meters
200 Yards

N

GDAŃSK

As you leave the Torture Chamber and Prison Tower, look to your left (100 yards away) to see a long, brick building with four fancy, uniform gables. This is the **Armory** (Zbrojownia)—one of the finest examples of Dutch Renaissance architecture anywhere. Though this part of the building appears to have the facades of four separate houses, it's a kind of urban camouflage to hide its real purpose from potential attackers. But there's at least one clue to what the building is really for: Notice the exploding cannonballs at the tops of the turrets. (We'll get a better look at the Armory from the other side, later in this walk.)

The round, pointy-topped tower next to the Armory is the **Straw Tower** (Baszta Słomiana). Gunpowder was stored here, and the roof was straw—so if it exploded, it would blow its top without destroying the walls.

• *Straight ahead, the final and fanciest gate between you and the Main Town is the...*

Golden Gate (Złota Brama)

While the other gates were defensive, this one's purely ornamental. The four women up top represent virtues that the people of Gdańsk should exhibit toward outsiders (left to right): Peace, Freedom, Prosperity, and Fame. The gold-lettered inscription, a psalm in medieval German, compares Gdańsk to Jerusalem: famous and important. Directly above the arch is the Gdańsk coat of arms: two white crosses under a crown on a red shield. We'll see this symbol all over town. Photographers love the view of the Main Town framed in this arch. Inside the arch, study the old photos showing the 1945 bomb damage. On the left is the glorious view you just enjoyed...

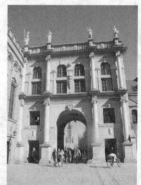

ravaged by war. And on the right is a heartbreaking aerial view of the city in 1945, when 80 percent of its buildings were in ruins.

• *Passing through the Golden Gate, you reach the Main Town's main drag.*

The Royal Way

Before you stretches ulica Długa (cleverly called the "Long Street"), the main promenade of what, 600 years ago, was the biggest and richest city in Poland (thanks to its profitable ties to the Hanseatic League of merchant cities). This promenade is nicknamed the "Royal Way" because (just as in Warsaw and Kraków) the king would follow this route when visiting town.

Walk half a block, and then look back at the Golden Gate.

The women on top of this side represent virtues the people of Gdańsk should cultivate in themselves (left to right): Wisdom, Piety, Justice, and Concord (if an arrow's broken, let's take it out of the quiver and fix it). The inscription—sharing a bit of wisdom as apropos today as it was in 1612—reads, "Concord makes small countries develop, and discord makes big countries fall." Gdańsk was cosmopolitan and exceptionally tolerant in the Middle Ages, attracting a wide range of people, including many who were persecuted elsewhere: Jews, Scots, Dutch, Flemish, Italians, Germans, and more. Members of each group brought with them strands of their culture, which they wove into the tapestry of this city—demonstrated by the eclectic homes along this street. Each facade and each gable were different, as nobles and aristocrats wanted to display their wealth. On my last visit, a traveler seeing this street for the first time gasped to me, "It's like stepping into a Fabergé egg."

During Gdańsk's Golden Age, these houses were taxed based on frontage (like the homes lining Amsterdam's canals)—so they were built skinny and deep. The widest houses belonged to the super-elite. Different as they are from the outside, every house had the same general plan inside. Each had three parts, starting with the front and moving back: First was a fancy drawing room, to show off for visitors. Then came a narrow corridor to the back rooms—often along the side of an inner courtyard. Because the houses had only a few windows facing the outer street, this courtyard provided much-needed sunlight to the rest of the house. The residential quarters were in the back, where the family actually lived: bedroom, kitchen, office. To see the interior of one of these homes, pay a visit to the interesting **Uphagen House** (at #12, on the right, a block and a half in front of the Golden Gate; described later).

This lovely street wasn't always so lively and carefree. At the end of World War II, the Royal Way was in ruins. That epic war actually began here, in what was then the "Free City of Danzig." Following World War I, nobody could decide what to do with this influential and multiethnic city, so rather than assign it to Germany or Poland, it was set apart as its own little autonomous statelet. In 1939, Danzig was 80 percent German-speaking—enough for Hitler to consider it his. And so, on September 1 of that year, the Nazis seized it in one day with relatively minor damage (though the attack on the Polish military garrison on the city's Westerplatte peninsula lasted a week).

But six years later, when the Soviets arrived (March 30, 1945), the city was left devastated. This was the first major, traditionally German city that the Red Army took on their march toward Berlin. And, while it was easy for the Soviets to seize the almost empty city, the commander then insisted that it be leveled,

Gdańsk History

Visitors to Gdańsk are surprised at how "un-Polish" the city's history is. In this cultural melting pot of German, Dutch, and Flemish merchants (with a smattering of Italians and Scots), Poles were only a small part of the picture until the city became exclusively Polish after World War II. However, in Gdańsk, cultural backgrounds traditionally took a back seat to the bottom line. Wealthy Gdańsk was always known for its economic pragmatism—no matter who was in charge, merchants here made money.

Gdańsk is Poland's gateway to the waters of Europe—where its main river (the Vistula) meets the Baltic Sea. The town was first mentioned in the 10th century, and was seized in 1308 by the Teutonic Knights (who called it "Danzig"). The Knights encouraged other Germans to settle on the Baltic coast, and gradually turned Gdańsk into a wealthy city. In 1361, Gdańsk joined the Hanseatic League, a trade federation of mostly Germanic merchant towns that provided mutual security. By the 15th century, Gdańsk was a leading member of this mighty network, which virtually dominated trade in northern Europe (and also included Toruń, Kraków, Lübeck, Hamburg, Bremen, Bruges, Bergen, Tallinn, Novgorod, and nearly a hundred other cities).

In 1454, the people of Gdańsk rose up against the Teutonic Knights, burning down their castle and forcing them out of the city. Three years later, the Polish king borrowed money from wealthy Gdańsk families to hire Czech mercenaries to take the Teutonic Knights' main castle, Malbork. In exchange, the Gdańsk merchants were granted special privileges, including exclusive export rights. Gdańsk now acted as a middleman for much of the trade passing through Polish lands, and paid only a modest annual tribute to the Polish king.

The 16th and 17th centuries were Gdańsk's Golden Age. Now a part of the Polish kingdom, the city had access to an enormous hinterland of natural resources to export—yet it maintained a privileged, semi-independent status. Like Amsterdam, Gdańsk became a progressive and booming merchant city. Its mostly Germanic and Dutch burghers imported Dutch, Flemish, and Italian architects to give their homes an appropriately Hanseatic flourish. At a time of religious upheaval in the rest of Europe, Gdańsk became known for its tolerance—a place that opened its doors to all visitors (many Mennonites and Scottish religious

building by building—in retaliation for all the pain the Nazis had caused in Russia. (Soviets didn't destroy nearby Gdynia—which they considered Polish, not German.) Soviet officers turned a blind eye as their soldiers raped and brutalized residents. An entire order of horrified nuns committed suicide by throwing themselves into the river.

It was only thanks to detailed drawings and photographs that

refugees emigrated here). It was also a haven for great thinkers, including philosopher Arthur Schopenhauer and scientist Daniel Fahrenheit (who invented the mercury thermometer).

Gdańsk declined, along with the rest of Poland, in the late 18th century, and became a part of Prussia (today's northern Germany) during the Partitions. But the people of Gdańsk—even those of German heritage—had taken pride in their independence, and weren't enthusiastic about being ruled from Berlin. After World War I, in a unique compromise to appease its complex ethnic makeup, Gdańsk did not fall under German or Polish control, but once again became an independent city-state: the Free City of Danzig (populated by 400,000 ethnic Germans and 15,000 Poles). The city, along with the so-called Polish Corridor connecting it to Polish lands, effectively cut off Germany from its northeastern territory. On September 1, 1939, Adolf Hitler started World War II when he invaded Gdańsk in order to bring it back into the German fold. Later, nearly 80 percent of the city was destroyed when the Soviets "liberated" it from Nazi control.

After World War II, Gdańsk officially became part of Poland, and was painstakingly reconstructed (mostly replicating the buildings of its Golden Age). In 1970, and again in 1980, the shipyard of Gdańsk witnessed strikes and demonstrations that would lead to the fall of European communism. Poland's great anti-communist hero and first post-communist president—Lech Wałęsa—is Gdańsk's most famous resident, and still lives here. When he flies around the world to give talks, he leaves via Gdańsk's "Lech Wałęsa Airport."

A city with a recent past that's both tragic and uplifting, Gdańsk celebrated its 1,000th birthday in 1997. Very roughly, the city has spent about 700 years as an independent entity, and about 300 years under Germanic overlords (the Teutonic Knights, Prussia, and the Nazis). But today, Gdańsk is decidedly its own city. And, as if eager to prove it, Gdańsk is making big improvements at a stunning pace: new museums (the European Solidarity Center), cultural facilities (the Shakespeare Theater), sports venues (a stadium that resembles a blob of amber, built for the 2012 Euro Cup tournament), and an ongoing surge of renovation and refurbishment that has the gables of the atmospheric Hanseatic quarter gleaming once again.

GDAŃSK

these buildings could be so carefully reconstructed. Notice the cheap plaster facades done in the 1950s—rough times under communism, in the decade after World War II. (Most of the town's medieval brick was shipped to Warsaw for a communist-sponsored "rebuild the capital first" campaign.) While the fine facades were restored, the buildings behind the facades were completely rebuilt to modern standards.

Just beyond Uphagen House, the **Cukiernia Sowa** ("The Owl," on the right at #13) is *the* place for cakes and coffee. Directly across the street, **Grycan** (at #73) has been a favorite for ice cream here for generations.

Just a few doors down, on the left, are some of the most striking **facades** along the Royal Way. The blue-and-white house with the three giant heads is from the 19th century, when the hot style was eclecticism—borrowing bits and pieces from various architectural eras. This was one of the few houses on the street that survived World War II.

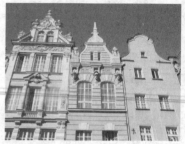

At the next corner on the right is the huge, blocky, red **post office,** which doesn't quite fit with the skinny facades lining the rest of the street. Step inside. With doves fluttering under an airy glass atrium, the interior's a class act. Directly across the street, the candy shop (**Ciuciu Cukier Artist**) is often filled with children clamoring to see lollipop-making demos. Step in and inhale a universal whiff of childhood.

A few doors farther down, on the left at #62, pop in to the **Millennium Gallery** amber shop (which would love to give you an educational amber polishing demo) to see the fascinating collection of old-timey photos, letting you directly compare Gdańsk's cityscape before and after the WWII destruction.

Above the next door, notice the colorful **scenes.** These are slices of life from 17th-century Gdańsk: drinking, talking, buying, playing music. The ship is a *koga,* a typical symbol of Hanseatic ports like Gdańsk.

A couple of doors down—still on the left—is **Neptun Cinema** (marked *KINO*). In the 1980s, this was the only movie theater in the city, and locals lined up for blocks to get in. Old-timers remember coming here with their grandparents to see a full day of cartoons. Now, as with traditional main-street cinemas in the US, this theater is threatened by the rising popularity of multiplexes outside the town center.

Across the street from the theater are the fancy facades of three houses belonging to the very influential medieval **Ferber family,** which produced many burghers, mayors, and even a bishop. On the house with the little dog over the door (#29), look for the heads in the circular medallions. These are Caesars of Rome. At the top of the building is Mr. Ferber's answer to the constant question, "Why build such an elaborate house?"—*PRO INVIDIA,* "For the sake of envy."

A few doors down, on the right, is Gdańsk's most scenically

situated milk bar, the recommended **Bar Mleczny Neptun.** Back in communist times, these humble cafeterias were subsidized to give workers an affordable place to eat out. To this day, they offer simple and very cheap grub.

Next door (at #35) is the **Russian Culture Center,** featuring Russian movies and art exhibits. With the dark past and the Polish support for Ukraine in the recent escalations of tensions there, this is a poignant address.

Before you stands the **Main Town Hall** (Ratusz Głównego Miasta) with its mighty brick clock tower. Consider climbing its observation tower and visiting its superb interior, which features ornately decorated meeting rooms for the city council (described later).

• *Just beyond the Main Town Hall, ulica Długa widens and becomes...*

The Long Market (Długi Targ)

Step from the Long Street into the Long Market, and do a slow, 360-degree spin to appreciate the amazing array of proud architecture here in a city center that rivals the magnificent Grand Place in Brussels. The centerpiece of this square is one of Gdańsk's most important landmarks, the statue of **Neptune**—god of the sea. He's a fitting symbol for a city that dominates the maritime life of Poland. Behind him is another fine museum, the **Artus Court.** Step up to the magnificent door and study the golden relief just above, celebrating the Vistula River (in so many ways the lifeblood of the Polish nation): Lady Vistula is exhausted after her heroic journey, and is finally carried by Neptune to her ultimate destination, the Baltic Sea. (This is just a preview of the ornate art that fills the interior of this fine building—described later.)

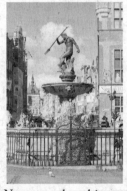

Midway down the Long Market (on the right, across from the Hard Rock Café) is a glass case with the **thermometer and barometer of Daniel Fahrenheit.** While that scientist was born here, he did his groundbreaking work in Amsterdam.

• *At the end of the Long Market is the...*

Green Gate (Zielona Brama)

This huge gate (named for the Green Bridge just beyond) was actually built as a residence for visiting kings...who usually preferred to stay back by Neptune instead (maybe because the river, just on the other side of this gate, stank). It might not have been good enough for kings and queens, but it's plenty fine for a former president—Lech Wałęsa's office is upstairs (see the plaque on the left side, *Biuro Lecha Wałęsy*). His windows, up in the gable, overlook the Long Market. A few steps down the skinny lane to the left is the endearing little **Historical Zone of the Free City of Gdańsk** museum (described later), which explains the inter-war period when "Danzig" was an independent and bicultural city-state.

• *Now go through the gate, walk out onto the Green Bridge, anchor yourself in a niche on the left, and look downstream.*

Riverfront Embankment

The Motława River—a side channel of the mighty Vistula—flows into the nearby Baltic Sea. This port was the source of Gdańsk's phenomenal Golden Age wealth. This embankment was jam-packed in its heyday, the 14th and 15th centuries. It was so crowded with boats that you hardly would have been able to see the water, and boats had to pay a time-based moorage fee for tying up to a post.

Look back at the Green Gate and notice that these bricks are much smaller than the locally made ones we saw earlier on this walk. These bricks are Dutch: Boats from Holland would come here empty of cargo, but with a load of bricks for ballast. Traders filled their ships with goods for the return trip, leaving the bricks behind.

The old-fashioned **galleons** and other tour boats moored nearby depart hourly for a fun cruise to Westerplatte (where, on September 1, 1939, Germans fired the first shots of World War II) and back.

Across the river is **Granary Island** (Spichrze), where grain was stored until it could be taken away by ships. Before World War II, there were some 400 granaries here. Today, much of the island is still in ruins while developers make their plans. Recently, the city ringed the island with an inviting boardwalk, which offers a restful escape from the city and fine views across the narrow river to the embankment. In the summer, sometimes they erect a big Ferris wheel here. And someday there will be several more rebuilt granaries in this area (likely mixed with modern buildings)—to match the ones you already see on either side of the bridge. The three rebuilt granaries downstream, in the distance on the next island, house exhibits for the National Maritime Museum (described later).

From your perch on the bridge, look down the embankment (about 500 yards, on the left) and find the huge wooden **Crane (Żuraw)** bulging over the water. This monstrous 15th-century crane—a rare example of medieval port technology—was once used for loading and repairing ships...beginning a shipbuilding tradition that continued to the days of Lech Wałęsa. The crane mechanism was operated by several workers scrambling around in giant hamster wheels. Treading away to engage the gears and pulleys, they could lift four tons up 30 feet, or two tons up 90 feet.

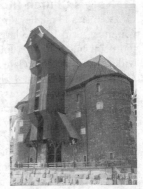

• *Walk along the embankment about halfway to the Crane, passing the lower embankment, with excursion boats heading to the Westerplatte WWII monument. Pause when you reach the big brick building with green window frames and a tower. This red-brick fort houses the* **Archaeological Museum** *(described later). Its collection includes the five ancient stones in a small garden just outside its door (on the left). These are the* **Prussian Hags**— *mysterious sculptures from the second century A.D. (each described in posted plaques).*

Turn left through the gate in the middle of the brick building. You'll find yourself on the most charming lane in town...

Mariacka Street

The calm, atmospheric "Mary's Street" leads from the embankment to St. Mary's Church. Stroll the length of it, enjoying the most romantic lane in Gdańsk. The **porches** extending out into the street, with access to cellars underneath, were a common feature in Gdańsk's Golden Age. For practical reasons, these were only restored on this street after the war. Notice how the porches are bordered with fine stone relief panels and gargoyles attached to storm drains. During a hard rainstorm, you'll understand why in Polish, these are called "pukers." Enjoy a little amber comparison-shopping. As you stroll up to the towering brick St. Mary's Church, imagine the entire city like this cobbled lane of proud merchants' homes, with street music, delightful facades, and brick church towers high above.

Look up at the church tower viewpoint—filled with people who hiked 409 steps for the view. Our next stop is the church, which you'll enter on the far side under the tower. Walk around the left side of the church, appreciating the handmade 14th-century bricks on the right and the plain post-WWII facades on the left. (Reconstructing the Royal Way was better funded. Here, the priority was simply getting people housed again.) In the distance is the fancy facade of the Armory (where you'll head after visiting the church).

• *But first, go inside...*

St. Mary's Church (Kościół Mariacki)

Of Gdańsk's 13 medieval red-brick churches, St. Mary's is the one you must visit. It's the largest brick church in the world—with a footprint bigger than a football field (350 feet long and 210 feet wide), it can accommodate 20,000 standing worshippers.

Cost and Hours: 4 zł, June-Sept Mon-Sat 9:00-18:30, Sun 13:00-18:30, closes progressively earlier off-season.

Visiting the Church: Inside, sit directly under the fine carved and painted 17th-century Protestant pulpit, midway down the nave, to get oriented.

Overview: Built from 1343 to 1502 by the Teutonic Knights (who wanted a suitable centerpiece for their newly captured main city), St. Mary's remains an important symbol of Gdańsk. The church started out Catholic, became Lutheran in the mid-1500s, and then became Catholic again after World War II. (Remember, Gdańsk was a Germanic city before World War II and part of the big postwar demographic shove, when Germans were sent west, and Poles from the east relocated here. Desperate, cold, and home-less, the new Polish residents moved into what was left of the German homes.) While the church was originally frescoed from top to bottom, the Lutherans whitewashed the entire place. Today, some of the 16th-century whitewash has been peeled back (behind the high altar—we'll see this area soon), revealing a bit of the orig-inal frescoes. The floor is paved with 500 gravestones of merchant families. Many of these were cracked when bombing sent the brick roof crashing down in 1945.

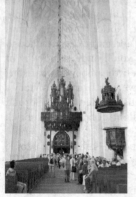

Most Gothic stone churches are built of stone in the basilica style—with a high nave in the middle, shorter aisles on the side, and flying buttresses to support the weight. (Think of Paris' Notre-Dame.) But since no handy source of stone is available locally, most Polish churches are built of brick, which won't work with the basilica design. So, like all Gdańsk churches, St. Mary's is a "hall church"—with three naves the same height, and no exterior buttresses.

Also like other Gdańsk churches, St. Mary's gave refuge to the Polish people after the communist government declared mar-tial law in 1981. When a riot broke out and violence seemed immi-nent, people flooded into churches, knowing that the ZOMO riot police wouldn't follow them inside.

Most of the church decorations are original. A few days before the Soviets arrived to "liberate" the city in 1945, locals—knowing what was in store—hid precious items in the countryside. Take some time now to see a few of the highlights.

• *From this seat, you can see most of what we'll visit in the church: As you face the altar, the astronomical clock is at 10 o'clock, the Ferber family medallion is at 1 o'clock, the Priests' Chapel is at 3 o'clock (under a tall colorful window), and the magnificent 17th-century organ is directly behind you (it's played at each Mass and during free concerts on Fri in summer).*

Pulpit: For Protestants, the pulpit is important. Designed as an impressive place from which to share the Word of God in the peoples' language, it's located mid-nave, so all can hear.

• *Opposite the pulpit is the moving...*

Priests' Chapel: The 1965 statue of Christ weeping commemorates 2,779 Polish chaplains executed by the Nazis because they were priests. See the grainy black-and-white photo of one about to be shot, above on the right.

• *Head up the nave to the...*

High Altar: The main altar, beautifully carved in 1517, is a triptych showing the coronation of Mary. She is surrounded by the Trinity: flanked by God and Jesus, with the dove representing the Holy Spirit overhead. The church's medieval stained glass was destroyed in 1945. Poland's biggest stained-glass window, behind the altar, is from 1980.

• *Start circling around the right side of the altar. Look right to find (high on a pillar) the big, opulent family marker.*

Ferber Family Medallion: The falling baby (under the crown) is Constantine Ferber. As a precocious child, li'l Constantine leaned out his window on the Royal Way to see the king's processional come through town. He slipped and fell, but landed in a salesman's barrel of fish. Constantine grew up to become the mayor of Gdańsk.

• *As you continue around behind the altar, search high above you, on the walls to your right, to spot those restored pre–Reformation frescoes. Directly behind the altar, under the big window, is the...*

Empty Glass Case: This case was designed to hold Hans Memling's *Last Judgment* painting, which used to be in this church, but is currently being held hostage by the National Museum. To counter the museum's claim that the church wasn't a good environment for such a precious work, the priest had this display case built—but that still wasn't enough to convince the museum to give the painting back. (You'll see a small replica of the painting in the rear of this church, but the real thing is in the National Museum.)

• *Now circle back the way you came to the area in front of the main altar, and proceed straight ahead into the transept. High on the wall to your right, look for the...*

GDAŃSK

Astronomical Clock: This 42-foot-tall clock is supposedly the biggest wooden clock in the world. Below it is an elaborate circular calendar that, like a medieval computer, calculates on which day each saint's festival day falls in different years (see the little guy on the left, with the pointer). Above are zodiac signs and the time (back then, the big hand was all you needed). Way up on top, Adam and Eve are naked and ready to ring the bell. Adam's been swinging his clapper at the top of the hour since 1473...but sadly, the clock is broken.

• *A few steps in front of the clock is a modern chapel with the...*

Memorial to the Polish Victims of the 2010 Plane Crash: The gold-shrouded Black Madonna honors the 96 victims of an air disaster that the killed much of Poland's government—including the president and first lady—during a terrible storm over Russia. The main tomb is for Maciej Płażyński, from Gdańsk, who was leader of the parliament. On the left, the jagged statue has bits of the wreckage, and lists each victim by name.

• *In a small chapel in the rear corner of the church—on the far right with your back to the high altar—you'll find the...*

Pietà and Memling Replica: The *pietà*, carved of limestone and painted in 1410, is by the Master of Gdańsk. In the same room is a musty old copy of Memling's *Last Judgment*—the exquisite original once graced this very chapel.

• *Next door are stairs leading to the...*

Church Tower: You can climb 409 steps to burn off some pierogi and earn a grand city view (5 zł, Mon-Sat 9:00-17:00, Sun 13:00-17:30). It's a long hike (and you'll know it—since every 10th step is numbered). But because the viewpoint is surrounded by a roof, the views are distant and may not be worth the effort. The first third is up a tight, medieval spiral staircase. Then you'll walk through the eerie, cavernous area between the roof and the ceiling, before huffing up steep concrete steps that surround the square tower (as you spiral up, up, up around the bells). Finally you'll climb a little metal ladder and pop out at the viewpoint.

• *Leaving the church, angle left and continue straight up ulica Piwna ("Beer Street") toward the sprightly facade of the Armory.*

The Gdańsk Armory (Zbrojownia)

The 1605 **Armory,** which we saw from a distance at the start of this walk, is one of the best examples of Dutch Renaissance architecture in Europe. Athena, the goddess of war and wisdom, stands in the center, amid motifs of war and ornamental pukers.

• *If you want to make your walk a loop, you're just a block away from where we started (to the left). But there's much more to see. Facing the Armory, turn right and start the second half of this walk.*

PART 2: THROUGH THE OLD TOWN TO THE SHIPYARDS

• *From here, we'll work our way out of the Main Town and head into the Old Town, toward Solidarity Square and the shipyards. Nearly all the way, we'll be walking along this street (which changes names a couple of times). Keep in mind that this part of the walk ends at the European Solidary Center's superb museum.*

From the Armory, head down Kołodziejska, which quickly becomes Węglarska. After two blocks (that is, one block before the big market hall), detour to the right down Świętojańska and use the side door to enter the brick church.

St. Nicholas Church (Kościół Św. Mikołaja)

Near the end of World War II, when the Soviet army reached Gdańsk on its march westward, they were given the order to burn all the churches. Only this one survived—because it happened to be dedicated to Russia's patron saint. As the best-preserved church in town, it has a more impressive interior than the others, with lavish black-and-gold Baroque altars.

• *Backtrack out to the main street and continue to the right, passing a row of seniors selling their grown and foraged edibles. Immediately after the church is Gdańsk's...*

Market Hall

Built in 1896 and renovated in 2005, Gdańsk's market hall is fun to explore. Appreciate the delicate steel-and-glass canopy overhead. This is a totally untouristy scene: You'll see everything from skintight *Polska* T-shirts, to wedding gowns, to maternity wear. The meat is downstairs, and the veggies are outside on the adjacent square. As this was once the center of a monastic community, the basement has the graves of medieval Dominican monks, which were exposed when the building was refurbished: Peer over the glass railing, and you'll see some of those scant remains.

Across the street from the Market Hall, a round, red-brick **tower,** part of the city's protective wall back in 1400, marks the end of the Main Town and the beginning of the Old Town.

• *Another block up the street, on the right, is the huge...*

St. Catherine's Church (Kościół Św. Katarzyny)

"Katy," as locals call it, is the oldest church in Gdańsk. In May of 2006, a carelessly discarded cigarette caused the church roof to burst into flames. Local people ran into the church and pulled everything outside, so nothing valuable was damaged; even the carillon bells were saved. However, the roof and wooden frame were totally destroyed. The people of Gdańsk were determined to rebuild this important symbol of the city. Within days of the fire, fundraising concerts were held to scrape together most of the money needed to raise the roof once more. Step inside. On the left side of the gate leading to the nave, photos show bomb damage. Farther in, on the left, are vivid photos of the more recent conflagration. The interior is evocative, with still-bare-brick walls that almost seem intentional—as if they're trying for an industrial-mod look.

• *The church hiding a block behind Katy—named for Catherine's daughter Bridget—has important ties to Solidarity, and is worth a visit. Go around the right side of Katy and skirt the parking lot to find the entrance.*

St. Bridget's Church (Kościół Św. Brygidy)

This was the home church of Lech Wałęsa during the tense days of the 1980s. The church and its priest, Henryk Jankowski, were particularly aggressive in supporting the ideals of Solidarity. Jankowski became a mouthpiece for the movement. In gratitude for the church's support, Wałęsa named his youngest daughter Brygida.

Cost and Hours: 2 zł, daily 10:00-18:00.

Visiting the Church: Head inside. For your visit, start at the high altar, then circle clockwise back to the entry.

The enormous, unfinished **high altar** is made entirely of amber—more than a thousand square feet of it. Features that are already in place include the Black Madonna of Częstochowa, a royal Polish eagle, and the Solidarity symbol (tucked below the Black Madonna). The structure, like a scaffold, holds pieces as they are completed and added to the ensemble. The video you may see playing overhead gives you a close-up look at the amber elements.

The wrought-iron gate of the adjacent **Chapel of Fatima** (right of main altar) recalls great battles and events in Polish history from 966 to 1939, with important dates boldly sparkling in gold. Some say the Polish Church is too political. But it was only through a politically engaged Church that this culture survived the Partitions of Poland over a century and a half, plus the brutal anti-religious policies of the communist period. The national soul of the Polish people— whether religious or not—is tied up in the Catholic faith.

Henryk Jankowski's tomb—a white marble box with red trim—is a bit farther to the right. Jankowski was a key hero during Solidarity times; the tomb proclaims him *Kapelan Solidarności*

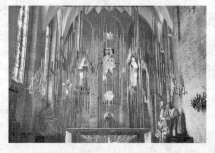

("Solidarity Chaplain"). But his public standing took a nosedive near the end of his life—thanks to ego-driven projects like his amber altar, as well as accusations of anti-Semitism and corruption. Forced to retire in 2007, Jankowski died in 2010. (An offering box is next to his tomb, if you'd like to donate to the amber altar project.)

In the rear corner, where a figure lies lifeless on the floor under a wall full of wooden crosses, is the tomb of Solidarity martyr **Jerzy Popiełuszko.** A courageous and famously outspoken Warsaw priest, in 1984 Popiełuszko was kidnapped, beaten, and murdered by the communist secret police. Notice that the figure's hands and feet are bound—as his body was found. The crosses are historic—each one was carried at various strikes against the communist regime. The communists believed they could break the spirit of the Poles with brutality—like the murder of Popiełuszko. But it only made the rebels stronger and more resolved to ultimately win their freedom. (Near the exit, on a monitor, a fascinating 12-minute video shows great moments of this church, with commentary by Lech Wałęsa himself.)

• *Return to the main street, turn right, and continue on. The big brick building ahead on the left, with the many windows, is the Great Mill. Walk past that and look down at the canal that once powered it.*

The Great Mill

This huge brick building dates from the 14th century. Look at the waterfalls and imagine standing here in 1400—with the mill's 18 wheels spinning 24/7, powering grindstones that produced 20 tons of flour a day. Like so much else here, the mill survived until 1945. Today the rebuilt structure houses a modern shopping mall.

The **park** just beyond the mill is worth a look. In the distance is the Old City Town Hall (Dutch Renaissance style, from 1595). The monument in the middle honors the 17th-century astronomer Jan Haweliusz. He's looking up at a giant, rust-colored wall with a map of the heavens. Haweliusz built the biggest telescopes of his era to better appreciate and understand the cosmos. Behind the mill stands the miller's home—its opulence indicates that, back in the Middle Ages, there was a lot of money in grinding. Just steps into the family-friendly park is a fountain that brings shrieks of joy to children on hot summer days. Watching families enjoy this park, I'm struck that these are good times for Poland—stability, one of the EU's healthiest economies, and

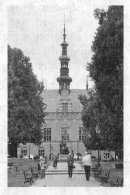

freedom. But next we walk through a stretch that, if you take away the colors, advertising, and smiles, reminds me of the dark days before 1989. And beyond that are the shipyards, where freedom from communism was born.

• To get to the **shipyards,** *keep heading straight up Rajska. You'll pass the modern Madison shopping mall. After another long block, jog right, passing to the right of the big, ugly, and green 1970s-era skyscraper. On your right—marked by the famous red sign on the roof—is today's* **Solidarity headquarters** *(which remains the strongest trade union in Poland, with 700,000 members, and is also active in many other countries). Just in front of the Solidarity building, you may see two big chunks of* **wall:** *a piece of the Berlin Wall and a stretch of the shipyard wall that Lech Wałęsa scaled to get inside and lead the strike. The message: What happened behind one wall eventually led to the fall of the other Wall.*

From here, hike on (about 100 yards) to the finale of this walk.

Solidarity Square and the Shipyards

Three tall crosses mark Solidarity Square and the rust-colored European Solidarity Center (with an excellent museum). For the exciting story of how Polish shipbuilders set in motion events that led to the end of the USSR, turn to page 542.

Sights in Gdańsk

MAIN TOWN (GŁÓWNE MIASTO)

The following sights are all in the Main Town, listed roughly in the order you'll see them on the self-guided walk of the Royal Way.

Gdańsk Historical Museum

The Gdańsk Historical Museum has four excellent branches: the Amber Museum, Uphagen House, Main Town Hall, and Artus Court. Along with St. Mary's Church (described on page 532), these are the four most important interiors in the Main Town. All have the same hours, but you must buy a separate ticket for each.

Cost and Hours: 10 zł apiece—except Main Town Hall, which is 12 zł; hours fluctuate, but typically open mid-June-mid-Sept Mon-Thu 9:00-16:00, Fri-Sat 10:00-18:00, Sun 10:00-16:00; mid-Sept-mid-June Tue 10:00-13:00, Wed-Sat 10:00-16:00, Thu until 18:00, Sun 11:00-16:00, closed Mon; last entry 30 minutes before closing.

Information: The museums share a phone number and website (central tel. 58-767-9100, www.mhmg.gda.pl).

All About Amber

Poland's Baltic seaside is known as the Amber Coast. You can see amber (*bursztyn*) in Gdańsk's Amber Museum and in shop windows everywhere. This fossilized tree resin originated here on the north coast of Poland 40 million years ago. It comes in as many different colors as Eskimos have words for snow: 300 distinct shades, from yellowish white to yellowish black, from opaque to transparent. (I didn't believe it either, until I toured Gdańsk's museum.) Darker-colored amber is generally mixed with ash and sand—making it more fragile, and generally less desirable. Lighter amber is mixed with gasses and air bubbles.

Amber has been popular since long before there were souvenir stands. Archaeologists have found Roman citizens (and their coins) buried with crosses made of amber. Almost 75 percent of the world's amber is mined in northern Poland, and it often simply washes up on the beaches after a winter storm. Some of the elaborate amber sculptures displayed at the museum are joined with "amber glue"—melted-down amber mixed with an adhesive agent. More recently, amber craftsmen are combining amber with silver to create artwork—a method dubbed the "Polish School."

Some Poles also believe amber is good for their health. A traditional cure for arthritis pain is to pour strong vodka over amber, let it set, and then rub it on sore joints. Other remedies call for mixing amber dust with honey or rose oil. It sounds superstitious, but users claim that it works.

▲Amber Museum (Muzeum Bursztynu)

Housed in a pair of connected brick towers (the former Prison Tower and Torture Chamber) just outside the Main Town's

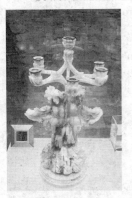

Golden Gate, this museum has two oddly contradictory parts. One shows off Gdańsk's favorite local resource, amber, while the other focuses on implements of torture (cost and hours above, overpriced 1.5-hour audioguide—25 zł). You'll follow the one-way route through four exhibits on amber (with lots of stairs), and then walk the rampart to the Prison Tower and the torture exhibit—with sound effects and mannequins used to demonstrate the grisly equipment. Exhibits are explained in English. For a primer before you visit, read the "All About Amber" sidebar.

▲Uphagen House (Dom Uphagena)

This interesting place at ulica Długa 12 is your chance to glimpse what's behind the colorful facades lining this street (see cost and hours earlier). It's the only grand Gdańsk mansion rebuilt as it was before 1945. The model near the entry shows the three parts: dolled-up visitors' rooms in front, a corridor along the courtyard, and private rooms in the back. The finely decorated salon was used to show off for guests. Most of this furniture is original (saved from WWII bombs by locals who hid it in the countryside). Passing into the dining room, note the knee-high paintings of hunting and celebrations. Along the passage to the back, each room has a theme: butterflies in the smoking room, then flowers in the next room, then birds in the music room. In the private rooms at the back, the decor is simpler. Downstairs, you'll pass through the kitchen, the pantry, and a room with photos of the house before the war, which were used to reconstruct what you see today.

▲▲Main Town Hall (Ratusz Głównego Miasta)

This landmark building contains remarkable decorations from Gdańsk's Golden Age (see cost and hours earlier). Inside you'll

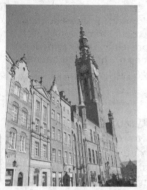

pass through an ornately carved wooden **door** from the 1600s into the lavish **Red Hall,** where the Gdańsk city council met during summer, then into the less impressive Winter Hall, and finally through another room into one with photos of **WWII damage.** Upstairs are some temporary exhibits and several examples of **Gdańsk-style furniture** (characterized by lots of ornamentation) and a coin collection, from the days when Gdańsk had the elite privilege of minting its own currency. Head upstairs to a fascinating exhibit about Gdańsk's time as a "free city" between the World Wars. Near the end of this room, you have the option to climb 293 concrete steps to the top of the **tower** for commanding city views (5 zł extra, mid-June-mid-Sept only).

▲▲Artus Court (Dwór Artusa)

In the Middle Ages, Gdańsk was home to many brotherhoods and guilds (like businessmen's clubs). For their meetings, the city provided this elaborately decorated hall, named for King Arthur—a

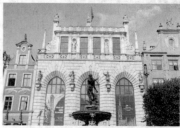

medieval symbol for prestige and power. Just as in King Arthur's Court, this was a place where powerful and important people came together. Of many such halls in Baltic Europe, this is the only original one that survives (cost and hours on page 538, dry and too-thorough audioguide-3 zł extra; in tall, white, triple-arched building behind Neptune statue at Długi Targ 43).

Other Museums in the Main Town
Historical Zone of the Free City of Gdańsk (Strefa Historyczna Wolne Miasto Gdańsk)

In a city so obsessed with its Golden Age and Solidarity history, this charming little collection illuminates a unique but often-overlooked chapter in the story of Gdańsk: The years between World Wars I and II, when—in an effort to find a workable compromise in this ethnically mixed city—Gdańsk was not part of Germany nor of Poland, but a self-governing "free city" *(wolne miasto)*. This modest museum earnestly shows off artifacts from the time—photos, stamps, maps, flags, promotional tourist leaflets, and other items from the free city, all marked with the Gdańsk symbol of two white crosses under a crown on a red shield. While some might find the subject obscure, this endearing collection is a treat for WWII history buffs. Be sure to borrow the English translations at the entrance.

Cost and Hours: 8 zł, Tue-Sun 12:00-17:00, until 18:00 May-Aug, closed Mon year-round, down the little alley just in front of the Green Gate at Warzywnicza 10A, tel. 58-320-2828, www.tpg. info.pl.

Archaeological Museum (Muzeum Archeologiczne)

This simple museum is worth a quick peek for those interested in archaeology. The ground floor has exhibits on excavated finds from Sudan, where the museum has a branch program. Upstairs, look for the distinctive urns with cute faces, which date from the Hallstatt Period and were discovered in slate graves around Gdańsk. Also upstairs are some Bronze and Iron Age tools; before-and-after photos of WWII Gdańsk; and a reconstructed 12th-century Viking-like Slavonic longboat. You can also climb the building's tower, with good views up Mariacka street toward St. Mary's Church.

Cost and Hours: Museum-8 zł (free on Sat), tower-5 zł; July-Aug Tue-Fri 9:00-17:00, Sat-Sun 10:00-17:00; Sept-June Tue and Thu-Fri 8:00-16:00, Wed 9:00-17:00, Sat-Sun 10:00-16:00; closed Mon year-round; ulica Mariacka 25, tel. 58-322-2100, www. archeologia.pl.

GDAŃSK

▲National Maritime Museum
(Narodowe Muzeum Morskie)

Gdańsk's history and livelihood are tied to the sea. This collection, spread among several buildings on either side of the river, examines all aspects of this connection. While nautical types may get a thrill out of the creaky, sprawling museum, most visitors find it little more than a convenient way to pass some time and enjoy a cruise across the river. The museum's lack of English information is frustrating; fortunately, some exhibits have descriptions you can borrow.

Cost and Hours: Each part of the museum has its own admission (6-8 zł). The Maritime Cultural Center is worth neither the time nor the money for grown-ups; I'd consider the 18-zł "karnet" combo-ticket that combines the other, better parts. It's open July-Aug daily 10:00-18:00; Sept-Oct and March-June Tue-Sun 10:00-16:00, closed Mon; Nov-Feb Tue-Sun 10:00-15:00, closed Mon; ulica Ołowianka 9, tel. 58-301-8611, www.cmm.pl.

SOLIDARITY AND THE GDAŃSK SHIPYARD

Gdańsk's single most memorable experience is exploring the shipyard (Stocznia Gdańska) that witnessed the beginning of the end of communism's stranglehold on Eastern Europe. Taken together, the sights in this area are worth ▲▲▲. Here, in the former industrial wasteland that Lech Wałęsa called the "cradle of freedom," this evocative site tells the story of the brave Polish shipyard workers who took on—and ultimately defeated—an Evil Empire. A visit to the Solidarity sights has two main parts: Solidarity Square (with the memorial and gate out in front of the shipyard), and the outstanding museum inside the European Solidarity Center.

Getting to the Shipyard: These sights cluster around Solidarity Square (Plac Solidarności), at the north end of the Old Town, about a 20-minute walk from the Royal Way. For the most interesting approach, follow "Part 2" of my self-guided walk (earlier), which ends here.

Background: After the communists took over Eastern Europe at the end of World War II, oppressed peoples throughout the Soviet Bloc rose up in different ways. The most dramatic uprisings—Hungary's 1956 Uprising and Czechoslovakia's 1968 "Prague Spring"—were brutally crushed under the treads of Soviet tanks. The formula for freedom that finally succeeded was a patient, nearly decade-long series of strikes and protests spearheaded by Lech Wałęsa and his trade union, called Solidarność— "Solidarity." (The movement also benefited from good timing, as it coincided with the *perestroika* and *glasnost* policies of the Soviet premier Mikhail Gorbachev.) While some American politicians might like to take credit for defeating communism, Wałęsa and his fellow workers were the ones fighting on the front lines, armed with nothing more than guts.

Solidarity Square (Plac Solidarności)

The seeds of August 1980 were sown a decade before. Since becoming part of the Soviet Bloc, the Poles staged frequent strikes, protests, and uprisings to secure their rights, all of which were put down by the regime. But the bloodiest of these took place in December of 1970—a tragic event memorialized by the "Monument of the Fallen Shipyard Workers," whose three crosses tower over what's now called Solidarity Square.

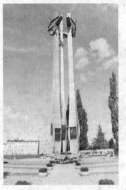

The 1970 strike was prompted by price hikes. The communist government set the prices for all products. As Poland endured drastic food shortages in the 1960s and 1970s, the regime frequently announced what it called "regulation of prices." Invariably, this meant an increase in the cost of essential foodstuffs. (To be able to claim "regulation" rather than "increase," the regime would symbolically lower prices for a few select items—but these were always nonessential luxuries, such as elevators and TV sets, which nobody could afford anyway.) The regime was usually smart enough to raise prices on January 1—when the people were fat and happy after Christmas, and too hung over to complain. But on December 12, 1970, bolstered by an ego-stoking visit by West German Chancellor Willy Brandt, Polish premier Władysław Gomułka increased prices. The people of Poland—who cared more about the price of Christmas dinner than relations with Germany—struck back.

A wave of strikes and sit-ins spread along the heavily industrialized north coast of Poland, most notably in Gdańsk, Gdynia, and Szczecin. Thousands of angry demonstrators poured through the gate of this shipyard, marched into town, and set fire to the Communist Party Committee building. In an attempt to quell the riots, the government-run radio implored the people to go back to work. On the morning of December 17, workers showed up at shipyard gates across northern Poland, and were greeted by the army and police. Without provocation, the Polish army opened fire on the workers. While the official death toll for the massacre stands at 44, others say the true number is much higher. The monument, with a trio of 140-foot-tall crosses, honors those lost to the regime that December.

Go to the middle of the **wall** behind the crosses, to the monument of the worker wearing a flimsy plastic work helmet,

Lech Wałęsa

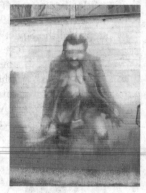

In 1980, the world was turned on its ear by a walrus-mustachioed shipyard electrician. Within three years, this seemingly run-of-the-mill Pole had precipitated the collapse of communism, led a massive 10-million-member trade union with enormous political impact, been named *Time* magazine's Man of the Year, and won a Nobel Peace Prize.

Lech Wałęsa was born in Popowo, Poland, in 1943. After working as a car mechanic and serving two years in the army, he became an electrician at the Gdańsk Shipyard in 1967. Like many Poles, Wałęsa felt stifled by the communist government, and was infuriated that a system that was supposed to be for the workers clearly wasn't serving them.

When the shipyard massacre took place in December of 1970 (see description on page 543), Wałęsa was at the forefront of the protests. He was marked as a dissident, and in 1976, he was fired. Wałęsa hopped from job to job and was occasionally unemployed. But he soldiered on, fighting for the creation of a trade union and building up quite a file with the secret police.

In August of 1980, Wałęsa heard news of the beginnings of the Gdańsk strike and raced to the shipyard. In an act that has

attempting to shield himself from bullets. Behind him is a list—pockmarked with symbolic bullet holes—of workers murdered on that day. *Lat* means "years old"—many teenagers were among the dead. The quote at the top of the wall is from St. John Paul II, who was elected pope eight years after this tragedy. The pope was known for his clever way with words, and this very carefully phrased quote—which served as an inspiration to the Poles during their darkest hours—skewers the regime in a way subtle enough to still be tolerated: "Let thy spirit descend, and renew the face of the earth—of *this* earth" (that is, Poland). Below that is the dedication: "They gave their lives so you can live decently."

Stretching to the left of this center wall are plaques representing labor unions from around Poland—and around the world (look for the Chinese characters)—expressing solidarity with these workers. To the right is an enormous Bible verse: "May the Lord give strength to his people. May the Lord bless his people with the gift of peace" (Psalms 29:11).

Inspired by the brave sacrifice of their true comrades, shipyard workers rose up here in August of 1980, formulating the "21 Points" of a new union called Solidarity. Their demands included

since become the stuff of legend, Wałęsa scaled the shipyard wall to get inside.

Before long, Wałęsa's dynamic personality won him the unofficial role of the workers' leader and spokesman. He negotiated with the regime to hash out the August Agreements, becoming a rock star-type hero during the so-called 16 Months of Hope...until martial law came crashing down in December of 1981. Wałęsa was arrested and interned for 11 months. After being released, he continued to struggle underground, becoming a symbol of anti-communist sentiment.

Finally, the dedication of Wałęsa and Solidarity paid off, and Polish communism dissolved—with Wałęsa rising from the ashes as the country's first post-communist president. But the skills that made Wałęsa a rousing success at leading an uprising didn't translate well to the president's office. Wałęsa proved to be a stubborn, headstrong politician, frequently clashing with the parliament and squabbling with his own party.

Wałęsa was defeated at the polls, by the Poles, in 1995, and when he ran again in 2000, he received a humiliating 1 percent of the vote. Poles say there are two Lech Wałęsas: the young, bombastic, working-class idealist Lech, at the forefront of the Solidarity strikes, who will always have a special place in their hearts; and the failed President Wałęsa, who got in over his head and tarnished his legacy.

the right to strike and form unions, the freeing of political prisoners, and an increase in wages. The 21 Points are listed in Polish on the panel at the far end of the right wall, marked *21 X TAK* ("21 times yes"). An unwritten precondition to any agreement was the right for the workers of 1980 to build a memorial to their comrades slain in 1970. The government agreed, marking the first time a communist regime ever allowed a monument to be built to honor its own victims. Wałęsa called it a harpoon in the heart of the communists. The towering monument, with three crucified anchors on top, was designed, engineered, and built by shipyard workers. In just four months after the historic agreement was signed, the monument was finished.

• *Now continue to the gate and peer through into the birthplace of Eastern European freedom.*

Gdańsk Shipyard (Stocznia Gdańska) Gate #2

When a Pole named Karol Wojtyła was elected pope in 1978—and visited his homeland in 1979—he inspired his 40 million countrymen to believe that impossible dreams can come true. Prices continued to go up, and the workers continued to rise up. By the summer of 1980, it was clear that the dam was about to break.

In August, Anna Walentynowicz—a Gdańsk crane opera-tor and known dissident—was fired unceremoniously just short of her retirement. This sparked a strike in the Gdańsk Shipyard (then called the Lenin Shipyard) on August 14, 1980. An elec-trician named Lech Wałęsa had been fired as an agitator years before and wasn't allowed into the yard. But on hearing news of the strike, Wałęsa went to the shipyard and climbed over the wall to get inside. The strike now had a leader.

These were not soldiers, nor were they idealistic flower chil-dren. The strike participants were gritty, salt-of-the-earth man-ual laborers: forklift operators, welders, electricians, machinists. Imagine being one of the 16,000 workers who stayed here for 18 days during the strike—hungry, cold, sleeping on sheets of Styrofoam, inspired by the new Polish pope, excited about

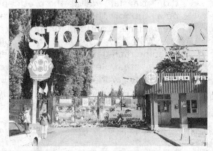

finally standing up to the regime...and terrified that at any moment you might be gunned down, like your friends had been a decade before. Workers, afraid to leave the shipyard, communi-cated with the outside world through this gate—wives and brothers showed up here and asked for a loved one, and those inside spread the word until the striker came forward. Occasionally, a truck pulled up inside the gate, with Lech Wałęsa standing atop its cab with a megaphone. Facing the thousands of people assembled outside the gate, Wałęsa gave progress reports on the negotiations and pleaded for supplies. The people of Gdańsk responded, bringing armfuls of bread and other food to keep the workers going. Solidarity.

During the strike, two items hung on the fence. One of them (which still hangs there today) was a picture of then Pope John Paul II—a reminder to believe in your dreams and have faith in God (and a reminder of the usefulness of a papal bully pulpit). The other item was a makeshift list of the strikers' 21 Points—demands scrawled in red paint and black pencil on pieces of plywood.

• *Walk around the right end of the gate and enter the former shipyard.*

The shipyard churned out over a thousand ships from 1948 to 1990, employing 16,000 workers. About 60 percent of these ships were exported to the USSR—and so, when the Soviet Bloc broke apart in the 1990s, they lost a huge market. Today the facilities employ closer to 1,200 workers...who now make windmills.

Before entering the museum, take a look around. Let me guess:

lots of construction? This part of the shipyard, long abandoned, is being redeveloped into a **"Young City"** (Młode Miasto)—envisioned as a new city center for Gdańsk, with shopping, restaurants, offices, and homes. Rusting shipbuilding equipment has been torn down, and old brick buildings are being converted into gentrified flats. The nearby boulevard called Nowa Wałowa will be the spine connecting this area to the rest of the city. Farther east, the harborfront will also be rejuvenated, creating a glitzy marina and extending the city's delightful waterfront people zone to the north (see www.ycgdansk.com). Fortunately, the shipyard gate, monument, and other important sites from the Solidarity strikes—now considered historical monuments—will remain.

• *The massive, rust-colored European Solidarity Center, which faces Solidarity Square, houses the museum where we'll learn the rest of the story.*

▲▲▲European Solidarity Center (Europejskie Centrum Solidarności)

Europe's single best sight about the end of communism is made even more powerful by its location: in the very heart of the place

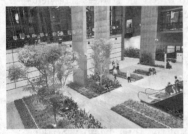

where those events occurred. Filling just one small corner of a huge, purpose-built educational facility, the permanent exhibition uses larger-than-life photographs, archival footage, actual artifacts, interactive touchscreens, and a state-of-the-art audioguide to eloquently tell the story of the end of Eastern European communism.

Cost and Hours: 17 zł, includes audioguide, daily 10:00-18:00, Sat-Sun until 20:00 May-Sept, last entry one hour before closing, Plac Solidarności 1, tel. 506-195-673, www.ecs.gda.pl.

❷ Self-Guided Tour: First, appreciate the architecture of the **building** itself. From the outside, it's designed to resemble the rusted hull of a giant ship—seemingly gloomy and depressing. But step inside to find an interior flooded with light, which cultivates a surprising variety of life—in the form of lush gardens that make the place feel like a very expensive greenhouse. You can interpret this symbolism a number of ways: Something that seems dull and dreary from the outside (the Soviet Bloc, the shipyards themselves, what have you) can be full of brightness, life, and optimism inside.

In the lobby, buy your ticket and pick up the essential, included audioguide. The exhibit has much to see, and some of it is arranged in a conceptual way that can be tricky to understand without a full grasp of the history. I've outlined the basics in this

self-guided tour, but the audioguide can illuminate more details—
including translations of films and eyewitness testimony from participants in the history.

• *The permanent exhibit fills seven lettered rooms—each with its own
theme—on two floors. From the lush lobby, head up the escalator and
into...*

The Birth of Solidarity (Room A): This room picks up right
in the middle of the dynamic story we just learned out on the
square. It's August of 1980, and the shipyard workers are rising
up. You step straight into a busy shipyard: punch clocks, workers'
lockers, and—up on the ceiling—hundreds of plastic helmets. A
big **map** in the middle of the room shows the extent of the shipyard in 1980. Inside the cab of the **crane**, you can watch an inter-
view with spunky Anna Walentynowicz, whose firing led to the
first round of strikes. Nearby stands a **truck**; Lech Wałęsa would
stand on top of the cab of a truck like this one to address the nervous locals who had amassed outside the shipyard gate, awaiting
further news.

In the middle of the room, carefully protected under glass, are
those original **plywood panels** onto which the strikers scrawled
their 21 demands, then lashed to the gate. Just beyond that, a giant
wall of photos and a map illustrate how the strikes that began
here spread like a virus across Poland. At the far end of the room,
behind the partition, stand **two tables** that were used during the
talks to end the strikes (each one with several actual items from
that era, under glass).

After 18 days of protests, the communist authorities finally
agreed to negotiate. On the afternoon of August 31, 1980,
the Governmental Commission and the Inter-Factory Strike
Committee (MKS) came together and signed the August
Agreements, which legalized Solidarity—the first time any communist government permitted a workers' union. As Lech Wałęsa
sat at a big table and signed the agreement, other union reps tape-
recorded the proceedings and played them later at their own factories to prove that the unthinkable had happened. Take a moment
to linger over the rousing **film** that plays on the far wall, which
begins with the strike, carries through with the tense negotiations that a brash young Lech Wałęsa held with the authorities,
and ends with the triumphant acceptance of the strikers' demands.
Lech Wałęsa rides on the shoulders of well-wishers out to the gate
to spread the good news.

• *Back by the original 21 demands, enter the next exhibit...*

The Power of the Powerless (Room B): This section traces
the roots of the 1980 strikes, which were preceded by several far
less successful protests. It all begins with a kiss: a giant photograph of Russian premier Leonid Brezhnev mouth-kissing the

Polish premier Edward Gierek, with the caption **"Brotherly Friendship."** Soviet premiers and their satellite leaders really did greet each other "in the French manner," as a symbolic gesture of their communist brotherhood.

Working your way through the exhibit, you'll see the door to a **prison cell**—a reminder of the intimidation tactics used by the Soviets in the 1940s and 50s to deal with their opponents as they exerted their rule over the lands they had liberated from the Nazis.

The typical **communist-era apartment** is painfully humble. After the war, much of Poland had been destroyed, and population shifts led to housing shortages. People had to make do with tiny space and ramshackle furnishings. Communist propaganda blares from both the radio and the TV.

A map shows **"red Europe"** (the USSR plus the satellites of Poland, Czechoslovakia, Hungary, and East Germany), and a **timeline** traces some of the smaller Soviet Bloc protests that led up to Solidarity: in East Germany in 1953, in Budapest and Poznań in 1956, the "Prague Spring" of 1968, and other 1968 protests in Poland.

In the wake of these uprisings, the communist authorities cracked down even harder. Peek into the **interrogation room,** with a wall of file cabinets and a lowly stool illuminated by a bright spotlight. (Notice that the white Polish eagle on the seal above the desk is missing its golden crown—during communism, the Poles were allowed to keep the eagle, but its crown was removed.)

The next exhibit presents a day-by-day rundown of the **1970 strikes,** from December 14 to 22, which resulted in the massacre of the workers who are honored by the monument in front of this building. A wall of mug shots gives way to exhibits chronicling the steady rise of dissent groups through the 1970s, culminating in the June 1976 protests in the city of Radom (prompted, like so many other uprisings, by unilateral price hikes).

• *Loop back through Room A, and proceed straight ahead into...*

Solidarity and Hope (Room C): While the government didn't take the August Agreements very seriously, the Poles did...and before long, 10 million of them—one out of every four, or effectively half of the nation's workforce—joined Solidarity. So began what's often called the **"16 Months of Hope."** Newly legal, Solidarity continued to stage strikes and make its opposition known. Slick Solidarity posters and children's art convey the childlike enthusiasm with which the Poles seized their hard-won kernels of freedom. The communist authorities' hold on the Polish people began to slip. Support and aid from the outside world poured in, but the rest of the Soviet Bloc looked on nervously, and the Warsaw Pact army assembled at the Polish border and glared at the uprisers. The threat of invasion hung heavy in the air.

• *Exiting this room, head up the staircase and into...*

At War with Society (Room D): You're greeted by a wall of TV screens delivering a stern message. On Sunday morning, December 13, 1981, the Polish head of state, **General Wojciech Jaruzelski**—wearing his trademark dark glasses—appeared on national TV and announced the introduction of **martial law.** Solidarity was outlawed, and its leaders were arrested. Frightened Poles heard the announcement and looked out their windows to see Polish Army tanks rumbling through the snowy streets. (On the opposite wall, see footage of tanks and heavily armed soldiers intimidating their countrymen into compliance.) Jaruzelski claimed that he imposed martial law to prevent the Soviets from invading. Today, many historians question whether martial law was really necessary—though Jaruzelski remained unremorseful through his death in 2014.

Continuing deeper into the exhibit, you come to a **prisoner transport.** Climb up inside to watch chilling scenes of riots, demonstrations, and crackdowns by the ZOMO riot police. In one gruesome scene, a demonstrator is quite intentionally—and practically in slow motion—run over by a truck. From here, pass through a gauntlet of *milicja* riot-gear shields to see the truck crashing through a gate. Overhead are the uniforms of miners from the **Wujek mine** who were massacred on December 16, 1981 (their names are projected on the pile of coal below).

Martial law was a tragic, terrifying, and bleak time for the Polish people. It didn't, however, kill the Solidarity movement, which continued its fight after going underground. Passing prison cells, you'll see a wall plastered with handmade, underground posters and graffiti. Notice how in this era, **Solidarity propaganda** is much more primitive; circle around the other side of the wall to see several presses that were actually used in clandestine Solidarity print shops during this time. The outside world sent messages of support as well as supplies—represented by the big wall of cardboard boxes. This approval also came in the form of a Nobel Peace Prize for Lech Wałęsa in 1983; you'll see video clips of his wife accepting the award on his behalf (Wałęsa feared that if he traveled abroad to claim it, he would not be allowed back into the country).

• *But even in these darkest days, there were glimmers of hope. Enter...*

The Road to Democracy (Room E): By the time the pope visited his homeland again in 1983, martial law had finally been lifted, and Solidarity—still technically illegal—was gaining momentum, gradually pecking away at the communists. Step into the small inner room with footage of the **pope's third pilgrimage** to his homeland, in 1987—by which time (thanks in no small part to his inspirational role in the ongoing revolution) the tide was turning.

Step into the room with the big, white **roundtable.** With the moral support of the pope and the entire Western world, the brave Poles were the first European country to throw off the shackles of communism when, in the spring of 1989, the "Roundtable Talks" led to the opening up of elections. (If you look through the view-finders of the TV cameras in the corners, you'll see footage of those meetings.) The government arrogantly called for parliamentary elections, reserving 65 percent of seats for themselves.

In the next room, you can see Solidarity's strategy in those **elections:** On the right wall are posters showing Lech Wałęsa with each of the candidates. Another popular "get out the vote" measure was the huge poster of Gary Cooper—an icon of America, which the Poles deeply respect and viewed as their friendly cousin across the Atlantic—except that, instead of a pistol, he's packing a ballot. Rousing reminders like this inspired huge voter turnout. The communists' plan backfired, as virtually every open seat went to Solidarity. It was the first time ever that opposition candidates had taken office in the Soviet Bloc. On the wall straight ahead, flashing a V-for-*wiktoria* sign, is a huge photo of Tadeusz Mazowiecki—an early leader of Solidarity, who became prime minister on June 4, 1989.

• *For the glorious aftermath, head into the final room.*

The Triumph of Freedom (Room F): This room is dominated by a gigantic **map of Eastern Europe.** A countdown clock on the right ticks off the departure of each one from communist clutches, as the Soviet Bloc "decomposes." You'll see how the success of Solidarity in Poland—and the ragtag determination of a scruffy band of shipyard workers right here in Gdańsk—inspired people all over Eastern Europe. By the winter of 1989, the Hungarians had opened their borders, the Berlin Wall had crumbled, and the Czechs and Slovaks had staged their Velvet Revolution. (Small viewing stations that circle the room reveal the detailed story for each country's own road to freedom.) Lech Wałęsa—the ship-yard electrician who started it all by jumping over a wall—became the first president of post-communist Poland. And a year later, in Poland's first true elections since World War II, 29 different parties won seats in the parliament. It was a free-election free-for-all.

In the middle of the room stands a white wall with **inspirational quotes** from St. John Paul II and Václav Havel—the Czech poet-turned-protester-turned-prisoner-turned-president—which are repeated in several languages. On the huge wall, the **Solidarity "graffiti"** is actually made up of thousands of little notes left behind by visitors to the museum. Feel free to grab a piece of paper and a pen and record your own reflections.

• *Finally, head downstairs and find the...*

John Paul II Room (Room G): Many visitors find that

touring this museum—with vivid reminders of a dramatic and pivotal moment in history that took place in our own lifetimes, which was brought about not by armies or presidents, but by everyday people—puts them in an emotional state of mind. Designed for silent reflection, this room overlooks the monument to those workers who were gunned down in 1970.

Shopping in Gdańsk

The big story in Gdańsk is amber *(bursztyn)*, a fossil resin available in all shades, shapes, and sizes (see the "All About Amber" sidebar, earlier). While you'll see amber sold all over town, the best place to browse and buy is along the atmospheric ulica Mariacka (between the Motława River and St. Mary's Church). This pretty street, with old-fashioned balconies and dozens of display cases, is fun to wander even if you're not a shopper. Other good places to buy amber are along the riverfront embankment and on ulica Długa. To avoid rip-offs—such as amber that's been melted and reshaped—always buy it from a shop, not from someone standing on the street. (But note that most shops also have a display case and salesperson out front, which are perfectly legit.) Prices everywhere are about the same, so rather than seeking out a specific place, just window-shop until you see what you want. Styles range from gaudy necklaces with huge globs of amber, to tasteful smaller pendants in silver settings, to cheap trinkets. All shades of amber—from near-white to dark brown—cost about the same, but you'll pay more for inclusions (bugs or other objects stuck in the amber).

Gdańsk also has several modern shopping malls, most of them in the Old Town or near the main train station. The walk between the Main Town and the Solidarity shipyard goes past some of the best malls (see page 535).

Eating in Gdańsk

In addition to traditional Polish fare, Gdańsk has some fine Baltic seafood. Herring *(śledź)* is popular here, as is cod *(dorsz)*. Natives brag that their salmon *(łosoś)* is better than Norway's. For a stiff drink, sample *Goldwasser* (similar to Goldschlager). This sweet and strong liqueur, flecked with actual gold, was supposedly invented here in Gdańsk. The following options are all in the Main Town, within three blocks of the Royal Way.

BUDGET RESTAURANTS IN THE CITY CENTER
These places are affordable, tasty, quick, and wonderfully convenient—on or very near the Royal Way (ulica Długa). They're worth considering even if you're not on a tight budget.

Bar pod Rybą ("Under the Fish") is nirvana for fans of baked potatoes *(pieczony ziemniak)*. They offer more than 20 variet- ies, piled high with a wide variety of toppings and sauces, from Mexican beef to herring to Polish cheeses. They also serve fish dishes with salad and potatoes, making this a cheap place to sam- ple local seafood. The tasteful decor—walls lined with old bottles, antique wooden hangers, and old street signs—is squeezed into a single cozy room packed with happy eaters. In the summer, order inside, and they'll bring your food to you at an outdoor table (pota- toes and fish dishes are each about 20-30 zł, daily 10:00-22:00, ulica Piwna 61, tel. 58-305-1307).

Bar Mleczny Neptun is your handiest milk-bar (communist- style budget cafeteria) option in the Main Town. A hearty meal of traditional Polish fare, including a drink, runs about 15-20 zł. This popular place has more charm than your typical institutional milk bar, including outdoor seating along the most scenic stretch of the main drag, and an upstairs dining room overlooking it all. The items on the counter are for display—point to what you want and they'll dish it up fresh (Mon-Fri 7:30-19:30, Sat-Sun 10:00-19:00, may have shorter hours off-season, free Wi-Fi, ulica Długa 33, tel. 58-301-4988).

Pijalnia Wódki i Piwa, part of a popular Polish chain, hides half a block behind the Hard Rock Café (on Kuśnierska). This lit- tle vodka-and-herring bar takes you back to the 1970s. Pop in to study the retro decor—ads from the 1970s and photos of the lines people routinely endured. The place is literally wallpapered with pages from the "Tribune of the Masses" newspaper infamous for its propaganda that passed for news. They play pop hits from the last years of communism. The menu is fun, accessible, and simple: 4 zł for vodka or other drinks, and 8 zł for herring or other bar nibbles (open daily 9:00-late).

Bar Turystyczny is misnamed—while it seems to harbor the illusion that it's for tourists, it has become beloved by locals as the central area's favorite milk bar. Easy to miss on the way between the Main Town and the Solidarity sights, it's always jammed (9-13-zł main dishes, Mon-Fri 8:00-18:00, Sat-Sun 9:00-17:00, Szeroka 8, tel. 58/301-6013).

ON THE RIVERFRONT EMBANKMENT

Perhaps the most appeal- ing dining zone in Gdańsk stretches along the riverfront embankment near the Crane. While these restaurants are mostly interchangeable, I've

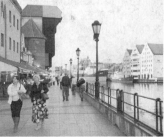

listed a few to consider, in the order you'll reach them as you walk north along the embankment.

Baryłka ("Barrel") is a simpler, more affordable alternative to some of the pricier places along here. While the outdoor seating is enticing, the elegant upstairs dining room, with windows overlooking the river, is also appealing (35-45-zł main dishes, daily 9:00-24:00, Długie Pobrzeże 24, tel. 58-301-4938).

Kamienica Goldwasser offers high-quality Polish and international cuisine. Choose between cozy, romantic indoor seating on several levels, or scenic outdoor seating (most main dishes 60-75 zł, daily 10:00-24:00, occasional live music, Długie Pobrzeże 22, tel. 58-301-8878).

Sushi 77, serving up a wide selection of surprisingly good sushi right next to the Crane, is a refreshing break from ye olde Polish food. Choose between the outdoor tables bathed in red light, or the mod interior (30-50-zł sushi sets, daily 12:00-23:00, Długie Pobrzeże 30, tel. 58-682-1823).

Past the Crane

About 100 yards past the Crane, near the old fish market (Targ Rybny), cluster several more options.

Lao Thai is a modern space right along the embankment selling surprisingly high-quality, yet still affordable, Thai cuisine (35-50-zł dishes, daily 12:00-22:00, ulica Targ Rybny 11, tel. 58/305-2525).

Targ Rybny/Fishmarkt ("The Fish Market") has less appealing outdoor seating that overlooks a park and parking lot. But the warm, mellow-yellow nautical ambience inside is pleasant, making this a good bad-weather option. It features classy but not stuffy service, with an emphasis on fish (most main dishes 40-55 zł, plus pricier seafood splurges, daily 10:00-23:00, ulica Targ Rybny 6C, tel. 58-320-9011).

Restauracja Kubicki, along the water just past the Hilton, has a long history (since 1918), but a recent remodel has kept the atmosphere—and its food—feeling fresh. This is a good choice for high-quality Polish and international food in a fun, sophisticated-but-not-stuffy interior that's a clever mix of old and new elements (30-55-zł main dishes, daily 12:00-23:00, Wartka 5, tel. 58-301-0050).

Sopot

Sopot (SOH-poht), dubbed the "Nice of the North," was a celebrated haunt of beautiful people during the 1920s and 1930s, and

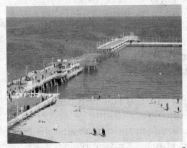

remains a popular beach getaway to this day.

Sopot was created in the late 19th century by Napoleon's doctor, Jean Georges Haffner, who believed Baltic Sea water to be therapeutic. By the 1890s, it had become a fashionable seaside resort. This gambling center boasted enough high-roller casinos to garner comparisons to Monte Carlo.

The casinos are gone, but the health resorts remain, and you'll still see more well-dressed people here per capita than just about anywhere in the country. While it's not quite Cannes, Sopot feels relatively high class, which is unusual in otherwise unpretentious Poland. But even so, a childlike spirit of summer-vacation fun pervades this St-Tropez-on-the-Baltic, making it an all-around enjoyable resort.

Cruisers see Sopot as a handy, pleasant place to kill time on their way back to their cruise ship in Gdynia. As it's halfway between Gdynia and Gdańsk, right on the train line, this is an easy stopover.

Orientation to Sopot

The main pedestrian drag, Monte Cassino Heroes street (ulica Bohaterów Monte Cassino), leads to the Molo, the longest pleasure pier in Europe. From the Molo, a broad, sandy beach stretches in each direction. Running parallel to the surf is a tree-lined, people-filled path made for strolling.

Tourist Information: Sopot's helpful TI is near the base of the Molo at Plac Zdrojowy 2 (look for blue *it* sign). Pick up the free map, info booklet, and events schedule (daily June-mid-Sept 9:00-20:00, mid-Sept-May 10:00-18:00, ulica Dworcowa 4, tel. 58-550-3783, www.sopot.pl).

Arrival in Sopot: From the SKM station, exit to the left and walk down the street. After a block, you'll see the PKP train station on your left. Continue on to the can't-miss-it main drag, ulica Bohaterów Monte Cassino (marked by the big red-brick church steeple). Follow it to the right, down to the seaside.

Sights in Sopot

▲Monte Cassino Heroes Street
(Ulica Bohaterów Monte Cassino)

Nicknamed "Monciak" (MOHN-chak) by locals, this in-love-with-life promenade may well be Poland's most manicured street (and is named in honor of the Polish soldiers who helped the Allies pry Italy's Monte Cassino monastery from Nazi forces during World War II). Especially after all the suburban and industrial dreck you passed through to get here, it's easy to be charmed by this pretty drag. The street is lined with happy tourists, trendy cafés, al fresco restaurants, movie theaters, and late-19th-century facades (known for their wooden balconies).

The most popular building along here (on the left, about halfway down) is the so-called **Crooked House** (Krzywy Domek), a trippy, Gaudí-inspired building that looks like it's melting. Hard-partying Poles prefer to call it the "Drunken House," and say that when it looks straight, it's time to stop drinking.

Molo (Pier)

At more than 1,600 feet long, this is Europe's longest wooden entertainment pier. While you won't find any amusement-park rides, you will be surrounded by vendors, artists, and Poles having the time of their lives. Buy a *gofry* (Belgian waffle topped with whipped cream and fruit) or an oversized cloud of *wata cukrowa* (cotton candy), grab your partner's hand, and stroll with gusto (7.50 zł, free Oct-April, open long hours daily, www.molo.sopot.pl).

Climb to the top of the Art Nouveau lighthouse for a waterfront panorama. Scan the horizon for sailboats and tankers. Any pirate ships? For a jarring reality check, look over to Gdańsk. Barely visible from the Molo are two of the most important sites in 20th-century history: the towering monument at Westerplatte, where World War II started, and the cranes rising up from the Gdańsk Shipyard, where Solidarity was born and European communism began its long goodbye.

In spring and fall, the Molo is a favorite venue for pole vaulting—or is that Pole vaulting?

The Beach

Yes, Poland has beaches. Nice ones. When I heard Sopot compared to places like Nice, I'll admit that I scoffed. But when I saw those stretches of inviting sand as far as the eye can see, I wished I'd packed my swim trunks. (You could walk from Gdańsk to Gdynia on beaches like this.) The sand is finer than anything I've seen in Croatia...though the water's not exactly crystal-clear. Most of the beach is public, except for a small private stretch in front of the Grand Hotel Sopot. Year-round, it's crammed with locals.

What If I Miss My Boat?

Remember that you can get help from the cruise line's port agent (listed on the destination information sheet distributed on the ship) and the local TI (see page 517). If the port agent suggests a costly solution (such as a private car with a driver), you may want to consider public transit.

Most train connections—including **Warnemünde,** Copenhagen, Amsterdam, and beyond—are via Berlin (4/day, 7-7.5 hours, transfer in Szczecin or Poznań). To research train schedules, see www.bahn.com. Overland connections to **Rīga** and **Tallinn** are time-consuming; for these and other points north and east, flying may be your best choice. Gdańsk's **Lech Wałęsa Airport** is well-connected to downtown by public bus #210, shuttle van, or taxi (tel. 58-348-1163, www.airport. gdansk.pl).

Local **travel agents** in Gdańsk can help you. For more advice on what to do if you miss the boat, see page 139.

At these northern latitudes, the season for bathing is brief and crowded.

Overlooking the beach next to the Molo is the **Grand Hotel Sopot.** It was renovated to top-class status recently, but its history goes way back. They could charge admission for room #226, a multiroom suite that has hosted the likes of Adolf Hitler, Marlene Dietrich, and Fidel Castro (but not all at the same time). With all the trappings of Sopot's belle époque—dark wood, plush upholstery, antique furniture—this room had me imagining Hitler sitting at the desk, looking out to sea, and plotting the course of World War II.

Polish Survival Phrases

Keep in mind a few Polish pronunciation tips: **w** sounds like "v," **ł** sounds like "w," **ch** is a back-of-your-throat "kh" sound (as in the Scottish "loch"), and **rz** sounds like the "zh" sound in "pleasure." The vowels with a tail (**ą** and **ę**) have a slight nasal "n" sound at the end, similar to French.

English	Polish	Pronunciation
Hello. (formal)	Dzień dobry.	jehn **doh**-brih
Hi. / Bye. (informal)	Cześć.	cheshch
Do you speak English? (asked of a man)	Czy Pan mówi po angielsku?	chih pahn **moo**-vee poh ahn-**gyehl**-skoo
Do you speak English? (asked of a woman)	Czy Pani mówi po angielsku?	chih **pah**-nee **moo**-vee poh ahn-**gyehl**-skoo
Yes. / No.	Tak. / Nie.	tahk / nyeh
I (don't) understand.	(Nie) rozumiem.	(nyeh) roh-**zoo**-myehm
Please. / You're welcome. / Can I help you?	Proszę.	**proh**-sheh
Thank you (very much).	Dziękuję (bardzo).	jehn-**koo**-yeh (**bard**-zoh)
Excuse me. / I'm sorry.	Przepraszam.	psheh-**prah**-shahm
(No) problem.	(Żaden) problem.	(**zhah**-dehn) **proh**-blehm
Good.	Dobrze.	**dohb**-zheh
Goodbye.	Do widzenia.	doh veed-**zay**-nyah
one / two / three	jeden / dwa / trzy	**yeh**-dehn / dvah / tzhih
four / five / six	cztery / pięć / sześć	**chteh**-rih / pyench / sheshch
seven / eight	siedem / osiem	**shyeh**-dehm / **oh**-shehm
nine / ten	dziewięć / dziesięć	**jeh**-vyench / **jeh**-shench
hundred / thousand	sto / tysiąc	stoh / **tih**-shants
How much?	Ile?	**ee**-leh
local currency	złoty (zł)	**zwoh**-tih
Write it.	Napisz to.	**nah**-peesh toh
Is it free?	Czy to jest za darmo?	chih toh yehst zah **dar**-moh
Is it included?	Czy jest to wliczone?	chih yehst toh vlee-**choh**-neh
Where can I find / buy...?	Gdzie mogę dostać / kupić...?	guh-**dyeh moh**-geh **doh**-statch / **koo**-peech
I'd like... (said by a man)	Chciałbym...	**khchaw**-beem
I'd like... (said by a woman)	Chciałabym...	**khchah**-wah-beem
We'd like...	Chcielibyśmy...	**khchehl**-ee-bish-mih
...a room.	...pokój.	**poh**-kooey
...a ticket to ___.	...bilet do ___.	**bee**-leht doh ___
Is it possible?	Czy jest to możliwe?	chih yehst toh mohzh-**lee**-veh
Where is...?	Gdzie jest...?	guh-**dyeh** yehst
...the train station	...dworzec kolejowy	**dvoh**-zhehts koh-leh-**yoh**-vih
...the bus station	...dworzec autobusowy	**dvoh**-zhehts ow-toh-boos-**oh**-vih
...the tourist information office	...informacja turystyczna	een-for-**maht**-syah too-ris-**titch**-nah
...the toilet	...toaleta	toh-ah-**leh**-tah
men / women	męska / damska	**mehn**-skah / **dahm**-skah
left / right / straight	lewo / prawo / prosto	**leh**-voh / **prah**-voh / **proh**-stoh
At what time...?	O której godzinie...?	oh kuh-**too**-ray gohd-**zhee**-nyeh
...does this open / close	...będzie otwarte / zamknięte	**bend**-zheh oht-**vahr**-teh / zahm-**knyehn**-teh
Just a moment.	Chwileczkę.	khvee-**letch**-keh
now / soon / later	eraz / niedługo / później	**teh**-rahz / nyed-**woo**-goh / **poozh**-nyey
today / tomorrow	dzisiaj / jutro	**jee**-shigh / **yoo**-troh

BERLIN
Germany

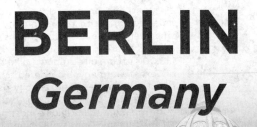

Germany Practicalities

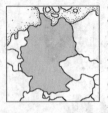

Germany (Deutschland) is energetic, efficient, and organized. It's Europe's muscleman, both economically and wherever people line up (Germans have a reputation for pushing ahead). At 138,000 square miles (about half the size of Texas), Germany is bordered by nine countries. The terrain gradually rises—from the flat lands of the north to the rugged Alps in the south. The European Union's most populous country and biggest economy, Germany is home to 82 million people—one-third Catholic and one-third Protestant. Germany is young compared with most of its European neighbors ("born" in 1871) but was a founding member of the EU. Germany's geographic diversity and cultural richness draw millions of visitors every year. While it's easy to fixate on the eerie Nazi remnants and chilling reminders of the Cold War, don't overlook Germany's lively squares, fine people zones, and many high-powered sights.

Money: 1 euro (€) = about $1.10. An ATM is called a *Geldautomat*. The local VAT (value-added sales tax) rate is 19 percent; the minimum purchase eligible for a VAT refund is €25 (for details on refunds, see page 134).

Language: The native language is German. For useful phrases, see page 640.

Emergencies: Dial 112 for police, medical, or other emergencies. In case of theft or loss, see page 125.

Time Zone: Germany is on Central European Time (the same as most of the Continent, one hour ahead of Great Britain, and six/nine hours ahead of the East/West Coasts of the US).

Embassies in Berlin: The **US embassy** is at Pariser Platz 2, tel. 030/83050; consular services at Clayallee 170 (tel. 030/8305-1200—consular calls answered Mon-Thu 14:00-16:00 only, germany.usembassy.gov). The **Canadian embassy** is at Leipziger Platz 17 (tel. 030/203-120, www.germany.gc.ca). Call ahead for passport services.

Phoning: Germany's country code is 49; to call from another country to Germany, dial the international access code (011 from the US/Canada, 00 from Europe, or + from a mobile phone), then 49, followed by the area code (without initial zero) and the local number. For calls within Germany, dial just the number if you are calling locally, and add the area code if calling long distance. To place an international call from Germany, dial 00, the code of the country you're calling (1 for US and Canada), and the phone number. For more tips, see page 1146.

Tipping: A gratuity is included in your bill at sit-down meals, so you don't need to tip further, but it's nice to round up your bill about 10 percent for great service. Tip a taxi driver by rounding up the fare a bit (pay €3 on an €2.85 fare). For more tips on tipping, see page 138.

Tourist Information: www.germany.travel

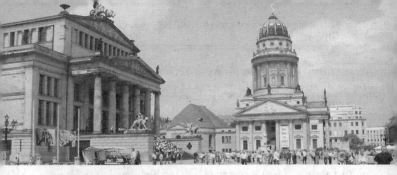

BERLIN
and the PORT of WARNEMÜNDE

Warnemünde • Rostock • Berlin

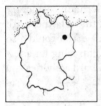

Berlin—Germany's historic and reunited capital—is one of Europe's great cities, and certainly deserves a place on any itinerary. But cruise ships visiting landlocked Berlin actually put in at the port town of Warnemünde (VAHR-neh-mewn-deh), three hours by train or bus to the north. At 150 miles from downtown Berlin, Warnemünde decisively wins the prize for "longest journey time from port." Even if you have a generous 12 to 14 hours in port (as many cruises do here), a visit to Berlin means you'll spend almost as much time in transit as you will in Berlin itself. This leads cruisers to the unavoidable question: To Berlin or not to Berlin?

This chapter covers detailed directions for getting from Warnemünde's cruise port to Berlin, and tips on how to spend your limited time in the city. But for those who don't want to make the trek, I've also suggested ideas for how to spend a day in Warnemünde and the neighboring city of Rostock.

TO BERLIN OR NOT TO BERLIN?
Your first decision is whether to make the long trip to the German capital. Make no mistake: By train, by tour bus, or by Porsche on the Autobahn, plan on at least three hours of travel time each way between your cruise ship at Warnemünde and Berlin—plus time spent sightseeing in Berlin and waiting for train connections.

Fortunately, Warnemünde's train station, which has some direct connections to Berlin, is a simple 5- to 10-minute walk from your ship. (Most trains from Warnemünde require an easy change in Rostock.) At www.bahn.com, you can check the times for trains from Warnemünde to "Berlin Hbf" (Hauptbahnhof, the city's main station) on the date you'll arrive, and look for return trains that will give you plenty of time to make the all-aboard. This will give you a realistic sense of how much time you would have in Berlin. A "Berlin On Your Own" cruise excursion, while more expensive than the train, may suit your schedule better and help you avoid the stress of train connections.

If you'd rather not make the trip, you can stick around the Warnemünde/Rostock area. Both towns were part of the communist former East Germany (DDR), which has left them with some less-than-charming architecture. But today **Warnemünde** is a fun, borderline-tacky seafront resort, with a vast sandy beach and a pretty harbor lined with low-impact diversions. And parts of the nearby city of **Rostock** (a 20-minute train ride away) verge on quaint—it has a fine old church, some museums, and a pedestrian core lined with shops and eateries that cater more to locals than to tourists.

Neither Warnemünde nor Rostock would be worth a special trip if you were putting together a "best of Germany" itinerary by train or car. But for a cruiser who doesn't want to bother with Berlin, I can think of worse places to spend a day. You could also treat this as a "half-day at sea"—enjoy nearby sightseeing for a few hours, then retreat to your ship for whatever onboard activities you haven't gotten around to yet.

PLANNING YOUR TIME
In Berlin

Remember, it takes at least six hours round-trip to go to and from Berlin. That likely leaves you with five or six hours in the city. Arriving by train at the Hauptbahnhof (Berlin's main train station), here's what I'd do:

• **Best of Berlin Walk:** This self-guided walk links the **Reichstag** and **Brandenburg Gate** with sights along **Unter den Linden** to **Alexanderplatz.** From the Hauptbahnhof, ride the U-Bahn or walk about 15 minutes (past grand governmental buildings) to the Reichstag. Ogle the exterior (or, if you've made reservations, ascend the dome—see page 595), then see the Brandenburg Gate, pause at the Memorial to the Murdered Jews of Europe, and follow my self-guided walk up Unter den Linden (considering a detour partway along to the Checkpoint Charlie Museum—see next). Allow 1.5 hours without stops, or—better—up to 3 hours if you fit in a few sights en route. The pleasant square called Gendarmenmarkt is worth the easy five-minute detour south of Unter den Linden (and is on the way to the 20th-century sights mentioned next).

From this sightseeing spine, you'll have to be selective. These are your top options:

• **Museum of the Wall at Checkpoint Charlie, Stretch of**

Wall, and Topography of Terror: If you're interested in Berlin's turbulent 20th-century history, consider detouring a few blocks south of Unter den Linden to this little pocket of sights. Allow an hour for the Checkpoint Charlie Museum, and another hour-plus for the surviving stretch of the Berlin Wall, Topography of Terror, and DDR Watchtower—history buffs should budget even more time.

• **Art Museums:** If you're primarily interested in art, consider spending some of your day at Museum Island (especially the Pergamon Museum, for ancient items—allow 1-2 hours, though note parts may be closed for renovation; and the Neues Museum, to see the bust of Nefertiti—allow 1 hour), or at the Kulturforum (the top museum here is the Gemäldegalerie, with Old Masters—allow 2 hours). These two museum zones are in different parts of town—ideally, choose one or the other.

• **Other Museums on Unter den Linden:** If you're staying on the Reichstag/Brandenburg Gate/Unter den Linden sightseeing spine outlined earlier, you may want to choose additional museums that are on the way. These include Museum Island (several branches, described earlier); the excellent German History Museum (allow at least 1 hour, likely more); or the quirky DDR Museum, for a look at communist-era East Germany (allow 1 hour).

• **Additional Sights in Berlin:** If you have a special interest, consider the Jewish Museum Berlin (allow 1-2 hours) or the Berlin Wall Memorial (allow 1.5 hours). Be aware that because they're not right along Unter den Linden, they'll eat up more transit time. If you're more interested in Berlin's thriving hipster street scene than in museums and history, you could stroll through Prenzlauer Berg (wander north from the Hackescher Markt S-Bahn station). On a very short visit, I'd skip western Berlin sights.

Don't be too ambitious. You'll have time for the Best of Berlin Walk and possibly one of the items listed above (two if you're quick). The key in Berlin is being selective—read my descriptions on the train ride in, make your choices, then hit the ground running.

In Warnemünde and Rostock

If the weather is nice, you could head to the beach in Warnemünde right away; otherwise, take the train to Rostock, see that town, then return to Warnemünde for an afternoon at the beach.

For a quick, targeted visit to Rostock, ride the tram to the Neuer Markt in the Old Town (allow 15 minutes or less), tour St. Mary's Church (allow 30 minutes), walk to University Square and poke around (allow 30 minutes), and consider visiting various museums and churches (none takes more than 30 minutes). On the way back to the station, history buffs will want to visit the Stasi

Documentation Center and Memorial (allow about one hour). All told, three or four hours are plenty to get a good taste of Rostock.

The Port of Warnemünde

Arrival at a Glance: Walk (5-10 minutes) to the train station to catch a train to Berlin (3 hours one-way, usually requires change in Rostock, infrequent—check schedules) or to Rostock (20 minutes, departures every 10 minutes). To stay in Warnemünde, you can walk to the beach and town center in 15-20 minutes. To reach Berlin, you can also spring for an "On Your Own" shuttle-bus excursion through your cruise line (more direct and reliable than the train, and generally only a bit more expensive).

Port Overview

Warnemünde is a pleasant former fishing town/seaside resort, situated at the mouth of the Warnow River. Though its port sprawls over a wide area, cruise ships put in at the most convenient location possible—a long pier immediately next to the train station and a short walk from the heart of town. Two main piers feed into empty-feeling terminal buildings.

Tourist Information: A small TI desk is in Pier 7 by Karl's. And the main branch of the TI is about a 10-minute walk away—just past the train station and Alter Strom canal (walking directions later). They hand out free maps and brochures about Warnemünde and Rostock, and try to convince cruisers to remain in the area instead of making the long trip into Berlin (TI open May-Oct Mon-Fri 9:00-18:00, Sat-Sun 10:00-15:00; Nov-April Mon-Fri 10:00-17:00, Sat 10:00-15:00, closed Sun; Am Strom 59, enter around the corner on Kirchenstrasse, tel. 0381/548-000, www.rostock.de).

Alternate Port: On the relatively rare occasions that Warnemünde's main cruise port is full, cruise ships put in across the river and harbor area, at the **Rostock passenger ferry terminal (Fährterminal).** From here, there's no direct connection into Warnemünde, but you're about halfway to Rostock; walk about 10 minutes to the suburban railway (S-Bahn) station called Seehafen, and ride the train into Rostock. Some cruise lines also provide a shuttle bus from this terminal into Rostock. From Rostock, you can connect to Berlin or to Warnemünde.

GETTING INTO TOWN

It's a very short stroll to the train station (with connections to Rostock or Berlin), and just a bit farther to Warnemünde's town center, TI, lone museum, and beach. Taxis aren't necessary in

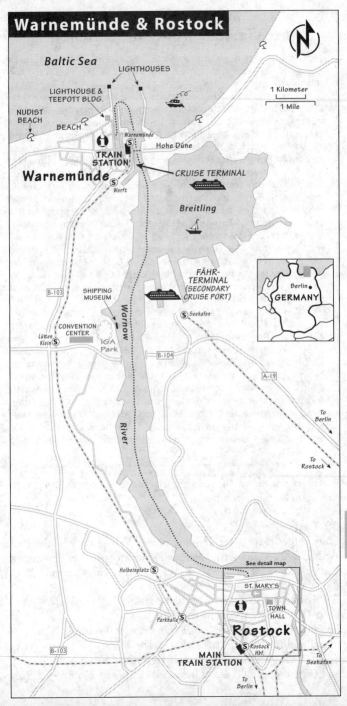

Warnemünde & Rostock

Baltic Sea

LIGHTHOUSES

LIGHTHOUSE & TEEPOTT BLDG.

NUDIST BEACH

BEACH

Warnemünde

Warnemünde

TRAIN STATION

Hohe Düne

CRUISE TERMINAL

Werft

Breitling

FÄHR-TERMINAL (SECONDARY CRUISE PORT)

Seehafen

B-103

SHIPPING MUSEUM

CONVENTION CENTER

Lütten Klein

IGA Park

Warnow

B-104

A-19

To Berlin

To Rostock

River

1 Kilometer

1 Mile

Berlin

GERMANY

BERLIN

See detail map

Holbeinplatz

ST. MARY'S

TOWN HALL

Rostock

Parkhalle

Rostock Hbf.

B-103

MAIN TRAIN STATION

To Seehafen

To Berlin

Excursions from Warnemünde

Most cruisers arriving in Warnemünde head into **Berlin** (3 hours each way by tour bus; some cruise lines charter a train for the journey).

For maximum freedom, consider a **Berlin On Your Own**-type excursion, which is simply a round-trip bus transfer to a central point in the city (often Gendarmenmarkt, just south of Unter den Linden). At around $150-200, this costs more than the round-trip train fare (around $115-135), but it saves you the stress of coordinating train schedules to get there and back in time.

For about double the price ($300-350), most cruise lines offer an **all-day trip** that includes transportation, a narrated bus ride around Berlin, and photo-op stops at major landmarks (these may include the Reichstag, Brandenburg Gate, Memorial to the Murdered Jews of Europe, Checkpoint Charlie, Gendarmenmarkt, Bebelplatz, or Potsdamer Platz—all of which are well worth seeing). Some tours also include more in-depth sightseeing stops at a sight or two and/or time on your own before returning to the ship. After transit time, if you have roughly six hours in Berlin, a two- to three-hour bus tour combined with about three hours of free time is a good day.

Carefully note which sights are included in your excursion. For example, cruisers interested in antiquities may appreciate a tour of the **Pergamon,** one of Europe's best museums for ancient sculpture. A **boat trip** on the Spree River through downtown Berlin provides a fine orientation to the city center. Some sights, however, are a waste of your time. **Charlottenburg Palace,** while pretty, ranks low on the list of European castles; it may be worth a drive-by, but its interior does not merit your precious time. And, while the distantly located **Allied Museum** tells the fascinating story of the early days of the Cold War here, I'd much rather spend an hour walking the streets where that history happened

Warnemünde unless you're in a hurry to reach Rostock or want to pay a premium to reach Berlin.

By Taxi

Only a few taxis meet arriving ships. While they'll highball estimates for various trips, the fair one-way price to downtown Rostock is €15-20. A ride all the way to Berlin costs around €250.

By Foot to the Train Station or into Downtown Warnemünde

Regardless of which cruise pier you arrive at, go through the terminal building, exit to the right, and walk with the train tracks on your left and the river on your right. Just watch for bull's-eye and *City* signs. You'll pass a hokey gift shop and an ultra-German

than reading about it in a museum.

A themed excursion is worth considering. Most cruise lines offer a guided tour to several actual sites of important **Nazi/WWII/Cold War** history. **Jewish heritage** excursions may visit the outstanding Jewish Museum, the sumptuous New Synagogue, and the poignant Memorial to the Murdered Jews of Europe.

For those who want to stay closer to the ship, there are several options—but be aware that cruise lines push these more for their proximity than for their sightseeing worthiness. Most common are guided visits of **Warnemünde** (walking tour, sometimes organ concert at the church) and **Rostock** (churches, Old Town, and city wall)—either separately or combined. Some Warnemünde and Rostock tours throw in a shopping stop in the village of Rövershagen or a visit to a local microbrewery. Nearby are **Bad Doberan** (with a red-brick Cistercian convent-turned-minster)—a visit here is often combined with a ride on the Molli narrow-gauge steam train to the seaside resorts of Heiligendamm and/or Kühlungsborn; **Wismar** (colorful Hanseatic port town oozing with red-brick buildings), sometimes combined with the even more striking town of **Lübeck; Güstrow Castle** (housing an art museum); and **Schwerin Castle** (a pretty Loire-style palace overlooking an idyllic lake). The Worst Possible Value award goes to the **Rostock On Your Own** "excursion," providing a round-trip bus ride to downtown Rostock and back for $60—more than 10 times the price of the easy train connection.

Other sights to consider include the palaces of Prussian royalty at **Potsdam** (opulent, but not uniquely so) and **Sachsenhausen Concentration Camp** (with a compelling documentation center of Nazi atrocities). However, since both of these are quite close to Berlin, they involve a long bus ride.

cafeteria (Pier 7 by Karl's), then a small car ferry across the river, and excursion boats to Rostock (€10 one-way, €14 round-trip, depart at least hourly, 45 minutes each way). About 50 yards beyond the car-ferry dock, look for signs on the left *(Tourist Information / Historischer Ortkern)* and follow them through the trees and into an underpass that goes beneath the train tracks. On the other side is the **train station** plaza. A departures board is overhead, and red-and-white ticket machines are to your left. To your right, you can follow signs for *DB Reiseagentur / Travelcenter* to enter the building with the ticket office (marked *Reiseagentur*). In the same building is the Crew Corner, offering Wi-Fi (free with purchase) and pay Internet access. For more on buying tickets to Rostock or Berlin, see the next section.

To continue into **town,** proceed through the station area

BERLIN

from where you popped out at
the underpass, and walk straight
ahead across the little bridge,
which gives you a good look at the
Alter Strom (old harbor). Once
over the bridge, continue straight
to find the TI, Heimatmuseum
(both on the left after one block),
and—one block farther—the big

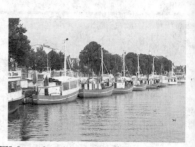

Kirchplatz (Church Square, with ATMs and a pharmacy). To reach
Warnemünde's beach, turn right just after the bridge and walk up
the waterfront street called Am Strom. Stroll along here for about
10 minutes, with pleasure craft on your right and cheesy seaside-
resort shops on your left. When the buildings end and you start
to see sand dunes, look left to find Warnemünde's trademark old
lighthouse and Teepott building (with the wavy roof). Going up
the stairs past the lighthouse, you'll come to Warnemünde's board-
walk-like beachfront promenade, with several beach access points
on your right. If you'd like to explore a bit on the way back to the
port, consider taking the lane that runs parallel to the old harbor a
block inland, Alexandrinenstrasse, lined with picturesque cottages.

By Train to Rostock or Berlin

From Warnemünde's little station, trains depart for both Rostock
and Berlin.

To reach **Rostock,** suburban trains (called S-Bahn, with the
green *S* symbol) depart every 10 minutes (about a 20-minute ride).
A one-way ticket costs just €1.90. There's also a €4.70 all-day ticket
that includes the round-trip journey between Warnemünde and
Rostock, plus trams within Rostock (if sightseeing in Rostock,
you'll probably take the tram from the train station into the town
center and back again—so this ticket saves you money). There are
multiple stops named Rostock on this line; you'll get off at Rostock
Hbf (Hauptbahnhof, the main station). For tips on getting into
the town center once you arrive in Rostock, see page 575.

For **Berlin,** train departures are sparse and can vary depending on the day of the week. Aim for the earliest train, likely around
8:00. Check the schedule at the Deutsche Bahn (German Railway)
website (www.bahn.com), at the Warnemünde train station ticket
office, or on one of the station's red-and-white ticket machines.
Most trains require a change in Rostock. And while you may see
more trains on the schedule, these require a second change, in the
town of Schwerin, and take about 30-40 minutes longer. Tickets
to Berlin cost roughly €45 each way, though deals may be available
(check www.bahn.com or ask at the train station). Your train will
arrive at Berlin's Hauptbahnhof (main train station). For more on

Services near the Port

There are few services directly at the port, but you'll find what you need a short walk away.

ATMs and Pharmacy: The nearest to the port are on Kirchplatz—the big, open square around Warnemünde's can't-miss-it church, just past the TI (from the train station, cross the bridge, continue straight on Kirchenstrasse, and you'll run right into it).

Internet Access: Inside the train station building is the Crew Corner (which is also open to the public). You can use their Wi-Fi (free with €5 purchase), or pay to use one of their cheap terminals (€4/hour; daily in summer 9:00-20:00).

arriving at this station—and how to get into town from there—see page 583. Be aware that train delays can occur, so don't cut it too close when planning your return ride to the ship.

Buying and Validating Tickets: You can buy train tickets at the red-and-white ticket machines at the platform. These have English instructions and take both cash (euros only) and credit cards. You can also buy tickets at the desk inside the station. If you buy your ticket at the machine, be sure to validate it in the orange box at the platform before boarding your train.

By Cruise-Line Excursion

In addition to fully guided excursions to Berlin, many cruise lines offer a transportation-only "On Your Own" option: An unguided bus ride from the pier in Warnemünde to Berlin and back at an appointed time, generally leaving you five or six hours in the capital. Some cruise lines even charter a train to make this trip. Although this is pricey (around $150-200 or more, compared to around $115-135 for a round-trip train ticket), it's worth think-ing about for the peace of mind it buys. Remember, if you're on a cruise-line trip and there's a traffic jam coming back, the ship will wait for you—but not so if you're returning on your own and your train is late. If one of the public train departures works perfectly for your trip, I'd opt for the train. But if the train times don't sync with your schedule, the "On Your Own" excursion could be well worth it for the additional hours it buys you in Berlin.

Your shuttle will likely drop you off at the delightful square called **Gendarmenmarkt,** just south of Unter den Linden in the very center of the Berlin (for a description of this square, see page 619). If you wind up here, you can walk two blocks up Charlottenstrasse and turn left on Unter den Linden to reach Brandenburg Gate and the Reichstag. Then, backtrack down Unter den Linden and continue all the way to Museum Island.

BERLIN

By Tour

Berlin Tours: Several Berlin tour companies pick up groups at the dock in Warnemünde for all-day tours of the city. Although a tour can be quite expensive on your own, when you divide the cost with fellow cruisers, it becomes affordable. **Ship2shore,** with top-quality guides and a dedication to personal service, offers Berlin day trips tailored to your interests starting at €99 per person (based on a minimum of 12 people; smaller groups also possible: €799/2 people, €880/3-4 people, €975/5-6 people, €1,099/6-11 people; tel. 030/243-58058, www.ship2shore.de, info@ship2shore.de). The **Original Berlin Walks** walking-tour company also runs excursions from Warnemünde into Berlin (€815 for up to 3 people in a minibus, €60/additional person up to a maximum of 7, see contact information on page 592).

Once you reach Berlin, there's a world of great walking tours, hop-on, hop-off bus tours, private guides for hire, and other sightseeing options. For details, see page 589.

Warnemünde, Rostock, and Environs Tours: If you want to stick closer to your ship, consider the **Friends of Dave Tours,** with itineraries focusing on Warnemünde and Rostock, Hanseatic history, or the royal Mecklenburg family. Dave is an endearing personality who includes all transportation costs, admissions, tips, drinks, and lunches in his tour price. When speaking to his groups (16 people max), Dave uses a comfortable "whisper system" to communicate in his low-key way via personal headphones. The full tour lasts 12 hours; the shorter version covering only Rostock and Warnemünde runs 9 hours (€120-135/person, tours run every day a cruise is in town, mobile 0174-302-1499, www.friendsofdavetours.com).

RETURNING TO YOUR SHIP

In planning your return from Berlin, be very clear on your ship's all-aboard time and work backward—allowing time for possible delays.

If you're meeting an "On Your Own" cruise-line **shuttle bus,** it'll pick you up wherever it dropped you off. Many stop at Gendarmenmarkt, a short walk south of Unter den Linden (down Charlottenstrasse) and within a block of two different U-Bahn stations (U6: Französische Strasse; U2 or U6: Stadtmitte).

If you're planning to ride the **train** back to Warnemünde, check the schedule carefully (www.bahn.com). Note that only a few trains depart for Warnemünde in the afternoon. Be sure that you'll arrive in Warnemünde with plenty of time to return to your ship (about a 5- to 10-minute walk from the Warnemünde train station).

Trains to Warnemünde depart from Berlin Hauptbahnhof.

The main east-west **S-Bahn** line zips you to the Hauptbahnhof from various points in town (including Friedrichstrasse, three blocks north of Unter den Linden; Hackescher Markt, a short walk north of Museum Island; and Alexanderplatz, at the end of Unter den Linden). From these stops, take any train going west, and hop off at Hauptbahnhof. You'll exit the S-Bahn on the top level of the station, but your Warnemünde train likely leaves from the bottom level, five stories below (confirm and ride the elevator down). This S-Bahn ride is covered by your ticket to Warnemünde. Alternatively, you could ride the **U-Bahn** line two stops from the Brandenburger Tor stop (but this ride is *not* covered by your train ticket). If you're in a rush, hail a **taxi** and say, "Hauptbahnhof."

Remember, you'll likely need to change trains in Rostock. From Rostock Hauptbahnhof (main station), local suburban trains (S-Bahn) depart for Warnemünde every 10 minutes, and the trip takes about 20 minutes (ride the train to the end of the line). At the Warnemünde station, go down the stairs between tracks 3 and 4 (labeled *Passaßgierkai*); walk through the trees, turn right, and follow the water to your awaiting ship.

If you get back to Warnemünde with time to spare, explore the town a bit. Walk along the old harbor (Alter Strom—just a 10- to 15-minute walk from your ship), poke around the cottages of the old center, or—with more time—head out to the beach.

See page 639 for help if you miss your boat.

Sights in Warnemünde

A pleasant old fishing town that managed to escape much of the ugliness of the DDR, Warnemünde feels like a tacky, unabashedly

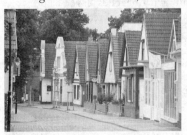

fun beachfront resort—like New Jersey's Atlantic City or England's Brighton or Blackpool...although on a much smaller scale. This town has more than its share of bars, fast-food joints, divey hotels, beachwear boutiques, and Euro-vacationers. Those who find Rostock dull and dreary believe Warnemünde (which is practically its suburb) the city's saving grace. While Warnemünde offers little in the way of culturally broadening sightseeing, it's a fun spot for a beachy break.

See "Getting into Town," earlier, for walking directions from the cruise port into town and its attractions. I've listed items here in the order you'll reach them as you approach them from your ship.

BERLIN

Old Harbor (Alter Strom)

Lined with colorful boats and fronted by bars, restaurants, hotels, and shops, this historic canal runs through the middle of Warnemünde. A boat-spotting stroll here is an entertaining way to while away some of your vacation time. From the seaward end of the canal, excursion boats try to lure you in for a one-hour cruise around the harbor and back (generally around €9, catering mostly to German tourists).

Warnemünde History Museum (Heimatmuseum)

This modest museum, tucked in a cute 18th-century house near the TI, traces the history of this modest burg from fishing village to seaside resort, and lets visitors walk through preserved historic rooms.

Cost and Hours: €3; April-Oct Tue-Sun 10:00-18:00, closed Mon; Nov-March Wed-Sun 10:00-18:00, closed Mon-Tue; Alexandrinenstrasse 31, tel. 0381/52667, www.heimatmuseum-warnemuende.de.

Lighthouse (Leuchtturm)

Strategically situated to watch over both the Old Harbor and the beach, Warnemünde's symbol is its 105-foot-tall, tile-clad lighthouse. Completed in 1898, the lighthouse sits next to the distinctively shaped (and aptly named) Teepott building. In the summer, you can climb to the tower's top for a view over Warnemünde and its beach.

Cost and Hours: €2, daily April-Oct 10:00-19:00, closed off-season.

The Beach (Badestrand)

Those who don't associate Germany with beaches haven't laid eyes on its Baltic seafront. Warnemünde has an incredibly broad, long stretch of white sand. While access to the beach is free, German holiday makers enjoy renting charming, almost whimsical, wicker cabana chairs called *Strandkörbe* for some shade and comfort (you'll find a big swathe of these at the lighthouse end of the beach; €3/hour, €11/day, €13/day for the front row facing the sea, €8 after 14:00). Eyeing this broad expanse of beach, it's easy to see how German imaginations could so easily be seized by David Hasselhof's *Baywatch*. At the far end of the beach, you may see the letters "FKK"—German code for "nude beach."

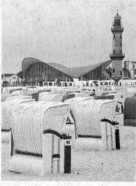

Rostock

Rostock, a regional capital with sprawling industrial ports and a tidy Old Town, clusters along the Warnow River about nine miles inland from the sea (and Warnemünde).

Dating back to medieval times, Rostock was an important shipping and shipbuilding town. It was a key player in the Hanseatic League, which connected it with trading partners from Scandinavia to Russia. Its university, founded in 1419, was the first of its kind in northern Europe and earned the city its nickname, "Light of the North." But the town declined in the 17th century after the Thirty Years' War and a big fire.

Later, the mid-20th century dealt the town a devastating one-two punch: First, because it had several important aircraft factories, it was leveled by WWII bombs. Second, in the postwar era, it fell on the eastern side of the Iron Curtain, and—although it was the DDR's primary industrial port—Rostock's communist caretakers did an architecturally questionable job of rebuilding. A few historic buildings are scattered around town, and it all feels quite well-kept, but on the whole it lacks the appeal of many German cities of its size. You get the feeling that if Rostock weren't next to a major cruise port, it would get virtually no tourism...and that would be just fine with everyone.

That said, the city does have a smattering of attractions for cruisers who'd like to do some real sightseeing during their day at

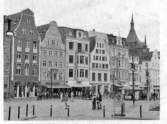

the port of Warnemünde. The hulking St. Mary's Church anchors an Old Town that's not quite old, but is where you'll find most of what there is to see: fragments of the old city walls (including an intact tower), a few museums and churches, and, above all, a workaday urban core where locals seem to go about their business oblivious to the big glitzy cruise ships that put in just down the river. The nondescript zone between the Old Town and train station hides a fascinating site for those interested in the Cold War: a former Stasi (communist secret police) prison block that's been converted into a museum and documentation center.

Orientation to Rostock

With about 200,000 inhabitants, Rostock sprawls along the Warnow River. But nearly everything worth seeing on a quick visit is in the compact Old Town (Altstadt), which is about a mile due

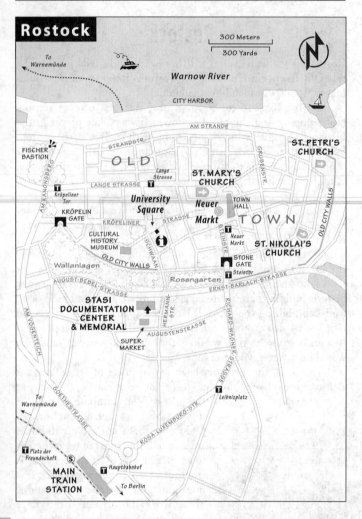

north of the Hauptbahnhof. There's little to see in the tidy residential area between the station and the Old Town, with one big exception: the Stasi Museum, which is a five-minute walk south of the Old Town and ring road.

Rostock's waterfront, severed from the Old Town by a busy highway, is dreary and dull—don't go there hoping for a charming, salty stroll.

TOURIST INFORMATION

Rostock's helpful TI is on University Square in the heart of the Old Town (May-Oct Mon-Fri 10:00-18:00, Sat-Sun 10:00-15:00; Nov-April Mon-Fri 10:00-17:00, Sat 10:00-15:00, closed Sun;

Universitätsplatz 6, tel. 0381/381-222, www.rostock.de).

Tours: The historical society based at the Kröpelin Gate leads one-hour walking tours of Rostock in English (€5, every day that a cruise is in town, departs from the gate at 11:00 and often at 13:00, tel. 0381/454-177 to confirm).

ARRIVAL IN ROSTOCK

Rostock is a 20-minute train ride from Warnemünde (for specifics on taking the train here, see page 568). Get off the train at the Rostock Hauptbahnhof (main train station, abbreviated Hbf). From here, it's a 15-minute walk or five-minute tram ride to the main square and Old Town.

To **walk,** head out the main door to the plaza in front of the station, and proceed straight ahead through the roundabout and up the big street called Rosa-Luxemburg-Strasse; bear left when this becomes Richard-Wagner-Strasse (just follow the tram tracks). You'll cross the ring road, pass the Steintor (Stone Gate of the old city fortifications), and carry on one long block to Neuer Markt and St. Mary's Church.

Taking the **tram** is simple: From the concourse connecting the tracks inside the station, follow the red tram icon signs to find the stairs leading down to the tram stop (marked *A*, indicating direction: city center). Buy a €1.90 ticket either at the machine near the tram stop (then stamp it on board) or at the machine on board (no additional stamp necessary). The ride is also covered if you bought the €4.70 all-day ticket (see page 568). Take tram #5 or #6, and ride it three stops to Neuer Markt.

Sights in Rostock

I've listed these sights in the order you'll likely visit them.

Neuer Markt (New Market Square)

The city's central gathering point, this square is an odd combination

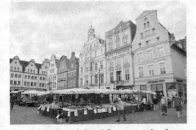

of beautiful historic buildings and blah communist-era construction. Highlights include the pretty, pink Town Hall (Rathaus) and the nicely reconstructed row of merchant houses facing it. The fountain in the middle of the square, from 2001, depicts Neptune and his four sons. And the big, hulking brick building overlooking it all is St. Mary's Church.

From Neuer Markt, you can tour the church, then head down the pedestrian shopping drag called Kröpeliner Strasse to

BERLIN

reach University Square, the Cultural History Museum, and the Kröpelin Gate—all described below.

▲St. Mary's Church (Marienkirche)

Dating from the 14th century (with WWII damage finally repaired in the 1990s), this is Rostock's main church. Inside, this

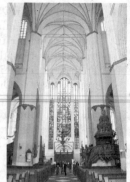

Gothic brick church is tall, white, and spacious—classic Lutheran. The church has some charming details that are worth lingering over—including memorials to generous supporters, a fine astronomical clock built in 1472, an intricately decorated bronze baptismal font, an elaborate Renaissance pulpit, a gorgeously adorned Baroque organ, and a striking stained-glass window from 1904 in the south portal ("Christ as Judge of the World").

Cost and Hours: €1.50 suggested donation; May-Sept Mon-Sat 10:00-18:00, Sun 11:15-17:00; Oct-April Mon-Sat 10:00-16:00, Sun 11:15-12:15.

Organ Performance: Mondays through Saturdays in summer (May-mid-Oct), a brief prayer service from 12:00 to 12:10 includes organ music. Music lovers who show up a few minutes early can meet the organist and go up into the loft to watch him play. In return, they ask that you make a donation and consider buying a CD.

University Square (Universitätsplatz)

From Neuer Markt, the lively, shop-lined Kröpeliner Strasse leads to this square. The TI is in the pretty yellow building on the left as you enter the square. The centerpiece *Fountain of Joy,* a communist-era creation (displaying a lightheartedness unusual for that time), sits in front of the university headquarters. Along the right side (as you face the fountain) are the so-called Five Gables—brick buildings with modern flourishes that were designed to echo the shape and style of the historic houses at these same addresses that were blown apart by WWII bombs. Around the left side of the fountain, past the mustard-yellow building with columns and through the brick gate, is a charming lane leading to the Cultural History Museum (described next).

When you're done exploring here, you can continue two more short blocks on Kröpeliner Strasse (out the far end of the square) to reach the Kröpelin Gate.

Cultural History Museum (Kulturhistorisches Museum)

This fine collection of historical items relating to Rostock is situated around a pleasant former cloister. Unfortunately, its near-total lack of English information makes the eclectic collection challenging to appreciate. The ground floor has local artifacts, a town model, grave markers, historic portraits of important Rostockers, and old wooden chests. Up on the first floor you'll find a particularly nice collection of old toys, porcelain and glassware, clocks, and coins. A small top-floor room shows off early 20th-century art. The museum also often has special exhibits. I consider this a free way to pass some time or get in out of the rain, though true historians or fans of dusty bric-a-brac may find something to get excited about.

Cost and Hours: Free, Tue-Sun 10:00-18:00, closed Mon, Klosterhof 7, tel. 0381/203-5901.

Kröpelin Gate (Kröpeliner Tor)

One of two surviving watchtowers from the old city wall, this picturesque gate (which strikes a medieval pose at the end of Kröpeliner Strasse) offers a disappointing little history exhibit and a view from the top that's not worth the 100 steps.

Cost and Hours: €1, daily 10:00-18:00, until 17:00 Nov-March, tel. 0381/121-6415.

Nearby: Next to the gate is a surviving stretch of the original town wall. This also marks the course of an inviting park that hems in the southern end of the Old Town. From the tram stop nearby, trams #5, #6, or E will take you back to the station.

More Churches

Two other historic churches, interesting for very different reasons, are on the eastern edge of the Old Town.

St. Nikolai's Church (Nikolaikirche), a few blocks east of Neuer Markt, is generally closed to the public, but it's worth taking a close look at its roofline from down below. Are those windows and balconies? During the communist period, the atheistic regime converted part of this church into an apartment complex. Although much of the building has been reclaimed for religious services, if you go to the church's front door, you'll still find a panel of doorbells for people who live here.

St. Petri's Church (Petrikirche), in the northeastern corner of town, overlooks the Alte Markt (Old Market Square). The empty-feeling, white, oh-so-Lutheran interior has little to distinguish it, but you can pay €3 to ride the elevator up to the tower for an okay view over town (which is blocked by fine mesh—making it impossible to get a good photo).

BETWEEN THE OLD TOWN AND THE TRAIN STATION

▲Stasi Documentation Center and Memorial

Hiding in a humdrum residential area, incongruously sharing a parking lot with a Penny supermarket, is a building that once

The Stasi (East German Secret Police)

To keep their subjects in line, the DDR government formed the Ministerium für Staatssicherheit (MfS, "Ministry for State Security")—nicknamed the Stasi. Modeled after the Soviet Union's secret police, the Stasi actively recruited informants from every walk of life, often intimidating them into cooperating by threatening their employment, their children's education, or worse. The Stasi eventually gathered an army of some 600,000 "unofficial employees" *(inoffizielle Mitarbeiter),* nearly 200,000 of whom were still active when communism fell in 1989. These "employees" were coerced into reporting on the activities of their coworkers, friends, neighbors, and even their own immediate family members.

Preoccupied with keeping track of "nonconformist" behavior, the Stasi collected whatever bits of evidence they could about suspects—including saliva, handwriting, odors, and voice recordings—and wound up with vast amounts of files. In late 1989, when it was becoming clear that communism was in its waning days, Stasi officials attempted to destroy their files—but barely had time to make a dent before government officials decreed that all documentation be preserved as evidence of their crimes. These days, German citizens can read the files that were once kept on them. (Locals struggle with the decision: Request a full view of their record—and see which friends and loved ones were reporting on them—or avoid the likely painful truth.) For a film that brilliantly captures the paranoid Stasi culture, see the 2006 Oscar-winner *The Lives of Others.*

held prisoners of the communist state. Today this former prison block has been converted into a museum and documentation cen-

ter about the crimes of the former regime—specifically, its secret police, known as the Stasi (see sidebar). Worth at least ▲▲ for those interested in the Cold War period in this part of Germany, the museum provides an opportunity to better understand some of Rostock's darkest days.

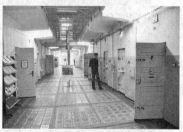

From 1960 to 1989, this prison held a total of 4,800 people (110 at a time) who were accused of crimes against the state—ranging from participating in protests to attempting to flee the country to simply telling a joke about the regime. Though this was thought to be a "pre-trial prison," some individuals were held here for up to a year and a half. With the help of English explanations and a free audioguide, you'll walk through the actual prison, peering into

cells; some contain exhibits about the Stasi, while others are preserved as they were when they held prisoners. Artifacts illustrate
the crimes and methods of the Stasi. For example, the jars with
yellow cloths are impregnated with a suspect's scent (they sweat
on a chair while being interrogated)—one bizarre example of the
many ways the Stasi kept tabs on those they were investigating.

Cost and Hours: Free; Tue-Fri 10:00-18:00, until 17:00 Nov-
Feb, Sat 10:00-17:00, closed Sun-Mon; Hermannstrasse 34b, tel.
0381/498-5651, www.bstu.bund.de.

Getting There: The prison, buried in a residential zone, is
a bit tricky to find, but it's marked with brown signs when you
get nearby—ideally, get a map locally (at the TI). The easiest
way to find it is to begin on University Square and head south
on Schwaansche Strasse. Passing through the park just south of
the Old Town, cross the ring road and continue straight as the
street becomes Hermannstrasse. Watch on the right for the Penny
supermarket; the prison block is directly across from the entrance.

BETWEEN ROSTOCK AND WARNEMÜNDE
IGA Park and Ship Building and Shipping Museum (Schiffbau- und Schifffahrtmuseum)

If you have ample time and are intrigued by all things maritime,
consider hopping off the S-Bahn on your way between Rostock
and Warnemünde to see this fine park loaded with kid-friendly
attractions (including mini-golf, Chinese and Japanese gardens,
flower gardens, a "miniature world," and more). You'll also find the
Shipping Museum—which fills five decks of a retired ship—and a
boat-building workshop that uses historical techniques.

Cost and Hours: Park-€1, park and museum-€4; park—daily
April-Oct 9:00-18:00, Nov-March 10:00-16:00; museum—daily
April-Oct 10:00-18:00; Nov-March 10:00-16:00, closed Mon; get
off the S-Bahn at the Rostock Lütten Klein stop and walk 15 minutes past the convention center toward the river, www.iga-park-
rostock.de.

Berlin

While it takes some effort to reach Berlin from Warnemünde, that effort is warranted. Berlin has emerged as one of Europe's top destinations: captivating, lively, fun-loving, all-around enjoyable—and easy on the budget. For the past two decades, Berlin has been a construction zone. Standing on ripped-up tracks and under a canopy of cranes, visitors witnessed the rebirth of a great European capital. Although construction continues, today the once-divided city is thoroughly woven back together.

Of course, Berlin is still largely defined by its tumultuous 20th century. The city was Hitler's capital during World War II, and in the postwar years, it became the front line of a new global war—one between Soviet-style communism and American-style capitalism. The East-West division was set in stone in 1961, when the East German government boxed in West Berlin with the Berlin Wall. The Wall stood for 28 years. In 1990, less than a year after the Wall fell, the two Germanys—and the two Berlins—officially became one. When the dust settled, Berliners from both sides of the once-divided city faced the monumental challenge of reunification.

When the Wall came down, the East was a decrepit wasteland and the West was a paragon of commerce and materialism. Since then, city planners have seized on the city's reunification and the return of the national government to make Berlin a great capital once again. A quarter-century later, the roles are reversed: It's eastern Berlin where you feel the vibrant pulse of the city, while western Berlin seems like yesterday's news. Berliners joke that they don't need to travel anywhere because their city's always changing. Spin a postcard rack to see what's new. A 10-year-old guidebook on Berlin covers a different city.

But even as the city busily builds itself into the 21st century, Berlin has made a point of acknowledging and remembering its past. A series of thought-provoking memorials installed throughout the city center—such as the Memorial to the Murdered Jews of Europe—directly confront some of Germany's most difficult history of the last century. Lacing these sights into your Berlin sightseeing is a way to learn from those horrific times.

As you appreciate the thrill of walking over what was the Wall and through the well-patched Brandenburg Gate, it's clear that history is not contained in some book; it's an evolving story in which we play a part. In Berlin, the fine line between history and current events is excitingly blurry.

But even for nonhistorians, Berlin is a city of fine experiences. Explore the fun and funky neighborhoods emerging in the former East, packed with creative hipster eateries and boutiques trying to one-up each other. Go for a cruise along the delightful Spree riverfront. In the city's world-class museums, walk through an enormous Babylonian gate amid rough-and-tumble ancient statuary, and peruse canvases by Dürer, Rembrandt, and Vermeer. Nurse a stein of brew in a rollicking beer hall, or dive into a cheap *Currywurst*.

Berlin today is like the nuclear fuel rod of a great nation. It's vibrant with youth, energy, and an anything-goes-and-anything's-possible buzz. As a booming tourist draw, Berlin now welcomes more visitors annually than Rome.

Orientation to Berlin

Berlin is huge, with 3.4 million people. Your time in the city will be short, so you'll need to prioritize. Most visitors focus on **eastern Berlin,** with the highest concentration of notable sights and colorful neighborhoods. Near the landmark Brandenburg Gate, you'll find the Reichstag building, Pariser Platz, and poignant memorials to the victims of Hitler (Jews, Roma and Sinti, and homosexuals). From the Brandenburg Gate, the famous Unter den Linden boulevard runs eastward through former East Berlin, passing the German History Museum and Museum Island (Pergamon Museum, Neues Museum, and Berlin Cathedral) on the way to Alexanderplatz (TV Tower). South of Unter den Linden are the delightful Gendarmenmarkt square, most Nazi sites (including the Topography of Terror), some good Wall-related sights (Museum of the Wall at Checkpoint Charlie and East Side Gallery), and the Jewish Museum. North of Unter den Linden are these worth-a-wander neighborhoods: Oranienburger Strasse (Jewish Quarter and New Synagogue), Hackescher Markt, and Prenzlauer Berg. Eastern Berlin's pedestrian-friendly Spree riverbank is also worth a stroll (or a river cruise).

With so much to see in eastern Berlin, and so little time, it's unlikely you'll venture into the city's other zones.

TOURIST INFORMATION

With any luck, you won't have to use Berlin's TIs—they're for-profit agencies working for the city's big hotels, which colors the information they provide. TI branches, appropriately called "info-stores," are unlikely to have the information you need (tel. 030/250-025, www.visitberlin.de). You'll find them at the **Hauptbahnhof** train station (daily 8:00-22:00, by main entrance on Europaplatz) and at the **Brandenburg Gate** (daily 9:30-19:00).

Skip the TI's €1 map, and instead browse the walking tour companies' brochures—many include nearly-as-good maps for

BERLIN

The History of Berlin

Berlin was a humble, marshy burg—its name perhaps derived from an old Slavic word for "swamp"—until prince electors from the Hohenzollern dynasty made it their capital in the mid-15th century. Gradually their territory spread and strengthened, becoming the powerful Kingdom of Prussia in 1701. As the leading city of Prussia, Berlin dominated the northern Germanic world—both militarily and culturally—long before there was a united "Germany."

The only Hohenzollern ruler worth remembering was Frederick the Great (1712-1786). The ultimate enlightened despot, he was both a ruthless military tactician (he consolidated his kingdom's holdings, successfully invading Silesia and biting off a chunk of Poland) and a cultured lover of the arts (he actively invited artists, architects, and other thinkers to his lands). "Old Fritz," as he was called, played the flute, spoke six languages, and counted Voltaire among his friends. Practical and cosmopolitan, Frederick cleverly invited to Prussia Protestants who were being persecuted elsewhere in Europe—including the French Huguenots and Dutch traders. Prussia became the beneficiary of these groups' substantial wealth and know-how. Frederick the Great left Berlin—and Prussia—a far more modern and enlightened place than he found it. Thanks largely to him, Prussia was well-positioned to become a magnet of sorts for the German unification movement in the 19th century.

When Germany first unified, in 1871, Berlin (as the main city of its most powerful constituent state, Prussia) was its natural capital. Even in the disarray of post-WWI Germany, Berlin thrived as an anything-goes, cabaret-crazy cultural capital of the Roaring '20s. During World War II, the city was Hitler's headquarters—and the place where the Führer drew his final breath. When the Soviet Army reached Berlin in 1945, the protracted fighting left the city in ruins.

free. If you take a walking tour, your guide is likely a better source of shopping and restaurant tips than the TI.

Museum Passes: The three-day, €24 **Museum Pass Berlin** gets you into more than 50 museums, including the national museums and most of the recommended biggies (though not the German History Museum), on three consecutive days (sold at the TI and participating museums). Sights covered by the pass include the Museum Island museums (Old National Gallery, Neues, Altes, Bode, and Pergamon), Gemäldegalerie, and the Jewish Museum Berlin, along with other more minor sights. As you'll routinely spend €10-14 per admission, this pays for itself if you'll be visiting multiple museums. However, you'd have to be a very busy sightseer to make the pass pay for itself on a brief visit.

The €18 **Museum Island Pass** (Bereichskarte Museumsinsel;

After World War II, Berlin was divided by the victorious Allied powers. The American, British, and French sectors became West Berlin, and the Soviet sector, East Berlin. In 1948 and 1949, the Soviets tried to starve the 2.2 million residents of the Western half in an almost medieval-style siege, blockading all roads in and out. But they were foiled by the Berlin Airlift, with the Western Allies flying in supplies from Frankfurt 24 hours a day for 10 months.

Years later, with the overnight construction of the Berlin Wall in 1961, an Iron (or, at least, concrete) Curtain literally cut through the middle of the city, completely encircling West Berlin. For details, see "The Berlin Wall (and Its Fall)" on page 626.

While the wild night when the Wall came down (November 9, 1989) was inspiring, Berlin still faced a fitful transition to reunification. Two cities—and countries—became one at a staggering pace. Reunification had its downside, and the Wall survives in the minds of some people. Some "Ossies" (impolite slang for Easterners) miss their security. Some "Wessies" miss their easy ride (military deferrals, subsidized rent, and tax breaks for living in an isolated city surrounded by the communist world). For free spirits, walled-in West Berlin was a citadel of freedom within the East.

But in recent years, the old East-West division has faded more and more into the background. Ossi-Wessi conflicts no longer dominate the city's political discourse. The city government has been eager to charge forward, with little nostalgia for anything that was associated with the East. Big corporations and the national government have moved in, and the dreary swath of land that was the Wall and its notorious "death strip" has been transformed (as the cash-starved city has been selling off lots of land to anyone determined to develop it). Berlin is a whole new city—and it's ready to welcome visitors.

does not include special exhibits) covers all the venues on Museum Island (otherwise €10-14 each) and is a good value if you're spending the day museum-hopping on the island.

ARRIVAL IN BERLIN
By Train at Berlin Hauptbahnhof
Trains from Warnemünde and Rostock arrive at Berlin's newest and grandest train station, Berlin Hauptbahnhof (main train station, a.k.a. "der Bahnhof," abbreviated Hbf). Europe's biggest, mostly underground train station is unique for its major lines coming in at right angles; this is where the national train system meets the city's S-Bahn train system.

The gigantic station can be intimidating, but it's laid out logically on five floors (which, confusingly, can be marked in different ways). Escalators and elevators connect the **main floor** (*Erdgeschoss*, EG, a.k.a level 0); the two **lower levels** (*Untergeschoss*, UG1 and UG2, a.k.a. levels -1 and -2); and the two **upper levels** (*Obersgeschoss*, OG1 and OG2, a.k.a. levels +1 and +2). Tracks 1-8—most often used by trains to

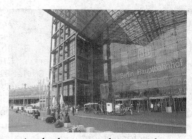

and from Rostock/Warnemünde—are in the lowest underground level (UG2), while tracks 11-16 (along with the S-Bahn, for connecting to other points in town) are on the top floor (OG2). Shops and services are concentrated on the three middle levels (EG, OG1, and UG1). The south entrance (toward the Reichstag and downtown, with a taxi stand) is marked *Washingtonplatz*, while the north entrance is marked *Europaplatz*.

Services: On the main floor (EG), you'll find the **TI** (facing the north/*Europaplatz* entrance, look left) and the **"Rail & Fresh WC"** facility (public pay toilets, near the Burger King and food court). Up one level (OG1) is a 24-hour **pharmacy.**

Train Information and Tickets: Before leaving the station, it's smart to reconfirm the schedule for trains back to Warnemünde—and, while you're at it, buy your ticket. The station has a Deutsche Bahn *Reisezentrum* information center on the first upper level (OG1/+1, open long hours daily). **EurAide** is an English-speaking information desk with answers to your questions about train travel around Europe. It's located at counter 12 inside the *Reisezentrum* on the first upper level (OG1/+1). It's American-run, so communication is simple (www.euraide.com).

Shopping: In addition to all those trains, the Hauptbahnhof is home to 80 shops with long hours—some locals call the station a "shopping mall with trains" (daily 8:00-22:00, only stores selling travel provisions are open Sun). The Kaisers supermarket (UG1, follow signs for tracks 1-2) is handy for assembling a picnic for your train ride.

Getting into Town: If you're in town for just a few hours, you'll likely want to head straight for the Brandenburg Gate, next to the Reichstag and at the start of Unter den Linden. You can **walk** (past big, governmental buildings) from the station to the Brandenburg Gate in about 15 minutes (use the exit marked *Washingtonplatz*, cut through the plaza to the footbridge, cross the river, and bear left past the boxy Bundestag building toward the glass dome of the Reichstag). To save time, ride the **subway:** The station's sole U-Bahn line—U55—goes only two stops, to the Brandenburger Tor station. The U-Bahn isn't covered by your train ticket, so you'll have to buy a ticket before hopping on; it's covered by the cheap €1.50 *Kurzstrecke Fahrschein* short-ride ticket (for details, see page 587).

To reach other points in town (or for a quick return to the station), consider the handy crosstown express **S-Bahn** train line. All S-Bahn trains are on tracks 15 and 16 at the top of the station (level OG2/+2). All trains on track 15 go east, stopping at Friedrichstrasse, Hackescher Markt (with connections to Prenzlauer Berg), Alexanderplatz, and Ostbahnhof (trains on track 16 go west, toward Bahnhof Zoo and Savignyplatz). Your train ticket or rail pass to the station covers your connecting S-Bahn ride into town; your outbound ticket includes the transfer via S-Bahn to the Hauptbahnhof.

HELPFUL HINTS

Medical Help: The US Embassy has a list of local English-speaking doctors (tel. 030/83050, germany.usembassy.gov).

Museum Tips: Some major Berlin museums are closed on Monday—if you're in town on that day, review hours carefully before making plans.

Addresses: Many Berlin streets are numbered with odd and even numbers on the same side of the street, often with no connection to the other side. To save steps, check the white street signs on curb corners; many list the street numbers covered on that side of the block.

Cold War Terminology: What Americans called "East Germany" was technically the German Democratic Republic—the Deutsche Demokratische Republik, or **DDR** (day-day-AIR). You'll still see those initials around what was once East Germany. The formal name for "West Germany" was the Federal Republic of Germany— the Bundesrepublik Deutschland (**BRD**)—and is the name now shared by all of reunited Germany.

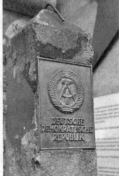

Internet Access: You'll find Wi-Fi at small Internet cafés all over the city. Friedrichstrasse and Hauptbahnhof train stations have coin-operated Internet terminals.

Berlin Souvenirs: If you're taken with the city's unofficial mascot, the *Ampelmännchen* (traffic-light man), you'll find a world of souvenirs slathered with his iconic red and green image at **Ampelmann Shops** (various locations, including along Unter den Linden at #35, near Gendarmenmarkt at Markgrafenstrasse 37, near Museum Island inside the

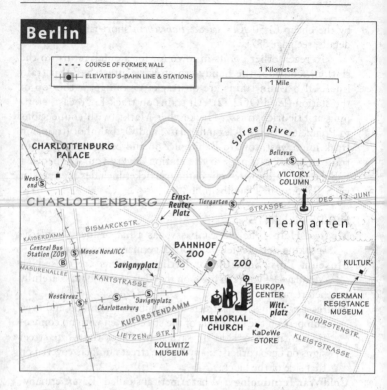

Berlin

- - - - COURSE OF FORMER WALL
—●— ELEVATED S-BAHN LINE & STATIONS

1 Kilometer
1 Mile

Spree River

CHARLOTTENBURG
PALACE

Bellevue Ⓢ

West
end Ⓢ

VICTORY
COLUMN

CHARLOTTENBURG

Ernst-
Reuter-
Platz

Tiergarten Ⓢ

STRASSE

DES 17. JUNI

Tiergarten

KAISERDAMM

BISMARCKSTR.

Central Bus
Station (ZOB) Ⓢ Messe Nord/ICC

BAHNHOF
ZOO

MASURENALLEE

Savignyplatz

KANTSTRASSE

ZOO

KULTUR-

Westkreuz Ⓢ

Ⓢ Savignyplatz

EUROPA
CENTER

GERMAN
RESISTANCE
MUSEUM

Charlottenburg

KURFÜRSTENDAMM

Witt.-
platz

KURFÜRSTENSTR.

LIETZEN. STR.

MEMORIAL
CHURCH

KaDeWe
STORE

KLEISTSTRASSE

KOLLWITZ
MUSEUM

DomAquarée mall, in the Hackesche Höfe, and at Potsdamer
Platz).

Shell Games: Believe it or not, there are still enough idiots on the
street to keep the con men with their shell games in business.
Don't be foolish enough to engage with any gambling on the
street.

Updates to This Book: For updates to this book, check www.
ricksteves.com/update.

GETTING AROUND BERLIN

Berlin's sights are spread far and wide. Right from the start, commit yourself to the city's fine public-transit system.

By Public Transit: Subway, Train, Tram, and Bus

Berlin's consolidated transit system uses the same ticket for
its many modes of transportation: U-Bahn (*Untergrund-Bahn,*
Berlin's subway), S-Bahn (*Stadtschnellbahn,* or "fast urban train,"
mostly aboveground and with fewer stops), *Strassenbahn* (trams),
and buses. For all types of transit, there are three lettered zones
(A, B, and C). Most of your sightseeing will be in zones A and B
(the city proper).

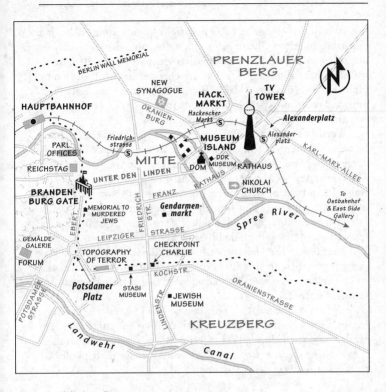

Ticket Options:

• The €2.60 **basic single** ticket *(Einzelfahrschein)* covers two hours of travel in one direction. It's easy to make this ticket stretch to cover several rides...as long as they're in the same direction.

• The €1.50 **short-ride** ticket *(Kurzstrecke Fahrschein)* covers a single ride of six bus stops or three subway stations (one transfer allowed). You can save a little bit on short-ride tickets by buying them in groups of four (€5.60).

• The €8.80 **four-trip** ticket *(4-Fahrten-Karte)* is the same as four basic single tickets at a small discount.

• The **day pass** *(Tageskarte)* is good until 3:00 the morning after you buy it (€6.70 for zones AB, €7.20 for zones ABC). The *Kleingruppenkarte* lets groups of up to five travel all day (€16.20 for zones AB, €16.70 for zones ABC).

Buying Tickets: You can buy U-Bahn/S-Bahn tickets from machines at stations. (They are also sold at BVG pavilions at train stations and the TI, from machines on board trams, and on buses from drivers, who'll give change.) *Erwachsener* means "adult"—anyone 14 or older. Don't be afraid of the ticket machines: First select the type of ticket you want, then load the coins or paper bills. (Coins work better, so keep some handy.) As you board the bus or tram, or enter the subway system, punch your ticket in a clock machine to validate it (or risk a €60 fine; for an all-day or multiday pass, stamp it only the first time you ride). Be sure to travel with a valid ticket. Tickets are checked frequently, often by plainclothes inspectors. Within Berlin, train tickets and rail passes are good only on S-Bahn connections from the train station when you arrive and to the station when you depart.

Transit Tips: The S-Bahn crosstown express is a river of public transit through the heart of the city, in which many lines converge on one basic highway. Get used to this, and you'll leap within a few minutes between key locations: Hauptbahnhof (all major trains in and out of Berlin), Friedrichstrasse (a short walk north of the heart of Unter den Linden), Hackescher Markt (Museum Island, restaurants, near Prenzlauer Berg), and Alexanderplatz (eastern end of my self-guided Best of Berlin Walk).

Sections of the U-Bahn or S-Bahn sometimes close temporarily for repairs. In this situation, a bus route often replaces the train (*Ersatzverkehr,* or "replacement transportation"; *zwischen* means "between").

Berlin's public transit is operated by BVG (except the S-Bahn, run by Deutsche Bahn). Schedules, including bus timetables, are available on the helpful BVG website (www.bvg.de). Get and use the excellent *Discover Berlin by Train and Bus* map-guide published by BVG (at subway ticket windows).

By Taxi

Cabs are easy to flag down, and taxi stands are common. A typical ride within town costs €8-10, and a crosstown trip (for example, Bahnhof Zoo to Alexanderplatz) will run about €15. Tariff 1 is for a *Kurzstrecke* ticket (see below). All other rides are tariff 2 (€3.40 drop plus €1.80/kilometer for the first 7 kilometers, then €1.28/kilometer after that). If possible, use cash—paying with a credit card comes with a hefty surcharge (about €4, regardless of the fare).

Money-Saving Taxi Tip: For any ride of less than two kilometers (about a mile), you can save several euros if you take advantage of the *Kurzstrecke* (short-stretch) rate. To get this rate, it's important that you flag the cab down on the street—not at or even near a taxi stand. Also, you must ask for the *Kurzstrecke* rate as soon as you hop in: Confidently say *"Kurzstrecke, bitte"* (KOORTS-shtreh-keh, BIT-teh), and your driver will grumble and flip the meter to a fixed €4 rate (for a ride that would otherwise cost €7).

Tours in Berlin

ON WHEELS
▲▲▲Hop-On, Hop-Off Buses

Several companies offer the same routine: a €15-17 circuit of the city with unlimited hop-on, hop-off privileges all day (about 15 stops at the city's major sights) on buses with cursory narration in English and German by a live, sometimes tired guide or a boring recorded commentary in whatever language you want to dial up. In season, each company has buses running at least four times per hour. They are cheap and great for photography—and Berlin really lends itself to this kind of bus-tour orientation. You can hop off at any major tourist spot (Potsdamer Platz, Museum Island, Brandenburg Gate, and so on). If possible, go with a live guide rather than the recorded spiel. When choosing seats, check the sun/shade situation—some buses are entirely topless, and others are entirely covered. My favorites are topless with a shaded covered section in the back (April-Oct daily 10:00-18:00, last bus leaves all stops at around 16:00, 2-hour loop; for specifics, look for brochures at the TI). Keep your ticket so you can hop off and on (with the same company) all day. Brochures explain extras offered by each company.

ON FOOT

Berlin's fascinating and complex recent history can be challenging to appreciate on your own, making the city an ideal place to explore with a walking tour, worth ▲▲▲. Equal parts historian and entertainer, a good Berlin tour guide makes the city's dynamic story come to life.

But unlike many other European countries, Germany has no regulations controlling who can give city tours. This can make guide quality hit-or-miss, ranging from brilliant history buffs who've lived in Berlin for years while pursuing their PhDs, to new arrivals who memorize a script and start leading tours after being in town for just a couple of weeks. In general you have the best odds of landing a great guide by using one of the more established companies I recommend in this section.

Most outfits offer walks that are variations on the same themes: general **introductory** walk, **Third Reich** walk (Hitler and Nazi sites), and day trips to Potsdam and the Sachsenhausen Concentration Camp Memorial (which you won't have time for on a quick port visit). Most in-city tours cost about €12-15 and last about three to four hours; public-transit tickets and entrances to sights are extra. I've included some basic descriptions for each company, but for details—including prices and specific schedules—see

BERLIN

Berlin at a Glance

▲▲▲German History Museum The ultimate swing through Germany's story. **Hours:** Daily 10:00-18:00. See page 611.

▲▲▲Pergamon Museum World-class museum of classical antiquities on Museum Island, partially closed through 2019 (including its famous Pergamon Altar). **Hours:** Daily 10:00-18:00, Thu until 20:00. See page 614.

▲▲▲Reichstag Germany's historic parliament building, topped with a modern dome you can climb (reservations required). **Hours:** Daily 8:00-24:00, last entry at 22:00. See page 594.

▲▲▲Brandenburg Gate One of Berlin's most famous landmarks, a massive columned gateway, at the former border of East and West. **Hours:** Always open. See page 600.

▲▲Memorial to the Murdered Jews of Europe Holocaust memorial with nearly 3,000 symbolic pillars, plus an exhibition about Hitler's Jewish victims. **Hours:** Memorial always open; information center open Tue-Sun 10:00-20:00, Oct-March until 19:00, closed Mon. See page 602.

▲▲Unter den Linden Leafy boulevard through the heart of former East Berlin, lined with some of the city's top sights. **Hours:** Always open. See page 604.

▲▲Neues Museum Egyptian antiquities collection and proud home of the exquisite 3,000-year-old bust of Queen Nefertiti. **Hours:** Daily 10:00-18:00, Thu until 20:00. See page 614.

▲▲Gendarmenmarkt Inviting square bounded by twin churches (one with a fine German history exhibit), a chocolate shop, and a concert hall. **Hours:** Always open. See page 619.

▲▲Topography of Terror Chilling exhibit documenting the Nazi perpetrators, built on the site of the former Gestapo/SS headquarters. **Hours:** Daily 10:00-20:00. See page 623.

▲▲Museum of the Wall at Checkpoint Charlie Kitschy but moving museum with stories of brave Cold War escapes, near the former site of the famous East-West border checkpoint; the surrounding street scene is almost as interesting. **Hours:** Daily 9:00-22:00. See page 625.

▲▲Jewish Museum Berlin Engaging, accessible museum celebrating Jewish culture, in a highly conceptual building. **Hours:** Daily 10:00-20:00, Mon until 22:00. See page 628.

▲▲**Gemäldegalerie** Germany's top collection of 13th-18th-century European paintings, featuring Holbein, Dürer, Cranach, Van der Weyden, Rubens, Hals, Rembrandt, Vermeer, Velázquez, Raphael, and more. **Hours:** Tue-Fri 10:00-18:00, Thu until 20:00, Sat-Sun 11:00-18:00, closed Mon. See page 622.

▲▲**Berlin Wall Memorial** A "docu-center" with videos and displays, several outdoor exhibits, and lone surviving stretch of an intact Wall section. **Hours:** Visitor Center April-Oct Tue-Sun 9:30-19:00, Nov-March until 18:00, closed Mon; outdoor areas accessible 24 hours daily. See page 631.

▲▲**Prenzlauer Berg** Lively, colorful neighborhood with hip cafés, restaurants, boutiques, and street life. **Hours:** Always open. See page 632.

▲**Pariser Platz** Historic square next to Brandenburg Gate, home to embassies and renowned Hotel Adlon. **Hours:** Always open. See page 601.

▲**Old National Gallery** German paintings, mostly from the Romantic Age. **Hours:** Tue-Sun 10:00-18:00, Thu until 20:00, closed Mon. See page 615.

▲**DDR Museum** Quirky collection of communist-era artifacts. **Hours:** Daily 10:00-20:00, Sat until 22:00. See page 617.

▲**Potsdamer Platz** The "Times Square" of old Berlin, long a postwar wasteland, now rebuilt with huge glass skyscrapers, an underground train station, and—covered with a huge canopy—the Sony Center mall. **Hours:** Always open. See page 621.

▲**Checkpoint Charlie** Famous Cold War crossing point between East and West Berlin, with a mock-up of the original American guard station and a streetside Berlin Wall photo exhibit. **Hours:** Always open. See page 624.

▲**New Synagogue** Largest prewar synagogue in Berlin, damaged in World War II, with a rebuilt facade and modest museum. **Hours:** March-Oct Sun-Mon 10:00-20:00, Tue-Thu 10:00-18:00, Fri 10:00-17:00—until 14:00 in March and Oct; Nov-Feb Sun-Thu 10:00-18:00, Fri 10:00-14:00; closed Sat year-round. See page 630.

▲**Kennedys Museum** Delightful exhibit recalls President John F. Kennedy's 1963 visit to Germany with great photos and video clips. **Hours:** Tue-Sun 11:00-19:00, closed Mon. See page 631.

BERLIN

the various websites or look for brochures in town (widely available at TIs, hotel reception desks, and many cafés and shops).

Brewer's Berlin Tours

Specializing in longer, more in-depth walks that touch on the entire span of Berlin's past, this company was started by the late, great Terry Brewer, who once worked for the British diplomatic service in East Berlin. Terry left the company to his guides, a group of historians who get very excited about Berlin. Their in-depth tours through the city are intimate, relaxed, and can flex with your interests. Their Best of Berlin introductory tour, billed at six hours, can last for eight (daily at 10:30). They also do a shorter 3.5-hour tour (free, tip expected, daily at 13:00) and an all-day Potsdam tour (Wed and Sat, May-Oct). All tours depart from Bandy Brooks ice-cream shop at the Friedrichstrasse S-Bahn station (tel. 030/2248-7435, mobile 0177-388-1537, www.brewersberlintours.com).

Insider Tour

This well-regarded company runs the full gamut of itineraries: introductory walk (daily), Third Reich, Cold War, Jewish Berlin, and so on. Their tours have two meeting points, in eastern and western Berlin; check their website for details (tel. 030/692-3149, www.insidertour.com).

Original Berlin Walks

Their flagship introductory walk, Discover Berlin, offers a good overview in four hours (daily year-round, meet at 10:00 at the taxi stand in front of the Bahnhof Zoo train station in western Berlin, April-Oct also daily at 13:30). They offer a Third Reich walking tour (4/week in summer) and themed walks on Jewish Life in Berlin, Cold War Berlin, and Queer Berlin (each 1/week April-Oct only). Ask about a discount with this book. All tours meet in front of the Bahnhof Zoo; the Discover Berlin and Jewish Life tours also have a second departure point opposite the Hackescher Markt S-Bahn station, outside the Weihenstephaner restaurant (tour info: tel. 030/301-9194, www.berlinwalks.de).

Alternative Berlin Tours

Specializing in cutting-edge street culture and art, this company emphasizes the bohemian chic that flavors the city's ever-changing urban scene. Their basic three-hour tour (daily at 11:00, 13:00, and 15:00) is tip-based; other tours cost €12-20 (all tours meet at Starbucks on Alexanderplatz under the TV Tower, mobile 0162-819-8264, www.alternativeberlin.com).

"Free" Tours

You'll see companies advertising supposedly "free" introductory tours all over town. Designed for and popular with students (free is good), it's a business model that has spread across Europe: English-speaking students (often Aussies and Americans) deliver a memorized script before a huge crowd lured in by the promise of a free tour. What the customers don't know is that the guide must turn over about €3 per person to the company, so tour leaders expect to be "tipped in paper" (€5 minimum per person is encouraged). The "free" intro tour is then used to push other tours that do charge a fee. While the guides can be highly entertaining, the better ones typically move on to more serious tour companies before long. These tours are fine for poor students with little interest in real history. But as with many things, when it comes to walking tours, you get what you pay for.

Local Guides

Berlin guides are generally independent contractors who work with the various tour companies (like those listed here). Many of them are Americans who came to town as students and history buffs, fell in love with the city, and now earn their living as guides. Some lead private tours on their own (generally charging around €50-60/hour or €200-300/day, confirm by email when booking). The following guides are all good: **Nick Jackson** (an archaeologist and historian who makes museums come to life, mobile 0171-537-8768, www.jacksonsberlintours.com); **Lee Evans** (makes 20th-century Germany a thriller, mobile 0177-423-5307, lee.evans@berlin.de); and **Bernhard Schlegelmilch** (mobile 0176-6422-9119, www.steubentoursberlin.com).

BY BIKE
Fat Tire Bike Tours

Choose among five different tours, which run (except where noted) from April through October (most €24, 4-6 hours, 6-10 miles): **City Tour** (March-Nov daily at 11:00, May-Sept also daily at 16:00, Dec-Feb Wed and Sat at 11:00), **Berlin Wall Tour** (Mon, Thu, Sat, and Sun at 10:30), **Third Reich Tour** (Wed, Fri, Sat, and Sun at 10:30), and **"Raw" Tour** (countercultural, creative aspects of contemporary Berlin, Tue, Fri, and Sun at 10:30). For any tour, meet at the TV Tower at Alexanderplatz (reserve ahead except for City Tour, tel. 030/2404-7991, www.fattirebiketours.com).

BY BOAT
Spree River Cruises

Several boat companies offer one-hour, €13 trips up and down the river. A relaxing hour on one of these boats can be time and money well spent. You'll listen to excellent English audioguides, see lots of wonderful new government-commissioned architecture, and enjoy the lively park action fronting the river. Boats leave from various

BERLIN

docks that cluster near the bridge at the Berlin Cathedral (just off Unter den Linden). I enjoyed the Historical Sightseeing Cruise from **Stern und Kreisschiffahrt** (mid-March-Nov daily 10:00-19:00, leaves from Nikolaiviertel Dock—cross bridge from Berlin Cathedral toward Alexanderplatz

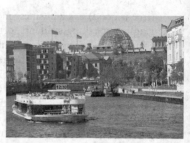

and look right, tel. 030/536-3600, www.sternundkreis.de). Confirm that the boat you choose comes with English commentary.

Sights in Berlin

The following sights are arranged roughly west to east, from the Reichstag down Unter den Linden to Alexanderplatz. I've linked these sights in a convenient, self-guided walk that I call the **"Best of Berlin"**—allow about 1.5 hours without stops for sightseeing (see map on page 606.) Adding tours of several sights can easily fill a whole day. Remember that reservations are required for the Reichstag dome, and you'd be wise to get a timed-entry ticket for the Pergamon Museum.

Also described here are sights to the south and north of Unter den Linden.

• *Start your walk in front of the Reichstag building in the big, grassy park called Platz der Republik, with its full-on view of the glass-domed...*

▲▲▲REICHSTAG

The parliament building—the heart of German democracy—has a short but complicated and emotional history. When it was inaugu-

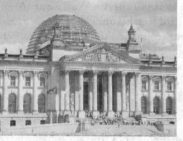

rated in the 1890s, the last emperor, Kaiser Wilhelm II, disdainfully called it the "chatting home for monkeys" *(Reichsaffenhaus).* It was placed outside the city's old walls—far from the center of real power, the imperial palace. But it was from the Reichstag that the German Republic was proclaimed in 1918. Look above the door, surrounded by stone patches from WWII bomb damage, to see the motto and promise: *Dem Deutschen Volke* ("To the German People").

In 1933, this symbol of democracy nearly burned down. The

Nazis—whose influence on the German political scene was on the rise—blamed a communist plot. A Dutch communist, Marinus van der Lubbe, was eventually convicted and guillotined for the crime. Others believed that Hitler himself planned the fire, using it as a handy excuse to frame the communists and grab power. Even though Van der Lubbe was posthumously pardoned by the German government in 2008, most modern historians concede that he most likely was guilty, and had acted alone—the timing was just incredibly fortuitous for the Nazis, who shrewdly used his deed to advance their cause.

The Reichstag was hardly used from 1933 to 1999. Despite the fact that the building had lost its symbolic value, Stalin ordered his troops to take the Reichstag from the Nazis no later than May 1, 1945 (the date of the workers' May Day parade in Moscow). More than 1,500 Nazi soldiers made their last stand here—extending World War II by two days. On April 30, after fierce fighting on its rooftop, the Reichstag fell to the Red Army.

For the building's 101st birthday in 1995, the Bulgarian-American artist Christo wrapped it in silvery gold cloth. It was then wrapped again—in scaffolding—and rebuilt by British architect Lord Norman Foster into the new parliamentary home of the Bundestag (Germany's lower house, similar to the US House of Representatives). In 1999, the German parliament convened here for the first time in 66 years. To many Germans, the proud resurrection of the Reichstag symbolizes the end of a terrible chapter in their country's history.

The **glass cupola** rises 155 feet above the ground. Its two sloped ramps spiral 755 feet to the top for a grand view. Inside the dome, a cone of 360 mirrors reflects natural light into the legislative chamber below. Lit from inside after dark, this gives Berlin a memorable nightlight. The environmentally friendly cone—with an opening at the top—also helps with air circulation, expelling stale air from the legislative chamber (no joke) and pulling in fresh, cool air.

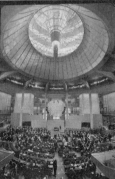

Cost and Hours: Free, but reservations required—see below, daily 8:00-24:00, last entry at 22:00, metal detectors, no big luggage allowed, Platz der Republik 1; S- or U-Bahn: Friedrichstrasse, Brandenburger Tor, or Bundestag; tel. 030/2273-2152, www.bundestag.de.

Reservations: To visit the dome, you'll need to **reserve online** (free); spots often book up several days in advance. Go

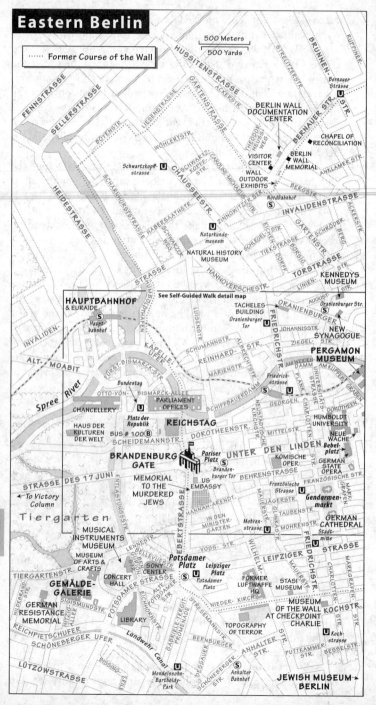

Eastern Berlin

...... Former Course of the Wall

500 Meters
500 Yards

FENNSTRASSE

SELLERSTRASSE

HEIDESTRASSE

HUSSITENSTRASSE

GARTENSTRASSE

ACKERSTR

BOYENSTR

LIESENSTRASSE

WOHLERTSTR.

SCHWARTZKOPF-STR.

CAROLINE-MICHAELIS-STR.

CHAUSSEESTR

Schwartzkopff-strasse U

SCHARNHORSTRASSE

SCHWARZER WEG

HABERSAATHSTR

ZINNOWITZER STR.

STRASSE

STREITZELSTR.

BRUNNEN STR.

RUPPINER

Bernauer Strasse

BERNAUER STR. U U

BERLIN WALL DOCUMENTATION CENTER

THEODOR-HEUSS-WEG

CHAPEL OF RECONCILIATION ◆

VISITOR CENTER

BERLIN WALL MEMORIAL ◆

WALL OUTDOOR EXHIBITS

ANKLAMER STR.

BERGSTR.

Nordbahnhof S

INVALIDENSTRASSE

EICHENDORFFSTR.

SCHLEGELSTR.

TIECKSTR.

BORSIG

ACKERSTR.

GARTENSTR.

SCHRÖDER

BERG

TORSTRASSE

STR.

KENNEDYS MUSEUM

HAUPTBAHNHOF & EURAIDE

Hauptbahnhof

INVALIDEN-STRASSE

ALT- MOABIT

Spree River

CHANCELLERY

HAUS DER KULTUREN DER WELT

STRASSE DES 17 JUNI

← To Victory Column

Tiergarten

TIERGARTENSTR.

GEMÄLDE-GALERIE

GERMAN RESISTANCE MEMORIAL

REICHPIETSCHUFER

SCHÖNEBERGER UFER

LÜTZOWSTRASSE

HUMBOLDTHAFEN

Naturkunde-museum

NATURAL HISTORY MUSEUM

HANNOVERSCHESTR.

LUISENSTR.

STRASSE

KAPELLE UFER

FÜRST-BISMARCK-STR.

OTTO-VON- BISMARCK-ALLEE

Bundestag

U

PARLIAMENT OFFICES

Platz der Republik

BUS #100 B

SCHEIDEMANNSTR.

REICHSTAG

BRANDENBURG GATE

MEMORIAL TO THE MURDERED JEWS

EBERTSTRASSE

PAULSTRASSE

MUSICAL INSTRUMENTS MUSEUM

MUSEUM OF ARTS & CRAFTS

CONCERT HALL

BENDLER

SIGISMUNDSTR.

HITZIGALLEE

STAUFFENBERGSTR.

LENNESTR.

BELLEVUESTR.

ALTE POTSDAMER STRASSE

POTSDAMER STRASSE

LINKSTR.

EICHHORNSTR.

LIBRARY

BISSINGZEILE

See Self-Guided Walk detail map

SCHUMANNSTR.

REINHARD-STR.

MARIENSTR.

ALBRECHTSTR.

FRIEDRICHSTR.

ZIEGEL

TACHELES BUILDING

Oranienburger Tor U

JOHANNISSTR.

AM WEIDEN-DAMM

Friedrich-strasse S

Oranienburger Str.

ORANIENBURGER STR.

ORANIENBURGER STR.

NEW SYNAGOGUE

PERGAMON MUSEUM

AM KUPFER-GRABEN

SCHIFFBAUERDAMM

GEORGEN-

PLANCK

CHARLOTTEN STR.

UNIVERSITÄTS STR.

DOROTHEEN-STR.

HUMBOLDT UNIVERSITY

NEUE WACHE

Bebel-platz

GERMAN STATE OPERA

KOMISCHE OPER

UNTER DEN LINDEN

Brandenburger Tor S

Pariser Platz

BEHRENSTRASSE

US EMBASSY

HANNAH-ARENDT-STR.

IN DEN MINISTER-GARTEN

Mohren-strasse U

VOSS-STR.

WILHELM STR.

Potsdamer Platz S

Leipziger Platz

Potsdamer Platz U

SONY CENTER

GABRIELE-TERGIT-PROMENADE

STRESEMANNSTR.

NIEDER-KIRCH-

BERNBURGER STR.

DESSAUER STR.

SCHÖNEBERGER STR.

Mendelssohn-Bartholdy-Park U

Anhalter Bahnhof S

Landwehr Canal

MITTELSTR.

NUSTADTISCHE KIRCHSTR.

DOROTHEENSTR.

MAUERSTR.

JÄGERSTR.

TAUBENSTR.

MOHRENSTR.

GLINKASTR.

Französische Strasse U

FRANZÖSISCHE STR.

Gendarmen-markt

GERMAN CATHEDRAL

Stadt-mitte U

LEIPZIGER STR.

FORMER LUFTWAFFE HQ

TOPOGRAPHY OF TERROR

ANHALTER STR.

DOROTHEEN

MARGRAFEN-STR.

FRANZÖSISCHE STR.

CHARLOTTENSTR.

FRIEDRICHSTR.

STRASSE

STASI MUSEUM

MUSEUM OF THE WALL AT CHECKPOINT CHARLIE

MAUERSTR.

PUTTKAMMER-STR.

KOCHSTR.

Koch-strasse U

BESSELSTR.

JEWISH MUSEUM BERLIN →

See Self-Guided Walk detail map

BERLIN

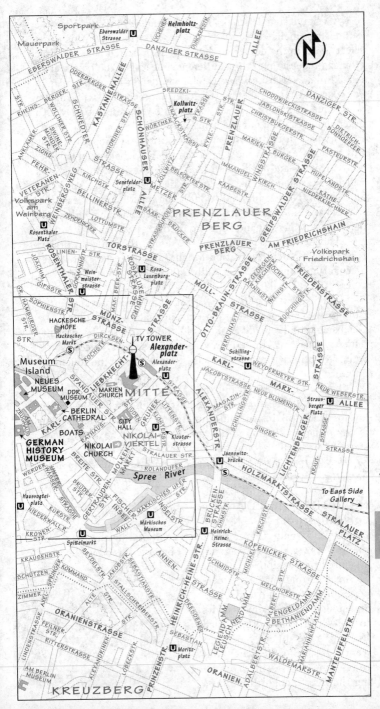

to www.bundestag.de, click "English" and—from the "Visit the Bundestag" menu—select "Online registration." On this page, select "Visit to the dome" to choose your preferred date and time (you can request up to three different time slots). You'll be sent an email link to a website where you'll enter details for each person in your party. After completing this form, another email will confirm your request, and a final email will contain your reservation (with a letter you must print out and bring with you).

If you're in Berlin without a reservation, try dropping by the tiny visitors center on the Tiergarten side of Scheidemannstrasse, across from Platz der Republik. A screen in its window shows which hourly slots still have tickets available (open daily April-Oct 8:00-20:00, Nov-March 8:00-18:00; you must book no less than 2 hours and no more than 2 days out; when booking, the whole party must be present and ID is required).

Another option for visiting the dome, though a bit pricey, is to make a lunch reservation for the rooftop restaurant, Käfer Dachgarten (lunches €22-25, daily 9:00-16:30 & 18:30-24:00, last access at 22:00, call 030/2262-9933 well in advance).

Getting In: Report a few minutes before your appointed time to the temporary-looking entrance facility in front of the Reichstag, and be ready to show ID and your reservation print-out. After passing through an airport-like security check, you'll wait with other visitors for a guard to take you to the Reichstag entrance.

Tours: Pick up the English **"Outlooks" flier** when you exit the elevator at the top of the Reichstag. The free GPS-driven **audioguide** explains the building and narrates the view as you wind up the spiral ramp to the top of the dome; the commentary starts automatically as you step onto the bottom of the ramp.

• *Facing the front of the Reichstag, you can take a short side-trip to the Spree River by circling around to the left of the building.*

NEAR THE REICHSTAG
Spree Riverfront

Admire the wonderful architecture incorporating the river into the people's world. It's a poignant spot because this river was once a symbol of division—the East German regime put nets underwater to stymie those desperate enough for freedom to swim to the West. When kings ruled Prussia, government buildings went right up to the water. But today, the city is incorporating the river thoughtfully into a

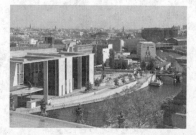

people-friendly cityscape. From the Reichstag, a delightful riverside path leads around the curve, past "beach cafés," to the riverbank behind the Chancellery. For a slow, low-impact glide past this zone, consider a river cruise, which starts from Museum Island (for more on these cruises, see page 593). The fine bridges symbolize the connection of East and West.

• *Back in front of the Reichstag, face the building and walk to the right. Near the road in front of the Reichstag, enmeshed in all the security apparatus and crowds, is a memorial of slate stones embedded in the ground.*

Memorial to Politicians Who Opposed Hitler

This row of slabs, which looks like a fancy slate bicycle rack, is a memorial to the 96 members of the Reichstag (the equivalent

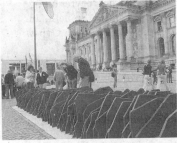

of our members of Congress) who were persecuted and murdered because their politics didn't agree with Chancellor Hitler's. They were part of the Weimar Republic, the weak and ill-fated attempt at post-WWI democracy in Germany. These were the people who could have stopped Hitler...so they became his first victims. Each slate slab memorializes one man—his name, party (mostly KPD—Communists, and SPD—Social Democrats), and the date and location of his death—generally in concentration camps. (*KZ* stands for "concentration camp.") They are honored here, in front of the building in which they worked.

• *Walk along the side of the Reichstag, on busy Scheidemannstrasse, toward the rear of the building. At the intersection with Ebertstrasse, cross to the right (toward the park). Along a railing is a small memorial of white crosses. This is the...*

Berlin Wall Victims Memorial

This monument commemorates some of the East Berliners who died trying to cross the Wall. Many of them perished within months of the Wall's construction on August 13, 1961. Most died

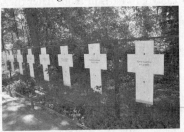

trying to swim the river to freedom. The monument used to stand right on the Berlin Wall behind the Reichstag. Notice that the last person killed while trying to escape was 20-year-old Chris Gueffroy, who died nine months before the Wall fell in 1989. (He was shot through the heart in no-man's land.) For more on the Wall, see "The Berlin Wall (and Its Fall)" sidebar on page 626.

• *Continue along Ebertstrasse (away from the Reichstag) for a few more steps and turn into the peaceful lane on the right (into Tiergarten park). Within a short distance, on your right, is the...*

Monument to the Murdered Sinti and Roma (Gypsies) of Europe

Unveiled in 2012, this memorial remembers the roughly 500,000 Sinti and Roma victims of the Holocaust. Enter through the rusty steel portal. On the other side is a circular reflecting pool surrounded by stone slabs, some containing the names of the death camps where hundreds of thousands of Sinti and Roma perished. In the water along the rim of the pool is the heart-wrenching poem "Auschwitz," by composer and writer Santino Spinelli, an Italian Roma. Dissonant music evoking the tragedy of the Gypsy genocide adds to the atmosphere.

• *Retrace your steps to Ebertstrasse and turn right, toward the busy intersection dominated by the imposing Brandenburg Gate. As you cross the street toward the gate, notice the double row of **cobblestones** beneath your feet—it goes about 25 miles around the city, marking where the Wall used to stand. Then walk under the gate that, for a sad generation, was part of a wall that divided this city.*

BRANDENBURG GATE AND NEARBY
▲▲▲Brandenburg Gate (Brandenburger Tor)

The historic Brandenburg Gate (1791) was the grandest—and is the last survivor—of 14 gates in Berlin's old city wall (this one led to the neighboring city of Brandenburg). The gate was the symbol of Prussian Berlin—and later the symbol of a divided Berlin. It's crowned by a majestic four-horse chariot, with the Goddess of Peace at the reins. Napoleon took this statue to the Louvre in Paris in 1806. After the Prussians defeated Napoleon and

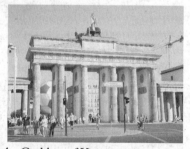

got it back (1813), she was renamed the Goddess of Victory.

The gate sat unused, part of a sad circle dance called the Wall, for more than 25 years. Now postcards all over town show the ecstatic day—November 9, 1989—when the world rejoiced at the sight of happy Berliners jamming the gate like flowers on a parade float. Pause a minute and think about struggles for freedom—past and present. (There's actually a special room built into the gate for this purpose.) Around the gate, look at the information boards with pictures of how this area changed throughout the 20th century. There's a TI within the gate (S-Bahn: Brandenburger Tor).

The gate sits on a major boulevard running east to west through Berlin. The western segment, called Strasse des 17 Juni (named for a workers' uprising against the DDR government on June 17, 1953), stretches for four miles from the Brandenburg Gate past the Victory Column to the Olympic Stadium. But we'll follow this city axis in the opposite direction, east, along Unter den Linden. The walk takes us into the core of old imperial Berlin and past the site where the palace of the Hohenzollern family, rulers of Prussia and then Germany, once stood. The palace is a phantom sight, long gone, but its occupants were responsible for just about all you'll see. Alexanderplatz, which marks the end of this walk, is near the base of the giant TV Tower hovering in the distance.

• *Pass all the way through the gate and stand in the middle of...*

▲Pariser Platz

"Parisian Square," so named after the Prussians defeated Napoleon in 1813, was once filled with important government buildings—all bombed to smithereens in World War II. For decades, it was an unrecognizable, deserted no-man's-land—cut off from both East and West by the Wall. But now it's rebuilt, and the banks, hotels, and embassies that were here before the bombing have reclaimed their original places—with a few additions, including a palace of coffee: Starbucks. The winners of World War II enjoy this prime real estate: The American, French, British, and Soviet (now Russian) embassies are all on or near this square.

As you face the gate, to your right is the French Embassy, and to your left is the **US Embassy.** This reopened in its historic pre-WWII location in 2008. The rebuilt building has been controversial: For safety's sake, Uncle Sam wanted more of a security zone around the building, but the Germans wanted to keep Pariser Platz a welcoming people zone. (Throughout the world, American embassies are the most fortified buildings in town.) The compromise: The extra security the US wanted is built into the structure.

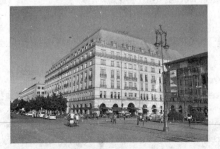

Easy-on-the-eyes barriers keep potential car bombs at a distance, and its front door is on the side farthest from the Brandenburg Gate.

Turn your back to the gate. On the right, jutting into the square, is the ritzy **Hotel Adlon,** long called home by visiting stars and

VIPs. In its heyday, it hosted such notables as Charlie Chaplin, Albert Einstein, and Greta Garbo. Damaged by the Russians just after World War II, the original hotel was closed with the construction of the nearby Wall in 1961 and later demolished. Today's grand Adlon was rebuilt in 1997. It was here that Michael Jackson shocked millions by dangling his baby, Blanket, over the railing (second balcony up).

• *Between the hotel and the US Embassy are two buildings worth a quick visit: the DZ Bank building (by Frank Gehry) and the glassy Academy of Arts. Enjoy the fun-loving scene on the square, and when you're ready to move on, work your way over to these two buildings; we'll enter both, then leave Pariser Platz through the Academy of Arts.*

DZ Bank Building: This building's architect, Frank Gehry, is famous for Bilbao's Guggenheim Museum, Prague's Dancing House, Seattle's Experience Music Project, Chicago's Millennium Park, and Los Angeles' Walt Disney Concert Hall. Gehry fans might be surprised at the bank building's low profile. Structures on Pariser Platz are designed so as not to draw attention away from the Brandenburg Gate. But to get your fix of wild and colorful Gehry, step into the lobby. Built in 2001 as an office complex and conference center, its undulating interior is like a big, slithery fish. Gehry explained, "The form of the fish is the best example of movement. I try to capture this movement in my buildings." For more of the architect's vision, read the nearby plaque.

• *Leaving the DZ Bank, turn right and head into the next building, the...*

Academy of Arts (Akademie der Künste): The glassy arcade is open daily (10:00-22:00, WC in basement, café serving light meals). Just past the café is the office where Albert Speer, Hitler's architect, planned the rebuilding of postwar Berlin into "Welthauptstadt Germania"—the grandiose "world capital" of Nazi Europe. Pass through the glass door to see Speer's favorite statue, *Prometheus Bound* (c. 1900). This is the kind of art that turned Hitler on: a strong, soldierly, vital man, enduring hardship for a greater cause. Anticipating the bombs, Speer had the statue bricked up in the basement here where it lay, undiscovered, until 1995.

This building provides a handy and interesting passage to the Holocaust memorial on the other side.

• *Exit the building out the back. Across the street, to the right, stretches the vast Holocaust memorial.*

▲▲Memorial to the Murdered Jews of Europe (Denkmal für die Ermordeten Juden Europas)

This Holocaust memorial, consisting of 2,711 gravestone-like pillars (called "stelae") and completed in 2005, was the first formal, German government-sponsored Holocaust memorial. Using the

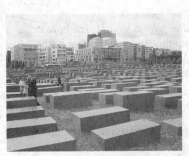

word "murdered" in the title was intentional and a big deal. Germany, as a nation, was officially admitting to a crime. Jewish-American architect Peter Eisenman won the competition for the commission.

Cost and Hours: The memorial is free and always open. The information center is open Tue-Sun 10:00-20:00, Oct-March until 19:00, closed Mon year-round; last entry 45 minutes before closing, S-Bahn: Brandenburger Tor or Potsdamer Platz, tel. 030/2639-4336, www.stiftung-denkmal. de. The €4 audioguide augments the experience.

Visiting the Memorial: The pillars, made of hollow concrete, stand in a gently sunken area, which can be entered from any side. The number of pillars isn't symbolic of anything; it's simply how many fit on the provided land. The pillars are all about the same size, but of differing heights. The memorial's location—where the Wall once stood—is coincidental. Nazi propagandist Joseph Goebbels' bunker was discovered during the work and left buried under the northeast corner of the memorial.

Once you enter the memorial, notice that people seem to appear and disappear between the columns, and that no matter where you are, the exit always seems to be up. The monument has been criticized because there's nothing intrinsically Jewish about it. Some were struck that there's no central gathering point or place for a ceremony. Like death, you enter it alone. There is no one intended interpretation. Is it a symbolic cemetery, or an intentionally disorienting labyrinth? It's up to the visitor to derive the meaning, while pondering this horrible chapter in human history.

After wandering through the memorial, go under the field of concrete pillars to the state-of-the-art **information center.** Inside, a thought-provoking exhibit (well-explained in English) studies the Nazi system of extermination and humanizes the victims, while also providing space for silent reflection.

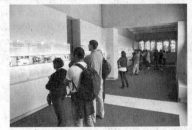

BERLIN

• *Wander through the gray pillars, but eventually emerge on the corner with the Information Center. Cross Hannah-Arendt-Strasse and go a half block farther. Walk alongside the rough parking lot (on the left side of street) to the info plaque over the...*

Site of Hitler's Bunker

More than six decades after the end of World War II, the bunker where Adolf Hitler killed himself lies hidden underneath a Berlin parking lot. While the Churchill War Rooms are a major sight in London, no one wants to turn Hitler's final stronghold into a major tourist attraction.

You're standing atop the buried remains of the *Führerbunker*. In early 1945, as Allied armies advanced on Berlin and Nazi Germany lay in ruins, Hitler and his staff retreated to a bunker complex behind the former Reich Chancellery. He stayed there for two months. It was here, as the Soviet army tightened its noose on the capital, that Hitler and Eva Braun, his wife of less than 48 hours, committed suicide on April 30, 1945. A week later, the war in Europe was over. The info board presents a detailed cutaway illustration of the bunker complex plus a timeline tracing its history and ultimate fate (the roof was removed and the bunker filled with dirt, then covered over).

• *From here, you can visit the next memorial (though a bit of a detour), or you can continue the walk. To do either, first head back to Hannah-Arendt-Strasse. To rejoin the walk, turn right, go one block, then head up Wilhelmstrasse back to Unter den Linden. To see the memorial, go left one block at Hannah-Arendt-Strasse, cross the street, and head down a path into Tiergarten park. There, look for a large, dark gray concrete box...*

Memorial to the Homosexuals Persecuted Under the National Socialist Regime

At this stark memorial find the small window through which you can watch a black-and-white film loop of same-sex couples kissing. The message: Life and love are precious, regardless of who we are. The law against homosexuality in Germany had been on the books since 1850, and Hitler enforced it with brutality. Signage by the sidewalk explains the memorial in English and German.

• *Now return to Unter den Linden by backtracking a couple of blocks down Hannah-Arendt-Strasse, then turning left on Wilhelmstrasse. Because Wilhelmstrasse was a main street of the German government during WWII, it was obliterated by bombs, and all its buildings are new today. The pedestrianized part of the street is home to the British Embassy. The fun, purple color of its wall is the colors of the Union Jack mixed together.*

When you get back on Unter den Linden, stand in the median, in front of Hotel Adlon.

SIGHTS ALONG UNTER DEN LINDEN

Unter den Linden, worth ▲▲, is the heart of the former East Berlin. In the good old days, this was one of Europe's grand boulevards. In the 15th century, this carriageway led from the palace to the hunting grounds (today's big Tiergarten). In the 17th century, Hohenzollern princes and princesses moved in and built their palaces here so they could be near the Prussian king.

Named centuries ago for its thousands of linden trees, this was the most elegant street of Prussian Berlin before Hitler's time,

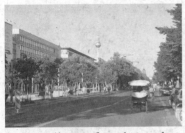

and the main drag of East Berlin after his reign. Hitler replaced the venerable trees—many 250 years old—with Nazi flags. Popular discontent drove him to replant the trees.

Today, Unter den Linden is no longer a depressing Cold War cul-de-sac, and its pre-Hitler strolling café ambience has returned. It is divided, roughly at Friedrichstrasse, into a business section, which stretches toward the Brandenburg Gate, and a cultural section, which spreads out toward Alexanderplatz. Frederick the Great wanted to have culture, mainly the opera and the university, closer to his palace and to keep business (read: banks) farther away, near the city walls.

• *Begin walking toward the giant TV Tower. In front of Hotel Adlon is the Brandenburger Tor S-Bahn station. Cover a bit of Unter den Linden underground by climbing down its steps and walking along the platform.*

Ghost Subway Station: The Brandenburger Tor S-Bahn station is one of Berlin's former ghost subway stations. During the Cold War, most underground train tunnels were simply blocked at the border. But a few Western lines looped through the East and then back into the West. To make a little hard Western cash, the Eastern government rented the use of these tracks to the West, but all but one of the stations in East Berlin were strictly off-limits. For 28 years, these stations were unused, as Western trains slowly passed through and passengers saw only

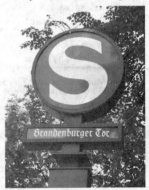

eerie DDR (East German) guards and lots of cobwebs. Literally within days of the fall of the Wall, these stations were reopened, and today they are a time warp, looking much as they did when built in 1931, with dreary old green tiles and original signage on ticket kiosks.

• *Walk along the track (the walls are lined with historic photos of the*

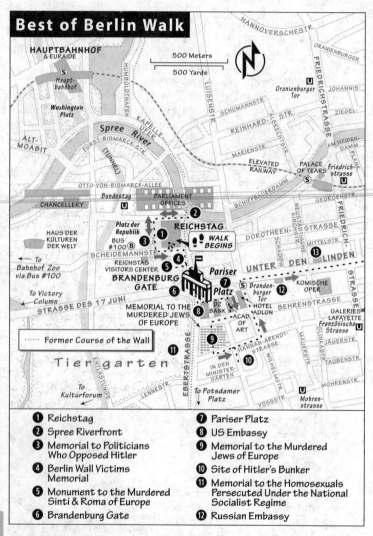

Best of Berlin Walk

1 Reichstag
2 Spree Riverfront
3 Memorial to Politicians Who Opposed Hitler
4 Berlin Wall Victims Memorial
5 Monument to the Murdered Sinti & Roma of Europe
6 Brandenburg Gate
7 Pariser Platz
8 US Embassy
9 Memorial to the Murdered Jews of Europe
10 Site of Hitler's Bunker
11 Memorial to the Homosexuals Persecuted Under the National Socialist Regime
12 Russian Embassy

Reichstag through the ages) and exit on the other side, to the right. You'll pop out at the Russian Embassy's front yard.

Russian Embassy: This was the first big postwar building project in East Berlin. It's built in the powerful, simplified Neoclassical style that Stalin liked. While not as important now as it was a few years ago, it's as immense as ever. It flies the Russian white, blue, and red. Find the hammer-and-sickle motif decorating the window frames—a reminder of the days when Russia was the USSR.

• *At the next intersection (Glinkastrasse), cross to the other side of Unter*

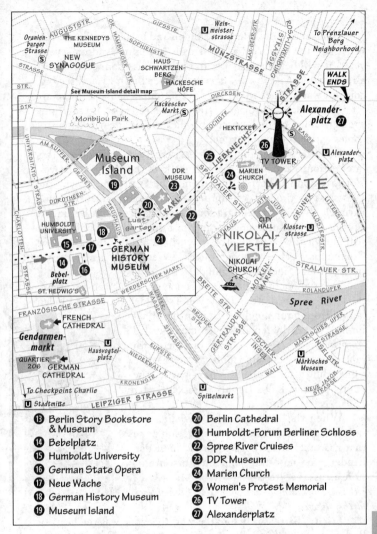

13 Berlin Story Bookstore & Museum	**20** Berlin Cathedral
14 Bebelplatz	**21** Humboldt-Forum Berliner Schloss
15 Humboldt University	**22** Spree River Cruises
16 German State Opera	**23** DDR Museum
17 Neue Wache	**24** Marien Church
18 German History Museum	**25** Women's Protest Memorial
19 Museum Island	**26** TV Tower
	27 Alexanderplatz

den Linden. At #40 is the entertaining...

Berlin Story Bookstore and Museum: Berlin Story is two shops side by side (on the left are Cold War souvenirs and the museum; on the right, the bookstore). The bookshop has just about the best range anywhere of English-language titles on Berlin (Mon-Sat 10:00-19:00, Sun 10:00-18:00). They have also created a beefy little museum covering the main points of modern Berlin history and a video about the Wall. It offers a vivid swing through the tumultuous story of this city (€5, or €4 with this book, includes good audioguide, daily 10:00-20:00, until 19:00 in Jan-Feb).

• *A few steps farther down is the...*

Intersection of Unter den Linden and Friedrichstrasse: This is perhaps the most central crossroads in Berlin. And for several years, it will be a mess as Berlin builds a new connection in its already extensive subway system. All over Berlin, you'll see big, colorful **water pipes** running aboveground. Wherever there are large construction projects, streets are laced with these drainage pipes. Berlin's high water table means that any new basement comes with lots of pumping out.

Looking at the jaunty DDR-style pedestrian lights at this intersection is a reminder that very little of the old East survives. Construction has been a theme since the Wall came down. The West lost no time in consuming the East; consequently, some have felt a wave of *Ost***-algia** for the old days of East Berlin. At election time, a surprising number of formerly East Berlin voters still opt for the extreme left party, which has ties to the bygone Communist Party—although the East-West divide is no longer at the forefront of most voters' minds.

One symbol of that communist era has been given a reprieve: the DDR-style pedestrian lights you'll see along Unter den Linden (and throughout much of the former East 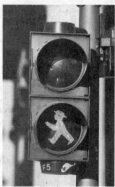 Berlin). The perky red and green men—called *Ampelmännchen*—were once threatened with replacement by far less jaunty Western-style signs. But, after a 10-year court battle, the wildly popular DDR signals were kept after all.

When the little green *Ampelmännchen* says you can go, cross the construction zone that has taken over this stretch of Unter den Linden, and note the Ampelmann souvenir store across the street.

• *Before continuing down Unter den Linden, look farther down...*

Friedrichstrasse: Before the war, this zone was the heart of Berlin. In the 1920s, Berlin was famous for its anything-goes love of life. This was the cabaret drag, a springboard to stardom for young and vampy entertainers like Marlene Dietrich. (Born in 1901, Dietrich starred in the first major German talkie—*The Blue Angel*—and then headed straight to Hollywood.) Over the last few years, this boulevard—lined with super-department stores (such as Galeries Lafayette) and big-time hotels (such as the Hilton and Regent)—is attempting to replace western Berlin's Ku'damm as the grand commerce-and-café boulevard of Berlin. More recently, western Berlin is retaliating with some new stores of its own. And so far, Friedrichstrasse gets little more than half the pedestrian traffic that Ku'damm gets in the West. Why? Locals complain that this area has no daily life—no supermarkets, not much ethnic street food, and so on.

Consider detouring to Galeries Lafayette, with its cool marble-and-glass, waste-of-space interior (Mon-Sat 10:00-20:00, closed Sun; check out the vertical garden on its front wall, belly up to its amazing ground-floor viewpoint, or have lunch in its recommended basement food court). The short walk there along Friedrichstrasse provides some of Berlin's most jarring old-versus-new architectural contrasts—be sure to look up as you stroll. If you continued down Friedrichstrasse, you'd wind up at sights listed under "South of Unter den Linden," on page 619—including **Checkpoint Charlie** (a 10-minute walk from here).

• *For now, continue down Unter den Linden a few more blocks, past the large equestrian statue of Frederick the Great, then turn right into...*

Bebelplatz

Walk to the center of the square, and find the glass window in the pavement. For centuries, up until the early 1700s, Prussia had been likened to a modern-day Sparta—it was all about its military. Voltaire famously said, "Whereas some states have an army, the Prussian army has a state." But Frederick the Great—who ruled from 1740 to 1786—established Prussia not just as a military power, but also as a cultural and intellectual heavyweight. This square was the center of the cultural capital that Frederick envisioned. His grand palace was just down the street (explained later).

Imagine that it's 1760. Pan around the square to see Frederick's

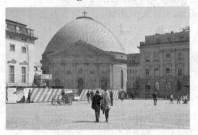

contributions to Prussian culture. Everything is draped with Greek-inspired Prussian pomp. Sure, Prussia was a modern-day Sparta. But Frederick also built an **"Athens on the Spree"**—an enlightened and cultured society.

To visually survey the square, start with the university across the street and spin counterclockwise:

Humboldt University, across Unter den Linden, is one of Europe's greatest. Marx and Lenin (not the brothers or the sisters) studied here, as did the Grimms (both brothers) and more than two dozen Nobel Prize winners. Einstein, who was Jewish, taught here until taking a spot at Princeton in 1932 (smart guy). Used-book merchants set up their tables in front of the university.

Turn 90 degrees to the left. The former **state library** (labeled *Juristische Fakultät*) is where Vladimir Lenin studied law during much of his exile from Russia. Bombed in WWII, the library was rebuilt by the East German government in the original style only because Lenin studied here. If you climb to the second floor of the library and go through the door opposite the stairs, you'll see a 1968 vintage stained-glass window depicting Lenin's life's work with almost biblical reverence. On the ground floor is Tim's Espressobar, a great little café with light food, student prices, and garden seating (€3 plates, Mon-Fri 8:00-20:00, Sat 9:00-17:00, closed Sun, handy WC).

Next to the library, the square is closed by one of Berlin's swankiest lodgings—**Hotel de Rome,** housed in a historic bank building with a spa and lap pool fitted into the former vault.

The round, Catholic **St. Hedwig's Church,** nicknamed the "upside-down teacup," is a statement of religious and cultural tolerance. The pragmatic Frederick the Great wanted to encourage the integration of Catholic Silesians after his empire annexed their region in 1742, and so the first Catholic church since the Reformation was built in Berlin. (St. Hedwig is the patron saint of Silesia, a region now shared by Germany, Poland, and the Czech Republic.) Like all Catholic churches in Berlin, St. Hedwig's is not on the street, but stuck in a kind of back lot—indicating inferiority to Protestant churches. You can step inside the church to see the cheesy DDR government renovation (generally daily until 17:00).

The **German State Opera** was bombed in 1941, rebuilt to bolster morale and to celebrate its centennial in 1943, and bombed again in 1945. It's currently undergoing an extensive renovation.

Now look down through the glass you're standing on: The room of empty bookshelves is a memorial repudiating the notorious Nazi **book burning.** It was on this square in 1933 that staff and students from the university threw 20,000 newly forbidden books (authored by Einstein, Hemingway, Freud, and T. S. Eliot, among others) into a huge bonfire on the orders of the Nazi propaganda minister, Joseph Goebbels. In fact, Goebbels himself tossed books onto the fire, condemning writers to the flames. He declared, "The era of extreme Jewish intellectualism has come to an end, and the German revolution has again opened the way for the true essence of being German."

The Prussian heritage of Frederick the Great was one of culture and enlightenment. Hitler chose this square to thoroughly squash those ideals, dramatically signaling that the era of tolerance and openness was over. A plaque nearby reminds us of the prophetic quote by the German poet Heinrich Heine. In 1820, he wrote, "Where they burn books, in the end they will also burn people." The Nazis despised Heine because he was a Jew who converted to Christianity. A century later, his books were among those that went up in flames on this spot.

This monument reminds us of that chilling event in 1933, while also inspiring vigilance against the anti-intellectual, scare-mongering forces of today that would burn the thoughts of people they fear to defend their culture from diversity.

• *Cross Unter den Linden to the university side. Just past the university is a Greek-temple-like building set in the small chestnut-tree-filled park. This is the...*

Neue Wache

This is the emperor's "New Guardhouse" (Neue Wache), from 1816. Converted by communist authorities in 1960 to a memorial

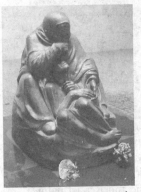

to the victims of fascism, the structure was transformed again, after the Wall fell, into a national memorial. Look inside, where a replica of the Käthe Kollwitz statue, *Mother with Her Dead Son*, is surrounded by thought-provoking silence. It marks the tombs of Germany's unknown soldier and an unknown concentration camp victim. The inscription in front reads, "To the victims of war and tyranny." Read the entire statement in English (on wall, left of entrance). The memorial, open to the sky, incorporates the elements—sunshine, rain, snow—falling on this modern-day *pietà*.

• *After the Neue Wache, the next building you'll see is Berlin's pink-yet-formidable Zeughaus (arsenal). Dating from 1695, it's considered the oldest building on the boulevard, and now houses the excellent...*

▲▲▲German History Museum (Deutsches Historisches Museum)

This fantastic museum is a two-part affair: the pink former Prussian arsenal building and the I. M. Pei-designed annex. The main building (fronting Unter den Linden) houses the permanent collection, offering the best look at German history under one roof, anywhere. The modern annex features good temporary exhibits surrounded by the work of a great contemporary architect. While this city has more than its share of hokey "museums" that slap together WWII and Cold War bric-a-brac, then charge too much for admission, this thoughtfully presented museum—with more than 8,000 artifacts telling not just the story of Berlin, but of all Germany—is clearly the top history museum in town.

Cost and Hours: €8, daily 10:00-18:00, Unter den Linden 2, tel. 030/2030-4751, www.dhm.de.

Audioguide: For the most informative visit, invest in the excellent €3 audioguide, with six hours of info to choose from.

Getting In: If the ticket-buying line is long at the main entrance, try circling around the back to the Pei annex (to reach it, head down the street to the left of the museum—called Hinter dem Giesshaus), where entry lines are usually shorter (but audioguides are available only at the main desk).

• *Continuing down Unter den Linden, you'll cross a bridge over the Spree River to reach...*

MUSEUM ISLAND (MUSEUMSINSEL)

This island is filled with some of Berlin's most impressive museums (all part of the Staatliche Museen zu Berlin). The earliest building—the Altes Museum—went up in the 1820s, and the rest of the complex began taking shape in the 1840s under King Friedrich Wilhelm IV, who envisioned the island as an oasis of culture and learning. The island's imposing Neoclassical buildings host five grand museums: the **Pergamon Museum** (classical antiquities; this is undergoing restoration and is only partially open till at least 2019); the **Neues Museum** ("New Museum," famous for its Egyptian collection with the bust of Queen Nefertiti); the **Old National Gallery** (Alte Nationalgalerie, 19th-century art, mostly German Romantic and Realist paintings); the **Altes Museum** ("Old Museum," more antiquities); and the **Bode Museum** (European statuary and paintings through the ages, coins, and Byzantine art).

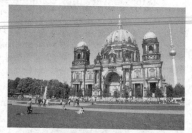

• *The museums of Museum Island are described in more detail below. On a short port visit, you may have time to sprint through one or two, but you'll have to be selective. Or, to see more of Berlin, bypass the museums and skip ahead.*

The Museums of Museum Island

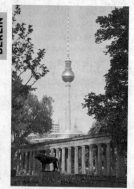

A formidable renovation is under way on Museum Island. When complete (it's hoped in 2019), a new visitors center—the James-Simon-Galerie—will link the Pergamon Museum with the Altes Museum, the Pergamon will get a fourth wing, tunnels will lace the complex together, and this will become one of the grandest museum zones in Europe. In the meantime, pardon their dust.

Cost: If you are visiting more than one museum, the €18 Museum Island

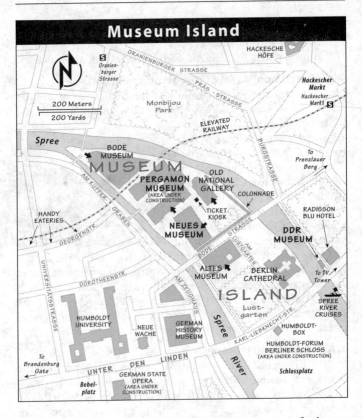

Museum Island

Pass combo-ticket—covering all five museums—is a far better value than buying individual entries (€10-14). All five museums are also included in the city's €24 Museum Pass Berlin (both passes described on page 582). Special exhibits are extra.

Hours: The Pergamon and Neues museums are open daily 10:00-18:00, with later hours on Thursday (until 20:00); the Old National Gallery, Bode Museum, and Altes Museum are open the same hours, except closed Monday.

When to Go: Mornings are busiest, and you're likely to find long lines any time of day on Saturday or Sunday. However, only the Pergamon Museum tends to have serious lines—for the other museums here, the timing of your visit isn't as critical.

Crowd-Beating Tips: Avoid the lines for the Pergamon Museum by purchasing a timed ticket online, or if you already have a Museum Pass Berlin or a Museum Island Pass (or plan to buy one), book a free timed-entry reservation (www.smb.museum). Both passes allow you to skip ticket-buying lines at the other museums on the island, but online booking is your only option for getting right to the head of the Pergamon's line.

Getting There: The nearest S-Bahn station is Hackescher Markt, about a 10-minute walk away.

Information: Tel. 030/266-424-242, www.smb.museum.

▲▲▲Pergamon Museum (Pergamonmuseum)

The star attraction of this world-class museum, part of Berlin's Collection of Classical Antiquities (Antikensammlung), is the fantastic and gigantic Pergamon Altar...which is off-limits to visitors until 2019, as the museum undergoes major renovation. But its Babylonian Ishtar Gate (slathered with glazed blue tiles from the sixth century B.C.) still makes it worth visiting, and its ancient Mesopotamian, Roman,

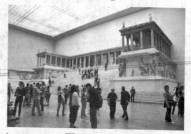

and early Islamic treasures are also impressive. The north wing is already closed (its Greek and Roman sculptures, plus some vases and bronze figurines, can be seen at the Altes Museum; the north wing's Hellenistic architecture and artworks, however, won't be seen again until 2019). Make ample use of the superb audioguide, included with admission—it will broaden your experience.

▲▲Neues (New) Museum

Oddly, Museum Island's so-called "new" museum features the oldest stuff around. There are three collections here: the Egyptian Collection (with the famous bust of Queen Nefertiti), the Museum of Prehistory and Early History, and some items from the Collection of Classical Antiquities (artifacts from ancient Troy—famously excavated by German adventurer Heinrich Schliemann—and Cyprus).

After being damaged in World War II and sitting in ruins for some 40 years, the Neues Museum has been gorgeously rebuilt. Everything is well-described by posted English information and the fine audioguide (included with admission), which celebrates new knowledge about ancient Egyptian civilization and offers fascinating insights into workaday Egyptian life as it describes the vivid papyrus collection, slice-of-life artifacts, and dreamy wax portraits decorating mummy cases (for more on the museum, see www.neues-museum.de).

The 3,000-year-old bust of **Queen Nefertiti** (the wife of King Akhenaton, c. 1340 B.C.) is the most famous piece of Egyptian art in Europe. (Note that she's had it with the paparazzi—photos of her are strictly *verboten*.) Called "Berlin's most beautiful woman," Nefertiti has all the right beauty marks: long neck, symmetrical face, and the perfect amount of makeup. And yet, she's not completely idealized. Notice the fine wrinkles that show she's human (though these only enhance her beauty). Like a movie star discreetly sipping a glass of wine at a sidewalk café, Nefertiti seems somehow more dignified in person. The bust never left its studio, but served as a master model for all other portraits of the queen. (That's probably why the left eye was never inlaid.) Stare at her long enough, and you may get the sensation that she's winking at you. Hey, beautiful!

▲Old National Gallery (Alte Nationalgalerie)

This gallery, behind the Neues Museum and Altes Museum, is designed to look like a Greek temple. Spanning three floors, it

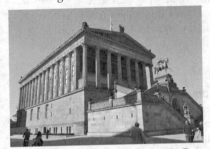

focuses on art (mostly paintings) from the 19th century: Romantic German paintings (which I find most interesting) on the top floor, and French and German Impressionists and German Realists on the first and second floors. You likely won't recognize any specific paintings, but it's still an enjoyable stroll through German culture from the century in which that notion first came to mean something. The included audioguide explains the highlights.

Bode Museum

At the "prow" of Museum Island, the Bode Museum (designed to appear as if it's rising up from the river) is worth a brief stop. Just inside, a grand statue of Frederick William of Brandenburg on horseback, curly locks blowing in the wind, welcomes you into the lonely halls of the museum. This fine building contains a hodgepodge of collections: Byzantine art, historic coins, ecclesiastical art, sculptures, and medals commemorating the fall of the Berlin Wall and German reunification. For a free, quick look at its lavish interior, climb the grand staircase to the charming café on the first floor.

Altes (Old) Museum

Perhaps the least interesting of the five museums, this building features the rest of the Collection of Classical Antiquities—namely, Etruscan, Roman, and Greek art. It also contains Greek and Roman sculptures, vases, and some bronze figurines from the currently closed north wing of the Pergamon Museum.

Other Sights on and near Museum Island

In addition to the five museums just described, Museum Island is home to the following sights. One more sight (the DDR Museum) sits just across the river.

BERLIN

Lustgarten

For 300 years, the island's big central square has flip-flopped between being a military parade ground and a people-friendly park, depending upon the political tenor of the time. During the revolutions of 1848, the Kaiser's troops dispersed a protesting crowd that had assembled here, sending demonstrators onto footpaths. Karl Marx later commented, "It is impossible to have a revolution in a country where people stay off the grass."

Hitler enjoyed giving speeches from the top of the museum steps overlooking this square. In fact, he had the square landscaped to fit his symmetrical tastes and propaganda needs.

In 1999, the Lustgarten was made into a park (read the history posted in the corner opposite the church). On a sunny day, it's packed with people relaxing and is one of Berlin's most enjoyable public spaces.

• *The huge church on Museum Island is the...*

Berlin Cathedral (Berliner Dom)

This century-old church's bombastic Wilhelmian architecture is a Protestant assertion of strength. (Aside from the cathedral, another big example of Wilhelmian architecture in Berlin is the Reichstag—which we saw earlier.) The church is most impressive from the outside, and there's no way to even peek inside without a pricey ticket.

Inside, the great reformers (Luther, Calvin, and company) stand around the brilliantly restored dome like stern saints guarding their theology. Frederick I (Frederick the Great's gramps) rests in an ornate tomb (right transept, near entrance to dome). The 270-step climb to the outdoor dome gallery is tough but offers pleasant, breezy views of the city at the finish line. The crypt downstairs is not worth a look.

Cost and Hours: €7 includes access to dome gallery, not covered by Museum Island ticket, Mon-Sat 9:00-20:00, Sun 12:00-20:00, until 19:00 Oct-March, closes early—around 17:30—on some days for concerts, interior closed but dome open during services, audioguide-€3, tel. 030/2026-9136, www.berliner-dom.de.

• *Kitty-corner across Unter den Linden from the Berlin Cathedral is a huge construction site, known as the...*

Humboldt-Forum Berliner Schloss

For centuries, this was the site of the Baroque palace of the Hohenzollern dynasty of Brandenburg and Prussia. Much of that palace actually survived World War II but was replaced by the communists with a blocky, Soviet-style "Palace" of the Republic—East Berlin's parliament building/entertainment complex and a showy symbol of the communist days. The landmark building fell into disrepair after reunification, and by 2009 had been dismantled.

After much debate about how to use this prime real estate, the German parliament decided to construct the Humboldt-Forum Berliner Schloss, a huge public venue filled with museums, shops, galleries, and concert halls behind a facade constructed in imitation of the original Hohenzollern palace. With a €1.2 billion price tag, many Berliners consider the reconstruction plan a complete waste of money. Funding disappointments are delaying the project and confusing the public. The latest news is that it should be finished by 2019.

In the meantime, the temporary **Humboldt-Box** has been set up. Until it gets in the way and has to be demolished, it will help the public follow the construction of the Humboldt-Forum.

• *Head to the bridge just beyond the Berlin Cathedral, with views of the riverbank. Consider...*

Cruising the Spree River

The recommended **Spree River boat tours** depart from the riverbank near the bridge by the Berlin Cathedral. For details, see page 593.

• *Before crossing the bridge (and leaving Museum Island), look down the river in the distance. To the right, the pointy twin spires of the 13th-century Nikolai Church mark the center of medieval Berlin. This* **Nikolaiviertel** *(Viertel means "quarter") was restored by the DDR and became trendy in the last years of communism. To the left is the gilded* **New Synagogue** *dome, rebuilt after WWII bombing (described on page 630).*

Now look down along the riverbank (directly across from the back-side of the Berlin Cathedral) for the...

▲DDR Museum

The exhibits here offer an interesting look at life in the former East Germany (DDR) without the negative spin most museums give. It's well-stocked with kitschy everyday items from the communist period, plus photos, video clips, and concise English explanations. The exhibits are interactive—you're encouraged to pick up and handle anything that isn't behind glass. Even the meals served in the attached restaurant are based on DDR-era recipes.

Cost and Hours: €7, daily 10:00-20:00, Sat until 22:00, just across the Spree from Museum Island at Karl-Liebknecht-Strasse 1, tel. 030/847-123-731, www.ddr-museum.de.

• *From the bridge, continue walking straight toward the TV Tower, down the big boulevard, which here changes its name to Karl-Liebknecht-Strasse.*

SIGHTS ALONG KARL-LIEBKNECHT-STRASSE

The first big building on the left after the bridge is the **Radisson Blu Hotel** and shopping center, with a huge aquarium in the center. The elevator goes right through the middle of a deep-sea world. (You can see it from the unforgettable Radisson hotel lobby—tuck in your shirt and walk past the guards with the confidence of a guest who's sleeping there.) It's a huge glass cylinder rising high above the central bar (best seen from the left corner as you enter). Here in the center of the old communist capital, it seems that capitalism has settled in with a spirited vengeance.

In the park immediately across the street (a big jaywalk from the Radisson) are grandfatherly statues of **Marx** and **Engels** (nicknamed the "old pensioners"). Surrounding them are stainless-steel monoliths with evocative photos illustrating the struggles of the workers of the world.

Farther along, where Karl-Liebknecht-Strasse intersects with Spandauer Strasse, look right to see the red-brick **city hall**. It was built after the revolutions of 1848 and arguably the first democratic building in the city.

Continue toward **Marien Church** (from 1270), with its spire mirroring the TV Tower. Inside, an artist's rendering helps you follow the interesting but very faded old "Dance of Death" mural that wraps around the narthex inside the door.

• *Immediately across the street from the church, detour a half-block down little Rosenstrasse to find a beautiful memorial set in a park.*

Women's Protest Memorial

This is a reminder of a successful and courageous protest against Nazi policies. In 1943, when "privileged Jews" (men married to Gentile women) were arrested, their wives demonstrated en masse on this street, home to Berlin's oldest synagogue (now gone). They actually won the freedom of their men. Note the Berliner on the bench nearby. As most Berliners did, he looks the other way, even when these courageous women demonstrated that you could speak up and be heard under the Nazis.

• *Back on Karl-Liebknecht-Strasse, look up at the 1,200-foot-tall...*

TV Tower (Fernsehturm)

Built (with Swedish know-how) in 1969 for the 20th anniversary of the communist government, the tower was meant to show the power of the atheistic state at a time when DDR leaders were having the crosses removed from church domes and spires. But when the sun hit the tower—the greatest spire in East Berlin—a huge cross was reflected on the mirrored ball. Cynics called it "God's Revenge." East Berliners dubbed the tower the "Tele-Asparagus." They joked that if it fell over, they'd have an elevator to the West.

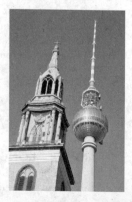

The tower has a fine view from halfway up, offering a handy city orientation and an interesting look at the flat, red-roofed sprawl of Berlin—including a peek inside the city's many courtyards, called *Höfe*. The retro tower is quite trendy these days, so it can be crowded (your ticket comes with an assigned entry time). Consider a kitschy trip to the observation deck for the view and lunch in its revolving restaurant (mediocre food, €12 plates, horrible lounge music, reservations smart for dinner, tel. 030/242-3333, www.tv-turm.de).

Cost and Hours: €13, daily March-Oct 9:00-24:00, Nov-Feb 10:00-24:00, www.tv-turm.de.

• *Walk four more minutes down the boulevard past the TV Tower and toward the big railway overpass.*

Walk under the train bridge and continue for a long half-block (passing the Galeria Kaufhof mall). Turn right onto a broad pedestrian street, and go through the low tunnel into the big square where blue U-Bahn station signs mark...

Alexanderplatz

This square was the commercial pride and joy of East Berlin. The Kaufhof department store (now Galeria Kaufhof) was the ultimate

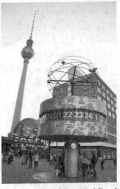

shopping mecca for Easterners. It, along with the two big surviving 1920s "functionalist" buildings, defined the square. Alexanderplatz is still a landmark, with a major U-Bahn/S-Bahn station. The once-futuristic, now-retro "World Time Clock," installed in 1969, is a nostalgic favorite and remains a popular meeting point.

Stop in the square for a coffee and to people-watch. You may see human hot-dog stands—hot-dog hawkers who wear ingenious harnesses that let them cook and sell tasty, cheap German sausages on the fly.

• *Our Best of Berlin Walk is finished. From here, you can hike back a bit to catch the riverboat tour or visit the Museum Island or German History museums, take in the sights south of Unter den Linden, or venture into the colorful Prenzlauer Berg neighborhood.*

SOUTH OF UNTER DEN LINDEN

The following sights—heavy on Nazi and Wall history—are listed roughly north to south (as you reach them from Unter den Linden).

▲▲Gendarmenmarkt

Many cruise-line shuttle buses from Warnemünde drop off and pick up at this delightful, historic square. The space is bounded by

BERLIN

twin churches, a tasty chocolate shop, and the Berlin Symphony's concert hall (designed by Karl Friedrich Schinkel, the man who put the Neoclassical stamp on Berlin and Dresden). In summer, it hosts a few outdoor cafés, *Biergarten*s, and sometimes concerts. Wonderfully symmetrical, the square is considered by

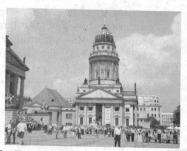

Berliners to be the finest in town (U6: Französische Strasse; U2 or U6: Stadtmitte; for eateries, see page 636).

The name of the square, which is part French and part German (after the *Gens d'Armes*, Frederick the Great's royal guard, who were headquartered here), reminds us that in the 17th century, a fifth of all Berliners were French émigrés—Protestant Huguenots fleeing Catholic France. Back then, Frederick the Great's tolerant Prussia was a magnet for the persecuted (and their money). These émigrés vitalized Berlin with new ideas and know-how...and their substantial wealth.

Of the two matching churches on Gendarmenmarkt, the one to the south (bottom end of square) is the **German Cathedral** (Deutscher Dom). This cathedral (not to be confused with the Berlin Cathedral on Museum Island) was bombed flat in the war and rebuilt only in the 1980s. It houses the thought-provoking Milestones, Setbacks, Sidetracks *(Wege, Irrwege, Umwege)* exhibit, which traces the history of the German parliamentary system—worth ▲. As the exhibit is designed for Germans rather than foreign tourists, there are no English descriptions—but you can follow the essential, excellent, and free 1.5-hour English audioguide (free entry, Tue-Sun 10:00-19:00, Oct-April until 18:00, closed Mon year-round, tel. 030/2273-0431).

The **French Cathedral** (Französischer Dom), at the north end of the square, offers a humble museum on the Huguenots (€2, Tue-Sun 12:00-17:00, closed Mon, enter around the right side) and a viewpoint in the dome up top (€3, daily April-Oct 10:00-19:00, Nov-March 10:00-18:00, last entry one hour before closing, 244 steps, enter through door facing square, tel. 030/2067-4690, www.franzoesischer-dom.de).

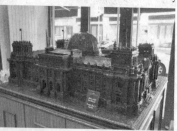

Fassbender & Rausch, on the corner near the German Cathedral, claims to be Europe's biggest chocolate store. The window

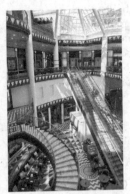

displays feature giant chocolate models of Berlin landmarks—Reichstag, Brandenburg Gate, Kaiser Wilhelm Memorial Church, and so on (Mon-Sat 10:00-20:00, Sun 11:00-20:00, corner of Mohrenstrasse at Charlottenstrasse 60, tel. 030/757-882-440).

Gendarmenmarkt is buried in what has recently emerged as Berlin's "Fifth Avenue" shopping district. For the ultimate in top-end shops, find the corner of Jägerstrasse and Friedrichstrasse and wander through the **Quartier 206** (Mon-Fri 10:30-19:30, Sat 10:00-18:00, closed Sun, www.quartier206.com). The adjacent, middlebrow **Quartier 205** has more affordable prices.

▲Potsdamer Platz

The "Times Square of Berlin," and possibly the busiest square in Europe before World War II, Potsdamer Platz was cut in two by the Wall and left a deserted no-man's-land for 40 years. Today, this immense commercial/residential/entertainment center, sit-

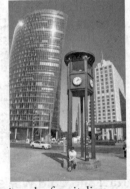

ting on a futuristic transportation hub, is home to the European headquarters of several big-league companies.

The new Potsdamer Platz was a vision begun in 1991, the year that Germany's parliament voted to relocate the seat of government to Berlin. Since then, Sony, Daimler, and other major corporations have turned the square once again into a city center. Like great Christian churches built upon pagan holy grounds, Potsdamer Platz—with its corporate logos flying high and shiny above what was the Wall—trumpets the triumph of capitalism.

Potsdamer Platz's centerpiece is the **Sony Center,** under a

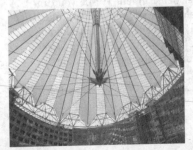

grand canopy (designed to evoke Mount Fuji). Office workers and tourists eat here by the fountain, enjoying the parade of people. The modern Bavarian Lindenbräu beer hall—the Sony boss wanted a *Brauhaus*—serves traditional food (€11-20, daily 11:00-24:00, big €12 salads, three-foot-long taster boards of eight different beers, tel.

BERLIN

030/2575-1280). Across the plaza, Josty Bar is built around a surviving bit of a venerable hotel that was a meeting place for Berlin's
rich and famous before the bombs (€12-20 meals, daily 8:00-
24:00, tel. 030/2575-9702). A huge **screen** above the Deutsche
Kinemathek museum (left of Starbucks) shows big sporting events
on special occasions. Otherwise it runs historic video clips of
Potsdamer Platz through the decades.

Kulturforum

Just west of Potsdamer Platz, Kulturforum rivals Museum Island
as the city's cultural heart, with several top museums and Berlin's
concert hall—home of the world-famous Berlin Philharmonic
orchestra. Of its sprawling museums, only the Gemäldegalerie is
a must (ride the S-Bahn or U-Bahn to Potsdamer Platz, then walk
along Potsdamer Platz).

▲▲Gemäldegalerie

Literally the "Painting Gallery," Germany's top collection of 13th-
through 18th-century European paintings (more than 1,400 canvases) is beautifully displayed in a building that's a work of art in
itself. The North Wing starts with German paintings of the 13th
to 16th century, including eight by Albrecht Dürer. Then come the
Dutch and Flemish—Jan van Eyck, Pieter Brueghel, Peter Paul
Rubens, Anthony van Dyck, Frans Hals, and Jan Vermeer. The
wing finishes with German, English, and French 18th-century
artists, such as Thomas Gainsborough and Antoine Watteau.
An octagonal hall at the end features an impressive stash of
Rembrandts. The South Wing is saved for the Italians—Giotto,
Botticelli, Titian, Raphael, and Caravaggio.

Cost and Hours: €10, Tue-Fri 10:00-18:00, Thu until 20:00,
Sat-Sun 11:00-18:00, closed Mon, audioguide included with entry,
clever little loaner stools, great salad bar in cafeteria upstairs,
Matthäikirchplatz 4, tel. 030/266-424-242, www.smb.museum.

Nazi and Cold War Sites

A variety of fascinating sites relating to Germany's tumultuous
20th century cluster south of Unter den Linden. While you can
see your choice of the following places in any order, I've linked
them by way of a short walk from Potsdamer Platz to Checkpoint
Charlie. (If you instead approach Checkpoint Charlie from Unter
den Linden via Friedrichstrasse, you'd likely visit these sights in
reverse order.)

• *From Potsdamer Platz, take a few steps down Stresemannstrasse
and detour left down Erna-Berger-Strasse to find a lonely concrete
watchtower.*

DDR Watchtower

This was one of many such towers built in 1966 for panoramic surveillance and shooting (note the rifle windows, allowing shots to be fired in 360 degrees). It was constantly manned by two guards who were forbidden to get to know each other (no casual chatting)—so they could effectively guard each other from escaping. This is one of only a few such towers still standing.

Cost and Hours: €3.50, open only sporadically, though officially daily 11:00-15:00.

• *Return to Stresemannstrasse, and continue south (away from Potsdamer Platz). As you round the corner turning left, you'll begin to see some...*

Fragments of the Wall

Surviving stretches of the Wall are rare in downtown Berlin, but you'll find a few in this area. On the left, as you turn from Erna-Berger-Strasse onto Stresemannstrasse, look carefully at the mod-

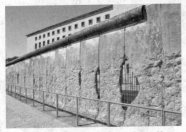

ern Ministry of the Environment (Bundesministerium für Umwelt) building; notice the nicely painted stretch of **inner wall** (inside the modern building constructed around it). The Wall was actually two walls, with a death strip in the middle (where Stresemannstrasse is today). Across the street, embedded in the sidewalk, you can see cobblestones marking the former path of the outer wall.

At the corner with Niederkirchnerstrasse, turn left and follow the cobbles in the sidewalk. After about a block (just beyond the Martin-Gropius-Bau museum), where the street becomes cobbled, an **original fragment** of the Berlin Wall stretches alongside the right side of the street.

• *Follow the Wall until it ends, at the intersection of Niederkirchnerstrasse and Wilhelmstrasse. Hook right around the end of the Wall to reach the...*

▲▲Topography of Terror (Topographie des Terrors)

Coincidentally, the patch of land behind the surviving stretch of Wall was closely associated with an even more deplorable regime: It was once the nerve center for the most despicable elements of the Nazi government, the Gestapo and the SS. This stark-gray, boxy building is one of the few memorial sites that focuses on the perpetrators rather than the victims of the Nazis. It's chilling but thought-provoking to see just how seamlessly and bureaucratically the Nazi institutions and state structures merged to become a well-oiled terror machine. There are few actual artifacts; it's mostly written explanations and photos, like reading a good textbook standing up. And, while you could read this story anywhere, to take this in atop the Gestapo headquarters is a powerful experience. The exhibit is a bit dense, but WWII historians (even armchair ones) will find it fascinating. The complex has two parts: indoors, in the modern boxy building, 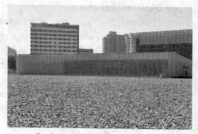 and outdoors, in the trench that runs along the surviving stretch of Wall.

Cost and Hours: Free, includes audioguide for outdoor exhibit, daily 10:00-20:00, outdoor exhibit closes at dusk, Niederkirchnerstrasse 8, tel. 030/254-5090, www.topographie.de.

• *Return to the intersection of Niederkirchnerstrasse and Wilhelmstrasse, and continue east, crossing Wilhelmstrasse. Niederkirchnerstrasse now becomes Zimmerstrasse, leading to Checkpoint Charlie. Along the way you'll pass several "Ost-algic" business ventures: vendors of DDR soft ice-cream, Trabi World (renting rides in iconic DDR tin-can cars), and the Wall Panorama Exhibition (not worth €10, as it's just huge photos). You'll wind up at...*

▲Checkpoint Charlie

This famous Cold War checkpoint was not named for a person, but for its checkpoint number—as in Alpha (#1, at the East-West German border, a hundred 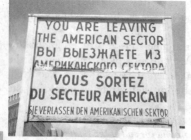 miles west of here), Bravo (#2, as you enter Berlin proper), and Charlie (#3, the best known because most foreigners passed through here). While the actual checkpoint has long since been dismantled, its former location is home to a fine museum and a mock-up of the original border crossing. The area has become a Cold War freak show and—as if celebrating the final victory of crass capitalism—is one of Berlin's worst tourist-trap zones. A McDonald's stands defiantly overlooking the former haunt of East German border guards. (For a more sober and intellectually redeeming look at the Wall's history, head for the Berlin Wall Memorial at Bernauer Strasse, described on page 631.)

The rebuilt **guard station** now hosts two actors playing American guards who pose for photos. Notice the larger-than-life **posters** of a young American soldier facing east and a young Soviet soldier facing west. (Look carefully at the "Soviet" soldier.

He was photographed in 1999, a decade after there were Soviet soldiers stationed here. He's a Dutch model. His uniform is a nonsensical pile of pins and ribbons with a Russian flag on his shoulder.)

A **photo exhibit** stretches up and down Zimmerstrasse, with great English descriptions telling the story of the Wall. While you could get this information from a book, it's certainly a different experience to stand here in person and ponder the gripping history of this place. A few yards away (on Zimmerstrasse), a **glass panel** describes the former checkpoint. From there, another double row of **cobbles** in Zimmerstrasse shows the former path of the Wall.

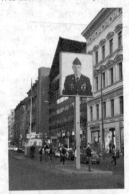

Warning: Here and in other places, hustlers charge an exorbitant €10 for a full set of Cold War-era stamps in your passport. Don't be tempted. Technically, this invalidates your passport—which has caused some tourists big problems.

• *Overlooking the chaos of the street scene is the...*

▲▲Museum of the Wall at Checkpoint Charlie (Mauermuseum Haus am Checkpoint Charlie)

While the famous border checkpoint between the American and Soviet sectors is long gone, its memory is preserved by one

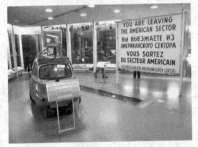

of Europe's most cluttered museums. During the Cold War, the House at Checkpoint Charlie stood defiantly—spitting distance from the border guards—showing off all the clever escapes over, under, and through the Wall. Today, while the drama is over and hunks of the Wall stand like trophies at its door, the museum survives as a living artifact of the Cold War days. The yellowed descriptions, which have scarcely changed since that time, tinge the museum with nostalgia. It's dusty, disorganized, and overpriced, with lots of reading involved, but all that just adds to this museum's borderline-kitschy charm.

Cost and Hours: €12.50, assemble 20 tourists and get in for €8.50 each, €3.50 audioguide, daily 9:00-22:00, U6 to Kochstrasse or U2 to Stadtmitte, Friedrichstrasse 43, tel. 030/253-7250, www. mauermuseum.de.

The Berlin Wall (and Its Fall)

The 96-mile-long "Anti-Fascist Protective Rampart," as it was called by the East German government, was erected almost overnight in 1961 to stop the outward flow of people from East to West (3 million had leaked out between 1949 and 1961). The Wall (*Mauer*) was actually two walls; the outer was a 12-foot-high concrete barrier whose rounded, pipe-like top (to discourage grappling hooks) was adorned with plenty of barbed wire. Sandwiched between the walls was a no-man's-land "death strip" between 30 and 160 feet wide. More than 100 sentry towers kept a close eye on the Wall. On their way into the death strip, would-be escapees tripped a silent alarm, which alerted sharpshooters.

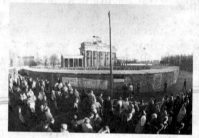

During the Wall's 28 years, border guards fired 1,693 times and made 3,221 arrests, and there were 5,043 documented successful escapes (565 of these were East German guards). At least 138 people died or were killed at the Wall while trying to escape.

As a tangible, almost too-apt symbol for the Cold War, the Berlin Wall got a lot of attention from politicians both East and West. Two of the 20th century's most repeated presidential quotes were uttered within earshot of the death strip. In 1963, US President John F. Kennedy professed American solidarity with the struggling people of Berlin: *"Ich bin ein Berliner."* A generation later in 1987, with the stiff winds of change already blowing westward from Moscow, President Ronald Reagan issued an ultimatum to his Soviet counterpart: "Mr. Gorbachev, tear down this wall."

The actual fall of the Wall had less to do with presidential proclamations than with the obvious failings of the Soviet system, a general thawing in Moscow (where Gorbachev introduced *perestroika* and *glasnost,* and declared that he would no longer employ force to keep Eastern European satellite states under Soviet rule), the brave civil-disobedience actions of many ordinary citizens behind the Wall—and a bureaucratic snafu.

By November of 1989, it was clear that change was in the air. Hungary had already opened its borders to the West that summer, making it next to impossible for East German authorities to keep people in. A series of anti-regime protests had swept nearby Leipzig a few weeks earlier, attracting hundreds of thousands of supporters. On October 7, 1989—on the 40th anniversary of the official creation of the DDR—East German premier Erich Honecker said, "The Wall will be standing in 50 and even in 100 years." He was only off by 99 years and 11 months. A similar rally in East Berlin's Alexanderplatz on November 4—with a half-million protesters chanting, *"Wir wollen raus!"* (We want

BERLIN

out!)—persuaded the East German politburo to begin a gradual process of relaxing travel restrictions.

The DDR's intention was to slightly crack the door to the West, but an inarticulate spokesman's confusion inadvertently threw it wide open. The decision was made on Thursday, November 9, to tentatively allow a few more Easterners to cross into the West—a largely symbolic reform that was intended to take place gradually, over many weeks. Licking their wounds, politburo members left town early for a long weekend. The announcement about travel restrictions was left to a spokesman, Günter Schabowski, who knew only what was on a piece of paper handed to him moments before he went on television for a routine press conference. At 18:54, Schabowski read the statement dutifully, with little emotion, seemingly oblivious to the massive impact of his own words: "exit via border crossings...possible for every citizen." Reporters, unable to believe what they were hearing, began to prod him about when the borders would open. Schabowski looked with puzzlement at the brief statement, shrugged, and offered his best guess: *"Ab sofort, unverzüglich."* ("Immediately, without delay.")

Schabowski's words spread like wildfire through the streets of both Berlins, its flames fanned by West German TV broadcasts (and Tom Brokaw, who had rushed to Berlin when alerted by NBC's bureau chief). East Berliners began to show up at Wall checkpoints, demanding that border guards let them pass. As the crowds grew, the border guards could not reach anyone who could issue official orders. (The politburo members were effectively hiding out.) Finally, around 23:30, a border guard named Harald Jäger at the Bornholmer Strasse crossing decided to simply open the gates. Easterners flooded into the West, embracing their long-separated cousins, unable to believe their good fortune. Once open, the Wall could never be closed again.

The carnival atmosphere of those first years after the Wall fell is gone, but hawkers still sell "authentic" pieces of the Wall, DDR flags, and military paraphernalia to gawking tourists. When it fell, the Wall was literally carried away by the euphoria. What managed to survive has been nearly devoured by decades of persistent "Wall-peckers."

Americans—the Cold War victors—have the biggest appetite for Wall-related sights, and a few bits and pieces remain for us to seek out. Berlin's best Wall sights are the Berlin Wall Memorial along Bernauer Strasse, with a long stretch of surviving Wall (near S-Bahn: Nordbahnhof; page 631), and the Museum of the Wall at Checkpoint Charlie (see page 625). Other stretches of the Wall still standing include the short section at Niederkirchnerstrasse/Wilhelmstrasse (near the Topography of Terror exhibit; page 623) and the longer East Side Gallery (near the Ostbahnhof; page 628).

BERLIN

More Sights South of Unter den Linden
▲▲Jewish Museum Berlin (Jüdisches Museum Berlin)

This museum is one of Europe's best Jewish sights. The highly conceptual building is a sight in itself, and the museum inside—an overview of the rich culture and history of Europe's Jewish community—is excellent, particularly if you take advantage of the informative and engaging audioguide. Rather than just reading dry texts, you'll feel as if this museum is fresh and alive—an exuberant celebration of the Jewish experience that's accessible to all. Even though the museum is in a nondescript residential neighborhood south of Checkpoint Charlie, it's well worth the trip.

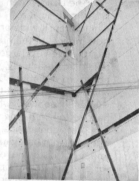

Cost and Hours: €8, daily 10:00-20:00, Mon until 22:00, last entry one hour before closing, closed on Jewish holidays. Tight security includes bag check and metal detectors. The excellent €3 audioguide—with four hours of commentary—is essential to fully appreciate the exhibits. Tel. 030/2599-3300, www.jmberlin.de.

Getting There: Take the U-Bahn to Hallesches Tor, find the exit marked *Jüdisches Museum,* exit straight ahead, then turn right on Franz-Klühs-Strasse. The museum is a five-minute walk ahead on your left, at Lindenstrasse 9.

Eating: The museum's restaurant, Café Schmus, offers good Jewish-style meals, albeit not kosher (daily 10:00-20:00, Mon until 22:00).

East Side Gallery

The biggest remaining stretch of the Wall is now the "world's longest outdoor art gallery." It stretches for nearly a mile and is covered with murals painted by artists from around the world. The murals (classified as protected monuments) got a facelift in 2009, when the city invited the original artists back to re-create their work for the 20th anniversary of the fall of the Wall. This segment of the Wall makes a poignant walk. For a quick look, take the S-Bahn to the Ostbahnhof station (follow signs to Stralauerplatz exit; once outside, TV Tower will be to your right; go left and at next corner look to your right—the Wall is across the busy street). The gallery is slowly being consumed by developers. If you walk the entire length of the East Side Gallery, you'll find a small Wall souvenir shop at the end and a bridge crossing the river to a subway station at Schlesisches Tor (in the colorful Turkish neighborhood of Kreuzberg). The bridge, a fine example of Brandenburg Neo-Gothic brickwork, has a neon "rock, paper, scissors" installment poking fun at the futility of the Cold War (visible only after dark).

NORTH OF UNTER DEN LINDEN

There are few major sights north of Unter den Linden, but this area has some of Berlin's trendiest, most interesting neighborhoods. I've listed these roughly from south to north, as you'd approach them from the city center and Unter den Linden. On a sunny day, a stroll (or tram ride) through these bursting-with-life areas can be as engaging as any museum in town.

Hackescher Markt

This area, in front of the S-Bahn station of the same name, is a great people scene. The brick trestle supporting the train track is a classic example of the city's Brandenburg Neo-Gothic brickwork. Most of the brick archways are now filled with hip shops, which have official—and newly trendy—addresses such as "S-Bahn Arch #9, Hackescher Markt." Within 100 yards of the S-Bahn station, you'll find recommended Turkish and Bavarian restaurants, walking-tour and pub-crawl departure points, and tram #M1 to Prenzlauer Berg. Also nearby are two fascinating examples of Berlin's traditional courtyards *(Höfe)*—one trendy and modern, the other retro-cool, with two fascinating museums.

Hackesche Höfe (a block in front of the Hackescher Markt S-Bahn station, at Rosenthaler Strasse 40) is a series of eight courtyards bunny-hopping through a wonderfully restored 1907 *Jugendstil* (German Art Nouveau) building. Berlin's apartments are organized like this—courtyard after courtyard leading off the main roads. This complex is full of trendy restaurants (including the recommended Turkish eatery, Hasir), theaters, and cinemas. Courtyard #5 is particularly charming, with a children's park, and an Ampelmann store (see page 585). This courtyard system is a wonderful example of how to make huge city blocks livable. Two decades after the Cold War, this area has reached the final evolution of East Berlin's urban restoration: total gentrification. These courtyards also offer a useful lesson for visitors: Much of Berlin's charm hides off the street front.

Haus Schwarzenberg, next door (at Rosenthaler Strasse 39), has a totally different feel. This rare surviving bit of East Berlin is owned by an artists' collective, with a bar, cinema (showing art films in their original language), an open-air art space (reminiscent of mid-1990s eastern Berlin), and the basement-level "Dead Chickens" gallery (with far-out hydro-powered art). Its Café Cinema is one of the last remaining '90s bohemian-chic bars. And within this amazing little zone you'll find two inspirational museums. **Museum of Otto Weidt's Workshop for the Blind**

BERLIN

(Museum Blindenwerkstatt Otto Weidt) vividly tells the amazing story of a Berliner heroically protecting blind and deaf Jews during World War II (free, daily 10:00-20:00). Otto Weidt employed them to produce brooms and brushes, and because that was useful for the Nazi war machine, he managed to finagle a special status for his workers. **Silent Heroes Memorial Center** (Gedenkstätte Stille Helden) is a well-presented exhibit celebrating the quietly courageous individuals who resisted the persecution of the Jews from 1933 to 1945 (free, daily 10:00-20:00).

Oranienburger Strasse

Oranienburger Strasse, a few blocks west of Hackescher Markt, is anchored by an important and somber sight, the New Synagogue (S-Bahn: Oranienburger Strasse). But the rest of this zone (roughly between the synagogue and Torstrasse) is colorful and quirky. The streets behind Grosse Hamburger Strasse flicker with atmospheric cafés, *Kneipen* (pubs), and art galleries.

▲New Synagogue (Neue Synagogue)

A shiny gilded dome marks the New Synagogue, now a museum and cultural center. Consecrated in 1866, this was once the biggest and finest synagogue in Germany, with seating for 3,200 worshippers and a sumptuous Moorish-style interior modeled after the Alhambra in Granada, Spain. It was desecrated by Nazis on Crystal Night (Kristallnacht) in 1938, bombed in 1943, and partially rebuilt in 1990. Only the 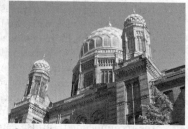 dome and facade have been restored—a window overlooks the vacant field marking what used to be the synagogue. On its facade, a small plaque—added by East Berlin Jews in 1966—reads "Never forget" *(Vergesst es nie)*. At that time East Berlin had only a few hundred Jews, but now that the city is reunited, the Jewish community numbers about 12,000.

Cost and Hours: Main exhibit-€3.50, dome-€2, temporary exhibits-€3, €7 combo-ticket covers everything, audioguide-€3; March-Oct Sun-Mon 10:00-20:00, Tue-Thu 10:00-18:00, Fri 10:00-17:00—until 14:00 in March and Oct; Nov-Feb Sun-Thu 10:00-18:00, Fri 10:00-14:00, closed Sat year-round; Oranienburger Strasse 28, enter through the low-profile door in the modern building just right of the domed synagogue facade, S-Bahn: Oranienburger Strasse, tel. 030/8802-8300 and press 1, www.cjudaicum.de.

BERLIN

▲The Kennedys Museum

This crisp, private enterprise (in a former Jewish girls' school building that survived the war) delightfully recalls John F. Kennedy's 1963 Germany trip with great photos and video clips as well as a photographic shrine to the Kennedy clan in America. Among the interesting mementos are old campaign buttons and posters, and JFK's notes with the phonetic pronunciation "Ish bin ein Bearleener." Jacqueline Kennedy commented on how strange it was that this—not even in his native language—was her husband's most quotable quote. The highlight: a theater where you can watch a newsreel of Kennedy's historic speech (20 minutes, plays continuously).

Cost and Hours: €5, Tue-Sun 11:00-19:00, closed Mon, from Oranienburger Strasse go a block up Tucholskystrasse and turn right to Auguststrasse 13, tel. 030/2065-3570, www.thekennedys. de.

Cold War Sights in the North
▲▲Berlin Wall Memorial (Gedenkstätte Berliner Mauer)

While tourists flock to Checkpoint Charlie, this memorial is Berlin's most substantial attraction relating to its gone-but-not-

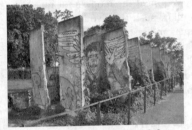

forgotten Wall. Exhibits line up along four blocks of Bernauer Strasse, stretching northeast from the Nordbahnhof S-Bahn station. You can enter two different museums (a Visitor Center and a Documentation Center, each with movies about the Wall) plus various open-air exhibits and

memorials, see several fragments of the Wall, and peer from an observation tower down into a preserved, complete stretch of the Wall system (as it was during the Cold War). To prepare for a visit here, read "The Berlin Wall (and Its Fall)" sidebar on page 626.

Cost and Hours: Free; Visitor Center and Documentation Center open April-Oct Tue-Sun 9:30-19:00, Nov-March until 18:00, closed Mon year-round; outdoor areas accessible 24 hours daily; Bernauer Strasse 111, tel. 030/4679-86666, www.berliner-mauer-gedenkstaette.de.

Getting There: Take the S-Bahn (line S-1, S-2, or S-25—all handy from Potsdamer Platz, Brandenburger Tor, or Friedrichstrasse) to the Nordbahnhof. The Nordbahnhof's underground hallways have history exhibits in English. Exit by following signs for *Bernauer Strasse*, and you'll pop out across the street from a long chunk of Wall and kitty-corner from the Visitor Center.

▲▲Prenzlauer Berg

Young, in-the-know locals agree that Prenzlauer Berg is one of Berlin's most colorful neighborhoods. The heart of this area, with a dense array of hip cafés, restaurants, boutiques, and street life, is roughly between Helmholtzplatz and Kollwitzplatz and along Kastanienallee (U2: Senefelderplatz and Eberswalder Strasse; or take the S-Bahn to Hackescher Markt and catch tram #M1 north). Similar outposts to the south—closer to Museum Island and Unter den Linden—cluster near the Hackescher Markt S-Bahn station; Rosenthaler Platz U-Bahn station; and Oranienburger Strasse (near the New Synagogue).

"Prenzl'berg," as Berliners call it, was largely untouched during World War II, but its buildings slowly rotted away under the communists. Then, after the Wall fell, it was overrun first with artists and anarchists, then with laid-back hipsters, energetic young families, and clever entrepreneurs who breathed life back into its classic old apartment blocks, deserted factories, and long-forgotten breweries. Years of rent control kept things affordable for its bohemian residents. But now landlords are free to charge what the market will bear, and the vibe is changing.

This is ground zero for Berlin's baby boom: Tattooed and pierced young moms and dads, who've joined the modern rat race without giving up their alternative flair, push their youngsters in designer strollers past trendy boutiques and restaurants. These days locals complain about cafés and bars catering to yuppies sipping prosecco, while working-class and artistic types are being priced out. But even though it has changed plenty, I find Prenzlauer Berg a celebration of life and a joy to stroll through.

Eating in Berlin

Don't be too determined to eat "Berlin-style." The city is known only for its mildly spicy sausage and for its street food (*Currywurst* and *Döner Kebab*—see the sidebar on the next page). Germans—especially Berliners—consider their food old-school; when they go out to eat, they're not usually looking for the "traditional local fare" many travelers are after. Nouveau German is California cuisine with scant memories of wurst, kraut, and pumpernickel. If the kraut is getting the wurst of you, take a break with some international or ethnic offerings—try one of the many Turkish, Italian, pan-Asian, and Balkan restaurants.

Colorful pubs—called *Kneipen*—offer light, quick, and easy meals and the fizzy local beer, *Berliner Weiss*. Ask for it *mit Schuss* for a shot of fruity syrup in your suds.

My recommendations are near the sightseeing core in eastern Berlin.

Berliner Street Fare

In Berlin, it's easy to eat cheap, with a glut of *Imbiss* snack stands, bakeries (for sandwiches), and falafel/kebab coun-

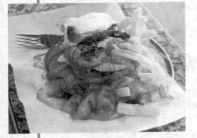

ters. Train stations have grocery stores, as well as bright and modern fruit-and-sandwich bars.

Sausage stands are everywhere (I've listed a couple of local favorites). Most specialize in **Currywurst,** created in Berlin after World War II, when a fast-food cook got her hands on some curry and Worcestershire

sauce from British troops stationed here. It's basically a grilled *Bockwurst*-type pork sausage smothered with curry sauce. *Currywurst* comes either *mit Darm* (with casing) or *ohne Darm* (without casing). If the casing is left on to grill, it gives the sausage a smokier flavor. (*Berliner Art*—"Berlin-style"—means that the sausage is boiled *ohne Darm*, then grilled.) Either way, the grilled sausage is then chopped into small pieces or cut in half (East Berlin style) and topped with sauce. While some places simply use ketchup and sprinkle on some curry powder, real *Currywurst* joints use tomato paste, Worcestershire sauce, and curry. With your wurst comes either a toothpick or small wooden fork; you'll usually get a plate of fries as well, but rarely a roll. You'll see *Currywurst* on the menu at some sit-down restaurants, but local purists say that misses the whole point: You'll pay triple and get a less authentic dish than you would at a street stand under elevated S-Bahn tracks.

Other good street foods to consider are *Döner Kebab* (Turkish-style skewered meat slow-roasted and served in a sandwich) and *Frikadelle* (like a hamburger patty; often called *Bulette* in Berlin).

For a quick, cheap, and tasty local hot dog, find one of the portable human hot-dog stands. Two companies, Grillrunner and Grillwalker, outfit their cooks in clever harnesses that let them grill and sell hot dogs from under an umbrella.

BERLIN

NEAR UNTER DEN LINDEN

While this government/commercial area is hardly a hot spot for eateries, I've listed a few places handy for your sightseeing, all a short walk from Unter den Linden.

Near Museum Island: Georgenstrasse, a block behind the Pergamon Museum and under the S-Bahn tracks, is lined with fun eateries filling the arcade of the train trestle—close to the sightseeing action but in business mainly for students from nearby

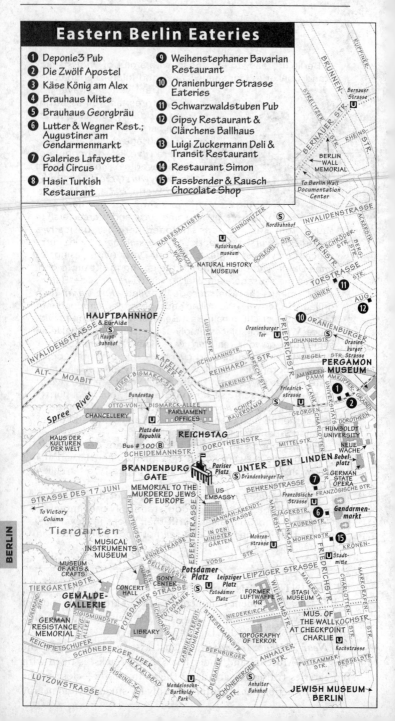

Eastern Berlin Eateries

1. Deponie3 Pub
2. Die Zwölf Apostel
3. Käse König am Alex
4. Brauhaus Mitte
5. Brauhaus Georgbräu
6. Lutter & Wegner Rest.; Augustiner am Gendarmenmarkt
7. Galeries Lafayette Food Circus
8. Hasir Turkish Restaurant
9. Weihenstephaner Bavarian Restaurant
10. Oranienburger Strasse Eateries
11. Schwarzwaldstuben Pub
12. Gipsy Restaurant & Clärchens Ballhaus
13. Luigi Zuckermann Deli & Transit Restaurant
14. Restaurant Simon
15. Fassbender & Rausch Chocolate Shop

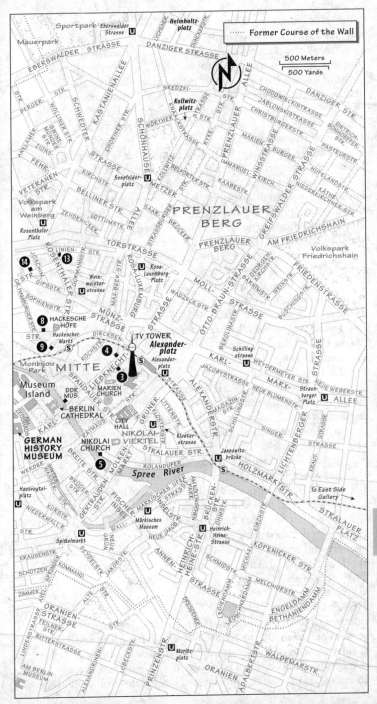

Sportpark
Mauerpark
EBERSWALDER STRASSE
Eberswalder Strasse
Helmholtz-platz
DANZIGER STRASSE
..... Former Course of the Wall

KASTANIENALLEE
SCHWEDTER STR.
WOLLINER STR.
BERGER STR.
ANKLAMER STR.
SWINE-MÜNDER STR.
ZIONS-
FEHR-
VETERANEN-STR.
Volkspark am Weinberg
Rosenthaler Platz

SCHÖNHAUSER
WÖRTHER-STRASSE
CHOR NER STR.
KIRCHSTR.
BELLINER STR.
ALLEE
ZEHDENICKER-
LOTTUMSTR.

500 Meters
500 Yards

N

SKEDZKI-
Kollwitz-platz

STRASSE
KOLLWITZ-
METZER
Senefelder-platz

RYKE STR.
BELFORTER STR.
RAABESTR.

PRENZLAUER STRASSE
PRENZLAUER BERG
WINSSTR.
IMMANUEL-KIRCH-

CHODOWIECKISTRASSE
JABLONSKISTRASSE
CHRISTBURGERSTR.
DIETRICH-BONHOEFER-STR.
PASTEURSTR.
MARIEN-BURGER STR.
GREIFSWALDER STRASSE
HUFELANDSTR.
NIEDERKIRCHNER STR.
KÄTHE-

AM FRIEDRICHSHAIN
Volkspark Friedrichshain
FRIEDENSTRASSE

DANZIGER STR.

PRENZLAUER BERG
MOLL-
STRASSE
OTTO-BRAUN-STRASSE
WADZECK STR.

ROSENTHALER STR.
LINIEN-STR.
JOACHIM-STR.
GIPSSTR.
SOPHIENSTR.
HACKESCHE HÖFE
Hackescher Markt
MONBIJOU Park
Museum Island
MITTE
DDR MUS.
BERLIN CATHEDRAL
GERMAN HISTORY MUSEUM

14 **13**
Wein-meister-strasse
MÜNZ-STRASSE
DIRCKSEN-
ROCHSTR.
8
9
4
3
LIEBKNECHT-
SPAND. STR.
MARIEN CHURCH
KARL-

TV TOWER
Alexander-platz
Alexanderplatz
S

Rosa-Luxemburg-Platz
MAX-BEER-STR.
ROSA-LUXEMBURG
TÖRSTRASSE

SCHILLING-STRASSE
BERLIN STR.
GRUNER-
LITTENSTR.
ALEXANDERSTR.
JACOBYSTRASSE
NEUE BLUMENSTR.
SCHILLINGSTR.
MAGAZIN-
SINGER-
KARL-MARX-

WEYDEMEYER STR.
NEUE WEBER STR.
Straus-berger Platz
ALLEE

STRASSE

BÜSCHING STR.
GEORGEN-
B. KIRCHG R.
BARNIMSTR.
WEINS TR.

LICHTENBERGER STRASSE
KRAUT STR.

NIKOLAI-VIERTEL
CITY HALL
NIKOLAI CHURCH
5
Kloster-strasse
STRALAUER STR.
ROLANDUFER
Spree River

Jannowitz-brücke
S
HOLZMARKT STR.

To East Side Gallery

STRALAUER PLATZ

BERLIN

BREITE STR.
MOLKEN MARKT
Hausvogtei-platz
U
NIEDERWALL.
KURSTR.
Spittelmarkt
U
GERTRAUDEN STR.
FISCHER INSEL
WALL-STR.
NEUE GRÜN.
SEYDEL STR.
JACOBSTR.
MÄRKISCHES UFER
INSELSTR.
NEUE JAKOB.
Märkisches Museum
Heinrich-Heine-Strasse
U

WERDER-
KRAUSENSTR.
SCHÜTZENSTR.
ZIMMER-
AXEL-SPRINGER-STR.
KOMMAND-
ALTE JAKOBSTR.
ANNEN-
HEINRICH-HEINE-STR.
STRASSE
SCHMIDSTR.
DRESDENER
LEGIENDAMM
LUCKAUER STR.
KÖPENICKER STR.
MICHAEL KIRCHSTR.
BRÜCKEN-STR.
ENGELDAMM
MELCHIORSTR.
BETHANIENDAMM

ORANIEN-STRASSE
FEILNER STR.
RITTERSTRASSE
LINDENSTRASSE
AM BERLIN MUSEUM
ALEXANDRINENSTR.
LÖBECKSTR.
PRINZENSTR.
U
Moritz-platz
ORANIEN- STRASSE
ADALBERTSTR.
WALDEMARSTR.

Humboldt University. **Deponie3** is a reliable Berlin *Kneipe* usually filled with students. Garden seating in the back is nice if you don't mind the noise of the S-Bahn passing directly above you. The interior is a cozy, wooden wonderland of a bar with several inviting spaces. They serve basic salads, traditional Berlin dishes, and hearty daily specials (€5-8 breakfasts, €8-13 lunches and dinners, open Mon-Fri daily from 10:00, under S-Bahn arch #87-88 at Georgenstrasse 5, tel. 030/2016-5740). For Italian food, a branch of **Die Zwölf Apostel** is nearby.

Near the TV Tower: **Käse König am Alex** is a wonderfully old-school eatery that's been serving traditional sauerkraut-type dishes to hungry locals since 1933 (with Prussian forks, flat to fit better into a soldier's mess kit). It's fast, the photo menu makes ordering fun, prices are great, and the waitresses are surly (€5-10 lunches and dinners, daily, free Wi-Fi, Panoramastrasse 1 under the TV Tower, tel. 030/8561-5220). Nearby, **Brauhaus Mitte** is a fun, tour-group-friendly DDR-era beer hall that makes its own beer and offers a menu of Berliner "specialties" and Bavarian dishes. They have decent salads and serve a four-beer sampler board (daily 11:00-24:00, across from the TV Tower at Karl-Liebknecht-Strasse 13, tel. 030/3087-8989).

In the Heart of Old Berlin's Nikolai Quarter: The *Nikolaiviertel* marks the original medieval settlement of Cölln, which would eventually become Berlin. The area was destroyed during the war but was rebuilt for Berlin's 750th birthday in 1987. The whole area has a cute, cobbled, and characteristic old town feel...Middle Ages meets Socialist Realism. Today, the district is pretty soulless by day but a popular restaurant zone at night. **Brauhaus Georgbräu** is a thriving beer hall serving homemade suds on a picturesque courtyard overlooking the Spree River. Eat in the lively and woody but mod-feeling interior, or outdoors with fun riverside seating—thriving with German tourists. It's a good place to try one of the few typical Berlin dishes: *Eisbein* (boiled ham hock) with sauerkraut and mashed peas with bacon (€11 with a beer and schnapps). The statue of St. George once stood in the courtyard of Berlin's old castle—until the Nazis deemed it too decadent and not "German" enough, and removed it (€7-14 plates, daily 12:00-24:00, 2 blocks south of Berlin Cathedral and across the river at Spreeufer 4, tel. 030/242-4244).

NEAR GENDARMENMARKT

South of Unter den Linden, the twin churches of Gendarmenmarkt seem to be surrounded by people in love with food. The lunch scene is thriving with upscale restaurants serving good cuisine at highly competitive prices to local professionals (see map on page 634 for locations). If in need of a quick-yet-classy lunch, stroll around the square and along Charlottenstrasse. For a quick bite, head to the cheap *Currywurst* stand behind the German Cathedral.

Lutter & Wegner Restaurant is well-known for its Austrian cuisine (*Schnitzel* and *Sauerbraten*) and popular with businesspeople. It's dressy, with fun sidewalk seating or a dark and elegant interior (€9-18 starters, €16-24 main dishes, daily 11:00-24:00, Charlottenstrasse 56, tel. 030/202-9540).

Augustiner am Gendarmenmarkt, next door to Lutter & Wegner, lines its sidewalk with trademark Bavarian white-and-blue-checkerboard tablecloths; inside, you'll find a classic Bavarian beer-hall atmosphere. Less pretentious than its neighbor, it offers good beer and affordable Bavarian classics in an equally appealing location (€6-12 light meals, €10-16 bigger meals, daily 10:00-24:00, Charlottenstrasse 55, tel. 030/2045-4020).

Galeries Lafayette Food Circus is a French festival of fun eateries in the basement of the landmark department store. You'll find a good deli and prepared-food stands, dishing up cuisine that's good-quality but not cheap (most options €10-15, cheaper €8-10 sandwiches and savory crêpes, Mon-Sat 10:00-20:00, closed Sun, Friedrichstrasse 76, U-Bahn: Französische Strasse, tel. 030/209-480).

BETWEEN THE RIVER AND PRENZLAUER BERG

All of these eateries are within a 10-minute walk of the Hackescher Markt S-Bahn station, in the area butting up against Prenzlauer Berg.

Near Hackescher Markt

Hasir Turkish Restaurant is your chance to dine with candles, hardwood floors, and happy Berliners savoring meaty Anatolian specialties. As Berlin is the world's largest Turkish city outside of Asia Minor, it's no wonder you can find some good Turkish restaurants here. But while most locals think of Turkish food as fast and cheap, this is a dining experience. The restaurant, in a courtyard next to the Hackesche Höfe shopping complex (see page 629), offers indoor and outdoor tables filled with an enthusiastic local crowd. The service can be a bit questionable, so bring some patience (€6-10 starters, €14-20 main dishes, large and splittable portions, daily 12:00-24:00, a block from the Hackescher Markt S-Bahn station at Oranienburger Strasse 4, tel. 030/2804-1616).

Weihenstephaner Bavarian Restaurant serves upmarket Bavarian traditional food for around €10-15 a plate; offers an atmospheric cellar, an inner courtyard, and a busy people-watching streetside terrace; and, of course, has excellent beer (daily 11:00-23:00, Neue Promenade 5 at Hackescher Markt, tel. 030/8471-0760).

BERLIN

On or near Oranienburger Strasse

Oranienburger Strasse, a few blocks west of Hackescher Markt, is busy with happy eaters. Restaurants on this stretch come with happy hours and lots of cocktails. **Aufsturz,** a lively pub, has a huge selection of beers and whisky and dishes up "traditional Berliner pub grub" to a young crowd (Oranienburger Strasse 67). **Amrit Lounge** is great if you'd like Indian food outdoors with an umbrellas-in-your-drink Caribbean ambience (€5 cocktails, €10-14 meals, long hours daily, Oranienburger Strasse 45). Next door is **QBA,** a fun Cuban bar and restaurant.

Schwarzwaldstuben, between Oranienburger Strasse and Rosenthaler Platz, is a Black Forest-themed pub—which explains the antlers, cuckoo clocks, and painting of a thick forest on the wall. It's friendly, with good service, food, and prices. The staff chooses the music (often rock or jazz), and the ambience is warm and welcoming. If they're full, you can eat at the long bar or at one of the sidewalk tables (€6-15 meals, daily 9:00-23:00, Tucholskystrasse 48, tel. 030/2809-8084).

Gipsy Restaurant serves good, cheap German and Italian dishes, including brats, pizza, and homemade cakes, in a bohemian-chic atmosphere (daily 12:30-23:00, at Clärchens Ballhaus, Auguststrasse 24, tel. 030/282-9295).

Near Rosenthaler Platz

Surrounding the U8: Rosenthaler Platz station, a short stroll or tram ride from the Hackescher Markt S-Bahn station, and an easy walk from the Oranienburger Strasse action, this busy neighborhood has a few enticing options.

Luigi Zuckermann is a trendy young deli with Israeli/New York style. It's a great spot to pick up a custom-made deli sandwich (choose your ingredients at the deli counter), hummus plate, salad, fresh-squeezed juice, or other quick, healthy lunch. Linger in the interior, grab one of the few sidewalk tables, or take your food to munch on the go (€5-8 meals, daily 8:00-24:00, Rosenthaler Strasse 67, tel. 030/2804-0644).

Transit is a stylish, innovative, affordable Thai/Indonesian/pan-Asian small-plates restaurant. Sit at one of the long shared tables and dig into a creative menu of €3 small plates and €8 big plates. Two people can make a filling meal out of three or four dishes (daily 11:00-24:00, Rosenthaler Strasse 68, tel. 030/2478-1645).

Restaurant Simon dishes up tasty Italian and German specialties—enjoy them either in the restaurant's simple yet atmospheric interior, or opt for streetside seating right on the park across the street (€8-12 main dishes, Mon-Sat 12:00-22:00, Fri-Sat until 23:00, Sun 17:00-22:00, Auguststrasse 53, at intersection with Kleine Auguststrasse, tel. 030/2789-0300).

What If I Miss My Boat?

Remember that you can get help from the cruise line's port agent (listed on the destination information sheet distributed on the ship) and the local TI (see page 581). If the port agent suggests a costly solution (such as a private car with a driver), you may want to consider public transit.

Rostock has a few long-distance overnight ferry connections to other cities, but these are sporadic and unlikely to reach where you're going. For the most part, you'll need to go by train to Berlin (3 hours) and connect from there to just about any other cruise port: to **Amsterdam** (and onward to **Zeebrugge, Paris/LeHavre,** or **London**); to **Copenhagen** (and onward to **Stockholm, Oslo,** and other Norwegian stops); to **Gdańsk;** and so on.

If you need to catch a **plane** to your next destination, you'll find an easy bus connection (bus #TXL) from either the Hauptbahnhof or Alexanderplatz to Tegel Airport.

Local **travel agents** in Warnemünde, Rostock, or Berlin can help you. For more advice on what to do if you miss the boat, see page 139.

BERLIN

German Survival Phrases

In the phonetics, ī sounds like the long i in "light," and bolded syllables are stressed.

English	German	Pronunciation
Good day.	Guten Tag.	**goo**-tehn tahg
Do you speak English?	Sprechen Sie Englisch?	**shprehkh**-ehn zee **ehgn**-lish
Yes. / No.	Ja. / Nein.	yah / nīn
I (don't) understand.	Ich verstehe (nicht).	ikh fehr-**shtay**-heh (nikht)
Please.	Bitte.	**bit**-teh
Thank you.	Danke.	**dahng**-keh
I'm sorry.	Es tut mir leid.	ehs toot meer līt
Excuse me.	Entschuldigung.	ehnt-**shool**-dig-oong
(No) problem.	(Kein) Problem.	(kīn) proh-**blaym**
(Very) good.	(Sehr) gut.	(zehr) goot
Goodbye.	Auf Wiedersehen.	owf **vee**-der-zayn
one / two	eins / zwei	īns / tsvī
three / four	drei / vier	drī / feer
five / six	fünf / sechs	fewnf / zehkhs
seven / eight	sieben / acht	**zee**-behn / ahkht
nine / ten	neun / zehn	noyn / tsayn
How much is it?	Wieviel kostet das?	**vee**-feel **kohs**-teht dahs
Write it?	Schreiben?	**shrī**-behn
Is it free?	Ist es umsonst?	ist ehs oom-**zohnst**
Included?	Inklusive?	in-kloo-**zee**-veh
Where can I buy / find...?	Wo kann ich kaufen / finden...?	voh kahn ikh **kow**-fehn / **fin**-dehn
I'd like / We'd like...	Ich hätte gern / Wir hätten gern...	ikh **heh**-teh gehrn / veer **heh**-tehn gehrn
...a room.	...ein Zimmer.	īn **tsim**-mer
...a ticket to ____.	...eine Fahrkarte nach ____.	**ī**-neh **far**-kar-teh nahkh
Is it possible?	Ist es möglich?	ist ehs **mur**-glikh
Where is...?	Wo ist...?	voh ist
...the train station	...der Bahnhof	dehr **bahn**-hohf
...the bus station	...der Busbahnhof	dehr **boos**-bahn-hohf
...the tourist information office	...das Touristen-informations-büro	dahs too-**ris**-tehn-in-for-maht-see-**ohns**-bew-roh
...the toilet	...die Toilette	dee toh-**leh**-teh
men	Herren	**hehr**-rehn
women	Damen	**dah**-mehn
left / right	links / rechts	links / rehkhts
straight	geradeaus	geh-**rah**-deh-**ows**
What time does this open / close?	Um wieviel Uhr wird hier geöffnet / geschlossen?	oom **vee**-feel oor veerd heer geh-**urf**-neht / geh-**shloh**-sehn
At what time?	Um wieviel Uhr?	oom **vee**-feel oor
Just a moment.	Moment.	moh-**mehnt**
now / soon / later	jetzt / bald / später	yehtst / bahld / **shpay**-ter
today / tomorrow	heute / morgen	**hoy**-teh / **mor**-gehn

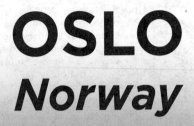

OSLO
Norway

Norway Practicalities

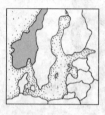

Norway (Norge) is stacked with super-latives—it's the most mountainous, most scenic, and most prosperous of all the Scandinavian countries. Perhaps above all, Norway is a land of intense natural beauty, its famously steep mountains and deep fjords carved out and shaped by an ancient ice age. Norway (148,700 square miles—just larger than Montana) is on the western side of the Scandinavian Peninsula, with most of the country sharing a border with Sweden to the east. Rich in resources like timber, oil, and fish, Norway has rejected joining the European Union, mainly to protect its fishing rights. Where the country extends north of the Arctic Circle, the sun never sets at the height of summer and never comes up in the deep of winter. The majority of Norway's 5 million people consider themselves Lutheran.

Money: 6 Norwegian kroner (kr, officially NOK) = about $1. An ATM is called a *minibank*. The local VAT (value-added sales tax) rate is 25 percent; the minimum purchase eligible for a VAT refund is 315 kr (for details on refunds, see page 134).

Language: The native language is Norwegian (the two official forms are Bokmål and Nynorsk). For useful phrases, see page 708.

Emergencies: Dial 112 for police, medical, or other emergencies. In case of theft or loss, see page 125.

Time Zone: Norway is on Central European Time (the same as most of the Continent, one hour ahead of Great Britain, and six/nine hours ahead of the East/West Coasts of the US).

Embassies in Oslo: The **US embassy** is at Henrik Ibsens Gate 48 (tel. 21 30 85 58, emergency tel. 21 30 85 40, http://norway.usembassy.gov). The **Canadian embassy** is at Wergelandsveien 7 (tel. 22 99 53 00, www.canada.no). Call ahead for passport services.

Phoning: Norway's country code is 47; to call from another country to Norway, dial the international access code (011 from the US/Canada, 00 from Europe, or + from a mobile phone), then 47, followed by the local number. For local calls within Norway, just dial the number as it appears in this book—whether you're calling from across the street or across the country. To place an international call from Norway, dial 00, the code of the country you're calling (1 for US and Canada), and the phone number. For more tips, see page 1146.

Tipping: Service is included at sit-down meals, but this goes to the owner, so for great service it's nice to round up your bill about 10 percent. Tip a taxi driver by rounding up the fare (pay 90 kr on an 85-kr fare). For more tips on tipping, see page 138.

Tourist Information: www.goscandinavia.com

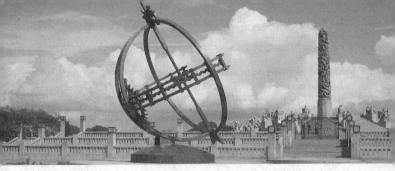

OSLO

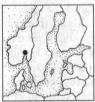

While Oslo is the smallest of the Scandinavian capitals, this brisk little city offers more sightseeing thrills than you might expect. As an added bonus, you'll be inspired by a city that simply has its act together.

Sights of the Viking spirit—past and present—tell an exciting story. Prowl through the remains of ancient Viking ships, and marvel at more peaceful but equally gutsy modern boats (the *Kon-Tiki, Ra, Fram,* and *Gjøa*). Dive into the traditional folk culture at the Norwegian open-air folk museum, and get stirred up by the country's heroic spirit at the Norwegian Resistance Museum.

For a look at modern Oslo, tour the striking City Hall, take a peek at sculptor Gustav Vigeland's people pillars, walk all over the Opera House, and celebrate the world's greatest peacemakers at the Nobel Peace Center.

Situated at the head of a 60-mile-long fjord, surrounded by forests, and populated by more than a half-million people, Oslo is Norway's cultural hub. For 300 years (1624-1924), the city was called Christiania, after Danish King Christian IV. With inde-

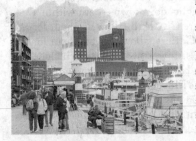

pendence, it reverted to the Old Norse name of Oslo. As an important port facing the Continent, Oslo has been one of Norway's main cities for a thousand years and the de facto capital since around 1300. Still, Oslo has always been small by European standards; in 1800, Oslo had 10,000 people, while cities such as Paris and London had 50 times as many.

Today the city sprawls out from its historic core to encompass nearly a million people in its metropolitan area—about one in five Norwegians. Oslo's port hums with international shipping and a sizeable cruise industry. Its waterfront, once traffic-congested and slummy, has already undergone a huge change and the extreme urban makeover is just starting. The vision: a five-mile people-friendly and traffic-free promenade stretching from east to west the entire length of its waterfront. Cars and trucks now travel in underground tunnels, upscale condos and restaurants are taking over, and the neighborhood has a splashy Opera House. Oslo seems to be constantly improving its infrastructure and redeveloping slummy old quarters along the waterfront into cutting-edge residential zones. The metropolis feels as if it's rushing to prepare for an Olympics-like deadline. But it isn't—it just wants to be the best city it can be.

You'll see a mix of grand Neoclassical facades and plain 1960s-style modernism, and a sprouting Nordic Manhattan-type skyline of skyscrapers nicknamed "the bar code buildings" for their sleek yet distinct boxiness. But overall, the feel of this major capital is green and pastoral—spread out, dotted with parks and lakes, and surrounded by hills and forests. For the visitor, Oslo is an all-you-can-see *smörgåsbord* of historic sights, trees, art, and Nordic fun.

PLANNING YOUR TIME

Oslo seems made-to-order for the cruise traveler who wants to see a lot in a single day on shore. While the city is spread out, its sightseeing highlights are concentrated in three zones (noted below). On a short port visit, I'd focus on two of these zones. If you're nervous about straying too far from your ship, all of the city-center sights listed here are reassuringly nearby, but some of Oslo's best sights are a bus, tram, or boat ride away. Logistically, it makes sense to start at the farthest-flung areas (Bygdøy or Vigeland Park), then work your way back toward the ship and do the city-center sights last.

• **City Center:** To get a look at today's Oslo, take my "Welcome to Oslo" self-guided walk (allow 30 minutes to sprint or an hour to linger). The two top sights downtown—both within a few steps of the walking route—are **City Hall** (allow one hour for a guided tour), and the **National Gallery** (allow about an hour for my self-guided tour). Lesser, but still worthwhile, sights include the **Nobel Peace Center, Opera House** (with hour-long guided tours), and **Norwegian Resistance Museum** (choose the ones that appeal to you, and allow 30-60 minutes each).

• **Vigeland Park:** This delightful people zone, populated by locals, tourists, and Gustav Vigeland's remarkable statues, is worth

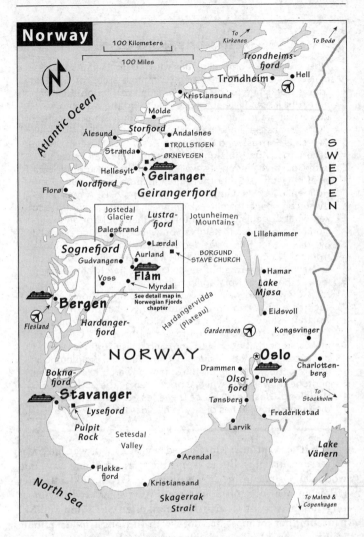

the 15-minute tram or bus ride west of downtown; once there, allow at least an hour to explore.

• **Bygdøy:** This "museum island" is most easily and scenically reached on a 10-minute ferry ride from Oslo's main harbor (carefully check return schedule to leave plenty of time to get back to your ship). Once here, you could spend all day at the many fine museums, ranging from an open-air folk museum to Viking ships to other Norwegian seafaring vessels (for full descriptions, see page 685 and choose your favorites; allow at least an hour per museum—and even more time for the spread-out Norwegian Folk Museum).

Excursions from Oslo

Most cruise lines offer activities within **Oslo** itself. As the city is user- and pedestrian-friendly (in most areas, and public transit works fine for others), I wouldn't pay for an excursion here. But if you'd like someone else to do the planning, various walking and bus tours lead you through the city center (Karl Johans Gate and harborfront area, including City Hall, Akershus Fortress, and Norwegian Resistance Museum), while others focus on the sights at Bygdøy (open-air museum—with Gol stave church—as well as Viking ship and other nautical museums). Still others may include a trip out to the Holmenkollen Ski Jump and surrounding hills. Any or all of these can be worthwhile—skim this chapter's descriptions to see what appeals to your interests, then look for an excursion that combines the sights you want to see. One place I'd avoid is the Ice Bar, a decidedly touristy venture a half-block from the National Museum. While it's entertaining, and can be refreshing on the rare hot day in Oslo, it's hardly an authentic look at the city or Norwegian culture.

A few excursions also include some out-of-town sights, such as a boat trip on the **Oslofjord** (which doesn't seem worth it—since you'll cruise in and out of the fjord on your ship anyway—unless you opt for a trip that's on a tall ship or makes stops that appeal to you) and a visit to the charming but super-touristy fjordside village of **Drøbak**. Train enthusiasts might enjoy a trip on the steam-powered **Krøderbanen** heritage railway line, while shoppers enjoy the 250-year-old **Hadeland Glassverk**. All of these less-urban options have their fans, but Oslo has plenty to fill a day.

• **Other Options:** Most one-day visitors will want to focus on these main sights. But to escape the tourist trail and delve into workaday Oslo, consider my walk to the **Grünerløkka district** (allow an hour or more round-trip). Avid skiers and Olympics pilgrims may want to visit **Holmenkollen Ski Jump and Ski Museum;** but for most, it's not worth the long trip (25-minute train ride plus 10-minute walk each way, and—on sunny days—a possible wait for the elevator to the top).

Sightsee Oslo Fjord from Your Ship: Oslo sits at the end of a long fjord. For many cruise itineraries, the hour approaching and the hour leaving Oslo is one of the most scenic parts of your cruise. Make a point to be on deck to enjoy the ride. About an hour out of town is a very narrow channel at Drøbak. This is famous among Norwegians as the place where they sank a big German warship at the start of World War II.

The Port of Oslo

Arrival at a Glance: It's easy to walk downtown from the two **Akershus** ports and the **Revierkai** port; **Filipstad** is farther out—still walkable, but more convenient by cruise-line shuttle bus. I'd avoid taxis, as the hefty $25 minimum makes even a short trip outrageously expensive.

Port Overview

Oslo has three main areas where cruise ships arrive. I've listed them more or less in order of usage. For now, each can moor one big ship. If there's one ship in town, it's likely at Akershus. The second would tie up at Vippetangen (just south of Akershus), the third at Revierkai, and the fourth at Filipstad. Though all of them are a walkable distance to and from downtown, getting there from Filipstad is easier with wheels. There's only one terminal building in Oslo, and that's at Akershus. The rest are just a place to tie up a big ship and for various buses to meet the cruisers. Most cruise lines provide a shuttle service from Filipstad only.

Akershus: Right on the harbor below Akershus Fortress, a short walk from the City Hall and town center, and the only port with a real terminal building, this is the handiest and most common entry point. There are technically two separate, adjacent berths here: **Søndre Akershuskai,** closer to town, and **Vippetangen,** a bit farther out (at the tip of the peninsula).

Revierkai: Around the east side of the Akershus Fortress peninsula, this port faces Oslo's new Opera House. Sights in the center are easily walkable from here.

Filipstad: Just west of downtown, next to the new Tjuvholmen development (around the far side of Aker Brygge from City Hall), this farther-out port is still walkable, but more convenient by cruise-line shuttle bus.

Expect Changes: Oslo's waterfront has been undergoing extensive development for the last few years, and work won't end anytime soon. Because much of this work also affects the cruise port areas, don't be surprised if some of the details in this section have changed. The long-term vision is for Filipstad to take more cruise traffic as the industry grows.

Tourist Information: The city's shiny new **Oslo Visitor Center** is in the Østbanehallen, the traditional-looking building right next to the train station (handy for those walking in from Revierkai). For more on the TI, see page 652.

OSLO

GETTING INTO TOWN

First I'll cover your taxi and tour options. Then I'll offer walking instructions from each of the ports. In general, from most ports you'll wind up at the City Hall/Aker Brygge area overlooking the harbor; however, if you're coming in from Revierkai, it's easier to visit the Opera House first, then head to the train station to take my "Welcome to Oslo" self-guided walk, which ends near City Hall/Aker Brygge.

By Taxi

A few taxis meet arriving ships, but they're very pricey and the city is workable without them. The 150-kr minimum (yes, that's a hefty $25) is enough to cover your trip into downtown from any of the cruise ports. A taxi to the museums at Bygdøy is also quite pricey, at around 300 kr (about $50) from downtown. Taxis can be a good value for groups. Minibus taxis are available and you are welcome to negotiate an hourly rate, but the city really lends itself to walking. I'd skip the big bill and make use of Oslo's fine public transportation. If you need a taxi but can't find one, call 02323.

By Tour

Various local tour options can be a good use of your time. Open Top Sightseeing's **hop-on, hop-off bus tours** meet arriving cruise ships at or near all ports and provide a good, affordable way to connect outlying sights, including Vigeland Park and Bygdøy. The tours can be a great value and super-convenient, and hopping off is always easy—but if you hit the timing wrong at popular stops like Vigeland Park, you may wait up to an hour for a chance to hop back on (all-day ticket-260 kr, credit card or Norwegian currency only, 19 stops, every 30 minutes, English headphone commentary, www.opentopsightseeing.no).

For other options in Oslo—including regular bus tours, fjord tours, walking tours, and local guides for hire—see "Tours in Oslo" on page 658.

By Foot from Each Port

The walking directions from each of Oslo's ports will get you close to the City Hall area at the head of the main harbor, which is also where most cruise-line shuttle buses drop off. This area is described in detail in the next section.

Akershus

By far the easiest place in town to arrive, the Akershus berths are within pleasant strolling distance of City Hall (10 minutes or less). From the **Søndre Akershuskai** berth, a bit closer to town, you can see the boxy twin towers of City Hall—just turn left from your

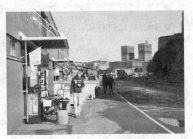

ship and head straight for it. The cruise terminal in front of this pier has lots of shops and a duty-free tax refund station (but no ATMs—for that, see "Services near City Hall and the Train Station" sidebar, later).

From **Vippetangen,** a bit farther out, it's still an easy walk (just 5 minutes longer). You may not be able to see City Hall from your ship—just walk with the water on your left. As you head into town, you'll pass the cruise terminal described earlier.

Revierkai

Around the east side of the Akershus peninsula, the Revierkai port faces Oslo's *other* big landmark: the strikingly modern Opera House, with its sloping roof leading right into the waters of the Oslofjord. If arriving here, you have several options: A fun first activity is to go for a stroll on the **Opera House** roof—to get there, simply walk to the end of the harbor and hook around to the right. (Their interesting tours are offered usually at 11:00, 12:00, and 14:00 in summer; see page 671.)

If you want to head to the **City Hall** area, several streets leading away from your ship can take you there; the most direct shot is along Rådhusgata, which is just beyond the giant, pink building with the towers. Walk along this street for about 15 minutes, and you'll pop out at City Hall.

If you want to begin with my self-guided walk—which ends near City Hall and shows you a lot more of downtown Oslo en route—head to the **train station:** First make your way to the Opera House. Then take the dark gray covered pedestrian bridge over the complicated intersection at the end of the harbor, and proceed straight ahead directly into the side door of Oslo's impressively modern train station. Continue straight up the escalators, turn left down the station's main hall, exit out the front, and start the walk (see page 660). From your ship to the station, figure about a 15-minute walk.

Filipstad

Located in an unappealing industrial port area just west of downtown, Filipstad is the only port that merits a shuttle bus, and cruises provide one (either free or about $8 each way). The shuttle will generally drop you at the harbor terminal at the Akershus dock (or at the Nobel Peace Center).

If you'd rather walk from Filipstad into town, it'll take you about 20 minutes to get from your ship to City Hall, but the stroll is far from interesting.

Services near City Hall and the Train Station

While Oslo has four places for ships to tie up, only Akershus has anything more than big cleats and a place for tour buses to meet their tourists. And the terminal at Akershus only has shops and a duty-free desk—no ATM or Wi-Fi. But once you're in town, resources abound. Assuming you'll enter town near City Hall or the train station, here are some services in each place.

ATMs: ATMs are easy to find behind the City Hall and around the train station.

Internet Access: The train station has free Wi-Fi and an Internet café.

Pharmacy: An Apotek 1 is between City Hall and Karl Johans Gate. There's a 24-hour pharmacy directly across the street and tram tracks from the train station's main entrance.

Years from now, when construction is finally completed around Filipstad and Tjuvholmen (a lively, cutting-edge residential zone across the little harbor from your ship), it'll be possible to cross directly from the port to Tjuvholmen and then it will be a quick, pleasant walk along Aker Brygge to reach the city center. But until then, you'll need to take the roundabout approach I've described below. Your ship's upper deck provides the perfect high-altitude vantage point for scouting your options before disembarking.

Exiting your ship at Filipstad, find your way to the port gate (at the far-left end of the big parking-lot zone at the pier). Continue straight out to the little roundabout and turn right, following the path out of the port area and the signs to *Sentrum*.

If you keep walking past the bus stop, you'll hit a foot/bike path that runs along a busy highway; turn right and follow this path into town. Reaching the next big roundabout, a hard right would get you to Tjuvholmen; to reach City Hall, continue straight (bearing right just slightly) along the busiest road, lined with new, modern buildings. Soon you'll see City Hall's boxy twin towers ahead. When you reach the cross-street called Dokkveien (with the tram tracks), you have a choice: To get to the harbor, turn right and take the road down to Aker Brygge and the Nobel Peace Center. If you'd rather head to the park near Karl Johans Gate in the heart of Oslo, go straight, and you'll pop out at the National Theater.

ARRIVING AT CITY HALL, AKER BRYGGE, AND THE HARBOR

No matter where your ship docks, you'll probably start your Oslo exploration in the harborfront zone in front of City Hall—with the Akershus Fortress on one side, and the Nobel Peace Center and Aker Brygge mall complex on the other. In addition to those four sightseeing options (all described later, under "Sights in Oslo"), here are some other choices:

To get oriented, you can follow the last parts of my "Welcome to Oslo" **self-guided walk,** starting with "City Hall" on page 669.

To reach the busy city center from the harborfront, circle around the City Hall building and go up the street directly behind it. You'll run into the inviting park that runs alongside Oslo's main drag, **Karl Johans Gate,** a short walk from the National Gallery and other sights.

From the harborfront, a boat trundles tourists across the bay to the sights at **Bygdøy** (boat and museums described on page 685).

If you'd like to zip to the **train station** area and the start of my self-guided walk (it ends near City Hall), you can take a tram. You'll find two tram stops (serving the same trams) in the zone in front of City Hall: The Aker Brygge stop is in front of the yellow Nobel Peace Center (to the right as you face the harbor), and the Rådhusplassen stop is at the far end of the City Hall complex, near the start of the Akershus Fortress area (look for the grass strip around the tracks, to the left as you face the harbor). From either tram stop, take tram #12 (direction: Disen) and ride it three stops to Jernbanetorget, the square in front of the train station.

You can also use tram #12 to reach **Vigeland Park.** Hop on at either of the stops mentioned above, going in the direction of Majorstuen, and get off at the Vigelandsparken stop.

If you'd like to do my **self-guided tram tour** (on trams #12 and #11), you don't have to go to the train station to start it—you can pick it up right here at either of the City Hall-area stops (get on tram #12, direction: Majorstuen). After turning into #11, this tram takes you to the station area (exit there to do my self-guided walk) and continues back to City Hall.

Enjoy Oslo!

RETURNING TO YOUR SHIP

To reach the cruise berths near **Akershus,** just head for City Hall and look for your ship (tram #12 brings you to the Rådhusplassen stop, between City Hall and your ship). To get back to **Revierkai,** make your way to the train station, exit out the side to cross the pedestrian walkway to the Opera House, and circle around the harbor to your ship (or, from the City Hall area, walk 10 minutes up Rådhusgata). Leave yourself plenty of time for the dull hike back to **Filipstad,** or—ideally—catch the cruise-line shuttle bus from Akershus pier or wherever it dropped you off.

If you have some time to kill before heading back, the lively people zone around City Hall and Aker Brygge is a fine place to spend it. Consider dropping in to the Nobel Peace Center to while away any remaining time before returning to your ship.

See page 706 for help if you miss your boat.

Oslo

Oslo is easy to manage. Its sights cluster around the main boulevard, Karl Johans Gate (with the Royal Palace at one end and the train station at the other), and in the Bygdøy (big-doy) district, a 10-minute ferry ride across the harbor. The city's other main sight, Vigeland Park (with Gustav Vigeland's statues), is about a mile behind the palace.

The monumental, homogenous city center contains most of the sights, but head out of the core to see the more colorful neighborhoods. Choose from Majorstuen and Frogner (chic boutiques, trendy restaurants), Grünerløkka (bohemian cafés, hipsters), and Grønland (multiethnic immigrants' zone).

Orientation to Oslo

TOURIST INFORMATION

The city's shiny new **Oslo Visitor Center** is in the Østbanehallen, the traditional-looking building right next to the central train station. Standing in the square (Jernbanetorget) by the tiger statue and facing the train station, you'll find the TI's entrance in the red-painted section between the station and Østbanehallen. You can also enter the TI from inside the train station (May-Sept daily 9:00-18:00, Oct-April daily 9:00-16:00, tel. 81 53 05 55, www.visitoslo.com).

At the TI, pick up these freebies: an Oslo map, the helpful public-transit map, the annual *Oslo Guide* (with plenty of details on sightseeing, shopping, and eating), and the *You Are Here Oslo* map and visitors guide (a young people's guide that's full of fun and off-beat ideas). For entertainment ideas and more, the free *What's On in Oslo* monthly has the most accurate record of museum hours and an extensive listing of happenings every day, such as special events, tours, and concerts. If you like to bike, ask about the public bike-rental system (100 kr/24 hours; you can rent a card from the TI to release simple one-speed bikes from racks around town).

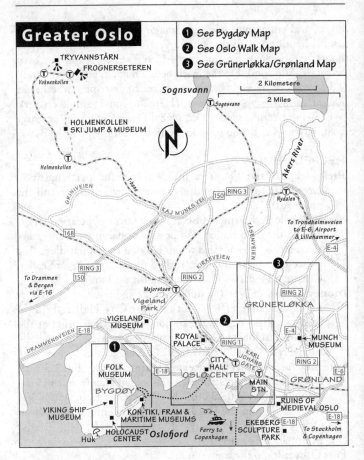

Greater Oslo

1 See Bygdøy Map
2 See Oslo Walk Map
3 See Grünerløkka/Grønland Map

TRYVANNSTÅRN
FROGNERSETEREN
Voksenkollen
HOLMENKOLLEN
SKI JUMP & MUSEUM
Holmenkollen
Sognsvann
Sognsvann
2 Kilometers
2 Miles
Akers River
GREINVEIEN
Tjana
KAJ MUNKS VEI
150 RING 3
Nydalen
To Trondheimsveien
to E-6, Airport
& Lillehammer
E-4
168
KIRKEVEIEN
RING 3
150
TÅSENVEIEN
To Drammen
& Bergen
via E-16
Majorstuen
RING 2
Vigeland
Park
GRÜNERLØKKA
3
VIGELAND
MUSEUM
E-18
DRAMMENSVEIEN
FOLK
MUSEUM
BYGDØY
1
ROYAL
PALACE
RING 1
2
CITY
HALL
OSLO CENTER
E-4
E-6
RING 2
MUNCH
MUSEUM
GRØNLAND
KARL
JOHANS
GATE
E-18
VIKING SHIP
MUSEUM
KON-TIKI, FRAM &
MARITIME MUSEUMS
MAIN
STN.
RUINS OF
MEDIEVAL OSLO
E-18
Huk
HOLOCAUST
CENTER
Oslofjord
Ferry to
Copenhagen
EKEBERG
SCULPTURE
PARK
E-18
To Stockholm
& Copenhagen

If you're traveling on, pick up the *Bergen Guide* and information for the rest of Norway, including the useful, annual *Fjord Norway Travel Guide*. Consider buying the Oslo Pass (described below).

Use It, a hardworking information center, is officially geared for those under age 26 but is generally happy to offer anyone its solid, money-saving, experience-enhancing advice (Mon-Fri 11:00-17:00, Sat 12:00-17:00, longer hours July-early Aug, closed Sun; Møllergata 3, look for *Ungdomsinformasjonen* sign, tel. 24 14 98 20, www.use-it.no). They offer these free services: Wi-Fi and Internet access, phone use, and luggage storage. Their free *You Are Here Oslo* guide—with practical info, maps, ideas on eating cheap, good nightspots, tips on picking up a Norwegian, the best beaches, and so on—is a must for young travelers and worthwhile for anyone curious about probing the Oslo scene.

Oslo Pass: This pass covers the city's public transit, ferry boats, and entry to nearly every major sight—all described in a useful handbook (320 kr/24 hours, 470 kr/48 hours, 590 kr/72 hours; big discounts for kids ages 4-15 and seniors age 67 and over, www.visitoslo.com). Do the math before buying; add up the individual costs of the sights you want to see to determine whether an Oslo Pass will save you money. (Here are some sample charges: one 24-hour transit pass-90 kr, Nobel Peace Center-90 kr, three boat museums at Bygdøy-270 kr, National Gallery-50 kr.)

HELPFUL HINTS

Pickpocket Alert: They're a problem in Oslo, particularly in crowds on the street and in subways and buses. To call the police, dial 112.

Street People and Drug Addicts: Oslo's street population loiters around the train station. While a bit unnerving to some travelers, locals consider this rough-looking bunch harmless. The police have pretty much corralled them to the square called Christian Frederiks Plass, south of the station.

Money: Banks in Norway don't change money. Use ATMs or Forex exchange offices (outlets near City Hall at Fridtjof Nansens Plass 6, at train station, and at Egertorget at the crest of Karl Johans Gate; hours vary by location but generally Mon-Fri 9:00-18:00, Sat 9:00-17:00, closed Sun).

Internet Access: @rctic Internet Café is pricey but central, located in the train station's main hall and above track 13 (60 kr/hour, daily 8:00-23:00). The TI near the train station has free Wi-Fi, and the **Use It** information center a block from Oslo Cathedral has free Wi-Fi and terminals, (see "Tourist Information," earlier).

Post Office: It's in the train station.

Pharmacy: Jernbanetorgets Vitus Apotek is open 24 hours daily (across from train station on Jernbanetorget, tel. 23 35 81 00).

Bike Rental: Viking Biking, run by Americans Curtis and Ben, rents bikes (125 kr/8 hours, 200 kr/24 hours, includes helmet, map, rain poncho, and lock, daily 9:30-18:00, Nedre Slottsgate 4, tel. 41 26 64 96, www.vikingbikingoslo.com; see "Tours in Oslo," later, for their guided bike tours).

Or use the public bike-rental system to grab basic **city bikes** out of locked racks at various points throughout town (100 kr/24 hours; get card at TI).

Updates to This Book: For updates to this book, check www.ricksteves.com/update.

GETTING AROUND OSLO

By Public Transit: Oslo's excellent transit system is made up of buses, trams, ferries, and a subway (*Tunnelbane,* or T-bane for

Sightseeing by Public Transit

With a transit pass or an Oslo Pass, take full advantage of the T-bane and the trams. Just spend five minutes to get a grip on the system, and you'll become amazingly empowered. Here are the only T-bane stations you're likely to use:

Jernbanetorget (central station, bus and tram hub, express train to airport)

Stortinget (top of Karl Johans Gate, near Akershus Fortress)

Nationaltheatret (National Theater, also a train station, express train to airport, near City Hall, Aker Brygge, Royal Palace)

Majorstuen (walk to Vigeland Sculpture Park, trendy shops on Bogstadveien)

Grønland (colorful immigrant neighborhood, cheap and fun restaurant zone, bottom of Grünerløkka district; the underground mall in the station is a virtual trip to Istanbul)

Holmenkollen (famous ski jump, city view)

Frognerseteren (highest point in town, jumping-off point for forest walks and bike rides)

Trams and buses that matter:

Trams #11 and **#12** ring the city (stops at central station, fortress, harborfront, City Hall, Aker Brygge, Vigeland Park, Bogstadveien, National Gallery, and Stortorvet)

Trams #11, #12, and **#13** to Olaf Ryes Plass (center of Grünerløkka district)

Trams #13 and **#19,** and **bus #31** (south and parallel to Karl Johans Gate to central station)

Bus #30 (Olaf Ryes Plass in Grünerløkka, train station, near Karl Johans Gate, National Theater, and Bygdøy, with stops at each Bygdøy museum)

short; see "Sightseeing by Public Transit" sidebar). Use the TI's free public transit map to navigate. The system runs like clockwork, with schedules clearly posted and followed. Many stops have handy electronic reader boards showing the time remaining before the next tram arrives (usually less than 10 minutes). **Ruter,** the public-transit information center, faces the train station under the glass tower; Mon-Fri 7:00-20:00, Sat-Sun 8:00-18:00, tel. 177 or 81 50 01 76, www.ruter.no.

Individual **tickets** work on buses, trams, ferries, and the T-bane for one hour (30 kr if bought at machines, transit office, Narvesen kiosks, convenience stores such as 7-Eleven or Deli de Luca, or via smartphone app—or 50 kr if bought on board). Other options include the **24-hour ticket** (90 kr; buy at machines, transit office, or via smartphone app; good for unlimited rides in 24-hour period) and the **Oslo Pass** (gives free run of entire system; described earlier). Validate your ticket or smartcard by holding it next to the card reader when you board.

Oslo at a Glance

▲▲▲**City Hall** Oslo's artsy 20th-century government building, lined with huge, vibrant, municipal-themed murals, best visited with included tour. **Hours:** Daily 9:00-18:00; 3 tours/day, tours run Wed only in winter. See page 669.

▲▲▲**National Gallery** Norway's cultural and natural essence, captured on canvas. **Hours:** Tue-Fri 10:00-18:00, Thu until 19:00, Sat-Sun 11:00-17:00, closed Mon. See page 674.

▲▲▲**Vigeland Park** Set in sprawling Frogner Park, with tons of statuary by Norway's greatest sculptor, Gustav Vigeland, and the studio where he worked (now a museum). **Hours:** Park—always open; Vigeland Museum—May-Aug Tue-Sun 10:00-17:00, Sept-April Tue-Sun 12:00-16:00, closed Mon year-round. See page 682.

▲▲▲**Norwegian Folk Museum** Norway condensed into 150 historic buildings in a large open-air park. **Hours:** Daily mid-May-mid-Sept 10:00-18:00, off-season park open Mon-Fri 11:00-15:00, Sat-Sun 11:00-16:00, but most historical buildings closed. See page 687.

▲▲**Norwegian Resistance Museum** Gripping look at Norway's tumultuous WWII experience. **Hours:** June-Aug Mon-Sat 10:00-17:00, Sun 11:00-17:00; Sept-May Mon-Fri 10:00-16:00, Sat-Sun 11:00-16:00. See page 673.

▲▲**Viking Ship Museum** An impressive trio of ninth-century Viking ships, with exhibits on the people who built them. **Hours:** Daily May-Sept 9:00-18:00, Oct-April 10:00-16:00. See page 688.

▲▲*Fram* **Museum** Captivating exhibit on the Arctic exploration ships *Fram* and *Gjøa*. **Hours:** June-Aug daily 9:00-18:00; May and Sept daily 10:00-17:00; Oct and March-April daily 10:00-16:00; Nov-Feb Mon-Fri 10:00-15:00, Sat-Sun 10:00-16:00. See page 689.

▲▲*Kon-Tiki* **Museum** Adventures of primitive *Kon-Tiki* and *Ra II* ships built by Thor Heyerdahl. **Hours:** Daily June-Aug 9:30-18:00, March-May and Sept-Oct 10:00-17:00, Nov-Feb 10:00-16:00. See page 690.

▲▲**Holmenkollen Ski Jump and Ski Museum** Dizzying vista and a schuss through skiing history. **Hours:** Daily June-Aug

9:00-20:00, May and Sept 10:00-17:00, Oct-April 10:00-16:00.
See page 696.

▲**Nobel Peace Center** Exhibit celebrating the ideals of the Nobel
Peace Prize and the lives of those who have won it. **Hours:** Mid-
May-Aug daily 10:00-18:00; Sept-mid-May Tue-Sun 10:00-18:00,
closed Mon. See page 670.

▲**Opera House** Stunning performance center that's helping revi-
talize the harborfront. **Hours:** Foyer and café/restaurant open
Mon-Fri 10:00-23:00, Sat 11:00-23:00, Sun 12:00-22:00; usually 3
tours/day of Opera House in summer. See page 671.

▲**Akershus Fortress Complex and Tours** Historic military base
and fortified old center, with guided tours, a ho-hum castle interior, and a couple of museums (including the excellent Norwegian
Resistance Museum, listed above). **Hours:** Park generally open
daily 6:00-21:00; usually 3 one-hour tours/day, fewer off-season.
See page 672.

▲**Norwegian Maritime Museum** Dusty cruise through Norway's
rich seafaring heritage. **Hours:** Mid-May-Aug daily 10:00-17:00;
Sept-mid-May Tue-Fri 10:00-15:00, Sat-Sun 10:00-16:00, closed
Mon. See page 691.

▲**Norwegian Holocaust Center** High-tech walk through rise
of anti-Semitism, the Holocaust in Norway, and racism today.
Hours: June-Aug daily 10:00-18:00, Sept-May Mon-Fri 10:00-
16:00, Sat-Sun 11:00-16:00. See page 691.

▲**Ekeberg Sculpture Park** Hilly, hikeable 63-acre forest park
dotted with striking contemporary art. **Hours:** Always open. See
page 697.

▲**Edvard Munch Museum** Works of Norway's famous
Expressionistic painter. **Hours:** Mid-June-Sept daily 10:00-17:00;
Oct-mid-June Wed-Mon 11:00-17:00, closed Tue. See page 697.

▲**Grünerløkka** Oslo's bohemian district, with bustling cafés and
pubs. **Hours:** Always open. See page 693.

▲**Aker Brygge and Tjuvholmen** Oslo's harborfront prome-
nade, and nearby trendy Tjuvholmen neighborhood with Astrup
Fearnley Museum, upscale galleries, shops, and cafés. **Hours:**
Always strollable. See page 672.

By Taxi: Taxis come with a 150-kr drop charge that covers you for three or four kilometers—about two miles (more on weekends). Taxis can be a good value if you're with a group. If you use a minibus taxi, you are welcome to negotiate an hourly rate. To get a taxi, wave one down, find a taxi stand, or call 02323.

Tours in Oslo

Oslo Fjord Tours

A fascinating world of idyllic islands sprinkled with charming vacation cabins is minutes away from the Oslo harborfront. For locals, the fjord is a handy vacation getaway. Tourists can get a glimpse of this island world by public ferry or tour boat. Cheap ferries regularly connect the nearby islands with downtown (free with Oslo Pass).

Several tour boats leave regularly from pier 3 in front of City Hall. Båtservice has a relaxing and scenic 1.5-hour hop-on, hop-off service, with recorded multilanguage commentary. It departs from the City Hall dock (185 kr, daily at 9:45, 11:15, 12:45, and 14:15; departs 30 minutes later from Opera House and one hour later from Bygdøy; tel. 23 35 68 90, www.boatsightseeing.com). They won't scream if you bring something to munch. They also offer two-hour fjord tours with lame live commentary (269 kr, 3-4/day late March-Sept).

Bus Tours

Båtservice, which runs the harbor cruises (above), also offers four-hour **bus tours** of Oslo, with stops at the ski jump, Bygdøy museums, and Vigeland Park (390 kr, 2/day mid-May-mid-Sept, departs next to City Hall, longer tours also available, tel. 23 35 68 90, www.boatsightseeing.com). HMK also does daily city bus tours (220 kr/2 hours, 350 kr/4 hours, departs next to City Hall, tel. 22 78 94 00, www.hmk.no). For details on **hop-on, hop-off bus tours,** see page 648.

Biking Tours

Viking Biking gives several different guided tours in English, including a three-hour Oslo Highlights Tour (250 kr, May-Sept daily at 13:00, Nedre Slottsgate 4, tel. 41 26 64 96, www.vikingbikingoslo.com). They also rent bikes; see "Helpful Hints," earlier.

Guided Walking Tour

Oslo Guideservice offers 1.5-hour historic "Oslo Promenade" walks from June through August (150 kr, free with Oslo Pass; Mon, Wed, and Fri at 17:30; leaves from sea side of City Hall, confirm departures at TI, tel. 22 42 70 20, www.guideservice.no).

OSLO

Local Guides

You can hire a private guide through **Oslo Guideservice** (2,000 kr/2 hours, tel. 22 42 70 20, www.guideservice.no); my guide Aksel had a passion for both history and his hometown of Oslo. Or try **Oslo Guidebureau** (prices start at 1,950 kr/3 hours, tel. 22 42 28 18, www.osloguide.no, mail@guideservice.no).

Oslo Tram Tour

Tram #12, which becomes tram #11 halfway through its loop (at Majorstuen), circles the city from the train station, lacing together many of Oslo's main sights. Apart from the practical value of being able to hop on and off as you sightsee your way around town (trams come by at least every 10 minutes), this 40-minute trip gives you a fine look at parts of the city you wouldn't otherwise see.

The route starts at the main train station, at the traffic-island tram stop located immediately in front of the transit office tower. The route makes almost a complete circle and finishes at Stortorvet (the cathedral square), dropping you off a three-minute walk from where you began the tour.

Starting out, you want tram #12 leaving from the second set of tracks, going toward Majorstuen. Confirm with your driver that the particular tram #12 you're boarding becomes tram #11 and finishes at Stortorvet; some of these may turn into tram #19 instead, which takes a different route. If yours becomes #19, simply hop out at Majorstuen and wait for the next #11. If #11 is canceled because of construction, leave #12 at Majorstuen and catch #19 through the center back to the train station, or hop on the T-bane (which zips every few minutes from Majorstuen to the National Theater—closest to the harbor and City Hall—and then to the station). Note that you can also begin this tour at either of the harborfront tram stops in front of City Hall (see page 651).

Here's what you'll see and ideas on where you might want to hop out:

From the **station,** you'll go through the old grid streets of 16th-century Christiania, King Christian IV's planned Renaissance town. After the city's 17th fire, in 1624, the king finally got fed up. He decreed that only brick and stone buildings would be permitted in the city center, with wide streets to serve as fire breaks.

You'll turn a corner at the **fortress** (Christiana Torv stop; get off here for the fortress and Norwegian Resistance Museum), then head for **City Hall** (Rådhus stop). Next comes the harbor and upscale **Aker Brygge** waterfront neighborhood (jump off at the Aker Brygge stop for the harbor and restaurant row). Passing the harbor, you'll see on the left a few old shipyard buildings that still

OSLO

survive. Then the tram goes uphill, past the **House of Oslo** (a mall of 20 shops highlighting Scandinavian interior design; Vikatorvet stop) and into a district of ugly 1960s buildings (when elegance was replaced by "functionality"). The tram then heads onto the street Norwegians renamed **Henrik Ibsens Gate** in 2006 to commemorate the centenary of Ibsen's death, honoring the man they claim is the greatest playwright since Shakespeare.

After Henrik Ibsens Gate, the tram follows Frognerveien through the chic **Frogner neighborhood.** Behind the fine old facades are fancy shops and spendy condos. Here and there you'll see 19th-century mansions built by aristocratic families who wanted to live near the Royal Palace; today, many of these house foreign embassies. Turning the corner, you roll along the edge of **Frogner Park** (which includes **Vigeland Park,** featuring Gustav Vigeland's sculptures), stopping at its grand gate (hop out at the Vigelandsparken stop).

Ahead on the left, a statue of 1930s ice queen Sonja Henie marks the arena where she learned to skate. Turning onto Bogstadveien, the tram usually becomes #11 at the Majorstuen stop. **Bogstadveien** is lined with trendy shops, restaurants, and cafés—it's a fun place to stroll and window-shop. (You could get out here and walk along this street all the way to the Royal Palace park and the top of Karl Johans Gate.) The tram veers left before the palace, passing the **National Historical Museum** and stopping at the **National Gallery** (Tullinløkka stop). As you trundle along, you may notice that lots of roads are ripped up for construction. It's too cold to fix the streets in winter, so, when possible, the work is done in summer. Jump out at **Stortorvet** (a big square filled with flower stalls and fronted by the cathedral and the big GlasMagasinet department store). From here, you're a three-minute walk from the station, where this tour began.

Welcome to Oslo Walk

This self-guided stroll, worth ▲▲, covers the heart of Oslo—the zone where most tourists find themselves walking—from the train station, up the main drag, and past City Hall to the harborfront. It takes a brisk 30 minutes if done nonstop.

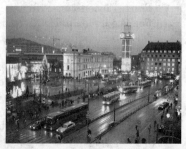

Train Station: Start at the plaza just outside the main entrance of Oslo's central train station (Oslo Sentralstasjon). The statue of the tiger prowling around out front alludes to the town's nickname of Tigerstaden ("Tiger Town"), and commemo-rates the 1,000th birthday of Oslo's founding, celebrated in the year 2000. In the 1800s, Oslo was considered an urban tiger, leav-ing its mark on the soul of simple country folk who ventured into the wild and crazy New York City of Norway. (These days, the presence of so many beggars, or *tigger*, has prompted the nickname "Tiggerstaden.")

With your back to the train station, look for the glass Ruter tower that marks the **public transit office;** from here, trams zip to City Hall (harbor, boat to Bygdøy), and the underground subway (T-bane, or *Tunnelbane*—look for the *T* sign to your right) goes to Vigeland Park (statues) and Holmenkollen. Tram #12—featured in the self-guided tram tour described earlier—leaves from directly across the street.

The green building behind the Ruter tower is a shopping mall called **Byporten** (literally, "City Gate," see big sign on roof-top), built to greet those arriving from the airport on the shuttle train. Oslo's 37-floor pointed-glass **skyscraper,** the Radisson Blu Plaza Hotel, looms behind that. Its 34th-floor SkyBar welcomes the public with air-conditioned views and pricey drinks (Mon-Sat 17:00-24:00, closed Sun). The tower was built with reflective glass so that, from a distance, it almost disappears. The area behind the Radisson—the lively and colorful "Little Karachi," centered along a street called Grønland—is where most of Oslo's immigrant pop-ulation settled. It's become a vibrant nightspot, offering a fun con-trast to the predictable homogeneity of Norwegian cuisine and culture.

Oslo allows hard-drug addicts and prostitutes to mix and mingle in the station area. Signs warn that this is a "monitored area," but victimless crimes proceed while violence is minimized. (Watch your purse and wallet here.)

• *Note that you are near the Opera House if you'd like to side-trip there now. Otherwise, turn your attention to Norway's main drag, called...*

Karl Johans Gate: This grand boulevard leads directly from the train station to the Royal Palace. The street is named for the French general Jean Baptiste Bernadotte, who was given a Swedish name, established the current Swedish dynasty, and ruled as a popular king (1818-1844) during the period after Sweden took Norway from Denmark.

Walk three blocks up Karl Johans Gate. This stretch is referred to as **"Desolation Row"** by locals because it has no soul, just shops greedily looking to devour tourists' money. If you visit in the snowy winter, you'll walk on bare concrete: Most of downtown Oslo's pedestrian streets are heated.

• *Hook right around the curved old brick structure of an old market and walk to the...*

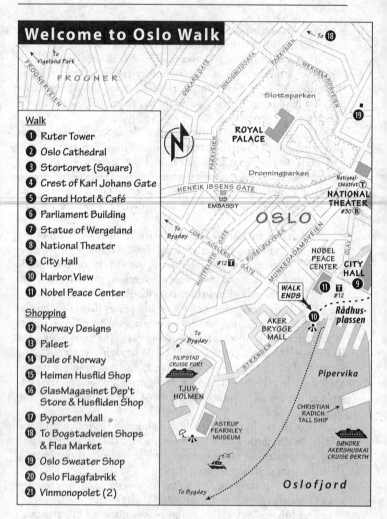

Welcome to Oslo Walk

Walk

1. Ruter Tower
2. Oslo Cathedral
3. Stortorvet (Square)
4. Crest of Karl Johans Gate
5. Grand Hotel & Café
6. Parliament Building
7. Statue of Wergeland
8. National Theater
9. City Hall
10. Harbor View
11. Nobel Peace Center

Shopping

12. Norway Designs
13. Paleet
14. Dale of Norway
15. Heimen Husflid Shop
16. GlasMagasinet Dep't Store & Husfliden Shop
17. Byporten Mall
18. To Bogstadveien Shops & Flea Market
19. Oslo Sweater Shop
20. Oslo Flaggfabrikk
21. Vinmonopolet (2)

Oslo Cathedral (Domkirke): This Lutheran church (daily 10:00-16:00) is the third cathedral Oslo has had, built in 1697 after the second burned down. It's where Norway commemorates its royal marriages and deaths. Seventy-seven deaths were mourned here following the tragic shootings and bombing of July 2011, when an anti-immigration fanatic named Anders Behring Breivik went berserk, setting off a car bomb in Oslo, killing eight, and then traveling to a Labor Party summer camp where he shot and killed 69 young people and counselors. In the grass in front of the cathedral, you may see a semipermanent memorial to the victims, consisting of a row of stones shaped like a heart.

Look for the cathedral's cornerstone (right of entrance), a

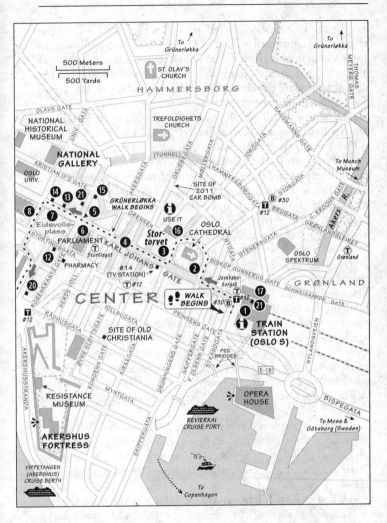

thousand-year-old carving from Oslo's first and long-gone cathedral showing how the forces of good and evil tug at each of us. Look high up on the tower. The tiny square windows midway up the copper cupola were once the lookout quarters of the fire watchman.

Step inside beneath the red, blue, and gold seal of Oslo and under an equally colorful ceiling (late Art Deco from the 1930s). The box above on the right is for the royal family. The fine Baroque pulpit and altarpiece date from 1700. The chandeliers are from the previous cathedral (which burned in the 17th century). The colorful windows in the choir (leading up to the altar) were made in 1910 by Emanuel Vigeland (Gustav's less-famous brother).

Leaving the church, stroll around to the right, behind the church. The **courtyard** is lined by a circa-1850 circular row of stalls from an old market. Rusty meat hooks now decorate the lamps of a peaceful café, which has quaint tables around a fountain. The atmospheric **Café Bacchus,** at the far left end of the arcade, serves food outside and in a classy café downstairs (light 150-200-kr meals, Mon-Fri 11:00-22:00, Sat 12:00-22:00, closed Sun, hamburgers, salads, good cakes, coffee, tel. 22 33 34 30).

• *The big square that faces the cathedral is called...*

Stortorvet: In the 17th century, when Oslo's wall was located about here, this was the point where farmers were allowed to enter and sell their goods. Today it's still lively as a flower and produce market (Mon-Fri). The statue shows Christian IV, the Danish king who ruled Norway around 1600, dramatically gesturing that-a-way. He named the city, rather immodestly, Christiania. (Oslo took back its old Norse name only in 1925.) Christian was serious about Norway. During his 60-year reign, he visited it 30 times (more than all other royal visits combined during 300 years of Danish rule). The big GlasMagasinet department store is a landmark on this square.

• *Return to Karl Johans Gate, and continue up the boulevard past street musicians, cafés, shops, and hordes of people. If you're here early in the morning (Mon-Fri), you may see a commotion at #14 (in the first block, on the left, look for the big 2 sign). This is the studio of a TV station (channel 2) where the Norwegian version of the* Today *show is shot, and as on Rockefeller Plaza, locals gather here, clamoring to get their mugs on TV.*

At the next corner, Kongens Gate leads left, past the 17th-century grid-plan town to the fortress. But we'll continue hiking straight up to the crest of the hill, enjoying some of the street musicians along the way. Pause at the wide spot in the street just before Akersgata to appreciate the...

Crest of Karl Johans Gate: Look back at the train station. A thousand years ago, the original (pre-1624) Oslo was located at the foot of the wooded hill behind the station (described later). Now look ahead to the Royal Palace in the distance, which was built in the 1830s "with nature and God behind it and the people at its feet." If the flag flies atop the palace, the king is in the country. Karl Johans Gate, a parade ground laid out in about 1850 from here to the palace—is now the axis of modern Oslo. Each May 17, Norway's Constitution Day, an annual children's parade turns this street into a sea of marching student bands and costumed young flag-wavers, while the royal family watches from the palace balcony. Since 1814, Norway has preferred peace. Rather than celebrating its military on the national holiday, it celebrates its children.

King Harald V and Queen Sonja moved back into the palace in 2001, after extensive (and costly) renovations. To quell the controversy caused by this expense, the public is now allowed inside to visit each summer with a pricey one-hour guided tour (95 kr, 3 English tours/day late June-mid-Aug, fills fast—buy tickets in advance online or at many convenience stores, such as the Narvesen kiosk near the palace, or by calling 81 53 31 33, www. kongehuset.no).

In the middle of the small square, the *T* sign marks a stop of the T-bane (Oslo's subway). W. B. Samson's bakery is a good place for a quick, affordable lunch, with a handy cafeteria line (WC in back); duck inside if just to be tempted by the pastries. Two traditional favorites are *kanelboller* (cinnamon rolls) and *skolebrød* ("school bread," with an egg-and-cream filling). From here, the street called Akersgata kicks off a worthwhile stroll past the site of the July 2011 bombing, the national cemetery, and through a parklike river gorge to the trendy Grünerløkka quarter (an hour-long walk, described on page 694).

People-watching is great along Karl Johans Gate, but remember that if it's summer, half of the city's regular population is gone—vacationing in their cabins or farther away—and the city center is filled mostly with visitors.

Hike two blocks down Karl Johans Gate, past the big brick Parliament building (on the left). On your right, seated in the square, is a statue of the 19th-century painter Christian Krohg. Continue down Karl Johans Gate. If you'd like to get a city view (and perhaps some refreshment), enter the glass doors at #27 and take the elevator to the eighth-floor roof-top bar, Etoile.

A few doors farther down Karl Johans Gate, just past the Freia shop (Norway's oldest and best chocolate), the venerable **Grand Hotel** (Oslo's celebrity hotel—Nobel Peace Prize winners sleep here) overlooks the boulevard.

• *Ask the waiter at the Grand Café—part of the Grand Hotel—if you can pop inside for a little sightseeing (he'll generally let you).*

Grand Café: This historic café was for many years the meeting place of Oslo's intellectual and creative elite (the playwright Henrik Ibsen was a regular here). Notice the photos and knickknacks on the wall. At the back of the café, a mural shows Norway's literary and artistic clientele—from a century ago—enjoying this fine hangout. On the far left, find Ibsen, coming in as he did every day at 13:00. Edvard Munch is on the right, leaning against the window, looking pretty drugged. Names are on the sill beneath the mural.

• *For a cheap bite with prime boulevard seating, continue past the corner to Deli de Luca, a convenience store with a super selection of takeaway food and a great people-watching perch. Across the street, a little*

Browsing

Oslo's pulse is best felt by strolling. Three good areas are along and near the central Karl Johans Gate, which runs from the train station to the palace (follow my self-guided "Welcome to Oslo" walk); in the trendy harborside Aker Brygge mall, a glass-and-chrome collection of sharp cafés, fine condos, and polished produce stalls (really lively at night, tram #12 from train station); and along Bogstadveien, a bustling shopping street with no-nonsense modern commerce, lots of locals, and no tourists (T-bane to Majorstuen and follow this street back toward the palace and tourist zone). While most tourists never get out of the harbor/Karl Johans Gate district, the real, down-to-earth Oslo is better seen elsewhere, in places such as Bogstadveien. The bohemian, artsy Grünerløkka district, described on page 694, is good for a daytime wander.

---

park faces Norway's...

Parliament Building (Stortinget): Norway's Parliament meets here (along with anyone participating in a peaceful protest outside). Built in 1866, the building seems to counter the Royal Palace at the other end of Karl Johans Gate. If the flag's flying, Parliament's in session. Today the king is a figurehead, and Norway is run by a unicameral Parliament and a prime minister. Guided tours of the Stortinget are offered for those interested in Norwegian government (free, 45 minutes; mid-June-Aug Mon-Fri at 10:00 and 13:00 in English, at 11:30 in Norwegian; line up at gate in front of the main entrance off Karl Johans Gate, tel. 23 31 35 96, www.stortinget.no).

• *Cross over into the park and stroll toward the palace, past the fountain. Pause at the...*

Statue of Wergeland: The poet Henrik Wergeland helped inspire the national resurgence of Norway during the 19th century. Norway won its independence from Denmark in 1814, but within a year it lost its freedom to Sweden. For nearly a century, until Norway won independence in 1905, Norwegian culture and national spirit was stoked by artistic and literary patriots like Wergeland. In the winter, the pool here is frozen and covered with children happily ice-skating. Across the street behind Wergeland stands the **National Theater** and statues of Norway's favorite playwrights: Ibsen and Bjørnstjerne Bjørnson. Across Karl Johans Gate, the pale yellow building is the first university building in Norway, dating from 1854. A block behind that is the National Gallery, with Norway's best collection of paintings (self-guided tour on page 676).

Take a moment here to do a 360-degree spin to notice how

quiet and orderly everything is. Many communities suffer from a "free rider" problem—which occurs when someone does something that would mess things up for all if everyone did it. (The transgressor believes his actions are OK because most people toe the line.) Norwegian society, with its heightened sense of social responsibility, doesn't experience this phenomenon.

• *Facing the theater, follow Roald Amundsens Gate left, to the towering brick...*

City Hall (Rådhuset): Built mostly in the 1930s with contributions from Norway's leading artists, City Hall is full of great

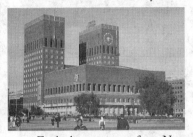

art and is worth touring (see page 669). The mayor has his office here (at the base of one of the two 200-foot towers), and every December 10, this building is where the Nobel Peace Prize is presented. For the best exterior art, circle the courtyard clockwise, studying the colorful woodcuts in the arcade. Each shows a scene from Norwegian mythology, well-explained in English: Thor with his billy-goat chariot, Ask and Embla (a kind of Norse Adam and Eve), Odin on his eight-legged horse guided by ravens, the swan maidens shedding their swan disguises, and so on. Circle to the right around City Hall, until you reach the front. The statues (especially the six laborers on the other side of the building, facing the harbor, who seem to guard the facade) celebrate the nobility of the working class. Norway, a social democracy, believes in giving respect to the workers who built their society and made it what it is, and these laborers are viewed as heroes.

• *Walk to the...*

Harbor: A decade ago, you would have dodged several lanes of busy traffic to get to Oslo's harborfront. But today, most cars cross underneath the city in tunnels. In addition, the city has made its town center relatively quiet and pedestrian-friendly by levying a traffic-discouraging 35-kr toll for every car entering town. (This system, like a similar one in London, subsidizes public transit and the city's infrastructure.)

At the water's edge, find the shiny metal plaque (just left of center) listing the contents of a sealed time capsule planted in 2000 out in the harbor in the little Kavringen lighthouse straight ahead (to be opened in 1,000 years). Go to the end of the stubby pier (on the right). This is the ceremonial "enter the city" point for momentous occasions. One such instance was in 1905, when Norway gained its independence from Sweden and a Danish prince sailed in from Copenhagen to become the first modern king of Norway.

OSLO

Another milestone event occurred at the end of World War II, when the king returned to Norway after the country was liberated from the Nazis.

• *Stand at the harbor and give it a sweeping counterclockwise look.*

Harborfront Spin-Tour: Oslofjord is a huge playground, with 40 city-owned, park-like islands. Big white cruise ships—a large part of the local tourist economy—dock just under the Akershus Fortress on the left. Just past the fort's impressive 13th-century ramparts, a statue of FDR grabs the shade. He's here in gratitude for the safe refuge the US gave to members of the royal family (including the young prince who is now Norway's king) during World War II—while the king and his government-in-exile waged Norway's fight against the Nazis from London.

Enjoy the grand view of City Hall. The yellow building farther to the left was the old West Train Station; today it houses the **Nobel Peace Center,** which celebrates the work of Nobel Peace Prize winners (see page 670). The next pier is the launchpad for harbor boat tours and the shuttle boat to the Bygdøy museums. A fisherman often moors his boat here, selling shrimp from the back.

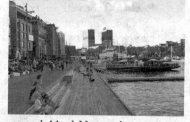

At the other end of the harbor, shipyard buildings (this was the former heart of Norway's once-important shipbuilding industry) have been transformed into **Aker Brygge**—Oslo's thriving restaurant/shopping/nightclub zone (see "Eating in Oslo").

Just past the end of Aker Brygge is a new housing development—dubbed Norway's most expensive real estate—called **Tjuvholmen.** It's anchored by the Astrup Fearnley Museum, an international modern art museum complex designed by renowned architect Renzo Piano (most famous for Paris' Pompidou Center; www.afmuseet.no). This zone is just one more reminder of Oslo's bold march toward becoming a city that is at once futuristic and people-friendly.

An ambitious urban renewal project called Fjord City (Fjordbyen)—which kicked off years ago with Aker Brygge, and led to the construction of Oslo's dramatic Opera House (see page 671)—is making remarkable progress in turning the formerly industrial waterfront into a flourishing people zone.

• *From here, you can stroll out Aker Brygge and through Tjuvholmen to a tiny public beach at the far end, tour City Hall, visit the Nobel Peace Center, hike up to Akershus Fortress, take a harbor cruise (see "Tours in Oslo," earlier), or catch a boat across the harbor to the museums at Bygdøy (from pier 3). The sights just mentioned are described in detail in the following section.*

Sights in Oslo

NEAR THE HARBORFRONT
▲▲▲City Hall (Rådhuset)

In 1931, Oslo tore down a slum and began constructing its richly decorated City Hall. It was finally finished—after a WWII

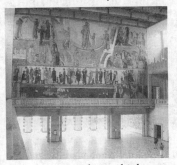

delay—in 1950 to celebrate the city's 900th birthday. Norway's leading artists all contributed to the building, an avant-garde thrill in its day. City halls, rather than churches, are the dominant buildings in Scandinavian capitals. The prominence of this building on the harborfront makes sense in this most humanistic, yet least churchgoing, northern end of the Continent. Up here, people pay high taxes, have high expectations, and are generally satisfied with what their governments do with their money.

Cost and Hours: Free, daily 9:00-18:00, free 50-minute guided tours daily at 10:00, 12:00, and 14:00 in summer, tours run Wed only in winter, free and fine WC, enter on Karl Johans Gate side, tel. 23 46 12 00.

Visiting City Hall: At Oslo's City Hall, the six statues facing the waterfront—dating from a period of Labor Party rule in Norway—celebrate the nobility of the working class. The art implies a classless society, showing everyone working together. The theme continues inside, with 20,000 square feet of bold and colorful Socialist Realist murals showing town folk, country folk, and people from all walks of life working harmoniously for a better society. The huge murals take you on a voyage through the collective psyche of Norway, from its simple rural beginnings through the scar tissue of the Nazi occupation and beyond. Filled with significance and symbolism—and well-described in English—the murals become even more meaningful with the excellent guided tours.

The main hall feels like a temple to good government, with its altar-like mural celebrating "work, play, and civic administration." The mural emphasizes Oslo's youth participating in community life—and rebuilding the country after Nazi occupation. Across the bottom, the slum that once cluttered up Oslo's harborfront is being cleared out to make way for this building. Above that, scenes show Norway's pride in its innovative health care and education systems. Left of center, near the top, Mother Norway rests on a church—reminding viewers that the Lutheran Church of Norway (the official state religion) provides a foundation for this society. On the right, four forms represent the arts; they illustrate how creativity springs from children. And in the center, the figure of Charity is surrounded by Culture, Philosophy, and Family.

The "Mural of the Occupation" lines the left side of the hall. It tells the story of Norway's WWII experience. Looking left to right, you'll see the following: The German blitzkrieg overwhelms the country. Men head for the mountains to organize a resistance movement. Women huddle around the water well, traditionally where news is passed, while Quislings (traitors named after the Norwegian fascist who ruled the country as a

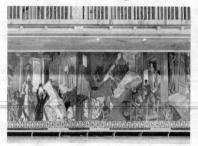

Nazi puppet) listen in. While Germans bomb and occupy Norway, a family gathers in their living room. As a boy clenches his fist (showing determination) and a child holds the beloved Norwegian flag, the Gestapo steps in. Columns lie on the ground, symbolizing how Germans shut down the culture by closing newspapers and the university. Two resistance soldiers are executed. A cell of resistance fighters (wearing masks and using nicknames so if tortured they can't reveal their compatriots' identities) plan a sabotage mission. Finally, prisoners are freed, the war is over, and Norway celebrates its happiest day: May 17, 1945—the first Constitution Day after five years under Nazi control.

While gazing at these murals, keep in mind that the Nobel Peace Prize is awarded in this central hall each December (though the general Nobel Prize ceremony occurs in Stockholm's City Hall). You can see videos of the ceremony and acceptance speeches in the adjacent Nobel Peace Center (see next).

Eating: Fans of the explorer Fridtjof Nansen might enjoy a coffee or beer across the street at Fridtjof, an atmospheric bar filled with memorabilia from Nansen's Arctic explorations. A model of his ship, the *Fram*, hangs from the ceiling, and 1894 photos and his own drawings are upstairs (Mon-Sat 12:00 until late, Sun 14:00-22:00, Nansens Plass 7, near Forex, tel. 93 25 22 30).

▲Nobel Peace Center (Nobels Fredssenter)

This thoughtful and thought-provoking museum, housed in the former West Train Station (Vestbanen), poses the question, "What is the opposite of conflict?" It celebrates the 800-some past and present Nobel Peace Prize winners with engaging audio and video exhibits and high-tech gadgetry (all with good English explanations). Allow time for reading about past prizewinners and listening to acceptance speeches by recipients from President Carter to Mother Theresa. Check out the astonishing interactive book detailing the life and work of Alfred Nobel, the Swedish inventor of dynamite, who initiated the prizes—perhaps to assuage his conscience.

Cost and Hours: 90 kr; mid-May-Aug daily 10:00-18:00; Sept-mid-May Tue-Sun 10:00-18:00, closed Mon; included English guided tours at 12:00 and 15:00, fewer in winter; Brynjulfs Bulls Plass 1, tel. 48 30 10 00, www.nobelpeacecenter.org.

▲Opera House

Opened in 2008, Oslo's striking Opera House is still the talk of the town and a huge hit. The building rises from the water on the city's eastern harbor, across the highway from the train station (use

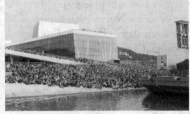

the sky-bridge). Its boxy, low-slung, glass center holds a state-of-the-art, 1,400-seat main theater with a 99-piece orchestra "in the pit" which can rise to put the orchestra "on the pedestal." The season is split between opera and ballet.

Information-packed 50-minute tours explain what makes this one of the greenest buildings in Europe and why Norwegian taxpayers helped foot the half-billion dollar bill for this project to make high culture (ballet and opera) accessible to the younger generation and a strata of society who normally wouldn't care. You'll see a workshop employing 50 people who hand-make costumes, and learn how the foundation of 700 pylons set 40 or 50 meters deep support the jigsaw puzzle of wood, glass, and 36,000 individual pieces of marble. The construction masterfully integrates land and water, inside and outside, nature and culture.

The jutting white marble planes of the Opera House's roof double as a public plaza. When visiting, you feel a need to walk all over it. The Opera House is part of a larger harbor-redevelopment plan that includes rerouting traffic into tunnels and turning a once-derelict industrial zone into an urban park.

Cost and Hours: Foyer and café/restaurant open Mon-Fri 10:00-23:00, Sat 11:00-23:00, Sun 12:00-22:00.

Tours: In summer, the Opera House offers sporadic foyer concerts (50 kr, generally at 13:00) and fascinating 50-minute guided tours of the stage, backstage area, and architecture (100 kr, usually 3 tours/day in English—generally at 11:00, 12:00, and 14:00, reserve by email at omvisninger@operaen.no or online at www.operaen.no, tel. 21 42 21 00).

Getting There: The easiest way to get to the Opera House is from the train station. Just follow signs for *Exit South/Utgang Syd* (standing in the main hall with the tracks to your back, it's to the left). Exiting the station, proceed straight ahead onto the pedestrian bridge (marked *Velkommen til Operaen*), which takes you effortlessly above traffic congestion to your goal.

▲Aker Brygge and Tjuvholmen

Oslo's harborfront was dominated by the Aker Brygge shipyard until it closed in 1986. Today this is the first finished part of a project (called Fjordbyen or Fjord City) that will turn the central stretch of Oslo's harborfront into a people-friendly park and culture zone. Aker Brygge is a stretch of trendy yacht-club-style restaurants facing a fine promenade—just the place to join in on a Nordic paseo on a balmy summer's eve.

The far end of Aker Brygge is marked by a big black anchor (from the German warship *Blücher*, sunk by Norwegian forces near Drøbak during the Nazi invasion on April 9, 1940). From there, a bridge crosses over into Tjuvholmen (named for the place they hung thieves back in the 17th century). This is a planned and future-esque community, with the trendiest and costliest apartments in town, lots of galleries, elegant shops and cafés, and the striking Astrup Fearnley Museum of Modern Art nearby. As you stroll through Tjuvholmen, admire how each building has its own personality.

Eating: Dining here is a great idea. Choose from many restaurants, or take advantage of the generous public benches, lounge chairs, and picnic tables that allow people who can't afford a fancy restaurant meal to enjoy the best seats of all (grocery stores are a block away from the harborfront views).

▲AKERSHUS FORTRESS COMPLEX

This park-like complex of sights scattered over Oslo's fortified old center is still a military base. (The Royal Guard is present because the castle is a royal mausoleum.) But the public is welcome, and as you dodge patrol guards and vans filled with soldiers, you'll see the castle, a prison, war memorials, the Norwegian Resistance Museum, the Armed Forces Museum, and cannon-strewn ramparts affording fine harbor views and picnic perches. There's an unimpressive changing of the guard daily at 13:30 (at the parade ground, deep in the castle complex). The park is generally open daily 6:00-21:00, but because the military is in charge here, times can change without warning. Expect bumpy cobblestone lanes and steep hills. To get here from the harbor, follow the stairs (which lead past the FDR statue) to the park.

Fortress Visitors Center: Located immediately inside the gate, the information center has an exhibit tracing the story of

Oslo's fortifications from medieval times through the environmental struggles of today. Stop here to pick up the fortress trail and site map, quickly browse through the museum, and consider catching a tour (see next; museum entry free, mid-June-mid-Aug Mon-Fri 10:00-17:00, Sat-Sun 11:00-17:00, shorter hours off-season, tel. 23 09 39 17, www.mil.no/felles/ak).

▲Fortress Tours

The 50-kr hour-long English walking tours of the grounds help you make sense of the most historic piece of real estate in Oslo (mid-June-mid-Aug 3/day, fewer off-season; depart from Fortress Visitors Center, call center at tel. 23 09 39 17 in advance to confirm times).

Akershus Castle

The first fortress here was built by Norwegians in 1299. It was
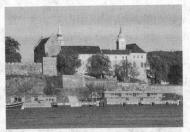
rebuilt much stronger by the Danes in 1640 so the Danish king (Christian IV) would have a suitable and safe place to stay during his many visits. When Oslo was rebuilt in the 17th century, many of the stones from the first Oslo cathedral were reused here, in the fortress walls.

Although it's one of Oslo's oldest buildings, the castle overlooking the harbor is mediocre by European standards; the big, empty rooms recall Norway's medieval poverty. From the old kitchen, where the ticket desk and gift shop are located, you'll follow a one-way circuit of rooms open to the public. Descend through a secret passage to the dungeon, crypt, and royal tomb. Emerge behind the altar in the chapel, then walk through echoing rooms including the Daredevil's Tower, Hall of Christian IV (with portraits of Danish kings of Norway on the walls), and Hall of Olav I. There are terrific harbor views (often filled with a giant cruise ship) from the rampart just outside.

Cost and Hours: 70 kr, includes audioguide with 45-minute tour and ghost story options; May-Aug Mon-Sat 10:00-16:00, Sun 12:30-16:00; Sept-April Sat-Sun 12:00-17:00 only, closed Mon-Fri; tel. 22 41 25 21.

▲▲Norwegian Resistance Museum
(Norges Hjemmefrontmuseum)

This fascinating museum tells the story of Norway's WWII experience: appeasement, Nazi invasion (they made Akershus their headquarters), resistance, liberation, and, finally, the return of the king.

OSLO

Cost and Hours: 50 kr; June-Aug Mon-Sat 10:00-17:00, Sun 11:00-17:00; Sept-May Mon-Fri 10:00-16:00, Sat-Sun 11:00-16:00; next to castle, overlooking harbor, tel. 23 09 31 38, www.forsvaretsmuseer.no.

Visiting the Museum: It's a one-way, chronological, can't-get-lost route. As you enter the museum, you're transported back to 1940, greeted by an angry commotion of rifles aimed at you. A German notice proclaiming, "You will submit or die" is bayonetted onto a gun in the middle.

You'll see propaganda posters attempting to get Norwegians to join the Nazi party, and the German ultimatum to which the king gave an emphatic "No." Various displays show secret radios, transmitters, underground newspapers, crude but effective home-made weapons, and the German machine that located clandestine radio stations. Exhibits explain how the country coped with 350,000 occupying troops; how airdrops equipped a home force of 40,000 ready to coordinate with the Allies when liberation was imminent; and the happy day when the resistance army came out of the forest, and peace and freedom returned to Norway.

The museum is particularly poignant because many of the patriots featured inside were executed by the Germans right outside the museum's front door; a stone memorial marks the spot. (At war's end, the traitor Vidkun Quisling was also executed at the fortress, but at a different location.) With good English descriptions, this is an inspirational look at how the national spirit can endure total occupation by a malevolent force. (Note: 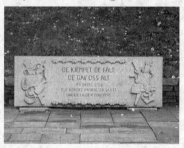 Copenhagen's Resistance Museum burned down and neutral Sweden didn't have a resistance.)

Armed Forces Museum (Forsvarsmuseet)

Across the fortress parade ground, a too-spacious museum traces Norwegian military history from Viking days to post-World War II. The early stuff is sketchy, but the WWII story is compelling.

Cost and Hours: Free, May-Aug Mon-Fri 10:00-16:00, Sat-Sun 11:00-17:00, shorter hours off-season, tel. 23 09 35 82.

DOWNTOWN MUSEUMS
▲▲▲National Gallery (Nasjonalgalleriet)

While there are many schools of painting and sculpture displayed in Norway's National Gallery, I suggest you focus on what's uniquely Norwegian. Paintings come and go in this museum

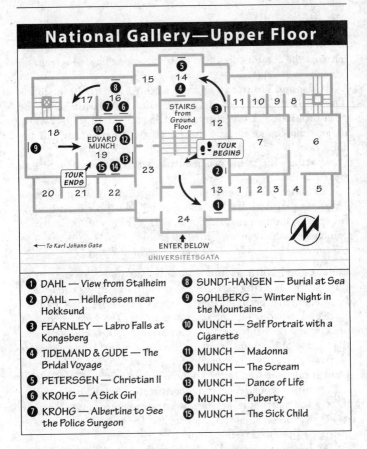

National Gallery—Upper Floor

15   14   5   4

8   16   7   6   17

STAIRS from Ground Floor

11   10   9   8   3   12

18   9

EDVARD MUNCH   10   11   12   13
19   15   14

TOUR ENDS

20   21   22   23

TOUR BEGINS   2

7   6

13   1   2   3   4   5

1

24

←—To Karl Johans Gate

ENTER BELOW
UNIVERSITETSGATA

1. DAHL — View from Stalheim
2. DAHL — Hellefossen near Hokksund
3. FEARNLEY — Labro Falls at Kongsberg
4. TIDEMAND & GUDE — The Bridal Voyage
5. PETERSSEN — Christian II
6. KROHG — A Sick Girl
7. KROHG — Albertine to See the Police Surgeon
8. SUNDT-HANSEN — Burial at Sea
9. SOHLBERG — Winter Night in the Mountains
10. MUNCH — Self Portrait with a Cigarette
11. MUNCH — Madonna
12. MUNCH — The Scream
13. MUNCH — Dance of Life
14. MUNCH — Puberty
15. MUNCH — The Sick Child

(pesky curators may have even removed some of the ones listed in the self-guided tour on the next page), but you're sure to see plenty that showcase the harsh beauty of Norway's landscape and people. A thoughtful visit here gives those heading into the mountains and fjord country a chance to pack along a little of Norway's cultural soul. Tuck these images carefully away with your goat cheese—they'll sweeten your explorations.

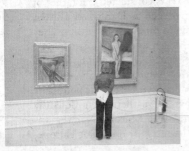

The gallery also has several Picassos, a noteworthy Impressionist collection, a Van Gogh self-portrait, and some Vigeland statues. Its many raving examples of Edvard Munch's work, including one of his famous *Scream* paintings, make a trip to the Munch Museum unnecessary for most (see page 697). It has about 50 Munch paintings in its collection, but only about a third are on display. Be prepared for changes, but don't worry—no matter what the curators decide to show, you won't have to scream for Munch's masterpieces.

Cost and Hours: 50 kr, free on Sun, Tue-Fri 10:00-18:00, Thu until 19:00, Sat-Sun 11:00-17:00, closed Mon, chewing gum prohibited, Universitets Gata 13, tel. 22 20 04 04, www.nasjonalmuseet.no. Pick up the guidebooklet to help navigate the collection.

Eating: The richly ornamented French Salon café offers an elegant break.

⊙ **Self-Guided Tour:** This easy-to-handle museum gives an effortless tour back in time and through Norway's most beautiful valleys, mountains, and fjords, with the help of its Romantic painters (especially Johan Christian Dahl).

• *Go up the stairs into Room 24 and turn left into Room 13.*

Landscape Paintings and Romanticism

Landscape painting has always played an important role in Norwegian art, perhaps because Norway provides such an awesome and varied landscape to inspire artists. The style reached its peak during the Romantic period in the mid-1800s, which stressed the beauty of unspoiled nature. (This passion for landscapes sets Norway apart from Denmark and Sweden.) After 400 years of Danish rule, the soul of the country was almost snuffed out. But with semi-independence and a constitution in the early 1800s, there was a national resurgence. Romantic paintings featuring the power of Norway's natural wonders and the toughness of its salt-of-the-earth folk came into vogue.

❶ **Johan Christian Dahl—*View from Stalheim* (1842):** This painting epitomizes the Norwegian closeness to nature. It shows a view very similar to the one that 21st-century travelers enjoy on the Norwegian fjords (see page 763): mountains, rivers, and farms clinging to hillsides. Painted in 1842, it's quintessential Romantic style. Nature rules—the background is as detailed as the foreground, and you are sucked in.

Johan Christian Dahl (1788-1857) is considered the father of Norwegian Romanticism. Romantics such as Dahl (and Turner, Beethoven, and Lord Byron) put emotion over rationality. They reveled in the power of nature—death and pessimism ripple through their work, though in this scene a double rainbow and a splash of sunlight give hope of a better day. The birch tree—standing boldly front and center—is a standard symbol for the politically downtrodden Norwegian people: hardy, weathered, but defiantly sprouting new branches. In the mid-19th century, Norwegians were awakening to their national identity. Throughout Europe, nationalism and Romanticism went hand in hand.

Find the farm buildings huddled near the cliff's edge, smoke rising from chimneys, and the woman in traditional dress tending her herd of goats, pausing for a moment to revel in the glory of nature. It reminds us that these farmers are hardworking, independent, small landowners. There was no feudalism in medieval Norway. People were poor...but they owned their own land. You can almost taste the goat cheese.

• *Look at the other works in Rooms 13 and 12. Dahl's paintings and those by his Norwegian contemporaries, showing heavy clouds and glaciers, repeat these same themes—drama over rationalism, nature pounding humanity. Human figures are melancholy. Norwegians, so close to nature, are fascinated by those plush, magic hours of dawn and twilight. The dusk makes us wonder: What will the future bring?*

In particular, focus on the painting to the left of the door in Room 13.

❷ **Dahl—*Hellefossen near Hokksund*** (1838): Another typical Dahl setting: romantic nature and an idealized scene. A fisherman checks on wooden baskets designed to catch salmon migrating up the river. In the background, a water-powered sawmill slices trees into lumber. Note another Dahl birch tree at the left, a subtle celebration of the Norwegian people and their labor.

• *Now continue into Room 12. On the right is...*

❸ **Thomas Fearnley—*Labro Falls at Kongsberg*** (1837): Man cannot control nature or his destiny. The landscape in this painting is devoid of people—the only sign of humanity is the jumble of sawn logs in the foreground. A wary eagle perched on one log seems to be saying, "While you can cut these trees, they'll always be mine."

• *Continue to the end of Room 12, and turn left into Room 14.*

❹ **Adolph Tidemand and Hans Gude—*The Bridal Voyage*** (1848): This famous painting shows the ultimate Norwegian scene:

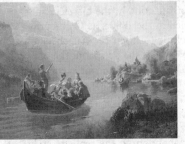 a wedding party with everyone decked out in traditional garb, heading for the stave church on the quintessential fjord (Hardanger). It's a studio work (not real) and a collaboration: Hans Gude painted the landscape, and Adolph Tidemand painted the people. Study their wedding finery. This work trumpets the greatness of both the landscape and Norwegian culture.

• *Also in Room 14, on the opposite wall, is an example of...*

OSLO

The Photographic Eye

At the end of the 19th century, Norwegian painters traded the emotions of Romanticism for more slice-of-life detail. This was the end of the Romantic period and the beginning of Realism. With the advent of photography, painters went beyond simple realism and into extreme realism.

❺ Eilif Peterssen—*Christian II* (1875): The Danish king signs the execution order for the man who'd killed the king's beloved mistress. With camera-like precision, the painter captures the whole story of murder, anguish, anger, and bitter revenge in the king's set jaw and steely eyes.

• *Go through Room 15 and into Room 16. Take time to browse the paintings.*

Vulnerability

Death, disease, and suffering were themes seen again and again in art from the late 1800s. The most serious disease during this period was tuberculosis (which killed Munch's mother and sister).

❻ Christian Krohg—*A Sick Girl* (1880): Christian Krohg (1852-1925) is known as Edvard Munch's inspiration, but to Norwegians, he's famous in his own right for his artistry and giant personality. This extremely realistic painting shows a child dying of tuberculosis, as so many did in Norway in the 19th century. The girl looks directly at you. You can almost feel the cloth, with its many shades of white.

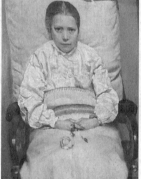

• *And just to the right of this painting, find...*

❼ Krohg—*Albertine to See the Police Surgeon* (c. 1885-1887): Krohg had a sharp interest in social justice. In this painting, Albertine, a sweet girl from the countryside, has fallen into the world of prostitution in the big city. She's the new kid on the Red Light block in the 1880s, as Oslo's prostitutes are pulled into the police clinic for their regular checkup. Note her traditional dress and the disdain she gets from the more experienced girls. Krohg has buried his subject in this scene. His technique requires the viewer to find her, and that search helps humanize the prostitute.

• *In Room 16 you may also find...*

❽ Carl Sundt-Hansen—*Burial at Sea* (1890): While Monet and the Impressionists were busy abandoning the realistic style, Norwegian artists continued to embrace it. In this painting, you're invited to participate. A dead man's funeral is attended by an ethnically diverse group of sailors and passengers, but only one is a woman—the widow. Your presence completes the half-circle at the on-deck ceremony. Notice how each person in the painting has his or her own way of confronting death. Their faces speak volumes about the life of toil here. A common thread in Norwegian art is the cycle—the tough cycle—of life. There's also an interest in everyday experiences. *Burial at Sea* may not always be on display. If it's not here, you may instead see a similar canvas, **Erik Werenskiold's** *A Peasant Burial* (1885).

• *Continue through Room 17 and into Room 18.*

Atmosphere

Landscape painters were often fascinated by the phenomena of nature, and the artwork in this room takes us back to this ideal from the Romantic Age. Painters were challenged by capturing atmospheric conditions at a specific moment, since it meant making quick sketches outdoors, before the weather changed yet again.

❾ Harald Sohlberg—*Winter Night in the Mountains* (1914):

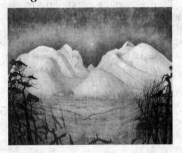

Harald Sohlberg was inspired by this image while skiing in the mountains in the winter of 1899. Over the years, he attempted to re-create the scene that inspired this remark: "The mountains in winter reduce one to silence. One is overwhelmed, as in a mighty, vaulted church, only a thousand times more so."

• *Follow the crowds into Room 19, the Munch room.*

Turmoil

Room 19 is filled with works by Norway's single most famous painter, Edvard Munch (see sidebar). Norway's long, dark winters and social isolation have produced many gloomy artists, but none gloomier than Munch. He infused his work with emotion and expression at the expense of realism. After viewing the paintings in general, take a look at these in particular (listed in clockwise order).

❿ Munch—*Self Portrait with a Cigarette* (1895): In this self-portrait, Munch is spooked, haunted—an artist working, immersed in an oppressive world. Indefinable shadows inhabit the background. His hand shakes as he considers his uncertain future. (Ironic, considering he created his masterpieces during this depressed period.) After eight months in a Danish clinic, he found peace—and lost his painting power. Afterward, Munch never again painted another strong example of what we love most about his art.

Edvard Munch (1863-1944)

Edvard Munch (pronounced "moonk") is Norway's most famous and influential painter. His life was rich, complex, and sad. His father was a doctor who had a nervous breakdown. His mother and sister both died of tuberculosis. He knew suffering. And he gave us the enduring symbol of 20th-century pain, *The Scream*.

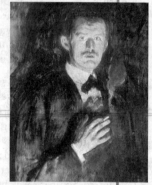

He was also Norway's most forward-thinking painter, a man who traveled extensively through Europe, soaking up the colors of the Post-Impressionists and the curves of Art Nouveau. He helped pioneer a new style—Expressionism—using lurid colors and wavy lines to "express" inner turmoil and the angst of the modern world.

After a nervous breakdown in late 1908, followed by eight months of rehab in a clinic, Munch emerged less troubled—but a less powerful painter. His late works were as a colorist: big, bright, less tormented...and less noticed.

⓫ **Munch—*Madonna* (1894-1895):** Munch had a tortured relationship with women. He never married. He dreaded and struggled with love, writing that he feared if he loved too much, he'd lose his painting talent. This painting is a mystery: Is she standing or lying? Is that a red halo or some devilish accessory? Munch wrote that he would strive to capture his subjects at their holiest moment. His alternative name for this work: *Woman Making Love*. What's more holy than a woman at the moment of conception?

⓬ **Munch—*The Scream* (1893):** Munch's most famous work

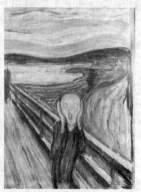

shows a man screaming, capturing the fright many feel as the human "race" does just that. The figure seems isolated from the people on the bridge—locked up in himself, unable to stifle his scream. Munch made four versions of this scene, which has become *the* textbook example of Expressionism. On one, he graffitied: "This painting is the work of a madman." He explained that the painting "shows today's society, reverberating within me...making me want to scream." He's sharing his internal angst. In fact, this Expressionist masterpiece is a breakthrough painting; it's angst personified.

🔞 **Munch—*Dance of Life* (1899-1900):** In this scene of five dancing couples, we glimpse Munch's notion of femininity. To him, women were a complex mix of Madonna and whore. We see Munch's take on the cycle of women's lives: She's a virgin (discarding the sweet flower of youth), a whore (a jaded temptress in red), and a widow (having destroyed the man, she is finally alone, aging, in black). With the phallic moon rising on the lake, Munch demonizes women as they turn men into green-faced, lusty monsters.

🔞 **Munch—*Puberty* (1894-1895):** One of the artist's most important non-*Scream* canvases reveals his ambivalence about women (see also his *Madonna*, earlier). This adolescent girl, grappling with her emerging sexuality, covers her nudity self-consciously. The looming shadow behind her—frighteningly too big and amorphous—threatens to take over the scene. The shadow's significance is open to interpretation—is it phallic, female genitalia, death, an embodiment of sexual anxiety...or Munch himself?

🔞 **Munch—*The Sick Child* (1896):** The death of Munch's sister in 1877 due to tuberculosis likely inspired this painting. The girl's face melts into the pillow. She's becoming two-dimensional, halfway between life and death. Everything else is peripheral, even her despairing mother saying good-bye. You can see how Munch scraped and repainted the face until he got it right.

• *Our tour is over, but there's more to see in this fine collection. Take a break from Nordic gloom and doom by visiting Rooms 15 and 23, with works by Impressionist and Post-Impressionist artists...even Munch got into the spirit with his Parisian painting, titled* Rue Lafayette. *You'll see lesser known, but still beautiful, paintings by non–Norwegian big names such as Picasso, Modigliani, Monet, Manet, Van Gogh, Gauguin, and Cézanne.*

National Historical Museum (Historisk Museum)

Directly behind the National Gallery and just below the palace is a fine Art Nouveau building offering an easy (if underwhelming) peek at Norway's history.

Cost and Hours: 50 kr, mid-May-mid-Sept Tue-Sun 10:00-17:00, mid-Sept-mid-May Tue-Sun 11:00-16:00, closed Mon year-round; Frederiks Gate 2, tel. 22 85 99 12, www.khm.uio.no.

Visiting the Museum: The ground floor offers a walk through the local history from prehistoric times. It includes the country's top collection of Viking artifacts, displayed in low-tech, old-school exhibits with barely a word of English to give it meaning. There's also some medieval church art. The museum's highlight is upstairs: an exhibit (well-described in English) about life in the Arctic for the Sami people (previously known to outsiders as Laplanders). In this overview of the past, a few Egyptian mummies and Norwegian coins through the ages are tossed in for good measure.

A PARK AND A MUSEUM
▲▲▲Vigeland Park

Within Oslo's vast Frogner Park is Vigeland Park, containing a lifetime of work by Norway's greatest sculptor, Gustav Vigeland (see sidebar). In 1921, he made a deal with the city. In return for a great studio and state support, he'd spend his creative life beautifying Oslo with this sculpture garden. From 1924 to 1943 he worked on-site, designing 192 bronze and granite statue groupings—600 figures in all, each nude and unique. Vigeland even planned the landscaping. Today the park is loved and respected by the people of Oslo (no police, no fences—and no graffiti). The Frognerbadet swimming pool is nearby in Frogner Park.

Cost and Hours: The garden is always open and free. The park is safe (cameras monitor for safety) and lit in the evening.

Getting There: Tram #12—which leaves from the central train station, Rådhusplassen in front of City Hall, Aker Brygge, and other points in town—drops you off right at the park gate (Vigelandsparken stop). Tram #19 (with stops along Karl Johans Gate) takes you to Majorstuen, a 10-minute walk to the gate (or you can change at Majorstuen to tram #12 and ride it one stop to Vigelandsparken).

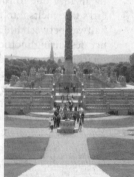
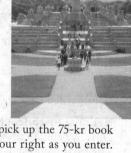

Visiting the Park: Vigeland Park is more than great art: It's a city at play. Appreciate its urban Norwegian ambience. The park is huge, but this visit is a snap. Here's a quick four-stop, straight-line, gate-to-monolith tour:

Enter the Park from Kirkeveien: For an illustrated guide and fine souvenir, pick up the 75-kr book in the Visitors Center (Besøkssenter) on your right as you enter.

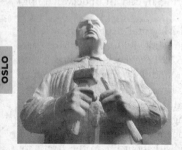

The modern cafeteria has sandwiches (indoor/outdoor seating, daily 9:00-20:30, shorter hours Sun and off-season), plus books, gifts, and WCs. Look at the statue of Gustav Vigeland (hammer and chisel in hand, drenched in pigeon poop) and consider his messed-up life. He lived with his many models. His

> ## Gustav Vigeland (1869-1943)
>
> As a young man, Vigeland studied sculpture in Oslo, then supplemented his education with trips abroad to Europe's art capitals. Back home, he carved out a successful, critically acclaimed career feeding newly independent Norway's hunger for homegrown art.
>
> During his youthful trips abroad, Vigeland had frequented the studio of Auguste Rodin, admiring Rodin's naked, restless, intertwined statues. Like Rodin, Vigeland explored the yin/yang relationship of men and women. Also like Rodin, Vigeland did not personally carve or cast his statues. Rather, he formed them in clay or plaster, to be executed by a workshop of assistants. Vigeland's sturdy humans capture universal themes of the cycle of life—birth, childhood, romance, struggle, child-rearing, growing old, and death.

marriages failed. His children entangled his artistic agenda. He didn't age gracefully. He didn't name his statues, and refused to explain their meanings. While those who know his life story can read it clearly in the granite and bronze, I'd forget Gustav's troubles and see his art as observations on the bittersweet cycle of life in general—from a man who must have had a passion for living.

Bridge: The 300-foot-long bridge is bounded by four granite columns: Three show a man fighting a lizard, the fourth shows a woman submitting to the lizard's embrace. Hmmm. (Vigeland was familiar with medieval mythology, where dragons represent man's primal—and sinful—nature.) But enough lizard love; the 58 bronze statues along the bridge are a general study of the human body. Many deal with relationships between people. In the middle, on the right, find the circular statue of a man and woman going round and round—perhaps the eternal attraction and love between the sexes. But directly opposite, another circle feels like a prison—man against the world, with no refuge. From the man escaping, look down at the children's playground: eight bronze infants circling a head-down fetus.

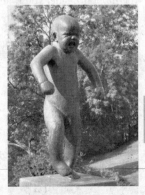

On your left, see the famous *Sinnataggen*, the hot-headed little boy. It's said Vigeland gave him chocolate and then took it away to get this reaction. The statues capture the joys of life (and, on a sunny day, so do the Norwegians filling the park around you).

Fountain: Continue through a rose garden to the earliest sculpture unit in the park. Six giants hold a fountain, symbolically toiling with the burden of life, as water—the source of life—cascades steadily around them. Twenty tree-of-life groups surround the fountain. Four clumps of trees (on each corner) show humanity's relationship to nature and the seasons of life: childhood, young love, adulthood, and winter.

Take a quick swing through life, starting on the right with youth. In the branches you'll see a swarm of children (Vigeland called them "geniuses"): A boy sits in a tree, boys actively climb while most girls stand by quietly, and a girl glides through the branches wide-eyed and ready for life...and love. Circle clockwise to the next stage: love scenes. In the third corner, life becomes more complicated: a sad woman in an

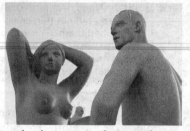

animal-like tree, a lonely child, a couple plummeting downward (perhaps falling out of love), and finally an angry man driving away babies. The fourth corner completes the cycle, as death melts into the branches of the tree of life and you realize new geniuses will bloom.

The 60 bronze reliefs circling the basin develop the theme further, showing man mixing with nature and geniuses giving the carousel of life yet another spin. Speaking of another spin, circle again and follow these reliefs.

The sidewalk surrounding the basin is a maze—life's long and winding road with twists, dead ends, frustrations, and, ultimately, a way out. If you have about an hour to spare, enter the labyrinth (on the side nearest the park's entrance gate, there's a single break in the black border) and follow the white granite path until (on the monolith side) you finally get out. (Tracing this path occupies

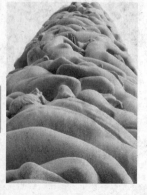

older kids, affording parents a peaceful break in the park.) Or you can go straight up the steps to the monolith.

Monolith: The centerpiece of the park—a teeming monolith of life surrounded by 36 granite groups—continues Vigeland's cycle-of-life motif. The figures are hunched and clearly earthbound, while Vigeland explores a lifetime of human relationships. At the center, 121 figures carved out of a single block of stone rocket skyward. Three stone carvers worked daily for 14 years, cutting Vigeland's full-size plaster model into the final 180-ton, 50-foot-tall erection.

Circle the plaza, once to trace the stages of life in the 36 statue groups, and a second time to enjoy how Norwegian kids relate to the art. The statues—both young and old—seem to speak to children.

Vigeland lived barely long enough to see his monolith raised. Covered with bodies, it seems to pick up speed as it spirals skyward. Some people seem to naturally rise. Others struggle not to fall. Some help others. Although the granite groups around the monolith are easy to understand, Vigeland left the meaning of the monolith itself open. Like life, it can be interpreted many different ways.

From this summit of the park, look a hundred yards farther, where four children and three adults are intertwined and spinning in the Wheel of Life. Now, look back at the entrance. If the main gate is at 12 o'clock, the studio where Vigeland lived and worked—now the Vigeland Museum—is at 2 o'clock (see the green copper tower poking above the trees). His ashes sit in the top of the tower in clear view of the monolith. If you liked the park, visit the Vigeland Museum (described next), a delightful five-minute walk away, for an intimate look at the art and how it was made.

▲▲Vigeland Museum

Filled with original plaster casts and well-described exhibits on his work, this palatial city-provided studio was Gustav Vigeland's

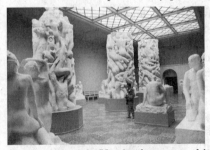

home and workplace. The high south-facing windows provided just the right light.

Vigeland, who had a deeply religious upbringing, saw his art as an expression of his soul. He once said, "The road between feeling and execution should be as short as possible." Here, immersed in his work, Vigeland supervised his craftsmen like a father, from 1924 until his death in 1943.

Cost and Hours: 60 kr; May-Aug Tue-Sun 10:00-17:00, Sept-April Tue-Sun 12:00-16:00, closed Mon year-round; bus #20 or tram #12 to Frogner Plass, Nobels Gate 32, tel. 23 49 37 00, www.vigeland.museum.no.

▲▲OSLO'S BYGDØY NEIGHBORHOOD

This thought-provoking and exciting cluster of sights is on a park-like peninsula just across the harbor from downtown. It provides

OSLO

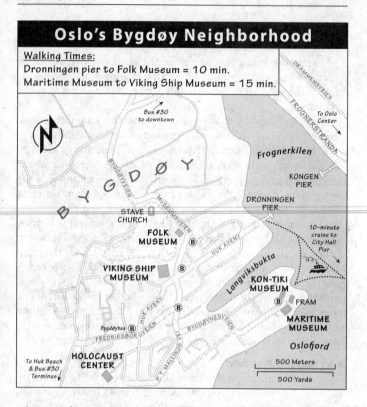

Oslo's Bygdøy Neighborhood

Walking Times:
Dronningen pier to Folk Museum = 10 min.
Maritime Museum to Viking Ship Museum = 15 min.

a busy and rewarding half-day (at a minimum) of sightseeing. Here, within a short walk, are six major sights (listed in order of importance):

• **Norwegian Folk Museum,** an open-air park with traditional log buildings from all corners of the country.

• **Viking Ship Museum,** showing off the best-preserved Viking longboats in existence.

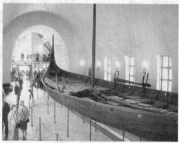

• **Fram Museum,** showcasing the modern Viking spirit with the *Fram*, the ship of Arctic-exploration fame, and the *Gjøa*, the first ship to sail through the Northwest Passage.

• **Kon-Tiki Museum,** starring the *Kon-Tiki* and the *Ra II*, in which Norwegian explorer Thor Heyerdahl proved that early civilizations—with their existing technologies—could have crossed the oceans.

• **Norwegian Maritime Museum,** interesting mostly to old salts, has a wonderfully scenic movie of Norway.

• **Norwegian Holocaust Center,** a high-tech look at the Holocaust in Norway and contemporary racism.

Getting There: Sailing from downtown to Bygdøy is fun, and it gets you in a seafaring mood. Ride the Bygdøy ferry—marked *Public Ferry Bygdøy Museums*—from pier 3 in front of City Hall (50 kr one-way; covered by Oslo Pass; mid-May-Aug daily 8:55-20:55, usually 3/hour; fewer sailings April and Sept; doesn't run Oct-March). Boats generally leave from downtown and from the museum dock at :05, :25, and :45 past each hour. In summer, avoid the nearby (much more expensive) tour boats. For a less memorable approach, you can take bus #30 (from train station or National Theater, direction: Bygdøy).

Getting Around Bygdøy: The Norwegian Folk and Viking Ship museums are a 10-minute walk from the ferry's first stop (Dronningen). The other boating museums (Fram, Kon-Tiki, and Maritime) are at the second ferry stop (Bygdøynes). The Holocaust Center is off Fredriksborgveien, about halfway between these two museum clusters. All Bygdøy sights are within a pleasant (when sunny) 15-minute walk of each other. The walk gives you a picturesque taste of small-town Norway.

City bus #30 connects the sights four times hourly in this order: Norwegian Folk Museum, Viking Ship Museum, Kon-Tiki Museum, Norwegian Holocaust Center. (For the Holocaust Center, you'll use the Bygdøyhus stop a long block away; tell the bus driver you want the stop for the "HL-Senteret.") The bus turns around at its final stop (Huk), then passes the sights in reverse order on its way back to the city center. Note that after 17:00, bus and boat departures are sparse. If returning to Oslo by ferry, get to the dock a little early—otherwise the boat is likely to be full, and you'll have to wait for the next sailing.

Eating at Bygdøy: Lunch options near the Kon-Tiki are a sandwich bar (relaxing picnic spots along the grassy shoreline) and a cafeteria (with tables overlooking the harbor). The Norwegian Folk Museum has a decent cafeteria inside and a fun little farmers' market stall across the street from the entrance. The Holocaust Center has a small café on its second floor.

▲▲▲Norwegian Folk Museum (Norsk Folkemuseum)

Brought from all corners of Norway, 150 buildings have been reassembled here on 35 acres. While Stockholm's Skansen was the first museum of this kind to open to the public (see page 271), this museum is a bit older, started in 1882 as the king's private collection (and the inspiration for Skansen).

Cost and Hours: 110 kr, daily mid-May-mid-Sept 10:00-18:00, off-season park open Mon-Fri 11:00-15:00, Sat-Sun 11:00-16:00 but most historical buildings closed, free lockers,

Museumsveien 10, bus #30 stops immediately in front, tel. 22 12 37 00, www.norskfolkemuseum.no.

Visiting the Museum: Think of the visit in three parts: the park sprinkled with old buildings, the re-created old town, and the folk-art museum. In peak season, the park is lively, with crafts-people doing their traditional things, barnyard animals roaming about, and costumed guides all around. (They're paid to happily answer your questions—so ask many.) The evocative Gol stave church, at the top of a hill at the park's edge, is a must-see (built in 1212 in Hallingdal and painstakingly reconstructed here). Across the park, the old town comes complete with apartments from various generations (including some reconstructions of people's actual homes) and offers an intimate look at lifestyles here in 1905, 1930, 1950, 1979, and even a modern-day Norwegian-Pakistani apartment.

The museum beautifully presents woody, colorfully painted folk art (ground floor), exquisite-in-a-peasant-kind-of-way folk costumes (upstairs), and temporary exhibits. Everything is thoughtfully explained in English. Don't miss the best Sami culture exhibit I've seen in Scandinavia (across the courtyard in the green building, behind the toy exhibit).

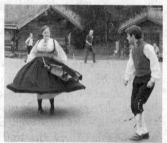

Upon arrival, pick up the site map and review the list of the day's activities, concerts, and guided tours. In summer, there are two guided tours in English per day; the Telemark Farm hosts a small daily fiddle-and-dance show; and a folk music-and-dance show is held each Sunday. The folk museum is most lively June through mid-August, when buildings are open and staffed. Otherwise, the indoor museum is fine, but the park is just a walk past lots of locked-up log cabins. If you don't take a tour, pick up a guidebook and ask questions of the informative attendants stationed in buildings throughout the park.

▲▲Viking Ship Museum (Vikingskiphuset)

In this impressive museum, you'll gaze with admiration at two finely crafted, majestic oak Viking ships dating from the 9th and 10th centuries, and the scant remains of a third vessel. Along with the two well-preserved ships, you'll see the bones of Vikings buried with these vessels and remarkable artifacts that may cause you to consider these notorious raiders in a different light. Over a thousand years ago, three things drove Vikings on their far-flung raids: hard economic times in their bleak homeland, the lure of prosperous and vulnerable communities to the south, and a mastery

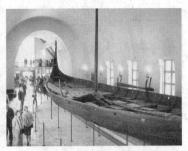

of the sea. There was a time when most frightened Europeans closed every prayer with, "And deliver us from the Vikings, Amen." Gazing up at the prow of one of these sleek, time-stained vessels, you can almost hear the screams and smell the armpits of those red-heads on the rampage.

Cost and Hours: 80 kr, daily May-Sept 9:00-18:00, Oct-April 10:00-16:00, Huk Aveny 35, tel. 22 13 52 80, www.khm.uio.no.

Visiting the Museum: Focus on the two well-preserved ships, starting with the *Oseberg,* from A.D. 834. With its ornate carving and impressive rudder, it was likely a royal pleasure craft. It seems designed for sailing on calm inland waters during festivals, but not in the open ocean.

The *Gokstad,* from A.D. 950, is a practical working boat, capable of sailing the high seas. A ship like this brought settlers to the west of France (Normandy was named for the Norsemen). And in such a vessel, explorers such as Eric the Red hopscotched from Norway to Iceland to Greenland and on to what they called Vinland—today's Newfoundland in Canada. Imagine 30 men hauling on long oars out at sea for weeks and months at a time. In 1892, a replica of this ship sailed from Norway to America in 44 days to celebrate the 400th anniversary of Columbus *not* discovering America.

The ships tend to steal the show, but don't miss the hall displaying **jewelry and personal items** excavated along with the ships. The ships and related artifacts survived so well because they were buried in clay as part of a gravesite. Many of the finest items were not actually Viking art, but goodies they brought home after raiding more advanced (but less tough) people. Still, there are lots of actual Viking items, such as metal and leather goods, that give insight into their culture. Highlights are the cart and sleighs, ornately carved with scenes from Viking sagas.

The museum doesn't offer tours, but it's easy to eavesdrop on the many guides leading big groups through the museum. Everything is well-described in English. You probably don't need the little museum guidebook—it repeats exactly what's already posted on the exhibits.

▲▲Fram Museum (Frammuseet)

This museum holds the 125-foot, steam- and sail-powered ship that took modern-day Vikings Roald Amundsen and Fridtjof Nansen deep into the Arctic and Antarctic, farther north and south than any vessel had gone before. For three years, the *Fram*—specially designed to survive the crushing pressures of a frozen-over sea—drifted, trapped in the Arctic ice. The museum was recently enlarged to include Amundsen's *Gjøa*, the first ship to sail through the Northwest Passage.

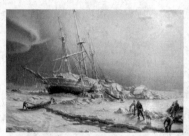

Cost and Hours: 100 kr; June-Aug daily 9:00-18:00; May and Sept daily 10:00-17:00; Oct and March-April daily 10:00-16:00; Nov-Feb Mon-Fri 10:00-15:00, Sat-Sun 10:00-16:00; Bygdøynesveien 36, tel. 23 28 29 50, www.frammuseum.no.

Visiting the Museum: Read the ground-floor displays, check out the videos below the bow of the ship, then climb the steps to the third-floor gangway to explore the *Fram*'s claustrophobic but fascinating interior. Also featured are a tent like the one Amundsen used, reconstructed shelves from his Arctic kitchen, models of the *Fram* and the motorized sled they used to traverse the ice and snow, and a "polar simulator" plunging visitors to a 15° Fahrenheit environment. A "Northern Lights Show," best viewed from the *Fram*'s main deck, is presented every 20 minutes.

Next, take the underground passageway to the adjacent A-frame building that displays the *Gjøa*, the motor- and sail-powered ship that Amundsen and a crew of six used from 1903 to 1906 to successfully navigate the Northwest Passage. Exhibits describe their ordeal as well as other Arctic adventures, such as Amundsen's 1926 airship (zeppelin) expedition from Oslo over the North Pole to Alaska. And pop in to the 100-seat cinema for a film about the polar regions (every 15 minutes).

▲▲Kon-Tiki Museum (Kon-Tiki Museet)

Next to the *Fram* is a museum housing the *Kon-Tiki* and the *Ra II*, the ships built by Thor Heyerdahl (1914-2002). In 1947, Heyerdahl and five crewmates constructed the *Kon-Tiki* raft out of balsa wood, using only pre-modern tools and techniques. They set sail from Peru on the tiny craft, surviving for 101 days on fish, coconuts, and sweet potatoes (which were native to Peru). About 4,300 miles later, they arrived in Polynesia. The point was to show that early South Americans could have settled Polynesia. (While Heyerdahl proved they could have, anthropologists doubt they did.) The *Kon-Tiki* story became a bestselling book and award-winning documentary (and helped spawn the "Tiki" culture craze in the US). In 1970, Heyerdahl's *Ra II* made a similar 3,000-mile journey from Morocco to Barbados to prove that Africans could have populated America. Both ships are well-displayed and described in English. Short clips from *Kon-Tiki*, the Oscar-winning 1950 documentary film, play in a small theater at the end of the exhibit.

Cost and Hours: 90 kr, daily June-Aug 9:30-18:00, March-May and Sept-Oct 10:00-17:00, Nov-Feb 10:00-16:00, Bygdøynesveien 36, tel. 23 08 67 67, www.kon-tiki.no.

▲Norwegian Maritime Museum (Norsk Sjøfartsmuseum)

If you like the sea, this museum is a salt lick, providing a wide-ranging look at Norway's maritime heritage. The collection was recently updated, with new exhibits such as "The Ship" ("Skipet"), tracing 2,000 years of maritime development, and "At Sea" ("Til Sjøs"), exploring what life is like on the ocean, from Viking days to the present. Don't miss the movie *The Ocean: A Way of Life*, included with your admission. It's a breathtaking widescreen film swooping you scenically over Norway's dramatic sea and fishing townscapes from here all the way to North Cape in a comfy theater (20 minutes, shown at the top and bottom of the hour, follow *Supervideografen* signs). And if you appreciate maritime art, the collection in the gallery should float your boat.

Cost and Hours: 80 kr, kids under 6 free; mid-May-Aug daily 10:00-17:00; Sept-mid-May Tue-Fri 10:00-15:00, Sat-Sun 10:00-16:00, closed Mon; Bygdøynesveien 37, tel. 24 11 41 50, www.marmuseum.no.

▲Norwegian Holocaust Center (HL-Senteret)

Located in the stately former home of Nazi collaborator Vidkun Quisling, this museum and study center offers a high-tech look at the racist ideologies that fueled the Holocaust. To show the Holocaust in a Norwegian context, the first floor displays historical documents about the rise of anti-Semitism and personal effects from Holocaust victims. Downstairs, the names of 760 Norwegian Jews killed by the Nazis are listed in a bright, white room. The *Innocent Questions* glass-and-neon sculpture outside shows an old-fashioned punch card, reminding viewers of how the Norwegian puppet government collected seemingly innocuous information before deporting its Jews. The *Contemporary Reflections* video is a reminder that racism and genocide continue today.

Cost and Hours: 50 kr, ask for free English audioguide or tablet, June-Aug daily 10:00-18:00, Sept-May Mon-Fri 10:00-16:00, Sat-Sun 11:00-16:00, Huk Aveny 56—take bus #30 to the Bygdøyhus stop, follow signs to *HL-Senteret*, tel. 22 84 21 00, www.hlsenteret.no.

GRÜNERLØKKA AND GRØNLAND DISTRICTS

The Grünerløkka district is trendy, and workaday Grønland is emerging as a fun spot. The Akers Rivers bisects Grünerløkka. You can connect the dots by taking the self-guided "Up Akers River and Down Grünerløkka Walk."

OSLO

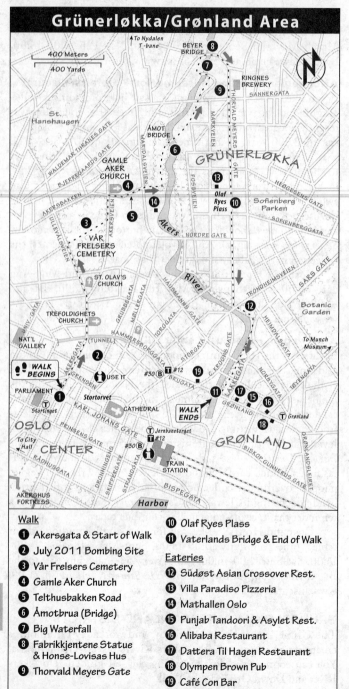

Grünerløkka/Grønland Area

400 Meters
400 Yards

To Nydalen
T-bane

BEYER
BRIDGE ❽
❼

RINGNES
BREWERY

❾

SANNERGATA

St.
Hanshaugen

ÅMOT
BRIDGE

❻

GRÜNERLØKKA

HEDGESENS GATE

GAMLE
AKER
CHURCH

❹

❶❸

Olaf
Ryes
Plass

Sofienberg
Parken

❺

❼❹

Akers

❿

SOFIENBERGGATA

❸

VÅR
FRELSERS
CEMETERY

NORDRE GATE

River

SARS GATE

ST. OLAV'S
CHURCH

Botanic
Garden

TREFOLDIGHETS
CHURCH

❿

To Munch
Museum

NAT'L
GALLERY

(TUNNEL)

HAMMERSPORGGATA

WALK
BEGINS

❷

USE IT

#30 Ⓑ Ⓣ #12

BRUGATA

❶❾

PARLIAMENT

❶

Stortinget

Stortorvet

CATHEDRAL

WALK
ENDS

❶❶

❶❼❶❺❶❻

GRØNLAND

❶❽

Ⓣ Grønland

OSLO
CENTER

To City
Hall

KARL JOHANS GATE

Ⓣ Jernbanetorget
Ⓣ #12

GRØNLAND

RÅDHUSGATA

TRAIN
STATION

BISPEGATA

AKERSHUS
FORTRESS

Harbor

Walk

❶ Akersgata & Start of Walk
❷ July 2011 Bombing Site
❸ Vår Frelsers Cemetery
❹ Gamle Aker Church
❺ Telthusbakken Road
❻ Åmotbrua (Bridge)
❼ Big Waterfall
❽ Fabrikkjentene Statue
   & Honse-Lovisas Hus
❾ Thorvald Meyers Gate

❿ Olaf Ryes Plass
❶❶ Vaterlands Bridge & End of Walk

Eateries

❶❷ Südøst Asian Crossover Rest.
❶❸ Villa Paradiso Pizzeria
❶❹ Mathallen Oslo
❶❺ Punjab Tandoori & Asylet Rest.
❶❻ Alibaba Restaurant
❶❼ Dattera Til Hagen Restaurant
❶❽ Olympen Brown Pub
❶❾ Café Con Bar

OSLO

Akers River

This river, though only about five miles long, powered Oslo's early industry: flour mills in the 1300s, sawmills in the 1500s, and Norway's Industrial Revolution in the 1800s. A walk along the river not only spans Oslo's history, but also shows the contrast the city offers. The bottom of the river (where this walk doesn't go)—bordered by the high-rise Oslo Radisson Blu Plaza Hotel and the "Little Pakistan" neighborhood of Grønland—has its share of drunks and drugs, reflecting a new urban reality in Oslo. Farther up, the river valley becomes a park as it winds past decent-size waterfalls and red-brick factories. The source of the river (and Oslo's drinking water) is the pristine Lake Maridal, situated at the edge of the Nordmarka wilderness. The idyllic recreation scenes along Lake Maridal are a favorite for nature-loving Norwegians.

▲Grünerløkka

The Grünerløkka district is the largest planned urban area in Oslo. It was built in the latter half of the 1800s to house the legions of workers employed at the factories powered by the Akers River. The first buildings were modeled on similar places built in Berlin. (German visitors observe that there's now more turn-of-the-20th-century Berlin here than in present-day Berlin.) While slummy in the 1980s, today it's trendy. Locals sometimes refer to it as "Oslo's Greenwich Village." Although that's a stretch, it is a bustling area with lots of cafés, good spots for a fun meal, and few tourists.

Getting There: Grünerløkka can be reached from the center of town by a short ride on tram #11, #12, or #13, or by taking the short but interesting walk described next.

▲Up Akers River and Down Grünerløkka Walk

While every tourist explores the harborfront and main drag of Oslo, few venture into this neighborhood that evokes the Industrial Revolution. Once housing poor workers, it now attracts hip professionals. A hike up the Akers River, finishing in the stylish Grünerløkka district, shines a truly different light on Oslo. Allow about an hour at a brisk pace, including a fair bit of up and down. Navigate with the TI's free city map and the map in this chapter. This walk is best during daylight hours.

Begin the walk by leaving Karl Johans Gate at the top of the hill, and head up **Akersgata**—Oslo's "Fleet Street" (lined with major newspaper companies). After two blocks, at Apotekergata, you may see the side street blocked off and construction work to the right. They're rebuilding after the horrific bombing of July 2011; the car bomb went off just a block to the right of here, on Grubbegata. Four buildings in the area suffered structural damage in the bombing. Continuing up Akersgata, the street name becomes Ullevålsveien as it passes those buildings. Norwegians are planning to build a memorial here in the near future.

Continuing past this somber site, you'll approach the massive brick Trefoldighets Church and St. Olav's Church before reaching the **Vår Frelsers (Our Savior's) Cemetery.** Enter the cemetery across from the Baby Shop store (where Ullevålsveien meets Wessels Gate).

Stop at the big metal map just inside the gate to chart your course through the cemetery: Go through the light-green

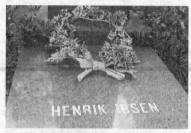

Æreslunden section— with the biggest plots and highest elevation—and out the opposite end (#13 on the metal map) onto Akersveien. En route, check out some of the tombstones of the illuminati and literati buried in the honorary Æreslunden section. They include Munch, Ibsen, Bjørnson, and many of the painters whose works you can see in the National Gallery (all marked on a map posted at the entrance). Exiting on the far side of the cemetery, walk left 100 yards up Akersveien to the church.

The Romanesque **Gamle Aker Church** (from the 1100s), the oldest building in Oslo, is worth a look inside (free, generally Mon-Thu 14:00-16:00, Fri 12:00-14:00). The church, which fell into ruins and has been impressively rebuilt, is pretty bare except for a pulpit and baptismal font from the 1700s.

From the church, backtrack 20 yards, head left at the playground, and go downhill on the steep **Telthusbakken Road** toward the huge, gray former grain silos (now student housing). The cute lane is lined with colorful old wooden houses: The people who constructed these homes were too poor to meet the no-wood fire-safety building codes within the city limits, so they built in what used to be suburbs. At the bottom of Telthusbakken, cross the busy Maridalsveien and walk directly through the park to the Akers River. The lively Grünerløkka district is straight across the river from here, but if you have 20 minutes and a little energy, detour upstream first and hook back down. Don't cross the river yet.

Walk along the riverside bike lane upstream through the river gorge park. Just above the first waterfall, cross **Åmotbrua,** the big white springy suspension footbridge from 1852 (moved here in 1958). Keep hiking uphill along the river. At the base of the next big waterfall, cross over again to the large brick buildings, hiking up the stairs to the **Beyer Bridge** (above the falls) and *Fabrikkjentene,* a statue of four women laborers. They're

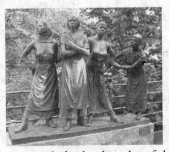

pondering the textile factory where they and 700 others toiled long and hard. This gorge was once lined with the water mills that powered Oslo through its 19th-century Industrial Age boom.

Look back (on the side you just left) at the city's two biggest, former textile factories. Once you could tell what color the fabric was being dyed each day by the color of the river. Just beyond them, between the two old factories, is a small white building housing the **Labor Museum** (Arbeidermuseet, free; late June-mid-Aug Tue-Sun 11:00-16:00, closed Mon; off-season Sat-Sun 11:00-16:00, closed Mon-Fri; borrow English handout). Inside you'll see old photos that humanize the life of laborers there, and an 1899 photo exhibit by Edvard Munch's sister, Inger Munch.

The tiny red house just over and below the bridge—the **Honse-Lovisas Hus** cultural center—makes a good rest-stop (Tue-Sun 11:00-18:00, closed Mon, coffee and wafels). Cross over to the red-brick Ringnes Brewery and follow **Thorvald Meyers Gate** down-hill directly into the heart of Grünerløkka. The main square, called **Olaf Ryes Plass,** is a happening place to grab a meal or drink (see "Eating," later). Trams take you from here back to the center.

• *To continue exploring, you could keep going straight and continue walking until you reach a T-intersection with a busy road (Trondheimsveien). From there (passing the recommended Südøst Asian Crossover Restaurant), you can catch a tram back to the center, or drop down to the riverside path and follow it downstream to Vaterlands bridge in the* **Grønland** *district. From here the train station is a five-minute walk down Stenersgata.*

Grønland

With the Industrial Revolution, Oslo's population exploded. The city grew from an estimated 10,000 in 1850 to 250,000 in 1900. The T-bane's Grønland stop deposits you in the center of what was the first suburb to accommodate workers of Industrial Age Oslo. If you look down side streets, you'll see fine 19th-century facades from this period. While the suburb is down-and-dirty like working-class and immigrant neighborhoods in other cities, Grønland is starting to emerge as a trendy place for eating out and after-dark fun. Locals know you'll get double the food and lots more beer for the kroner here (see "Eating," later). If you'd enjoy a whiff of Istanbul, make a point to wander through the underground commercial zone at the Grønland station (easy to visit even if you're not riding the T-bane).

OUTER OSLO
▲▲Holmenkollen Ski Jump and Ski Museum

The site of one of the world's oldest ski jumps (from 1892), Holmenkollen has hosted many championships, including the 1952 Winter Olympics. To win the privilege of hosting the 2011 World Ski Jump Championship, Oslo built a bigger jump to match modern ones built elsewhere. This futuristic, cantilevered, Olympic-standard **ski jump** has a tilted elevator that you can ride to the top (on a sunny day, you may have to wait your turn for the elevator). Stand right at the starting gate, just like an athlete, and get a feel for this daredevil sport. The jump empties into a 30,000-seat amphitheater, and if you go when it's clear, you'll see one of the best possible views of Oslo. While the view is exciting from the top, even more exciting is watching thrill-seekers rocket down the course on a zip-line from the same lofty perch (600 kr per trip).

As you ponder the jump, consider how modern athletes continually push the boundaries of their sport. The first champion here in 1892 jumped 21 meters (nearly 69 feet). In 1930 it took a 50-meter jump to win. In 1962 it was 80 meters, and in 1980 the champ cracked 100 meters. And, most recently, a jump of 140 meters (459 feet) took first place.

The **ski museum,** a must for skiers, traces the evolution of the sport, from 4,000-year-old rock paintings to crude 1,500-year-old wooden sticks to the slick and quickly evolving skis of modern times, including a fun exhibit showing the royal family on skis. You'll see gear from Roald Amundsen's famous trek to the South Pole, including the stuffed remains of Obersten (the Colonel), one of his sled dogs.

Cost and Hours: 120-kr ticket includes museum and viewing platform at top of jump; daily June-Aug 9:00-20:00, May and Sept 10:00-17:00, Oct-April 10:00-16:00; tel. 22 92 32 64, www.holmenkollen.com or www.skiforeningen.no.

Simulator: To cap your Holmenkollen experience, step into the simulator and fly down the ski jump and ski in a virtual downhill race. My legs were exhausted after the five-minute terror. This simulator (or should I say stimulator?) costs 60 kr. It's located at the lower level of the complex, near the entry of the ski museum. Outside, have fun watching a candid video of those shrieking inside.

Getting There: T-bane line #1 gets you out of the city, through the hills, forests, and mansions that surround Oslo, and to the jump (direction: Frognerseteren). From the Holmenkollen station, you'll hike steeply up the road 15 minutes to the ski jump. (Getting back is just 5 minutes. Note T-bane departure times before you leave.)

Nearby: For an easy downhill jaunt through the Norwegian forest, with a woodsy coffee or meal break in the middle, stay on the T-bane past Holmenkollen to the end of the line (Frognerseteren) and walk 10 minutes downhill to the recommended **Frognerseteren Hovedrestaurant,** a fine traditional eatery with a sod roof, reindeer meat on the griddle, and a city view (see page 707). Continue on the same road another 20 minutes downhill to the ski jump, and then to the Holmenkollen T-bane stop. The **Holmenkollen Restaurant,** described on page 707, is just a few steps above the T-bane stop and offers a similar view and better food and prices, but without the pewter-and-antlers folk theme.

▲Ekeberg Sculpture Park and Ruins of Medieval Oslo

The buzz in Oslo is its modern sculpture park (opened in 2013), with striking art sprinkled through a forest with grand city views. There's lots of climbing. The park has a long story, from evidence of the Stone Age people who chose to live here 7,000 years ago to the memory of its days as a Nazi military cemetery in World War II.

Getting There: The park, always open and free, is a 10-minute tram ride southeast of the center (catch tram #18 or #19 from station, platform E). From the Ekebergparken tram stop, climb uphill to the visitors center with its small museum (30 kr), where you can join a guided walk in English (150 kr, 90 minutes, Mon-Sat at 13:00, Sun at 14:00), or just pick up a map and start your hike.

▲Edvard Munch Museum (Munch Museet)

The only Norwegian painter to have had a serious impact on European art, Munch (pronounced "moonk") is a surprise to many who visit this fine museum, located one mile east of Oslo's center. The emotional, disturbing, and powerfully Expressionistic work of this strange and perplexing man is arranged chronologically. You'll see an extensive collection of paintings, drawings, lithographs, and photographs. (Note that Oslo's centrally located National Gallery, which also displays many of Munch's most popular works, is a better alternative for those who just want to see a dozen great Munch paintings, including "The Scream," without leaving the city center.)

The Munch Museum was in the news in August of 2004, when two Munch paintings, *Madonna* and a version of his famous *Scream,* were brazenly stolen right off the walls in broad daylight. Two men in black hoods simply entered through the museum café, waved guns at the stunned guards and tourists, ripped the paintings off the wall, and sped off in a black Audi station wagon. Happily, in 2006, the thieves were caught and the stolen paintings recovered. Today they are on display again, behind glass and with heightened security.

Cost and Hours: 95 kr; mid-June-Sept daily 10:00-17:00; Oct-mid-June Wed-Mon 11:00-17:00, closed Tue; 25-kr audioguide,

OSLO

guided tours in English daily July-Aug at 13:00, T-bane or bus #60 to Tøyen, Tøyengata 53, tel. 23 49 35 00, www.munch.museum.no. For more on Munch, see page 680.

Shopping in Oslo

Shops in Oslo are generally open 10:00-18:00 or 19:00. Many close early on Saturday and all day Sunday. Shopping centers are open Monday through Friday 10:00-21:00, Saturday 9:00-18:00, and are closed Sunday. Remember, when you make a purchase of 315 kr or more, you can get the 25 percent tax refunded when you leave the country if you hang on to the paperwork (see page 134). Here are a few favorite shopping opportunities many travelers enjoy, but not on Sunday, when they're all closed.

Norway Designs, just outside the National Theater, shows off the country's sleek, contemporary designs in clothing, kitch-enware, glass, textiles, jewelry—and high prices (Stortingsgata 12, T-bane: Nationaltheatret, tel. 23 11 45 10).

Paleet is a mall in the heart of Oslo, with 30 shops on three levels and a food court in the basement (Karl Johans Gate 37, tel. 23 08 08 11).

Dale of Norway, considered Norway's biggest and best maker of traditional and contemporary sweaters, offers its complete collection at this "concept store" (Karl Johans Gate 45, tel. 97 48 12 07).

Heimen Husflid has a superb selection of authentic Norwegian sweaters, *bunads* (national costumes), traditional jewelry, and other Norwegian crafts (top quality at high prices, Rosenkrantz Gate 8, tel. 23 21 42 00).

GlasMagasinet is one of Oslo's oldest and fanciest department stores (top end, good souvenir shop, near the cathedral at Stortorvet 9, tel. 22 82 23 00).

The Husfliden Shop, in the basement of the GlasMagasinet department store (listed previously), is popular for its Norwegian-made sweaters, yarn, and colorful Norwegian folk crafts (tel. 22 42 10 75).

The Oslo Sweater Shop has competitive prices for Norwegian-made sweaters (in Radisson Blu Scandinavia Hotel at Tullinsgate 5, tel. 22 11 29 22).

Byporten, the big, splashy mall adjoining the central train station, is filled with youthful and hip shops, specialty stores, and eateries (Jernbanetorget 6, tel. 23 36 21 60).

The street named **Bogstadveien** is considered to have the city's trendiest boutiques and chic, high-quality shops (stretches from behind the Royal Palace to Majorstuen near Vigeland Park).

Oslo's Flea Market makes Saturday morning a happy day for those who brake for garage sales (at Vestkanttorvet, March-Nov only, two blocks east of Frogner Park at the corner of Professor Dahl's Gate and Neubergsgate).

Oslo Flaggfabrikk sells quality flags of all shapes and sizes, including the long, pennant-shaped *vimpel*, seen fluttering from flagpoles all over Norway (875 kr for 11.5-foot *vimpel*—dresses up a boat or cabin wonderfully, near City Hall at Hieronymus Heyerdahlsgate 1, entrance on Tordenskioldsgate—on the other side of the block, tel. 22 40 50 60).

Vinmonopolet stores are the only places where you can buy wine and spirits in Norway. The most convenient location is at the central train station. Another location, not far from Stortinget, is at Rosenkrantzgate 11. The bottles used to be kept behind the counter, but now you can actually touch the merchandise. Locals say it went from being a "jewelry store" to a "grocery store." (Light beer is sold in grocery stores, but strong beer is still limited to Vinmonopolet shops.)

Eating in Oslo

EATING CHEAPLY

How do the Norwegians afford their high-priced restaurants? They don't eat out much. This is one city in which you might just settle for simple or ethnic meals—you'll save a lot and miss little. Many menus list small and large plates. Because portions tend to be large, choosing a small plate or splitting a large one makes some otherwise pricey options reasonable. You'll notice many locals just drink free tap water, even in fine restaurants. For a description of Oslo's classic (and expensive) restaurants, see the TI's *Oslo Guide* booklet.

Picnic for lunch. Basements of big department stores have huge, first-class supermarkets with lots of alternatives to sandwiches. The little yogurt tubs with cereal come with collapsible spoons. Wasa crackers and meat, shrimp, or cheese spread in a tube are cheap and pack well. The central station has a Joker supermarket with long hours (Mon-Fri 6:00-23:00, Sat 8:00-23:00, Sun 9:00-23:00).

You'll save 12 percent by getting takeaway food from a restaurant rather than eating inside. (The VAT on takeaway food is 12 percent; restaurant food is 24 percent.) Fast-food restaurants ask if you want to take away or not before they ring up your order on the cash register. Even McDonald's has a two-tiered price list.

Oslo is awash with little budget eateries (modern, ethnic, fast food, pizza, department-store cafeterias, and so on). **Deli de Luca,** a cheery convenience store chain, notorious for having a store on every key corner in Oslo, is a step up from the similarly ubiquitous

Norwegian Cuisine

Traditionally, Norwegian cuisine doesn't rank very high in terms of excitement value. But the typical diet of meat, fish, and potatoes is definitely evolving to incorporate more diverse products, and the food here is steadily improving. Fresh produce, colorful markets, and efficient supermarkets abound in Europe's most expensive corner.

In this land of farmers and fishermen, you'll find raw ingredients like potatoes, salmon, or beef in traditional recipes. Norway's national dish is *Fårikål,* a lamb or mutton stew with cabbage, peppercorns, and potatoes. It's served with lingonberry jam and lefse—a soft flatbread made from potatoes, milk, and flour. This dish is so popular that the last Thursday in September is *Fårikål* day in Norway. Norwegian grandmothers prepare this hearty stew by throwing together the basic ingredients with whatever leftovers are lying around the kitchen. There's really no need for a recipe, so every stew turns out differently—and every grandma claims hers is the best.

Because of its long, cold winters, Norway relies heavily on the harvesting and preservation of fish. Smoked salmon, called *røkt laks,* is prepared by salt-curing the fish and cold-smoking it, ensuring the temperature never rises above 85°F. This makes the texture smooth and almost raw. *Bacalao* is another favorite: salted and dried cod that is soaked in water before cooking. You'll often find *bacalao* served with tomatoes and olives.

Some Norwegians serve lutefisk around Christmas time, but you'll rarely see this salty, pungent dish on the menu. Instead, try the more pleasant *fiskekake,* a small white fish cake made with cream, eggs, milk, and flour. You can find these patties year-round. For a break from the abundance of seafood, try local specialties such as reindeer meatballs, or pork-and-ground beef meat cakes called *kjøttkaker.* True to Scandinavian cuisine, *kjøttkaker* are usually slathered in a heavy cream sauce.

Dessert and coffee after a meal are essential. *Bløtkake,* a popular delight on Norway's Constitution Day (May 17), is a layered cake drizzled with strawberry juice, covered in whipped cream, and decorated with fresh strawberries. The cloudberry *(multe),* which grows in the Scandinavian tundra, makes a unique jelly that tastes delicious on vanilla ice cream, or even whipped into a rich cream topping for heart-shaped waffles. Norwegians are proud of their breads and pastries, and you'll never be too far from a bakery that sells an almond-flavored *kringle* or a cone-shaped *krumkake* cookie filled with whipped cream.

OSLO

7-Elevens. Most are open 24/7, selling sandwiches, pastries, sushi, and to-go boxes of warm pasta or Asian noodle dishes. You can fill your belly here for about 80 kr. Some outlets (such as the one at the corner of Karl Johans Gate and Rosenkrantz Gate) have seating on the street or upstairs. Beware: Because this is still a *convenience* store, not everything is well-priced. Convenience stores—while convenient—charge double what supermarkets do.

KARL JOHANS GATE STRIP

Strangely, **Karl Johans Gate** itself—the most Norwegian of boulevards—is lined with a strip of good-time American chain eateries and sports bars where you can get ribs, burgers, and pizza, including T.G.I. Fridays and the Hard Rock Cafe. **Egon Restaurant** offers a daily 110-kr all-you-can-eat pizza deal (available Tue-Sat 11:00-18:00, Sun-Mon all day). Each place comes with great sidewalk seating and essentially the same prices.

Grand Café is perhaps the most venerable place in town. At lunchtime, they set up a sandwich buffet (150-kr single-sandwich, 315-kr all-you-like). Lunch plates are 150-200 kr. Reserve a window, and if you hit a time when there's no tour group, you're suddenly a posh Norwegian (daily 11:00-23:00, Karl Johans Gate 31, tel. 23 21 20 18).

Deli de Luca, just across from the Grand Café, offers good-value food and handy seats on Karl Johans Gate. For a fast meal with the best people-watching view in town, you may find yourself dropping by here repeatedly (for 60 kr you can get a calzone, or a portion of chicken noodles, beef noodles, or chicken vindaloo with rice—ask to have it heated up, open 24/7, Karl Johans Gate 33, tel. 22 33 35 22).

United Bakeries, next to the Paleet mall, is a quiet bit of Norwegian quality among sports bars, appreciated for its salads, light lunches, and fresh pastries (seating inside and out, Mon-Fri 7:00-20:00, Sat 9:00-20:00, Sun 9:00-16:00).

Kaffistova, a block off the main drag, is where my thrifty Norwegian grandparents always took me. And it remains almost unchanged since the 1970s. This alcohol-free cafeteria still serves simple, hearty, and typically Norwegian (read: bland) meals for a good price (140-kr daily specials, Mon-Fri 10:00-21:00, Sat-Sun 11:00-19:00, Rosenkrantz Gate 8, tel. 23 21 42 10).

Theatercaféen, since 1900 *the* place for Norway's illuminati to see and be seen (note the celebrity portraits adorning the walls), is a swanky splurge steeped in Art Nouveau elegance (175-195-kr starters, 200-375-kr main dishes, 655-kr three-course meal, Mon-Sat 11:00-23:00, Sun 15:00-22:00, in Hotel Continental at Stortingsgata 24, across from National Theater, tel. 22 82 40 50).

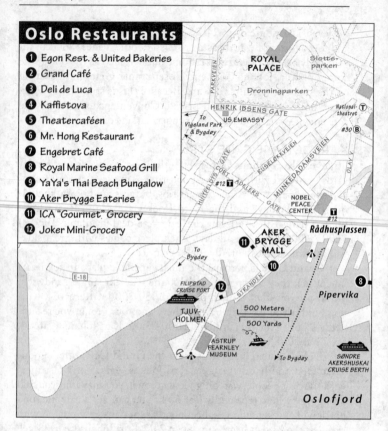

Oslo Restaurants

1. Egon Rest. & United Bakeries
2. Grand Café
3. Deli de Luca
4. Kaffistova
5. Theatercaféen
6. Mr. Hong Restaurant
7. Engebret Café
8. Royal Marine Seafood Grill
9. YaYa's Thai Beach Bungalow
10. Aker Brygge Eateries
11. ICA "Gourmet" Grocery
12. Joker Mini-Grocery

Mr. Hong Restaurant is a busy Asian eatery serving fish, duck, chicken, pork, and beef dishes and an all-day, all-you-can-eat grill buffet (165-240-kr main dishes, 200-kr buffet, Mon-Fri 14:00-23:00, Sat 13:00-23:30, Sun 14:00-22:00, Stortingsgata 8, entrance on Rosenkrantz Gate, tel. 22 42 20 08).

EATING IN THE SHADOW OF THE FORTRESS

Engebret Café is a fine old restaurant in a 17th-century building in the Christiania section of town below the fortress. Since 1857 it's been serving old-fashioned Norse food (reindeer is always on the menu) in a classic old Norwegian setting, with outdoor dining in spring and summer (250-350-kr main dishes, Mon-Fri 11:30-23:00, Sat in summer 13:00-23:00, closed Sun and July, Bankplassen 1, tel. 22 82 25 25).

Royal Marine Seafood Grill is a good bet for affordable dining on the harborfront. All seats are outside, where you'll enjoy nice views and sunsets on the Oslofjord. In contrast to the Aker Brygge scene, this is a casual place under the castle with nothing

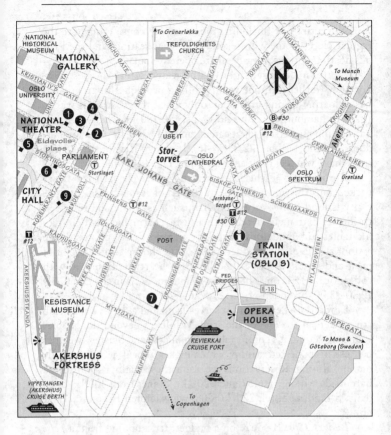

trendy about it (150-180-kr salads, burgers, fish-and-chips, 200-kr seafood dishes, daily May-Aug 14:00-22:00, closed Sept-April, Akershusstranda 5, tel. 22 08 03 00).

YaYa's Thai Beach Bungalow is a welcome change from Norwegian bland. The tiki-bar decor is infectious, the menu is fun and accessible, and the food is surprisingly authentic—I slurped up every morsel of my green curry pork. Don't be surprised if your dinner is accompanied by the sounds and lights of an hourly tropical thunderstorm (100-kr starters, 170-kr main dishes, vegetarian options, daily 16:00-22:00, Fri-Sat until 23:00, between the Parliament building and City Hall at Øvre Vollgate 13, tel. 22 83 71 10).

HARBORSIDE DINING IN AKER BRYGGE

Aker Brygge, the harborfront mall, is popular with businesspeople and tourists. While it isn't cheap, its inviting cafés and restaurants with outdoor, harborview tables make for a memorable waterfront meal. Before deciding where to eat, you might want to walk the entire lane (including the back side), considering both the regular places (some with second-floor view seating) and the various floating options. Nearly all are open for lunch.

Lekter'n Lounge, right on the water, offers the best harbor view (rather than views of strolling people). This trendy bar has a floating dining area open only when the weather is warm. It serves hamburgers, fish-and-chips, 150-180-kr salads, mussels, and shrimp buckets. Budget eaters can split a 160-kr pizza (all outdoors, Stranden 3, tel. 22 83 76 46). If you go just for drinks, the sofas make you feel right at home and a DJ adds to the ambience.

Rorbua, the "Fisherman's Cabin," is a lively yet cozy eatery tucked into this mostly modern stretch of restaurants. The specialty is food from Norway's north, such as whale and reindeer. Inside, it's extremely woody with a rustic charm and candlelit picnic tables surrounded by harpoons and old B&W photos. Grab a stool at one of the wooden tables, and choose from a menu of meat-and-potato dishes (200-300 kr). A hearty daily special with coffee for 165 kr is one of the best restaurant deals in the city (daily 12:30-23:00, Stranden 71, tel. 22 83 64 84).

Lofoten Fiskerestaurant serves fish amid a dressy yacht-club atmosphere at the end of the strip. While it's beyond the people-watching action, it's comfortable even in cold and blustery weather because of its heated atrium, which makes a meal here practically outdoor dining. Reservations are a must, especially if you want a harborside window table (lunch-200 kr, dinner from 300 kr, open daily, Stranden 75, tel. 22 83 08 08, www.lofoten-fiskerestaurant. no).

Budget Tips: If you're on a budget, try a hotdog from a *pølse* stand or get a picnic from a nearby grocery store and grab a bench along the boardwalk. The **ICA "Gourmet"** grocery store—in the middle of the mall a few steps behind all the fancy restaurants—has salads, warm take-away dishes (sold by the weight), and more (turn in about midway down the boardwalk, Mon-Fri 8:00-22:00, Sat 9:00-20:00, closed Sun). Farther down, the **Joker mini-grocery** (just over the bridge and to the right on Lille Stranden in Tjuvholmen) is open until 22:00.

TRENDY DINING AT THE BOTTOM OF GRÜNERLØKKA

These spots are located on the map on page 692.

Südøst Asian Crossover Restaurant, once a big bank, now fills its vault with wine (which makes sense, given Norwegian alcohol prices). Today it's popular with young Norwegian professionals as a place to see and be seen. It's a fine mix of Norwegian-chic woody ambience inside with a trendy menu, and a big riverside terrace outdoors with a more casual menu. Diners enjoy its chic setting, smart service, and modern creative Asian fusion cuisine (200-kr dinner plate, 300-kr dinner menu, daily 16:00-24:00, at bottom of Grünerløkka, tram #11, #12, or #17 to Trondheimsveien 5, tel. 23 35 30 70).

Olaf Ryes Plass, Grünerløkka's main square (and the streets nearby), is lined with inviting eateries and has a relaxed, bohemian-chic vibe. The top side of the square (near Villa Paradiso Pizzeria) has several pubs selling beer-centric food to a beer-centric crowd. To get here, hop on tram #11, #12, or #13 to Olaf Ryes Plass.

Villa Paradiso Pizzeria serves Oslo's favorite pizza. Youthful and family-friendly, it has a rustic interior and a popular terrace overlooking the square and people scene (120-180-kr pizza, Olaf Ryes Plass 8, tel. 22 35 40 60).

Mathallen Oslo is a former 19th-century factory, spiffed up and morphed into a neighborhood market with a mix of produce stalls and enticing eateries all sharing food-circus-type seating in the middle (Tue-Sun until late, closed Mon, on the river, 5-minute walk from Olaf Ryes Plass).

EATING CHEAP AND SPICY IN GRØNLAND

The street called Grønland leads through this colorful immigrant neighborhood (a short walk behind the train station or T-bane: Grønland; see the map on page 692). After the cleanliness and orderliness of the rest of the city, the rough edges and diversity of people here can feel like a breath of fresh air. Whether you eat here or not, the street is fun to explore. In Grønland, backpackers and immigrants munch street food. Cheap and tasty *börek* (feta, spinach, mushroom) is sold hot and greasy to go for 25 kr.

Punjab Tandoori is friendly and serves hearty meals (70-100-kr, lamb and chicken curry, tandoori specials). I like eating outside here with a view of the street scene (daily 11:00-23:00, Grønland 24).

Alibaba Restaurant is clean, simple, and cheap for Turkish food. They have good indoor or outdoor seating (139-kr fixed-price meal Mon-Thu only, open daily 12:30-22:30, corner of Grønlandsleiret and Tøyengata at Tøyengata 2, tel. 22 17 22 22).

Asylet is more expensive and feels like it was here long before Norway ever saw a Pakistani. This big, traditional eatery—like a Norwegian beer garden—has a rustic, cozy interior and a cobbled backyard filled with picnic tables (150-240-kr plates and hearty dinner salads, daily 11:00-24:00, Grønland 28, tel. 22 17 09 39).

Dattera Til Hagen feels like a college party. It's a lively scene filling a courtyard with picnic tables and benches under strings of colored lights. If it's too cold, hang out inside. Locals like it for the tapas, burgers, salads, and Norwegian microbrews on tap (180-kr plates, Grønland 10, tel. 22 17 18 61).

OSLO

What If I Miss My Boat?

Remember that you can get help from the cruise line's port agent (listed on the destination information sheet distributed on the ship) and the local TI (see page 652). If the port agent suggests a costly solution (such as a private car with a driver), you may want to consider public transit.

Trains connect Oslo easily to **Bergen** and **Stavanger. Flåm** is an easy bus or train ride off the main Oslo-Bergen line. Trains are also likely your best option for **Copenhagen** and **Stockholm;** for other points on the continent (such as **Amsterdam, Warnemünde/Berlin,** or **Zeebrugge/Brussels**), you'll probably connect through Copenhagen (for train connections, see www.bahn.com). To reach **Tallinn, Helsinki,** or **St. Petersburg** (only if you already have a visa), your best option is likely a train to Stockholm, then take the boat from there.

Another option for reaching **Copenhagen** is the overnight boat operated by DFDS Seaways (Danish tel. 00 45 33 42 30 10, www.dfdsseaways.us).

If you need to catch a **plane** to your next destination, you can ride an express train to Oslo's airport (lufthavn), also called Gardermoen (tel. 91 50 64 00, www.osl.no). Some discount airlines use smaller airports that are farther out: Rygge Airport (near the city of Moss, 40 miles south of Oslo, tel. 69 23 00 00, www.en.ryg.no) or Sandefjord Airport Torp (70 miles south of Oslo, tel. 33 42 70 00, www.torp.no).

Local **travel agents** in Oslo can help you. For more advice on what to do if you miss the boat, see page 139.

Olympen Brown Pub is a dressy dining hall that's a blast from the past. You'll eat in a spacious, woody saloon with big dark furniture, faded paintings of circa-1920 Oslo lining the walls, and huge chandeliers. It's good for solo travelers, because sharing the long tables is standard practice. They serve hearty 200-kr plates and offer a huge selection of beers. Traditional Norwegian cuisine is served downstairs, while upstairs on the rooftop, the food is grilled (daily 11:00-2:00 in the morning, Grønlandsleiret 15, tel. 22 17 28 08).

Café Con Bar is a trendy yuppie eatery on the downtown edge of Grønland. Locals consider it to have the best burgers in town (150 kr). While the tight interior seating is very noisy, the sidewalk tables are great for people-watching (160-kr daily specials, 150-190-kr main dishes, Mon-Sat 10:00-late, Sun 12:00-late, kitchen closes at 23:00, where Grønland hits Brugata).

NEAR THE SKI JUMP, HIGH ON THE MOUNTAIN

Frognerseteren Hovedrestaurant, nestled high above Oslo (and 1,400 feet above sea level), is a classy, sod-roofed old restaurant. Its terrace, offering a commanding view of the city, is a popular stop for famous apple cake and coffee. The café is casual and less expensive, with indoor and outdoor seating (90-kr sandwiches and cold dishes, 140-190-kr entrées, Mon-Sat 11:00-22:00, Sun 11:00-21:00). The elegant view restaurant is pricier (375-395-kr plates, Mon-Fri 12:00-22:00, Sat 13:00-22:00, Sun 13:00-21:00, reindeer specials, tel. 22 92 40 40).

The **Holmenkollen** restaurant, just below the ski jump and a few steps above the Holmenkollen T-bane stop, is a practical alternative to the Frognerseteren restaurant. It serves better food at better prices with a similarly grand Oslo fjord view, but without the folk charm.

You can combine a trip into the forested hills surrounding the city with lunch and get a chance to see the famous Holmenkollen Ski Jump up close (see page 696).

Norwegian Survival Phrases

Norwegian can be pronounced quite differently from region to region. These phrases and phonetics match the mainstream Oslo dialect, but you'll notice variations. Vowels can be tricky: *å* sounds like "oh," *æ* sounds like a bright "ah" (as in "apple"), and *u* sounds like the German *ü* (purse your lips and say u). Certain vowels at the ends of words (such as *d* and *t*) are sometimes barely pronounced (or not at all). In some dialects, the letters *sk* are pronounced "sh." In the phonetics, ī sounds like the long i in "light," and bolded syllables are stressed.

English	Norwegian	Pronunciation
Hello. (formal)	God dag.	goo dahg
Hi. / Bye. (informal)	Hei. / Ha det.	hī / hah deh
Do you speak English?	Snakker du engelsk?	**snahk**-kehr dew **eng**-ehlsk
Yes. / No.	Ja. / Nei.	yah / nī
Please.	Vær så snill.	vayr soh sneel
Thank you (very much).	(Tusen) takk.	(**tew**-sehn) tahk
You're welcome.	Vær så god.	vayr soh goo
Can I help you?	Kan jeg hjelpe deg?	kahn yī **yehl**-peh dī
Excuse me.	Unnskyld.	**ewn**-shuld
(Very) good.	(Veldig) fint.	(**vehl**-dee) feent
Goodbye.	Farvel.	fahr-**vehl**
one / two	en / to	ayn / toh
three / four	tre / fire	treh / **fee**-reh
five / six	fem / seks	fehm / sehks
seven / eight	syv / åtte	seev / **oh**-teh
nine / ten	ni / ti	nee / tee
hundred	hundre	**hewn**-dreh
thousand	tusen	**tew**-sehn
How much?	Hvor mye?	voor **mee**-yeh
local currency: (Norwegian) crown	(Norske) kroner	(**norsh**-keh) **kroh**-nehr
Where is...?	Hvor er...?	voor ehr
...the toilet	...toalettet	toh-ah-**leh**-teh
men	menn / herrer	mehn / **hehr**-rehr
women	damer	**dah**-mehr
water / coffee	vann / kaffe	vahn / **kah**-feh
beer / wine	øl / vin	uhl / veen
Cheers!	Skål!	skohl
The bill, please.	Regningen, takk.	**rī**-ning-ehn tahk

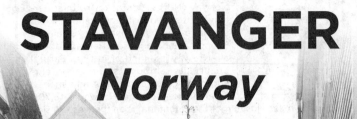

STAVANGER
Norway

Norway Practicalities

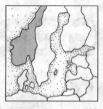

Norway (Norge) is stacked with super-latives—it's the most mountainous, most scenic, and most prosperous of all the Scandinavian countries. Perhaps above all, Norway is a land of intense natural beauty, its famously steep mountains and deep fjords carved out and shaped by an ancient ice age. Norway (148,700 square miles—just larger than Montana) is on the western side of the Scandinavian Peninsula, with most of the country shar-ing a border with Sweden to the east. Rich in resources like timber, oil, and fish, Norway has rejected joining the European Union, mainly to protect its fishing rights. Where the country extends north of the Arctic Circle, the sun never sets at the height of summer and never comes up in the deep of win-ter. The majority of Norway's 5 million people consider them-selves Lutheran.

Money: 6 Norwegian kroner (kr, officially NOK) = about $1. An ATM is called a *minibank*. The local VAT (value-added sales tax) rate is 25 percent; the minimum purchase eligible for a VAT refund is 315 kr (for details on refunds, see page 134).

Language: The native language is Norwegian (the two official forms are Bokmål and Nynorsk). For useful phrases, see page 708.

Emergencies: Dial 112 for police, medical, or other emergen-cies. In case of theft or loss, see page 125.

Time Zone: Norway is on Central European Time (the same as most of the Continent, one hour ahead of Great Britain, and six/nine hours ahead of the East/West Coasts of the US).

Embassies in Oslo: The **US embassy** is at Henrik Ibsens Gate 48 (tel. 21 30 85 58, emergency tel. 21 30 85 40, http://norway.usembassy.gov). The **Canadian embassy** is at Wergelandsveien 7 (tel. 22 99 53 00, www.canada.no). Call ahead for passport services.

Phoning: Norway's country code is 47; to call from another country to Norway, dial the international access code (011 from the US/Canada, 00 from Europe, or + from a mobile phone), then 47, followed by the local number. For local calls within Norway, just dial the number as it appears in this book—whether you're calling from across the street or across the country. To place an international call from Norway, dial 00, the code of the country you're calling (1 for US and Canada), and the phone number. For more tips, see page 1146.

Tipping: Service is included at sit-down meals, but this goes to the owner. For great service, it's nice to round up your bill about 10 percent to reward your server. Tip a taxi driver by rounding up the fare (pay 90 kr on an 85-kr fare). For more tips on tipping, see page 138.

Tourist Information: www.goscandinavia.com

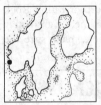

STAVANGER

This burg of about 125,000 is a mildly charming (if unspectacular) waterfront city whose streets are lined with unpretentious shiplap cottages that echo its perennial ties to the sea. Stavanger feels more cosmopolitan than most small Norwegian cities, thanks in part to its oil industry—which brings multinational workers (and their money) into the city. Known as Norway's festival city, Stavanger hosts several lively events, including jazz in May (www.maijazz.no), Scandinavia's biggest food festival in July (www.gladmat.no), and chamber music in August (www.icmf.no).

From a sightseeing perspective, Stavanger barely has enough to fill a day: The Norwegian Petroleum Museum is the only big-time sight in town. The city's fine cathedral is worth a peek. But for most visitors, the main reason to come to Stavanger is to use it as a launch pad for side-tripping to Lysefjord and/or the famous, iconic Pulpit Rock: an eerily flat-topped peak thrusting up from the fjord, offering perfect, point-blank views deep into the Lysefjord.

PLANNING YOUR TIME

Stavanger is a small town with enjoyable ambience, but it lacks big sights; you'll probably look for ways to kill time rather than run out of it. The one big exception is a side-trip to the Lysefjord and/or Pulpit Rock, which can eat up the better part of your day in port (but may not be possible, depending on your cruise arrival and departure schedule).

If you stick around town, take your pick from these options—noting that some may not open until well after your ship docks.

• **Cathedral:** This is worth a quick look (easy to see in less than 30 minutes).

• **Norwegian Petroleum Museum:** The city's main museum deserves at least an hour, or two hours if you want to watch all the movies (or are traveling with kids who'd enjoy the interactive features).

• **Other Museums:** Stavanger's many small museums can round out your day, but none of them demands more than 30 to 60 minutes.

• **Strolling Town:** Spend whatever time you have left exploring, especially the atmospheric lanes of Gamle Stavanger and Kirkegata, the main drag through town.

With relatively little else to do in Stavanger, many visitors choose to use this day for a side-trip to the **Lysefjord** and/or **Pulpit Rock.** Handy fjord excursion boats leave from the harbor, near where the cruise ships put in. Ideally, do some homework and confirm schedules before you arrive, so you know which company (if any) has a trip that fits with your ship's arrival and departure.

Excursion Alert: Before joining a Lysefjord or Pulpit Rock excursion run by anyone other than your cruise line, be absolutely clear on the return time—and before you book, make sure the guide knows what time you need to be back.

The Port of Stavanger

Arrival at a Glance: It's simple: Just walk along the harbor into the town center (5-15 minutes, depending on where you're docked).

Port Overview

Cruise ships dock on either side of Stavanger's central harbor (Vågen), an inlet between Gamle Stavanger (the old town) and the city-center peninsula. Ships dock either along the west side of the harbor, an embankment called **Strandkaien;** or along the east side, called **Skagenkaien.** When more ships are in town, they dock farther out along these embankments; the walk to the end of the harbor and the town center can

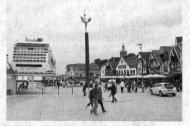

take anywhere from 5 minutes (from the nearest berths) to 15 minutes (from the farthest).

Tourist Information: There's no TI at the cruise port itself, but it's a short walk to the main branch, overlooking the plaza in front of the cathedral (see "Tourist Information" on page 716).

Excursions from Stavanger

The one cruise-line excursion that's worth considering is to the **Lysefjord,** across the bay, and the iconic **Pulpit Rock** that overlooks it. You can do a similar trip on your own, but your options are limited, and it's tricky to coordinate schedules with your cruise's arrival and departure. If you've always wanted to see Pulpit Rock, and this is your best chance, an excursion may be the right choice.

Otherwise, various excursions cobble together sights in and around Stavanger, including the Petroleum Museum, the Sverd i Fjell monument ("Swords in Mountain," honoring a historic A.D. 872 battle), an Iron Age farm, a cheese factory, the charming and well-preserved Utstein Abbey (often with a musical recital), a pile of prehistoric avalanche boulders called Gloppedalsura, and a drive to Byrkjelandsvatnet Lake. Any of these can be interesting, and—as there's little to see in Stavanger itself—they can be a nice way to get out into the countryside. The cruise around Stavanger Archipelago is pointless (offering little to see beyond what you'll see coming and going on your cruise ship).

GETTING INTO TOWN

Stavanger is extremely cruiser-friendly. From either embankment, you can just stroll along the harbor into town, following the handy directional signs you pass along the way. Specifics for each pier are below. The route's so walkable that taxis don't bother meeting cruise ships, and there's no point taking public transportation. You'll see **hop-on, hop-off buses** at the dock, but in this small and compact city, they're unlikely to be useful (204 kr/day, 10 stops, every 20 minutes).

From Strandkaien

Arriving at Strandkaien, you face rows of pointy-topped, white, wooden houses climbing the hill (Gamle Stavanger).

Exiting your ship, turn left and walk along the waterfront. On your way, you'll pass the Norwegian Emigration Center (closed to visitors), then the Maritime Museum (with free Wi-Fi in the lobby). If you need cash, also keep an eye out for the Fokus Bank, with an ATM inside. Circling around the end of the harbor, head up through the small market plaza to reach the cathedral and, facing it, the TI.

Note that Gamle Stavanger is directly above the Strandkaien embankment—just head up any narrow cobbled lane to find it. This makes for a handy place to kill any remaining time before boarding your ship.

STAVANGER

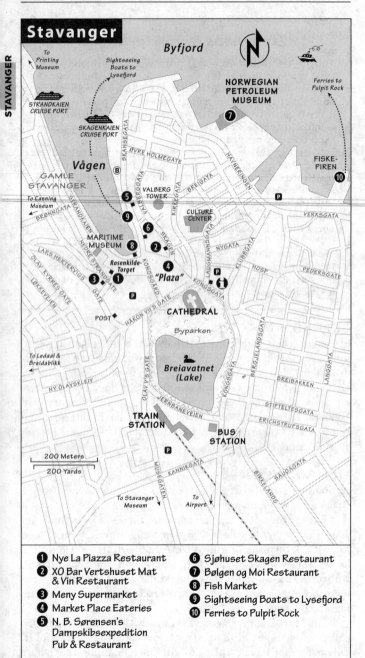

Stavanger

Byfjord

To Printing Museum

Sightseeing Boats to Lysefjord

NORWEGIAN PETROLEUM MUSEUM

❼

Ferries to Pulpit Rock

STRANDKAIEN CRUISE PORT

SKAGENKAIEN CRUISE PORT

Vågen

ØVRE HOLMEGATE

SKANSEGATA

FISKE-PIREN

❿

GAMLE STAVANGER

Ⓑ

VALBERGGATA

VALBERG TOWER

KIRKEGATA

BREIGATA

HAVNERINGEN

To Canning Museum

BRØNNGATA

❺

CULTURE CENTER

Ⓟ

VERKSGATA

STRANDKAIEN

❾

SKAGEN

NYGATA

LAUGMANNSGATA

KLUBBGATA

HOSP

PEDERSGATA

LARS HERTERVIGS GATE

MARITIME MUSEUM

❻

❽

❷

Rosenkilde-Torget

NEDRE STRANDGT

OLAV KYRRES GATE

LØKKEVEIEN

❸

❶

KONGSGT

❹

"Plaza"

Ⓟ

Ⓟ

KONGSGATA

Ⓟ

Ⓘ

CATHEDRAL

POST

HAKON VII's GATE

Byparken

BERGJELANDSGATA

To Ledaal & Breidablikk

OLAV V's GATE

Breiavatnet (Lake)

KONGSGATA

BREIBAKKEN

LANGGATA

NY OLAVSKLEIV

JERNBANEVEIEN

STIFTELSEGATA

TRAIN STATION

BUS STATION

ERICHSTRUPSGATA

SAUDAGATA

200 Meters

200 Yards

Ⓟ

MUSÉGATEN

KANNIKGATA

BIRKELANDS

To Stavanger Museum

To Airport

---

❶ Nye La Piazza Restaurant

❷ XO Bar Vertshuset Mat & Vin Restaurant

❸ Meny Supermarket

❹ Market Place Eateries

❺ N. B. Sørensen's Dampskibsexpedition Pub & Restaurant

❻ Sjøhuset Skagen Restaurant

❼ Bølgen og Moi Restaurant

❽ Fish Market

❾ Sightseeing Boats to Lysefjord

❿ Ferries to Pulpit Rock

Services in Stavanger

Take the short walk into the heart of town, where you'll find the following:

ATMs: The closest locations to each dock are noted under "Getting into Town," earlier; the most central option is at the SpareBank overlooking the market square, facing the cathedral and TI.

Internet Access: The TI can tell you the password for their free Wi-Fi connection. There's also free Wi-Fi in the lobby of the Maritime Museum, along Strandkaien. For Internet terminals, try the library up the street from the TI.

Pharmacy: The handiest is Apotek 1, inside the Torgterrassen mall facing the market plaza just below the cathedral and TI (Mon-Fri 9:00-20:00, Sat 9:00-19:00, closed Sun).

From Skagenkaien

Exiting your ship, turn right and walk along the harborfront, passing the departure point for excursion boats to the Lysefjord. You'll quickly arrive at the end of the harbor; from here, you can angle up through the market square to reach the cathedral and TI. If you need cash, look for an ATM at the entrance to the 7-Eleven and another in the SpareBank at the top of the square.

RETURNING TO YOUR SHIP

Just walk—you can see your ship from almost anywhere in town. Remember, if you have time to kill on your way back, you could wander the pretty Gamle Stavanger zone just above Strandkaien, or use the free Wi-Fi inside the Maritime Museum (also along Strandkaien). See page 721 for help if you miss your boat.

Orientation to Stavanger

The most scenic and interesting parts of Stavanger surround its harbor. Here you'll find the Maritime Museum, lots of shops and restaurants (particularly around the market plaza and along Kirkegata, which connects the cathedral to the Petroleum Museum), the indoor fish market, and a produce market (Mon-Fri 9:00-18:00, Sat 9:00-16:00, closed Sun). The artificial Lake Breiavatnet—bordered by Kongsgaten on the east and Olav V's Gate on the west—separates the train and bus stations from the harbor.

TOURIST INFORMATION

The helpful staff at the TI can help you plan your time in Stavanger, and can also give you hiking tips and day-trip information. Pick up a free city guide and map (June-Aug daily 9:00-20:00; Sept-May Mon-Fri 9:00-16:00, Sat 9:00-14:00, closed Sun; Domkirkeplassen 3, tel. 51 85 92 00, www.regionstavanger.com).

Sights in Stavanger

▲Stavanger Cathedral (Domkirke)

While it's hardly the most impressive cathedral in Scandinavia, Stavanger's top church—which overlooks the town center on a small ridge—has a harmoni-ous interior and a few intrigu-ing details worth lingering over. Good English information throughout the church brings meaning to the place.

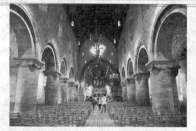

Cost and Hours: 30-kr until 15:30, free after 15:30, open June-Aug daily 11:00-19:00, free and open shorter hours off-season, tel. 51 84 04 00, www.kirken. stavanger.no.

Visiting the Church: St. Swithun's Cathedral (its official name) was originally built in 1125 in a Norman style, with basket-handle Romanesque arches. After a fire badly damaged the church in the 13th century, a new chancel was added in the pointy-arched Gothic style. You can't miss where the architecture changes about three-quarters of the way up the aisle. On the left, behind the bap-tismal font, notice the ivy-lined railing on the stone staircase; this pattern is part of the city's coat of arms. And nearby, appreciate the colorful, richly detailed "gristle Baroque"-style pulpit (from 1658). Notice that the whole thing is resting on Samson's stoic shoul-ders—even as he faces down a lion.

Stroll the church, perusing its several fine "epitaphs" (tomb markers), which are paintings in ornately decorated frames. Go on a scavenger hunt for two unique features; both are on the sec-ond columns from the back of the church. On the right, at the top facing away from the nave, notice the stone carvings of Norse mythological figures: Odin on the left, and a wolf-like beast on the right. Although the medieval Norwegians were Christians, they weren't ready to entirely abandon all of their pagan traditions. On the opposite column, circle around the base and look at ankle level, facing away from the altar. Here you see a grotesque sculpture that looks like a fish head with human hands. Notice that its head has been worn down. One interpretation is that early worshippers would ritualistically put their foot on top of it, as if to push the evil back to the underworld. Mysteriously, both of these features are one-offs—you won't find anything like them on any other column in the church.

▲▲Norwegian Petroleum Museum (Norsk Oljemuseum)

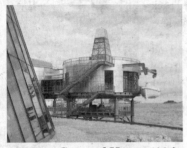

This entertaining, informative museum—dedicated to the discovery of oil in Norway's North Sea in 1969 and the industry built up around it—offers an unapologetic look at the country's biggest moneymaker. With half of Western Europe's oil reserves, the formerly poor agricultural nation of Norway is the Arabia of the North, and a world-class player. It's ranked third among the world's top oil exporters, producing 1.6 million barrels a day.

Cost and Hours: 100 kr; June-Aug daily 10:00-19:00; Sept-May Mon-Sat 10:00-16:00, Sun 10:00-18:00; tel. 51 93 93 00, www.norskolje.museum.no. The small museum shop sells various petroleum-based products. The museum's Bølgen og Moi restaurant, which has an inviting terrace over the water, serves lunch and dinner (see listing under "Eating in Stavanger," later).

Visiting the Museum: The exhibit describes how oil was formed, how it's found and produced, and what it's used for. You'll see models of oil rigs, actual drill bits, see-through cylinders that you can rotate to investigate different types of crude, and lots of explanations (in English) about various aspects of oil. Interactive exhibits cover everything from the "History of the Earth" (4.5 billion years displayed on a large overhead globe, showing how our planet has changed—stay for the blast that killed the dinosaurs), to day-to-day life on an offshore platform, to petroleum products in our lives (though the peanut-butter-and-petroleum-jelly sandwich is a bit much). Kids enjoy climbing on the model drilling platform, trying out the emergency escape chute at the platform outside, and playing with many other hands-on exhibits.

Several included movies delve into specific aspects of oil: The kid-oriented "Petropolis" 3-D film is primitive but entertaining and informative, tracing the story of oil from creation to extraction. Other movies (in the cylindrical structures outside) highlight intrepid North Sea divers and the construction of an oil platform. Each film is 12 minutes long, and runs in English at least twice hourly.

Even the museum's architecture was designed to echo the foundations of the oil industry—bedrock (the stone building),

STAVANGER

slate and chalk deposits in the sea (slate floor of the main hall), and the rigs (cylindrical platforms). While the museum has its fair share of propaganda, it also has several good exhibits on the environmental toll of drilling and consuming oil.

Gamle Stavanger

Stavanger's "old town" centers on Øvre Strandgate, on the west side of the harbor. Wander the narrow, winding, cobbled back lanes, with tidy wooden houses, oasis gardens, and flower-bedecked entranceways. Peek into a workshop or gallery to find ceramics, glass, jewelry, and more. Many shops are open roughly daily 10:00-17:00, coinciding with the arrival of cruise ships (which loom ominously right next to this otherwise tranquil zone).

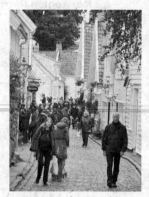

Museum Stavanger (M.U.S.T.)

This "museum" is actually 10 different museums scattered around town. The various branches include the **Stavanger Museum,** featuring the history of the city and a zoological exhibit (Muségate 16); the **Maritime Museum** (Sjøfartsmuseum), near the bottom end of Vågen harbor (Nedre Strandgate 17-19); the **Norwegian Canning Museum** (Norsk Hermetikkmuseum—the *brisling,* or herring, is smoked the first Sunday of every month and mid-June–mid-Aug Tue and Thu—Øvre Strandgate 88A); **Ledaal,** a royal residence and manor house (Eiganesveien 45); and **Breidablikk,** a wooden villa from the late 1800s (Eiganesveien 40A). The **Printing Museum** is closed but is slated to reopen by 2016.

Cost: You can buy one 100-kr ticket to cover all of them, or you can pay 70 kr for any individual museum (if doing at least two, the combo-ticket is obviously the better value). Note that a single 70-kr ticket gets you into the Maritime Museum, Canning Museum, and Printing Museum (when open), which are a three-for-one sight. You can get details and buy tickets at any of the museums; handiest is the Maritime Museum right along the harbor.

Hours: Museum hours vary but generally open mid-June–mid-Aug daily 10:00 or 11:00-16:00; off-season Tue-Sun 11:00-16:00, closed Mon, except Ledaal and Breidablikk—these are open Sun only in winter; www.museumstavanger.no.

DAY TRIPS TO LYSEFJORD AND PULPIT ROCK

The nearby Lysefjord is an easy day trip. Those with more time (and strong legs) can hike to the top of the 1,800-foot-high Pulpit Rock (Preikestolen). The dramatic 270-square-foot plateau atop the rock gives you a fantastic view of the fjord and surrounding mountains. The TI has brochures for several boat tour companies and sells tickets.

Warning: Remember, timing a Pulpit Rock trip that coincides with your cruise-ship departure is risky business. Be absolutely clear on your trip's return time and your ship's all-aboard time—and don't cut it close, just in case.

Boat Tour of Lysefjord

Rødne Clipper Fjord Sightseeing offers three-hour round-trip excursions from Stavanger to Lysefjord (including a view of Pulpit Rock—but no stops). Conveniently, their boats depart from the main Vågen harbor in the heart of town (east side of the harbor, in front of Skansegata, along Skagenkaien; 450 kr; mid-May-mid-Sept daily at 10:00 and 14:00, also Thu-Sat at 12:00 July-Aug; early May and late Sept daily at 12:00 Oct-April Wed-Sun only at 11:00; tel. 51 89 52 70, www.rodne.no). A different company, **Norled,** also runs similar trips, as well as slower journeys up the Lysefjord on a "tourist car ferry" (www.norled.no).

Ferry and Bus to Pulpit Rock

Hiking up to the top of Pulpit Rock is a popular outing that will take the better part of a day; plan on at least four hours of hiking (two hours up, two hours down), plus time to linger at the top for photos, plus round-trip travel from Stavanger (about an hour each way by a ferry-and-bus combination)—eight hours minimum should do it. The trailhead is easily reached in summer by public transit or tour package. Then comes the hard part: the hike to the top. The total distance is 4.5 miles and the elevation gain is roughly 1,000 feet. Pack a lunch and plenty of water, and wear good shoes.

Two different companies sell ferry-and-bus packages to the trailhead from Stavanger. Ferries leave from the Fiskepiren boat terminal to Tau; buses meet the incoming ferries and head to Pulpit Rock cabin or to Preikestolen Fjellstue, the local youth hostel. Be sure to time your hike so that you can catch the last bus leaving Pulpit Rock cabin for the ferry (confirm time when booking your ticket). These trips generally go daily from mid-May through mid-September; weekends only in April, early May, and late September; and not at all from October to March (when the ferry stops running). As the details tend to change from year to year, confirm all schedule details with the TI or the individual companies: **Tide Reiser** (240 kr, best options for an all-day round-trip are departures at 8:40 or 9:20, return bus from trailhead corresponds with ferry to Stavanger, tel. 55 23 88 87, www.tidereiser. com) and **Boreal** (150 kr for the bus plus 92 kr for the ferry—you'll buy the ferry ticket separately, best options depart at 8:40 or 9:20, last return bus from trailhead to ferry leaves at 19:55, tel. 51 56 41 00, www.pulpitrock.no).

Rødne Clipper Fjord Sightseeing (listed earlier) may run a handy trip in July and August that begins with a scenic Lysefjord cruise, then drops you off at Oanes to catch the bus to the Pulpit Rock hut trailhead; afterwards, you can catch the bus to Tau for the ferry return to Stavanger. It's similar to the options described above, but adds a scenic fjord cruise at the start. To confirm this is still going and get details, contact Rødne (750 kr plus 46 kr for return ferry to Stavanger, tel. 51 89 52 70, www.rodne.no).

Eating in Stavanger

For information on Norwegian cuisine, see page 700.

CASUAL DINING

Nye La Piazza, just off the harbor, has an assortment of pasta and other Italian dishes, including pizza, for 150-200 kr (100-kr lunch special, 300-320-kr meat options, Mon-Sat 13:00-23:00, Sun 13:00-22:00, Rosenkildettorget 1, tel. 51 52 02 52).

XO Bar Vertshuset Mat & Vin, in an elegant setting, serves up big portions of traditional Norwegian food and pricier contemporary fare (300-400 kr, light meals-150-190 kr, open Mon-Wed 11:00-23:30, Thu-Sat 11:00-1:30, a block behind main drag along harbor at Skagen 10 ved Prostebakken, mobile 91 00 03 07).

Meny is a large supermarket with a good selection and a fine deli for super-picnic shopping (Mon-Fri 9:00-20:00, Sat until 18:00, closed Sun, in Straen Senteret shopping mall, Lars Hertervigs Gate 6, tel. 51 50 50 10).

Market Plaza Eateries: The busy square between the cathedral and the harbor is packed with reliable Norwegian chain restaurants. If you're a fan of **Deli de Luca, Peppes Pizza,** or **Dickens Pub,** you'll find all of them within a few steps of here.

DINING ALONG THE HARBOR WITH A VIEW

The harborside street of Skansegata is lined with lively restaurants and pubs, and most serve food. Here are a couple of options:

N. B. Sørensen's Dampskibsexpedition has a lively pub on the first floor (225-340 kr for pasta, fish, meat, and vegetarian dishes; Mon-Wed 11:00-24:00, Sat 11:00-late, Sun 13:00-23:00, Skagenkaien 26). The restaurant is named after an 1800s company that shipped from this building, among other things, Norwegians heading to the US. Passengers and cargo waited on the first floor, and the manager's office was upstairs. The place is filled with emigrant-era memorabilia.

Sjøhuset Skagen, with a woodsy interior, invites diners to

What If I Miss My Boat?

Remember that you can get help from the cruise line's port agent (listed on the destination information sheet distributed on the ship) and the local TI (see page 716). If the port agent suggests a costly solution (such as a private car with a driver), you may want to consider public transit.

You can catch the bus to **Bergen** (http://kystbussen. no) or the train to **Oslo** (www.nsb.no). For **Flåm,** it's probably best to take the bus to Bergen, then a boat or train to the Sognefjord. For any points **outside Norway,** you'll most likely connect through Oslo. To research train schedules, see www. bahn.com.

If you need to catch a **plane** to your next destination, Stavanger's Sola Airport is a nine-mile bus ride outside the city (tel. 67 03 10 00, www.avinor.no).

Local **travel agents** in Stavanger can help you. For more advice on what to do if you miss the boat, see page 139.

its historic building for lunch or dinner. The building, from the late 1700s, housed a trading company. Today, you can choose from local seafood specialties with an ethnic flair, as well as plenty of meat options (180-195-kr lunches, 230-400-kr dinners, Mon-Sat 11:30-23:00, Sun 13:00-21:30, Skagenkaien 16, tel. 51 89 51 80).

Bølgen og Moi, the restaurant at the Petroleum Museum, has fantastic views over the harbor (lunch: 190-kr lunch special, 190-250-kr main dishes, served Mon 11:00-16:00, Kjeringholmen 748, tel. 51 93 93 53).

BERGEN
Norway

Norway Practicalities

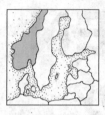

Norway (Norge) is stacked with superlatives—it's the most mountainous, most scenic, and most prosperous of all the Scandinavian countries. Perhaps above all, Norway is a land of intense natural beauty, its famously steep mountains and deep fjords carved out and shaped by an ancient ice age. Norway (148,700 square miles—just larger than Montana) is on the western side of the Scandinavian Peninsula, with most of the country sharing a border with Sweden to the east. Rich in resources like timber, oil, and fish, Norway has rejected joining the European Union, mainly to protect its fishing rights. Where the country extends north of the Arctic Circle, the sun never sets at the height of summer and never comes up in the deep of winter. The majority of Norway's 5 million people consider themselves Lutheran.

Money: 6 Norwegian kroner (kr, officially NOK) = about $1. An ATM is called a *minibank*. The local VAT (value-added sales tax) rate is 25 percent; the minimum purchase eligible for a VAT refund is 315 kr (for details on refunds, see page 134).

Language: The native language is Norwegian (the two official forms are Bokmål and Nynorsk). For useful phrases, see page 708.

Emergencies: Dial 112 for police, medical, or other emergencies. In case of theft or loss, see page 125.

Time Zone: Norway is on Central European Time (the same as most of the Continent, one hour ahead of Great Britain, and six/nine hours ahead of the East/West Coasts of the US).

Embassies in Oslo: The **US embassy** is at Henrik Ibsens Gate 48 (tel. 21 30 85 58, emergency tel. 21 30 85 40, http://norway.usembassy.gov). The **Canadian embassy** is at Wergelandsveien 7 (tel. 22 99 53 00, www.canada.no). Call ahead for passport services.

Phoning: Norway's country code is 47; to call from another country to Norway, dial the international access code (011 from the US/Canada, 00 from Europe, or + from a mobile phone), then 47, followed by the local number. For local calls within Norway, just dial the number as it appears in this book—whether you're calling from across the street or across the country. To place an international call from Norway, dial 00, the code of the country you're calling (1 for US and Canada), and the phone number. For more tips, see page 1146.

Tipping: Service is included at sit-down meals, but this goes to the owner, so for great service, it's nice to round up your bill about 10 percent. Tip a taxi driver by rounding up the fare (pay 90 kr on an 85-kr fare). For more tips on tipping, see page 138.

Tourist Information: www.goscandinavia.com

BERGEN

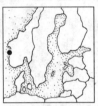

Bergen is permanently salted with robust cobbles and a rich sea-trading heritage. Norway's capital in the 13th century, Bergen's wealth and importance came thanks to its membership in the heavyweight medieval trading club of merchant cities called the Hanseatic League. Bergen still wears her rich maritime heritage proudly—nowhere more scenically than the colorful wooden warehouses that make up the picture-perfect Bryggen district along the harbor.

Protected from the open sea by a lone sheltering island, Bergen is a place of refuge from heavy winds for the giant working boats that serve the North Sea oil rigs. (Much of Norway's current affluence is funded by the oil it drills just offshore.) Bergen is also one of the most popular cruise-ship ports in northern Europe, hosting about 300 ships a year and up to five ships a day in peak season. Each morning is rush hour, as cruisers hike past the fortress and into town.

Bergen gets an average of 80 inches of rain annually (compared to 30 inches in Oslo). A good year has 60 days of sunshine. Bring along a light rain-jacket.

With 240,000 people, Bergen has big-city parking problems and high prices, but visitors sticking to the old center find it charming. Enjoy Bergen's salty market, then stroll the easy-on-foot old quarter, with cute lanes of delicate old wooden houses. From downtown Bergen, a funicular zips you up little Mount Fløyen for a bird's-eye view of this sailors' town. A foray into the countryside takes you to a variety of nearby experiences: a dramatic cable-car ride to a mountaintop perch (Ulriken643); a scenic

---

Excursions from Bergen

There's little reason to take an excursion here, as Bergen's top sights are easy to reach and appreciate on your own from the cruise ports. Most **Bergen** excursions include a walking tour around town (including Bryggen), often with tours of Håkon's Hall and Rosenkrantz Tower, and sometimes the funicular trip up Mount Fløyen. Outside town, excursions typically bundle Edvard Grieg's Home at **Troldhaugen** (at Nordås Lake) with **Fantoft Stave Church.** These sights are time-consuming to link by public transportation, so if you're dying to see them, an excursion may be worthwhile. Another excursion covers the ornately decorated, wooden **Villa Lysøen,** the former home of Ole Bull (built on its own little island). While it's inter-esting, it's also fairly distant (about a 30-minute bus ride each way); I'd rather save time for sights in Bergen itself.

---

stave church (Fantoft); and the home of Norway's most beloved composer, Edvard Grieg, at Troldhaugen.

PLANNING YOUR TIME

Bergen is compact, with several good sightseeing options that can be visited quickly.

• **Bryggen Walking Tour:** In summer (June-Aug), plan your day around this excellent 1.5-hour guided tour in English, which leads you through the historic, wooden Bryggen Hanseatic quar-ter and includes short visits to the top two museums, noted below (daily at 11:00 and 12:00, smart to reserve ahead in July). If the tour's not running when you're in town, you can still visit the sights on your own.

• **Bryggens Museum:** This fine archaeological museum focuses on early Bryggen history. Allow one hour.

• **Hanseatic Museum:** Explore the fascinating, still-furnished interior of one of Bryggen's historic wooden houses. Allow one hour.

• **Fløibanen Funicular:** This seven-minute trip takes you to bird's-eye views over town from atop Mount Fløyen. Allow 30-45 minutes round-trip, more if you want to hike down.

• **Other Sights in Town:** Many of Bergen's lesser attrac-tions—including Håkon's Hall/Rosenkrantz Tower at the for-tress, Fortress Museum, Theta Museum, cathedral, and Leprosy Museum—can be seen in 30 minutes each (though the hall and tower at the fortress are best if you have an hour to spare for the guided tour). The branches of the Kode Art Museum (conveniently located next to where some cruise-line shuttle buses drop off) could keep an art lover busy for hours, but a brief walk through

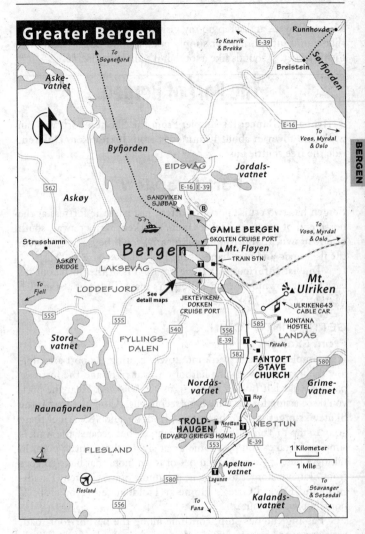

the main collection can take less than an hour. The aquarium and Gamle Bergen (Old Bergen) take longer to reach; I'd skip these unless you have a special interest.

• **Out-of-Town Sights:** If you're feeling adventurous and want to get out of town, you can head out to the **Ulriken643 Cable Car,** Edvard Grieg's Home at **Troldhaugen,** or **Fantoft Stave Church**—but each requires a bus or tram ride (figure about an hour each way from downtown Bergen to Troldhaugen or the church, less for the cable car).

For one busy day in Bergen, I'd take the walking tour (including visits to the Bryggens and Hanseatic Museums), ride up to

Mount Fløyen, and wrap up my visit with any of the other sights that sound intriguing—or simply poke around Bryggen and the Fish Market. It sounds like a lot, but it's all easily doable.

The Port of Bergen

Arrival at a Glance: It's simple: From the **Skolten** port, you can walk into town in about 10 minutes; from **Jekteviken/Dokken,** ride the free shuttle bus.

Port Overview

Bergen has two cruise ports: **Skolten,** just past the fortress at the north end of town; and **Jekteviken/Dokken,** farther away, south of downtown. If your ship gets in early, you'll be setting up with the fishermen and merchants at the Fish Market.

Tourist Information: There are no TIs at the ports, but it's easy to get downtown to visit Bergen's main TI (right at the Fish Market; see page 731).

GETTING INTO TOWN
From Skolten

It's a simple and scenic **walk** into town. Exiting the port area, follow the busy road with the harbor on your right and the fortress/park on your left (follow traffic signs for *Sentrum*). Near the port, you'll see a stop for the City Sightseeing bus. Along the road is the Skutevikstorget stop for buses #3, #4, #5, #6, and #83. All of these go one stop to Torget, in the town center—but because the walk is simple and takes you past some great sights, there's little point in taking a bus. If you're headed out of town, note that bus #83 goes from Skutevikstorget to stops near Fantoft Stave Church (Paradis stop) and Edvard Grieg's Home at Troldhaugen (Hop stop; 2/hour, about 30 minutes).

Passing the bus stop, continue along the harborfront road, crossing over to the fortress side at the crosswalk. Very shortly you'll pass the side entrance into the fortress complex, which is also the starting point of my self-guided walk.

If you want to skip the walk for now and head straight downtown, just keep walking, and you'll be there (at the Fish Market, with the TI nearby) in about five more minutes. If you need cash, look for the ATM two short blocks after the fortress—on the left, at the Windfjord sweater and souvenir shop.

From Jekteviken/Dokken

This arrival point is in a drab, sprawling industrial port just south of downtown. Although it's only a 20-minute walk to the center,

Services in Bergen

Services are virtually nonexistent at the ports. But since both ports are easily connected to downtown, you can find what you need there.

ATMs: Various ATMs are scattered around the city-center zone near the Fish Market. On your way into town from the Skolten port, the first ATM you'll pass is at the **Windfjord** sweater and souvenir shop, two blocks past the fortress on the harborside road.

Internet Access: The **TI** (near the Fish Market) has a strong, fast, free Wi-Fi connection; the password is posted on the wall. For terminals with Internet access, see page 735.

Pharmacy: Two handy options are right downtown, near all the sightseeing: **Boots Apotek** is just a half-block in front of the funicular station to Mount Fløyen (Mon-Fri 9:00-17:00, Sat 10:00-16:00, closed Sun, Vetrlidsallmenningen 11). **Apotek 1** is inside the Galleriet Shopping Mall, facing the Seafarers' Monument on the main square, Torgallmenningen (Mon-Fri 9:00-21:00, Sat 9:00-18:00, closed Sun).

the port authority (which doesn't want tourists wandering around all the big containers) provides a **free shuttle bus** to the center. This convenient service takes you to a stop along the south side of Lille Lungegårdsvann, the cute manmade lake in the city center. Stepping off the bus, you'll be on the street called Rasmus Meyers Allé, which is right in front of the four branches of the Kode Art Museums (described on page 751). From here, it's a pleasant and easy 10-minute walk to the Fish Market, TI, harbor, and most sightseeing: First, walk with the lake on your right. At the end of the lake, you'll reach the park called Byparken (the terminus for the Bybanen tram to Fantoft Stave Church and Edvard Grieg's Home at Troldhaugen is nearby). Continue through the park, straight past the pretty pavilion, and up the long square called Ole Bulls Plass. This is the finishing point of my self-guided walk (consider doing it in reverse from here; or, if you take the walk later, it'll lead you back here and to the bus). Head halfway up Ole Bulls Plass (passing the fountain of the namesake violinist) to the big, bluish stone slab. Turn right and head up another long, broad square, Torgallmenningen; at the end of this, you'll pass the blocky Seafarers' Monument. The Fish Market, TI, and Bryggen are just beyond it.

By Taxi

There's little need for a taxi from **Skolten,** thanks to its easy proximity to town. But if you want to take one, plan on 70-80 kr to points downtown. Likewise, taxis aren't necessary for the

Jekteviken/Dokken port, since the free shuttle takes you straight downtown. But if you need to take a taxi, plan on around 110 kr between the port and downtown.

If taxis aren't waiting at the port, call 07000 or 08000 to summon one.

By Tour

Remember: If you're in town in June, July, or August, I highly recommend taking the **Bryggen Walking Tour** to get oriented (departs at 11:00 and 12:00; details on page 732).

Hop-on, hop-off bus tours meet arriving ships at Skolten; if arriving at Jekteviken/Dokken, you can ride the shuttle bus into town and catch the bus tour at Byparken (150 kr/24 hours, 2/hour; for more details, see page 733). But in this compact and walkable city, these bus tours don't make much sense (unless the weather is miserable and you just want a once-over-lightly look at the town).

For more information on this and other local tour options in Bergen, see "Tours in Bergen" on page 732.

RETURNING TO YOUR SHIP

To **Skolten,** it's an easy walk around the fortress (just walk with the harbor on your left). If you have time to kill before "all aboard," you can browse through Bryggen (which is a quick 10-minute walk from your ship) or tour the fortress sights (even closer).

To return to **Jekteviken/Dokken,** catch the shuttle bus right where it dropped you, in front of the Kode Art Museums by the little lake along Rasmus Meyers Allé; my self-guided walk leads you there. If you've got time to kill, take a quick spin through the museums.

See page 760 for help if you miss your boat.

Bergen

Bergen clusters around its harbor—nearly everything listed in this chapter is within a few minutes' walk. The busy Torget (the square with the Fish Market) is at the head of the harbor. As you face the sea from here, Bergen's TI is at the left end of the Fish Market. The town's historic Hanseatic Quarter, Bryggen (BREW-gun), lines the harbor on the right. Express boats to the Sognefjord (Balestrand and Flåm) dock at the harbor on the left.

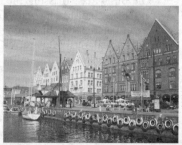

Charming cobbled streets surround the harbor and climb the encircling hills. Bergen's popular Fløibanen funicular climbs high above the city to the top of Mount Fløyen for the best view of the town. Surveying the surrounding islands and inlets, it's clear why this city is known as the "Gateway to the Fjords."

Orientation to Bergen

TOURIST INFORMATION

The centrally located TI is upstairs in the long, skinny, modern, Torghallen market building, next to the Fish Market (June-Aug daily 8:30-22:00; May and Sept daily 9:00-20:00; Oct-April Mon-Sat 9:00-16:00, closed Sun; handy budget eateries downstairs and in Fish Market; tel. 55 55 20 00, www.visitbergen.com).

The TI covers Bergen and western Norway; provides information and tickets for tours; has a fjord information desk; and maintains a very handy events board listing today's slate of tours, concerts, and other events. Pick up this year's edition of the free *Bergen Guide*, which has a fine map and lists all sights, hours, and special events. This booklet can answer most of your questions. If you need assistance and there's a line, take a number. They also have free Wi-Fi (password posted on wall). For a short visit, it's not worth buying the Bergen Card, which covers trams, buses, and most museums (200 kr/24 hours, sold at TI).

HELPFUL HINTS

Museum Tours: Many of Bergen's sights are hard to appreciate without a guide. Fortunately, several include a wonderful and intimate guided tour with admission. Make the most of the following sights by taking advantage of their included tours: Håkon's Hall and Rosenkrantz Tower, Bryggens Museum, Hanseatic Museum, Leprosy Museum, Gamle Bergen, and Edvard Grieg's Home.

Internet Access: The **TI** offers free, fast Wi-Fi (look for the password posted on the wall), but no terminals. The **Bergen Public Library,** next door to the train station, has free terminals in their downstairs café (30-minute limit, Mon-Thu 10:00-18:00, Fri 10:00-16:00, Sat 10:00-15:00, closed Sun, Strømgaten 6, tel. 55 56 85 60). The church-run **Kafe Magdalena,** just off the harbor at Kong Oscars Gate 5, has two free terminals.

GETTING AROUND BERGEN

Most in-town sights can easily be reached by foot; only the aquarium and Gamle Bergen (and farther-flung sights such as the Fantoft Stave Church, Edvard Grieg's Home at Troldhaugen, and the Ulriken643 cable car) are more than a 10-minute walk from the TI.

By Bus: City buses cost 41 kr per ride (pay driver in cash), or 31 kr per ride if you buy a single-ride ticket from a machine or convenience stores such as Narvesen, 7-Eleven, Rimi, and Deli de Luca. The best buses for a Bergen joyride are #6 (north along the coast) and #11 (into the hills).

By Tram: Bergen's recently built light-rail line (Bybanen) is a convenient way to visit Edvard Grieg's Home or Fantoft Stave Church. The tram begins next to Byparken (on Kaigaten, between Bergen's little lake and Ole Bulls Plass), then heads to the train station and continues south. Buy your 31-kr ticket from the machine prior to boarding (to use a US credit card, you'll need to know your PIN code). You can also buy single-ride tickets at Narvesen, 7-Eleven, Rimi, and Deli de Luca stores. You'll get a gray *minikort* pass. Validate the pass when you board by holding it next to the card reader (watch how other passengers do it). Ride it about 20 minutes to the Paradis stop for Fantoft Stave Church (don't get off at the "Fantoft" stop, which is farther from the church); or continue to the next stop, Hop, to hike to Troldhaugen.

By Ferry: The *Beffen,* a little orange ferry, chugs across the harbor every half-hour, from the dock a block south of the Bryggens Museum to the dock—directly opposite the fortress—a block from the Nykirken church (20 kr, Mon-Fri 7:30-16:00, plus Sat May-Aug 11:00-16:00, never on Sun, 3-minute ride). The *Vågen* ferry runs from the Fish Market every half-hour to a dock near the aquarium (50 kr one-way, daily June-Aug 10:00-17:30, off-season 10:00-16:00, 10-minute ride). These short "poor man's cruises" have good harbor views.

By Taxi: For a taxi, call 07000 or 08000 (they're not as expensive as you might expect).

Tours in Bergen

▲▲▲Bryggen Walking Tour

This tour of the historic Hanseatic district is one of Bergen's best activities. Local guides take visitors on an excellent 1.5-hour walk in English through 900 years of Bergen history via the old Hanseatic town (20 minutes in Bryggens Museum, 20-minute visit to the medieval Hanseatic Assembly Rooms, 20-minute walk through Bryggen, and 20 minutes in Hanseatic Museum). Tours leave from the Bryggens Museum (next to the Radisson Blu Royal Hotel). When you consider that the price includes entry tickets to all three sights, the

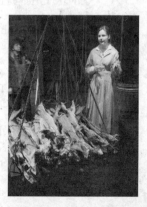

tour more than pays for itself (120 kr, June-Aug daily at 11:00 and 12:00, maximum 30 in group, no tours Sept-May, tel. 55 58 80 10, bryggens.museum@bymuseet.no). While the museum visits are a bit rushed, your tour ticket allows you to re-enter the museums for the rest of the day. The 11:00 tour can sell out, especially in July; to be safe, you can call, email, or drop by ahead to reserve a spot.

Local Guide
Sue Lindelid is a British expat who has spent more than 25 years showing visitors around Bergen (800 kr/2-hour tour, 900 kr/3 or more people; 1,000 kr/3-hour tour, 1,200 kr/3 or more people; mobile 90 78 59 52, suelin@hotmail.no).

▲Bus Tours
The TI sells tickets for various bus tours, including a 2.5-hour Grieg Lunch Concert tour that goes to Edvard Grieg's Home at Troldhaugen—a handy way to reach that distant sight (250 kr, discount with Bergen Card, includes 30-minute concert but not lunch, June-mid-Sept daily at 11:30, departs from TI).

Hop-On, Hop-Off Buses
City Sightseeing links most of Bergen's major sights and also stops at the Skolten cruise port, but doesn't go to Fantoft Stave Church, Troldhaugen, or Ulriken643 cable car. If your sightseeing plans don't extend beyond the walkable core of Bergen, skip the bus and save some kroner (150 kr/24 hours, late May-Aug 9:00-16:30, 2/hour, also stops right in front of Fish Market, mobile 97 78 18 88, www.citysightseeing-bergen.net).

▲Harbor Tour
The *White Lady* leaves once daily at 11:00 (summer only) from the Fish Market for a 1.5-hour cruise. The ride is both scenic and informative, with a relaxing sun deck and good—if scant—recorded narration (150 kr, June-Aug). A daily four-hour afternoon fjord trip is also available (500 kr, June-Aug, tel. 55 25 90 00, www.whitelady.no).

Tourist Train
The tacky little "Bergen Express" train departs from in front of the Hanseatic Museum for a 55-minute loop around town (150 kr, 2/hour in peak season, otherwise hourly; runs daily May 10:00-16:00, June-Aug 10:00-19:00, Sept 10:00-15:00; headphone English commentary).

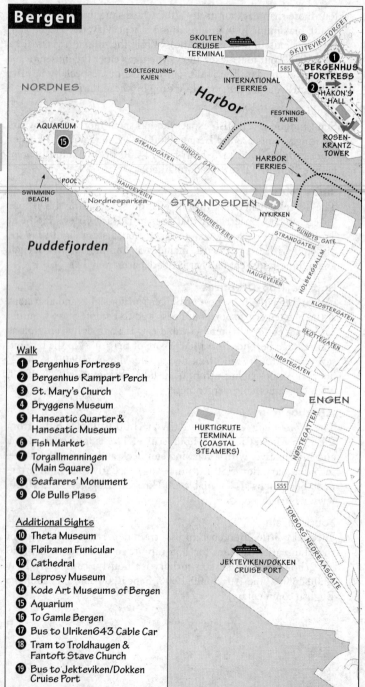

Bergen

SKOLTEN
CRUISE
TERMINAL

SKOLTEGRUNNS-
KAIEN

INTERNATIONAL
FERRIES

SKUTEVIKSTORGET

B

585

❶ BERGENHUS
FORTRESS

❷ HÅKON'S
HALL

NORDNES

Harbor

FESTNINGS-
KAIEN

ROSEN-
KRANTZ
TOWER

AQUARIUM

❶⑮

STRANDGATEN

C. SUNDTS GATE

HARBOR
FERRIES

POOL

HAUGEVEIEN

SWIMMING
BEACH

Nordnesparken

STRANDSIDEN

NYKIRKEN

C. SUNDTS GATE

Puddefjorden

NORDNESVEIEN

STRANDGATEN

HOLBERGSALLM

HAUGEVEIEN

KLOSTERGATEN

SKOTTEGATEN

NØSTEGATEN

ENGEN

HURTIGRUTE
TERMINAL
(COASTAL
STEAMERS)

NØSTEGATTEN

555

TORBORG NEDREAASGATE

JEKTEVIKEN/DOKKEN
CRUISE PORT

Walk
❶ Bergenhus Fortress
❷ Bergenhus Rampart Perch
❸ St. Mary's Church
❹ Bryggens Museum
❺ Hanseatic Quarter &
   Hanseatic Museum
❻ Fish Market
❼ Torgallmenningen
   (Main Square)
❽ Seafarers' Monument
❾ Ole Bulls Plass

Additional Sights
⑩ Theta Museum
⑪ Fløibanen Funicular
⑫ Cathedral
⑬ Leprosy Museum
⑭ Kode Art Museums of Bergen
⑮ Aquarium
⑯ To Gamle Bergen
⑰ Bus to Ulriken643 Cable Car
⑱ Tram to Troldhaugen &
   Fantoft Stave Church
⑲ Bus to Jekteviken/Dokken
   Cruise Port

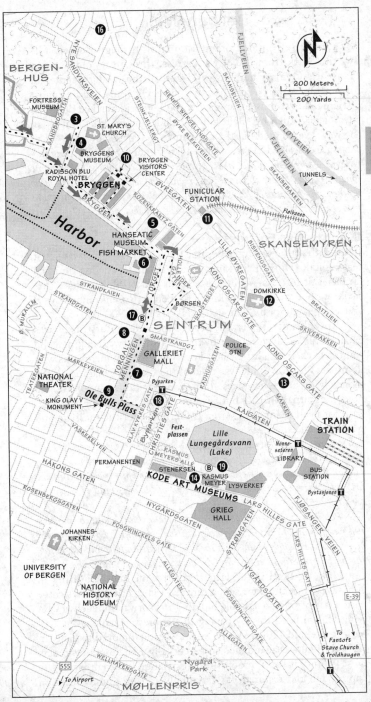

Bergen Walk

For a quick self-guided orientation stroll through Bergen, follow this walk from the city's fortress, through its old wooden Hanseatic Quarter and Fish Market, to the modern center of town. This walk is also a handy sightseeing spine, passing most of Bergen's best museums; ideally, you'll get sidetracked and take advantage of their excellent tours (included with admission) along the way. I've pointed out the museums you'll pass en route—all of them are described in greater detail later, under "Sights in Bergen."

• *Begin where Bergen did, at its historic fortress. From the harborfront road, 50 yards before the stone tower with the water on your left, veer up the ramp behind the low stone wall on the right, through a gate, and into the fortress complex. Stand before the stony skyscraper.*

❶ Bergenhus Fortress

In the 13th century, Bergen became the Kingdom of Norway's first real capital. (Until then, kings would circulate, staying on royal farms.) This fortress—built in the 1240s and worth ▲—was a garrison, with a tower for the king's residence (Rosenkrantz Tower) and a large hall for his banquets (Håkon's Hall).

Rosenkrantz Tower, the keep of the 13th-century castle, was expanded in the 16th century by the Danish-Norwegian king, who wanted to exercise a little control over the German merchants who dominated his town. He was tired of the Germans making all the money without paying taxes. This tower—with its cannon trained not on external threats but toward Bryggen—while expensive, paid for itself many times over as Germans got the message and paid their taxes.

• *Step through the gate (20 yards to the right of the tower) marked 1728 and into the courtyard of the Bergenhus Fortress. In front of you stands Håkon's Hall with its stepped gable. Tours for both the hall and the tower leave from the building to the right of Håkon's Hall (for details, see page 746).*

Pop into the museum lobby to enjoy a free exhibit about the massive 1944 explosion of the German ammunition ship in the harbor. For the best view of Håkon's Hall, walk through the gate and around the building to the left. Stand on the rampart between the hall and the harbor.

Håkon's Hall is the largest secular medieval building in Norway. When the pope sent a cardinal to perform Håkon's coronation, there was no suitable building in Norway for such a VIP. King Håkon fixed that by having this impressive banqueting hall built in the mid-1200s. When Norway's capital moved to Oslo, in 1299, the hall was abandoned and eventually used for grain storage. For a century it had no roof. In the Romantic 19th century, it was appreciated and restored. It's essentially a giant, grand reception hall used today as it was eight centuries ago: for banquets.

• *Continue walking along the rampart (climbing some steps and going about 100 yards past Håkon's Hall) to the far end of Bergenhus Fortress, where you find a statue of a king and a fine harbor view.*

❷ Bergenhus Rampart Perch and Statue of King Håkon VII

The cannon on the ramparts here illustrates how the fort protected this strategic harbor. The port is busy with both cruise ships and support ships for the nearby North Sea oil rigs. Long before this modern commerce, this is where the cod fishermen of the north met the traders of Europe. Beyond the ships is an island protecting Bergen from the open sea.

The statue is of the beloved King Håkon VII (1872-1957), grandfather of today's king. While exiled in London during World War II, King Håkon kept up Norwegian spirits through radio broadcasts. The first king of modern Norway (after the country won its independence from Sweden in 1905), he was a Danish prince married to Queen Victoria's granddaughter—a savvy monarch who knew how to play the royalty game.

Continuing around Håkon's Hall, follow the linden tree-lined lane. On the left, a massive concrete structure disguised by ivy looms as if evil. It was a German bunker built during the Nazi occupation—easier now to ignore than dismantle.

Twenty yards ahead on the right is a rare set of free public toilets.

• *You've now returned to the tower and circled the castle grounds. Before leaving, consider taking one of the guided tours of the hall and tower that leave at the top of each hour (described in "Sights in Bergen," later). Head back down the ramp, out to the main road, and continue with the harbor on your right. (After a block, history buffs could follow* Bergenhus *signs, up the street to the left, to the free and fascinating* **Fortress Museum**—*with its collection of Norwegian military history and Nazi occupation exhibits.) Proceed one more block along the harbor until you reach the open, park-like space on your left. Walk 100 yards (just past the handy Rema 1000 supermarket) to the top of this park, where you'll see...*

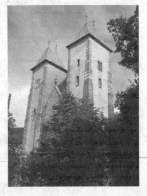

❸ St. Mary's Church (Mariakirken)

Dating from the 12th century, this is Bergen's oldest building in continuous use. It's closed for a couple of years while a 100-million-kroner

Bergen at a Glance

▲▲▲**Bryggen Walking Tour** Wonderful 1.5-hour tour of the historic Hanseatic district that covers 900 years of history and includes short visits to the Bryggens Museum, Hanseatic Assembly Rooms, and Hanseatic Museum, plus a walk through Bryggen. **Hours:** June-Aug daily at 11:00 and 12:00. See page 732.

▲▲**Bryggens Museum** Featuring early bits of Bergen (1050-1500), found in a 1950s archaeological dig. **Hours:** Mid-May-Aug daily 10:00-16:00; Sept-mid-May Mon-Fri 11:00-15:00, Sat 12:00-15:00, Sun 12:00-16:00. See page 748.

▲▲**Hanseatic Museum** Small museum highlighting Bryggen's glory days, located in an old merchant house furnished with artifacts from the time German merchants were tops in trading—most interesting with included tour. **Hours:** Daily May-Sept 9:00-17:00; Oct-April Tue-Sat 11:00-14:00, Sun 11:00-16:00, closed Mon. See page 748.

▲▲**Fløibanen Funicular** Zippy lift to top of Mount Fløyen for super views of Bergen, islands, and fjords, with picnic ops, an eatery, playground, and hiking trails. **Hours:** Mon-Fri 7:30-23:00, Sat-Sun 8:00-23:00. See page 749.

Leprosy Museum Former hospital for lepers, with small exhibit and worthwhile free tour offered on the top of every hour. **Hours:** Mid-May-Aug daily 11:00-15:00, closed Sept-mid-May. See page 750.

▲**Harbor Tour** Scenic 1.5-hour cruise, with recorded narration, leaving from the Fish Market. **Hours:** June-Aug at 11:00. See page 733.

▲**Fish Market** Lively market with cheap seafood eateries and free samples. **Hours:** Daily 7:00-19:00; Sept-May Mon-Sat 7:00-16:00, closed Sun. See page 743.

▲**Bergenhus Fortress: Håkon's Hall and Rosenkrantz Tower** Fortress with a 13th-century medieval banquet hall, a climbable

renovation is under way. This stately church of the Hanseatic merchants has a dour stone interior, enlivened by a colorful, highly decorated pulpit.

In the park below the church, find the statue of Snorri Sturluson. In the 1200s, this Icelandic scribe and scholar wrote down the Viking sagas. Thanks to him, we have a better understanding of this Nordic era. A few steps to the right, look through the window of the big modern building at an archaeological site

tower offering a history exhibit and views, and a worthwhile, included tour. **Hours:** Mid-May-Aug—hall open daily 10:00-16:00, tower open daily 9:00-16:00; Sept-mid-May—hall open daily 12:00-15:00, tower open Sun only 12:00-15:00. See page 746.

▲**Kode Art Museums of Bergen** Collection spread among four neighboring lakeside buildings: Lysverket (international and Norwegian artists), Rasmus Meyer (Norwegian artists, including Munch), Stenersen (contemporary art), and Permanenten (decorative arts). **Hours:** Daily 11:00-17:00, closed Mon mid-Sept-mid-May. See page 751.

▲**Aquarium** Well-presented sea life, with a walk-through "shark tunnel" and feeding times at the top of most hours in summer. **Hours:** Daily May-Aug 10:00-18:00, Sept-mid-Oct daily 10:00-16:00, mid-Oct-April Tue-Sun 10:00-16:00, closed Mon. See page 751.

▲**Gamle Bergen (Old Bergen)** Quaint gathering of 50 homes and shops dating from 18th to 20th century, with guided tours of museum interiors at the top of the hour. **Hours:** Mid-May-Aug daily 9:00-16:00, closed Sept-mid-May. See page 751.

Near Bergen
▲▲**Edvard Grieg's Home**, **Troldhaugen** Home of Norway's greatest composer, with artifacts, tours, and concerts. **Hours:** Daily May-Sept 9:00-18:00, Oct-April 10:00-16:00. See page 752.

▲**Ulriken643 Cable Car** A quick ride up to the summit of Ulriken, Bergen's tallest mountain, with nonstop views, a restaurant, and hiking trails. **Hours:** Daily 9:00-21:00, off-season 9:00-17:00. See page 752.

Fantoft Stave Church Replica of a 12th-century wooden church in atmospheric wooded setting. **Hours:** Mid-May-mid-Sept daily 10:30-18:00, interior closed off-season. See page 754.

showing the oldest remains of Bergen—stubs of the 12th-century trading town's streets tumbling to the harbor before land reclamation pushed the harbor farther out.

• *The window is just a sneak peek at the excellent* ❹ *Bryggens Museum, which provides helpful historical context for the Hanseatic Quarter we're about to visit (see listing later, under "Sights in Bergen"). The museum's outstanding Bryggen Walking Tour is your best bet for seeing this area (June–Aug daily at 11:00 and 12:00, see "Tours in*

Bryggen's History

Pretty as Bryggen is today, it has a rough-and-tumble history. A horrific plague decimated the population and economy of Norway in 1350, killing about half of its people. A decade later, German merchants arrived and established a Hanseatic trading post, bringing order to that rustic society. For the next four centuries, the port of Bergen was essentially German territory.

Bergen's old German trading center was called "the German wharf" until World War II (and is now just called "the wharf," or "Bryggen"). From 1370 to 1754, German merchants controlled Bergen's trade. In 1550, it was a Germanic city of 1,000 workaholic merchants—surrounded and supported by some 5,000 Norwegians.

The German merchants were very strict and lived in a harsh, all-male world (except for Norwegian prostitutes). This wasn't a military occupation, but a mutually beneficial economic partnership. The Norwegian cod fishermen of the far north shipped their dried cod to Bergen, where the Hanseatic merchants marketed it to Europe. Norwegian cod provided much of Europe with food (a source of easy-to-preserve protein) and cod oil (which lit the lamps until about 1850).

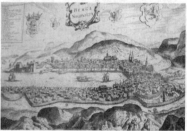

While the city dates from 1070, little survives from before the last big fire in 1702. In its earlier heyday, Bergen was one of the largest wooden cities in Europe. Congested wooden buildings, combined with lots of small fires (to provide heat and light in this cold and dark corner of Europe), spelled disaster for Bergen. Over the centuries, the city suffered countless fires, including 10 devastating ones. Back then, it wasn't a question of *if* there would be a fire, but *when* there would be a fire—with major blazes every 20 or so years. Each time the warehouses burned, the merchants would

Bergen," earlier). Continue down to the busy harborfront. On the left is the most photographed sight in town, the Bryggen quarter. To get your bearings, first read the "Bryggen's History" sidebar; if it's nice out, cross the street to the wharf and look back for a fine overview of this area. (Or, in the rain, huddle under an awning.)

❺ Bergen's Hanseatic Quarter (Bryggen)

Bergen's fragile wooden old town is its iconic front door. The long "tenements" (rows of warehouses) hide atmospheric lanes that creak and groan with history.

Remember that while we think of Bergen as "Norwegian,"

toss the refuse into the bay and rebuild. Gradually, the land crept out, and so did the buildings. (Looking at the Hanseatic Quarter from the harborfront, you can see how the buildings have settled. The foundations, composed of debris from the many fires, settle as they rot.)

After 1702, the city rebuilt using more stone and brick, and suffered fewer fires. But this one small wooden quarter was built after the fire, in the early 1700s. To prevent future blazes, the Germans forbade all fires and candles for light or warmth except in isolated and carefully guarded communal houses behind each tenement. It was in these communal houses that apprentices studied, people dried out their soggy clothes, hot food was cooked, and the men drank and partied. When there was a big banquet, one man always stayed sober—a kind of designated fire watchman.

Flash forward to the 20th century. One of the biggest explosions of World War II occurred in Bergen's harbor on April 20, 1944. An ammunition ship loaded with 120 tons of dynamite blew up just in front of the fortress. The blast leveled entire neighborhoods on either side of the harbor (notice the ugly 1950s construction opposite the fortress) and did serious damage to Håkon's Hall and Rosenkrantz Tower. How big was the blast? There's a hut called "the anchor cabin" a couple of miles away in the mountains. That's where the ship's anchor landed. The blast is considered to be accidental, despite the fact that April 20 happened to be Hitler's 55th birthday and the ship blew up about 100 yards away from the Nazi commander's headquarters (in the fortress).

After World War II, Bryggen was again slated for destruction. Most of the locals wanted it gone—it reminded them of the Germans who had occupied Norway for the miserable war years. Then excavators discovered rune stones indicating that the area predated the Germans. This boosted Bryggen's approval rating, and the quarter was saved. Today this picturesque and historic zone is the undisputed tourist highlight of Bergen.

Bryggen was German—the territory of *Deutsch*-speaking merchants and traders. (The most popular surname in Bergen is the German name Hanson—"son of Hans.") From the front of Bryggen, look back at the Rosenkrantz Tower. The little red holes at its top mark where cannons were once pointed at the German quarter by Norwegian royalty who wanted a slice of all that trade revenue in taxes. The threat was countered by German grain—without which the Norwegians would starve.

Notice that the first six houses are perfectly straight; they were built in the 1980s to block the view of a modern hotel behind. The more ramshackle stretch of 11 houses beyond date from the early 1700s. Each front hides a long line of five to ten businesses.

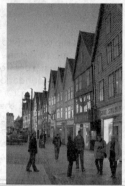

• *To wander into the heart of this woody medieval quarter, head down Bredsgården, the lane a couple of doors before the shop sign featuring the anatomically correct unicorn. We'll make a loop to the right: down this lane nearly all the way, under a passage into a square (with a well, a vibrant outdoor restaurant, and a big wooden cod), and then back to the harbor down a parallel lane. Read the information below, then explore, stopping at the big wooden cod.*

Bit by bit, Bryggen is being restored using medieval techniques and materials. As you explore, you may stumble upon a rebuilding project in action.

Strolling through Bryggen, you feel swallowed up by history. Long rows of planky buildings (medieval-style double tenements) lean haphazardly across narrow alleys. The last Hanseatic merchant moved out centuries ago, but this is still a place of (touristy) commerce. You'll find artists' galleries, T-shirt boutiques, leather workshops, atmospheric restaurants, fishing tackle shops, sweaters, sweaters, sweaters...and trolls.

Turning right at the top of the lane, you enter a lively cobbled square. On the far side is that big wooden cod (next to a well), a reminder that the economic foundation of Bergen—the biggest city in Scandinavia until 1650 and the biggest city in Norway until 1830—was this fish. The stone building behind the carved cod was one of the fireproof cookhouses serving a line of buildings that stretched to the harbor. Today it's the Hetland Gallery, filled with the entertaining work of a popular local artist famous for fun caricatures of the city. Facing the same square is the Bryggen visitors center, worth peeking into.

• *Enjoy the center and the shops. Then return downhill to the harborfront, turn left, and continue the walk.*

Half of Bryggen (the brick-and-stone stretch to your left between the old wooden facades and the head of the bay) was torn down around 1900. Today the stately buildings that replaced it—far less atmospheric than Bryggen's original wooden core—are filled with tacky trinket shops and touristy splurge restaurants.

Head to the lone wooden red house at the end of the row, which houses the **Hanseatic Museum.** This highly recommended museum is your best chance to get a peek inside one of those old wooden tenements.

• *The Fish Market is just across the street. Before enjoying that, we'll circle a few blocks inland and around to the right.*

The red-brick building (with frilly white trim, stepped gable, and a Starbucks) is the old meat market. It was built in 1877, after hygiene was discovered and the meat was moved inside from today's Fish Market. At the intersection just beyond, look left (uphill past the meat market) to see the Fløibanen station. Ahead, on the right, is an unusually classy McDonald's in a 1710 building that was originally a bakery.

But let's look at Norwegian fast food: Across the street, Söstrene Hagelin is a celebration of white and fishy cuisine—very Norwegian. A few steps uphill, the tiny red shack flying the Norwegian flags is the popular 3-Kroneren hotdog stand (described in "Eating in Bergen," later). Review the many sausage options.

BERGEN

At the McDonald's, wander the length of the cute lane of 200-year-old buildings. Called Hollendergaten, its name comes from a time when the king organized foreign communities of traders into various neighborhoods; this was where the Dutch lived. The curving street marks the former harborfront—these buildings were originally right on the water.

Hooking left, you reach the end of Hollendergaten. Turn right back toward the harborfront. Ahead is the grand stone Børsen building (now Matbørsen, a collection of trendy restaurants), once the stock exchange. Step inside to enjoy its 1920s Art Deco-style murals celebrating Bergen's fishing heritage.

• *Now, cross the street and immerse yourself in Bergen's beloved Fish Market.*

❻ Fish Market (Fisketorget)

A fish market has thrived here since the 1500s, when fishermen rowed in with their catch and haggled with hungry residents.

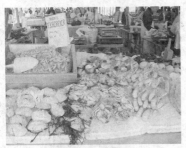

While it's now become a food circus of eateries selling fishy treats to tourists—no local would come here to actually buy fish—this famous market is still worth ▲, offering lots of smelly photo fun and free morsels to taste (June-Aug daily 7:00-19:00, less lively on Sun; Sept-May Mon-Sat 7:00-16:00, closed Sun). Many stands sell premade smoked-salmon (laks) sandwiches, fish soup, and other snacks ideal for a light lunch (confirm prices before ordering). To try Norwegian jerky, pick up a bag of dried cod snacks (*torsk*).

• *Watch your wallet: If you're going to get pickpocketed in Bergen, it'll likely be here. When done exploring, with your back to the market, hike a block to the right (note the pointy church spire in the distance and the*

The Hanseatic League, Blessed by Cod

Middlemen in trade, the clever German merchants of the Hanseatic League ruled the waves of northern Europe for 500 years (c. 1250-1750). These sea-traders first banded together in a Hanse, or merchant guild, to defend themselves against pirates. As they spread out from Germany, they established trading posts in foreign lands, cut deals with local leaders for trading rights, built boats and wharves, and organized armies to protect ships and ports.

By the 15th century, these merchants had organized more than a hundred cities into the Hanseatic League, a free-trade zone that stretched from London to Russia. The League ran a profitable triangle of trade: Fish from Scandinavia was exchanged for grain from the eastern Baltic and luxury goods from England and Flanders. Everyone benefited, and the German merchants—the middlemen—reaped the profits.

At its peak in the 15th century, the Hanseatic League was the dominant force—economic, military, and political—in northern Europe. This was an age when much of Europe was fragmented into petty kingdoms and dukedoms. Revenue-hungry kings and robber-baron lords levied chaotic and extortionist tolls and duties. Pirates plagued shipments. It was the Hanseatic League, rather than national governments, that brought the stability that allowed trade to flourish.

Bergen's place in this Baltic economy was all about cod—a form of protein that could be dried, preserved, and shipped anywhere. Though cursed by a lack of natural resources, the city

---

big blocky stone monument dead ahead) into the modern part of town and a huge wide square. Pause at the intersection just before crossing into the square, about 20 yards before the blocky monument. Look left to see Mount Ulriken with its TV tower. A cable car called Ulriken643 takes you to its 2,110-foot summit. (Shuttle buses leave from this corner, at the top and bottom of the hour, to its station; for summit details, see page 752.) Now, walk up to that big square monument and meet some Vikings.

❼ Seafarers' Monument

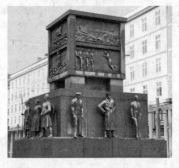

Nicknamed "the cube of goat cheese" for its shape, this 1950 monument celebrates Bergen's contact with the sea and remembers those who worked on it and died in it. Study the faces: All social classes are represented. The statues relate to the scenes depicted in the reliefs above. Each side represents a century (start

was blessed with a good harbor conveniently located between the rich fishing spots of northern Norway and the markets of Europe. Bergen's port shipped dried cod and fish oil southward and imported grain, cloth, beer, wine, and ceramics.

Bryggen was one of four principal Hanseatic trading posts (Kontors), along with London, Bruges, and Novgorod. It was the last Kontor opened (c. 1360), the least profitable, and the final one to close. Bryggen had warehouses, offices, and living quarters. Ships docked here were unloaded by counterpoise cranes. At its peak, as many as a thousand merchants, journeymen, and apprentices lived and worked here.

Bryggen was a self-contained German enclave within the city. The merchants came from Germany, worked a few years here, and retired back in the home country. They spoke German, wore German clothes, and attended their own churches. By law, they were forbidden to intermarry or fraternize with the Bergeners, except on business.

The Hanseatic League peaked around 1500, then slowly declined. Rising nation-states were jealous of the Germans merchants' power and wealth. The Reformation tore apart old alliances. Dutch and English traders broke the Hanseatic monopoly. Cities withdrew from the League and Kontors closed. In 1754, Bergen's Kontor was taken over by the Norwegians. When it closed its doors on December 31, 1899, a sea-trading era was over, but the city of Bergen had become rich...by the grace of cod.

with the Vikings and work clockwise): 10th century—Vikings, with a totem pole in the panel above recalling the pre-Columbian Norwegian discovery of America; 18th century—equipping Europe's ships; 19th century—whaling; 20th century—shipping and war. For the 21st century, see the real people—a cross-section of today's Norway—sitting at the statue's base. Major department stores (Galleriet, Xhibition, and Telegrafen) are all nearby.

• *The monument marks the start of Bergen's main square...*

❽ Torgallmenningen

Allmenningen means "for all the people." Torg means "square." And, while this is the city's main gathering place, it was actually created as a firebreak. The residents of this wood-built city knew fires were inevitable. The street plan was designed with breaks, or open spaces like this square, to help contain the destruction. In 1916, it succeeded in stopping a fire, which is why it has a more modern feel today.

Walk the length of the square to the far end marked by an angled slab of blue stone (quarried in Brazil). This is a monument to King Olav V, who died in 1991. This is a popular meeting point: Locals like to say, "Meet you at the Blue Stone." It marks the center of a park-like swath known as...

❾ Ole Bulls Plass

This drag leads from the National Theater (above on right) to a little lake (below on left).

Detour a few steps up for a better look at the **National Theater,** built in Art Nouveau style in 1909. Founded by violinist Ole Bull in 1850, this was the first theater to host plays in the Norwegian language. After 450 years of Danish and Swedish rule, 19th-century Norway enjoyed a cultural awakening, and Bergen became an artistic power. Ole Bull collaborated with the playwright Henrik Ibsen. Ibsen commissioned Edvard Grieg to compose the music for his play *Peer Gynt.* These three lions of Norwegian culture all lived and worked right here in Bergen.

Head downhill on the square to a delightful fountain featuring a **statue of Ole Bull** in the shadow of trees. Ole Bull was an 1800s version of Elvis. A pop idol and heartthrob in his day, Ole Bull's bath water was bottled and sold by hotels, and women fainted when they heard him play violin. Living up to his name, he fathered over 40 children.

From here, the park spills farther downhill to a cast-iron pavilion given to the city by Germans in 1889, and on to the little manmade lake (Lille Lungegårdsvann), which is circled by an enjoyable path. This green zone is considered a park and is cared for by the local parks department.

• *If you're up for a lakeside stroll, now's your chance. Also notice that alongside the lake (to the right as you face it from here) is a row of buildings housing the enjoyable **Kode Art Museums**. And to the left of the lake are some fine residential streets (including the picturesque, cobbled Marken); within a few minutes' walk are the **Leprosy Museum** and the **cathedral**.*

Sights in Bergen

CENTRAL BERGEN

Several museums listed here—including the Bryggens Museum, Håkon's Hall, Rosenkrantz Tower, Leprosy Museum, and Gamle Bergen—are part of the Bergen City Museum (Bymuseet) organization. If you buy a ticket to any of them, you can pay half-price at any of the others simply by showing your ticket.

▲Bergenhus Fortress:
Håkon's Hall and Rosenkrantz Tower

The tower and hall, sitting boldly out of place on the harbor just beyond Bryggen, are reminders of Bergen's importance as the first permanent capital of Norway. Both sights feel vacant and don't really speak for themselves; the included guided tours, which provide a serious introduction to Bergen's history, are essential for grasping their significance.

Cost and Hours: Hall and tower—90 kr for both (or 60 kr each), includes a guided tour; mid-May-Aug—hall open daily 10:00-16:00, tower open daily 9:00-16:00; Sept-mid-May—hall open daily 12:00-15:00, tower open Sun only 12:00-15:00; tel. 55 31 60 67, free WC.

Visiting the Hall and Tower: The hall and the tower are described in my "Bergen Walk," earlier. Consider them as one sight and start with Håkon's Hall (mid-May-Aug tours leave daily from the building to the right of Håkon's Hall at the top of the hour, last one departs at 15:00; few tours off-season). Tours include both buildings.

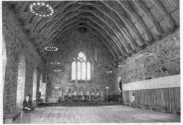

Håkon's Hall, dating from the 13th century, is the largest secular medieval building in Norway. Built as a banqueting hall, that's essentially what it is today. While it's been rebuilt, the ceiling's design is modeled after grand wooden roofs of that era. Beneath the hall is a whitewashed cellar.

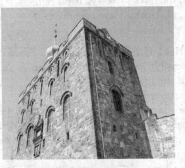

Rosenkrantz Tower, the keep of a 13th-century castle, is today a stack of barren rooms connected by tight spiral staircases, with a good history exhibit on the top two floors and a commanding view from its rooftop. In the 16th century, the ruling Danish-Norwegian king enlarged the tower and trained its cannon on the German-merchant district, Bryggen, to remind the merchants of the importance of paying their taxes.

Fortress Museum (Bergenhus Festningmuseum)

This humble museum (which functioned as a prison during the Nazi occupation), set back a couple of blocks from the fortress, will interest historians with its thoughtful exhibits about military history, especially Bergen's WWII experience (look for the Norwegian Nazi flag). You'll learn about the resistance movement in Bergen (including its underground newspapers), the role of women in the Norwegian military, and Norwegian troops who have served with UN forces in overseas conflicts.

Cost and Hours: Free, daily 11:00-17:00, ask to borrow a translation of the descriptions at the entrance, just behind Thon Hotel Bergen Brygge at Koengen, tel. 55 54 63 87.

▲▲Bryggens Museum

This modern museum explains the 1950s archaeological dig to uncover the earliest bits of Bergen (1050-1500). Brief English explanations are posted. From September through May, when there is no tour, consider buying the good museum guidebook (25 kr).

Cost and Hours: 70 kr; in summer, entry included with Bryggen Walking Tour described earlier; mid-May-Aug daily 10:00-16:00; Sept-mid-May Mon-Fri 11:00-15:00, Sat 12:00-15:00, Sun 12:00-16:00; inexpensive cafeteria; in big, modern building just beyond the end of Bryggen and the Radisson Blu Royal Hotel, tel. 55 58 80 10, www.bymuseet.no.

Visiting the Museum: The manageable, well-presented permanent exhibit occupies the ground floor. First up are the foundations from original wooden tenements dating back to the 12th century (displayed right where they were excavated) and a giant chunk of the hull of a 100-foot-long, 13th-century ship that was found here. Next, an exhibit (roughly shaped like the long, wooden double-tenements outside) shows off artifacts and explains lifestyles from medieval Bryggen. Behind that is a display of items you might have bought at the medieval market. You'll finish with exhibits about the church in Bergen, the town's role as a royal capital, and its status as a cultural capital. Upstairs are two floors of temporary exhibits.

▲▲Hanseatic Museum (Hanseatiske Museum)

This little museum offers the best possible look inside the wooden houses that are Bergen's trademark. Its creaky old rooms—with hundred-year-old cod hanging from the ceiling—offer a time-tunnel experience back to Bryggen's glory days. It's located in an atmospheric old merchant house furnished with dried fish, antique ropes, an old oxtail (used for wringing spilled cod-liver oil back into the bucket), sagging steps, and cupboard beds from the early 1700s—one with a medieval pinup girl. You'll explore two upstairs levels, fully furnished and with funhouse floors. The place still feels eerily lived-in; neatly sorted desks with tidy ledgers seem to be waiting for the next workday to begin.

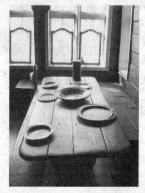

Cost and Hours: 70 kr; entry

included with Bryggen Walking Tour; daily May-Sept 9:00-17:00; Oct-April Tue-Sat 11:00-14:00, Sun 11:00-16:00, closed Mon; Finnegården 7a, tel. 55 54 46 96 or 55 54 46 90, www.museumvest. no.

Tours: There are scant English explanations, but it's much better if you take the good, included 45-minute guided tour (3/day in English—call to confirm, mid-May-mid-Sept only, times displayed just inside door). Even if you tour the museum with the Bryggen Walking Tour, you're welcome to revisit (using the same ticket) and take this longer tour.

Theta Museum

This small museum highlights Norway's resistance movement. You'll peek into the hidden world of a 10-person cell of coura-geous students, whose group—called Theta—housed other fight-ers and communicated with London during the Nazi occupation in World War II. It's housed in Theta's former headquarters—a small upstairs room in a wooden Bryggen building.

Cost and Hours: 30 kr, June-Aug Tue, Sat, and Sun 14:00-16:00, closed Mon, Wed-Fri, and Sept-May, Enhjørningsgården.

▲▲Fløibanen Funicular

Bergen's popular funicular climbs 1,000 feet in seven minutes to the top of Mount Fløyen for the best view of the town, sur-

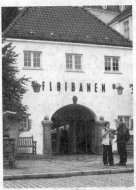

rounding islands, and fjords all the way to the west coast. The top is a popular pic-nic or pizza-to-go spot, perfect for enjoy-ing the sunset (Peppes Pizza is tucked behind the Hanseatic Museum, a block away from the base of the lift). The Fløien Folkerestaurant, at the top of the funicular, offers affordable self-service food all day in season. Behind the station, you'll find a playground and a fun giant troll photo op. The top is also the starting point for many peaceful hikes.

You'll buy your funicular ticket at the base of the Fløibanen (notice the photos in the entry hall of the construction of the funicular and its 1918 grand opening).

If you'll want to hike down from the top, ask for the *Fløyen Hiking Map* when you buy your ticket; you'll save 50 percent by purchasing only a one-way ticket up. From the top, walk behind the station and follow the signs to the city center. The top half of the 30-minute hike is a gravelly lane through a forest with fine views. The bottom is a paved lane through charming old wooden homes. It's a steep descent. To save your knees, you could ride the lift most of the way down and get off at the Promsgate stop to wander through the delightful cobbled and shiplap lanes (note that only the :00 and :30 departures stop at Promsgate).

Cost and Hours: 85 kr round-trip, 43 kr one-way, Mon-Fri 7:30-23:00, Sat-Sun 8:00-23:00, departures 4/hour—on the quarter-hour most of the day, runs continuously if busy, tel. 55 33 68 00, www.floibanen.no.

Cathedral (Domkirke)

Bergen's main church, dedicated to St. Olav (the patron saint of

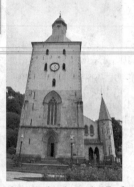

Norway), dates from 1301. Drop in to enjoy its stoic, plain interior with stuccoed stone walls and a giant wooden pulpit. Sit in a hard, straight-backed pew and just try to doze off. Like so many old Norwegian structures, its roof makes you feel like you're huddled under an overturned Viking ship. The church is oddly lopsided, with just one side aisle. Before leaving, look up to see the gorgeous wood-carved organ over the main entrance. In the entryway, you'll see portraits of each bishop dating all the way back to the Reformation.

Cost and Hours: Free; mid-June-mid-Aug Mon-Fri 10:00-16:00, Sun 9:30-13:00, closed Sat; shorter hours off-season.

Leprosy Museum (Lepramuseet)

Leprosy is also known as "Hansen's Disease" because in the 1870s a Bergen man named Armauer Hansen did groundbreaking work

in understanding the ailment. This unique museum is in St. Jørgens Hospital, a leprosarium that dates back to about 1700. Up until the 19th century, as much as 3 percent of Norway's population had leprosy. This hospital—once called "a graveyard for the living" (its last patient died in 1946)—has

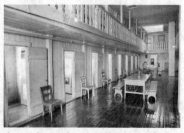

a meager exhibit in a thought-provoking dorm for the dying. It's most worthwhile if you read the translation of the exhibit (borrow a copy at the entry) or take the free tour (at the top of each hour). As you leave, if you're interested, ask if you can see the medicinal herb garden out back.

Cost and Hours: 70 kr, mid-May-Aug daily 11:00-15:00, closed Sept-mid-May, between train station and Bryggen at Kong Oscars Gate 59, tel. 55 96 11 55, www.bymuseet.no.

▲Kode Art Museums of Bergen (Kunstmuseene i Bergen)

If you need to get out of the rain (and you enjoyed the National Gallery in Oslo), check out this collection, filling four neighboring buildings facing the lake along Rasmus Meyers Allé. The Lysverket building has an eclectic cross-section of both international and Norwegian artists. The Rasmus Meyer branch specializes in Norwegian artists and has an especially good Munch exhibit. The Stenersen building has installations of contemporary art, while the Permanenten building has decorative arts. Small description sheets in English are in each room.

Many visitors focus on the **Lysverket** ("Lighthouse"; from outside, enter through Door 4), featuring an easily digestible collection. The ground floor includes an extensive display of works by Nikolai Astrup (1880-1928), who depicts Norway's fjords with bright colors and Expressionistic flair. One flight up is a great collection of J. C. Dahl and his students, who captured the majesty of Norway's natural wonders (look for Adelsteen Normann's impressive, photorealistic view of Romsdalfjord).

Cost and Hours: 100 kr, daily 11:00-17:00, closed Mon mid-Sept-mid-May, Rasmus Meyers Allé 3, tel. 55 56 80 00, www.kunstmuseene.no.

▲Aquarium (Akvariet)

Small but fun, this aquarium claims to be the second-most-visited sight in Bergen. It's wonderfully laid out and explained in English. Check out the view from inside the "shark tunnel" in the tropical shark exhibit.

Cost and Hours: 250 kr, kids-150 kr, daily May-Aug 10:00-18:00, Sept-mid-Oct daily 10:00-16:00, mid-Oct-April Tue-Sun 10:00-16:00, closed Mon, feeding times at the top of most hours in summer, cheery cafeteria with light sandwiches, Nordnesbakken 4, tel. 40 10 24 20, www.akvariet.no.

Getting There: It's at the tip of the peninsula on the south end of the harbor—about a 20-minute walk or short ride on bus #11 from the city center. Or hop on the handy little *Vågen* "Akvariet" ferry that sails from the Fish Market to near the aquarium (50 kr one-way, 80 kr round-trip, 2/hour, June-Aug 10:00-17:30, off-season until 16:00).

Nearby: The lovely park behind the aquarium has views of the sea and a popular swimming beach.

▲Gamle Bergen (Old Bergen)

This Disney-cute gathering of 50-some 18th- through 20th-century homes and shops was founded in 1934 to save old buildings from destruction as Bergen modernized. Each of the buildings was moved from elsewhere in Bergen and reconstructed here. Together, they create a virtual town that offers a cobbled look at the old life. It's free to wander through the town and park to enjoy the facades of the historic buildings, but to get into the 20 or so museum buildings, you'll have to join a tour (departing on the hour 10:00-16:00).

Cost and Hours: Free entry, 80-kr tour (in English) required for access to buildings, mid-May-Aug daily 9:00-16:00, closed Sept-mid-May, tel. 55 39 43 04, www.bymuseet.no.

Getting There: Take any bus heading west from Bryggen (such as #6, direction: Lønborglien) to Gamle Bergen (stop: Nyhavnsveien). You'll get off after the tunnel at a freeway pull-out and walk 200 yards, following signs to the museum. Any bus heading back into town takes you to the center (buses come by every few minutes). With the easy bus connection, there's no reason to taxi.

NEAR BERGEN
▲Ulriken643 Cable Car

It's amazingly easy and quick to zip up six minutes to the 643-meter-high (that's 2,110 feet) summit of Ulriken, the tallest mountain near Bergen. Stepping out of the cable car, you enter a different world, with views stretching to the ocean. A chart clearly shows the many well-marked and easy hikes that fan out over the vast rocky and grassy plateau above the tree line (circular walks of various lengths,

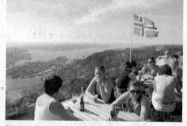

a 40-minute hike down, and a 4-hour hike to the top of the Fløibanen funicular). For less exercise, you can simply sunbathe, crack open a picnic, or enjoy the Ulriken restaurant.

Cost and Hours: 150 kr round-trip, 90 kr one-way, 8/hour, daily 9:00-21:00, off-season 9:00-17:00, tel. 53 64 36 43, www.ulriken643.no.

Getting There: It's about three miles southeast of Bergen. From the Fish Market, you can take a blue double-decker shuttle bus that includes the cost of the cable-car ride (250 kr, ticket valid 24 hours, May-Sept daily 9:00-17:00, 2/hour, departs from the corner of Torgallmenningen and Strandgaten, buy ticket as you board or at TI). Alternatively, the public bus stops 200 yards from the lift station.

▲▲Edvard Grieg's Home, Troldhaugen

Norway's greatest composer spent his last 22 summers here (1885-1907), soaking up inspirational fjord beauty and composing many of his greatest works. Grieg fused simple Norwegian folk

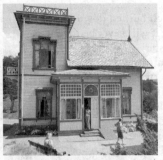

tunes with the bombast of Europe's Romantic style. In a dreamy Victorian setting, Grieg's "Hill of the Trolls" is pleasant for anyone and essential for Grieg fans. You can visit his house on your own, but it's more enjoyable if you take the included 20-minute tour. The house and adjacent museum are full of memories and artifacts, including the composer's Steinway. The walls are festooned with photos of the musical and literary superstars of his generation. When the hugely popular Grieg died in 1907, 40,000 mourners attended his funeral. His little studio hut near the water makes you want to sit down and modulate.

Cost and Hours: 90 kr, includes guided tour in English, daily May-Sept 9:00-18:00, Oct-April 10:00-16:00, café, tel. 55 92 29 92, www.troldhaugen.com.

Grieg Lunch Concert: Troldhaugen offers a great guided tour/concert package that includes a shuttle bus from the Bergen TI to the doorstep of Grieg's home on the fjord (departs 11:30), an hour-long tour of the home, a half-hour concert (Grieg's greatest piano hits, at 13:00), and the ride back into town (you're back in the center by 14:00). Your guide will narrate the ride out of town as well as take you around Grieg's house (250 kr, daily June-mid-Sept). Lunch isn't included, but there is a café on site, or you could bring a sandwich along. While the tour rarely sells out, try to drop by the TI earlier that day to reserve your spot.

Getting to Troldhaugen: It's six miles south of Bergen. The **tram** drops you a long 20-minute walk away from Troldhaugen.

Catch the tram in the city center at its terminus near Byparken (between the lake and Ole Bulls Plass), ride it for about 25 minutes, and get off at the stop called Hop. Walk in the direction of Bergen (about 25 yards), cross at the crosswalk, and follow signs to Troldhaugen.

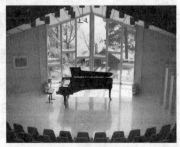

Part of the way is on a pedestrian/bike path; you're halfway there when the path crosses over a busy highway. If you want to make the 13:00 lunchtime concert, leave Bergen at 12:00.

To avoid the long walk from the tram stop, consider the Grieg Lunch Concert package (described earlier).

Fantoft Stave Church

This huge, preserved-in-tar stave church burned down in 1992. It was rebuilt and reopened in 1997, but it will never be the same. Situated in a quiet forest next to a mysterious stone cross, this replica of a 12th-century wooden church is bigger, though no better, than others covered in this book. But it's worth a look if you're in the neighborhood, even after-hours, for its atmospheric setting.

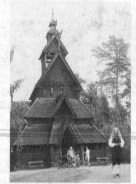

Cost and Hours: 50 kr, mid-May-mid-Sept daily 10:30-18:00, interior closed off-season, no English information, tel. 55 28 07 10, www.fantoftstavkirke.com.

Getting There: It's three miles south of Bergen on E-39 in Paradis. Take the tram (from Byparken, between the lake and Ole Bulls Plass) or bus #83 (from Torget, by the Fish Market) to the Paradis stop (not the "Fantoft" stop). From Paradis, walk uphill to the parking lot on the left, and find the steep footpath to the church.

Shopping in Bergen

Most shops are open Mon-Fri 9:00-17:00, Thu until 19:00, Sat 9:00-15:00, and closed Sunday. Many of the tourist shops at the harborfront strip along Bryggen are open daily—even during holidays—until 20:00 or 21:00.

Ting (Things) offers a fun alternative to troll shopping, with contemporary housewares and quirky gift ideas (daily 10:00-22:30, at Bryggen 13, a block past the Hanseatic Museum, tel. 55 21 54 80).

Husfliden is a shop popular for its handmade goodies and reliably Norwegian sweaters (fine variety and quality but expensive, just off Torget, the market square, at Vågsallmenninge 3, tel. 55 54 47 40).

The Galleriet Mall, a shopping center on Torgallmenningen, holds six floors of shops, cafés, and restaurants. You'll find a pharmacy, photo shops, clothing, sporting goods, bookstores, mobile-phone shops, and a basement grocery store (Mon-Fri 9:00-21:00, Sat 9:00-18:00, closed Sun).

Eating in Bergen

Bergen has numerous choices: restaurants with rustic, woody atmosphere, candlelight, and steep prices (main dishes around 300 kr); trendy pubs and cafés that offer good-value meals (100-190 kr);

cafeterias, chain restaurants, and ethnic eateries with less ambience where you can get quality food at lower prices (100-150 kr); and take-away sandwich shops, bakeries, and cafés for a light bite (50-100 kr).

You can always get a glass or pitcher of water at no charge, and fancy places give you free seconds on potatoes—just ask. Remember, if you get your food to go, it's taxed at a lower rate and you'll save 12 percent.

SPLURGE IN BRYGGEN

You'll pay a premium to eat here, but you'll have a memorable meal in a pleasant setting. If it's beyond your budget, remember that you

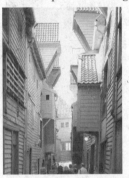

can fill up on potatoes and drink tap water to dine for exactly the price of the plate.

Bryggeloftet & Stuene Restaurant, in a brick building just before the wooden stretch of Bryggen, is a vast eatery serving seafood, vegetarian, and traditional meals. Upstairs feels more elegant and less touristy than the main floor—if there's a line downstairs, just head on up (150-180-kr lunches, 200-350-kr dinners, Mon-Sat 11:00-23:30, Sun 13:00-23:30, try reserving a view window upstairs—no reservations for outside seating, #11 on Bryggen harborfront, tel. 55 30 20 70).

NEAR THE FISH MARKET

Pygmalion Restaurant has a happy salsa vibe, with local art on the walls and a fun, healthy international menu. It's run with creativity and passion by Sissel. Her burgers are a hit, and there are always good vegetarian options, hearty salads, and pancakes (80-kr wraps, 180-kr burgers, 150-200-kr main plates, daily 11:00-22:00, two blocks inland from the Fish Market at Nedre Korskirkealmenning 4, tel. 55 31 32 60).

CHARACTERISTIC PLACES NEAR OLE BULLS PLASS

Bergen's "in" cafés are stylish, cozy, small, and open very late—a great opportunity to experience its yuppie scene. Around the cinema on Neumannsgate, there are numerous ethnic restaurants, including Italian, Middle Eastern, and Chinese.

Pingvinen Pub ("The Penguin") is a homey place in a charming neighborhood, serving traditional Norwegian home cooking to an enthusiastic local clientele. The pub has only indoor seating, with a long row of stools at the bar and five charming, living-room-cozy tables—a great setup for solo diners. For Norwegian fare in a completely untouristy atmosphere, this is a good, affordable

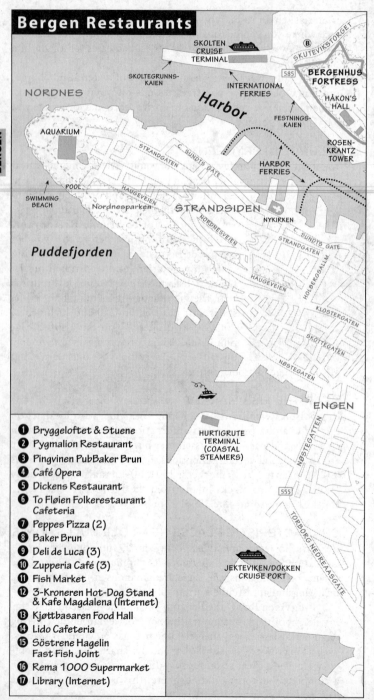

Bergen Restaurants

1. Bryggeloftet & Stuene
2. Pygmalion Restaurant
3. Pingvinen PubBaker Brun
4. Café Opera
5. Dickens Restaurant
6. To Fløien Folkerestaurant Cafeteria
7. Peppes Pizza (2)
8. Baker Brun
9. Deli de Luca (3)
10. Zupperia Café (3)
11. Fish Market
12. 3-Kroneren Hot-Dog Stand & Kafe Magdalena (Internet)
13. Kjøttbasaren Food Hall
14. Lido Cafeteria
15. Söstrene Hagelin Fast Fish Joint
16. Rema 1000 Supermarket
17. Library (Internet)

BERGEN

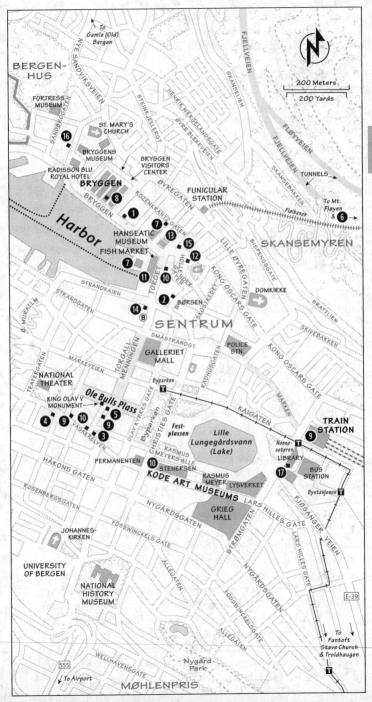

option. Their seasonal menu (reindeer in the fall, whale in the spring) is listed on the board (160-220-kr main dishes, nightly until 22:00, Vaskerelven 14 near the National Theater, tel. 55 60 46 46).

Café Opera, with a playful-slacker vibe and chessboards for the regulars, is the hip budget choice for its loyal, youthful following. With two floors of seating and tables out front across from the theater, it's a winner (light 60-80-kr sandwiches until 16:00, 100-200-kr dinners, daily 10:00-24:00, Engen 18, tel. 55 23 03 15).

Dickens is a lively, checkerboard-tiled, turn-of-the-century-feeling place. The window tables in the atrium are great for people-watching, as is the fine outdoor terrace, but you'll pay higher prices for the view (200-kr lunches, 250-300-kr dinners, daily 11:00-23:00, Kong Olav V's Plass 4, tel. 55 36 31 30).

ATOP MOUNT FLØYEN, AT THE TOP OF THE FUNICULAR

Fløien Folkerestaurant Cafeteria offers meals indoors and out with a panoramic view. It's self-service with sandwiches for around 60 kr and a 139-kr soup buffet (May-Aug daily 10:00-22:00, Sept-April Sat-Sun only 12:00-17:00, tel. 55 33 69 99).

GOOD CHAIN RESTAURANTS

You'll find these chain restaurants in Bergen and throughout Norway. All are open long hours daily. In good weather, enjoy a takeout meal with sun-worshipping locals in Bergen's parks.

Peppes Pizza has cold beer and good pizzas (medium size for 1-2 people-200-220 kr, large for 2-3 people-220-300 kr, takeout possible; consider the Thai Chicken, with satay-marinated chicken, pineapple, peanuts, and coriander). There are six Peppes in Bergen, including one behind the Hanseatic Museum near the Fløibanen funicular station and another inside the Zachariasbryggen harborfront complex, next to the Fish Market (with views over the harbor).

Baker Brun makes 50-70-kr sandwiches, including wonderful shrimp baguettes and pastries such as *skillingsbolle*—cinnamon rolls—warm out of the oven. Their branch in the Bryggen quarter is a prime spot for a simple, inexpensive bite (open from 7:00, seating inside or takeaway).

Deli de Luca is a cut above other takeaway joints, adding sushi, noodle dishes, and calzones to the normal lineup of sandwiches. While a bit more expensive than the others, the variety and quality are appealing (open 24/7, 60-kr sandwiches and calzones, branches in train station and near Ole Bulls Plass at Torggaten 5, branch with indoor seating on corner of Engen and Vaskerelven, tel. 55 23 11 47).

Zupperia is a lively, popular chain that offers burgers, salads, Norwegian fare, and Asian dishes for 75 to 150 kr; their Thai soup is a local favorite. For a lighter meal, order off the lunch menu (120-150 kr) any time of day (daily 12:00-22:00, but Nordahl Bruns location closed Mon). Branches are across from the Fish Market at Market 13, near the National Theater at Vaskerelven 12, and between Ole Bulls Plass and the lake (Nordahl Bruns Gate 9).

BUDGET BETS NEAR THE FISH MARKET

The Fish Market has lots of stalls bursting with salmon sandwiches, fresh shrimp, fish-and-chips, and fish cakes. For a tasty, memorable, and inexpensive Bergen meal, assemble a seafood picnic here (ask for prices first; June-Aug daily 7:00-19:00; Sept-May Mon-Sat 7:00-16:00, closed Sun). Also be sure to peruse the places next door in the ground floor of the TI building, Torghallen.

3-Kroneren, your classic hot-dog stand, sells a wide variety of sausages (various sizes and flavors—including reindeer). The well-described English menu makes it easy to order your choice of artery-clogging guilty pleasures (20-kr tiny weenie, 55-kr medium-size weenie, 75-kr jumbo, open daily from 11:00 until 5:00 in the morning, you'll see the little hot-dog shack a block up Kong Oscars Gate from the harbor, Kenneht is the boss). Each dog comes with a free little glass of fruit punch.

Kjøttbasaren, upstairs in the restored meat market of 1887, is a genteel-feeling food hall with stalls selling groceries such as meat, cheese, bread, and olives, plus *lefse*, reindeer sausage, and goat cheese—a great opportunity to assemble a bang-up picnic (Mon-Fri 10:00-17:00, Thu until 18:00, Sat 9:00-16:00, closed Sun). You can picnic at top or bottom of the Fløibanen funicular, just up the street.

Lido Cafeteria offers basic, affordable food with great harbor and market views, better ambience than most self-service places, and a museum's worth of old-town photos on the walls. For cold items (such as 50-100-kr open-face sandwiches and desserts), grab what you want, pay the cashier, and find a table. For hot dishes (120-170-kr Norwegian standards, including one daily special discounted to 110 kr), get a table, order and pay at the cashier, and they'll bring your food to you (120-kr salad bar, Mon-Fri 10:00-19:00, Sat and Sun 10:00-18:00; second floor at Torgallmenningen 1a, tel. 55 32 59 12).

Söstrene Hagelin Fast Fish Joint is an easygoing eatery that's cheerier than its offerings—a dreary extravaganza of Norway's white cuisine. It's all fish here: fish soup, fish burgers, fish balls, fish cakes, and even fish pudding (meals for around 60 kr, Mon-Sat 10:00-22:00, Sun 12:00-18:00, Kong Oscars Gate 2).

Kafe Magdalena, a humble little community center just two

BERGEN

blocks off the Fish Market, is run by the church and staffed by volunteers. While it's designed to give Bergen's poor citizens an inviting place to enjoy, everyone's welcome (it's a favorite of local guides). There's little choice here; the menu is driven by what's available to the mission cheap (40-kr daily plate, 70 kr for bigger meal served after 13:30, nice cheap open-face sandwiches, waffles, coffee, Mon-Fri 11:00-16:00, closed Sat-Sun, Kong Oscars Gate 5). They have two computer terminals with Internet access and free Wi-Fi.

PICNICS AND GROCERIES

While you'll be tempted to drop into 7-Eleven-type stores, you'll pay for the convenience. Pick up your groceries for half the price at a real supermarket. The **Rema 1000 supermarket,** just across from the Bryggens Museum and St. Mary's Church, is particularly handy (Mon-Fri 7:00-23:00, Sat 8:00-21:00, closed Sun).

NORWEGIAN FJORDS

Norway Practicalities

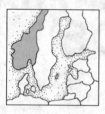

Norway (Norge) is stacked with super-latives—it's the most mountainous, most scenic, and most prosperous of all the Scandinavian countries. Perhaps above all, Norway is a land of intense natural beauty, its famously steep mountains and deep fjords carved out and shaped by an ancient ice age. Norway (148,700 square miles—just larger than Montana) is on the western side of the Scandinavian Peninsula, with most of the country sharing a border with Sweden to the east. Rich in resources like timber, oil, and fish, Norway has rejected joining the European Union, mainly to protect its fishing rights. Where the country extends north of the Arctic Circle, the sun never sets at the height of summer and never comes up in the deep of winter. The majority of Norway's 5 million people consider themselves Lutheran.

Money: 6 Norwegian kroner (kr, officially NOK) = about $1. An ATM is called a *minibank*. The local VAT (value-added sales tax) rate is 25 percent; the minimum purchase eligible for a VAT refund is 315 kr (for details on refunds, see page 134).

Language: The native language is Norwegian (the two official forms are Bokmål and Nynorsk). For useful phrases, see page 708.

Emergencies: Dial 112 for police, medical, or other emergencies. In case of theft or loss, see page 125.

Time Zone: Norway is on Central European Time (the same as most of the Continent, one hour ahead of Great Britain, and six/nine hours ahead of the East/West Coasts of the US).

Embassies in Oslo: The **US embassy** is at Henrik Ibsens Gate 48 (tel. 21 30 85 58, emergency tel. 21 30 85 40, http://norway.usembassy.gov). The **Canadian embassy** is at Wergelandsveien 7 (tel. 22 99 53 00, www.canada.no). Call ahead for passport services.

Phoning: Norway's country code is 47; to call from another country to Norway, dial the international access code (011 from the US/Canada, 00 from Europe, or + from a mobile phone), then 47, followed by the local number. For local calls within Norway, just dial the number as it appears in this book—whether you're calling from across the street or across the country. To place an international call from Norway, dial 00, the code of the country you're calling (1 for US and Canada), and the phone number. For more tips, see page 1146.

Tipping: Service is included in your bill at sit-down meals, but goes to the owner, so for great service it's nice to round up about 10 percent. Tip a taxi driver by rounding up the fare (pay 90 kr on an 85-kr fare). For more tips on tipping, see page 138.

Tourist Information: www.goscandinavia.com

NORWEGIAN FJORDS

Flåm, the Sognefjord, and Norway in a Nutshell • Geirangerfjord

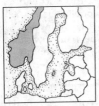

While Oslo and Bergen are fine cities, Norway is first and foremost a place of unforgettable natural beauty—and its greatest claims to scenic fame are its deep, lush fjords. Three million years ago, an ice age made this land as inhabitable as the center of Greenland. As the glaciers advanced and cut their way to the sea, they gouged out long grooves—today's fjords. The entire west coast of the country is slashed by stunning fjords.

Various Norwegian cruise ports offer a taste of fjord scenery

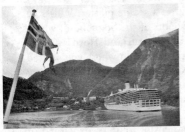

(Oslo, Bergen, and Stavanger are all situated on or near fjords), but many cruises also head for two particularly scenic and accessible fjords unencumbered by big cities: the Sognefjord (at the village of Flåm) and the Geirangerfjord. Flåm is the hub for a well-coordinated web of train, boat, and bus connections—appropriately nicknamed the "Norway in a Nutshell" route—that let you see some of Norway's best scenery efficiently on your own. Geirangerfjord, more remote, works best by excursion. I've covered each of these fjords separately in this chapter.

FLÅM, THE SOGNEFJORD, AND NORWAY IN A NUTSHELL

Among the fjords, the Sognefjord—Norway's longest (120 miles) and deepest (1 mile)—is tops. The seductive Sognefjord has tiny but tough ferries, towering canyons, and isolated farms and

Excursions from Flåm

Cruise lines push their own version of the **Norway in a Nutshell** loop, sometimes billed as "Best of Flåm"; you'll likely take some of the same boats, buses, and trains that are available to the public (though some legs may be chartered). If you're willing and able to figure out the Nutshell on your own (using this chapter's step-by-step tips), you'll save money. But if you'd just prefer to let someone else do the planning, an excursion can be worthwhile.

Other excursion options from Flåm include various individual legs of the Nutshell, such as the **Flåmsbana** mountain train up to Myrdal and back, or a cruise on the **Nærøyfjord.** You may also be offered a **kayak trip** on the Aurlandsfjord (near Flåm). All of these are easy to book on your own. However, a few farther-flung options are more challenging to reach by public transit, and worth considering by excursion: a bus trip to a **mountain farm** (Otternes) or a visit to **Borgund Stave Church** (doable but time-consuming by public bus).

In general, with various options possible on your own, I'd consider an excursion from Flåm only if you want to visit an out-of-the-way destination, or if you simply don't want to hassle with booking your own trip.

villages marinated in the mist of countless waterfalls.

While the port town of Flåm itself has modest charms, a series of well-organized and spectacular bus, train, and ferry connections— together called "Norway in a Nutshell"—lays Norway's beautiful fjord country before you on a scenic platter. With the Nutshell, you'll delve into two offshoots of the Sognefjord, which make an upside-down "U" route: the Aurlandsfjord and the Nærøyfjord. This trip brings you right back to where you started 6.5 hours earlier—after cruising Norway's narrowest fjord, riding a bus along an impossibly twisty and waterfall-lined road, taking the train across the mountainous spine of the country, then dropping back down to sea level on yet another super-scenic train. All connections are conveniently designed for tourists, explained in English, and described in this chapter.

This region enjoys mild weather for its latitude, thanks to the warm Gulf Stream. (When it rains in Bergen, it just drizzles here.) But if the weather is bad—don't fret. I've often arrived to gloomy weather, only to enjoy sporadic splashes of brilliant sunshine all day long.

Recently the popularity of the Nutshell route has skyrocketed among both cruise-ship and land-based travelers. And the 2005 completion of the longest car tunnel in the world (15 miles between Flåm and Lærdal) rerouted the main E-16 road between

Bergen and Oslo through this idyllic fjord corner. All of this means that July and August come with a crush of crowds, dampening some of the area's magic. Unfortunately, many tourists are overcome by Nutshell tunnel-vision, and spend so much energy scurrying between boats, trains, and buses that they forget to simply enjoy the fjords. Relax—you're on vacation.

PLANNING YOUR TIME

There's very little to do in Flåm itself. If you're here for a full day, splurge and do the Nutshell loop (unless you're on a tight budget or your cruise schedule doesn't allow it, in which case you can still do one or two of the segments). Here are your options:

• **Norway in a Nutshell Round-Trip:** Outlined step-by-step in this chapter, this ultimate boat, bus, and train journey takes 6.5 hours.

• **"Poor Man's Nutshell":** If your schedule doesn't allow the full Nutshell, you could cobble together its two best parts (connected by a 20- to 25-minute bus ride): the two-hour Nærøyfjord cruise and the 2.5-hour round-trip on the Flåmsbana. This one-two punch lets you see the best of the Nutshell.

• **Flåmsbana Mountain Train Only:** From Flåm, you can take a round-trip on the Flåmsbana train steeply into the mountains, then back down into the valley. Allow an hour each way on the train, plus time at the top station, Myrdal (not much to see—basically killing time before the return train). Warning: Morning trains sell out quickly, particularly when multiple cruise ships are in town; to book a morning ticket, order online in advance or get off your ship as quickly as possible and make a beeline to the train ticket office.

• **Nærøyfjord Cruise Only:** While the first half of the Flåm-Gudvangen cruise is redundant with your cruise ship's sail-away, the second half takes you to a fjord too skinny for big ships: the Nærøyfjord. From Gudvangen, you can zip back to Flåm on the bus (20-25 minutes), or cruise all the way back (2.25 hours). Allow about three hours round-trip if returning by bus, or about five hours round-trip if cruising both ways.

• **Flåm:** If you have time to kill in Flåm, you'll find there's little to do other than shopping or dipping into the Railway Museum. Consider renting a boat for a ride on the fjord, taking one of the high-speed boat tours with FjordSafari, or going for a hike in the local area (the TI hands out a map suggesting local walks).

• **Borgund Stave Church:** One of Norway's finest stave churches sits 35 miles from Flåm. While visiting the church itself takes an hour or so, the whole excursion by public bus from Flåm takes around four hours round-trip (and there's only one possible connection per day—see page 771). That's a long way to go just to

Services near the Port

Though it's a small town, Flåm has much of what you need. Most of Flåm's services are in a modern cluster of buildings in and around the train station, including the TI, train ticket desk, public WC, cafeteria, an ATM, and souvenir shops.

Grocery Store: The Co-op grocery, near the cruise dock, has a basic pharmacy and post office inside (Mon-Sat 9:00-20:00, shorter hours off-season, closed Sun year-round).

Pharmacy: There's no real pharmacy in Flåm, but you will find some basics in the **Co-op** grocery store (noted above). The nearest pharmacy is in **Lærdal** (just east, through the world's longest tunnel); if you're doing the Nutshell route, note that there's a pharmacy in **Voss** (Vitus Apotek, a 5-minute walk into town from the train station and a few doors down from the TI, facing the town church at Vangsgatan 22D, Mon-Fri 8:30-17:00, Sat 9:00-15:00, closed Sun).

Car Rental: There's only one rental car in Flåm, and you'll find it at Heimly Pensjonat just around the harbor (tel. 57 63 23 00, www.heimly.no, post@heimly.no).

see a church—but it's one of the best examples anywhere of this uniquely Norwegian church architecture (and includes a museum).

• **Outlying Sights:** Several intriguing sights lie outside of Flåm, not easily reachable by public transportation. These include Otternes Farms and other fjordside villages (such as Undredal). While it's possible to reach these by renting a car, a better option is likely the package tours offered by Sognefjorden Sightseeing & Tours (described on page 770).

In this destination (even more than others), it really pays to do some homework and decide what you want to do before you step off the ship. Smart travelers will buy the Nutshell package or the Flåmsbana mountain train tickets in advance (described later under "Orientation to the Nutshell"). Otherwise, line up early to be one of the first ashore (especially if tendering)—you won't regret it, as those few extra minutes might help you beat the crowds to the TI and train ticket office. Both offices open at 8:15 (though the line forms earlier); the first Flåmsbana train departs at 8:35; the first fjord cruise leaves at 9:00. That leaves you a fairly narrow window to make your plans. Double- and triple-check connections with posted schedules, the TI, the train station ticket-sellers, and so on. Connections are generally coordinated to work efficiently together, and the people you'll meet along the way are typically patient about explaining things to nervous tourists.

The Port of Flåm

Arrival at a Glance: It's simple: From your ship or tender, it's a very short stroll to the train station and boat dock. The key is doing your homework and getting an early start.

Port Overview

Little Flåm has space for one big cruise ship to **dock** at its pier; stepping off your ship, you'll turn left, go through the port gate, and walk between the water and a row of shops to reach the train station area.

Entering the train station through the door facing the pier, you'll find the TI on your right and the train ticket office on your left. If you're doing the whole Nutshell, go to the TI first and buy their package. If you're doing only the Flåmsbana train—or want to piece together your own Nutshell route—go to the train ticket office to get your Flåmsbana ticket (and, while you're at it, reserve a seat on the Voss-Myrdal train trip). The electronic board above the ticket office notes which, if any, of today's Flåm-Myrdal train departures are sold out. Farther into the station are the Sognefjorden Sightseeing & Tours office, a gift shop, and a cafeteria.

If multiple ships are in town, some will anchor in the harbor and **tender** passengers to the pier right in front of the train station.

Tourist Information: Flåm's TI is inside its train station—just look for the green-and-white *i* sign.

Strategies: Remember, time is of the essence here. If you want to venture beyond Flåm, disembark as quickly as possible and head for the TI to sort through your options and buy tickets.

RETURNING TO YOUR SHIP

It's easy—you can see your ship from anywhere in Flåm. But just in case, see page 782 for help if you miss your boat.

Flåm

Flåm (pronounced "flome")—at the head of the Aurlandsfjord—feels more like a transit junction than a village. But its striking setting, easy transportation connections, and touristy bustle make it a popular springboard for exploring the nearby area.

Orientation to Flåm

The train station has most of the town services (see sidebar). The boat dock for fjord cruises is just beyond the end of the tracks. Surrounding the station are a Co-op grocery and a smattering of hotels, travel agencies, and touristy restaurants. Aside from a few scattered farmhouses and some homes lining the road, there's not much of a town here. (The extremely sleepy old town center—where tourists rarely venture, and which you'll pass on the Flåmsbana train—is a few miles up the river, in the valley.)

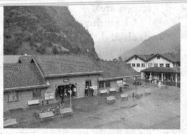

TOURIST INFORMATION

At the TI inside the train station, you can purchase your boat tickets—or the entire Nutshell package—and load up on handy brochures (daily May and late Sept 8:15-16:00, June-mid-Sept 8:15-20:00, closed Oct-April, tel. 57 63 21 06, www.visitflam.com or www.alr.no). The TI hands out a variety of useful items: an excellent flyer with a good map and up-to-date schedules for public transit options; a diagram of the train-station area, identifying services available in each building; and a map of Flåm and the surrounding area, marked with suggested walks and hikes, starting from right in town. Answers to most of your questions can be found posted on the walls and from staff at the counter. Bus schedules, boat and train timetables, maps, and more are photocopied and available for your convenience.

Sights in and near Flåm

ALONG THE WATERFRONT

Flåm's village activities are all along or near the pier.

The **Flåm Railway Museum** (Flåmsbana Museet), sprawling through the long old train station alongside the tracks, has surprisingly good exhibits about the history of the train that connects

Flåm to the main line up above. You'll find good English explanations, artifacts, re-creations of historic interiors (such as a humble schoolhouse), and an old train car. It's the only real museum in town and a good place to kill time while waiting for your boat or train (free, daily 9:00-17:00, until 20:00 in summer).

A pointless and overpriced **tourist train** does a 45-minute loop around Flåm (95 kr).

The pleasantly woody **Ægir Bryggeri,** a microbrewery designed to resemble an old Viking longhouse, offers tastes of its five beers (135 kr).

Consider renting a boat to go out on the peaceful waters of the fjord. You can paddle near the walls of the fjord and really get a sense of the immensity of these mountains. You can rent rowboats, motorboats, and paddleboats at the little marina across the harbor. If you'd rather have a kayak, **Njord** does kayak tours, but won't rent you one unless you're certified (tel. 91 32 66 28, www.njord.as).

But the main reason people come to Flåm is to leave it—see some options next.

OUTSIDE FLÅM

With a day in Flåm, the best choice is the Norway in a Nutshell trip, described on page 774. Otherwise any of the following are possible—and reachable, to an extent, by public transit. But, as many options are time-consuming, you'll need to be selective.

▲▲Flåmsbana Mountain Railway

This historic rail line picturesquely links fjordside Flåm with mountaintop Myrdal. It can be done either round-trip, or one-way as part of the Norway in a Nutshell trip. Note: Because this is such an easy and fast way to reach grand views from Flåm, many of your fellow passengers head straight for the Flåmsbana mountain train. If you can wait to do it later in the day, you'll enjoy fewer crowds. But you should still buy your tickets as early as possible, as even the later trains can sell out on busy days. For details on the train, see page 776.

▲▲▲Cruising Nærøyfjord

The most scenic fjord I've seen anywhere in Norway is about an hour from Flåm (basically the last half of the 2-hour Flåm-Gudvangen trip). Your cruise ship passes the mouth of the Nærøyfjord, but for a closer look, you can take the **Fjord 1 ferry,** described on page 778 as part of the Norway in a Nutshell trip (4.5-hour round-trips departing Flåm in peak season at 9:00, 11:00, and 13:20, 400 kr; faster to return from Gudvangen to Flåm by 25-minute bus; for details on both options, see page 778).

Or you can consider two other Flåm-based options:

Sognefjorden Sightseeing & Tours: This private company runs trips from Flåm to Gudvangen and back to Flåm, using their own boats and buses (rather than the public ones on the "official" Nutshell route). If the Nutshell departures don't work for you, consider these trips as an alternative. Their main offering, the World Heritage Cruise, is a boat trip up the Nærøyfjord with a return by bus (365 kr, 3 hours, multiple departures daily mid-May–mid-Sept). They also do a variation on this trip with a 45-minute stop in the village of Undredal for lunch and a goat-cheese tasting (495 kr, June–Aug only); a bus trip up to the Stalheim Hotel for the view (290 kr, or combined with return from Gudvangen by boat for 510 kr); a bus ride up to the thrilling Stegastein viewpoint (a concrete-and-wood viewing pier sticking out from a mountainside high above Aurland, 190 kr, mid-May–mid-Sept); and more. For details, drop by their office inside the Flåm train station, call 57 66 00 55, or visit www.visitflam.com/sognefjorden.

▲▲**FjordSafari to Nærøyfjord**: FjordSafari takes little groups out onto the fjord in small, open Zodiac-type boats with an English-speaking guide. Participants wear full-body weather suits, furry hats, and spacey goggles (making everyone on the boat look like crash-test dummies). As the boat rockets across the water, you'll be thankful for the gear, no matter what the weather. Their two-hour Flåm-Gudvangen-Flåm tour focuses on the Nærøyfjord, and gets you all the fjord magnificence you can imagine (610 kr). Their three-hour tour is the same as the two-hour tour, except that it includes a stop in Undredal, where you can see goat cheese being made, taste the finished product, and wander that sleepy village (720 kr, several departures daily June–Aug, fewer off-season, kids get discounts, tel. 99 09 08 60, www.fjordsafari.no, Maylene). Their 1.5-hour "mini" tour costs 510 kr and just barely touches on the Nærøyfjord...so what's the point?

▲Flåm Valley Bike Ride or Hike

For the best single-day, non-fjord activity from Flåm, take the Flåmsbana train to Myrdal, then hike or mountain-bike along the road (half gravel, half paved) back down to Flåm (2-3 hours by bike, gorgeous waterfalls, great mountain scenery, and a cute church with an evocative graveyard, but no fjord views).

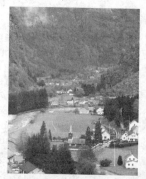

Walkers can just hike the best two hours from Myrdal to Blomheller, and catch the train from there into the valley. Or, without riding the train, you can simply walk up the valley 2.5 miles to the church and a little farther to a waterfall.

Whenever you get tired hiking up or down the valley, you can hop on the next train. Pick up the helpful map with this and other hiking options (ranging from easy to strenuous) at the Flåm TI.

Cyclists can rent good mountain bikes from the bike-rental cabin next to the Flåm train station (daily June-Sept 8:00-20:00, 50 kr/hour, 250 kr/day, includes helmet). It costs 100 kr to take a bike to Myrdal on the train.

▲▲Otternes Farms

This humble but magical cluster of four centuries-old farms is about three miles from Flåm (easy for drivers; a decent walk or bike

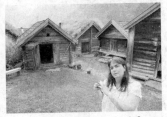

ride otherwise). It's perched high on a ridge, up a twisty gravel road midway between Flåm and the tiny town of Aurland. Laila Kvellestad runs this low-key sight, valiantly working to save and share traditional life as it was back when butter was the farmers' gold. (That was before emigration decimated the workforce, coinage replaced barter, and industrialized margarine became more popular than butter—all of which left farmers to eke out a living relying only on their goats and the cheese they produce.) Until 1919 the only road between Aurland and Flåm passed between this huddle of 27 buildings, high above the fjord. First settled in 1522, farmers lived here until the 1990s. Laila gives 45-minute English tours through several time-warp houses and barns at 10:00, 12:00, 14:00, and 16:00 (50-kr entry plus 30 kr for guided tour, June-mid-Sept daily 10:00-17:00, tel. 48 12 51 38, www.otternes.no). It's wise to call first to confirm tour times and that it's open. For an additional 70 kr, Laila serves a traditional snack of pancakes and coffee or tea with your tour. Or, book in advance for a 175-kr full lunch featuring locally sourced specialties such as *rømmegrøt* (porridge) and meatballs.

▲▲Borgund Stave Church

About 16 miles east of Lærdal, in the village of Borgund, is Norway's most-visited and one of its best-preserved stave churches. Borgund's church comes with one of this country's best stave-church history museums, which beautifully explains these icons of medieval Norway.

Cost and Hours: 75 kr, buy tickets in museum across street, daily June-Aug 8:00-20:00, May and Sept 10:00-17:00, closed Oct-April. The museum has a shop and a fine little cafeteria serving filling and tasty lunches (70-kr soup with bread, tel. 57 66 81 09, www.stavechurch.com).

Getting There: A bus departs Flåm around midday

(direction: Lillehammer) and heads for the church, with a return bus departing Borgund in midafternoon (170-kr round-trip, get ticket from driver, about 1.5 hours each way with about 1 hour at the church, bus runs daily May-Sept, tell driver you want to get off at the church).

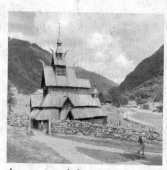

Visiting the Church: Dating from around 1180, the interior features only a few later additions, including a 16th-century pulpit, 17th-century stone altar, painted decorations, and crossbeam reinforcements.

The oldest and most authentic item in the church is the stone baptismal font. In medieval times, priests conducting baptisms would go outside to shoo away the evil spirits from an infant before bringing it inside the church for the ritual. (If infants died before being baptized, they couldn't be buried in the churchyard, so parents would put their bodies in little coffins and hide them under the church's floorboards to get them as close as possible to God.)

Explore the dimly lit interior, illuminated only by the original, small, circular windows up high. Notice the X-shaped crosses of St. Andrew (the church's patron), carvings of dragons, and medieval runes.

Eating in Flåm

Dining options are expensive and touristy. Don't aim for high cuisine here—go practical. Almost all eateries are clustered near the train station. Hours can be unpredictable, flexing with the season, but you can expect these to be open daily in high season.

The **Flåmsbrygga** complex, sprawling through a long building toward the fjord from the station, includes a hotel, the affordable **Furukroa Caféteria** (daily 8:00-20:00 in season, cafeteria with 50-65-kr cold sandwiches, 100-150-kr fast-food meals, and 200-225-kr pizzas), and the pricey **Flåmstova Restaurant** (235-kr lunch buffet, 325-kr dinner buffet, plus other menu options at dinner). Next door is their fun, Viking-longhouse-shaped brewpub, **Ægir Bryggeri** (daily 17:00-22:00, local microbrews, 200-300-kr Viking-inspired meals). **Toget Café,** with seating in old train cars, prides itself on using as many locally sourced and organic ingredients as possible (65-75-kr sandwiches, 160-195-kr main dishes). **Bakkastova Kafe,** at the other end of town, feels cozier; it's in a traditional Norwegian red cabin just above the Fretheim Hotel, with a view terrace, and serves sandwiches, salads, and authentic Norwegian fare (daily 10:00-18:00).

The Facts on Fjords

The process that created the majestic Sognefjord began during an ice age about three million years ago. A glacier up to 6,500 feet thick slid downhill at an inch an hour, following a former river valley on its way to the sea. Rocks embedded in the glacier gouged out a steep, U-shaped valley, displacing enough rock material to form a mountain 13 miles high. When the climate warmed up, the ice age came to an end. The melting glaciers retreated and the sea level rose nearly 300 feet, flooding the valley now known as the Sognefjord. The fjord is more than a mile deep, flanked by 3,000-foot mountains—for a total relief of 9,300 feet. Waterfalls spill down the cliffs, fed by runoff from today's glaciers. Powdery sediment tinges the fjords a cloudy green, the distinct color of glacier melt.

Why are there fjords on the west coast of Norway, but not, for instance, on the east coast of Sweden? The creation

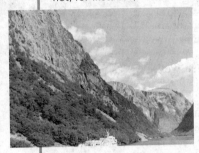

of a fjord requires a setting of coastal mountains, a good source of moisture, and a climate cold enough for glaciers to form and advance. Due to the earth's rotation, the prevailing winds in higher latitudes blow from west to east, so chances of glaciation are ideal where there is an ocean to the west of land with coastal mountains. When the winds blow east over the water, they pick up a lot of moisture, then bump up against the coastal mountain range, and dump their moisture in the form of snow—which feeds the glaciers that carve valleys down to the sea.

You can find fjords along the northwest coast of Europe—including western Norway and Sweden, Denmark's Faroe Islands, Scotland's Shetland Islands, Iceland, and Greenland; the northwest coast of North America (from Puget Sound in Washington state north to Alaska); the southwest coast of South America (Chile); the west coast of New Zealand's South Island; and on the continent of Antarctica.

As you travel through Scandinavia, bear in mind that, while we English-speakers use the word "fjord" to mean only glacier-cut inlets, Scandinavians often use it in a more general sense to include bays, lakes, and lagoons that weren't formed by glacial action.

Norway in a Nutshell

The most exciting single-day trip you could make from Flåm is this circular boat/bus/train jaunt through fjord country.

Orientation to the Nutshell

From Flåm, the basic idea is this: Begin with a cruise on two arms of the Sognefjord, ride a bus up from the fjord to join Norway's main train line, and ride that train to catch a different train steeply back down to Flåm and the fjord. Each of these steps is explained in the self-guided tour, later. Transportation along the Nutshell route is carefully coordinated. If any segment of your journey is delayed, the transportation for the next segment will wait for you (because everyone on board is catching the same connection).

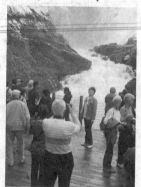

Information: Local TIs are well-informed about your options, and sell tickets for various segments of the trip. At TIs and train stations, look for souvenir-worthy brochures with photos, descriptions, and exact times. However, the suggested "day plan" schedules the TI hands out don't necessarily include *all* options. (For example, on my last visit, their suggested Nutshell day would have made me spend nearly two hours in dull Voss; I figured out a connection cutting that layover in half, and getting me back to Flåm with two hours to spare before my ship's departure.)

Timing: In the summer (late June-late Aug), the connections are most convenient, the weather is most likely to be good... and the route is at its most crowded. Outside of this time, sights close and schedules become more challenging. It's easy to confirm schedules, connections, and prices locally or online (www.ruteinfo.net).

Eating: Options along the route aren't great—on the Nutshell I'd consider food just as a source of nutrition and forget about fine dining. You can buy some food on the fjord cruises (50-75-kr hot dogs, burgers, and pizza) and the express train line (50-100-kr hot meals, 150-kr daily specials). Depending on the timing of your layovers, Myrdal, Voss, or Flåm are your best lunch-stop options (the Myrdal and Flåm train stations have decent cafeterias, and other eateries surround the Flåm and Voss stations)—although you won't have a lot of time there if you're making the journey all in one day. Your best bet is to pack picnic meals and munch en

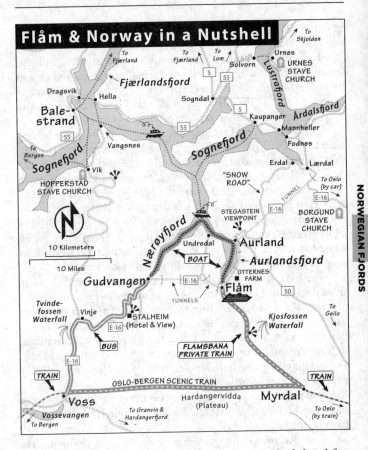

Flåm & Norway in a Nutshell

To Skjolden

To Fjærland
To Fjærland
To Lom
Urnes
Solvorn
URNES STAVE CHURCH

Fjærlandsfjord

Dragsvik
Hella
Sogndal

Bale-strand
Kaupanger
Ärdalsfjord
Mannheller
Fodnes

Vangsnes
Sognefjord
Sognefjord
Erdal
Lærdal

To Bergen
Sognefjord
Vik
To Oslo (by car)

HOPPERSTAD STAVE CHURCH
"SNOW ROAD"
TUNNEL
E-16
BORGUND STAVE CHURCH

N
STEGASTEIN VIEWPOINT

10 Kilometers
Nærøyfjord
Undredal
Aurland

10 Miles
Aurlandsfjord

BOAT
OTTERNES FARM
Gudvangen
E-16
Flåm
50

TUNNELS
To Geilo

Tvinde-fossen Waterfall
Vinje
STALHEIM (Hotel & View)
Kjosfossen Waterfall

BUS
E-16
FLAMSBANA PRIVATE TRAIN

TRAIN
E-16
OSLO-BERGEN SCENIC TRAIN
TRAIN

Voss
Hardangervidda (Plateau)
Myrdal

Vossevangen
To Granvin & Hardangerfjord
To Oslo (by train)
To Bergen

route. Or consider discreetly raiding your cruise ship's breakfast buffet. (As this is frowned upon, don't tell them I suggested it.)

With a Package Deal or On Your Own?: You can either buy the Nutshell loop as a package deal, or you can buy tickets for each leg individually. As the cost is nearly the same, the main reason to buy tickets on your own is if you're a student or a senior (and therefore eligible for discounts). Or, if the suggested route doesn't work for your itinerary, you can consider mixing and matching schedules to come up with a better plan.

Package Deal: To do the Nutshell as a round-trip loop from Flåm, you'll pay 840 kr, which covers all of the tickets and reservations you need. Sold by Fjord Tours (tel. 81 56 82 22, www.fjordtours.no), the Nutshell package can be purchased in advance. It's possible to get tickets at the TI in Flåm—but advance booking allows you to avoid the crowds waiting for the TI to open the morning of your arrival. If your cruise visits Bergen or Oslo before landing in Flåm, you can purchase the package at the train station in either city. To follow my recommended route, ask for a round-trip from Flåm "starting by fjord-cruise boat."

Individual Tickets: If you're booking tickets individually, be aware that certain legs can sell out during busy times and should be booked online in advance: the Voss-Myrdal train (intercity express only) and the Flåmsbana (Myrdal-Flåm) mountain train. You can book both online at www.nsb.no.

The **Voss-Myrdal train** is one segment of Norway's busiest train line, stretching from Bergen to Oslo. Intercity express trains that go this entire distance often sell out, especially in July and August. However, the schedule I recommend uses a local train that doesn't continue all the way to Oslo—it rarely sells out and can't even be booked online. First determine whether you're taking an intercity train (*fjerntog*, all the way from Bergen to Oslo) or a local train (*lokaltog*, runs only in this region). Then, if you are on an intercity train, reserve the Voss-Myrdal segment in advance, as soon as your itinerary is set—ideally at least a week ahead.

The **Flåmsbana train** departures are greatly affected by cruise ships docked in Flåm. Morning departures from Flåm to Myrdal can sell out, and late-morning or early-afternoon trains from Myrdal back to Flåm can be jammed. At other times, you can just buy your ticket on the spot at either the Myrdal or Flåm stations, or from the conductor on the train (same price). If you plan to wait and purchase it at the train station in Flåm, go there immediately when you get off your ship.

You can purchase your **fjord-cruise** ticket on the boat or from the TI in Flåm, and buy tickets for the **Gudvangen bus** on board from the driver.

Last Resort: If one or more of the needed segments are booked up, hope is not lost. If you buy your Nutshell package from the TI, they may have access to segments that are already sold out for those booking individually. And, in a pinch, the Sognefjorden Sightseeing & Tours company has trips that don't use the official Nutshell vehicles. In some cases you can ride their private boat one-way for the same price as the official Nutshell boat—potentially even at a time more convenient to your schedule than the official options. Carefully quiz the TI about this as you're sorting through your options.

DOING THE NUTSHELL ON YOUR OWN

While your cruise line may push overpriced package deals for doing the Nutshell loop, a savvy cruiser can do exactly the same thing on their own for a fraction of the price. However, to do it smoothly, you'll need to do a little homework (plan out your day ahead of time), get an early start, and stay organized. Once under way, you'll have a blast.

Nutshell Worksheet

Use this worksheet for making the most of your time in port. Fill in the times based on schedules for the current year; even if the TI and train ticket office are closed when you arrive (both open at 8:15), use the schedules posted outside to sort this out, so you know what to ask for once you get in:

Nutshell Leg	Depart	Arrive
Your ship arrives in Flåm	N/A	_____
Boat from Flåm to Gudvangen	_____	_____
Bus from Gudvangen to Voss	_____	_____
Train from Voss to Myrdal	_____	_____
Flåmsbana train from Myrdal to Flåm	_____	_____
All aboard in Flåm	_____	N/A

Whether you can do the entire Norway in a Nutshell route if arriving by cruise ship depends on what time your ship arrives and departs. Also, be aware that if more than one ship comes to Flåm in a day, some passengers will have to tender ashore—potentially pushing back your landfall substantially.

Nutshell Schedule

It's smart to buy the Nutshell package in advance. But if you haven't, head directly to the TI (inside the train station—see directions on page 767, opens at 8:15) to confirm your plans and buy your package, before any of the segments sell out. If all goes well, you may even have a few minutes to kill in Flåm before you hop on your fjord-cruise boat.

Here's a suggested schedule for a cruiser who arrives in Flåm at 8:00 (or earlier) and departs at 17:00 (or later). These times are based on 2014 peak-season schedules; it's crucial to reconfirm that this plan will work for your schedule.

Nutshell Leg	Depart	Arrive
Boat from Flåm to Gudvangen	9:00	11:25
Bus from Gudvangen up to Voss	11:40	12:55
Train from Voss to Myrdal	13:10	14:00
Flåmsbana train from Myrdal to Flåm	14:40	15:40

Self-Guided Tour of the Nutshell Loop

If you're doing the full loop on your own, here are step-by-step instructions.

▲▲▲Flåm-Gudvangen Fjord Cruise

From **Flåm,** scenic sightseeing boats ply the fjord's waters around the corner to **Gudvangen.** With minimal English narration, the boat takes you close to the goats, sheep, waterfalls, and awesome cliffs.

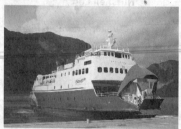

There are two boat companies to choose from: Fjord 1—the boat included in the Nutshell package—and Sognefjorden—a private company. Between them, there are departures about hourly from Flåm to Gudvangen. Beware: The first ticket desk you hit in Flåm's visitors center is the Sognefjorden boat desk, and they'll sell you a boat ticket implying it's your only option.

Fjord 1 is the public ferry with cars and lots of open space. The Sognefjorden boat (same price, route, and journey time) is more of a sightseeing boat rather than a public car and post boat—but it's mostly closed in.

I much prefer the Fjord 1 boat because I like to be in the open air, I enjoy hanging out on the car deck, and the Gudvangen-Voss Nutshell bus connection in Gudvangen is immediate and reliable.

You'll cruise up the lovely **Aurlandsfjord,** motoring by the town of **Aurland,** pass the town of **Undredal,** and hang a left at the stunning **Nærøyfjord.** The cruise ends at the apex of the Nærøyfjord, in **Gudvangen.**

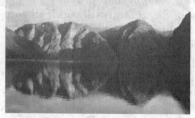

The trip is breathtaking in any weather. For the last hour, as you sail down the Nærøyfjord, camera-clicking tourists scurry around struggling to get a photo that will catch the magic. Waterfalls turn the black cliffs into bridal veils, and you can nearly reach out and touch the cliffs of the Nærøyfjord. It's the world's narrowest fjord: six miles long and as little as 820 feet wide and 40 feet deep. On a sunny day, the ride is one of those fine times—like when you're high on the tip of an Alp—when a warm camaraderie spontaneously combusts between the strangers who've come together for the experience.

Cost: For the whole route (Flåm-Gudvangen), you'll pay 300 kr one-way (150 kr for students with ISIC cards; 450 kr round-trip).

Schedule: In summer (May-Sept), boats run four to five times each day in both directions. Specific departure times can vary, but generally boats leave Flåm at 9:00, 13:20, 15:10, and 18:00 (with an additional 11:00 departure from late June to late August) and leave Gudvangen at 10:30, 11:45, 15:45, and 17:40 (with an additional 13:30 departure from late June to late August). Frequency drops off-season. The trip takes about two hours and 15 minutes. Your only concern is that the Nutshell bus may not meet the last departure of day (check locally); the worst-case scenario is that you'd need to catch the regular commuter bus to Voss, which makes more stops and doesn't take the razzle-dazzle Stalheimskleiva corkscrew road.

Reservations: Don't bother. Just buy your ticket in Flåm as soon as you know which boat you want.

Other Ways to Cruise Nærøyfjord: Consider a thrilling ride on a little inflatable FjordSafari speedboat (described under "Outside of Flåm"; see page 770).

Returning from Gudvangen to Flåm: To head from Gudvangen directly back to Flåm, you can ride a bus that cuts through a tunnel to get there in substantially less time than the two-hour return boat (about 25 minutes, 50-65 kr). Some buses depart from right in front of the boat dock, with others leaving from a stop out on the main E-16 highway (an easy 5-minute walk from the boat—just walk straight ahead off the boat and up the town's lone road, past its few houses, until you reach the big cross street; the bus stop is just across this road). While the specific schedule is often in flux, a bus always leaves soon after each boat arrives from Flåm—just ask around for where to catch it.

▲Gudvangen-Voss Bus

Nutshellers get off the boat at Gudvangen and take the 25-mile bus ride to Voss. Gudvangen is little more than a boat dock and giant tourist kiosk. If you want, you can browse through the grass-roofed souvenir stores and walk onto a wooden footbridge—then catch your bus. Buses meet each ferry, or will show up soon. While some buses—designed for commuters rather than sightseers—take the direct route to Voss, buses tied to the Nutshell schedule take a super-scenic detour via Stalheim (described below). If you're a waterfall junkie, sit on the left.

First the bus takes you up the **Nærøydal** and through a couple of long tunnels. Then you'll take a turnoff to drive past the landmark **Stalheim Hotel** for the first of many spectacular views back into fjord country. Though the hotel dates from 1885, there's been an inn here since about 1700, where the royal mailmen would change horses. The hotel is geared for tour groups (genuine trolls sew the pewter buttons on the sweaters), but the priceless view from the backyard is free.

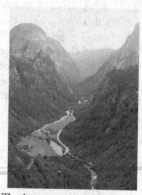

Leaving the hotel, the bus wends its way down a road called **Stalheimskleiva,** with a corkscrew series of switchbacks flanked by a pair of dramatic waterfalls. With its 18 percent grade, it's the steepest road in Norway.

After winding your way down into the valley, you're back on the same highway. The bus goes through those same tunnels again, then continues straight on the main road through pastoral countryside to Voss. You'll pass a huge lake, then follow a crystal-clear, surging river. Just before Voss, look to the right for the wide **Tvindefossen waterfall,** tumbling down its terraced cliff.

Cost: 100 kr, pay on board.

Reservations: Not necessary.

Voss

The Nutshell bus from Gudvangen drops you at the Voss train station. A plain town in a lovely lake-and-mountain setting, Voss lacks the striking fjordside scenery of Flåm, Aurland, or Undredal,

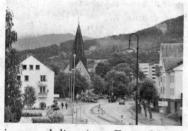

and is basically a home base for summer or winter sports (Norway's Winter Olympics teams often practice here). Voss surrounds its fine, 13th-century church with workaday streets—busy with both local shops and souvenir stores—stretching in several directions. Fans of American football may want to see the humble monument to player and coach Knute Rockne, who was born in Voss in 1888; look for the metal memorial plaque on a rock near the train station.

Voss' helpful **TI** is a five-minute walk from the train station—just head toward the church (June-Aug daily 8:00-19:00; Sept-May Mon-Sat 8:30-17:00, closed Sun; facing the church in the center of town at Vangsgatan 20, mobile 40 61 77 00, www.visitvoss.no).

▲Voss-Myrdal Train

Although this train line stretches super-scenically all the way from Oslo to Bergen, you'll only do a brief, 40-minute segment right in the middle. Even on this short stretch, you'll see deep woods and lakes, as well as barren, windswept heaths and glaciers.

The tracks were begun in 1894 to link Stockholm and Bergen, but Norway won its independence from Sweden in 1905, so the line served to link the two main cities in the new country—Oslo and Bergen. The entire railway, an amazing engineering feat completed in 1909, is 300 miles long; peaks at 4,266 feet, which, at this Alaskan latitude, is far above the tree line; goes under 18 miles of snow sheds; trundles over 300 bridges; and passes through 200 tunnels in just under 7 hours.

For the best views, sit on the right-hand side of the train. After passing above sprawling Voss, the train goes through two long tunnels and above canyons. You'll enjoy raging-river-and-waterfalls views, then pass over a lake that's very close to the tree line—vegetation clears out and the landscape looks nearly lunar.

Arriving at Myrdal, hop out of the train and simply cross the platform for your awaiting Flåm-bound train. (If it's not there, it will be shortly.)

Cost: The Voss-Myrdal segment costs 120 kr.

Schedule: Local *(lokaltog)* and intercity trains *(fjerntog,* all the way from Bergen to Oslo) run from Voss to Myrdal three to five times per day. They both cost the same, but the local takes about 10 minutes longer (for a total travel time of 50 minutes).

Reservations: Local trains (recommended) are less likely to fill up, and you can't book them online. In peak season, it's smart to book intercity express trains at least a week in advance at www. nsb.no.

▲▲Myrdal-Flåm Train (Flåmsbana)

The little 12-mile spur line leaves the Oslo-Bergen line at Myrdal (2,800 feet), which is nothing but a scenic high-altitude train junction with a decent cafeteria. From Myrdal, the Flåmsbana train winds down to Flåm (sea level) through 20 tunnels (more than

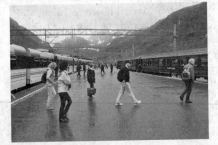

three miles' worth) in 55 thrilling minutes. It's party time on board, and the engineer even stops the train for photos at the best waterfall, Kjosfossen. According to a Norwegian legend, a temptress lives behind these falls and tries to lure men to the rocks with her singing...look

What If I Miss My Boat?

Remember that you can get help from the cruise line's port agent (listed on the destination information sheet distributed on the ship) and the local TI (see page 767). If the port agent suggests a costly solution (such as a private car with a driver), you may want to consider public transit.

If you get left behind, don't panic: You're right in the heart of the well-trafficked Norway in a Nutshell route. Use this chapter's tips to connect up to the main **Oslo-Bergen** train line to reach either of those cities. For **Stavanger,** head to Bergen to catch the bus (http://kystbussen.no)—likely faster—or to Oslo to catch the train (www.nsb.no). Flåm is also connected to Bergen by express boat (tel. 51 86 87 00, www.norled.no).

If you need to catch a **plane** to your next destination, you'll probably be best off heading to the airports in Oslo (Gardermoen Airport, tel. 91 50 64 00, www.osl.no) or Bergen (Flesland Airport, tel. 67 03 15 55, www.avinor.no/bergen).

Local **travel agents** in Flåm can help you.

For more advice on what to do if you miss the boat, see page 139.

NORWEGIAN FJORDS

out for her...and keep a wary eye on your partner.

The train line is an even more impressive feat of engineering when you realize it's not a cogwheel train—it's held to the tracks only by steel wheels, though it does have five separate braking systems. Before boarding, pick up the free, multilingual souvenir pamphlet with lots of info on the trip (or see www.flaamsbana.no). Video screens onboard and sporadic English commentary on the loudspeakers explain points of interest, but there's not much to say—it's all about the scenery.

If you're choosing seats, you'll enjoy slightly more scenery if you sit on the left going down.

Cost: 320 kr one-way, 420 kr round-trip. You can buy tickets at the Flåmsbana stations in Myrdal or Flåm, on the train (same price), or online at www.nsb.no.

Schedule: The train departs in each direction nearly hourly.

Reservations: On trains going from Myrdal down to Flåm, you can always squeeze in, even if it's standing-room only. However, morning trains ascending from Flåm to Myrdal (when there are several cruise ships in port) can sell out. This is a concern only for those wanting to leave Flåm to Myrdal in the morning. If that's you, buy your ticket in advance online or right when the Flåm ticket office opens (at 8:15).

Geirangerfjord

The nine-mile-long, 2,000-foot-deep Geirangerfjord (geh-RAHN-gher-fyord), an offshoot of the long Storfjord, snakes like an S-shaped serpent between the cut-glass peaks of western Norway. Tucked amid cliffs one observer termed "the most preposterous mountains on the entire west coast," the Geirangerfjord is simply stunning. Cruising in—and back out again—you'll drift past steep cliffs and cover-girl waterfalls, such as the famous "Seven Sisters" cascades that tumble 800 feet down a long, craggy swath of gray granite. Facing them is a waterfall dubbed "The Suitor," which sputters endlessly in a futile attempt to impress the seven maidens across the way. (Supposedly the waterfall forms a bottle shape, because perennial rejection has driven the would-be suitor to drink.) And, while any Norwegian fjord waterfall looks like a bridal veil to me, Geirangerfjord actually has one named "The Bridal Veil."

All of this beauty makes Geirangerfjord a magnet for cruise ships, about 200 of which (carrying some 330,000 passengers) call at the town of Geiranger during their relatively short season. When even just one big ship is in town, the population of this village of about 250 hardy Norwegians can increase more than tenfold...things get very crowded.

While the town tries hard to entertain all those visitors, there's only so much to do in this sleepy corner of the fjord. And, compared with Flåm, Geiranger doesn't have the public-transit connections that provide an easy and scenic loop trip without your own wheels. No trains or lifts bring you up into the mountains. Instead, to gain some altitude and reach the famous views—which I highly recommend—you'll have to book a tour (either through your cruise line or a local company), hike steeply up, or pay for a steeply priced taxi.

About half of the cruises that visit the Geirangerfjord make two stops: First comes a "technical call" in the village of Hellesylt, partway along the fjord; second, an hour or two later, there's a call at the village of Geiranger, at the fjord's endpoint. The "technical call" in Hellesylt means that only passengers who have paid the cruise line for an excursion are allowed off the ship at this point. (While adventurous travelers may be tempted to get off here to poke around, then make their way by public ferry up the fjord to Geiranger, this is typically not permitted.)

PLANNING YOUR TIME

For many cruisers, the best part about the Geirangerfjord is the sail-in and sail-away. If you expect good weather in the morning,

NORWEGIAN FJORDS

Excursions at Geirangerfjord

Of all the ports of call described in this book, Geirangerfjord may be the one where excursions are most worth considering. This is both because of the unique "technical call" arrangement many ships have at Hellesylt (which means paying for an excursion buys you an extra hour or two on land); and because there's relatively little to see in Geiranger town itself, while there's fantastic scenery from up above that's difficult to reach affordably on your own, but easy to reach on an excursion. While Geiranger-based tour operators can get you to many of the worthwhile outlying sights, others—including the fantastic Trollstigen mountain road—are easily accessible only by excursion.

Itineraries starting from **Geiranger town** may include a stop at the Geiranger Fjord Center, the Flydalsjuvet and Dalsnibba viewpoints, and a variety of waterfalls and mountain farms. Some excursions include a guided hike (after a bus ride to the trailhead) up to Storsæter Waterfall, which you can actually walk behind. Other trips head up the Ørnevegen ("Eagle Road") for more views, and some longer trips continue all the way to Trollstigen. You may also be offered kayak tours, RIB (rigid inflatable boat) tours, or mountain-bike trips, all of which can also be booked directly through local agencies (details in this chapter).

If your cruise includes a "technical call" at **Hellesylt,** you'll have the option to pay for an excursion that boards a bus there and drives (gradually) across the mountains to meet your ship in Geiranger, at the far end of the fjord. En route, the tour stops off at Hornindal Lake (Europe's deepest at more than 1,600 feet), the Nordfjord (at the town of Stryn), villages, waterfalls, and more; the final stretch takes you past the Dalsnibba and Flydalsjuvet viewpoints on the way back to your ship. Because it's a one-way journey, this option gives you the maximum Norwegian scenery for your time in this region—but note that it leaves you with very little time back in Geiranger before "all aboard."

it's worth getting up early just to experience your ship plying the fjord's glassy waters when it's relatively quiet (the beauty crescendos about an hour before your call time in Geiranger). If you prefer to sleep in, you'll see the same scenery on the way out—but, as weather here can change on a dime, I'd take advantage of any clearing that you get.

To make the most of your Geiranger visit, consider your options before you arrive. Assuming you don't want to purchase a cruise-line excursion but still want to see some of the area (such as mountain farms and high-altitude viewpoints), your best bet is to book a tour through a local company. As these can fill up

---

Services near the Port of Geiranger

Many of these services are either at the TI (right next to the tender dock) or at the Joker grocery store (marked *Dagligvarer/Grocerie/Lebensmittel*, facing the marina on a lonesome jetty a quick walk around the harbor to the right as you get off your tender).

ATMs: Geiranger's **ATM** *(minibank)* is outside the front door of the Joker grocery store.

Internet Access: You can get online at the TI, as well as at Café Olé, Laizas Café, and Hotel Union.

Pharmacy: The Joker grocery stocks basic pharmacy items; there's no full-service pharmacy in Geiranger town or nearby (the nearest—Storfjord Apotek—is in Stranda, halfway out the fjord; tel. 70 26 08 11).

---

quickly, decide on your priorities and head straight for the ticket office when you get off your tender (better yet, book in advance).

If you just stick around the town of Geiranger, you'll quickly exhaust all of its sightseeing options. The Geiranger Fjord Center, which can be seen in about an hour, is a 30-minute uphill hike from the port (including a few minutes to dip into the church and enjoy the views). After that, it's just strolling, shopping, hiking, or renting a kayak or bike.

If you're fit and adventurous, and have plenty of time, you could ride a sightseeing boat to the fjord below the remote farm called Skageflå. It takes about an hour to hike up, up, up to the farm, after which you can either hike three to four hours all the way back to Geiranger, or walk back down to the fjord and catch a boat to town (be sure to arrange a pickup time in advance with your tour boat company).

The Port of Geiranger

Arrival at a Glance: You'll step off the tender in the heart of town.

Port Overview

It's very simple. Cruise ships tender passengers in to a dock in the harborfront core of town. Stepping off your tender, look right to spot the TI. Nearby are the town bus stop, the boat dock for local ferries, souvenir shops, and eateries. Partway along the harbor to the right is the Joker grocery store, with various services (ATM, post office, and more—see sidebar).

Geiranger is basically a one-street town. That street passes the harbor (with the cruise tender dock), then twists up a hill alongside a waterfall, passing the town church, the big Hotel Union, and the Geiranger Fjord Center. Along the waterfront you'll find more hotels, the Joker grocery store, and a campground.

Tourist Information: Geiranger's TI is right along the harborfront—look for the green-and-white *i* sign (open long hours daily in summer, Wi-Fi, Internet terminals, WCs, tel. 70 26 30 99, www.visitalesund-geiranger.com). The TI also has a desk for Geiranger Fjordservice (described below).

Taxis: If you need a taxi, ask at the TI or call Geiranger Taxi (tel. 40 00 37 41, www.geirangertaxi.no). Here are some sample round-trip fares (for up to 4 people) for trips into the surrounding countryside:

Flydalsjuvet or Ørnesvingen ("Eagle Bend") viewpoint (45 minutes): 700 kr

Flydalsjuvet and Dalsnibba viewpoints combined (2 hours): 1,600 kr

Trollstigen scenic road (4 hours): 3,500 kr

Tours in Geiranger

As public transportation isn't practical for reaching the countryside splendor near the Geirangerfjord, locally based tour operators are your most cost-effective way to enjoy maximum fjord beauty in your limited time in port. As the various options tend to sell out when big ships are in port, it's smart either to prebook (best choice), or to head from your tender straight to the ticket office.

Geiranger Fjordservice, the dominant operation (with a convenient office right inside the Geiranger town TI), offers tours and excursions out on the fjord and up into the hills (www.geirangerfjord.no). They do sightseeing boat trips (with the option of hopping off for a steep hike up to a mountain farm), speedy RIB tours (one-hour ride on a rigid inflatable boat, 500 kr, hourly departures), panoramic bus rides, fishing trips, helicopter rides, bike tours, and more. Their **scenic bus tour** to the mountain viewpoints at Dalsnibba and Flydalsjuvet helps you efficiently reach the famous Geiranger views (290 kr, 2 hours; mid-June-Aug daily at 9:30 and 12:30; sporadically off-season). Their **"Fjord Country Highlights"** tour takes you in the opposite direction, up the "Eagle Road" to Ørnesvingen, tranquil lakes, and a remote cabin (250 kr, 2.75 hours, runs sporadically—check schedule online). For a more flexible alternative, their **hop-on, hop-off bus** loops you around to a variety of famous panoramic viewpoints—including Ørnesvingen and Flydalsjuvet—giving you a few minutes at each one (200 kr, 1.5-hour loop, 5/day). For any tour, you can book ahead online, then bring your voucher to their desk in the TI to pick up your boarding pass.

Kayak More Tomorrow runs all-day kayak tours up and down the Geirangerfjord (1,150 kr, departs daily in season at 9:00, be clear on return time, tel. 95 11 80 62, www.kayakmoretomorrow. com). They also offer stand-up paddleboarding lessons and rent kayaks.

Sights on and near Geirangerfjord

IN GEIRANGER
Geiranger Town
This functional little burg, with a waterfall tumbling through its middle, is magnificently set, if not quite "charming." With time to kill in Geiranger, stroll around the harbor, consider a hike into the surrounding hills, and maybe rent a kayak at the campground. To stretch your legs and see the two real "sights" in town, huff steeply up the main street to dip into the small, octagonal town church (with great views from its front yard) and to visit the Geiranger Fjord Center.

Geiranger Fjord Center (Norsk Fjordsenter)
Overlooking Geiranger's rushing waterfall at the top of town, this modern facility has interactive exhibits that illuminate both the geology and the hardscrabble lifestyles of Norway's fjords. You'll see replicas of typical fjordland homes, and learn about the traditional steamships that tied fjordside communities together when nothing else did.

Cost and Hours: 110 kr, May-Aug daily 10:00-18:00, until 15:00 off-season, a 30-minute walk out of town up the main road, across the road and waterfall from the big Hotel Union, tel. 70 26 38 10, www.verdsarvfjord.no.

Kayaking
Slicing through still fjord waters on a sea kayak can be an indelible Norwegian memory (and one that's worth booking ahead). You can rent kayaks at **Kayak More Tomorrow,** based at Geiranger Camping right along the waterfront (single kayak-150 kr/hour, double kayak-300 kr/hour, long hours daily in season, just around the harbor past Joker grocery, tel. 95 11 80 62, www. kayakmoretomorrow.com). They also offer stand-up paddleboarding and lead kayak-plus-hiking tours. **Geiranger Fjordservice** offers kayak tours, but their base is inconveniently located at Grande Camping (on a little lip of land nearly two miles out the fjord from Geiranger)—they can come pick you up in town for an additional fee (695 kr, 3-hour tour); see company details and contact info under "Tours in Geiranger," earlier.

Mountain Biking

Geiranger Adventure drops you off at a high mountain road so you can coast back down to the fjord (4/day in summer, tel. 47 37 97 71). They also rent bikes and cars.

Hiking

Ask the TI for advice about various hikes into the countryside around Geiranger (they sell "Rambling Maps"). Given the village's precarious position—bullied onto a narrow lip of land surrounded by vertical cliffs—expect a steep walk.

NEAR GEIRANGER

Most of these sights are best seen either with a cruise-ship excursion or on a tour run by a local company (for options, see earlier). While a public ferry does connect Geiranger to Hellesylt in about an hour (departs about every 1.5 hours, www.fjord1.no), it's unlikely you'll have time to take it on your short port visit—and it's redundant with your ship's sail-away anyway.

Hellesylt

The best way to see this village, which sits at the opposite end of the Geirangerfjord from Geiranger town—is if you pay for a cruise-line excursion that disembarks here. But even if you don't make it, you're not missing much; aside from the huge waterfall thundering furiously through its middle, Hellesylt is a sleepy village used primarily as a springboard for the grand scenery that stretches to its east.

Viewpoints and Mountain Drives

From Geiranger, highway 63 twists northward up out of the fjord toward Eidsdal. Corkscrewing up 11 switchbacks, this so-called Ørnevegen ("Eagle Road") was built in 1955 to connect remote little Geiranger to the rest of Norway through the frigid winter months. At the highest hairpin (around 2,000 feet), the viewpoint called Ørnesvingen ("Eagle Bend") offers breathtaking Geirangerfjord panoramas. As the road isn't practical by public transit, you're best off reaching it with a tour, an excursion, or a taxi.

To the south, highway 63 scrambles up out of the Geirangerfjord to two other fantastic viewpoints, offering *the* quintessential Geiranger panoramas. The road first passes **Flydalsjuvet** (a modern viewpoint platform, just a few miles out of Geiranger, that stares straight down a 260-foot-deep gorge to the fjord) before summiting at **Dalsnibba** (high above the tree line at nearly 5,000 feet, more distant views of the fjord, accessible only on the three-mile Nibbevegen toll road off of highway 63, www.dalsnibba.no). Various bus tour itineraries combine these

What If I Miss My Boat?

Remember that you can get help from the cruise line's port agent (listed on the destination information sheet distributed on the ship) and the local TI (see page 786). If the port agent suggests a costly solution (such as a private car with a driver), you may want to consider public transit.

If you're stuck in the town of Geiranger, you can ride a direct bus to **Oslo** (8.5 hours, summer only, www.nettbuss. no). To reach **Bergen,** first take the public ferry to Hellesylt (1 hour), where you can hop on the main bus line to Bergen (8 hours, www.ruteinfo.net).

The closest airport to Geiranger is about a three-hour bus ride away, in the city of Ålesund; from here, you can fly to **Oslo, Bergen,** and other Norwegian towns (www.avinor.no/en/airport/alesund-airport).

Local **travel agents** in Geiranger can help you. For more advice on what to do if you miss the boat, see page 139.

two grand viewpoints efficiently.

Yet another popular scenic road, **Trollstigen,** is farther from Geiranger proper but often included in cruise-line excursions. Connecting the fjord to the town of Åndalsnes, to the north, this famous "Troll's Ladder" (highway 63 past the Ørnevegen) traverses 11 switchbacks and provides perhaps the most spectacular scenery in this land of oh-so-spectacular scenery.

Shelf Farms

Because the cliffs rise directly from the deep—leaving precious few patches for fjordside settlements—any relatively flat surface high on the mountain wall seems occupied by a tidy, lonesome, and aptly named "shelf farm." Most of these, next to impossible to cultivate amid short summers, brutally cold winters, and a constant threat of rockslides, were active well into the 20th century but are now abandoned. A few have been turned into open-air museums that teach visitors about intrepid Norwegian fjord lifestyles. Two popular farms, both perched about 800 feet above the fjord waters, are **Knivsflå** (next to the Seven Sisters falls) and **Skageflå** (directly across the fjord). While visiting these on your own is impractical with a short day in port, various local tour companies offer boat rides from Geiranger to the fjord wall, where you get off and hike up to the farms (figure about an hour if you're in shape). When booking your boat ride, be sure to arrange a pickup time for your return to Geiranger. Alternatively, you can hike (about 3-4 hours) from Skageflå back to Geiranger. Guided visits of the farms are sometimes available—check with your tour company.

AMSTERDAM
The Netherlands

Netherlands Practicalities

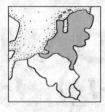

The Netherlands (Nederland)—sometimes referred to by its nickname, "Holland"—is Europe's most densely populated and also one of its wealthiest and best-organized countries. Occupying a delta near the mouth of three large rivers, for centuries the Netherlands has battled the sea, reclaiming low-lying lands and converting marshy estuaries into fertile farmland. The Netherlands has 16.8 million people: 80 percent are Dutch, and half have no religious affiliation. Despite its small size (16,000 square miles—about twice the size of New Jersey), the Netherlands boasts the planet's 23rd-largest economy. It also has one of Europe's lowest unemployment rates, relying heavily on foreign trade through its port at Rotterdam (Europe's largest).

Money: 1 euro (€) = about $1.10. An ATM is called a *geldautomaat*. The local VAT (value-added sales tax) rate is 21 percent; the minimum purchase eligible for a VAT refund is €50 (for details on refunds, see page 134).

Language: The native language is Dutch. For useful phrases, see page 858.

Emergencies: Dial 112 for police, medical, or other emergencies. In case of theft or loss, see page 125.

Time Zone: The Netherlands is on Central European Time (the same as most of the Continent—one hour ahead of Great Britain, and six/nine hours ahead of the East/West Coasts of the US).

Embassies in the Netherlands: The **US consulate** in Amsterdam is at Museumplein 19 (tel. 020/575-5309, after-hours emergency tel. 070/310-2209, http://amsterdam.usconsulate.gov). In The Hague, the **US embassy** is at Lange Voorhout 102 (tel. 070/310-2209, http://netherlands.usembassy.gov), and the **Canadian embassy** is at Sophialaan 7 (tel. 070/311-1600, www.canada.nl). Call ahead for passport services.

Phoning: The Netherland's country code is 31; to call from another country to the Netherlands, dial the international access code (011 from the US/Canada, 00 from Europe, or + from a mobile phone), then 31, followed by the area code (without initial zero) and the local number. For calls within the Netherlands, dial just the number if you are calling locally, and add the area code if calling long distance. To place an international call from the Netherlands, dial 00, the code of the country you're calling (1 for US and Canada), and the phone number. For more tips, see page 1146.

Tipping: As service is included at sit-down meals, you don't need to tip further, though it's nice to round up your bill about 5-10 percent for good service. Round up taxi fares a bit (pay €5 on a €4.50 fare). For more tips on tipping, see page 138.

Tourist Information: www.holland.com

AMSTERDAM

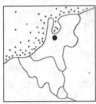

Amsterdam still looks much like it did in the 1600s—the Dutch Golden Age—when it was the world's richest city, an international sea-trading port, and the cradle of capitalism. Wealthy, democratic burghers built a city upon millions of pilings, creating a wonderland of canals lined with trees and townhouses topped with fancy gables. Immigrants, Jews, outcasts, and political rebels were drawn here by its tolerant atmosphere, while painters such as young Rembrandt captured that atmosphere on canvas.

Today's Amsterdam is a progressive place of 820,000 people and almost as many bikes. It's a city of good living, cozy cafés, great art, street-corner jazz, stately history, and a spirit of live and let live.

Amsterdam also offers the Netherlands' best people-watching. The Dutch are unique, and observing them is a sightseeing experience all in itself. They're a handsome and healthy people, and among the world's tallest. They're also open and honest—I think of them as refreshingly blunt—and they like to laugh. As connoisseurs of world culture, they appreciate Rembrandt paintings, Indonesian food, and the latest French film—but with an un-snooty, blue-jeans attitude.

Be warned: Amsterdam, a bold experiment in freedom, may box your Puritan ears. For centuries, the city has taken a tolerant approach to things other places try to forbid. Traditionally, the city attracted sailors and businessmen away from home, so it was profitable to allow them to have a little fun. In the 1960s, Amsterdam became a magnet for Europe's hippies. Since then, it's become a world capital of alternative lifestyles. Stroll through any neighborhood and see things that are commonplace here but rarely found elsewhere. Prostitution is allowed in the Red Light District, while "smartshops" sell psychedelic drugs and marijuana is openly sold and smoked. (The Dutch aren't necessarily more tolerant or decadent than the rest of us—just pragmatic and looking for smart solutions.)

Approach Amsterdam as an ethnologist observing a strange culture. It's a place where carillons chime quaintly from spires towering above coffeeshops where yuppies go to smoke pot. Take it all in, then pause to watch the clouds blow past stately old gables— and see the Golden Age reflected in a quiet canal.

PLANNING YOUR TIME

Although Amsterdam does have a few must-see museums, its best attraction is its own carefree ambience. The city's a joy on foot— and a breezier and faster delight by bike. For sightseers who want to do more than relax, these are the top choices:

• **Rijksmuseum:** You can see the highlights of this world-class collection of Dutch Masters in about an hour and a half.

• **Van Gogh Museum:** The planet's best collection of this beloved Dutch artist's work demands at least an hour to see.

• **Anne Frank House:** This evocative sight, in the actual home where Jewish refugees were hidden from the Nazis, is worth an hour.

• **Other Museums:** Depending on your interests, consider the **Stedelijk Museum** (art since 1945), **Amsterdam Museum** (city history), **Amstelkring Museum** ("Our Lord in the Attic" hidden church), and **Dutch Resistance Museum** (ingenuity of anti-Nazi agitators). Each of these merits an hour.

• **Canal Cruise:** A one-hour boat trip offers a fine orientation to the city.

• **Explore Neighborhoods:** Of Amsterdam's many colorful and characteristic neighborhoods, the most popular to explore are the **Jordaan** (an upscale-hipster residential zone at the western edge of downtown) and the **Red Light District** (a fascinating, in-your-face look at legalized prostitution, southeast of Central Station). Allow an hour of strolling apiece.

The two great art museums (Rijks and Van Gogh) cluster near the south end of the town center, so you can tackle things in a geographically logical order: From Central Station, zip to the museums by tram. Then work your way back toward the station (and the cruise terminal), detouring to the Anne Frank House and other sights that interest you as time allows.

Reservations: Amsterdam's top sights—Rijksmuseum, Van Gogh Museum, Anne Frank House—suffer from long lines. It's essential to purchase your tickets for these ahead of time—especially for Anne Frank House, which limits advance reservations

> ## Excursions from Amsterdam
>
> It's easy to do everything in **Amsterdam** on your own, thanks to the Dutch public transportation system and the fact that everyone here speaks English—even the tram drivers. But for those who want more help, you'll find various excursions advertised by your cruise line: bus tours; town walking tours; canal cruises; guided visits to the Van Gogh Museum, Anne Frank House, and Rijksmuseum; diamond-themed tours (including a visit to Gassan Diamonds); and Jewish heritage tours (including a visit to the Jewish Historical Museum and important neighborhoods). All of these sights are easily visited on your own—and in many cases far cheaper for independent travelers. For example, a brief bus tour with a canal cruise offered through a cruise line might cost $50-60, while going with a local company offering an essentially identical cruise costs less than $20.
>
> While Amsterdam is both grand and accessible, big cities aren't for everyone. Various cruise excursions focus on small-town and countryside sights. If you're here during the flower festival at **Keukenhof** (mid-March–mid-May), it's worth touring the remarkable flower gardens there—and a bit tricky by public transportation. Similarly, the beautiful Dutch countryside and villages are challenging to link on your own with limited time; excursion itineraries generally include some combination of the idyllic **Waterland** towns of Edam, Volendam, Marken, and/or Broek; the open-air museum (with great windmills) of **Zaanse Schans;** and the reclaimed land of **Beemster Polder.** And in this little country, you can even do a "Grand Tour of Holland" in one short day, with brief stops in the charming town of **Delft** and the bustling city of **The Hague.** If you'd like to see a lot of the Netherlands in a little time, these excursions are worth doing for the efficiency they provide. But most people find plenty in Amsterdam to keep them entertained.

AMSTERDAM

(easiest online; for details, see "Advance Tickets for Major Sights" on page 800). When booking your appointment times, use these guidelines:

• Rijksmuseum: Open tickets good for entry at any time; plan to arrive about one hour after your scheduled disembarkation.

• Van Gogh Museum: About two hours after your Rijksmuseum arrival (assuming you'll see the Rijksmuseum very quickly).

• Anne Frank House: About three hours after your Van Gogh appointment (allowing time for lunch, exploring, and strolling to the Anne Frank House).

So, if your ship arrives at 8:00, arrive at the Rijksmuseum around 9:00, book Van Gogh for 11:00, and book Anne Frank for 14:00. (If you'd prefer more time to savor the Rijksmuseum, push back your Van Gogh and Anne Frank reservations.)

Alternatively, you can spring for a sightseeing pass (described on page 800); for example, the €55 Museumkaart lets you skip the ticket line at the Rijksmuseum and you'll wait in a shorter line at the Van Gogh Museum. This won't save you money on a short visit, but it will save you time (and avoid the hassle and tight time-table of reserving individual entrances).

The Port of Amsterdam

Arrival at a Glance: Amsterdam's cruise terminal is a three-minute tram ride or 15-minute walk to the central train station, with connections by tram, bus, or boat to anywhere in the city (see map on page 828). If Amsterdam's terminal is full, a few ships dock at the Felison Terminal in IJmuiden, which has a shuttle to the city (www.felisonterminal.nl).

Port Overview

Passenger Terminal Amsterdam (PTA)—an ultra-modern facil-ity with a roof that looks like a glass whale—is just minutes away from the center of Amsterdam. Inside the terminal, you'll find an information desk, lockers, an ATM, and shops.

Tourist Information: When ships arrive, the Port of Amsterdam staffs an information desk on the ground floor of the terminal—ask for their map for cruisers. The main Amsterdam TI is right in front of nearby Central Station (for details, see page 800).

GETTING INTO TOWN

A fleet of taxis wait right outside the terminal, but they're expen-sive; meanwhile, trams are easy, cheap, and fast. If you're ready to pretend you're an Amsterdammer, there's even a bike-rental facil-ity a few steps away.

From the Cruise Terminal to Central Station

It's easy to reach Central Station, either by tram or by foot.

By Tram: Amsterdam's public transit system waits just outside the cruise terminal door. Exiting the terminal, follow the *Town Center* sign and use the crosswalk to cross the busy portside street. You'll see a tram stop with an electric sign reading *Centraal Station* and displaying the arrival time for the next tram. Take tram #26 just one stop to the end of the line, Central Station (runs every 4-8 minutes, trip takes 3 minutes). A one-hour tram ticket costs €2.80; if you'll be taking more than two transit journeys on your visit, buy a €7.50 one-day transit pass, good for all trams and buses (for either ticket, pay the conductor in cash).

By Foot: From the cruise terminal, it's just 15 minutes by foot to Amsterdam's Central Station: As you leave the terminal, follow the *Town Center* sign, turn right at the busy road, and walk past the shops, hotel, and concert hall (Muziekgebouw Bimhuis). Continue walking with the water on your right—you'll see the glass-and-steel arch of the station's roof. You'll end up walking between the station and the water; when you come to a major crosswalk (on your left), follow the crowds crossing the street to enter the lower level of Central Station.

From Central Station to Other Parts of Town

The portal connecting Amsterdam to the world is the aptly named Central Station (Amsterdam Centraal). The station is packed with shops, eateries (including handy Albert Heijn "to go" supermarkets), ATMs, Internet access, and a pharmacy (see "Services near the Port of Amsterdam" on page 798). Through at least 2015, expect the station and the plaza in front of it to be a construction zone and in a state of some flux.

If you arrive by tram, you'll get off at the Centraal Station stop, in front of the station. If you walk here from the cruise terminal, you'll enter the station through its "back door"—just take the main corridor all the way through (crossing under all the platforms) and follow *Centrum* signs to pop out in front.

The plaza at the station's front is a local transit hub with convenient access to trams, buses, and metro. Orient yourself, standing with your back to the station: Straight ahead, just past the canal, is Damrak street, leading to Dam Square (10-minute walk). To your left are the TI and GVB public-transit offices. Farther to your left is a bike rental place: MacBike (in the station building, see page 804.)

Just beyond the taxis are platforms for the city's blue-and-white **trams,** which come along frequently, ready to take you anywhere your feet won't (buy ticket or pass from conductor; if you bought a tram ticket for the ride from the cruise terminal, it's good for an hour and can be used for a connecting tram ride to wherever you're headed). The following trams are most useful for your sightseeing and depart from the west side of Stationsplein (with the station behind you, they're to your right): Trams #2 (marked *Nieuw Sloten*) and #5 (marked *A'veen Binnenhof*) head south from here to Dam Square, then Leidseplein, then Museumplein—with the **Van Gogh** and **Rijks museums;** tram #1 (marked *Osdorp*) also goes to Leidseplein.

To reach the **Anne Frank House,** it's about a 20-minute walk, or you can ride tram #13, #14, or #17 to the Westermarkt

Services near the Port of Amsterdam

ATMs: The Travelex ATM by the revolving door as you leave the cruise terminal may not have the best rates; ideally, wait to use the banks of ATMs inside Central Station.

Internet Access: It's easy at cafés all over town, but the best place for serious surfing is the towering **Central Library,** which has hundreds of fast terminals and Wi-Fi (Openbare Bibliotheek Amsterdam, daily 10:00-22:00). It's very close to the cruise terminal: Turn right when you leave the terminal, walk with the water on your right, turn left at the first bike/pedestrian path that goes under the train tracks, and follow that path to a modern building facing the inner harbor. The library also has a great view and a comfy cafeteria. The **café** across the street from Central Station (in the white building next to the TI) has pay Internet access and Wi-Fi. **"Coffeeshops,"** which sell marijuana, usually also offer Internet access—letting you surf with a special bravado.

Pharmacy: For over-the-counter remedies, try **Hema** on the main floor of Central Station. For prescriptions, head for **BENU Apotheek** on Dam Square (Mon-Fri 8:00-17:30, Sat 10:00-17:00, Sun 12:00-17:00, Damstraat 2, tel. 020/624-4331). Farther afield, the shop named **DA** (Dienstdoende Apotheek) has all the basics—shampoo and toothpaste— as well as a pharmacy counter hidden in the back (Mon-Sat 9:00-22:00, Sun 11:00-22:00, Leidsestraat 74-76 near where it meets Keizersgracht, tel. 020/627-5351).

Other Services: There are pay **lockers** on the cruise terminal's first floor. AmsterBike **bike rentals** is in the parking garage under the Mövenpick Hotel next door; they offer electric bikes and bike tours as well as regular rentals (daily 9:00-18:00 except closed Wed in winter, tel. 020/419-9063, www.amsterbike.eu; more bike rental options are near Central Station—see page 804). There are also cafés, souvenir shops, and even a Segway rental office next to the terminal.

stop, about a block south of the museum's entrance.

A variety of **canal boat tours** depart from in front of the station (for details, see page 805).

By Taxi

A taxi ride to the Rijksmuseum or Van Gogh Museum costs about €16. For more on taxis, see page 805.

The red line of Amsterdam's hop-on, hop-off **Canal Bus** stops at the cruise terminal on its way through scenic canals to the Rijksmuseum and Van Gogh Museum, Leidseplein, and back to Central Station. As you exit the terminal, you'll see the *Canal Bus* sign and dock at the end of the narrow inlet between the buildings and the highway (€24/24-hour pass, ticket also good on green and orange lines, about 2/hour in summer, less frequent off-season, tel. 020/217-0500, www.canal.nl). Other canal boat options (including cheaper one-hour orientation tours) depart from in front of Central Station. For more on all of the options, see page 805.

By Tour

For information on local tour options in Amsterdam—including local guides for hire, walking tours, and bus or boat tours—see "Tours in Amsterdam" on page 806.

RETURNING TO YOUR SHIP

From Central Station, take tram #26 one stop to Muziekgebouw Bimhuis. As you face the station's main entrance, the tram stop is on the right—it will be marked *IJburg*.

If you have some extra time before heading back, check out the public library for its view, cheap Internet access, and cafeteria (near the cruise terminal and described in the "Services near the Port of Amsterdam" sidebar).

See page 852 for help if you miss your boat.

Amsterdam

Amsterdam's Central Station (Amsterdam Centraal), on the north edge of the city, is your starting point, with the TI, bike rental, and trams branching out to all points. The street called Damrak is the main north-south axis, connecting Central Station with Dam Square (people-watching and hangout center) and its Royal Palace. From this main street, the city spreads out like a fan, with 90 islands, hundreds of bridges, and a series of concentric canals—named Singel (the original moat), Herengracht (Gentleman's Canal), Keizersgracht (Emperor's Canal), and Prinsengracht (Prince's Canal)—that were laid out in the 17th century, Holland's Golden Age. Amsterdam's major sights are all within walking distance of Dam Square.

To the east of Damrak is the oldest part of the city (today's Red Light District), and to the west is the newer part, where you'll find the Anne Frank House and the peaceful Jordaan neighborhood. Museums and the bustling square, Leidseplein, are at the southern edge of the city center.

Orientation to Amsterdam

TOURIST INFORMATION

The Dutch name for a TI is "VVV," pronounced "fay fay fay." Amsterdam's main TI, located across the street from Central Station, is centrally located, but it's crowded and inefficient, and the free maps are poor quality (Mon-Sat 9:00-17:00, Sun 10:00-16:00). The TI sells a good city map (€2.50), walking-tour brochures (€3), skip-the-line museum tickets (though it's easier buying these online), and the *Time Out Amsterdam* entertainment guide (€3). Inside Central Station, the GWK Currency Exchange offices (though not officially TIs) can answer basic tourist questions, with shorter lines (daily 9:00-22:00).

ADVANCE TICKETS AND SIGHTSEEING CARDS

You can avoid long ticket lines (common from late March-Oct) at the **Rijksmuseum, Van Gogh Museum,** and **Anne Frank House** by booking tickets in advance or getting a sightseeing pass. (If you're visiting off-season, it's less important to worry about line-skipping options, especially if you use my other crowd-beating tips.)

Since there's no single option that's best for every sight, here's the scoop:

Advance Tickets: It's easy to buy tickets online for the three major museums through each museum's website, generally with no extra booking fee. You just print out your ticket and bring it to the ticket-holder's line for a quick entry. You can also buy advance tickets at TIs (though lines there can be long). Because advance reservations for the Anne Frank House are limited, you should buy your ticket as soon as you're sure of your itinerary.

Sightseeing Passes: On a brief cruise visit, I'd skip all the passes (and make individual reservations at the sights instead), or splurge on the Museumkaart solely for the ability to skip some lines.

The **Museumkaart** (€55) sightseeing pass covers many museums throughout the Netherlands for a year (though it doesn't include public transit like the I amsterdam Card). It pays for itself if you visit six museums. While that's unlikely on your short port visit, the ability to skip lines at some sights might still be worth the hefty price. But you can't bypass the line at the Anne Frank House (to avoid waiting, you must make an online reservation), and at the Van Gogh Museum, you'll need to queue up, though at a much shorter line than ticket-buyers. The Museumkaart is sold at participating museums. Buy it at a less-crowded one to avoid lines (e.g., the Royal Palace on Dam Square). For a full list of included sights, see www.amsterdam.info/museums/museumkaart.

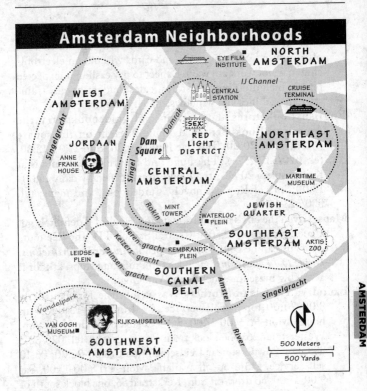

Amsterdam Neighborhoods

The **I amsterdam Card** is probably not worth the cost on a brief port visit, even though it includes a canal boat ride and a transportation pass. But it does not cover the Rijksmuseum or Anne Frank House, and it only lets you skip lines at the Van Gogh Museum (€47/24 hours, €57/48 hours, or €67/72 hours). You can check the list of sights at www.iamsterdamcard.com. Another pass you'll see advertised, the **Holland Pass,** is not worth it.

HELPFUL HINTS

Theft Alert: Tourists are considered green and rich, and the city has more than its share of hungry thieves—especially in the train station, on trams, in and near crowded museums, at places of drunkenness, and at the many hostels. Wear your money belt. If there's a risk you'll be out late high or drunk, leave all valuables on your cruise ship or in your hotel. Blitzed tourists are easy targets for petty theft.

Street Smarts: Beware of silent transportation—trams, electric mopeds, and bicycles—when walking around town. Don't walk on tram tracks or pink/maroon bicycle paths. Before you step off any sidewalk, do a double- or triple-check in both directions to make sure all's clear.

Cash Only: Thrifty Dutch merchants, who hate paying the unusually high fees charged by credit-card companies here, often refuse US credit cards (and cards without an electronic chip may not work anyway). Expect to pay cash in unexpected places, including grocery stores, cafés, budget hotels, train-station machines and windows, and at some museums.

English Bookstores: For fiction and guidebooks, try the **American Book Center** at Spui 12, right on the square (Mon 12:00-20:00, Tue-Sat 10:00-20:00, Sun 11:00-18:30, tel. 020/535-2575). The huge and helpful **Scheltema** is at Koningsplein 20 near the Leidsestraat (generally daily 10:00-19:00; lots of English novels, guidebooks, and maps; tel. 020/523-1411).

Maps: Given the city's maze of streets and canals, I'd definitely get a good city map (€2.50 at Central Station TI). The free tourist maps can be confusing, except for *Amsterdam Museums: Guide to 44 Museums* (includes tram info and stops, ask for it at the big museums, such as the Van Gogh).

Laundry: Try **Clean Brothers Wasserij** in the Jordaan (daily 8:00-20:00 for €7 self-service, €9 drop-off—ready in an hour—Mon-Fri 9:00-17:00, Sat 9:00-18:00, no drop-off Sun, Westerstraat 26, one block from Prinsengracht, tel. 020/627-9888) or **Powders,** near Leidseplein (daily 8:00-22:00, €6-10 self-service, €13 drop-off available Mon- Fri 8:00-17:00, Sat 9:00-15:00, no drop-off Sun, Kerkstraat 56, one block south of Leidsestraat, mobile 06-8140-4069).

Updates to This Book: For updates to this book, check www.ricksteves.com/update.

GETTING AROUND AMSTERDAM

Amsterdam is big, and you'll find the trams handy. The longest walk a tourist would make is an hour from Central Station to the Rijksmuseum. When you're on foot, be extremely vigilant for silent but potentially painful bikes, trams, and crotch-high bollards.

By Tram, Bus, and Metro

Amsterdam's public-transit system includes trams, buses, and an underground metro. Of these, trams are most useful for most tourists.

Paper Tickets: Within Amsterdam, a single transit ticket (called a single-use or disposable OV-chipkaart) costs €2.80 and is good for one hour on the tram, bus, and metro, including transfers. Passes good for unlimited transportation are available for 24 hours (€7.50), 48 hours (€12), 72 hours (€16.50), and 96 hours (€21). Given how expensive single tickets are, think about buying a pass before you buy that first ticket.

The easiest way to buy a ticket or pass is to simply board a tram or bus and pay the conductor (whose station is usually at the rear of the tram; no extra fee). Tickets and passes are also available at metro-station vending machines (which take cash but not US credit cards unless they have a chip), at GVB public-transit offices, and at TIs.

The entire country's public-transit network operates on a system with a multiple-use OV-Chipkaart. However, this system works best for locals and isn't practical for short-time visitors (it requires a nonrefundable €7.50 deposit plus a €2.50 fee to cash out, and can only be reloaded at train stations)—on a brief cruise visit, don't bother.

Information: For more on riding public transit, visit the helpful GVB public-transit information office in front of Central Station (Mon-Fri 7:00-21:00, Sat-Sun 10:00-18:00). Its free, multilingual *Public Transport Amsterdam Tourist Guide* includes a transit map and explains ticket options and tram connections to all the sights. Everything is also explained in English on their helpful website at www.gvb.nl.

Riding the Trams: Board the tram at any entrance not marked with a red/white "do not enter" sticker. If you need a

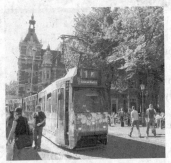

ticket or pass, pay the conductor (in a booth at the back); if there's no conductor, pay the driver in front. You must always "check in" as you board by scanning your ticket or pass at the pink-and-gray scanner, and "check out" by scanning it again when you get off. The scanner will beep and flash a green light after a successful scan. Be careful not to accidentally scan your ticket or pass twice while boarding, or it becomes invalid. Checking in and out is very important, as controllers do pass through and fine violators. To open the door when you reach your stop, press a green button on one of the poles near an exit.

Trams #2 *(Nieuw Sloten)* and #5 *(A'veen Binnenhof)* travel the north-south axis, from Central Station to Dam Square to Leidseplein to Museumplein (Van Gogh and Rijksmuseum). Tram #1 (marked *Osdorp*) also runs to Leidseplein. At Central Station, these three trams depart from the west side of station's plaza (with the station behind you, they're to your right).

If you get lost in Amsterdam, remember that most of the city's trams take you back to Central Station, and all drivers speak English.

Buses and Metro: Tickets and passes work on buses and the metro just as they do on the trams—scan your ticket or pass to "check in" as you enter and again to "check out" when you leave. The metro system is scant—used mostly for commuting to the suburbs—but it does connect Central Station with some sights east of Damrak (Nieuwmarkt-Waterlooplein-Weesperplein). The glacial speed of the metro-expansion project is a running joke among cynical Amsterdammers.

By Bike

Everyone—bank managers, students, pizza delivery boys, and police—uses this mode of transport. It's by far the smartest way to travel in a city where 40 percent of all traffic rolls on two wheels. You'll get around town by bike faster than you can by taxi. One-speed bikes, with *"brrringing"* bells, rent for about €10 per day at any number of places. For information on bike tours, see 807.

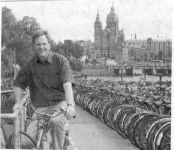

MacBike, with thousands of bikes, is the city's bike-rental powerhouse—you'll see their bright-red bikes all over town (they do stick out a bit). It has a huge and efficient outlet at Central Station (€7.50/3 hours, €9.75/24 hours, €15.75/48 hours, €21.75/72 hours, more for 3 gears and optional insurance, 25 percent discount with I amsterdam Card; either leave €50 deposit plus a copy of your passport, or leave a credit-card imprint; free helmets, daily 9:00-17:45; at east end of station—on the left as you're leaving; tel. 020/620-0985, www.macbike.nl). They have two smaller satellite stations at Leidseplein (Weteringschans 2) and Waterlooplein (Nieuwe Uilenburgerstraat 116). Return your bike to the station where you rented it. MacBike sells several pamphlets outlining bike tours with a variety of themes in and around Amsterdam for €1-2.

Lock Your Bike: Bike thieves are bold and brazen in Amsterdam. Bikes come with two locks and stern instructions to use both. The wimpy ones go through the spokes, whereas the industrial-strength chains are meant to be wrapped around the actual body of the bike and through the front wheel, and connected to something stronger than any human. (Note the steel bike-hitching racks sticking up all around town, called "staples.") Follow your rental agency's locking directions diligently. If you're sloppy, it's an expensive mistake and one that any "included" theft insurance won't cover.

Biking Tips: As the Dutch believe in fashion over safety, no one here wears a helmet. They do, however, ride cautiously, and so should you: Use arm signals, follow the bike-only traffic signals, stay in the obvious and omnipresent bike lanes, and yield to traffic on the right. Fear oncoming trams and tram tracks. Carefully cross tram tracks at a perpendicular angle to avoid catching your tire in the rut. Warning: Police ticket cyclists just as they do drivers. Obey all traffic signals, and walk your bike through pedestrian zones. Fines for biking through pedestrian zones are reportedly €30-50. Leave texting-while-biking to the locals. A handy bicycle route-planner can be found at www.routecraft.com (select "bike-planner," then click the British flag for English).

By Boat

While the city is great on foot, bike, or tram, you can also get around Amsterdam by boat. **Rederij Lovers** boats shuttle tourists on a variety of routes covering different combinations of the city's top sights. Their Museum Line, for example, costs €18 and stops near the Hermitage, Rijksmuseum/Van Gogh Museum, and Central Station (at least every 45 minutes, 6 stops, 2 hours). Sales booths in front of Central Station (and the boats) offer free brochures listing museum hours and admission prices. Most routes come with recorded narration and run daily 10:00-17:30 (tel. 020/530-1090, www.lovers.nl).

The similar **Canal Bus** is actually a hop-on, hop-off boat, offering 16 stops—including one at the cruise terminal—on three different boat routes (€24/24-hour pass, discounts when booking online, departures daily 9:45-18:30, until 20:45 on Fri-Sun April-Oct, leaves near Central Station and Rederij Lovers dock, tel. 020/217-0500, www.canal.nl).

If you're simply looking for a floating, nonstop tour, the regular canal tour boats (without the stops) give more information, cover more ground, and cost less (see "Tours in Amsterdam," next).

For do-it-yourself canal tours and lots of exercise, Canal Bus also rents "canal bikes" (a.k.a. paddleboats) at several locations: near the Anne Frank House, near the Rijksmuseum, near Leidseplein, and where Leidsestraat meets Keizersgracht (€8/1 hour, €11/1.5 hours, €14/2 hours, prices are per person, daily July-Aug 10:00-22:00, Sept-June 10:00-18:00).

By Taxi

For short rides, Amsterdam is a bad town for taxis. Given the good tram system and ease of biking, I use taxis less in Amsterdam than in just about any other city in Europe. The city's taxis have a high drop charge (about €7) for the first two kilometers (e.g., from Central Station to the Mint Tower), after which it's €2.12 per kilometer. You can wave them down, find a rare taxi stand, or call one (tel. 020/777-7777). All taxis are required to have meters. You'll also see **bike taxis,** particularly near Dam Square and Leidseplein. Negotiate a rate for the trip before you board (no meter), and they'll wheel you wherever you want to go (estimate €1/3 minutes, no surcharge for baggage or extra weight, sample fare from Leidseplein to Anne Frank House: about €6).

Tours in Amsterdam

BY BOAT
▲▲Canal Boat Tours

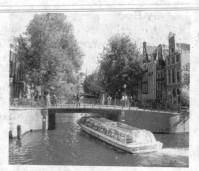

These long, low, tourist-laden boats leave continually from several docks around town for a relaxing, if uninspiring, one-hour introduction to the city (with recorded headphone commentary). Select a boat tour based on your proximity to its starting point. Tip: Boats leave only when full, so jump on a full boat to avoid waiting at the dock. Choose from one of these three companies:

Rederij P. Kooij is cheapest (€10, 3/hour in summer 10:00-22:00, 2/hour in winter 10:00-17:00, at corner of Spui and Rokin streets, about 10 minutes from Dam Square, tel. 020/623-3810, www.rederijkooij.nl).

Blue Boat Company's boats depart from near Leidseplein (€15; every half-hour April-Sept 10:00-18:00, hourly Oct-March 10:00-17:00; 1.25 hours, Stadhouderskade 30, tel. 020/679-1370, www.blueboat.nl).

Holland International offers a standard one-hour trip and a variety of longer tours from the docks opposite Central Station (€15.50, 1-hour "100 Highlights" tour with recorded commentary, daily 4/hour 9:00-18:00, 2/hour 18:00-22:00; Prins Hendrikkade 33a, tel. 020/217-0500, www.hir.nl).

ON FOOT
Free City Walk

New Europe Tours "employs" native, English-speaking students to give irreverent and entertaining three-hour walks (using the same "free tour, ask for tips, sell their other tours" formula popular in so many great European cities). While most guides lack a local's deep understanding of Dutch culture, not to mention professional training, they're certainly high-energy. This long walk covers a lot of the city with an enthusiasm for the contemporary pot-and-prostitution scene (free but tips expected, daily at 11:15 and 14:15, www.neweuropetours.eu). They also offer paid tours (Red Light District—€12, daily at 19:00; coffeeshop scene—€12, daily at 15:00; Amsterdam by bike—€18.50, includes bike, daily at 12:00). Their walking tours leave from the National Monument on Dam Square; the bike tour leaves from Central Station.

Adam's Apple Tours
Frank Sanders' walking tour offers a two-hour, English-only look at the historic roots and development of Amsterdam. You'll have a small group of generally 5-6 people and a caring guide, starting off at Central Station and ending up at Dam Square (€25; May-Sept daily at 10:00, 12:30, and 15:00 based on demand; call 020/616-7867 to confirm times and book, www.adamsapple.nl). Frank is happy to tailor a private walk to your interests.

Private Guide
Albert Walet is a likeable, hardworking, and knowledgeable local guide who enjoys personalizing tours for Americans interested in knowing his city. Al specializes in history, architecture, and water management, and exudes a passion for Amsterdam (€70/2 hours, €120/4 hours, up to 4 people, on foot or by bike, mobile 06-2069-7882, abwalet@yahoo.com).

BY BIKE
Guided Bike Tours
Yellow Bike Guided Tours offers city bike tours of either two hours (€21, daily at 10:30) or three hours (€25, daily at 13:30), which both include a 20-minute break. They also offer a four-hour, 15-mile tour of the dikes and green pastures of the countryside (€31.50, lunch extra, includes 45-minute break, April-Oct daily at 10:30). All tours leave from Nieuwezijds Kolk 29, three blocks from Central Station (reservations smart, tel. 020/620-6940, www.yellowbike.nl). If you'd prefer a private guide, contact Albert Walet, listed earlier.

Joy Ride Bike Tours is a creative little company run by Americans Sean and Allison Cody. They offer group tours designed to show you all of the clichés—cheese, windmills, and clogs—as you pedal through the pastoral polder land in 4.5 hours (€30, April-Sept Thu-Mon, meet at 10:15 and depart precisely at 10:30, no tours Tue-Wed, groups limited to 15 people and no kids under 13 years). They also offer private tours tailored to your interests (€125/2 people plus €25/person after that). Helmets, rain gear, and saddlebags are provided free. All tours must be booked in advance; tours meet behind the Rijksmuseum next to the Cobra Café (mobile 06-4361-1798, www.joyridetours.nl).

Amsterdam at a Glance

▲▲▲**Rijksmuseum** Best collection anywhere of the Dutch Masters—Rembrandt, Hals, Vermeer, and Steen—in a spectacular setting. **Hours:** Daily 9:00-17:00. See page 810.

▲▲▲**Van Gogh Museum** More than 200 paintings by the angst-ridden artist. **Hours:** Daily 9:00-18:00, Fri until 22:00 March-Oct, Sat until 22:00 July-Aug and Oct. See page 814.

▲▲▲**Anne Frank House** Young Anne's hideaway during the Nazi occupation. **Hours:** April-Oct daily 9:00-21:00, Sat and July-Aug until 22:00; Nov-March daily 9:00-19:00, Sat until 21:00. See page 820.

▲▲**Stedelijk Museum** The Netherlands' top modern-art museum, recently and extensively renovated. **Hours:** Daily 10:00-18:00, Thu until 22:00. See page 817.

▲▲**Vondelpark** City park and concert venue. **Hours:** Always open. See page 819.

▲▲**Amsterdam Museum** City's growth from fishing village to trading capital to today, including some Rembrandts and a playable carillon. **Hours:** Daily 10:00-17:00. See page 823.

▲▲**Amstelkring Museum** Catholic church hidden in the attic of a 17th-century merchant's house. **Hours:** Mon-Sat 10:00-17:00, Sun and holidays 13:00-17:00. See page 825.

▲▲**Red Light District Walk** Women of the world's oldest profession on the job. **Hours:** Best from noon into the evening; avoid late at night. See page 825.

▲▲**Netherlands Maritime Museum** Rich seafaring story of the Netherlands, told with vivid artifacts. **Hours:** Daily 9:00-17:00. See page 827.

▲▲**Hermitage Amsterdam** Russia's Tsarist treasures, on loan from St. Petersburg. **Hours:** Daily 10:00-17:00. See page 831.

▲▲**Dutch Resistance Museum** History of the Dutch struggle against the Nazis. **Hours:** Tue-Fri 10:00-17:00, Sat-Mon 11:00-17:00. See page 833.

▲**Museumplein** Square with art museums, street musicians, crafts, and nearby diamond demos. **Hours:** Always open. See page 818.

▲**Leidseplein** Lively square with cafés and street musicians. **Hours:** Always open, best on sunny afternoons. See page 819.

▲**Royal Palace** Lavish former city hall that takes you back to the Golden Age of the 17th century. **Hours:** Daily 11:00-17:00 when not closed for official ceremonies. See page 823.

▲**Begijnhof** Quiet courtyard lined with picturesque houses. **Hours:** Daily 8:00-17:00. See page 823.

▲**Hash, Marijuana, and Hemp Museum** All the dope, from history and science to memorabilia. **Hours:** Daily 10:00-23:00. See page 826.

▲**Rembrandt's House** The master's reconstructed house, displaying his etchings. **Hours:** Daily 10:00-18:00. See page 829.

▲**Diamond Tours** Offered at shops throughout the city. **Hours:** Generally daily 9:00-17:00. See page 830.

▲**Jewish Historical Museum** The Great Synagogue and exhibits on Judaism and culture, with Portuguese Synagogue across the street. **Hours:** Daily 11:00-17:00. See page 831.

▲**Dutch Theater** Moving memorial in former Jewish detention center. **Hours:** Daily 11:00-17:00. See page 832.

▲**Tropical Museum** Re-creations of tropical-life scenes. **Hours:** Tue-Sun 10:00-17:00, closed Mon. See page 833.

AMSTERDAM

Sights in Amsterdam

One of Amsterdam's delights is that it has perhaps more small specialty museums than any other city its size. From marijuana to Old Masters, you can find a museum to suit your interests.

For tips on how to save time otherwise spent in the long ticket-buying lines of the big three museums—the Anne Frank House, Van Gogh Museum, and Rijksmuseum—see "Advance Tickets and Sightseeing Cards" on page 800.

Most museums require baggage check—usually free (often in coin-op lockers where you get your coin back).

The following sights are arranged by neighborhood for handy sightseeing.

SOUTHWEST AMSTERDAM

▲▲▲Rijksmuseum

At Amsterdam's Rijksmuseum ("Rijks" rhymes with "bikes"), Holland's Golden Age shines with the best collection anywhere of the Dutch Masters—from Vermeer's quiet domestic scenes and Steen's raucous family meals, to Hals' snapshot portraits and Rembrandt's moody brilliance.

The 17th century saw the Netherlands at the pinnacle of its power. The Dutch had won their independence from Spain, trade and shipping boomed, wealth poured in, the people were understandably proud, and the arts flourished. This era was later dubbed the Dutch Golden Age. With no church bigwigs or royalty around to commission big canvases in the Protestant Dutch Republic, artists had to find different patrons—and they discovered the upper-middle-class businessmen who fueled Holland's capitalist economy. Artists painted their portraits and decorated their homes with pretty still lifes and unpreachy, slice-of-life art.

This delightful museum—recently much improved after a long renovation—offers one of the most exciting and enjoyable art experiences in Europe. As if in homage to Dutch art and history, the Rijksmuseum lets you linger over a vast array of objects and paintings, appreciating the beauty of everyday things.

Cost and Hours: €17.50, not covered by I amsterdam Card, daily 9:00-17:00, last entry 30 minutes before closing, audioguide-€5, tram #2 or #5 from Central Station to Rijksmuseum stop; info tel. 020/674-7047 or switchboard tel. 020/674-7000, www.rijksmuseum.nl. The entrance is off the passageway that tunnels right through the center of the building.

Avoiding Crowds: The museum is most crowded on weekends and holidays, and there's always a peak midday crush around noon. Avoid crowds by coming on Monday or Tuesday, and plan your visit for either first thing in the morning or later in the day (it's least crowded after 15:00). You can reserve tickets in advance at www.rijksmuseum.nl. If you're staying overnight in Amsterdam before or after a cruise, you may be able to buy your ticket through your hotel. The ticket is good any time (no entry time specified). A Museumkaart pass also lets you skip the line.

Visiting the Museum: After showing your ticket (and perhaps renting a videoguide), follow the crowds up the stairway to the top (second) floor, where you emerge into the **Great Hall.** With its stained-glass windows, vaulted ceiling, and murals of Golden Age explorers, it feels like a cathedral to Holland's middle-class merchants. Gaze down the long adjoining hall to the far end, with the "altarpiece" of this cathedral—Rembrandt's *Night Watch.* Now, follow the flow of the crowds toward it, into the **Gallery of Honor.** This grand space was purpose-built to hold the Greatest Hits of the Golden Age, by the era's biggest rock stars: Frans Hals, Vermeer, Jan Steen, and Rembrandt.

Frans Hals (c. 1582-1666) was the premier Golden Age portrait painter. Merchants hired him the way we'd hire a wedding photographer. With a few quick strokes, Hals captured not only the features, but also the personality. In *A Militiaman Holding a Berkemeyer* (a.k.a. *The Merry Drinker,* c. 1628-1630), you're greeted by a jovial man in a black hat, capturing the earthy, exuberant spirit of the Dutch Golden Age. Notice the details—the happy red face of the man offering us a *berkemeyer* drinking glass, the sparkle in his eyes, the lacy collar, the decorative belt buckle, and so on. Rather than posing his subject, making him stand for hours saying "cheese," Hals tried to catch him at a candid moment. He often painted common people, fishermen, and barflies, such as this one. He had to work quickly to capture the serendipity of the moment. Hals used a stop-action technique, freezing the man in mid-gesture, with the rough brushwork creating a blur that suggests the man is still moving.

Johannes Vermeer (1632-1675) is the master of tranquility and stillness. He creates a clear and silent pool that is a world in itself. Most of his canvases show interiors of Dutch homes, where Dutch women engage in everyday activities, lit by a side window. The Rijksmuseum has the best collection of Vermeers in the world—four of them. (There are only some 34 in captivity.) But each is a small jewel worth lingering over.

Vermeer's *The Milkmaid* (c. 1660) brings out the beauty in everyday things. The subject is ordinary—a kitchen maid—but you could look for hours at the tiny details and rich color tones. These are everyday objects, but they glow in a diffused light: the crunchy crust, the hanging basket, even the rusty nail in the wall with its tiny shadow. In paintings such as *Woman Reading a Letter* (c. 1663), Vermeer's placid scenes often have an air of mystery. The woman is reading a letter. From whom? A lover? A father on a two-year business trip to Indonesia? Not even taking time to sit down, she reads intently, with parted lips and a bowed head. It must be important. (She looks pregnant, adding to the mystery, but that may just be the cut of her clothes.) Again, Vermeer has framed a moment of everyday life. But within this small world are hints of a wider, wilder world—the light coming from the left is obviously from a large window, giving us a whiff of the life going on outside. The map hangs prominently, reminding us of travel, and perhaps of where the letter is from.

Jan Steen (c. 1625-1679, pronounced "yahn stain"), the Norman Rockwell of his day, painted humorous scenes from the lives of the lower classes. As a tavern owner, he observed society firsthand. Find the painting *Adolf and Catharina Croeser* (a.k.a. *The Burgomaster of Delft and His Daughter*, 1655). Steen's well-dressed burgher sits on his front porch, when a poor woman and child approach to beg, putting him squarely between the horns of a moral dilemma. On the one hand, we see his rich home, well-dressed daughter, and a vase of flowers—a symbol that his money came from morally suspect capitalism. On the other hand, there are his poor fellow citizens and the church steeple, reminding him of his Christian duty. In *The Merry Family* (1668), the family is eating, drinking, and singing like there's no tomorrow. The broken eggshells and scattered cookware symbolize waste and extravagance. The neglected proverb tacked to the fireplace reminds us that children will follow in the footsteps of their parents. Dutch Golden Age families were notoriously lenient with their kids. Even today, the Dutch describe a rowdy family as a "Jan Steen household."

Rembrandt van Rijn (1606-1669) is the greatest of all Dutch painters. Whereas most painters specialized in one field—portraits, landscapes, still lifes—Rembrandt excelled in them all. The son of a Leiden miller who owned a waterwheel on the Rhine ("van Rijn"), Rembrandt took Amsterdam by storm with his famous painting *The Anatomy Lesson of Dr. Nicolaes Tulp* (1632, currently in The Hague's Mauritshuis Royal Picture Gallery). The commissions poured in for official portraits, and he was soon wealthy and married. But Holland's war with England (1652-1654) devastated the art market, and Rembrandt's free-spending ways forced him to declare bankruptcy (1656)—the ultimate humiliation in success-oriented Amsterdam. The commissions came more slowly. The money ran out. His mother died. He had to auction off his paintings and furniture to pay debts. He moved out of his fine house to a cheaper place on Rozengracht. His bitter losses added a new wisdom to his work. In his last years, his greatest works were his self-portraits, showing a tired, wrinkled man stoically enduring life's misfortunes. His death effectively marked the end of the Dutch Golden Age.

Start with *Isaac and Rebecca* (a.k.a. *The Jewish Bride*, c. 1665-1669). The man gently draws the woman toward him. She's comfortable enough with him to sink into thought, and she reaches up unconsciously to return the gentle touch. They're young but wizened. This uncommissioned portrait (its subjects remain unknown) is a truly human look at the relationship between two people in love.

At the far end of the Gallery of Honor is the museum's star masterpiece—*The Night Watch* (a.k.a. *The Militia Company of Captain Frans Banninck Cocq*, 1642). This is Rembrandt's most famous—though not necessarily greatest—painting. Created in 1642, when he was 36, it was one of his most important commissions: a group portrait of a company of Amsterdam's Civic Guards to hang in their meeting hall. It's an action shot. With flags waving and drums beating, the guardsmen (who, by the 1640s, were really only an honorary militia of rich bigwigs) spill onto the street from under an arch in the back. These guardsmen on the move epitomize the proud, independent, upwardly mobile Dutch.

Why is *The Night Watch* so famous? Compare it with other, less famous group portraits nearby, where every face is visible and everyone is well-lit, flat, and flashbulb-perfect. By contrast, Rembrandt rousted the Civic Guards off their fat duffs. By adding movement and depth to an otherwise static scene, he took posers and turned them into warriors. He turned a simple portrait into great art.

Now backtrack a few steps to the Gallery of Honor's last alcove to find Rembrandt's *Self-Portrait as the Apostle Paul* (1661). Rembrandt's many self-portraits show us the evolution of a great painter's style, as well as the progress of a genius's life. For Rembrandt, the two were intertwined. In this somber, late self-portrait, the man is 55 but he looks 70. With a lined forehead, a bulbous nose, and messy hair, he peers out from under several coats of glazing, holding old, wrinkled pages. His look is...skeptical? Weary? Resigned to life's misfortunes? Or amused? (He's looking at us, but not *just* at us—remember that a self-portrait is done staring into a mirror.)

This man has seen it all—success, love, money, fatherhood, loss, poverty, death. He took these experiences and wove them into his art. Rembrandt died poor and misunderstood, but he remained very much his own man to the end.

The Rest of the Rijks: Most visitors are here to see the Golden Age art, but the museum has much, much more. The Rijks is dedicated to detailing Dutch history from 1200 until 2000, with upward of 8,000 works on display. There's everything from an

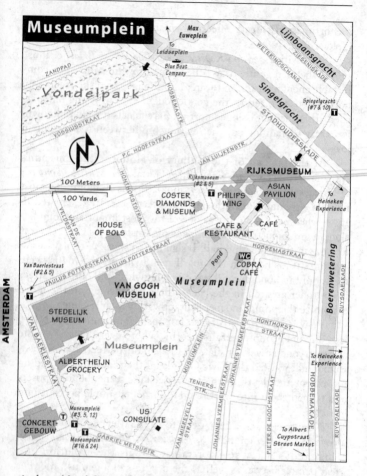

airplane (third floor, in the 20th-century exhibit) to women's fashion and Delftware (lower level). The Asian Art Pavilion shows off 365 objects from Indonesia—a former Dutch colony—as well as items from India, Japan, Korea, and China. (The bronze Dancing Shiva, in Room 1 of the pavilion, is considered one of the best in the world.)

▲▲▲Van Gogh Museum

The Van Gogh Museum (we say "van GO," the Dutch say "van *hock*") is a cultural high even for those not into art. Located near the Rijksmuseum, the museum houses the 200 paintings owned by Vincent's younger brother, Theo. It's a user-friendly stroll through the work and life of one enigmatic man. If you like brightly colored landscapes in the Impressionist style, you'll like this museum. If you enjoy finding deeper meaning in works of art, you'll really love it. The mix of Van Gogh's creative genius, his tumultuous life, and the traveler's determination to connect to it makes this museum as much a walk with Vincent as with his art.

Cost and Hours: €17, more for special exhibits, free for those under 18 and for those with one ear, daily 9:00-18:00, Fri until 22:00 March-Oct, Sat until 22:00 July-Aug and Oct, tel. 020/570-5200, www.vangoghmuseum.nl.

New Entrance: Because the museum is opening a new main entrance in 2015, expect some changes to the entry procedure and the exhibits.

Avoiding Lines: Skip the wait in the ticket-buying line by purchasing advance tickets online (www.vangoghmuseum.nl) or at the TI. Museumkaart holders queue up at a shorter line than ticket buyers. The I amsterdam Card admits you immediately.

Visiting the Museum: The core of the museum is on the first

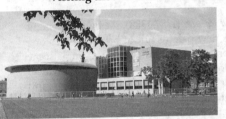

floor. The galleries proceed roughly chronologically, through the changes in Vincent van Gogh's life (1853-1890). The paintings are divided into five periods—the Netherlands, Paris, Arles, St-Rémy, and Auvers-sur-Oise—proceeding clockwise around the floor.

You could see Vincent van Gogh's canvases as a series of suicide notes—or as the record of a life full of beauty...perhaps too full of beauty. He attacked life with a passion, experiencing highs and lows more intensely than the average person. The beauty of the world overwhelmed him; its ugliness struck him as only another dimension of beauty. He tried to absorb the full spectrum of experience, good and bad, and channel it onto a canvas. The frustration of this overwhelming task drove him to madness. If all this is a bit overstated—and I guess it is—it's an attempt to show the emotional impact that Van Gogh's works have had on many people, me included.

Here are some highlights in the first-floor collection. Start with his stark, dark early work in **the Netherlands (1880-1885).** These dark, gray canvases show us the hard, plain existence of the people and town of Nuenen, in the rural southern Netherlands. The style is crude—Van Gogh couldn't draw very well and would never become a great technician. The paint is laid on thick, as though painted with Nuenen mud. The main subject is almost always dead center, with little or no background, so there's a claustrophobic feeling. We are unable to see anything but the immediate surroundings. For example, *The Potato Eaters* (1885) is set in a dark, cramped room lit only by a dim lamp, where poor workers help themselves to a steaming plate of potatoes. They've earned it. Their hands are gnarly, their faces kind. Vincent deliberately wanted the canvas to be potato-colored.

Vincent then moved from rural, religious, poor Holland to the City of Light—**Paris (March 1886–Feb 1888).** The sun begins to break through, lighting up everything he paints. His canvases are more colorful and the landscapes more spacious, with plenty of open sky, giving a feeling of exhilaration after the closed, dark world of Nuenen.

In the cafés and bars of Paris' bohemian Montmartre district, Vincent met the revolutionary Impressionists. At first, Vincent copied from the Impressionist masters. He painted garden scenes like Claude Monet, café snapshots like Edgar Degas, "block prints" like the Japanese masters, and self-portraits like...nobody else.

In his *Self-Portrait as a Painter* (1887–1888), the budding young artist proudly displays his new palette full of bright new colors, trying his hand at the Impressionist technique of building a scene using dabs of different-colored paint. In *Red Cabbages and Onions* (1887), Vincent quickly developed his own style: thicker paint; broad, swirling brushstrokes; and brighter, clashing colors that make even inanimate objects seem to pulsate with life.

Despite his new sociability, Vincent never quite fit in with his Impressionist friends. He wanted peace and quiet, a place where he could throw himself into his work completely. So he headed for a town in the sunny south of France—**Arles (Feb 1888–May 1889).** After the dreary Paris winter, the colors of springtime overwhelmed him. The blossoming trees inspired him to paint canvas after canvas, drenched in sunlight. One fine example is *The Yellow House* (a.k.a. *The Street*, 1888). Vincent rented this house with the green shutters. (He ate at the pink café next door.) Look at that blue sky! He painted in a frenzy, working feverishly to try and take it all in. His unique style evolved beyond Impressionism—thicker paint, stronger outlines, brighter colors (often applied right from the paint tube), and swirling brushwork that makes inanimate objects pulse and vibrate with life.

He invited his friend Paul Gauguin to join him, envisioning a sort of artists' colony in Arles. He spent months preparing a room upstairs for Gauguin's arrival. He painted *Sunflowers* (1889) to brighten up the place. Vincent saw sunflowers as his signature subject, and he painted a half-dozen versions of them, each a study in intense yellow. He said he wanted the colors to shine "like stained glass."

Gauguin arrived. At first, he and Vincent got along great. But then things went sour. They clashed over art, life, and their prickly personalities. On Christmas Eve 1888, Vincent went ballistic.

Enraged during an alcohol-fueled argument, he pulled out a razor and waved it in Gauguin's face. Gauguin took the hint and quickly left town. Vincent was horrified at himself. In a fit of remorse and madness, he mutilated his own ear and presented it to a prostitute.

The people of Arles realized they had a madman on their hands. A doctor diagnosed "acute mania with hallucinations," and the local vicar talked Vincent into admitting himself to a mental hospital in **St-Rémy (May 1889-1890).** In the hospital, Vincent continued to paint whenever he was well enough. We see a change from bright, happy landscapes to more introspective subjects. The colors are less bright and more surreal, the brushwork even more furious. The strong outlines of figures are twisted and tortured, such as in *The Garden of Saint Paul's Hospital* (a.k.a. *Leaf Fall*, 1889). A solitary figure (Vincent?) winds along a narrow, snaky path as the wind blows leaves on him. The colors are surreal—blue, green, and red tree trunks with heavy black outlines. A road runs away from us, heading nowhere.

Vincent moved north to **Auvers-sur-Oise (May-July 1890),** a small town near Paris where he could stay under a doctor friend's supervision. *Wheat Field with Crows* (1890) is one of the last paintings Vincent finished. We can try to search the wreckage of his life for the black box explaining what happened, but there's not much there. His life was sad and tragic, but the record he left is one not of sadness, but of beauty—intense beauty.

The windblown wheat field is a nest of restless energy. Scenes like this must have overwhelmed Vincent with their incredible beauty—too much, too fast, with no release. The sky is stormy and dark blue, almost nighttime, barely lit by two suns boiling through the deep ocean of blue. The road starts nowhere, leads nowhere, disappearing into the burning wheat field. Above all of this swirling beauty fly the crows, the dark ghosts that had hovered over his life since Nuenen.

On July 27, 1890, Vincent left his room, walked out to a nearby field, and put a bullet through his chest. He stumbled back to his room, where he died two days later, with Theo by his side.

The Rest of the Museum: You'll find more paintings by Van Gogh on the second floor (level 2). The third floor has work by fellow painters, those who influenced Vincent and those who were influenced by him. In the basement auditorium (level -1), a 15-minute video gives a basic introduction to Van Gogh. Temporary exhibitions are found in the Kurokawa Wing.

▲▲Stedelijk Museum

The Netherlands' top modern-art museum is filled with a fun, far-out, and refreshing collection that includes post-1945 experimental and conceptual art as well as works by Picasso, Chagall, Cézanne,

Kandinsky, and Mondrian. The Stedelijk (STAYD-eh-lik), like the Rijksmuseum, also boasts a newly spiffed-up building, which now flaunts an architecturally daring entry facing Museumplein (near the Van Gogh Museum).

Before entering, notice the architecture of the modern section (aptly nicknamed "the bathtub") abutting the original older building. Once inside, pick up the current map and envision the museum's four main sections: the permanent collection 1850-1950 (ground floor, right half), design (ground floor, left half), permanent collection 1950-2000 (first floor), and the various temporary exhibits (scattered about, usually some on each floor). Each room comes with thoughtful English descriptions. (And if you're into marijuana, I can't think of a better space than the Stedelijk in which to enjoy its effects.)

Cost and Hours: €15, daily 10:00-18:00, Thu until 22:00, top-notch gift shop, Paulus Potterstraat 13, tram #2 or #5 from Central Station to Van Baerlestraat, tel. 020/573-2911, www.stedelijk.nl. The fine €5 audioguide covers both the permanent and temporary exhibits.

▲Museumplein

Bordered by the Rijks, Van Gogh, and Stedelijk museums, and the Concertgebouw (classical music hall), this park-like square is interesting even to art haters. Amsterdam's best acoustics are found underneath the Rijksmuseum, where street musicians perform everything from chamber music to Mongolian throat singing. Mimes, human statues, and crafts booths dot the square. Skateboarders career across a concrete tube, while locals enjoy a park bench or a coffee at the Cobra Café (playground nearby). And the city's marketing brilliance—the climbable "I amsterdam" letters—awaits as mostly young visitors grab their selfies.

Nearby is **Coster Diamonds,** a handy place to see a diamond-cutting and polishing demo (free, frequent, and interesting 30-minute tours followed by sales pitch, popular for decades with tour groups, prices marked up to include tour guide kickbacks, daily 9:00-17:00, Paulus Potterstraat 2-6, tel. 020/305-5555, www.costerdiamonds. com). The end of the tour leads you straight into their Diamond Museum, which is worthwhile only for those who have a Museumkaart (which covers entry) or feel the need to see even more diamonds (€8.50, daily 9:00-17:00, tel. 020/305-5300, www.diamantmuseumamsterdam.nl). The tour at **Gassan**

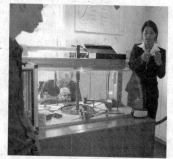

Diamonds is free and better (see page 830), but Coster is convenient to the Museumplein scene.

Heineken Experience

This famous brewery, having moved its operations to the suburbs, has converted its old headquarters into a slick, Disneyesque beerfest—complete with a beer-making simulation ride. The self-guided "experience" also includes do-it-yourself music videos, photo ops that put you inside Heineken logos and labels, and no small amount of hype about the Heineken family and the quality of their beer. It's a fun trip—like an hour at a beer lover's amusement park—if you can ignore the fact that you're essentially paying for 60 minutes of advertising. Note that this place is a huge hit with twentysomething travelers.

Cost and Hours: €18, includes two drinks, daily 11:00-19:00, Fri-Sun until 20:30, longer hours July-Aug, last entry 90 minutes before closing; tram #16, #24, or #25 to Stadhouderskade; an easy walk from Rijksmuseum, Stadhouderskade 78, tel. 020/523-9222, www.heinekenexperience.com.

▲▲Vondelpark

This huge, lively city park is popular with the Dutch—families with little kids, romantic couples, strolling seniors, and hipsters sharing blankets and beers. It's a favored venue for free summer concerts. On a sunny afternoon, it's a hedonistic scene that seems to say, "Parents...relax." The park's 'T Blauwe Theehuis ("The Blue Tea House") is a delightful spot to nurse a drink and take in the scene; see page 845.

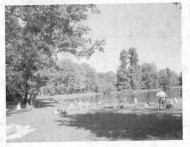

SOUTHERN CANAL BELT

▲Leidseplein

Brimming with cafés, this people-watching mecca is an impromptu stage for street artists, accordionists, jugglers, and unicyclists. It's particularly bustling on sunny afternoons. After dark, it's a vibrant tourists' nightclub center. Stroll nearby Lange Leidsedwarsstraat (one block north) for a taste-bud tour of ethnic eateries, from Greek to Indonesian.

Rembrandtplein

One of the city's premier nightlife spots is the leafy Rembrandtplein (and the adjoining Thorbeckeplein). Rembrandt's statue stands here, along with a jaunty group of life-size statues giving us *The Night Watch* in 3-D—step into the ensemble for a photo-op. Several late-night dance clubs keep the area lively into the wee hours. Utrechtsestraat is lined with upscale shops and restaurants. Nearby Reguliersdwarsstraat (a street one block south of Rembrandtplein) is a center for gay and lesbian nightclubs.

WEST AMSTERDAM
▲▲▲Anne Frank House

A pilgrimage for many, this house offers a fascinating look at the hideaway of young Anne during the Nazi occupation of the Netherlands. Anne, her parents, an older sister, and four others spent a little more than two years in a "Secret Annex" behind her father's business. While in hiding, 13-year-old Anne kept a diary chronicling her extraordinary experience. The thoughtfully designed exhibit offers thorough coverage of the Frank family, the diary, the stories of others who hid, and the Holocaust. Though the eight Jews were eventually discovered, and all but one died in concentration camps, their story has an uplifting twist—the diary of Anne Frank, an affirmation of the human spirit that cannot be crushed.

Cost and Hours: €9, not covered by I amsterdam Card; April-Oct daily 9:00-21:00, Sat and July-Aug until 22:00; Nov-March daily 9:00-19:00, Sat until 21:00; last entry 30 minutes before closing, often less crowded right when it opens or after 18:00, no baggage check, no large bags allowed inside, Prinsengracht 267, near Westerkerk, tel. 020/556-7100, www.annefrank.org.

Avoiding Lines: Expect long ticket-buying lines from opening to closing during summer months, and during midday hours off-season. If you don't have a ticket, try arriving right when the museum opens or after 18:00.

To skip the lines, book a timed-entry ticket online (€9.50, www.annefrank.org) as soon as you're sure of your itinerary. With your ticket in hand, you can bypass the line and ring the buzzer at the low-profile door marked *Entrance: Reservations Only*.

Museumkaart holders (who get in free) can pay €0.50 to reserve an entry time online. Even if you don't have the card yet, choose the Online Ticket Sales option to select a time, then present your confirmation at the "reservations only" door. If you haven't purchased your Museumkaart yet, you can buy one right there.

Visiting the Museum: We'll walk through the rooms where Anne Frank, her parents, her sister, and four other Jews hid for 25 months in the Secret Annex, its entrance concealed by a bookcase. Begin in the **first-floor offices** where Otto Frank ran a successful business called Opekta, selling spices and pectin for making jelly. Photos and displays show Otto with some of his colleagues.

AMSTERDAM

During the Nazi occupation, while the Frank family hid in the back of the building, these brave people kept Otto's business running, secretly bringing supplies to the Franks. Upstairs in the **second-floor warehouse,** two models show the two floors where Anne, her family, and four others lived. All told, eight people lived in a tiny apartment smaller than 1,000 square feet.

In July of 1942, the family and four fellow Jews went into hiding. Otto handed over the keys to the business to his "Aryan" colleagues, sent a final postcard to relatives, gave the family cat to a neighbor, spread rumors that they were fleeing to Switzerland, and prepared his family to "dive under" (*onderduik,* as it was called).

At the back of the second floor warehouse is the clever hidden passageway into the Secret Annex. Though not exactly a secret (since it's hard to hide an entire building), the annex was a typical back-house *(achterhuis),* a common feature in Amsterdam buildings, and the Nazis had no reason to suspect anything on the premises of the legitimate Opekta business.

Pass through the bookcase entrance into **Otto, Edith, and Margot's Room.** The room is very small, even without the furniture. Imagine yourself and two fellow tourists confined here for two years. Pencil lines on the wall track Margot's and Anne's heights, marking the point at which these growing lives were cut short.

Next is **Anne Frank's Room.** Pan the room clockwise to see some of the young girl's idols in photos and clippings she pasted there herself: American actor Robert Stack, the future Queen Elizabeth II as a child, matinee idol Rudy Vallee, figure-skating actress Sonja Henie, and, on the other wall, actress Greta Garbo, actor Ray Milland, Renaissance man Leonardo da Vinci, and actress Ginger Rogers.

Out the window (which had to be blacked out) is the back courtyard, which had a chestnut tree and a few buildings. These things, along with the Westerkerk bell chiming every 15 minutes, represented the borders of Anne's "outside world."

Ascend the steep staircase—silently—to the **Common Living Room.** This was also the kitchen and dining room. Otto Frank was well off, and early on, the annex was well-stocked with food. Later, as war and German restrictions plunged Holland into poverty and famine, they survived on canned foods and dried kidney beans. At night, the living room became a sleeping quarters.

The next space is **Peter van Pels' Room.** Initially, Anne was cool toward Peter, but after two years together, a courtship developed, and their flirtation culminated in a kiss. The **staircase** (no visitor access) leads up to where they stored their food. Anne loved to steal away here for a bit of privacy. At night they'd open a hatch to let in fresh air. From here we leave the Secret Annex, passing displays as we return to the Opekta storeroom and offices in the front house.

On August 4, 1944, a German policeman accompanied by three Dutch Nazis pulled up in a car, politely entered the Opekta office, and went straight to the bookcase entrance. No one knows who tipped them off. Eventually the Franks were sent to Auschwitz, a Nazi extermination camp in Poland (see the transport list, which includes "Anneliese Frank"). On the platform at Auschwitz, they were "forcibly separated from each other" (as Otto later reported) and sent to different camps. Anne and Margot were sent to Bergen-Belsen. They both died of typhus in March of 1945, only weeks before the camp was liberated. The other Secret Annex residents—except Otto—were gassed or died of disease.

The Rest of the Museum: The Otto Frank Room has a 1967 video of Anne's father talking about how the diaries were discovered in the annex. Downstairs you can see Anne's three diaries, which were published after the war. Other displays tell the story of those who helped the Franks, those who survived, and the Anne Frank legacy.

The Anne Frank Foundation is obviously concerned that we learn from Europe's Nazi nightmare. It was Otto Frank's dream that visitors come away from the Anne Frank House with an indelible impression—and a better ability to apply these lessons to our contemporary challenges. He wrote: "The task that Anne entrusted to me continually gives me new strength to strive for reconciliation and for human rights all over the world."

Westerkerk

Located near the Anne Frank House, this landmark Protestant church has an appropriately barren interior, Rembrandt's body buried somewhere under the pews, and Amsterdam's tallest steeple.

While the church is free to visit, the Westerkerk tower is climbable only with a guided tour. The English-language, 30-minute tour takes you on a 185-step climb, rewarding you with a look at the carillon and grand city views. Tours are limited to six people; to reserve a spot, come in person on the same day or call.

Cost and Hours: Church entry free, generally April-Sept Mon-Sat 11:00-15:00, closed Sun and Oct-March; tower-€8 by tour only, April-Oct Mon-Sat 10:00-18:00, May-Aug until 20:00, closed Sun and Nov-March; tours leave on the half-hour, last tour leaves 30 minutes before closing; Prinsengracht 281, tel. 020/624-7766, www.westerkerk.nl.

CENTRAL AMSTERDAM, NEAR DAM SQUARE
▲Royal Palace (Koninklijk Huis)

This palace was built as a lavish city hall (1648-1655), when Holland was a proud new republic and Amsterdam was the richest city on the planet—awash in profit from trade. The building became a "Royal Palace" when Napoleon installed his brother Louis as king (1806). After Napoleon's fall, it continued as a royal residence for the Dutch royal family, the House of Orange. Today, it's one of King Willem-Alexander's official residences, with a single impressive floor open to the public. Visitors can gawk at a grand hall and stroll about 20 rooms branching off from it, all of them lavishly decorated with chandeliers, paintings, statues, and furniture that reflect Amsterdam's former status as the center of global trade.

Cost and Hours: €10, includes audioguide, daily 11:00-17:00 but often closed for official business, last entry 30 minutes before closing, tel. 020/620-4060, www.paleisamsterdam.nl.

▲Begijnhof

Stepping into this tiny, idyllic courtyard in the city center, you escape into the charm of old Amsterdam. (Please be considerate of the people who live around the courtyard, and don't photograph the residents or their homes.) Notice house #34, a 500-year-old wooden structure (rare, since repeated fires taught city fathers a trick called brick). Peek into the hidden Catholic church, dating from the time when post-Reformation Dutch Catholics couldn't worship in public. It's opposite the English Reformed church, where the Pilgrims worshipped while waiting for their voyage to the New World—marked by a plaque near the door.

Cost and Hours: Free, daily 8:00-17:00, on Begijnensteeg lane, just off Kalverstraat between #130 and #132, pick up flier at office near entrance, www.ercadam.nl.

▲▲Amsterdam Museum

Housed in a 500-year-old former orphanage, this creative museum traces the city's growth from fishing village to world trade center to hippie haven. The key is to not get lost somewhere in the 17th century as you navigate the meandering maze of rooms. The museum tries hard to make the city's history engaging and fun (almost too hard—it dropped "history" from its name for fear of putting people off). But the story of Amsterdam is indeed engaging and fun, and this is the only museum in town designed to tell it.

Start with the easy-to-follow "DNA" section, which hits the historic highlights from 1000 to 2000. The city was built atop pilings in marshy soil (the museum stands only four feet above sea level). By 1500, they'd built a ring of canals and established the sea trade. The Golden Age (1600s) is illustrated by fine paintings of citizens, including Rembrandt's portrait of his wife Saskia.

AMSTERDAM

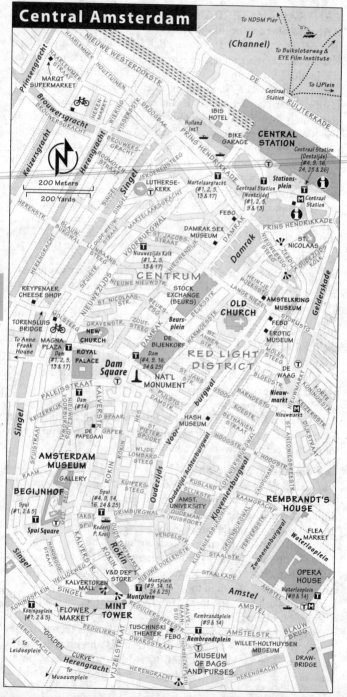

Central Amsterdam

IJ (Channel)

To NDSM Pier

To Buiksloterweg & EYE Film Institute

To IJPlein

Centraal Station

CENTRAL STATION

RUIJTERKADE

NIEUWE WESTERDOKSTR.

HAARLEMMER

HAARLEMMERSTR.

HOUTTUINEN

DE

Prinsengracht

Keizersgracht

Herengracht

Singel

MARQT SUPERMARKET

Brouwersgracht

BROUWERSGRACHT

ROOMOLENSTRAAT

IBIS HOTEL

Holland Int'l

BIKE GARAGE

PRINS HENDRIKKADE

Centraal Station (Oostzijde) (#4, 9, 16, 24, 25 & 26)

Stationsplein

Centraal Station

Centraal Station (Westzijde) (#1, 2, 5, 9 & 13)

LUTHERSE-KERK

Martelaargracht (#1, 2, 5, 13 & 17)

MARTELAARSGRACHT

JEROENSTEEG

200 Meters

200 Yards

FEBO

DAMRAK SEX MUSEUM

PRINS HENDRIKKADE

ST. NICOLAAS

GELDERSKADE

OUDEZIJDS KOLK

Voorburgwal

Nieuwezijds Kolk (#1, 2, 5, 13 & 17)

ST. JACOBS STRAAT

NIEUWENDIJK

DAMRAK

Damrak

HEINTJE

ZEEDIJK

NIEUWEBRUGSTEEG

LANGE NIEZEL

CENTRUM

NIEUWE NIEUWSTR.

STOCK EXCHANGE (BEURS)

OLD CHURCH

AMSTELKRING MUSEUM

REYPENAER CHEESE SHOP

ST. NICOLAASSTR.

GRAVENSTR.

BEURS PSG.

Beursplein

WARMOESSTR.

FEBO

EROTIC MUSEUM

STORMSTG.

MOLENSTEEG

TORENSLUIS BRIDGE

MAGNA PLAZA

NEW CHURCH

ZOUTSTEEG

DE BIJENKORF

Dam (#4, 9, 16, 24 & 25)

ST. ANNENSTR.

RED LIGHT

ST. JANSSTR.

DISTRICT

DE WAAG

Nieuwmarkt

KORTE KONINGSSTR.

To Anne Frank House

ROYAL PALACE

Dam Square

NAT'L MONUMENT

Dam (#1, 2, 5, 13 & 17)

PIJLSTG.

DAMSTR.

WARMOESSTR.

BARNDESTG.

Nieuwmarkt

NIEUWMARKT

KEIZERSSTR.

PALEISSTRAAT

Dam (#14)

KALVERSTR.

SPAAR.

NES

HASH MUSEUM

KOESTR.

BETHANIEN-STRAAT

ST. ANTONIESBREESTR.

DIJKSTRAAT

Singel

KEIZERSRIJK

NIEUWEZIJDS VOORBURGWAL

ST. PIETER-SPOORT

Voor-burgwal

HOOGSTR.

DE PAPEGAAI

GAPER.

WIJDE LOMBARD-STEEG

N. HOOGSTR.

RUSLAND

SLIJKSTR.

ZANDSTR.

AMSTERDAM MUSEUM

GALLERY

ROKIN

KUIPERS-STEEG

Oudezijds Achterburgwal

KLOVENIERSBURGWAL

RAAMGRACHT

REMBRANDT'S HOUSE

BEGIJNHOF

Spui (#1, 2 & 5)

RAAM

Spui (#4, 9, 14, 16, 24 & 25)

GRIMBURGWAL

AMST. UNIVERSITY

OUDE-MANHUISPOORT

GROENBURGWAL

ZWANENBURGWAL

FLEA MARKET

Waterlooplein

Spui Square

TAKSTR.

Rederij P. Kooij

OUDE TURFMARKT

NIEUWE DOELENSTR.

VENDELSTR.

VERVERSTR.

STAALSTR.

OPERA HOUSE

Waterlooplein (#9 & 14)

Singel

KALVERSTR.

ROKIN

Amstel

V&D DEP'T STORE

Muntplein (#9, 14, 16, 24 & 25)

STAALKADE

Zwanenburgwal

KALVERTOREN MALL

HANDBOOGSTRAAT

HEILIGEWEG

SINGEL

Muntplein

MINT TOWER

Rembrandtplein (#9 & 14)

Rembrandtplein

DRAW-BRIDGE

Koningsplein (#1, 2 & 5)

Koningsplein

FLOWER MARKET

REGULIERSBREESTR.

TUSCHINSKI THEATER

FEBO

WILLET-HOLTHUYSEN MUSEUM

AMSTEL

BLAUW BRUG

To Leidseplein

"GOLDEN

REGULIERS

HALVE

AMSTELSTR.

CURVE"

Herengracht

REGULIERSDWARSSTRAAT

VIJZELSTRAAT

MUSEUM OF BAGS AND PURSES

HERENGRACHT

To Museumplein

HERENGRACHT

The 1800s brought modernization and new technologies, like the bicycle. After the gloom of World War II, Amsterdam emerged to become the "Capital of Freedom." The museum's free pedestrian corridor—lined with old-time group portraits—is a powerful teaser.

Cost and Hours: €11, daily 10:00-17:00, one-hour audioguide-€4, pleasant restaurant, next to Begijnhof at Kalverstraat 92, tel. 020/523-1822, www.ahm.nl. This museum is a fine place to buy the Museumkaart (for details, see page 800).

RED LIGHT DISTRICT
▲▲Amstelkring Museum
Although Amsterdam has long been known for its tolerant attitudes, 16th-century politics forced Dutch Catholics to worship discreetly. At this museum near Central Station, you'll find a fascinating, hidden Catholic church filling the attic of three 17th-century merchants' houses.

For two centuries (1578-1795), Catholicism in Amsterdam was illegal but tolerated (like pot in the 1970s). When hardline Protestants took power in 1578, Catholic churches were vandalized and shut down, priests and monks were rounded up and kicked out of town, and Catholic kids were razzed on their way to school. The city's Catholics were forbidden to worship openly, so they gathered secretly to say Mass in homes and offices. In 1663, a wealthy merchant built Our Lord in the Attic (Ons' Lieve Heer op Solder), one of a handful of places in Amsterdam that served as a secret parish church until Catholics were once again allowed to worship in public. This unique church—embedded within a townhouse in the middle of the Red Light District—comes with a little bonus: a rare glimpse inside a historic Amsterdam home straight out of a Vermeer painting. Don't miss the silver collection and other exhibits of daily life from 300 years ago.

Cost and Hours: €8, includes audioguide, Mon-Sat 10:00-17:00, Sun and holidays 13:00-17:00, no photos, Oudezijds Voorburgwal 40, tel. 020/624-6604, www.opsolder.nl.

▲▲Red Light District Walk
Europe's most popular ladies of the night tease and tempt here, as they have for centuries, in several hundred display-case windows around Oudezijds Achterburgwal and Oudezijds Voorburgwal, surrounding the Old Church (Oude Kerk, described later). If you're in town only for the day, the area still offers a fascinating stroll. If you're spending the night in Amsterdam before or after your cruise, this neighborhood is a fascinating walk in the early evening—but drunks and druggies make the streets uncomfortable late at night after the gawking tour groups leave (about 22:30).

AMSTERDAM

The neighborhood, one of Amsterdam's oldest, has hosted prostitutes since 1200. Prostitution is entirely legal here, and the prostitutes are generally entrepreneurs, renting space and running their own businesses, as well as filling out tax returns and even paying union dues. Popular prostitutes net about €500 a day (for what's called "S&F" in its abbreviated, printable form, charging €30-50 per customer).

Sex Museums

Amsterdam has three sex museums: two in the Red Light District and another one a block in front of Central Station on Damrak street. While visiting one can be called sightseeing, visiting more than that is harder to explain. The one on Damrak is the cheapest and most interesting. Here's a comparison:

The **Damrak Sex Museum** tells the story of pornography from Roman times through 1960. Every sexual deviation is revealed in various displays. The museum includes early French pornographic photos; memorabilia from Europe, India, and Asia; a Marilyn Monroe tribute; and some S&M displays (€4, not covered by Museumkaart, daily 9:30-23:00, Damrak 18, a block in front of Central Station, tel. 020/622-8376).

The **Erotic Museum** in the Red Light District is five floors of uninspired paintings, videos, old photos, and sculpture (€7, not covered by Museumkaart, daily 11:00-24:00, along the canal at Oudezijds Achterburgwal 54, tel. 020/624-7303).

Red Light Secrets Museum of Prostitution is a pricey look at the world's oldest profession. If you're wondering what it's like to sit in those red booths, watch the video taken from the prostitute's perspective as "johns" check you out. The exhibit is much smaller than the others (€7.50, not covered by Museumkaart, daily 12:00-24:00, Oudezijds Achterburgwal 60, tel. 020/662-5300).

Old Church (Oude Kerk)

This 14th-century landmark—the needle around which the Red Light District spins—has served as a reassuring welcome-home symbol to sailors, a refuge to the downtrodden, an ideological battlefield of the Counter-Reformation, and, today, a tourist sight with a dull interior.

Cost and Hours: €7.50, Mon-Sat 10:00-18:00, Sun 13:00-17:30, free carillon concerts Tue and Sat at 16:00, tel. 020/625-8284, www.oudekerk.nl. It's 167 steps to the top of the church tower (€7, April-Sept Thu-Sat only 13:00-17:00, visits leave every half-hour).

Marijuana Sights in the Red Light District

Three related establishments cluster together along a canal in the Red Light District. The **Hash, Marijuana, and Hemp Museum,** worth ▲, is the most worthwhile of the three; it shares a ticket with the less substantial **Hemp Gallery.** Right nearby is **Cannabis College,** a free nonprofit center that's "dedicated to ending the global war against the cannabis plant through public education." For more information, see "Smoking in Amsterdam" on page 850.

Cost and Hours: Museum and gallery-€9, daily 10:00-23:00, Oudezijds Achterburgwal 148, tel. 020/624-8926, www. hashmuseum.com. College entry free, daily 11:00-19:00, Oudezijds Achterburgwal 124, tel. 020/423-4420, www.cannabiscollege.com.

NORTHEAST AMSTERDAM
NEMO (National Center for Science and Technology)

This kid-friendly science museum is a city landmark. Its distinctive copper-green building juts up from the water like a sinking ship.

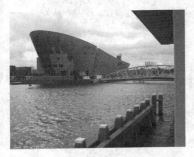

Several floors feature exhibits that allow kids (and adults) to explore topics such as light, sound, and gravity, and play with bubbles, topple giant dominoes, and draw with lasers.

Up top is a restaurant with a great city view, as well as a sloping terrace that becomes a popular "beach" in summer, complete with lounge chairs and a lively bar. On the bottom floor is a cafeteria offering €5 sandwiches.

Cost and Hours: €15, June-Aug daily 10:00-17:30, Sept-May generally closed Mon, tel. 020/531-3233, www.e-nemo.nl. The roof terrace—open until 19:00 in the summer—is generally free.

Getting There: It's above the entrance to the IJ tunnel at Oosterdok 2. From Central Station, you can walk there in 15 minutes, or take bus #22 or #48 to the Kadijksplein stop.

▲▲Netherlands Maritime Museum
(Nederlands Scheepvaartmuseum)

This huge, kid-friendly collection of model ships, maps, and sea-battle paintings fills the 300-year-old Dutch Navy Arsenal (cleverly located a little ways from the city center, as this was where they stored the gunpowder). The "Paintings" rooms illustrate how ships changed from sail to steam, and how painting styles changed from realistic battle scenes to Romantic seascapes to Impressionism and Cubism.

The "Navigational Instruments" section has quadrants (a wedge-shaped tool you could line up with the horizon and the stars to determine your location), compasses, and plumb lines. In "Ornamentation," admire the busty gals that adorned the prows of

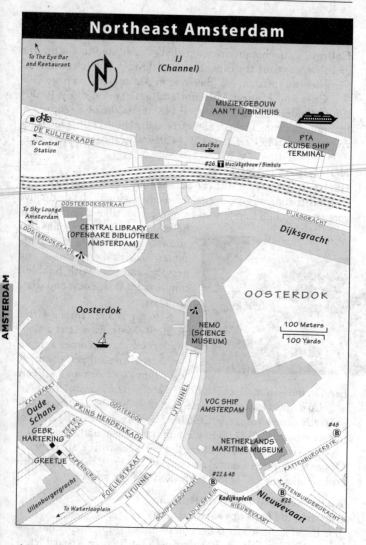

Northeast Amsterdam

To The Eye Bar
and Restaurant

IJ
(Channel)

N

MUZIEKGEBOUW
AAN 'T IJ/BIMHUIS

PTA
CRUISE SHIP
TERMINAL

DE RUIJTERKADE

To Central
Station

Canal Bus

#26 T Muziekgebouw / Bimhuis

OOSTERDOKSSTRAAT

To Sky Lounge
Amsterdam

DIJKSGRACHT

Dijksgracht

CENTRAL LIBRARY
(OPENBARE BIBLIOTHEEK
AMSTERDAM)

OOSTERDOKSKADE

OOSTERDOK

Oosterdok

NEMO
(SCIENCE
MUSEUM)

100 Meters

100 Yards

VOC SHIP
AMSTERDAM

KALKMARKT

Oude
Schans

PRINS HENDRIKKADE

OOSTERDOK

#48
B

PEPER-
STRAAT

GEBR.
HARTERING

NETHERLANDS
MARITIME MUSEUM

GREETJE

KATTENBURGERSTR.

KAPENBURG

IJTUNNEL

FOELIESTRAAT

#22 & 48
B

KATTENBURGERGRACHT

#22
B

Kadijksplein

Nieuwevaart

Uilenburgergracht

To Waterlooplein

SCHIPPERSGRACHT

KADIJKSPLEIN

NIEUWEVAART

AMSTERDAM

ships, and learn of their symbolic meaning for superstitious sailors.

Downstairs on the first floor, see "Yacht Models" through the ages, from early warships to today's luxury vessels. The section on "Atlases" (i.e., maps) shows how human consciousness expanded as knowledge of the earth grew. The west wing is more kid-oriented and less meaty, with an exhibit on whales and a friendly look at the Golden Age.

The finale is a chance to explore below the decks of an old tall-masted ship, a replica of the *Amsterdam*, a 18th-century cargo ship. Given the Dutch seafaring heritage, this is an appropriately important and impressive place.

Cost and Hours: €15 covers both museum and ship, both open daily 9:00-17:00, bus #22 or #48 from Central Station to Kattenburgerplein 1, tel. 020/523-2222, www.scheepvaartmuseum.nl.

SOUTHEAST AMSTERDAM

To reach the following sights from the train station, take tram #9 or #14. All of these sights (except the Tropical Museum) are close to one another and can easily be connected into an interesting walk—or, better yet, a bike ride. Several of the sights in southeast Amsterdam cluster near the large square, Waterlooplein, dominated by the modern opera house.

Waterlooplein Flea Market

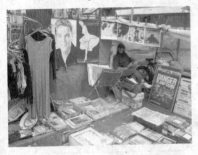

For more than a hundred years, the Jewish Quarter flea market has raged daily except Sunday (at the Waterlooplein metro station, behind Rembrandt's House). The long, narrow park is filled with stalls selling cheap clothes, hippie stuff, old records, tourist knickknacks, and garage-sale junk.

▲Rembrandt's House (Museum Het Rembrandthuis)

A middle-aged Rembrandt lived here from 1639 to 1658 after his wife's death, as his popularity and wealth dwindled down to obscurity and bankruptcy. As you enter, ask when the next etching or painting demonstration is scheduled and pick up the excellent audioguide.

Start with the video on Rembrandt's life—his rise, peak, and fall—then tour the rooms. The house is reconstructed and filled with period objects (not his actual belongings) that re-create what his bankruptcy inventory of 1656 said he owned. You'll see his well-equipped kitchen and big entrance hall. His art cabinet is filled with odd curios collected by this eccentric genius—shells, books, classical busts, and a Baroque-era jackalope. In his large studio, imagine him at work, creating *The Night Watch*, *The Portrait of Maria Trip*, and numerous self-portraits (seen at the Rijksmuseum). You can attend an

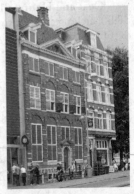

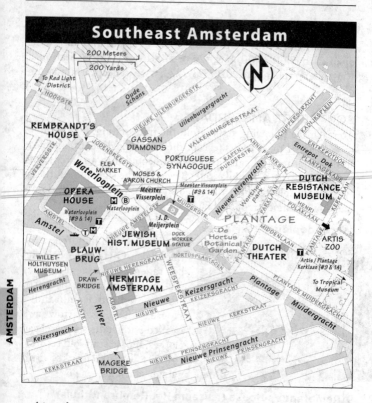

Southeast Amsterdam

etching demonstration and ask the printer to explain the etching process (drawing in soft wax on a metal plate that's then dipped in acid, inked up, and printed). For the finale, enjoy several rooms of original Rembrandt etchings. You're not likely to see a single Rembrandt painting, but the master's etchings are marvelous and well-described. I came away wanting to know more about the man and his art.

Cost and Hours: €12.50, includes audioguide, daily 10:00-18:00, etching and painting demonstrations almost hourly between 11:00 and 15:00, Jodenbreestraat 4, tel. 020/520-0400, www.rembrandthuis.nl.

▲Diamonds

Many shops in this "city of diamonds" offer tours. These tours come with two parts: a chance to see experts behind magnifying glasses polishing the facets of precious diamonds, followed by a visit to an intimate sales room to see (and perhaps buy) a mighty shiny yet very tiny souvenir.

The handy and professional **Gassan Diamonds** facility fills a huge warehouse one block from Rembrandt's House. A visit here plops you in the big-tour-group fray (notice how each tour group has a color-coded sticker so they know which guide gets the commission on what they buy). You'll get a sticker, join a free 15-minute tour to see a polisher at work, and hear a general explanation of the process. Then you'll have an opportunity to sit down and have color and clarity described and illustrated with diamonds ranging in value from

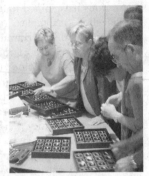

$100 to $30,000. Before or after, you can have a free cup of coffee in the waiting room across the parking lot (daily 9:00-17:00, Nieuwe Uilenburgerstraat 173-175, tel. 020/622-5333, www.gassan. com, handy WC). Another company, **Coster**, also offers diamond demos. They're not as good as Gassan's, but convenient if you're near the Rijksmuseum (described on page 810).

▲▲Hermitage Amsterdam

The famous Hermitage Museum in St. Petersburg, Russia (described on page 387), loans art to Amsterdam for a series of rotating, and often exquisitely beautiful, special exhibits in the Amstelhof, a 17th-century former nursing home that takes up a whole city block along the Amstel River.

Why is there Russian-owned art in Amsterdam? The Hermitage collection in St. Petersburg is so vast that they can only show about 5 percent of it at any one time. Therefore, the Hermitage is establishing satellite collections around the world. The one here in Amsterdam is the biggest, filling the large Amstelhof.

Cost and Hours: Generally €15, but price varies with exhibit; daily 10:00-17:00, come later in the day to avoid crowds, audioguide-€4, mandatory free bag check, café, Nieuwe Herengracht 14, tram #9 from the train station, recorded info tel. 020/530-7488, www.hermitage.nl.

▲Jewish Historical Museum (Joods Historisch Museum)

This interesting museum tells the story of the Netherlands' Jews through three centuries, serving as a good introduction to Judaism and Jewish customs and religious traditions.

Originally opened in 1932, the museum was forced to close during the Nazi years. Recent renovations have joined four historic former synagogues together into one modern complex. Your ticket also includes the Portuguese Synagogue a half-block away.

The centerpiece of the museum is the Great Synagogue. First see its ground floor (for an overview of Jewish culture), then go upstairs to the women's gallery (for history from 1600 to 1900). Next comes the 20th century (housed in the former New Synagogue) and the grim era of the Nazi occupation, which decimated the community. Personal artifacts—chairs, clothes—tell the devastating history in a very real way. Downstairs (in the Aanbouw Annex) are temporary exhibits, generally showing the work of Jewish artists from around the world. Then, with the same ticket, finish your visit by crossing the street to the Portuguese Synagogue, with its treasury.

Cost and Hours: €12, includes Portuguese Synagogue, more for special exhibits, ticket also covers Dutch Theater—see next listing; museum daily 11:00-17:00, Portuguese Synagogue daily 10:00-16:00, last entry 30 minutes before closing; free audioguides cover the Great Synagogue and Portuguese Synagogue, displays all have English explanations, children's museum, Jonas Daniel Meijerplein 2, tel. 020/531-0310, www.jhm.nl. The museum has a modern, minimalist, kosher café.

▲Dutch Theater (Hollandsche Schouwburg)

Once a lively theater in the Jewish neighborhood, and today a moving memorial, this building was used as an assembly hall for local Jews destined for Nazi concentration camps. On the wall, 6,700 family names pay tribute to the 104,000 Jews deported and killed by the Nazis. Some 70,000 victims spent time here, awaiting transfer to concentration camps. Upstairs is a small history exhibit with a model of the ghetto, plus photos and memorabilia (such as shoes and letters) of some victims, putting a human face on the staggering numbers. Television monitors show actual footage of the Nazis rounding up Amsterdam's Jews. 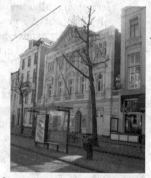 You can also see a few costumes from the days when the building was a theater. While the exhibit is small, it offers plenty to think about. Back in the ground-floor courtyard, notice the hopeful messages that visiting school groups attach to the wooden tulips.

Cost and Hours: Covered by €12 Jewish Historical Museum ticket, daily 11:00-17:00, last entry 30 minutes before closing, Plantage Middenlaan 24, tel. 020/531-0380, www. hollandscheschouwburg.nl.

▲▲Dutch Resistance Museum (Verzetsmuseum)

This is an impressive look at how the Dutch resisted (or collaborated with) their Nazi occupiers from 1940 to 1945. You'll see

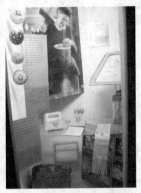

propaganda movie clips, study forged ID cards under a magnifying glass, and read about ingenious and courageous efforts—big and small—to hide local Jews from the Germans and undermine the Nazi regime.

The museum does a good job of presenting the Dutch people's struggle with a timeless moral dilemma: Is it better to collaborate with a wicked system to effect small-scale change—or to resist outright, even if your efforts are doomed to fail? You'll learn why some parts of Dutch society opted for the former, and others for the latter.

Cost and Hours: €10 includes audioguide; Tue-Fri 10:00-17:00, Sat-Mon 11:00-17:00, English descriptions, no flash photos, mandatory and free bag check, tram #9 from station or #14 from Dam Square, Plantage Kerklaan 61, tel. 020/620-2535, www.verzetsmuseum.org.

▲Tropical Museum (Tropenmuseum)

As close to the Third World as you'll get without lots of vaccinations, this imaginative museum offers wonderful re-creations of tropical life and explanations of Third World problems (largely created by Dutch colonialism and the slave trade). Ride the elevator to the top floor, and circle your way down through this immense collection, opened in 1926 to give the Dutch people a peek at their vast colonial holdings. Don't miss the display case where you can see and hear the world's most exotic musical instruments. The Ekeko cafeteria serves tropical food.

Cost and Hours: €12.50, Tue-Sun 10:00-17:00, closed Mon, tram #9 to Linnaeusstraat 2, tel. 020/568-8200, www.tropenmuseum.nl.

Shopping in Amsterdam

Amsterdam brings out the browser even in those who were not born to shop. Amsterdam has lots of one-of-a-kind specialty stores, street markets, and specific streets and neighborhoods worthy of a browse. Poke around and see what you can find. For information on shopping, pick up the TI's *Shopping in Amsterdam* brochure.

Ten general markets, open six days a week (generally 9:30-17:00, closed Sun), keep folks who brake for garage sales pulling U-turns. Markets include **Waterlooplein** (the flea market, described later), the huge **Albert Cuyp** street market (in the De Pijp District near the Rijksmuseum), and various flower markets (such as the Singel canal **Flower Market** near the Mint Tower).

Most shops in the center are open 10:00-18:00 (later on Thu—typically until 20:00 or 21:00); the businesslike Dutch know no siesta, but many shopkeepers take Sundays and Monday mornings off.

Department Stores

When you need to buy something but don't know where to go, two chain stores are handy for everything from inexpensive clothes and notebooks to food and cosmetics. **Hema** is at Kalverstraat 212, in the Kalvertoren mall, and at Central Station. **Vroom & Dreesmann (V&D),** with its great La Place cafeteria, is at Kalverstraat 203.

The **De Bijenkorf** department store, towering high above Dam Square, is Amsterdam's top-end option and worth a look even if you're not shopping. It sparkles with name brands, which are actually independent stores operating under the Bijenkorf roof. The entire fifth floor is a ritzy self-service cafeteria with a fine rooftop terrace.

Shopping Zones

Amsterdam has four top shopping areas—all equally good, but each with a different flavor: The Nine Little Streets (touristy, tidy, and central); Haarlemmerstraat/Haarlemmerdijk (emerging, borderline-edgy neighborhood of creative, unpretentious shops); Staalstraat (postcard-cute, short-and-sweet street tucked just away from the tourist crowds); and the Jordaan (mellow residential zone with a smattering of fine shops).

The Nine Little Streets (De Negen Straatjes): This handy central zone—hemmed in by a grid plan between Dam Square and the Jordaan—is home to a diverse array of shops mixing festive, inventive, nostalgic, practical, and artistic items. Trendy cafés dot the area. While not quite as artsy or funky as it once was, this zone remains a very convenient place to browse. Walking west from the Amsterdam Museum/Spui Square or south from the Anne Frank House puts you right in the thick of things; see the map on page 838. For a preview, see www.theninestreets.com.

Haarlemmerstraat/Haarlemmerdijk: A bit grotty until recently, the area just west of Central Station has morphed into a thriving and trendy string of shops, cafés, and restaurants. It has arguably the most inspired and eclectic assortment of shops in Amsterdam—a browse here is a fun chance to spot new trends, and maybe to pick up some local clothes and goods (vintage and casual young fashions abound). The former dike along what was Amsterdam's harborfront provides the high spine of this neighborhood. From the Singel canal near Central Station, this lively drag leads a half-mile west along a colorful string of lanes, all the way to Haarlem Gate, a triumphal arch built in the 1840s.

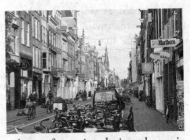

Staalstraat: This lively street, boasting more than its share of creative design shops, is tucked in a youthful area just east of the university zone (see map on page 824). **Retro & Chic** sells vintage, while the **Juggle** shop is a fun spot to browse for all of your juggling needs. **Droog,** despite a name that evokes controlled substances, is actually a "destination" design store that is half gallery (with cutting-edge installations) and half shop (selling a bumper crop of clever kitchen and household gadgets you never knew you desperately wanted). Nearby is the bustling **Waterlooplein flea market.**

The Jordaan: Once a working-class district, this colorful old neighborhood is now upscale—a veritable wonderland of funky shops. **Rozengracht,** the wide street just southwest of the Anne Frank House, has several eclectic shops. **Antiekcentrum Amsterdam** isn't just an antique mall—it's a sprawling warren of display cases crammed with historic bric-a-brac (including lots of smaller items, easily packed home), and all of it for sale. You'll find everything from old helmets and medals to vintage blue tiles (closed Tue, Elandsgracht 109, www.antiekcentrumamsterdam.nl). The cross-street **Hazenstraat** has a fine assortment of art galleries and other shops. **Eerste** and **Tweede Egelantierssdwarsstraat,** both lined with great restaurants and recommended in "Eating in Amsterdam," also have some fun shops mixed in.

Eating in Amsterdam

Amsterdam has a thriving restaurant scene. In this international city, there's something for every taste. While I've listed options, one good strategy is simply to pick an area and wander.

Along the main tourist spine, the sloppy food ghetto thrives around Leidseplein; if you want to eat with a bunch of rowdy Aussies in a very touristy zone, wander along Leidseplein's "Restaurant Row" (on Leidsedwarsstraat). The area around Spui Square and that end of Spuistraat is also trendy, though not as noisy. For fewer crowds, better food and service, and far more charm, head a few blocks west, into the Jordaan district, which has its own, more authentically Dutch "Restaurant Row" (on Tweede Egelantierssdwarsstraat). For a local take on restaurants, check out this food blog: www.dutchgrub.com.

Note that many of my listings are lunch-only (usually termed "café" rather than "restaurant")—good for a handy bite near major sights. Similarly, many top restaurants serve only dinner. Before trekking across town to any of my listings, check the hours.

Before you leave Amsterdam, try to have a drink at a brown café; see page 848.

CENTRAL AMSTERDAM

You'll likely have lunch at some point in the city's core, but you'll find a better range of more satisfying choices in the Jordaan area of West Amsterdam (described later). For the locations of these eateries, see the "West/Central Amsterdam Restaurants" map on page 839.

On and near Spui

Gartine is a hidden gem, filling a rustic and relaxed but border-line-elegant little space tucked just off the tourist-thronged Spui and Rokin zones. It's a calm and classy spot for a good lunch (€6-9 open-faced sandwiches, €16-20 high tea, Wed-Sun 10:00-18:00, closed Mon-Tue, Taksteeg 7, tel. 020/320-4132).

Restaurant Kantjil en de Tijger is a lively, modern place with a plain and noisy ambience, full of happy, youthful eaters who know a good value. The food is purely Indonesian; the waiters are happy to explain your many enticing options. Their three *rijsttafels* (traditional "rice tables" with about a dozen small courses) range from €25 to €33 per person. Though they are designed for two people, three people can make a meal by getting a *rijsttafel* for two plus a soup or light dish (daily 12:00-23:00, reservations smart, mostly indoor with a little outdoor seating, Spuistraat 291, tel. 020/620-0994, www.kantjil.nl).

Kantjil to Go is a tiny take-out bar serving up inexpensive Indonesian fare. Their printed menu explains the mix-and-match plan (€6 for medium, €7.50 for large, daily 12:00-21:00, a half-block off Spui Square at Nieuwezijds Voorburgwal 342, behind the restaurant listed above, tel. 020/620-3074). Split a large box, grab a bench on the charming Spui Square around the corner, and you've got perhaps the best cheap, hot meal in town.

Pannenkoekenhuis Upstairs is a tight, tiny (just four tables), characteristic perch up some extremely steep stairs, where Arno and Ali cook and serve delicious €6-12 pancakes throughout the afternoon. They'll tell you that I discovered this place long before Anthony Bourdain did (Tue-Fri 12:00-19:00, closed Mon, Grimburgwal 2, tel. 020/626-5603).

Restaurant d'Vijff Vlieghen, in spite of being called "The Seven Flies," is a dressy Dutch museum of a restaurant with an interior right out of a Rembrandt painting. It's a romantic splurge, offering Dutch, French, and international cuisine (€23-27 main courses, €36 three-course dinner, nightly 18:00-22:00, Spuistraat 294, tel. 020/530-4060).

Singel 404, just across the Singel canal from Spui and near the Nine Little Streets, is a popular café serving €4-7 sandwiches on bread, bagels, and flatbread (daily 10:30-19:00, food served until 18:00, Singel 404, tel. 020/428-0154).

Café 't Gasthuys, a brown café, is a good canalside choice in this part of town (Grimburgwal 7, described on page 849).

Atrium University Cafeteria feeds travelers and students from Amsterdam University for great prices, but only on weekdays (€7 meals, Mon-Fri 11:00-15:00 & 17:00-19:30, closed Sat-Sun; from Spui, walk west down Landebrug Steeg past recommended Café 't Gasthuys three blocks to Oudezijds Achterburgwal 237, then go through arched doorway on the right; tel. 020/525-3999).

Café Luxembourg is a venerable old bistro with a very tired interior and tables (some in a heated veranda) looking right out on Spui Square. The food's basic, but it's easy and friendly with nice Belgian beer on tap. If it's a burger you want, try their Luxemburger (€10-15 salads and sandwiches, €16-20 main dishes, daily 9:00-23:00, Spui 24, tel. 020/620-6264).

Near Rokin and the Mint Tower

De Jaren Café ("The Years") is chic yet inviting, and clearly a favorite with locals. Upstairs is a minimalist restaurant with a top-notch salad bar and canal-view deck. Downstairs is a modern café, great for light lunches (soups, salads, and sandwiches served all day and evening) or just coffee over a newspaper. On a sunny day, the café's canalside patio is a fine spot to nurse a drink; this is also a nice place to go just for a drink and to enjoy the spacious Art Deco setting (daily 9:30-24:00, a long block up from Muntplein at Nieuwe Doelenstraat 20, tel. 020/625-5771).

La Place Cafeteria, on the ground floor of the V&D department store, has an abundant, colorful array of fresh, appealing, self-serve food. A multistory eatery that seats 300, it has a small outdoor terrace upstairs. Explore before you make your choice. This bustling spot has a lively market feel, with everything from made-on-the-spot stir-fry, to fresh juice, to veggie soups, and much more (€5 pizza and sandwiches, Sun-Mon 11:00-19:00, Tue-Wed 10:00-19:30, Thu-Sat 10:00-21:00, at the end of Kalverstraat near Mint Tower, tel. 020/622-0171). For fast and healthy take-out food (such as sandwiches, yogurt, and fruit cups), try the bakery on the department store's ground floor.

Marks and Spencer, up the street from V&D's La Place, has an enticing mini-grocery on the ground floor selling packaged

AMSTERDAM

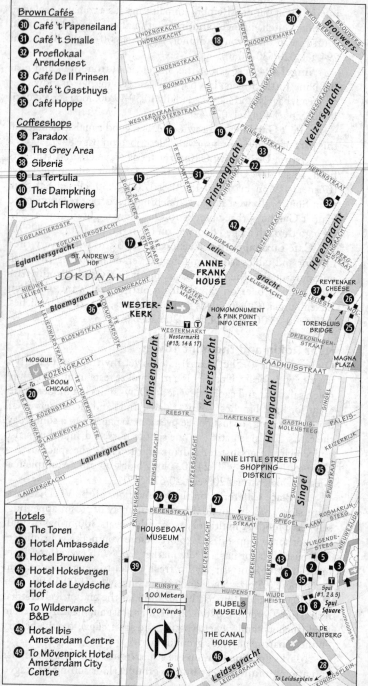

Brown Cafés
30 Café 't Papeneiland
31 Café 't Smalle
32 Proeflokaal Arendsnest
33 Café De II Prinsen
34 Café 't Gasthuys
35 Café Hoppe

Coffeeshops
36 Paradox
37 The Grey Area
38 Siberië
39 La Tertulia
40 The Dampkring
41 Dutch Flowers

Hotels
42 The Toren
43 Hotel Ambassade
44 Hotel Brouwer
45 Hotel Hoksbergen
46 Hotel de Leydsche Hof
47 To Wildervanck B&B
48 Hotel Ibis Amsterdam Centre
49 To Mövenpick Hotel Amsterdam City Centre

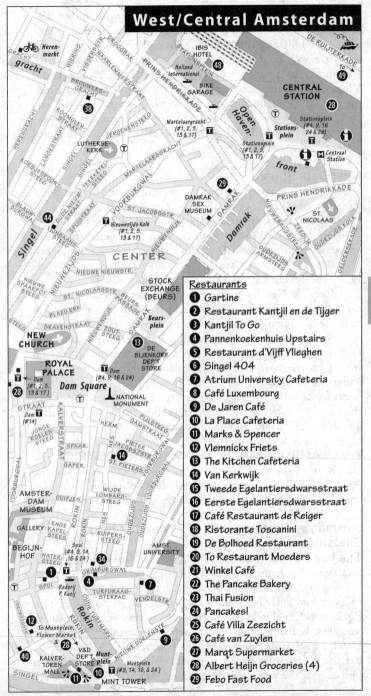

AMSTERDAM

West/Central Amsterdam

Restaurants

1. Gartine
2. Restaurant Kantjil en de Tijger
3. Kantjil To Go
4. Pannenkoekenhuis Upstairs
5. Restaurant d'Vijff Vlieghen
6. Singel 404
7. Atrium University Cafeteria
8. Café Luxembourg
9. De Jaren Café
10. La Place Cafeteria
11. Marks & Spencer
12. Vlemnickx Friets
13. The Kitchen Cafeteria
14. Van Kerkwijk
15. Tweede Egelantiersdwarsstraat
16. Eerste Egelantiersdwarsstraat
17. Café Restaurant de Reiger
18. Ristorante Toscanini
19. De Bolhoed Restaurant
20. To Restaurant Moeders
21. Winkel Café
22. The Pancake Bakery
23. Thai Fusion
24. Pancakes!
25. Café Villa Zeezicht
26. Café van Zuylen
27. Marqt Supermarket
28. Albert Heijn Groceries (4)
29. Febo Fast Food

sandwiches, salads, and other prepared meals with an upscale-English flair (€4-6 meals, Mon 10:00-20:00, Tue-Sat 9:00-20:00, Thu until 21:00, Sun 11:00-20:00, Kalverstraat 226).

Fries: While Amsterdam has no shortage of *Vlaamse frites* ("Flemish fries") stands, locals and in-the-know visitors head for **Vlemnickx,** an unpretentious hole-in-the-wall *frites* counter hiding just off the main Kalverstraat shopping street. They sell only fries, with a wide variety of sauces—they call themselves *"de sausmeesters"* (Sun-Mon 12:00-19:00, Tue-Sat 11:00-19:00, Thu until 20:00, Voetboogstraat 31).

Near Dam Square

Eateries along Damrak are touristy, overpriced, and dreary. But if you need a meal in this area, these listings are good options.

The Kitchen Cafeteria at De Bijenkorf fills the top floor of Amsterdam's swankiest department store with delightful, tasty self-service options, from Dutch to Asian to salads and burgers. It's modern and spacious, with a great outdoor terrace (daily 10:00-19:30, Thu-Fri until 20:30, Dam 1, tel. 088-245-9080).

Along the Nes: The narrow, relatively quiet street called Nes, running south from Dam Square and paralleling Rokin one block to the east, is fun to browse. It's home to several small theaters and restaurants, among them the popular **Van Kerkwijk,** an unpretentious but quirky eatery that has a loyal following. There's no written menu—your server relays the day's offerings of freshly prepared and reasonably priced international dishes. They don't take reservations and there's often a line; pass the time with a drink in the bar (€6 lunches, €8 lunch salads, €11-20 main courses at dinner, daily 11:00-23:00, Nes 41, tel. 020/620-3316).

WEST AMSTERDAM, IN THE JORDAAN DISTRICT

Nearly all of these places are within a few scenic blocks of the Anne Frank House, providing handy lunches in the city's most charming neighborhood. For locations, see the map on page 839.

Jordaan's "Restaurant Row": Tweede (2nd) Egelantierssdwarsstraat

The Jordaan's trendiest street (sometimes spelled Anjeliersdwarsstraat) is home to a variety of tempting places to eat. This is a youthful and exuberant scene, with high-energy eateries that spill out into lively brick-sidewalk seating. Stroll its length from Egelantiers Canal to Westerstraat to survey your options: Japanese pancakes, Italian trattoria, fancy burgers, ice cream, and a classic Dutch *eetcafé,* **Café Sonneveld** (which serves basic €10-20 meals, but has great tables facing the most delightful intersection in Jordaan—at the very start of the street). Many of these places are quite popular; as you stroll, consider reserving a spot for a return dinner visit.

La Oliva is a very well-regarded tapas bar that lays out a tantalizing array of Northern Spanish (Basque and Cantabrian) *pintxos* in a hip environment. As you'll likely share several small plates, your bill can add up fast (€11-16 small plates, €23-27 big plates, daily 13:00-24:00, at #122, tel. 020/320-316).

La Perla has a big, busy wood-fired oven surrounded by a few humble tables, with a more formal dining room across the street and—best of all—sidewalk tables on one of the liveliest intersections in the Jordaan (€12-14 pizzas, daily 12:00-24:00, locations face each other at #14 and #53—take your pick, tel. 020/624-8828).

Eerste (1st) Egelantierssdwarsstraat: This smaller street, one block parallel to "Restaurant Row," has a few more choices but lacks the main drag's bustle. The block just before Westerstraat has the highest concentration of good choices—Indian, tapas, and more. **Kinnaree Thai Restaurant,** with a modern ambience, features delicious, freshly prepared Thai cuisine served by an attentive waitstaff (€15 dishes, daily 17:30-22:00, at #14). **Los Pilones** next door, owned by a pair of brothers, serves surprisingly authentic Mexican food (€18 meals, at #6).

Elsewhere in the Jordaan

Café Restaurant de Reiger must offer the best cooking of any *eetcafé* in the Jordaan. Famous for its fresh ingredients, ribs, and delightful bistro ambience, it's part of the classic Jordaan scene. The daily specials (€18-20) on the chalkboard always include a meat, fish, and vegetarian dish. They're proud of their fresh fish and French-Dutch cuisine. The café, which is crowded late and on weekends, takes no reservations. Come early and have a drink at the bar while you wait (€10 starters, €20 main courses, Tue-Sun 17:00-24:00, closed Mon, Nieuwe Leliestraat 34, tel. 020/624-7426).

Café 't Smalle, a recommended brown café, is also a good place for a light lunch (Egelantiersgracht 12, described on page 849).

Ristorante Toscanini is an upmarket Italian place that's always packed. With a lively, spacious ambience and great Italian cuisine, this place is a treat—if you can get a seat. Reservations are essentially required. Eating with the local, in-the-know crowd and the busy open kitchen adds to the fun energy (€10-14 first courses, €16-25 main courses, Mon-Sat 18:00-22:30, closed Sun, deep in the Jordaan at Lindengracht 75, tel. 020/623-2813, http://restauranttoscanini.nl).

De Bolhoed Vegetarian Restaurant has serious vegetarian and vegan food in a colorful setting that Buddha would dig, with a clientele that appears to dig Buddha. Just inhaling here brings you inner peace (big splittable portions, €17 dinners, light lunches, daily 12:00-22:00, dinner starts at 17:00, Prinsengracht 60, tel. 020/626-1803).

Restaurant Moeders is a celebration of motherhood with a homey menu and a mismatched world of tables, chairs, plates and silverware—all donated by neighbors at the grand opening. The tight interior feels like a family rec room, and tables spill out onto the street overlooking a canal. The fun, accessible menu features Dutch and international home cooking. Make a reservation before taking the long walk out here (€8 starters, €15-20 main courses, every day is Mothers' Day from 17:00, Rozengracht 251, tel. 020/626-7957, www.moeders.com).

Winkel, the North Jordaan's canalside hangout, is a sloppy and youthful favorite serving simple bar food. It has a borderline-hipster vibe, with a rustic interior and great casual tables on the big open square. It's busy on Monday mornings, when the Noordermarkt flea market is underway. But Amsterdammers come from across town all week for the *appeltaart*. Rather than eat a meal here, I'd come to enjoy the square and a slice of pie (€11-14 plates, Mon-Sat 8:00-late, Sun 10:00-late, Noordermarkt 43, tel. 020/623-0223).

Between Dam Square and the Jordaan

The Pancake Bakery has long been a favorite of backpackers, youth hostelers, and people who just want a pancake for dinner. They offer a fun and creative menu with lots of hearty €10-15 savory pancakes (including a rainbow of international-themed options—kind of like a pizza place, but with pancakes) and €7-10 dessert pancakes. The scene feels like a bar, with a quieter zone upstairs (daily 9:00-21:30, American breakfasts until noon, two blocks north of the Anne Frank House at Prinsengracht 191, tel. 020/625-1333).

In the Nine Little Streets District: This popular shopping zone also has several appealing eateries. Comparison-shop for what looks best, or try one of my recommendations. **Thai Fusion,** despite the name, serves straight-up, top-quality Thai food in a sleek black-and-white room wedged neatly in the middle of the Nine Little Streets action (€14-18 main courses, daily 16:30-22:30, good veggie options, Berenstraat 8, tel. 020/320-8332). **Pancakes!** is a fresh and modern-feeling little eatery serving up savory and sweet pancakes from an inviting location in the heart of the Nine Little Streets (€6-10 pancakes, daily 10:00-18:30, Berenstraat 38, tel. 020/528-9797).

On "Big Head Square" (Torensluis Bridge): Two cafés face the atmospheric, canal-spanning "Big Head Square" (with the landmark statue of Multatuli's massive noggin). While neither is as atmospheric as a true brown café, they compensate with particularly scenic outdoor tables and longer menus. **Café Villa Zeezicht** has the better interior, with all the romantic feel of a classic Old World café. The interior is crammed with tiny tables topped by tall candlesticks, and wicker chairs outside gather under a wisteria-covered awning. The menu is uninventive—decent pastas, burgers, and salads for €10-15. Come here instead for their famous *appeltaart* and for the great people-watching on Torensluis bridge (daily 9:00-21:30, Torensteeg 7, tel. 020/626-7433). Across the street, **Café van Zuylen** is bigger and feels more upscale. It owns the most scenic outdoor tables, right out on the bridge. In bad weather you can sit in the glassed-in front room or the cozier and classier back room (farther down Torensteeg). They have Dutch and Belgian beers on tap (open long hours daily, Torensteeg 4, tel. 020/639-1055).

SOUTHERN CANAL BELT

Stroll through the colorful cancan of eateries on Lange Leidsedwarsstraat, the "Restaurant Row" just off Leidseplein, and choose your favorite (but don't expect intimacy or good value). Nearby, busy Leidsestraat offers plenty of starving-student options (between Prinsengracht and Herengracht) offering fast and fun food for around €5 a meal. To escape the crowds without too long a walk from Leidseplein, wander a few blocks away from the hubbub to one of these options.

Buffet van Odette, an elegant little restaurant with a feminine twinkle, serves Mediterranean and Italian cuisine with lots of farm-fresh, seasonal vegetables. It seems just perfect: healthy, unpretentious, very romantic, and peaceful. They have a few tables outside facing a picturesque canal (€10-15 lunch plates, €12 buffet salad at lunch, dinner-€8-14 starters and €15-19 main courses, always vegetarian option and fish, Wed-Mon 10:00-21:00, closed Tue, Prinsengracht 598, tel. 020/423-6034).

De Balie Grand Café is a venerable ground-floor eatery in part of a former prison complex—now home to galleries and concert venues. While just a block off the touristy Leidseplein, you'll feel as if you're in a parallel, tourist-free world. They serve salads, sandwiches, and simple plates, and your bill helps support culture and progressive thinking—peruse the program of events at your table. Dinner (€8 starters, €18 mains) is served from 17:30 to 21:30 (open daily for lunch and dinner, great local beers, free Wi-Fi, Kleine-Gartmanplantsoen 10, tel. 020/553-5130).

South of Rembrandtplein: **Tempo Doeloe Indonesian Restaurant,** proudly and purely Indonesian, is renowned. Tourists pack their 50 seats, so it can be hot and crowded (€32 *rijsttafel,* €38 giant *rijsttafel,* price is per person, Mon-Sat 18:00-22:00, closed Sun, several blocks south of Rembrandtplein at Utrechtsestraat 75, reservations smart, tel. 020/625-6718, www.tempodoeloerestaurant.nl).

SOUTHWEST AMSTERDAM

The area surrounding Amsterdam's museum quarter is one of the city's most upscale, with swanky broad boulevards, the top-of-the-line fashion street (P. C. Hooftstraat), and exclusive homes. While a few eateries are within just a few steps of the big museums, my less-touristy picks are generally within a 10-minute walk and have better food and service. These restaurants are good for a lunch or early dinner combined with museum-going—none is worth going out of your way for.

The Seafood Bar—modern, slick, and extremely popular—features a tasty array of seafood. The decor is white-subway-tile trendy, and the food focuses on fresh and sustainable dishes with a Burgundian flair. You can try dropping by, but it's best to reserve during mealtimes (€8-12 sandwiches, €13-18 fish-and-chips, €15-23 main courses and oysters, daily 12:00-22:00, Van Baerlestraat 5, between the Rijksmuseum and Vondelpark, tel. 020/670-8355, www.theseafoodbar.nl).

Sama Sebo Indonesian Restaurant is considered one of the best Indonesian restaurants in town. It's a venerable local favorite for *rijsttafel,* with a waitstaff that seems to have been on board since Indonesia was still a colony. I prefer the energy in the casual "bodega" to the more formal restaurant (and only in the bodega will they serve the smaller €18 lunch plate for dinner). Their 17-dish, €32 classic *rijsttafel* spread is as good as any. At lunch the €18 *bami goreng* or *nasi goreng* (fried noodles or rice) is a feast of its own (Mon-Sat 12:00-15:00 & 17:00-22:00, closed Sun, reservations smart for dinner, P.C. Hooftstraat 27, between the Rijksmuseum and Vondelpark, tel. 020/662-81460, www.samasebo.nl).

Café Gruter, with a classic brown café interior and great seating on a little square, is a neighborhood hangout—away from the center's tourism in a ritzy residential zone with fashion boutiques and leafy squares (lunch daily 11:00-16:00, also serves dinner, open very late, Willemsparkweg 73, tel. 020/679-6252). Ride tram #2 to the Jacob Obrechtstraat stop—one tram stop beyond the Van Gogh Museum—near a gateway to Vondelpark.

Renzo's is a tempting Italian delicatessen, where you can buy good sandwiches or prepared pasta dishes and *antipasti* (priced by weight, can be heated up; about €5-7 for a meal). Get your food to go, or pay a bit more to sit at one of the tables in the tiny interior, with more seating upstairs (house wine-€2.50/glass, or buy a bottle for the take-away price to enjoy with your meal, daily 11:00-21:00, Van Baerlestraat 67, between the Rijksmuseum and Vondelpark, tel. 020/763-1673).

Café Loetje has a rollicking neighborhood-beer-hall feel. Of the three dining zones, the interior is least interesting; head instead for the glassed-in winter garden (in bad weather) or the sprawling outdoor tables (in good weather). In addition to beer, they slam out good, affordable pub grub (€9-16 meals, daily 11:00 until late, Johannes Vermeerstraat 52, several blocks southeast of Museumplein, tel. 020/662-8173).

In De Pijp: This neighborhood—southeast of the Rijksmuseum—is best known for its thriving Albert Cuyp market. And although the market stalls are typically wrapped up by about 17:00, the restaurants in this area stay busy late into the evening. **Restaurant Bazar,** right in the center of the market action, offers a memorable and fun budget eating experience. Converted from a church, it has spacious seating and mod belly-dance music, and is filled with young locals enjoying good, cheap Middle Eastern and North African cuisine (€8.50 daily plate, delicious €13 couscous, €16 main dishes, daily 11:00 until late, Albert Cuypstraat 182, tel. 020/675-0544, http://bazaramsterdam.nl).

Frans Halsstraat: This pleasant tree-and-restaurant-lined street connects the De Pijp market action and the Rijksmuseum. Browse along here to see what looks good. **De Waaghals Vegetarian Restaurant** is a local favorite for its top-quality organic produce and appealing dining room, where red tables lead to peek-a-boo views of the back garden (€12-18 main courses, daily 17:00-21:30, Frans Halsstraat 29, tel. 020/679-9609).

In Vondelpark: 'T Blauwe Theehuis ("The Blue Tea House") is a venerable meeting point where, since the 1930s, all generations have come for drinks and light meals. The setting, deep in Vondelpark, is like a Monet painting. Sandwiches are served at tables outside, inside, and on the rooftop from 11:00 to 16:00, drinks and apple pie are served all day, and pot smoking—while discreet—is as natural here as falling leaves (daily 9:00-22:00 in summer, Vondelpark 5, tel. 020/662-0254). **Café Gruter,** listed earlier, is just outside Vondelpark.

CHEAP AND FAST EATS

To dine cheaply yet memorably alongside the big spenders, grab a meal to go, then find a bench on a lively neighborhood square or along a canal. Sandwiches *(broodjes)* of delicious cheese on fresh bread are cheap at snack bars, delis, and *broodjes* shops. Ethnic restaurants—many of them Indonesian or Surinamese, and seemingly all named with varying puns on "Wok"—serve inexpensive, splittable carryout meals. Middle Eastern fast-food stands and diners abound, offering a variety of meats wrapped in pita bread.

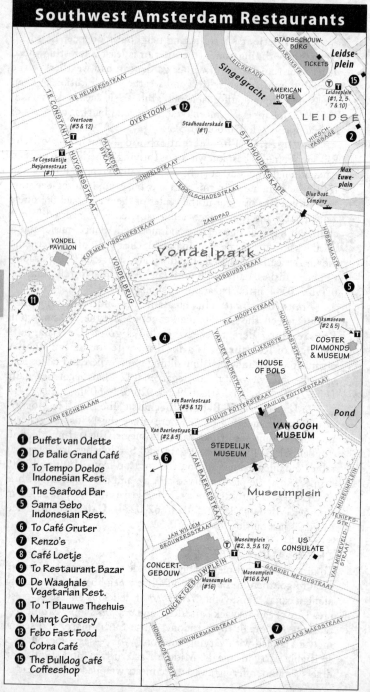

Southwest Amsterdam Restaurants

1. Buffet van Odette
2. De Balie Grand Café
3. To Tempo Doeloe Indonesian Rest.
4. The Seafood Bar
5. Sama Sebo Indonesian Rest.
6. To Café Gruter
7. Renzo's
8. Café Loetje
9. To Restaurant Bazar
10. De Waaghals Vegetarian Rest.
11. To 'T Blauwe Theehuis
12. Marqt Grocery
13. Febo Fast Food
14. Cobra Café
15. The Bulldog Café Coffeeshop

STADSSCHOUW-BURG
Leidse-plein
TICKETS
Singelgracht
AMERICAN HOTEL
Leidseplein (#1, 2, 5, 7 & 10)
LEIDSE
Overtoom (#3 & 12)
OVERTOOM
Stadhouderskade (#1)
HIRSCH PASSAGE
1e Constantijn Huygensstraat (#1)
Max Euwe-plein
Blue Boat Company
VONDEL PAVILION
Vondelpark
To
Rijksmuseum (#2 & 5)
COSTER DIAMONDS & MUSEUM
P.C. HOOFTSTRAAT
HOUSE OF BOLS
van Baerlestraat (#3 & 12)
Pond
van Baerlestraat (#2 & 5)
VAN GOGH MUSEUM
STEDELIJK MUSEUM
To
Museumplein
US CONSULATE
JAN WILLEM BROUWERSSTRAAT
Museumplein (#2, 3, 5 & 12)
CONCERT-GEBOUW
Museumplein (#16)
Museumplein (#16 & 24)
GABRIEL METSUSTRAAT
WOUWERMANSTRAAT
NICOLAAS MAESSTRAAT

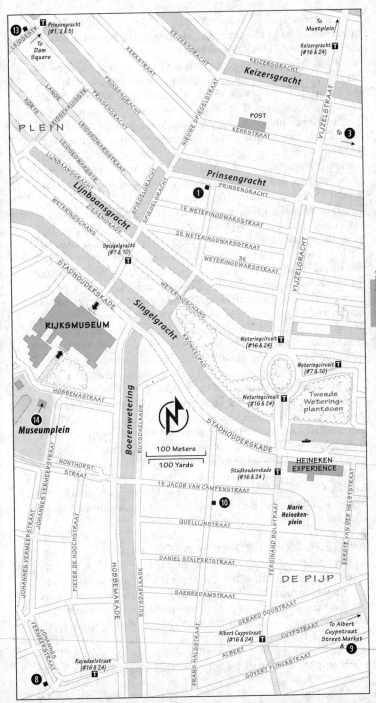

AMSTERDAM

Supermarkets: To stock up on picnic items, you'll find mini-markets all around town. For the location of the following chains, see the maps on pages 839 and 846.

I like **Marqt,** an elegant picnicker's dream, with the freshest organic produce and plenty of prepared foods. This chain is making a bold step into a cashless future and accepts only credit cards. It's worth a look even if you're just browsing (your magnetic-strip card will work fine, daily 9:00-21:00). You'll find locations in the Nine Little Streets district (along Keizersgracht, at Wolvenstraat 34) and in the emerging Haarlemmerdijk zone west of the train station (Haarlemmerstraat 165). Another Marqt is several blocks from Vondelpark and Leidseplein (Overtoom 21). And there's one south of Rembrandtplein (Utrechtsestraat 17).

Albert Heijn grocery stores are more traditional, cheaper, take cash, and are all over town (daily 8:00-22:00). They have great deli sections with picnic-perfect takeaway salads and sandwiches. Helpful, central locations are near Dam Square behind the Royal Palace (Nieuwezijds Voorburgwal 226), near the Mint Tower (Koningsplein 4), on Leidsestraat (at Koningsplein, on the corner of Leidsestraat and Singel), and inside Central Station (at the far end of the passage under the tracks). Be aware that none of their stores accepts US credit cards: Bring cash, and don't get in the checkout lines marked *PIN alleen.*

Dutch Fried Fast Food: **Febo** is an Amsterdam junk-food institution, catering mainly to late-night drinkers looking for greasy fried foods to soak up the booze. A wall of self-service, coin-op windows provides piping-hot gut bombs: fried cheese, burgers, croquettes, and so on (change machine on wall). While many diners turn up their noses, a certain breed of locals swears by their slogan—*De lekkerste!* (The tastiest!). You'll find branches all over town, including a handy one at Leidsestraat 94, just north of Leidseplein; another at Damrak 6; in the Red Light District (facing the Old Church across the canal at Oudezijds Voorburgwal 33); and another near Rembrandtplein and the Tuschinski Theater (Reguliersbreestraat 38).

AMSTERDAM'S "BROWN" CAFÉS

Be sure to experience the Dutch institution of the *bruin* café (brown café)—so called for the typically hardwood decor and nicotine-stained walls. (While smoking was banned several years ago—making these places even more inviting to nonsmokers—the prior pigmentation persists.) Exemplifying the *gezellig* (cozy) quality that the Dutch hold dear, these are convivial hangouts, where you can focus on conversation while slowly nursing a drink. Like a British pub, the corner brown café is the neighborhood's living room.

In the North Jordaan: **Café 't Papeneiland** is a classic brown café with Delft tiles, an evocative old stove, and a stay-awhile perch overlooking a canal with welcoming benches (daily 10:00-24:00, drinks but almost no food—€3.50-cheese or liverwurst sandwiches, €4.30-apple pie, overlooking northwest end of Prinsengracht at #2, tel. 020/624-1989).

Buried Deep in the Jordaan: **Café 't Smalle** is extremely charming, with three zones: canalside (literally—on a little barge in the canal), inside around the bar, and up some steep stairs in a quaint little back room. The café is open late, and serves simple meals from 11:00 to 17:30 (salads, soup, and fresh sandwiches; plenty of fine €3-4 Belgian beers on tap, interesting wines by the glass; at Egelantiersgracht 12—where it hits Prinsengracht, tel. 020/623-9617).

Between Central Station and the Jordaan: **Proeflokaal Arendsnest** is the ideal brown café experience for beer lovers. Awash in wonderful old-fashioned decor, it displays the day's 30 rotating Belgian beers "on tap/on draft" on a big chalkboard (daily 14:00-24:00, Herengracht 90, tel. 020/421-2057). **Café De II Prinsen,** dating from 1910, feels more local. It's relaxed and convivial, with a few outdoor tables facing a particularly pretty canal and a lively shopping street (Dutch beers on tap, daily 12:00-24:00, Prinsenstraat 27, tel. 020/428-4488).

Near Central Station: Fittingly for this neighborhood at the edge of the Red Light District, **Proeflokaal de Ooievaar** ("Pelican") feels like a grubby sailors' tavern—which is exactly what it was (open long hours daily, at the corner of the Red Light District facing Central Station at Sint Olofspoort 1, look for the pelican on the sign, tel. 020/420-9004).

Near Rokin: **Café 't Gasthuys** offers a long bar, a lovely secluded back room, peaceful canalside seating, and sometimes slow service (€6-10 lunch plates, €11-15 main courses, cheeseburgers are a favorite, daily 12:00-16:30 & 17:30-22:00, Grimburgwal 7—from the Rondvaart Kooij boat dock, head down Langebrugsteeg, and it's one block down on the left, tel. 020/624-8230).

On Spui Square: **Café Hoppe** is a classic drinking bar that's as brown as can be. They have a good selection of traditional drinks and *jenevers* (gins), sandwiches at lunch (€6-7, 12:00-17:00), a packed interior, and fun stools outside to oversee the action on Spui (Mon-Thu 14:00-24:00, Fri-Sun 12:00-24:00, Spui 18, tel. 020/420-4420).

Smoking in Amsterdam

MARIJUANA (A.K.A. CANNABIS)

For tourists from lands where you can do hard time for lighting up, the open use of marijuana here can feel either somewhat disturbing, or exhilaratingly liberating...or maybe just refreshingly sane. Several decades after being legalized in the Netherlands, marijuana causes about as much excitement here as a bottle of beer.

Marijuana Laws and "Coffeeshops"

Throughout the Netherlands, you'll see "coffeeshops"—cafés selling marijuana, with display cases showing various joints or baggies for sale.

Rules and Regulations: The retail sale of marijuana is strictly regulated, and proceeds are taxed. The minimum age for purchase is 18, and coffeeshops can sell up to five grams of marijuana per person per day. It's also illegal for these shops (or anyone) to advertise marijuana. In fact, in many places, the prospective customer has to take the initiative, and ask to see the menu. In some coffeeshops, you actually have to push and hold down a button to see an illuminated menu—the contents of which look like the inventory of a drug bust.

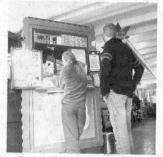

Shops sell marijuana and hashish both in prerolled joints and in little baggies. Joints are generally sold individually (€3-5, depending on the strain you choose), though some places sell only small packs of three or four joints. Baggies generally contain a gram and go for €8-15. The better pot, though costlier, can actually be a better value, as it takes less to get high—and it's a better high. But if you want to take it easy, as a general rule, cheaper is milder.

Each coffeeshop is allowed to keep an inventory of about a pound of pot in stock: The tax authorities don't want to see more than this on the books at the end of each accounting cycle, and a shop can lose its license if it exceeds this amount. A popular shop—whose supply must be replenished five or six times a day—simply has to put up with the hassle of constantly taking small deliveries. A shop can sell a ton of pot with no legal problems, as long as it maintains that tiny stock and just refills it as needed. The reason? Authorities want shops to stay small and not become export bases.

Smoking Tips: The Dutch (like most Europeans) are accustomed to mixing tobacco with marijuana—but any place that caters to Americans will have joints without tobacco; you just have to ask specifically for a "pure" joint. Shops have loaner bongs and inhalers, and dispense rolling papers like toothpicks. While it's good style to ask first, as long as you're a paying customer (e.g., you buy a cup of coffee), you can generally pop in to any coffeeshop and light up, even if you didn't buy your pot there.

Tourists who haven't smoked pot since their college days are famous for overindulging in Amsterdam. Coffeeshop baristas nickname tourists about to pass out "Whitey"—the color their faces turn just before they hit the floor. They warn Americans (who aren't used to the strength of the local stuff) to try a lighter leaf. If you do overdo it, the key is to eat or drink something sweet to avoid getting sick. Cola is a good fast fix, and coffeeshop staff keep sugar tablets handy. They also recommend trying to walk it off.

Don't ever buy pot on the street in Amsterdam. Well-established coffeeshops are considered much safer, and coffeeshop owners have an interest in keeping their trade safe and healthy. They're also generally very patient in explaining the varieties available.

COFFEESHOPS

Most of downtown Amsterdam's coffeeshops feel grungy and foreboding to American travelers who aren't part of the youth-hostel crowd.

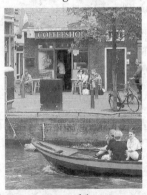

The neighborhood places (and those in small towns around the countryside) are much more inviting to people without piercings, tattoos, and favorite techno artists. I've listed a few places with a more pub-like ambience for Americans wanting to go local, but within reason. For locations, see the map on page 838 in the "Eating in Amsterdam" section.

Paradox is the most *gezellig* (cozy) coffeeshop I found—a mellow, graceful place. The managers, Ludo and Wiljan, and their staff are patient with descriptions and happy to walk you through all your options. This is a rare coffeeshop that serves light meals (single tobacco-free joints-€3, loaner bongs, games, Wi-Fi, daily 10:00-20:00, two blocks from Anne Frank House at Eerste Bloemdwarsstraat 2, tel. 020/623-5639).

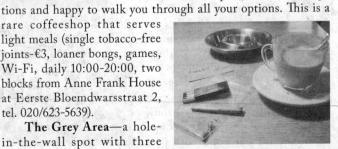

The Grey Area—a hole-in-the-wall spot with three

What If I Miss My Boat?

Remember that you can get help from the cruise line's port agent (listed on the destination information sheet distributed on the ship) and the local TI (see page 804). If the port agent suggests a costly solution (such as a private car with a driver), you may want to consider public transit.

Amsterdam is well-connected by train to a variety of cruise ports, including **Zeebrugge** (via Brussels), **Le Havre** (via Paris), **Southampton** and **Dover** (Eurostar via Brussels/London, then train onward to either port), **Copenhagen, Warnemünde** (via Berlin), and beyond.

If you need to catch a **plane** to your next destination, it's an easy train ride from downtown Amsterdam to Schiphol Airport. For more information, see the next section.

Local **travel agents** in Amsterdam can help you. For more advice on what to do if you miss the boat, see page 139.

---

tiny tables—is a cool, welcoming, and smoky place appreciated among local aficionados as a perennial winner of Amsterdam's Cannabis Cup awards. Judging by the autographed photos on the wall, many famous Americans have dropped in (say hi to Willie Nelson). You're welcome to just nurse a bottomless cup of coffee (daily 12:00-20:00, they close relatively early out of consideration for their neighbors, between Dam Square and Anne Frank House at Oude Leliestraat 2, tel. 020/420-4301).

Siberië Coffeeshop is a short walk from Central Station, but feels cozy, with a friendly canalside ambience. Clean, big, and bright, this place has the vibe of a mellow Starbucks and plays host to the occasional astrology reading (daily 11:00-23:00, Fri-Sat until 24:00, Wi-Fi for customers, helpful staff, English menu, Brouwersgracht 11, tel. 020/623-5909).

La Tertulia is a sweet little mother-and-daughter-run place with pastel decor and a cheery terrarium atmosphere (Tue-Sat 11:00-19:00, closed Sun-Mon, sandwiches, brownies, games, Prinsengracht 312).

The Bulldog Café is the high-profile, leading touristy chain of coffeeshops. These establishments are young but welcoming, with reliable selections. They're pretty comfortable for green tourists wanting to just hang out for a while. The flagship branch, in a former police station right on Leidseplein, is very handy, offering alcohol upstairs, pot downstairs, and fun outdoor seating on a

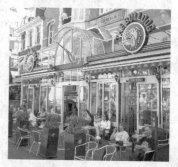

heated patio (daily 10:00-24:00, later on weekends, Leidseplein 17—see map on page 846, tel. 020/625-6278). Their original café still sits on the canal near the Old Church in the Red Light District.

The Dampkring is a rough-and-ready constant party. It's a high-profile, busy place, filled with a young clientele and loud music, but the owners still take the time to explain what they offer (daily 10:00-24:00, close to Spui at Handboogstraat 29, tel. 020/638-0705).

Dutch Flowers, conveniently located near Spui Square on Singel canal, has a very casual "brown café" ambience, with a mature set of regulars. A couple of tables overlooking the canal are perfect for enjoying the late-afternoon sunshine (daily 10:00-23:00, on the corner of Heisteeg and Singel at Singel 387, tel. 020/624-7624).

Starting or Ending Your Cruise in Amsterdam

If your cruise begins and/or ends in Amsterdam, you'll want some extra time here; for most travelers, one extra day (beyond your cruise departure day) is a minimum to see the highlights of this grand city. For a longer visit here, pick up my *Rick Steves Amsterdam & the Netherlands* guidebook.

Airport Connections

SCHIPHOL AIRPORT

Schiphol (SKIP-pol) Airport is located about 10 miles southwest of Amsterdam's city center (airport code: AMS, toll tel. 0900-0141, from other countries dial +31-20-794-0800, www.schiphol.nl).

Though Schiphol officially has four terminals, it's really just one big building. You could walk it end to end in about 20 minutes (but allow some time to pass through security checkpoints between certain terminals). All terminals have ATMs, banks, shops, bars, and free Wi-Fi. An inviting shopping and eating zone called Holland Boulevard runs between Terminals 2 and 3.

Baggage-claim areas for all terminals empty into the same arrival zone, called Schiphol Plaza. Here you'll find a busy **TI** (near Terminal 2, daily 7:00-22:00), a train station, and bus stops for getting into the city.

To get train information or buy a ticket, take advantage of the **"Train Tickets and Services" counter** (Schiphol Plaza ground level, just past Burger King). They have an easy info desk and generally short lines—so transactions here tend to be much quicker than at Amsterdam's Central Station ticket desks.

Getting from Schiphol Airport to Downtown and the Cruise Terminal

Direct **trains** to Amsterdam's Central Station run frequently (4-6/hour, 15 minutes, €5). The cruise terminal is an easy tram ride—just one stop—from the station. In front of Central Station, look for the tram stop marked *IJburg* (on the right, as you face the station). From here, catch tram #26 and ride it one stop to Muziekgebouw Bimhuis, which is right in front of the terminal.

The Connexxion **shuttle bus** departs from lane A7 in front of the airport and takes you directly to most hotels or to the cruise terminal (which is right next to the Mövenpick Hotel Amsterdam City Centre). There are three different routes, so ask the attendant which one works best for your destination (2/hour, 20 minutes, €17 one-way, €27 round-trip, some routes may cost a couple euros more). For trips from Amsterdam to Schiphol, reserve at least two hours ahead (tel. 088-339-4741, www.airporthotelshuttle.nl).

Public bus #197 (departing from lane B9 in front of the airport) is only handy for those going to the Leidseplein district (€5, buy ticket from driver).

By **taxi**, allow about €60-70 to the cruise terminal or downtown Amsterdam.

Getting from the Cruise Terminal to the Airport

If your cruise ends in Amsterdam and you're flying out of Schiphol Airport, it's an easy connection (I'd skip the taxi, which charges a hefty €60-70 to the airport). First, ride tram #26 from in front of the cruise terminal one stop, to Central Station (for details, see page 800). Then head inside the train station and take a train to Schiphol Airport (4-6/hour, 15 minutes, €5).

Hotels in Amsterdam

If you need a hotel in Amsterdam before or after your cruise, here are a few to consider. Amsterdam is a tough city for budget accommodations, and any hotel room under €140 (or B&B room under €100) will have rough edges. Still, you can sleep well and safely in a great location for €100 per double.

Some national holidays merit making reservations far in advance. Amsterdam is jammed during tulip season (late March-mid-May), conventions, festivals, and on summer weekends. During peak season, some hoteliers won't take weekend bookings for those staying fewer than two or three nights.

Canalside rooms can come with great views—and early-morning construction-crew noise. If you're a light sleeper, ask the hotelier for a quiet room in the back. Smoking is illegal in hotel rooms throughout the Netherlands. Canal houses were built tight. They have steep stairs with narrow treads; few have elevators. If steep stairs are potentially problematic, book a hotel with an elevator.

STATELY CANALSIDE HOTELS IN WEST AMSTERDAM

Both of these hotels, a half-mile apart, face historic canals. They come with lovely lobbies (some more ornate than others) and rooms that can feel like they're from another century. This area oozes elegance and class, and it is fairly quiet at night.

$$$ The Toren is a chandeliered, historic mansion with a pleasant, canalside setting and a peaceful garden for guests out back. Run by Eric and Petra Toren, this smartly renovated, super-romantic hotel is classy yet friendly, with 38 rooms in a great location on a quiet street two blocks northeast of the Anne Frank House. The capable staff is a great source of local advice. The gilt-frame, velvet-curtained rooms are an opulent splurge (tiny Sb-€115, Db-€200, deluxe Db-€250, third person-€40, prices bump way up during conferences and decrease in winter, breakfast buffet-€14, air-con, elevator, guest computer, Wi-Fi, Keizersgracht 164, tel. 020/622-6033, www.thetoren.nl, info@thetoren.nl). To get the best prices, check their website for the "daily rate," book direct, and in the "remarks" field, ask for the 10 percent Rick Steves cash discount.

$$$ Hotel Ambassade, lacing together 59 rooms in a maze of connected houses, is elegant and fresh, sitting aristocratically on Herengracht. The staff is top-notch, and the public areas (including a library and a breakfast room) are palatial, with antique furnishings and modern art (Sb-€220, Db-€280, more expensive deluxe canal-view doubles and suites, Tb-€245-325, extra bed-€60, ask for Rick Steves discount when booking, see website for specials, breakfast-€17.50, air-con, elevator, guest computer, Wi-Fi, Herengracht 341, tel. 020/555-0222, www.ambassade-hotel.nl, info@ambassade-hotel.nl, Roos—pronounced "Rose").

SIMPLER CANALSIDE HOTELS

These places have basic rooms—some downright spare, none plush. Both of them, however, offers a decent night's sleep in a lovely area of town.

$$ Hotel Brouwer—woody and old-time homey—has a tranquil yet central location on the Singel canal. Renting eight rooms with canal views, old furniture, and soulful throw rugs, it's

AMSTERDAM

so popular that it's often booked three or four months in advance—reserve as soon as possible (Sb-€78, Db-€128, Tb-€160, cash only, small elevator, guest computer, Wi-Fi, located between Central Station and Dam Square, near Lijnbaanssteeg at Singel 83, tel. 020/624-6358, www.hotelbrouwer.nl, akita@hotelbrouwer.nl).

$$ Hotel Hoksbergen is well-run and welcoming, with a peaceful canalside setting. Helpful, hands-on owners Tony and Jay rent 14 rooms with newly remodeled bathrooms (Db-€105, Tb-€143, five Qb apartments-€165-198, fans, Wi-Fi, Singel 301, tel. 020/626-6043, www.hotelhoksbergen.com, info@hotelhoksbergen.nl).

CHARMING B&BS IN SOUTHERN CANAL BELT

The area around Amsterdam's rip-roaring nightlife center (Leidseplein) is colorful, comfortable, and convenient. These canalside mom-and-pop places are within a five-minute walk of rowdy Leidseplein, but generally are in quiet and typically Dutch settings. Within walking distance of the major museums, and steps off the tram line, this neighborhood offers a perfect mix of charm and location.

$$ Hotel de Leydsche Hof, a hidden gem located on a canal, doesn't charge extra for its views. Its four large rooms are a symphony in white, some overlooking a tree-filled backyard, others a canal, but be prepared for lots of stairs. Frits and Loes give their big, elegant, old building a stylish air. Breakfast is served in the grand canal-front room (Db-€130-150, cash only, 2-night minimum, guest computer, Wi-Fi, Leidsegracht 14, tel. 020/638-2327, mobile 06-3099-2744, www.freewebs.com/leydschehof, loespiller@planet.nl).

$$ Wildervanck B&B, run by Helene and Sjoerd Wildervanck with the help of their three girls, offers two tastefully decorated rooms in an elegant 17th-century canal house (big Db on first floor-€140, Db with twin beds on ground floor-€125, extra bed-€35, 2-night minimum, breakfast in their pleasant dining room, Wi-Fi, just west of Leidsestraat at Keizersgracht 498, tel. 020/623-3846, www.wildervanck.com, info@wildervanck.com).

NEAR THE TRAIN STATION AND CRUISE TERMINAL

$$$ Hotel Ibis Amsterdam Centre, located next door to Central Station, is a modern, efficient, 363-room place. It offers a central location, comfort, and good value, without a hint of charm (Db-€141-160 Nov-Aug, Db-€200 Sept-Oct, breakfast-€16, check website for deals, book long in advance—especially for Sept-Oct, air-con, elevators, pay guest computer, Wi-Fi; facing Central Station, go left toward the multistory bicycle garage to Stationsplein 49; tel. 020/721-9172, www.ibishotel.com, h1556@

accor.com). When business is slow, usually in midsummer, they occasionally rent rooms to same-day drop-ins for around €110.

To sleep right next door to the cruise terminal, consider the **$$$ Mövenpick Hotel Amsterdam City Centre** (www.moeven pick-hotels.com)—but keep in mind that this location is less practical for getting to anywhere other than your ship.

Nightlife in Amsterdam

On summer evenings, people flock to the main squares for drinks at outdoor tables. Leidseplein is the liveliest square, surrounded by theaters, restaurants, and nightclubs. The slightly quieter Rembrandtplein (with adjoining Thorbeckeplein and nearby Reguliersdwarsstraat) is the center of gay clubs and nightlife. Spui features a full city block of bars. And Nieuwmarkt, on the east edge of the Red Light District, is a bit rough, but is probably the least touristy. The Red Light District (particularly Oudezijds Achterburgwal) is less sleazy in the early evening, and almost carnival-like as the neon lights come on and the streets fill with tour groups. But it starts to feel scuzzy after about 22:30. The **brown cafés** recommended on page 849 are ideal after-hours hangouts. For entertainment and nightlife information, the TI's website, www.iamsterdam.com, has good English listings for upcoming events (click on "What to do," then "What's on"). Newsstands sell *Time Out Amsterdam* and Dutch newspapers (Thu editions generally list events). Several museums—including the Anne Frank House, Van Gogh Museum, Hermitage Amsterdam, and Stedelijk—stay open late on certain days (see hours in "Amsterdam at a Glance" on page 808).

AMSTERDAM

Dutch Survival Phrases

Most people speak English, but if you learn the pleasantries and key phrases, you'll connect better with the locals. To pronounce the guttural Dutch "g" (indicated in phonetics by *h*), make a clear-your-throat sound, similar to the "ch" in the Scottish word "loch."

English	Dutch	Pronunciation
Hello.	*Hallo.*	**hah**-loh
Good day.	*Dag.*	da*h*
Good morning.	*Goedemorgen.*	**hoo**-deh-mor-*h*ehn
Good afternoon.	*Goedemiddag.*	**hoo**-deh-mid-da*h*
Good evening.	*Goedenavond.*	**hoo**-dehn-ah-fohnd
Do you speak English?	*Spreekt u Engels?*	shpraykt oo **eng**-ehls
Yes. / No.	*Ja. / Nee.*	yah / nay
I (don't) understand.	*Ik begrijp (het niet).*	ik beh-**hripe** (heht neet)
Please. (can also mean "You're welcome")	*Alstublieft.*	**ahl**-stoo-bleeft
Thank you.	*Dank u wel.*	dahnk oo vehl
I'm sorry.	*Het spijt me.*	heht spite meh
Excuse me.	*Pardon.*	**par**-dohn
(No) problem.	*(Geen) probleem.*	(hayn) **proh**-blaym
Good.	*Goede.*	**hoo**-deh
Goodbye.	*Tot ziens.*	toht zeens
one / two	*een / twee*	ayn / t'vay
three / four	*drie / vier*	dree / feer
five / six	*vijf / zes*	fife / zehs
seven / eight	*zeven / acht*	**zay**-fehn / ah*t*
nine / ten	*negen / tien*	**nay**-hehn / teen
What does it cost?	*Wat kost het?*	vaht kohst heht
Is it free?	*Is het vrij?*	is heht fry
Is it included?	*Is het inclusief?*	is heht in-**kloo**-seev
Can you please help me?	*Kunt u alstublieft helpen?*	koont oo **ahl**-stoo-bleeft **hehl**-pehn
Where can I buy / find...?	*Waar kan ik kopen / vinden...?*	var kahn ik **koh**-pehn / **fin**-dehn
I'd like / We'd like...	*Ik wil graag / Wij willen graag...*	ik vil hrah / vy **vil**-lehn hrah
...a room.	*...een kamer.*	ayn **kah**-mer
...a train / bus ticket to ____.	*...een trein / bus kaartje naar ____.*	ayn trayn / boos **kart**-yeh nar ____
...to rent a bike.	*...een fiets huren.*	ayn feets **hoo**-rehn
Where is...?	*Waar is...?*	var is
...the train / bus station	*...het trein / bus station*	heht trayn / boos **staht**-see-ohn
...the tourist info office	*...de VVV*	deh fay fay fay
...the toilet	*...het toilet*	heht **twah**-leht
men / women	*mannen / vrouwen*	**mah**-nehn / **frow**-ehn
left / right	*links / rechts*	links / re*h*ts
straight ahead	*rechtdoor*	**reh**t-dor
What time does it open / close?	*Hoe laat gaat het open / dicht?*	hoo laht *h*aht heht **oh**-pehn / di*h*t
now / soon / later	*nu / straks / later*	noo / strahks / **lah**-ter
today / tomorrow	*vandaag / morgen*	**fahn**-da*h* / **mor**-hehn

BRUGES & BRUSSELS

Belgium

Belgium Practicalities

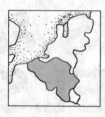

Travelers are often pleasantly surprised by Belgium—a charming, welcoming, and underrated land that produces some of Europe's best beer, creamiest chocolates, most beloved comic strips, and tastiest french fries. Squeezed between Germany, France, and the Netherlands, Belgium has 10.5 million people packed into nearly 12,000 square miles (similar to Maryland)—making it the second most densely populated country in Europe (after the Netherlands). About three-quarters of the population is Catholic. Belgium is a culturally, linguistically, and politically divided country, with 60 percent of the population speaking Dutch...but an economy dominated by French speakers. The capital city of Brussels is important internationally as the capital of the European Union—more than 25 percent of the people living there are foreigners.

Money: €1 (euro) = about $1.40. The local VAT (value-added sales tax) rate is 21 percent; the minimum purchase eligible for a VAT refund is €125.01 (for details on refunds, see page 134).

Language: The official languages are Dutch (also called Flemish), French, and German. For useful phrases, see pages 640, 928, and 1141.

Emergencies: Dial 112 for police, medical, or other emergencies. In case of theft or loss, see page 125.

Time Zone: Belgium is on Central European Time (the same as most of the Continent, one hour ahead of Great Britain, and six/nine hours ahead of the East/West Coasts of the US).

Embassies in Brussels: The **US embassy** is at Boulevard du Régent 27 (tel. 02-811-4300, after-hours emergency tel. 02-811-4000, http://belgium.usembassy.gov). The **US consulate** is next door to the embassy at Boulevard du Régent 25. The **Canadian embassy** is at Avenue de Tervueren 2 (tel. 02-741-0611, www.ambassade-canada.be). Call ahead for passport services.

Phoning: Belgium's country code is 32; to call from another country to Belgium, dial the international access code (011 from the US/Canada, 00 from Europe, or + from a mobile phone), then 32, followed by the local number (drop the initial zero). For local calls within Belgium, just dial the number as it appears in this book—whether you're calling from across the street or across the country. To place an international call from Belgium, dial 00, the code of the country you're calling (1 for US and Canada), and the phone number. For more tips, see page 1146.

Tipping: The bill for sit-down meals already includes a tip, though for good service it's nice to round up about 5-10 percent. Round up taxi fares a bit (pay €3 on an €2.85 fare). For more tips on tipping, see page 138.

Tourist Information: www.visitbelgium.com

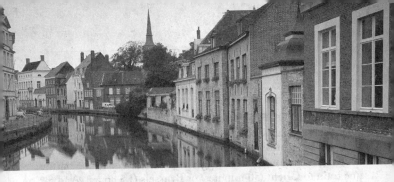

BRUGES, BRUSSELS,
and the PORT of ZEEBRUGGE

Zeebrugge • Bruges • Brussels • Ghent

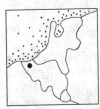

Belgium's port of Zeebrugge is the gateway to this entire, small country: With several hours in port, you could visit nearly any point within its borders. Most cruisers, however, set their sights on two places in particular: Bruges, a charming, quintessentially medieval town; and Brussels, the bustling capital of Belgium and of Europe.

With pointy, gilded architecture, stay-a-while cafés, vivid time-tunnel art, and dreamy canals dotted with swans, **Bruges** (pronounced "broozh") is a heavyweight sightseeing destination, as well as a joy. Where else can you ride a bike along a canal, munch mussels and wash them down with the world's best beer, savor heavenly chocolate, and see Flemish Primitives and a Michelangelo, all within 300 yards of a bell tower that jingles every 15 minutes? And do it all without worrying about a language barrier?

Six hundred years ago, **Brussels** was just a nice place to stop and buy a waffle on the way to Bruges. With no strategic importance, it was allowed to grow as a free trading town. Today it's a city of one million people, the capital of Belgium, the headquarters of NATO, and the seat of the European Union.

If neither of these options fits the bill, consider the midsize city of **Ghent,** which lies halfway between Brussels and Bruges—both geographically and in spirit. This charming university city offers historic, art-packed churches as well as cutting-edge museums.

Cruise lines often advertise their Zeebrugge stop as "Brussels," but I recommend setting your sights on Bruges instead. Bruges is not only much closer and easier to reach from your ship, but—thanks to its user-friendliness and overall charm—it's all-around the more preferable destination.

PLANNING YOUR TIME

From Zeebrugge, it's a breeze (short walk, 10- to 15-minute tram ride to the town of Blankenberge, then 15-minute train ride) to zip into **Bruges**. If you prefer a bigger city, you can continue on the same train to **Ghent** (50 minutes) or **Brussels** (1.5 hours). And for WWI history buffs, the famous **Flanders Fields** are also nearby. With one day in port, you'll need to choose just one of these; for tips on each, see below.

Note: On Mondays, most museums—including major ones in both Bruges (Groeninge, Memling) and Brussels (Royal Museums, BELvue, Musical Instruments, Comic Strip)—are closed.

In Bruges

With a day in Bruges, I'd do the following (ranked here by importance, and in a smart chronological order):

• **Bruges City Walk:** Stroll through town visiting the Markt (Market Square), the Basilica of the Holy Blood, the City Hall's Gothic Room, the Church of Our Lady, and the Begijnhof (allow 2 hours total); if your energy holds up, climb the bell tower on the Markt (add 30-45 minutes).

• **Groeninge Museum:** This fine collection of 15th-century Flemish art takes about an hour to see.

• **Memling Museum:** With a quirky collection of medieval medical trades, plus some paintings by Hans Memling, this deserves an hour.

• **Canal Cruise:** This relaxing and scenic trip takes 30 minutes.

• **De Halve Maan Brewery Tour:** If you have an hour to spare (see schedule on page 882), this tour offers a good taste of Belgian beer.

In Brussels

As a much bigger city, Brussels simply takes more time to get around. But several key sights are in the downtown core. Riding the train to the Central Station, you're within walking distance of these options:

• **Grand Place:** My self-guided tour of Brussels' spectacular main square includes a peek at the famous *Manneken-Pis* statue. Allow two hours.

• **Royal Museums:** For an excellent art collection, head to the Upper Town for the Old Masters, Fin de Siècle, and René Magritte Museums (allow an hour to quickly see the highlights of the Old Masters/Fin de Siècle collections, plus another hour for Magritte).

• **BELvue Museum:** This concise overview of Belgian history, next to the Royal Museums, is worth an hour.

• **Other Museums:** If the options noted above aren't appealing, consider Brussels' good Musical Instruments Museum or Comic Strip Center (allow an hour apiece).

In Ghent

From Ghent's Sint-Pieters Station, it's a 15-minute tram ride into the heart of town. On a short visit, I'd stroll the historic center, tour the Cathedral of St. Bavo (with its grand Van Eyck altarpiece; allow about an hour), and—depending on your interests—visit the castle or Design Museum (each deserves about an hour).

In Flanders Fields

This spread-out area is best seen on an excursion or with a taxi from the port (Taxi Snel; see page 866). If you'd like to try it on your own, consider this: Take the coastal tram to Ostend, rent a car, and tour the WWI battlefields and museums near Ypres. Figure 50 minutes by coastal tram from Zeebrugge to Ostend, then an hour each way to drive between Ostend and Ypres.

The Port of Zeebrugge

Arrival at a Glance: From your ship, you'll ride a shuttle bus to the port gate, walk (10 minutes) to a tram stop, then ride the tram 10-15 minutes to the Blankenberge train station. From there, hourly trains zip to Bruges (15 minutes), Ghent (50 minutes), and Brussels (1.5 hours).

Port Overview

Zeebrugge (ZAY-brew-gah), 10 miles north of Bruges, is a little village with a gigantic port (Europe's ninth busiest).

The sprawling port zone has two cruise berths, but no terminal building. Larger cruise ships use **Swedish Quay** (Zweedse Kaai), which pokes straight up into the main harbor. Smaller cruise ships use **Maritime Station** (Zeestation), across the harbor along Leopold II-Dam. From these berths, a free shuttle bus brings you to either the port gate or a local tram stop.

Tourist Information: The Zeebrugge TI—open only in summer—is in a red beachside building three blocks from the Strandwijk tram stop, at the intersection of Sint-Thomas Morusstraat and Zeedijk (daily July-Aug 10:00-13:30 &

14:00-18:00, Zeedijk 25, tel. 050-444-646). Otherwise, the most convenient TI is in Blankenberge, near the train station (April-Sept daily 9:00-11:45 & 13:30-17:00, until 19:00 July-Aug; Oct-March Mon-Sat 9:00-11:45 & 13:30-17:00, Sun 10:00-13:00; Koning Leopold III Plein, tel. 050-412-227, www.blankenberge.be).

Sights in Zeebrugge: Zeebrugge is a **beach town** as well as a North Sea port. If you'd rather just soak up some sun, grab your towel and a swimsuit and head for the Zeebrugge Strandwijk tram stop. (If you arrive at Maritime Station, your shuttle bus drops you right there; from Swedish Quay, walk to the Zeebrugge Kerk tram stop—directions given below—and then ride two stops.) From the Zeebrugge Strandwijk stop, go toward the white church, and walk past it along an arbor-covered walkway. At the next street, turn left. At the next intersection, turn right and head for the sand. A small building has showers, WCs, and a summer-only TI that loans bikes (daily July-Aug 10:00-13:30 & 14:00-18:00). Beach cafés and restaurants are nearby.

GETTING INTO TOWN

A free shuttle bus takes you from your ship to the port gate or a tram stop. While a few taxis are generally standing by to hustle passengers to Bruges, public transit is nearby.

By Public Transportation

Belgium's coastal tram takes you from the port into the town of Blankenberge, with a TI, shops, a pharmacy, and (most important) frequent, direct trains to Bruges, Ghent, and Brussels.

Note: Although Zeebrugge does have its own train stations, they are inconvenient for cruisers and offer only milk-run connections to Bruges. Zeebrugge is also linked by bus to Bruges, but the schedule is infrequent. It's smartest to take the coastal tram all the way to Blankenberge's well-connected station.

From the Port Gate to Blankenberge Train Station

The coastal tram (Kusttram) runs every 20 minutes and is covered by a €3 ticket (good for up to one hour)—pay the driver, then validate your ticket in the yellow machine. If you'll also be taking public transit in Bruges, it's smart to buy a day pass for €7 (validate it each time you board, day pass valid only on De Lijn transport in Brussels; tram info: toll tel. 070-220-200, www.delijn.be).

Which tram stop you use depends on whether you arrive at Swedish Quay or Maritime Station.

From **Swedish Quay,** turn right as you leave the port gate and walk 10 minutes along the highway into Zeebrugge. The Zeebrugge Kerk stop for the coastal tram is right in front of

Excursions from Zeebrugge

Just about anything you'd want to see is doable on your own from Zeebrugge using public transportation—with the notable exception of Flanders Fields.

The most popular excursion options are tours to either charming, manageable Bruges or big, bustling Brussels. The Bruges excursion usually includes a walking tour around the Old Town. The Brussels excursion generally includes a tour that's part by bus and part on foot. Given the size and relative ease of reaching Bruges, seeing that city on your own is a no-brainer; for Brussels, less adventurous travelers may want to consider an excursion.

Other popular choices include the pleasant university town of Ghent (halfway between Bruges and Brussels); the big, fashion-oriented port city of Antwerp (including a visit to the Cathedral of Our Lady, decorated with several works by native son Peter Paul Rubens); or a trip to the town of Ypres and the surrounding World War I battlefields known as Flanders Fields. For something lower-impact, some cruise lines offer a relaxing canalside bike ride between Bruges and the neighboring hamlet of Damme.

Any of these tours may include a few Belgian clichés: canal boat ride, chocolate workshop, sampling a Belgian waffle, or beer tasting. Yes, these things are touristy—but they're also undeniably fun and tasty. Enjoy them.

the church. Take any tram going in direction: Oostende or De Panne—use the closest platform (don't cross the tracks).

From **Maritime Station,** your shuttle bus drops you off very near the tram's Zeebrugge Strandwijk stop. Just board the tram going in direction: Oostende or De Panne.

Ride the tram to **Blankenberge Station** (about 14 minutes, a video screen inside the tram displays the next stop). The Blankenberge TI is right behind the tram stop in a building facing a large square (Koning Leopold III Plein). From the tram, cross the street to reach the train station.

From Blankenberge Train Station to Bruges, Ghent, and Brussels

Every train leaving Blankenberge goes through Bruges—just take the next train. Most trains leave at :10 past the hour, arriving in **Bruges** in 15 minutes (€3 one-way), then continuing on to **Ghent** (€8.50 one-way, 50 minutes total, get off at Gent-Sint-Pieters station), then **Brussels** (€16.10 one-way, 1.5 hours total, get off at Brussel-Centraal/Bruxelles-Central station, www.belgianrail.be). Only local debit cards work in the ticket machines, so you'll need to use the station's ticket office, which takes US credit cards.

Services near the Port of Zeebrugge and in Blankenberge

ATMs: Two ATMs are a short distance from the Zeebrugge Kerk stop for the coastal tram, about a 15-minute walk from the port gate: Leaving the port area from Swedish Quay, turn right and walk along the coastal road. Once in town, pass the church and tram stop and continue along the tram tracks. At the next major intersection, there's a KBC bank on the left and a BNP Paribas bank on the right. If you're taking the tram to Blankenberge, you'll find ATMs at the train station there.

Internet Access: The Blankenberge library has free Wi-Fi and Internet access (Mon-Fri 14:00-18:00, Sat 10:00-13:00, closed Sun, near the train station at Onderwijsstraat 17, tel. 050-415-978, http://bibliotheek.blankenberge.be).

Pharmacy: The most convenient pharmacy is in Blankenberge. Ride the tram to Blankenberge's train station, cross the large square, and turn right up the pedestrian shopping street called Kerkstraat. You'll see a neon green cross about 100 feet up the street for Apotheek Spaens (Mon-Tue and Thu-Sat 9:00-12:00 & 14:00-18:30, closed Wed and Sun, staff speaks English, Kerkstraat 83, tel. 050-411-141). In Zeebrugge, Apotheek Havendam, near the beach, is open only on weekdays (Mon-Fri 9:00-12:30 & 14:00-18:45, closed Sat-Sun, Brusselstraat 34, tel. 050-545-514).

Grocery: If you want to buy a picnic or stock up on snacks, you'll find a Spar grocery store on the main street by the Zeebrugge Kerk tram stop (daily, Kustlaan 94, tel. 050-544-686).

By Cruise-Line Shuttle Bus

Some cruise lines provide a shuttle bus from the dock all the way to Blankenberge's train station (generally for a fee).

By Taxi

Taxis queue up just outside the port gate. Fares are expensive—most cabs charge at least €50 one-way for a trip to Bruges. It's best to arrange for a taxi in advance; try Taxi Snel, which has a standard rate of €50 between Zeebrugge and Bruges (tel. 050-363-649, mobile 0478-353-535, www.taxisnel.be). A taxi from the port to the train station in Blankenberge costs about €20.

Here are some likely fares for one-way journeys to farther destinations: Brussels—€225; Ghent—€140; Ypres (Flanders Fields)—€180.

By Tour

For information on local tour options in Bruges—including local guides for hire, walking tours, and bus tours—see "Tours in Bruges" on page 872. For Brussels, see page 896.

RETURNING TO YOUR SHIP

Coming by train from Bruges, Ghent, or Brussels, simply ride the train back to Blankenberge (you can't miss it—it's the end of the line). Once you arrive in Blankenberge, leave the station, cross the street, and take the tram in the direction of Knokke. If your ship is at **Maritime Station,** jump off at the Zeebrugge Strandwijk stop to catch the cruise-line shuttle bus. If your ship is at **Swedish Quay,** stay on the tram until the Zeebrugge Kerk stop (with a large brick church right next to the platform). From here, it's a 10-minute walk back to the cruise port gate and your shuttle bus. If you're in a hurry, you can spring for a cab (€20) from the Blankenberge train station to the dock.

See page 927 for help if you miss your boat.

Bruges

Right from the start, Bruges was a trading center. In the 11th century, the city grew wealthy on the cloth trade. By the 14th century, Bruges' population was 35,000, as large as London's. As the middleman in the sea trade between northern and southern Europe, it was one of the biggest cities in the world and an economic powerhouse. In addition, Bruges had become the most important cloth market in northern Europe.

In the 15th century, while England and France were slugging it out in the Hundred Years' War, Bruges was the favored residence of the powerful Dukes of Burgundy—and at peace. Commerce and the arts boomed. The artists Jan van Eyck and Hans Memling had studios here.

But by the 16th century, the harbor had silted up and the economy had collapsed. The Burgundian court left, Belgium became a minor Habsburg possession, and Bruges' Golden Age abruptly ended. For generations, Bruges was known as a mysterious and dead city. In the 19th century, a new port, Zeebrugge, brought renewed vitality to the area. And in the 20th century, tourists discovered the town.

Today, Bruges prospers because of tourism: It's a uniquely well-preserved Gothic city and a handy gateway to Europe. It's no secret, but even with the crowds, it's the kind of place where you don't mind being a tourist.

BRUGES & BRUSSELS

Orientation to Bruges

The tourist's Bruges is less than one square mile, contained within a canal (the former moat). Nearly everything of interest and importance is within a convenient cobbled swath between the train station and the Markt (Market Square; a 20-minute walk). Most tourists are concentrated in the triangle formed by the Markt, Burg Square, and the Church of Our Lady; outside of that tight zone, the townscape is sleepy and relatively uncrowded.

TOURIST INFORMATION

The main TI, called **In&Uit** ("In and Out"), is in the big, red concert hall on the square called 't Zand (daily 10:00-18:00, take a number from the touch-screen machines and wait, 't Zand 34, tel. 050-444-646, www.brugge.be, toerisme@brugge.be). They have three terminals with free Internet access and printers.

Other TI branches include one at the **train station** (Mon-Fri 10:00-17:00, Sat-Sun 10:00-14:00) and one on the **Markt,** sharing a building with the Historium museum (daily 10:00-17:00, Markt 1).

ARRIVAL AT BRUGES TRAIN STATION

Travelers stepping out the door of the Bruges train station are greeted by a taxi stand and a roundabout with center-bound buses

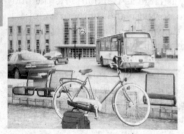

circulating through every couple of minutes. Coming in, you'll see the bell tower that marks the main square (Markt, the center of town). The station has a TI, ATMs, and lockers.

The best way to get to the town center is by **bus.** Buses #1, #3, #4, #6, #11, #13, #14, and #16 go to the Markt (all marked *Centrum*). Simply hop on, pay €2 (€1.20 if you buy in advance at Lijnwinkel shop just outside the train station), and you're there in four minutes (get off at third stop—either Markt or Wollestraat). A **taxi** from the train station to downtown is about €8.

It's a 20-minute **walk** from the station to the Markt: Cross the busy street and canal in front of the station, head up Oostmeers, and turn right on Zwidzandstraat. You can rent a **bike** at the station, but other bike-rental shops are closer to the center (see "Helpful Hints," next).

HELPFUL HINTS

Blue Monday: If you're in Bruges on a Monday, when several museums are closed, consider the following activities or attractions: the bell-tower climb on the Markt, Begijnhof, De Halve Maan Brewery tour, Basilica of the Holy Blood, City Hall's Gothic Room, Bruges Beer Museum, Historium, chocolate shops and museum, and Church of Our Lady. You can also join a boat, bus, or walking tour, or rent a bike and pedal into the countryside.

Museum Pass: The main TI on 't Zand and the city museums sell a "Museumpas" **combo-ticket** for €20 (valid for 3 days at 16 locations). Because the Groeninge and Memling museums cost €8 each, you'll save money with this pass if you plan to see at least one other covered sight.

Market Days: Bruges hosts markets on Wednesday morning (on the Markt) and Saturday morning ('t Zand). On good-weather Saturdays, Sundays, and public holidays, a flea market hops along Dijver in front of the Groeninge Museum. The Fish Market sells souvenirs daily and seafood Wednesday through Saturday mornings until 13:00.

Internet Access: There are free computer terminals at the **TI** on 't Zand. **Call Shop,** just a block off the Markt, is the most central of the city's many "telephone shops" offering Internet access (daily 9:00-20:00, Philipstockstraat 4).

Post Office: It's on the Markt near the bell tower (Mon-Fri 9:00-18:00, Sat 9:30-15:00, closed Sun, tel. 050-331-411).

Bike Rental: Bruges Bike Rental is central and cheap, with friendly service and long hours (€3.50/hour, €5/2 hours, €7/4 hours, €10/day, show this book to get student rate—€8/day, no deposit required—just ID, daily 10:00-22:00, free city maps and child seats, behind the far-out iron facade at Niklaas Desparsstraat 17, tel. 050-616-108, Bilal). **Fietsen Popelier Bike Rental** is also good (€4/hour, €8/4 hours, €12/day, no deposit required, daily 10:00-19:00, sometimes open later in summer, free Damme map, Mariastraat 26, tel. 050-343-262). **Koffieboontje Bike Rental** is just under the bell tower on the Markt (€4/hour, €9/day, €20/day for tandem, these prices for Rick Steves readers, daily 9:00-22:00, free city maps and child seats, Hallestraat 4, tel. 050-338-027). **Fietspunt Brugge** is a huge outfit at the train station (7-speed bikes, €12/24-hours, €7/4 hours, free maps, Mon-Fri 7:00-19:30, Sat-Sun 9:00-21:30, just outside the station and to the right as you exit, tel. 050-396-826).

Best Town View: The bell tower overlooking the Markt rewards those who climb it with the ultimate Bruges view.

Updates to This Book: For updates to this book, check ricksteves.com/update.

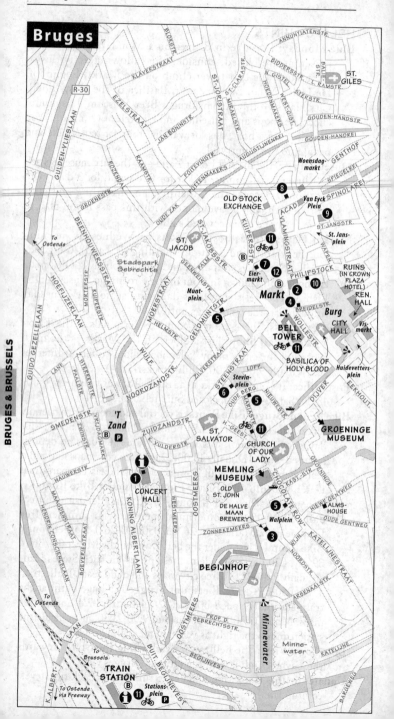

Bruges

R-30

To Ostende

ST. GILES

OLD STOCK EXCHANGE

Van Eyck Plein

ST. JACOB

St. Jansplein

ST. JANSSTR.

RUINS (IN CROWN PLAZA HOTEL)

REN. HALL

Eiermarkt

Markt

Burg

CITY HALL

Vismarkt

BELL TOWER

BASILICA OF HOLY BLOOD

Huidevettersplein

Stevinplein

GROENINGE MUSEUM

'T Zand

ST. SALVATOR

CHURCH OF OUR LADY

MEMLING MUSEUM

ALMSHOUSE

Concert Hall

OLD ST. JOHN

DE HALVE MAAN BREWERY

Walplein

BEGIJNHOF

Minnewater

TRAIN STATION

Stationsplein

To Ostende

To Brussels

To Ostende via Freeway

Stadspark Sebrechte

Muntplein

Woensdagmarkt

BRUGES & BRUSSELS

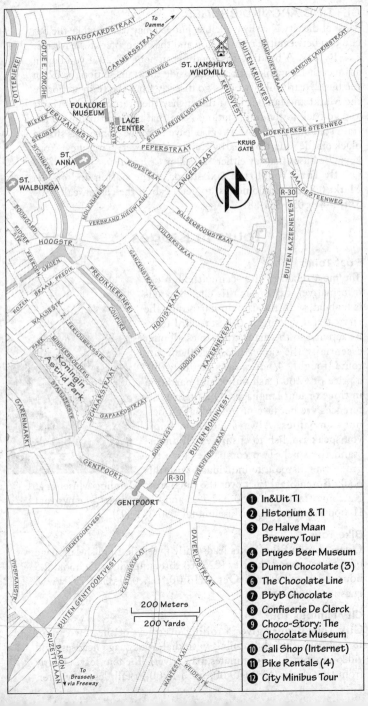

1. In&Uit TI
2. Historium & TI
3. De Halve Maan Brewery Tour
4. Bruges Beer Museum
5. Dumon Chocolate (3)
6. The Chocolate Line
7. BbyB Chocolate
8. Confiserie De Clerck
9. Choco-Story: The Chocolate Museum
10. Call Shop (Internet)
11. Bike Rentals (4)
12. City Minibus Tour

GETTING AROUND BRUGES

Most of the city is easily walkable, but you may want to take the bus or a taxi between the train station and the city center at the Markt.

By Bus: A bus ticket is good for an hour (€1.20 if you buy in advance at Lijnwinkel shop just outside the train station, or €2 on the bus). Nearly all city buses go directly from the train station to the Markt and fan out from there; they then return to the Markt and go back to the train station. Note that buses returning to the train station from the Markt also leave from the library bus stop, a block off the square on nearby Kuiperstraat (every 5 minutes). Your key: Use buses that say either *Station* or *Centrum*.

By Taxi: You'll find taxi stands at the station and on the Markt (€8/first 2 kilometers; to get a cab in the center, call 050-334-444 or 050-333-881).

Tours in Bruges

Boat Tours

The most relaxing and scenic (though not informative) way to see this city of canals is by boat, with the captain narrating. The city carefully controls this standard tourist activity, so the many companies all offer essentially the same thing: a 30-minute route (roughly 4/hour, daily 10:00-17:00), a price of €7.60 (cash only), and narration in three or four languages. Qualitative differences are because of individual guides, not companies. Always let them know you speak English to ensure you'll understand the spiel. Two companies give the group-rate discount to individuals with this book: **Boten Stael** (just over the canal from Memling Museum at Katelijnestraat 4, tel. 050-332-771) and **Gruuthuse** (Nieuwstraat 11, opposite Groeninge Museum, tel. 050-333-393).

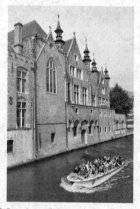

Bike Tour

QuasiMundo Bike Tours leads daily five-mile English-language bike tours around the city (€25, €3 discount with this book, 2.5 hours, departs March-Oct at 10:00, tel. 050-330-775, www.quasimundo.com).

City Minibus Tour

City Tour Bruges gives a rolling overview of the town in an 18-seat, two-skylight minibus with dial-a-language headsets and video support (€16, 50 minutes, pay driver). The tour leaves hourly from the Markt (10:00-19:00, until 18:00 in fall, less in winter, tel. 050-355-024, www.citytour.be). The narration, though clear, is slow-moving and a bit boring. But the tour is a lazy way to cruise past virtually every sight in Bruges.

Walking Tours

Your Bruges is enthusiastically run by Andy. His entertaining two-hour walks focus on Bruges' back streets, less-discovered sights, and a few silly legends and stories. This is more affordable than hiring your own guide, since Andy charges per person—with no minimum—and may collect several of my readers into a small group (€10/person, cheaper for groups of more than 10, typically available afternoons and weekends, arrange in advance, tel. 0468-174-700, yourbruges@gmail.com).

The **TI** also arranges walks through the core of town (€9, 2 hours, daily July-Aug, Sat-Sun only mid-April-June and Sept-Oct, depart from TI on 't Zand Square at 14:30—just drop in a few minutes early and buy tickets at the TI desk). Though earnest, the tours are heavy on history and given in two languages, so they may be less than peppy. Still, to propel you beyond the pretty gables and canal swans of Bruges, they're good medicine.

Local Guides

Daniëlle Janssens gives two-hour walks for €80, three-hour walks for €120, and full-day tours of Bruges and Brussels for €210 (mobile 0476-493-203, www.tourmanagementbelgium.be, tmb@skynet.be). You can also hire a guide through the **TI** (typically €70/2-hour tour, reserve at least one week in advance, for contact information see "Tourist Information," earlier).

Horse-and-Buggy Tour

The buggies around town can take you on a clip-clop tour (€36, 35 minutes; price is per carriage, not per person; buggies gather in Minnewater, near entrance to Begijnhof, and on the Markt). When divided among four or five people, this can be a good value.

Sights in Bruges

ON OR NEAR THE MARKT

▲Markt (Market Square)

The crossroads of Bruges is one of the most enjoyable town squares in Belgium—and in this country, that's really saying something. In Bruges' heyday as a trading center, a canal came right up to this square. And today it's still the heart of the modern city. The square is ringed by the frilly post office, enticing restaurant terraces, great old gabled buildings, and the iconic bell tower. Under the bell tower are two great Belgian-style french-fry stands. The streets spoking off this square are lined with tempting eateries and

Bruges at a Glance

▲▲Bell Tower Overlooking the Markt, with 366 steps to a worthwhile view and a carillon close-up. **Hours:** Daily 9:30-17:00. See page 874.

▲▲Burg Square Historic square with sights and impressive architecture. **Hours:** Always open. See page 875.

▲▲Groeninge Museum Top-notch collection of mainly Flemish art. **Hours:** Tue-Sun 9:30-17:00, closed Mon. See page 876.

▲▲Church of Our Lady Tombs and church art, including Michelangelo's *Madonna and Child*. **Hours:** Mon-Sat 9:30-17:00, Sun 13:30-17:00. See page 878.

▲▲Memling Museum at St. John's Hospital Art by the greatest of the Flemish Primitives. **Hours:** Tue-Sun 9:30-17:00, closed Mon. See page 879.

▲▲Begijnhof Benedictine nuns' peaceful courtyard and Beguine's House museum. **Hours:** Courtyard open daily 6:30-18:30; museum open Mon-Sat 10:00-17:00, Sun 14:00-17:00, shorter hours off-season. See page 881.

▲▲De Halve Maan Brewery Tour Fun tour that includes beer. **Hours:** April-Oct Mon-Fri tours approximately on the hour

shops. Most city buses run from near here to the train station—use the library bus stop, a block down Kuiperstraat from the Markt.

▲▲Bell Tower (Belfort)

Most of this bell tower has presided over the Markt since 1300, serenading passersby with cheery carillon music. The octagonal lantern was added in 1486, making it 290 feet high—that's 366 steps. The view is worth the climb...and probably even the pricey admission. Some mornings and summer evenings, you can sit in the courtyard or out on the square to enjoy a carillon concert.

Cost and Hours: €8, daily 9:30-17:00, 16:15 last-entry time strictly enforced—best to show up before 16:00, pay WC in courtyard.

▲Historium

I despise the Disneyfication of Europe, but this glitzy sight right on the Markt is actually

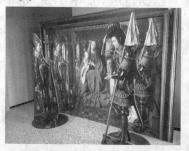

10:00-17:00, Sat-Sun until 18:00; Nov-March Mon-Fri 10:00 and 15:00 only, Sat 10:00-17:00, Sun 11:00-16:00. See page 882.

▲**Markt** Main square that is the modern heart of the city, with carillon bell tower. **Hours:** Always open. See page 873.

▲**Historium** Glitzy multimedia exhibit that re-creates the sights, sounds, and even smells of 1430s Bruges. **Hours:** Daily 10:00-18:00. See page 874.

▲**Basilica of the Holy Blood** Romanesque and Gothic church housing a relic of the blood of Christ. **Hours:** Daily 9:30-12:00 & 14:00-17:00; Nov-March closed on Wed afternoon. See page 875.

▲**City Hall** Beautifully restored Gothic Room from 1400, plus the Renaissance Hall. **Hours:** Daily 9:30-17:00, Renaissance Hall closed 12:30-13:30. See page 876.

▲**Bruges Beer Museum** History of Belgian beer and the brewing process, with tastings. **Hours:** Daily 10:00-17:00. See page 883.

▲**Choco-Story: The Chocolate Museum** The delicious story of Belgium's favorite treat. **Hours:** Daily 10:00-17:00. See page 884.

entertaining—and it takes a genuine interest in history. It's pricey and cheesy—sort of "Pirates of the Belgian-ean" (or maybe "Hysterium")—but it immerses you in the story of Bruges in a way a textbook cannot.

Cost and Hours: €11, daily 10:00-18:00, last entrance one hour before closing, includes audioguide, may be too creepy for kids, Markt 1, tel. 050-270-311, www.historium.be.

▲▲Burg Square

This opulent, prickly spired square is Bruges' civic center, the historic birthplace of Bruges, and the site of the ninth-century castle of the first count of Flanders. It's home to the Basilica of the Holy Blood and City Hall (described next). Today, it's an atmospheric place to take in an outdoor concert while surrounded by six centuries of architecture.

▲Basilica of the Holy Blood

Originally the Chapel of Saint Basil, this church is famous for its relic of the blood of Christ, which, according to tradition, was brought to Bruges in 1150 after the Second Crusade. The lower chapel is dark and solid—a fine example of Romanesque style. The upper chapel (separate entrance, climb the stairs) is decorated Gothic. An interesting treasury museum is next to the upper chapel.

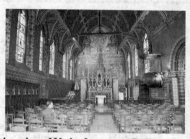

Cost and Hours: Church-free, treasury-€2, daily 9:30-12:00 & 14:00-17:00; Nov-March closed on Wed afternoon; Burg Square, tel. 050-336-792, www.holyblood.com.

▲City Hall (Stadhuis)

This complex houses several interesting sights, including a room full of old town maps and paintings, and the highlight—the grand, beautifully restored **Gothic Room** from 1400, starring a painted and carved wooden ceiling adorned with hanging arches. Your ticket also covers the less impressive **Renaissance Hall** (Brugse Vrije), next door and basically just one ornate room with a Renaissance chimney (separate entrance—in corner of square at Burg 11a).

Cost and Hours: €4; daily 9:30-17:00, Renaissance Hall closed 12:30-13:30, last entry 30 minutes before closing; includes audioguide, tel. 050-448-711, www.brugge.be.

SOUTH OF THE MARKT

Also in this area is the De Halve Maan Brewery, with an excellent beer tour (described later, under "Experiences in Bruges").

▲▲Groeninge Museum

This museum houses a world-class collection of mostly Flemish art, from Memling to Magritte. While there's plenty of worthwhile modern art, the highlights are the vivid and pristine Flemish Primitives. (In Flanders, "Primitive" simply means "before the Renaissance.") Flemish art is shaped by its love of detail, its merchant patrons' egos, and the power of the Church. Lose yourself in the halls of Groeninge: Gaze across 15th-century canals, into the eyes of reassuring Marys, and through town squares littered with leotards, lace, and lopped-off heads.

Cost and Hours: €8, more for special exhibits; Tue-Sun 9:30-17:00, closed Mon; Dijver 12, tel. 050-448-743, www.brugge.be/musea.

Visiting the Museum: The collection fills 10 rooms on one easy floor, arranged chronologically from the 15th to the 20th century. I'd head right to Rooms 2-4 for the following paintings—the core of the collection.

Jan van Eyck's *Virgin and Child with Canon Joris van der*

Paele (1436) is his masterpiece. Van Eyck, the world's first and greatest oil painter, brings Mary and the saints down from heaven and into a typical (rich) Bruges home. He strips off their haloes, banishes all angels, and pulls the plug on heavenly radiance. If this is a religious painting, then where's God? God's in the details, from the bishop's damask robe and Mary's wispy hair to the folds in Jesus' baby fat.

Van Eyck's *Portrait of Margareta van Eyck* (1439) is a simple portrait, but revolutionary—one of history's first individual portraits that wasn't of a saint, a king, a duke, or a pope, and wasn't part of a religious work. It signals the advent of humanism, celebrating the glory of ordinary people. Van Eyck proudly signed the work on the original frame, with his motto saying he painted it *"als ik kan" (ALC IXH KAN)*..."as good as I can."

Rogier van der Weyden's *St. Luke Drawing the Virgin's Portrait* (c. 1435) shows off this fine artist's skill. Van der Weyden, the other giant among the Flemish Primitives, adds the human touch to Van Eyck's rather detached precision. Baby Jesus can't contain his glee, wiggling his fingers and toes, anticipating lunch. Meanwhile, St. Luke (the patron saint of painters) looks on intently with a sketch pad in his hand, trying to catch the scene. These small gestures, movements, and facial expressions add an element of human emotion that later artists would amplify.

Van der Weyden's *Duke Philip the Good* (c. 1450) depicts the tall, lean, elegant, and charismatic duke who transformed Bruges from a commercial powerhouse to a cultural one. In 1425, Philip moved his court to Bruges, making it the de facto capital of a Burgundian empire stretching from Amsterdam to Switzerland. He's wearing the gold-chain necklace of the Order of the Golden Fleece, a distinguished knightly honor he gave himself. As a lover of painting, hunting, fine clothes, and many mistresses, Philip was a role model for Italian princes, such as Lorenzo the Magnificent— the *uomo universale*, the Renaissance Man.

Hans Memling's *The Moreel Triptych* (1484) is perhaps the art world's first group portrait, and everything about it celebrates the family of Willem Moreel, the wealthy two-term mayor of Bruges.

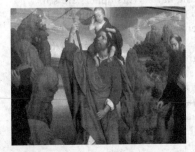

The true stars of the triptych are not the saints in the central panel but the earth-bound mortals who paid for it. Moreel (left panel) kneels in devotion along with his five sons (and St. William, who was Willem's patron saint). Barbara (right) kneels with their 13 daughters (and her patron saint, Barbara).

Saints and mortals mingle in a unique backdrop that's both down-to-earth (the castle, plants, and St. Barbara's stunning dress) and ethereal (the weird rock formations and unnaturally pristine light). Memling's motionless, peaceful world invites meditation. It was perfect for where the triptych originally stood—in the Moreel burial chapel.

The Rest of the Museum: Breeze through the final rooms to get a quick once-over of Flemish art after Bruges' Golden Age. As Bruges declined into a cultural backwater, its artists simply copied the trends going on elsewhere: Italian-style Madonnas, British-style aristocrat portraits, French-Realist landscapes, Impressionism, and thick-paint Expressionism.

After fast-forwarding through the centuries, pause (in Rooms 9 and 10) to appreciate a couple of Belgium's 20th-century masters—Paul Delvaux and René Magritte.

▲▲Church of Our Lady (Onze-Lieve-Vrouwekerk)

The church stands as a memorial to the power and wealth of Bruges in its heyday, featuring Michelangelo's delicate statue of

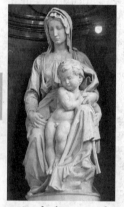

the *Madonna and Child*. If you like tombs and church art, pay to wander through the apse, but note that the church is undergoing a major, years-long renovation, during which different parts of the interior will be closed to visitors.

Cost and Hours: The rear of the church is free to the public. To get into the main section costs €6; Mon-Sat 9:30-17:00, Sun 13:30-17:00, Mariastraat, tel. 050-448-711, www.brugge.be/musea.

Visiting the Church: Enter and stand in the back to admire the Church of Our Lady. Its 14th- and 15th-century stained glass was destroyed by iconoclasts, so the church is lit more brightly today than originally. Like most of Belgium, it is Catholic. The medieval-style screen divided the clergy from the commoners who gathered here in the nave. Worshippers are still attended by 12 Gothic-era statues of apostles, each with his symbol and a grandiose Baroque wooden pulpit, with a roof that seems to float in midair.

Head for the church's highlight, the *Madonna and Child* by **Michelangelo.** You'll pay and pass through the turnstile, then enter the chapel with the small marble statue (1504), said to be the only Michelangelo statue to leave Italy in the sculptor's lifetime (thanks to the wealth generated by Bruges' cloth trade). It was bought in Tuscany by a wealthy Bruges businessman, who's buried in the same chapel (to the right).

Next visit the **tombs at the high altar.** The reclining statues mark the tombs of the last local rulers of Bruges: Mary of Burgundy, and her father, Charles the Bold. The dog and lion at their feet are symbols of fidelity and courage. Underneath the tombs are the actual excavated gravesites with mirrors to help you enjoy the well-lit, centuries-old tomb paintings.

Bruges residents would stand before these tombs and ponder the great decline of their city. In 1482, when 25-year-old Mary of Burgundy tumbled from a horse and died, she left behind a toddler son and a husband who was heir to the Holy Roman Empire. Beside her lies her father, Charles the Bold, who also died prematurely, in war. Their twin deaths meant Bruges belonged to Austria, and would soon be swallowed up by the empire and ruled from Vienna by Habsburgs—who didn't understand or care about its problems. Trade routes shifted, and goods soon flowed through Antwerp, then Amsterdam, as Bruges' North Sea port silted up. The city was eventually mothballed. The sleeping beauty of Flemish towns was later discovered by modern-day tourists to be remarkably well-pickled, which explains its current affluence.

The Rest of the Church: The wooden balcony to the left of the painted altarpiece is part of the Gruuthuse mansion next door, providing the noble family with prime seats for Mass.

In a side chapel in the apse you'll see excavations that turned up fascinating grave paintings on the tombs below and near the altar. Dating from the 14th and 15th centuries, these show Mary represented as Queen of Heaven (on a throne, carrying a crown and scepter) and Mother of God (with the baby Jesus on her lap). Since Mary is in charge of advocating with Jesus for your salvation, she's a good person to have painted on the wall of your tomb.

▲▲Memling Museum at St. John's Hospital (Sint Janshospitaal)

The former monastery/hospital complex has a fine collection in what was once the monks' church. It contains several much-loved paintings by the greatest of the Flemish Primitives, Hans Memling. His *St. John Altarpiece* triptych is a highlight, as is the miniature, gilded-oak shrine to St. Ursula.

Cost and Hours: €8, Tue-Sun 9:30-17:00, closed Mon, last entry 30 minutes before closing, includes good audioguide, across the street from the Church of Our Lady, Mariastraat 38, tel. 050-448-713, www.brugge.be/musea.

Visiting the Museum: After showing your ticket, enter a vast hall. The building itself, which has housed a hospital since 1188, is impressive, with stout wood pillars and brick walls. This hall was lined with beds filled with the sick and dying. Nuns served as nurses. At the far end was the high altar, which once displayed Memling's *St. John Altarpiece* (which we'll see). Bedridden patients could gaze on this peaceful, colorful vision and gain a moment's comfort from their agonies.

Browse the hall's displays of medical implements. It's clear that medicine of the day was well-intentioned but very crude. In many ways, this was less a hospital than a hospice, helping the dying make the transition from this world to the next. Religious art (displayed throughout the museum) was therapeutic, addressing the patients' mental and spiritual health.

Continue through the displays and head through the wooden doorway to the black-and-white tiled room where **Memling's paintings** are displayed. A large triptych (three-paneled altarpiece) dominates the space—the **St. John Altarpiece** (a.k.a. *The Mystical Marriage of St. Catherine*, 1474). The piece was dedicated to the hospital's patron saints, John the Baptist and John the Evangelist (see the inscription along the bottom of the frame), but Memling broadened the focus to take in a vision of heaven and the end of the world.

In the central panel, Mary, with Baby Jesus on her lap, sits in a canopied chair, crowned by hovering blue angels. It's an imaginary gathering of conversing saints *(sacra conversazione)*, though nobody in this meditative group is saying a word. In the left panel, even the gruesome beheading of John the Baptist becomes serene under Memling's gentle brush.

On the right, John sits on a high, rocky bluff. Overhead, in a rainbow bubble, God appears on his throne, resting his hand on a sealed book. A lamb steps up to open the seals, unleashing the awful events at the end of time. Standing at the bottom of the rainbow, an angel in green gestures to John and says, "Write this down." John picks up his quill, but he pauses, absolutely transfixed, experiencing the Apocalypse now.

In a glass case nearby, you'll find another Memling masterpiece, the **St. Ursula Shrine** (c. 1489). On October 21, 1489, the mortal remains of St. Ursula were brought here to the church and placed in this gilded oak shrine, built specially for the occasion and decorated with paintings by Memling. Ursula, yet another Christian martyred by the ancient Romans, became a sensation in the Middle Ages when builders in Germany's Cologne unearthed a huge pile of bones believed to belong to her and her 11,000 slaughtered cohorts. Look carefully at the "roof" of the church-shaped shrine, and you'll see Ursula, holding the arrow with which she was martyred.

In the small adjoining room, find more Memlings, including the **Diptych of Martin van Nieuwenhove** (1489). Three-dimensional effects—borrowed from the Italian Renaissance style—enliven this two-panel devotional painting. Both Mary and Child and the 23-year-old Martin, though in different panels, inhabit the same space within the painting. If you line up the paintings' horizons (seen in the distance, out the room's windows), you'll see that both panels depict the same room—with two windows at the back and two along the right wall.

Want proof? In the convex mirror on the back wall (just to the left of Mary), the scene is reflected back at us, showing Mary and Martin from behind, silhouetted in the two "windows" of the picture frames. Apparently, Mary makes house calls, appearing right in the living room of the young donor Martin.

Memling's bread-and-butter was portraits created for families of wealthy businessmen. *Portrait of a Young Woman* (1480) takes us right back to that time. The young woman looks out of the frame as if she were looking out a window. Her hands rest on the "sill," with the fingertips sticking over. Memling accentuates her fashionably pale complexion and gives her the pensive, sober expression of a medieval saint. Still, she keeps her personality, with distinct features like her broad nose, neck tendons, and realistic hands. What's she thinking? (My guess: "It's time for a waffle.")

▲▲Begijnhof

Begijnhofs were built to house women of a lay Catholic order, called Beguines. Though obedient to a mother superior, they did

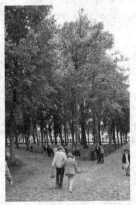

not take the vows of a nun. They spent their days deep in prayer, spinning wool, making lace, teaching, and caring for the sick. The Beguines' ranks swelled during the Golden Age, when so many women were widowed or unwed due to the hazards of war and overseas trade. The order of Beguines offered such women a dignified place to live and work. When the order died out, many *begijnhofs* were taken over by towns for subsidized housing. Today, single religious women live in the small homes. Benedictine nuns live in a building on the far side.

Cost and Hours: Courtyard-free, daily 6:30-18:30; museum-€2, Mon-Sat 10:00-17:00, Sun 14:00-17:00, shorter hours off-season, English explanations, museum is left of entry gate; tel. 050-330-011.

Visiting the Begijnhof: There are several sights here. You can tour the simple **museum** to get a sense of Beguine life. It's a typical Beguine residence—kitchen, dining room, bedroom—with period furniture (spinning wheel, foot warmer). Don't miss the bedroom out back across the tiny cloister. The "Liturgical Center" is little more than a gift shop.

In the **church,** enjoy the peaceful interior, with its carved pulpit and tombstones on the floor. The altar has corkscrew columns and a painting of the Beguines' patron, St. Elizabeth. On the right wall is an 800-year-old golden statue of Mary. The rope that dangles from the ceiling is yanked by a nun to announce a sung vespers service. The Benedictine nuns gather at 11:55, proceed through the garden, and sing and chant a capella in the choir of the church. The public is welcome for this service.

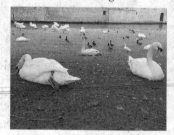

Nearby: Just south of the Begijnhof is the waterway called **Minnewater,** an idyllic world of flower boxes, canals, and swans.

Experiences in Bruges

While Bruges has some top-notch museums, many of its charms are more experiential.

BEER

Hoisting a glass of beer is a quintessential ▲▲▲ Bruges experience. The city offers a wide variety of places to sample brews (see listings on page 890), one of the most accessible and enjoyable brewery tours in Belgium, and an interesting museum on beer.

▲▲De Halve Maan Brewery Tour

Belgians are Europe's beer connoisseurs, and this handy tour is a great way to pay your respects. The brewery makes the only beers

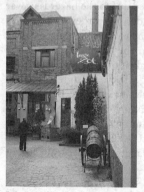

brewed in Bruges: Brugse Zot ("Fool from Bruges") and Straffe Hendrik ("Strong Henry"). The happy gang at this working-family brewery gives entertaining and informative 45-minute tours in two languages (lots of steep steps but a great rooftop panorama). Avoid crowds by visiting at 11:00. Their bistro, where you'll drink your included beer, serves quick, hearty lunch plates.

Cost and Hours: €7.50 tour includes a beer; tours run April-Oct Mon-Fri approximately on the hour 10:00-17:00, Sat-Sun until 18:00; Nov-March Mon-Fri 10:00 and 15:00 only, Sat 10:00-17:00, Sun 11:00-16:00; check the chalkboard for the schedule when you arrive; tours can fill up; Walplein 26, tel. 050-444-223, www.halvemaan.be.

▲Bruges Beer Museum

With a red-carpet entrance just off the Markt, this ode to beer's frothy history overlooks the square from the top of the post office. Head up three flights of stairs to the museum's entrance, where you'll get an iPad and headphones to tour the exhibit and learn about the history of beer-making. The most interesting section is on the top floor, where you can run your hands through raw hops, yeast, and barley while getting a step-by-step guide to modern brewing.

When you've had your historical fill, saunter down to the bar and trade the iPad for three tokens good for your choice of tasting-size beers from a rotating list of 15 local drafts. The bar offers Markt views and is also open to the public (ticket not required).

Cost and Hours: €11 ticket includes three tastings, daily 10:00-17:00, Breidelstraat 3, tel. 0479-359-567, www.bruges beermuseum.com.

CHOCOLATE

Bruggians are connoisseurs of fine chocolate. You'll be tempted by chocolate-filled display windows all over town. While Godiva is the best big-factory/high-price/high-quality brand, there are plenty of smaller family-run places in Bruges that offer exquisite handmade chocolates. All of the following chocolatiers are proud of their creative varieties and welcome you to assemble a 100-gram assortment of five or six chocolates.

A rule of thumb when buying chocolate: Bruges' informal "chocolate mafia" keeps the price for midrange pralines quite standard, at about €24 per kilogram (or €2.40 for 100 grams). Swankier and "gastronomical" places (like The Chocolate Line or BbyB) charge significantly more, but only aficionados may be able to tell the difference. On the other hand, if a place is priced well *below* this range, be suspicious: Quality may suffer.

By the way, if you're looking for value, don't forget to check the supermarket shelves. Try Côte d'Or Noir de Noir for a simple bar of pure dark chocolate that won't flatten in your luggage.

▲Chocolate Shops

Katelijnestraat, which runs south from the Church of Our Lady, is "Chocolate Row," with a half-dozen shops within a few steps. For locations, see the map on page 871.

Dumon: Perhaps Bruges' smoothest, creamiest chocolates are at Dumon, just off the Markt (a selection of 5 or 6 chocolates are a deal at €2.30/100 grams). Nathalie Dumon runs the store with Madame Dumon still dropping by to help make their top-notch chocolate daily and sell it fresh. Try a small mix-and-match box to sample a few out-of-this-world flavors, and come back for more

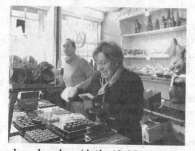

of your favorites. The original location is just north of the Markt at Eiermarkt 6 (Wed-Mon 10:00-18:00, closed Tue, old chocolate molds on display in basement, tel. 050-346-282). A bigger, glitzier Dumon branch at Simon Stevinplein 11 has a full coffee and hot chocolate bar (daily 10:00-18:30, tel. 050-333-360). A third, less-interesting branch is farther south, at Walstraat 6.

The Chocolate Line: Locals and tourists alike flock to The Chocolate Line (pricey at €5.60/100 grams) to taste the *gastronomique* varieties concocted by Dominique Person—the mad scientist of chocolate. His unique creations mix chocolate with various, mostly savory, flavors. Even those that sound gross can be surprisingly good (be adventurous). The kitchen—busy whipping up 80 varieties—is on display in the back. Enjoy the window display, refreshed monthly (daily 9:30-18:00 except Sun-Mon opens at 10:30, between Church of Our Lady and the Markt at Simon Stevinplein 19, tel. 050-341-090).

BbyB: This chichi, top-end chocolate gallery (whose name stands for "Babelutte by Bartholomeus," for the Michelin-starred restaurateur who owns it) lines up its pralines in a minimalist display case like priceless jewels, each type identified by number. If you don't mind—or actually enjoy—the pretense, the chocolates are top-notch (about €4 for a 5-flavor sleeve, €9 for a sleek 10-flavor sampler box; Tue-Fri 10:00-12:00 & 13:00-18:00, Sat 10:00-18:00, closed Sun-Mon; Sint-Amandsstraat 39, tel. 050-705-760, www.bbyb.be).

Confiserie De Clerck: Third-generation chocolatier Jan sells his handmade chocolates for just €1.20/100 grams, making this one of the best deals in town. Some locals claim his chocolate's just as good as at pricier places, while others insist that any chocolate this cheap must be subpar—taste it and decide for yourself. The time-warp candy shop is so delightfully old-school, you'll want to visit one way or the other (Mon-Wed and Fri-Sat 10:00-19:00, closed Thu and Sun, Academiestraat 19, tel. 050-345-338).

▲Choco-Story: The Chocolate Museum

With lots of artifacts well-described in English, this kid-friendly museum fills you in on the production of truffles, bonbons, hollow figures, and solid bars of chocolate. Head up the stairs by the gigantic chocolate egg to follow the chronological exhibit, tracing 4,000 years of chocolate history. The finale is downstairs in the "demonstration room," where—after a 10-minute cooking demo—you get a taste.

Cost and Hours: €8, ticket includes chocolate bar; daily 10:00-17:00, last entry 45 minutes before closing; where Wijnzakstraat meets Sint Jansstraat at Sint Jansplein, 3-minute walk from the Markt; tel. 050-612-237, www.choco-story-brugge.be.

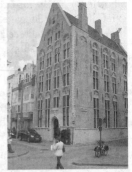

Lace Center (Kant Centrum)

This lace museum and school lets you learn about lace-making and then see lace actually being made.

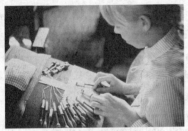

Observe as ladies toss bobbins madly while their eyes go bad.

Cost and Hours: €5, Mon-Sat 10:00-17:00, closed Sun, demonstrations usually 14:00-17:00, Balstraat 16 (see location on map on page 871), www. kantcentrum.eu.

Nearby: Nearly across the street from the Lace Center is a lace shop with a good reputation, **'t Apostelientje** (Tue 13:00-17:00, Wed-Sat 9:30-12:15 & 13:15-17:00, Sun 10:00-13:00, closed Mon, Balstraat 11, tel. 050-337-860, mobile 0495-562-420).

BIKING

The Dutch word for bike is *fiets* (pronounced "feets"). And though Bruges' sights are close enough for easy walking, the town is a treat for bikers. A bike quickly gets you into dreamy back lanes without a hint of tourism. Take a peaceful ride through the town's nooks and crannies and around the outer canal. Ask at the rental shop for maps and ideas (see "Bike Rental" on page 869 for more info).

Shopping in Bruges

Souvenir shoppers will find plenty of options. Shops are generally open from 10:00 to 18:00 and closed Sundays.

WHAT TO BUY

Chocolate: A box of Belgian pralines is at the top of most souvenir shoppers' lists; see my tips and recommended chocolate shops on page 883.

Beer: Another consumable souvenir is Belgian beer—either a bottle (or three) for later in your trip, or a prized brew checked carefully in your luggage home. In addition to the pubs listed earlier—a few of which sell bottles to go—the streets of Bruges are lined with bottle shops. At some, you can buy the correct glass that's designed to go with each type of beer (it's a fragile item to pack, but purists insist). Options include the touristy souvenir store **2Be** (described below) or **The Bottle Shop,** which sells 600 different beers by the bottle and has a staff that enjoys helping visitors navigate the many choices (daily 10:00-18:30, just south of the Markt at Wollestraat 13, tel. 050-349-980).

Lace: This is a popular item, but very expensive; 't Apostelientje, described on page 885, is one good option (and conveniently located nearly across the street from the Lace Center).

WHERE TO SHOP

Souvenir shops abound on the streets that fan out from the Markt and the ones heading southwest, toward the Church of Our Lady. **2Be,** in a classic old brick mansion overlooking a canal a block south of the Markt, is huge, obvious, and grotesquely touristy...but well-stocked with a wide variety of tacky and not-so-tacky Belgian souvenirs: Tintin, Smurfs, beer, and chocolates. The "beerwall" at the entrance shows off over a thousand types of Belgian brew; their cellar is filled with a remarkably well-stocked bottle shop; and their pub has several rotating draft beers you can enjoy on a relaxing terrace floating over a perfect canal (daily 10:00-19:00, Wollestraat 53, tel. 050-611-222, www.2-be.biz).

More colorful are the shops along **Geldmuntstraat** (which becomes **Noordzandstraat**). Along this atmospheric drag— with perhaps Bruges' most enjoyable window-shopping—are smaller, more expensive chains and upscale boutiques (including L'Heroine, highlighting Belgian designers at Noordzandstraat 32); housewares shops (such as Cook & Serve, a fun kitchen gadgets shop, at Geldmuntstraat 16); and the popular Da Vinci gelato shop (see listing on page 892).

For the highest concentration of tourists (and, consequently, the highest concentration of souvenir, chocolate, lace, and *wafel* shops), head down **Katelijnestraat,** which runs south from the Church of Our Lady and the Memling Museum. While you'll find no great values here, it's convenient for souvenir shopping.

Eating in Bruges

Bruges doesn't really have any specialties all its own, but restaurants here excel at all the predictable Belgian dishes: mussels cooked a variety of ways (one order can feed two), fish dishes, grilled meats, and french fries. The town's two indigenous beers are the prizewinning Brugse Zot, a golden ale, and Straffe Hendrik, a potent, bitter triple ale.

RESTAURANTS

Rock Fort is a chic spot with a modern, fresh coziness and a high-powered respect for good food. Two young chefs, Peter Laloo and Hermes Vanliefde, give their French cuisine a creative, gourmet twist. At the bar they serve a separate tapas menu. This place is a winner (€6-12 tapas, great pastas and salads,

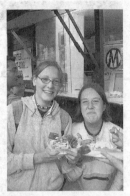

€15 lunch special, beautifully presented €17-34 dinner plates, €40 five-tapas special, fancy €49 fixed-price four-course meal, open Mon-Fri 12:00-14:30 & 18:30-23:00, closed Sat-Sun, reservations recommended, Langestraat 15, tel. 050-334-113, www.rock-fort. be).

Bistro in den Wittenkop, very Flemish, is a stylishly small, laid-back, old-time place specializing in local favorites for dinner. It's a classy spot to enjoy hand-cut fries, which go particularly well with Straffe Hendrik beer (€37 three-course meal, €21-26 plates, Mon-Sat 18:00-21:30, closed Sun, reserve ahead, terrace in summer, Sint Jakobsstraat 14, tel. 050-332-059, www.indenwittenkop. be).

Bistro den Amand, with a plain interior and a few outdoor tables, exudes unpretentious quality the moment you step in. In this mussels-free zone, Chef An is enthusiastic about stir-fry and vegetables, as her busy wok and fun salads prove. Portions are splittable and there are always good vegetarian options. The creative dishes—some with a hint of Asian influence—are a welcome departure from Bruges' mostly predictable traditional restaurants. It's on a bustling pedestrian lane a half-block off the Markt (€35 three-course meal, €18-25 plates; Mon-Tue and Thu-Sat 12:00-14:15 & 18:00-21:00, closed Wed and Sun; Sint-Amandstraat 4, tel. 050-340-122, www.denamand.be, An Vissers and Arnout Beyaert).

Tom's Diner is a trendy, cozy little candlelit bistro in a quiet, cobbled residential area a 10-minute walk from the center. Young chef Tom gives traditional dishes a delightful modern twist, such as his signature Flemish meat loaf with rhubarb sauce. If you want to flee the tourists and experience a popular neighborhood joint, this is it—the locals love it. Reserve before you make the trip (€16-23 plates, Tue-Sat 12:00-14:00 & 18:00-23:00, closed Sun-Mon, north of the Markt near Sint-Gilliskerk at West-Gistelhof 23, tel. 050-333-382, www.tomsdiner.be).

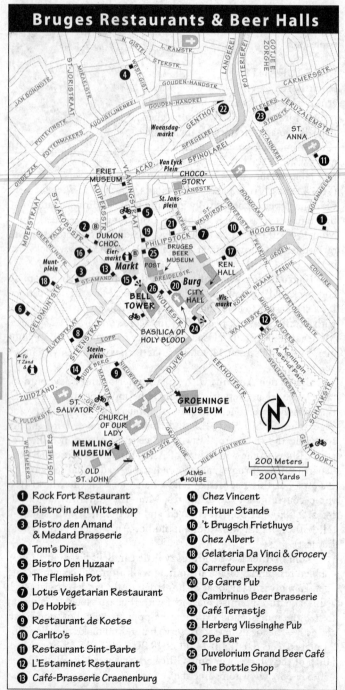

Bruges Restaurants & Beer Halls

1. Rock Fort Restaurant
2. Bistro in den Wittenkop
3. Bistro den Amand & Medard Brasserie
4. Tom's Diner
5. Bistro Den Huzaar
6. The Flemish Pot
7. Lotus Vegetarian Restaurant
8. De Hobbit
9. Restaurant de Koetse
10. Carlito's
11. Restaurant Sint-Barbe
12. L'Estaminet Restaurant
13. Café-Brasserie Craenenburg
14. Chez Vincent
15. Frituur Stands
16. 't Brugsch Friethuys
17. Chez Albert
18. Gelateria Da Vinci & Grocery
19. Carrefour Express
20. De Garre Pub
21. Cambrinus Beer Brasserie
22. Café Terrastje
23. Herberg Vlissinghe Pub
24. 2Be Bar
25. Duvelorium Grand Beer Café
26. The Bottle Shop

Bistro Den Huzaar is classy but affordable, serving big portions of Belgian classics. The long dining room stretches back on well-worn wooden floors with white-tablecloth elegance. It's dignified but relaxed (€17-20 main dishes, €35 fixed-price meal, Fri-Tue 12:00-14:30 & 18:00-20:30, closed Wed-Thu, 5-minute walk north of the Markt at Vlamingstraat 36, tel. 050-333-797).

The Flemish Pot is a busy eatery where enthusiastic chefs Mario and Rik cook up a traditional menu of vintage Flemish specialties—from beef and rabbit stew to eel—served in little iron pots and skillets. Seating is tight and cluttered, the tourist-oriented menu can be pricey, and service can be spotty. But you'll enjoy huge portions, refills from the hovering "fries angel," cozy atmosphere, and a good selection of local beers (€32-35 three-course meals, €22-29 plates, daily 12:00-22:00, reservations smart, just off Geldmuntstraat at Helmstraat 3, tel. 050-340-086, www. devlaamschepot.be).

Lotus Vegetarian Restaurant serves serious lunch plates (€14 *plat du jour* offered daily), salads, and homemade chocolate cake in a pleasantly small, bustling, and upscale setting. To keep carnivorous companions happy, they also serve several very good, organic meat dishes (Mon-Fri from 11:45, last orders at 14:00, closed Sat-Sun, just north of Burg Square at Wapenmakersstraat 5, tel. 050-331-078).

De Hobbit, featuring an entertaining dinner menu, is always busy with happy eaters. It's nothing fancy, just good, basic food served in a fun, crowded, traditional grill house (daily 18:00-23:00, family-friendly, Kemelstraat 8, reservations smart, tel. 050-335-520, www.hobbitgrill.be).

Restaurant de Koetse is handy for central, good-quality, local-style food. The feeling is traditional, a bit formal (stuffy even), and dressy, yet accessible. The cuisine is Belgian and French, with an emphasis on grilled meat, seafood, and mussels (€25 lunch menu Mon-Sat, €36 three-course meals, €20-30 plates include vegetables and a salad, Fri-Wed 12:00-14:30 & 18:00-22:00, closed Thu, non-smoking section, Oude Burg 31, tel. 050-337-680, Piet).

Carlito's is a good choice for basic Italian fare. Their informal space, with whitewashed walls and tea-light candles, is two blocks from Burg Square (€9-15 pizzas and pastas, daily 12:00-14:30 & 18:00-22:30, patio seating in back, Hoogstraat 21, tel. 050-490-075).

Restaurant Sint-Barbe, on the eastern edge of town, is a homey little neighborhood place where Evi serves classy Flemish dishes made from local ingredients in a fresh, modern space on two floors (€12 soup-and-main lunch, €14-22 main courses, Thu-Mon 11:30-14:00 & 18:00-22:00, closed Tue-Wed, food served until 21:00, St. Annaplein 29, tel. 050-330-999).

L'Estaminet is a youthful, jazz-filled eatery. Don't be intimidated by its lack of tourists. Local students flock here for the Tolkien-chic ambience, hearty €10 spaghetti, and big meal-size salads. This is Belgium—it serves more beer than wine. For outdoor dining under an all-weather canopy, enjoy the relaxed patio facing peaceful Astrid Park (Fri-Wed 11:30-24:00, Thu 16:00-24:00, Park 5, tel. 050-330-916).

Restaurants on the Markt: Most tourists seem to be eating on the Markt with the bell tower high overhead and horse carriages clip-clopping by. The square is ringed by tourist traps with aggressive waiters expert at getting you to consume more than you intended. Still, if you order smartly, you can have a memorable meal or drink here on one of the finest squares in Europe at a reasonable price. Consider **Café-Brasserie Craenenburg,** with a straightforward menu, where you can get pasta and beer for €15 and spend all the time you want ogling the magic of Bruges (daily 7:30-23:00, Markt 16, tel. 050-333-402). While it's overpriced for dining, it can be a fine place to savor a before- or after-meal drink with the view.

Cheaper Restaurants Just off the Markt: For a similar but less expensive array of interchangeable, tourist-focused eateries, head a few steps off the Markt up **Sint-Amandstraat** (through the gap between Café Craenenburg and the clock tower). You'll pop out into a pleasant little square with lots of choices. The best of these is **Bistro den Amand** (recommended earlier), but if that's full or closed, this is a fine place to browse for something else. **Medard Brasserie,** also on this square, serves the cheapest hot meal in town—hearty meat spaghetti (big plate-€4, huge plate-€6.50, sit inside or out, Mon-Tue and Thu-Sat 12:00-20:00, closed Wed and Sun, Sint Amandstraat 18, tel. 050-348-684).

PUBS AND BEER HALLS

My best budget-eating tip for Bruges: Stop into one of the city's bars for a simple meal and a couple of world-class beers with great Bruges ambience. Among these listings, Cambrinus puts more emphasis on its food; Café Terrastje and Herberg Vlissinghe have a small selection of still-substantial meals; and De Garre has lighter food and snacks. The bar at 2Be and the Duvelorium Grand Beer Café aren't good places to eat; go to these to focus on the beer.

Just off the Markt: De Garre (deh-HAHR-reh) is a good place to gain an appreciation for Belgian beer culture. Rather than a noisy pub scene, it has a dressy, sit-down-and-focus-on-your-friend-and-the-fine-beer vibe. Beer pilgrims flock here, as it's the only place on earth that sells the Tripel van de Garre beer on tap. As it's 12 percent alcohol, there's a three-Tripel limit...and many tourists find that the narrow alley out front provides much-needed support as they start their stumble back home (daily 12:00-24:00, later on weekends, additional seating up tiny staircase, off Breidelstraat between Burg and the Markt, on tiny Garre alley, tel. 050-341-029).

Rollicking Beer Brasserie: **Cambrinus** is a touristy but enjoyable *bierbrasserie*. Bright, tight, and boisterous, it serves 400 types of beer and good pub grub. It's more high-spirited and accessible than some of Bruges' traditional, creaky old beer halls (€15-22 main dishes, daily 11:00-23:00, reservations smart, Philipstockstraat 19, tel. 050-332-328, www.cambrinus.eu/english.htm).

In the **Gezellig** *Quarter, Northeast of the Markt:* These pubs are tucked in the wonderfully *gezellig* (cozy) quarter that follows the canal past Jan Van Eyckplein, northeast of the Markt. Just walking out here is a treat, as it gets you away from the tourists. **Café Terrastje** is a cozy pub serving light meals. Enjoy the subdued ambience inside, or relax on the front terrace overlooking the canal and heart of the *gezellig* district (€6-8 sandwiches, €10-18 dishes; food served Fri-Mon 12:00-15:00 & 18:00-21:00, open until 23:30; Tue 12:00-18:00; closed Wed-Thu; corner of Genthof and Langerei, tel. 050-330-919, Ian and Patricia). **Herberg Vlissinghe** is the oldest pub in town (1515). Bruno keeps things basic and laid-back, serving simple plates (lasagna, grilled-cheese sandwiches, and famous €10 angel-hair spaghetti) and great beer in the best old-time tavern atmosphere in town. This must have been the Dutch Masters' rec room. The garden outside comes with a *boules* court—free for guests to watch or play (Wed-Sat 11:00-24:00, Sun 11:00-19:00, closed Mon-Tue, Blekersstraat 2, tel. 050-343-737).

Beer with a View: Though it's tucked in back of a tacky tourist shop, the bar at **2Be** serves several local beers on tap and boasts a fine scenic terrace over a canal (see page 886). **Duvelorium Grand Beer Café** is pricey but picturesque. It's located upstairs from the Historium, with a spiny Gothic terrace overlooking the bustle on the Markt. As it's operated by the big beer producer Duvel, choices are more limited than some local watering holes (eight beers on tap, plus lots of bottles), and the prices are high—but it's worth paying extra for the view (same hours as Historium—see listing on page 874, you can enter the pub without paying for the museum, last orders at 19:00).

SWEETS AND QUICK EATS
Belgian Fries
Belgian french fries *(frieten)* are a treat. Proud and traditional *frituur*s serve tubs of fries and various local-style shish kebabs. Belgians dip their *frieten* in mayonnaise or other flavored sauces, but ketchup is there for the Yankees. I encourage you to skip the

BRUGES & BRUSSELS

ketchup and have a sauce adventure.

On the Markt: For a quick, cheap, and scenic snack, hit a *frituur* and sit on the steps or benches overlooking the Markt (convenient benches are about 50 yards past the post office). Twin take-away fry carts are on the square at the base of the bell tower (daily

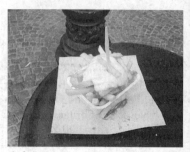

10:00-24:00). I find the cart on the left better quality and more user-friendly.

Elsewhere: **Chez Vincent,** with pleasant outdoor tables on a terrace facing St. Salvator's Cathedral along the lively Steenstraat shopping drag, is a cut above. It's understandably popular for using fresh, local ingredients to turn out tasty fries and all manner of other fried and grilled Belgian tasties: burgers, sausages, meatballs, croquettes, and so on (€3-5 fries and basics, Wed-Fri 12:00-14:30 & 17:30-20:00, Sat-Sun 12:00-20:00, closed Mon-Tue, Sint-Salvatorskerkhof 1, tel. 050-684-395).

't Brugsch Friethuys, a block off the Markt, is handy for fries you can sit down and enjoy. Its forte is greasy, deep-fried Flemish fast food. The €13.30 "Big Hunger menu" comes with all the traditional gut bombs (daily 11:00-late, at the corner of Geldmuntstraat and Sint Jakobsstraat, Luc will explain your options).

Picnics

A handy location for groceries is the **Carrefour Express** mini-supermarket, just off the Markt on Vlamingstraat (daily 8:00-19:00); for a slightly wider selection, **Delhaize-Proxy** is just up Geldmuntstraat (Mon-Sat 9:00-19:00, closed Sun, Noordzandstraat 4).

Belgian Waffles and Ice Cream

You'll see waffles sold at restaurants and take-away stands. One of Bruges' best is also one of its most obvious: **Chez Albert,** on Breidelstraat connecting the Markt and Burg Square, is pricey, but the quality is good and—thanks to the tourist crowds—turnover is quick, so the waffles are fresh (daily 10:00-18:00, at #18).

Gelateria Da Vinci, the local favorite for homemade ice cream, has creative flavors and a lively atmosphere. As you approach, you'll see a line of happy lickers. Before ordering, ask to sample the Ferrero Rocher (chocolate, nuts, and crunchy cookie) and plain yogurt (daily 11:00-22:00, later in summer, Geldmuntstraat 34, tel. 050-333-650, run by Sylvia from Austria).

Brussels

Six hundred years ago, Brussels was just a nice place to stop and buy a waffle on the way to Bruges. With no strategic importance,

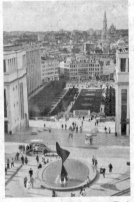

it was allowed to grow as a free trading town. Today it's the capital of Belgium, the headquarters of NATO, and the seat of the European Union. It's also a fascinating and vibrant city in its own right, with fun-to-explore neighborhoods, good sightseeing, an impressive selection of restaurants, and a quirky Flemish/French mix.

The Brussels of today reflects its past. The city enjoyed a Golden Age of peace and prosperity (1400-1550) when many of its signature structures were built. In the late 1800s, Brussels had another growth spurt, fueled by industrialization, wealth taken from the Belgian Congo, and the exhilaration of the country's recent independence (1830). The "Builder King" Leopold II erected grand monuments and palaces. Then, in 1992, EU countries signed the Treaty of Maastricht, and sleepy Brussels suddenly was thrust into the spotlight as the unofficial capital of the new Europe. It started a frenzy of renovation, infrastructure projects, foreign visitors, and world attention.

In Brussels, people speak French. Bone up on *bonjour* and *s'il vous plaît* (see the French survival phrases on page 1141). The Bruxellois are cultured and genteel—even a bit snobby compared to their more earthy Flemish cousins. The whole feel of the town is urban French, not rural Flemish. And yet you may notice an impish sparkle and *joie de vivre*, as evidenced by their love of comic strips (giant comic-strip panels are painted on buildings all over town) and their civic symbol: a statue of a little boy peeing.

Brussels is the cutting edge of modern Europe, but still clothed in its Old World garments. Stroll the Grand Place, snap a selfie with the *Manneken-Pis*, and watch diplomats at work at the EU assembly halls. Then grab some mussels, fries, and a hearty Belgian beer, and watch the sun set behind the Town Hall's lacy steeple.

Orientation to Brussels

Central Brussels is surrounded by a ring of roads (which replaced the old city wall) called the Pentagon. (Romantics think it looks more like a heart.) All the sights I mention are within this ring.

The epicenter holds the main square (the Grand Place), the TI, and Central Station (all within three blocks of one another).

What isn't so apparent from maps is that Brussels is a city divided by altitude. A ridgeline that runs north-south splits the town into the Upper Town (east half, elevation 200 feet) and Lower Town (west, at sea level), with Central Station in between.

Brussels' bilingual street signs, combined with the near-complete lack of a regular grid plan, can make navigating the city confusing. It's easy to get turned around. I rely heavily on a good map (such as the TI's) when exploring this town.

TOURIST INFORMATION

Brussels has two competing TIs (indicative of Belgium's latent Walloon-Flemish tension). The TI at Rue du Marché aux Herbes 63 covers **Brussels and Flanders** (April-Sept Mon-Sat 9:00-18:00, Sun 10:00-17:00, shorter hours off-season; three blocks down-hill from Central Station, tel. 02-504-0390, www.visitflanders. com, fun Europe store nearby). They offer free Wi-Fi and several Internet terminals.

The other TI, which focuses on just the **city of Brussels,** is inside the Town Hall on the Grand Place (daily April-Nov 9:00-18:00, shorter hours off-season; tel. 02-513-8940, www. visitbrussels.be).

Sightseeing Deals: Brussels does not offer a must-have sight-seeing pass. The **Brussels Card,** sold at TIs, is unlikely to pay for itself if you are in town for less than a day (www.brusselscard.be). The TIs also offer a discount deal called **Must of Brussels,** which could save you a few euros (www.mustofbrussels.com).

ARRIVAL AT BRUSSELS CENTRAL TRAIN STATION

Brussels has three stations: Centraal/Central, Midi/Zuid/South, and Nord/Noord/North. Central Station, nearest to the sights, is a short walk from the Grand Place and is by far the easiest for arriving sightseers (pay close attention and ask your conductor for help to ensure you get off at the right stop). The station has handy services: a small grocery store, fast food, waiting rooms, and luggage lockers (between tracks 3 and 4).

You can walk from Central Station to the Grand Place in about five minutes: Following signs inside the station for *Marché aux Herbes/Grasmarkt,* you'll be directed through the Galerie Horta shopping mall, where you'll ride an escalator down, pass a Smurf shop, and pop out 50 yards from the little square called "Agora." At the far end of this square, turn left to reach the Grand Place, or continue straight ahead to find the big Brussels and Flanders TI on your left.

Hop-on, hop-off tourist buses depart from Central

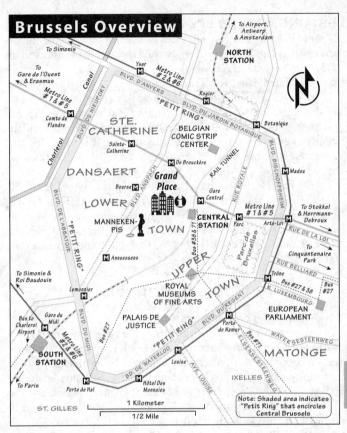

Brussels Overview

To Simonis

To Airport, Antwerp & Amsterdam

NORTH STATION

To Gare de l'Ouest & Erasmus

Yser

Metro Line #2 & #6

BLVD. D'ANVERS

Comte de Flandre

Metro Line #1 & #5

Canal

BLVD. DE NIEUPORT

"PETIT RING"

Rogier

BLVD. DU JARDIN BOTANIQUE

Botanique

Charleroi

STE. CATHERINE

Sainte-Catherine

BELGIAN COMIC STRIP CENTER

BLVD. BISCHOFFSHEIM

Madou

De Brouckère

DANSAERT

Bourse

BLVD. AITBACH

Grand Place

Gare Central

RUE ROYALE

Metro Line #1 & #5

To Stokkel & Herrmann-Debroux

LOWER

TOWN

CENTRAL STATION

Arts-Loi

RUE DE LA LOI

MANNEKEN-PIS

Bus #88 & 71

Parc

To Cinquantenaire Park

Anneessens

UPPER

Parc de Bruxelles

RUE BELLIARD

To Simonis & Roi Baudouin

Lemonnier

TOWN

ROYAL MUSEUMS OF FINE ARTS

Trône

Bus #27 & 38

Bus #27

Bus to Charleroi Airport

Gare du Midi

BLVD. DU MIDI

Bus #27

PALAIS DE JUSTICE

BLVD. DU RÉGENT

R. LUXEMBOURG

EUROPEAN PARLIAMENT

Metro Line #2 & #6

"PETIT RING"

Porte de Namur

Bus #71

WAVERSESTEENWEG

SOUTH STATION

BD. DE WATERLOO

Louise

AVE. LOUISE

IJZELENSTEENWEG

MATONGE

To Paris

Porte de Hal

Hôtel Des Monnaies

IXELLES

ST. GILLES

1 Kilometer

1/2 Mile

Note: Shaded area indicates "Petit Ring" that encircles Central Brussels

BRUGES & BRUSSELS

Station—handy if you want an easy way to get oriented to the city (see "Tours in Brussels," later).

HELPFUL HINTS

Sightseeing Schedules: Brussels' most important museums are closed on Monday. Of course, the city's single best sight—the Grand Place—is always open. You can also enjoy a bus tour any day of the week.

Internet Access: The **Brussels and Flanders TI** (listed earlier) offers free Wi-Fi, as well as free use of their Internet terminals (15-minute limit). There's also an **Internet café** in a dreary urban area between the Grand Place and Ste. Catherine (also cheap calls and printing, calling cabins downstairs, computer terminals upstairs, daily 9:30-23:15, 18 Rue Marché aux Poulets).

Updates to This Book: For updates to this book, check www. ricksteves.com/update.

GETTING AROUND BRUSSELS

Most of central Brussels' sights can be reached on foot. But public transport is handy for climbing to the Upper Town (buses #38 or #71, from near Central Station).

By Métro, Bus, and Tram: A single €2.10 ticket is good for one hour on all public transportation. Buy individual tickets at newsstands, in Métro stations (vending machines accept credit cards or coins), or (for €0.40 extra) from the bus driver. Validate your ticket when you enter a bus by feeding it into one of the breadbox-size machines. Transit info: tel. 02-515-2000, www. mivb.be.

By Taxi: Cabbies charge a €2.40 drop fee, as well as €1.70 per additional kilometer. Convenient taxi stands near the Grand Place are at the Bourse and the "Agora" square (Rue du Marché aux Herbes). In the Upper Town, try Place du Grand Sablon. To call a cab, try **Taxi Bleu** (tel. 02-268-0000) or **Autolux** (tel. 02-512-3123).

Tours in Brussels

Hop-On, Hop-Off Bus Tours

Two companies—**City Tours** and **CitySightseeing/Open Tours**—offer nearly identical 1.5-hour loops with (mediocre) recorded narration on double-decker buses that go topless on sunny days. You can hop on and off for 24 hours with one ticket. The handiest starting points are at Central Station and the Bourse. Each charges about €20-22 and runs about twice hourly (roughly April-Oct daily 10:00-16:00, Sat until 17:00; Nov-March daily 10:00-15:00, Sat until 16:00; City Tours—tel. 02-513-7744, www.brussels-city-tours.com; CitySightseeing/Open Tours—tel. 02-466-1111, www.citysightseeingbrussel.be).

Bus Tours

City Tours also offers a typical three-hour guided bus tour (in up to five languages), providing an easy way to get the grand perspective on Brussels. You start with a walk around the Grand Place, then jump on a tour bus (€26, year-round daily at 10:00, depart from their office a block off Grand Place at Rue du Marché aux Herbes 82; you can buy tickets there at a TI; tel. 02-513-7744, www.brussels-city-tours.com).

Local Guides

You can hire a private guide through **Visit Brussels** (€117/3 hours, €216/full day, tel. 02-548-0448, guides@visitbrussles.be; I enjoyed the guiding of Didier Rochette). **Claude and Dominique Janssens** are a father-and-son team who lead tours both in Brussels and to other Belgian cities, including Bruges, Ghent, and

Antwerp (€120/3 hours, €240/full day plus €25 for lunch, Claude's mobile 0485-025-423, Dominique's mobile 0486-451-155, www. discover-b.be, claude@discover-b.be). **Daniëlle Janssens,** who is based in Bruges, offers a full-day tour of Brussels for €210 (for contact info, see "Local Guides" on page 873).

Grand Place Walk

Like most European cities, Brussels has a main square, but few are as "Grand" as this one. From its medieval origins as a market for a small village, the Grand Place has grown into a vast public space enclosed by Old World buildings with stately gables. Today, the "Place" is *the* place to see Europe on parade. Visitors come to bask in the ambience, sample chocolate, and relax with a beer at an outdoor café.

This walk allows all that, but also goes a bit beyond. We'll take in the spectacular (if heavily touristed) square, browse an elegant shopping arcade, run the frenetic gauntlet of "Restaurant Row," stand at the center of modern Brussels at the Bourse, and end at the grand finale (he said with a wink): the one-of-a-kind *Manneken-Pis*. Allow two hours for this walk.

• *Begin this walk standing on Brussels' very grand main square.*

❶ The Grand Place

This colorful cobblestone square is the heart—historically and geographically—of heart-shaped Brussels. As the town's market square for 1,000 years, this was where farmers and merchants sold their wares in open-air stalls, enticing travelers from the main east-west highway across Belgium, which ran a block north of the square. Today, shops and cafés sell chocolates, *gaufres* (waffles), beer, mussels, fries, *dentelles* (lace), and flowers (for details on cafés and chocolate shops on the Grand Place, see the sidebar on page 906).

Pan the square to get oriented. Face the Town Hall with its skyscraping spire. One TI is on your right, under the Town Hall's arches, while another TI is one block behind you; "Restaurant Row" is another block beyond that. To your right, a block away (downhill), is the Bourse building. The Upper Town is to your left, rising up the hill beyond the Central Station. Over your left shoulder a few blocks away is St. Michael's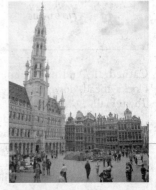

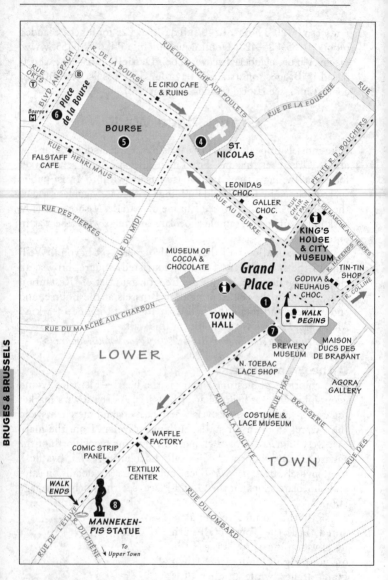

Cathedral. And most important? The *Manneken-Pis* is three blocks ahead, down the street that runs along the left side of the Town Hall.

The **Town Hall** (Hôtel de Ville) dominates the square with its 300-foot-tall tower, topped by a golden statue of St. Michael slaying a devil. Built in the 1400s, this was where the city council met to rule this free trading town. Brussels proudly maintained its self-governing independence while dukes, kings, and clergymen ruled

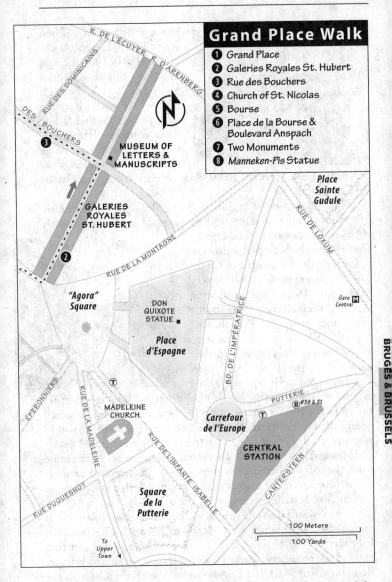

Grand Place Walk

1 Grand Place
2 Galeries Royales St. Hubert
3 Rue des Bouchers
4 Church of St. Nicolas
5 Bourse
6 Place de la Bourse & Boulevard Anspach
7 Two Monuments
8 Manneken-Pis Statue

BRUGES & BRUSSELS

much of Europe. You can step into the Town Hall courtyard for a little peace (but the building's interior is only open by tour—€5, English tours offered Wed at 15:00, Sun at 10:00 and 14:00, no Sun tours Oct-March).

Opposite the Town Hall is the impressive, gray **King's House** (Maison du Roi), which now houses the **City Museum.** It's gone through several incarnations in its 800-year history. First it was the medieval square's bread market—hence, the building's Dutch

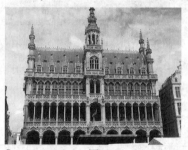

name—Broodhuis. Then (early 1500s) it became the regional office for the vast Habsburg empire of Charles V—hence, its French name—Maison du Roi. The lacy, prickly Gothic facade dates from the late-1800s, when it was renovated to be the City Museum (€4, Tue-Sun 10:00-17:00, Thu until 20:00, closed Mon, www.museedelaville debruxelles.be).

The fancy smaller buildings giving the square its uniquely grand medieval character are former **guild halls** (now mostly shops and restaurants), their impressive gabled roofs topped with statues. Once the home offices for the town's different professions (brewers, bakers, and *Manneken-Pis* corkscrew makers), they all date from shortly after 1695—the year French king Louis XIV's troops took the high ground east of the city, sighted their cannons on the Town Hall spire, and managed to level everything around it (4,000 mostly wooden buildings) without ever hitting the spire itself. As a matter of pride, these Brussels businessmen rebuilt their offices better than ever, completing everything within seven years. They're in stone, taller, and with ornamented gables and classical statues. While they were all built at about the same time, the many differences in styles reflect the independent spirit of the people and the many cultural influences that converged in this crossroads trading center.

The **Swan House** (#9, just to the left of the Town Hall) once housed a bar where Karl Marx and Friedrich Engels met in February of 1848 to write their *Communist Manifesto*. Later that year, when the treatise sparked socialist revolution around Europe, Belgium exiled Marx and Engels. Today, the once-proletarian bar is one of the city's most expensive restaurants. Next door (#10) was and still is the brewers' guild, now housing the **Brewery Museum** (€5, includes a local beer, daily 10:00-17:00, www.belgian brewers.be).

• *Exit the Grand Place next to Godiva (from the northeast, or uphill, corner of the square), and go north one block on Rue de la Colline. Along the way, you'll pass a popular **Tintin boutique** (at #9). It sells merchandise of the popular Belgian comic-strip hero to both kids and* *adults who grew up with him. Continue to Rue du Marché aux Herbes, which was once the main east-west highway through Belgium. The little park-like square just to your right—a modest gathering place with market stalls—is nicknamed "Agora" (after the nearby covered shopping area). Looking to the right, notice that it's all uphill from here to the Upper Town, another four blocks (and 200-foot elevation gain) beyond. Straight ahead, you enter the arcaded shopping mall called...*

❷ Galeries Royales St. Hubert

Built in 1847, Europe's oldest still-operating shopping mall served as the glass-covered model that inspired many other shopping

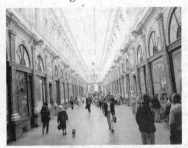

galleries in Paris, London, and beyond. It celebrated the town's new modern attitude (having recently gained its independence from the Netherlands). Built in an age of expansion and industrialization, the mall demonstrated efficient modern living, with elegant apartments upstairs above trendy shops, theaters, and cafés.

Even today, people live in the upstairs apartments.

Looking down the arcade (233 yards long), you'll notice that it bends halfway down, designed to lure shoppers farther. Its iron-and-glass look is still popular, but the decorative columns, cameos, and pastel colors evoke a more elegant time. It's Neo-Renaissance, like a pastel Florentine palace.

• *Midway down the mall, where the two sections bend (and where you'll find the interesting little Museum of Letters and Manuscripts, €7, closed Mon, www.mlmb.be), turn left and exit the mall onto...*

❸ Rue des Bouchers

Yikes! During meal times, this street is absolutely crawling with

tourists browsing through wall-to-wall, midlevel-quality restaurants. Brussels is known worldwide for its food, serving all kinds of cuisine, but specializing in seafood (particularly mussels). You'll have plenty to choose from along the table-clogged "Restaurant Row." To get an idea of prices, compare their posted *menùs*—the fixed-price, several-course meal offered by most restaurants. But don't count on getting a good value—better restaurants are just a few steps away (for specifics, see page 913).

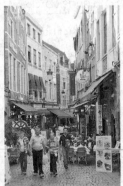

Brussels at a Glance

▲▲▲**Grand Place** Main square and spirited heart of the Lower Town, surrounded by mediocre museums and delectable chocolate shops. **Hours:** Always open. See page 897.

▲▲▲**Royal Museums of Fine Arts of Belgium** Museums displaying Old Masters (14th-18th century), turn-of-the-century art (19th-20th centuries), and works by the prominent Belgian Surrealist painter René Magritte. **Hours:** Tue-Sun 10:00-17:00, closed Mon, Magritte Museum open Wed until 20:00. See page 910.

▲▲*Manneken-Pis* World-famous statue of a leaky little boy. **Hours:** Always peeing. See page 905.

▲▲**BELvue Museum** Interesting Belgian history museum with a focus on the popular royal family. **Hours:** Tue-Fri 9:30-17:00, July-Aug until 18:00, Sat-Sun 10:00-18:00, closed Mon. See page 913.

▲**City Museum** Costumes worn by the *Manneken-Pis* statue and models of Brussels' history. **Hours:** Tue-Sun 10:00-17:00, Thu until 20:00, closed Mon. See page 899.

▲**Costume and Lace Museum** World-famous Brussels lace, as well as outfits, embroidery, and accessories from the 17th-20th centuries. **Hours:** Tue-Sun 10:00-17:00, closed Mon. See page 905.

▲**St. Michael's Cathedral** White-stone Gothic church where Belgian royals are married and buried. **Hours:** Mon-Fri 7:00-18:00, Sat-Sun 8:30-18:00. See page 907.

▲**Belgian Comic Strip Center** Homage to hometown heroes including the Smurfs, Tintin, and Lucky Luke. **Hours:** Tue-Sun 10:00-18:00, closed Mon. See page 907.

▲**Musical Instruments Museum** Exhibits with more than 1,500 instruments, complete with audio. **Hours:** Tue-Fri 9:30-17:00, Sat-Sun 10:00-17:00, closed Mon. See page 912.

▲**Town Hall** Focal point of the Grand Place, with arresting spire but boring interior. **Hours:** Tours depart Wed at 15:00, Sun at 10:00 and 14:00, no Sun tours Oct-March. See page 898.

The first intersection, with Petite Rue des Bouchers, is the heart of the restaurant quarter, which sprawls for several blocks around. The street names reveal what sorts of shops used to stand here—butchers *(bouchers)*, herbs, chickens, and cheese.

• *At this intersection, turn left onto Petite Rue des Bouchers and walk straight back to the Grand Place. (You'll see the Town Hall tower ahead.) At the Grand Place, turn right (west) on Rue au Beurre. Comparison-shop a little more at the Galler and Leonidas chocolate stores and pass by the little "Is it raining?" fountain. At the intersection with Rue du Midi is the...*

❹ Church of St. Nicolas

Since the 12th century, there's been a church here. Inside, along the left aisle, see rough stones in some of the arches from the early church. Outside, notice the barnacle-like shops, such as De Witte Jewelers, built right into the church. The church was rebuilt 300 years ago with money provided by the town's jewelers. As thanks, they were given these shops with apartments upstairs. Close to God, this was prime real estate. And jewelers are still here.

• *Just beyond the church, you run into the back entrance of a big Neoclassical building.*

❺ The Bourse (Stock Exchange) and Art Nouveau Cafés

The stock exchange was built in the 1870s in the Historicist style—a mix-and-match, Neo-everything architectural movement. Plans are in the works for the former stock exchange to host a big beer museum. The **ruins** under glass on the right side of the Bourse are from a 13th-century convent; there's a small museum inside.

Several **historic cafés** huddle around the Bourse. To the right (next to the covered ruins) is the woody **Le Cirio,** with its delightful circa-1900 interior. Around the left side of the Bourse is the **Falstaff Café,** which is worth a peek inside. Some Brussels cafés, like the Falstaff, are still decorated in the early 20th-century Art Nouveau style. Ironwork columns twist and bend like flower stems, and lots of Tiffany-style stained glass and mirrors make them light and spacious. Slender, elegant, willowy Gibson Girls decorate the wallpaper, while waiters in bowties glide by.

• *Circle around to the front of the Bourse, toward the busy Boulevard Anspach.*

❻ Place de la Bourse and Boulevard Anspach

Brussels is the political nerve center of Europe (with as many lobbyists as Washington, DC), and the city sees several hundred demonstrations a year. When the local team wins a soccer match or some political group wants to make a statement, this is where people flock to wave flags and honk horns.

It's also where the old town meets the new. To the right along Boulevard Anspach are two shopping malls and several first-run movie theaters. Rue Neuve, which parallels Anspach, is a bustling pedestrian-only shopping street.

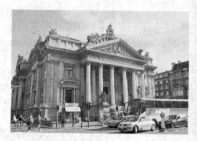

• *Now return to the Grand Place.*

From the Grand Place to the *Manneken-Pis*

• *Leave the Grand Place kitty-corner, heading south down the street running along the left side of the Town Hall, Rue Charles Buls (which soon changes its name to Stoofstraat). Just five yards off the square, under the arch, are* ❼ *two monuments honoring illustrious Brussels notables.*

The first monument features a beautiful young man—an Art Nouveau allegory of knowledge and science (which brings illumination, as indicated by the Roman oil lamp)—designed by Victor Horta. It honors **Charles Buls,** mayor from 1888 to 1899. If you enjoyed the Grand Place, thank him for saving it. He stopped King Leopold II from blasting a grand esplanade from Grand Place up the hill to the palace.

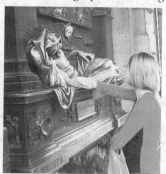

A few steps farther you'll see tourists and locals rubbing a **brass statue** of a reclining man. This was **Alderman Evrard 't Serclaes,** who in 1356 bravely refused to surrender the keys of the city to invaders, and so was tortured and killed. Touch him, and his misfortune becomes your good luck. Judging by the reverence with which locals treat this ritual, I figure there must be something to it.

From here, the street serves up a sampler of typical Belgian products. A half-block farther (on the left), the **N. Toebac Lace Shop** shows off some fine lace. Brussels is perhaps the best-known city for traditional lace making, and this shop still sells handmade pieces in the old style: lace clothing,

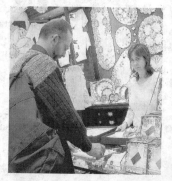

doilies, tablecloths, and ornamental pieces. The shop gives travelers with this book a 15 percent discount. For more on lace, visit the **Costume and Lace Museum,** which is a block away and just around the corner (€4, Tue-Sun 10:00-17:00, closed Mon, www.museeducostumeetdeladentelle.be).

A block farther down the street is the recommended, always popular **Waffle Factory,** where €2-3 gets you a freshly made takeaway "Belgian" waffle .

Cross busy Rue du Lombard and step into the **Textilux Center** (Rue du Lombard 41, on the left) for a good look at Belgian tapestries—both traditional wall-hangings and modern goods, such as tapestry purses and luggage in traditional designs.

Continuing down the street, notice a **mural** on the wall ahead, depicting that favorite of Belgian comic heroes, Tintin, escaping down a fire escape. Tintin is known and beloved by virtually all Europeans. His dog is named Snowy, Captain Haddock keeps an eye out for him, and the trio is always getting into misadventures. Dozens of these building-sized comic-strip panels decorate Brussels, celebrating the Belgians' favorite medium.

• *Follow the crowds, noticing the excitement build, because in another block you reach the...*

❽ *Manneken-Pis*

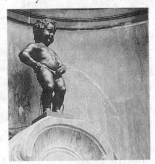

Even with low expectations, this bronze statue is smaller than you'd think—the little squirt's under two feet tall, practically the size of a newborn. Still, the little peeing boy is an appropriately low-key symbol for the unpretentious Bruxellois. The statue was made in 1619 to provide drinking water for the neighborhood. Notice that the baby, sculpted in Renaissance style, actually has the musculature of a man instead of the pudgy limbs of a child. The statue was knighted by the occupying King Louis XV—so French soldiers had to salute the eternally pissing lad when they passed.

As it's tradition for visiting VIPs to bring the statue an outfit, and he also dresses up for special occasions, you can often see the *Manneken* peeing through a colorful costume. A sign on the fence lists the month's festival days and how he'll be dressed. For example, on January 8, Elvis Presley's birthday, he's an Elvis impersonator; on Prostate Awareness Day, his flow is down to a slow drip. He can also be hooked up to a keg to pee wine or beer.

There are several different legends about the story behind *Manneken*—take your pick: He was a naughty boy who peed

BRUGES & BRUSSELS

Tasty Treats Around the Grand Place

Brussels' grand square (and the surrounding area) offers plenty of places to sample Belgium's culinary specialties.

Cafés: Mussels in Brussels, Belgian-style fries, yeasty local beers, waffles...if all you do here is plop down at a café on the square, try some of these specialties, and watch the world go by—hey, that's a great afternoon in Brussels.

The outdoor cafés are casual and come with fair prices (a decent Belgian beer costs €4.50, and a really good one is more like €5-7—with no cover or service charge). Have a seat, and a waiter will serve you. The half-dozen or so cafés on the downhill side of the square are all roughly equal in price and quality for simple drinks and foods—check the posted menus. As they are generally owned by breweries, you won't have a big selection of beers.

Choco-Crawl: The best chocolate shops all lie along the north (uphill) side of the square, starting with Godiva at the high end (higher in both altitude and price). The cost goes down slightly as you descend to the other shops. Each shop has a mouth-watering display case of chocolates and sells 100-gram mixes (six or so pieces) for about €5, or individual pieces for about €1 (for more on buying chocolate in Belgium, see page 883).

Godiva is synonymous with fine Belgian chocolate. Now owned by a Turkish company, Godiva still has its management and the original factory (built in 1926) in Belgium. This store, at Grand Place 22, was Godiva's first (est. 1937). The almond and honey goes way beyond almond roca.

Neuhaus, a few doors down at #27, has been encouraging local chocoholics since 1857. Their main store is in the Galeries Royales St. Hubert. Neuhaus publishes a good little pamphlet explaining its products. The "caprice" (toffee with vanilla crème) tastes like Easter. Neuhaus claims to be the inventor of the praline.

Galler, just off the square at Rue au Beurre 44, is homier and less famous because it doesn't export. Still family-run, it proudly serves the less sugary dark chocolate. The new top-end choice, 85 percent pure chocolate, is called simply "Black 85"—and worth a sample if you like chocolate without the sweetness. Galler's products are well-described in English.

Leonidas, four doors down at Rue au Beurre 34, is where cost-conscious Bruxellois get their fix, sacrificing 10 percent in quality to nearly triple their take (machine-made, only €2.20/100 grams). White chocolate is their specialty. If all the chocolate has made you thirsty, wash it down with **250 Beers,** next to Leonidas.

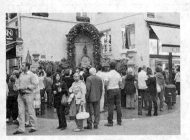

inside a witch's house, so she froze him. A rich man lost his son and declared, "Find my son, and we'll make a statue of him doing what he did when found." Or—the locals' favorite version—the little tyke loved his beer, which came in handy when a fire threatened the wooden city: He bravely put it out.

Want the truth? The city commissioned the *Manneken* to show the freedom and joie de vivre of living in Brussels—where happy people eat, drink...and drink...and then pee.

Sights in Brussels

The Grand Place and its sights may be Brussels' top attraction (described in the self-guided walk, earlier), but the city also offers a variety of museums, big and small, to fill your time here.

EAST OF THE GRAND PLACE
▲St. Michael's Cathedral

One of Europe's classic Gothic churches, built between roughly 1200 and 1500, Brussels' cathedral is made from white stone and topped by twin towers. For nearly 1,000 years, it's been the most important church in this largely Catholic country. (Whereas the Netherlands went in a Protestant direction in the 1500s, Belgium remains 80 percent Catholic—although only about 20 percent attend Mass.)

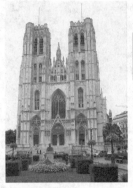

Cost and Hours: Free, but small fees to visit the underwhelming crypt and treasury, Mon-Fri 7:00-18:00, Sat-Sun 8:30-18:00.

▲Belgian Comic Strip Center
(Centre Belge de la Bande Dessinée)

Belgians are as proud of their comics as they are of their beer, lace, and chocolates. Something about the comic medium resonates with the wry and artistic-yet-unpretentious Belgian sensibility. Belgium has produced some of the world's most popular comic characters, including the Smurfs, Tintin, and Lucky Luke. You'll find these, and many less famous local comics, at the Comic Strip Center. It's not a wacky, lighthearted place, but a serious museum about a legitimate artistic medium. Most of the cartoons are in

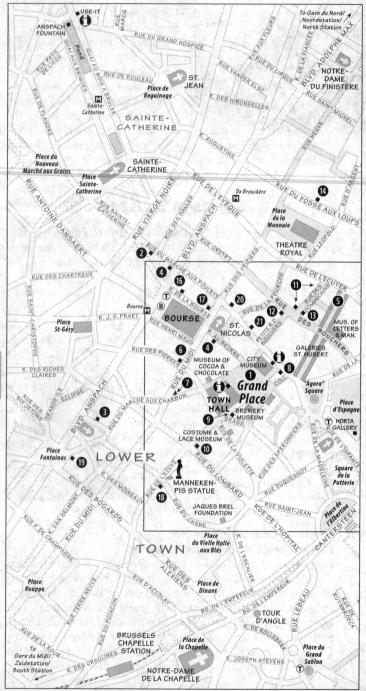

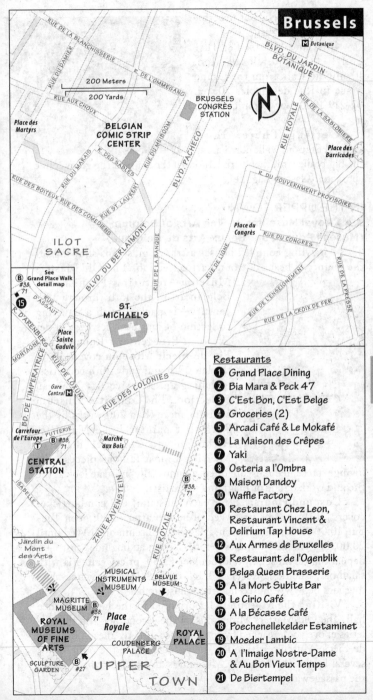

Brussels

Ⓜ Botanique

Restaurants

1. Grand Place Dining
2. Bia Mara & Peck 47
3. C'Est Bon, C'Est Belge
4. Groceries (2)
5. Arcadi Café & Le Mokafé
6. La Maison des Crêpes
7. Yaki
8. Osteria a l'Ombra
9. Maison Dandoy
10. Waffle Factory
11. Restaurant Chez Leon, Restaurant Vincent & Delirium Tap House
12. Aux Armes de Bruxelles
13. Restaurant de l'Ogenblik
14. Belga Queen Brasserie
15. A la Mort Subite Bar
16. Le Cirio Café
17. A la Bécasse Café
18. Poechenellekelder Estaminet
19. Moeder Lambic
20. A l'Imaige Nostre-Dame & Au Bon Vieux Temps
21. De Biertempel

French and Dutch, but descriptions come in English.

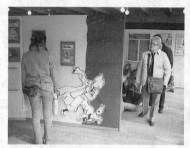

Cost and Hours: €8, Tue-Sun 10:00-18:00, closed Mon, 10-minute walk from the Grand Place to Rue des Sables 20, tel. 02-219-1980, www.comicscenter. net.

Getting There: From Central Station, walk north along the big boulevard, then turn left down the stairs at the giant comic character (Gaston Lagaffe).

IN THE UPPER TOWN
▲▲▲Royal Museums of Fine Arts of Belgium (Musées Royaux des Beaux-Arts de Belgique)

This sprawling complex houses a trio of museums showing off the country's best all-around art collection. The **Old Masters**

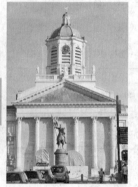

Museum—featuring Flemish and Belgian art of the 15th through 18th century—is packed with a dazzling collection of masterpieces by Van der Weyden, Bruegel, and Rubens. The **Fin-de-Siècle Museum** covers art of the late 19th and early 20th centuries, including an extensive Art Nouveau collection. The **Magritte Museum** contains more than 200 works by the Surrealist painter René Magritte. Although you won't see many of Magritte's most famous pieces, this lovingly presented museum offers an unusually intimate look at the life and work of one of Belgium's top artists.

Cost and Hours: €8 for each museum, €13 combo-ticket covers all three, free first Wed of month after 13:00; open Tue-Sun 10:00-17:00, closed Mon, Magritte Museum open Wed until 20:00, last entry 30 minutes before closing; audioguides cost €4-5 depending on museum, tour booklet-€2.50, pricey cafeteria with salad bar, Rue de la Régence 3, tel. 02-508-3211, www.fine-arts-museum.be, www.musee-magritte-museum.be.

Visiting the Museum: Get oriented in the large entrance hall. The Old Masters Museum is on the second floor (in the galleries above you), reached by the staircase directly ahead. The Fin-de-Siècle Museum is through the passageway to the right, down several levels. The Magritte Museum is also to the right, through the passageway.

• *Go up to the second floor and start with the Flemish masters in the...*

Old Masters Museum: Art history fans will appreciate this richly creative collection, which encompasses the Flemish Primitives as well as the fertile periods of the Flemish Renaissance and Baroque. Here are just of few of the highlights:

Rogier van der Weyden's *Portrait of Anthony of Burgundy* (c. 1456-1465) shows one of the artist's many portraits. Capitalist Flanders in the 1400s was one of the richest, most cultured, and progressive areas in Europe, rivaling Florence and Venice. Van der Weyden (c. 1399-1464) was its official portrait painter. He faithfully rendered life-size, lifelike portraits of wealthy traders, bankers, and craftsmen. Here he captures the wrinkles in Anthony's neck and the faint shadow his chin casts on his Adam's apple.

Hans Memling's *Martyrdom of St. Sebastian* (c. 1475) depicts a serene Sebastian filled with arrows by a serene firing squad in a serene landscape. The well-dressed archers and saint freeze this moment in the martyrdom so the crowd can applaud the colorful costumes and painted cityscape backdrop. Memling (c. 1430-1494) is clearly a master of detail, and the calm faces, beautiful textiles, and hazy landscape combine to create a surprisingly meditative mood for a martyrdom.

Pieter Bruegel I the Elder's *The Census at Bethlehem* (1566) shows one of the artist's signature landscapes filled with crowds of peasants in motion. In this painting, perched at treetop level, you have a bird's-eye view over a snow-covered village near Brussels. Into the scene rides a woman on a donkey led by a man—it's Mary and husband Joseph hoping to find a room at the inn (or at least a manger), because Mary's going into labor. Bruegel (c. 1527-1569) brings Mary down to earth, and places Jesus' birth in the humble here and now.

In **Peter Paul Rubens'** *The Ascent to Calvary* (c. 1636), life-size figures scale this 18-foot-tall canvas on the way to Christ's Crucifixion. The scene ripples with motion, from the windblown clothes to steroid-enhanced muscles to billowing flags and a troubled sky. By hiring top-notch assistants, Rubens (1577-1640) could crank out large altarpieces such as this for the area's Catholic churches.

Jacques-Louis David's *The Death of Marat* (1793) seems a scene ripped from the day's headlines. Jean-Paul Marat—a crusading French journalist—has been stabbed to death in his bathtub by a conservative fanatic. With his last strength, he pens a final, patriotic, "Vive la Révolution" message to his fellow patriots. Jacques-Louis David (1748-1825), one of Marat's fellow revolutionaries, immediately set to work painting a tribute to his fallen comrade. He makes it a secular pietà, with the brave writer portrayed as a martyred Christ.

BRUGES & BRUSSELS

• *Return to the ground-floor entrance hall to find the passageway to the...*

Fin-de-Siècle Museum: Brussels likes to think of itself as the capital of Art Nouveau and the crossroads of Europe, and this newly remodeled space presents a convincing case. Covering the period from the mid-19th century to the early 20th century, it shows the many cultural trends that converged in Brussels to create great art. The collection features a handful of high-powered paintings by notable Impressionists, Post-Impressionists, Realists, and Symbolists (Seurat, Gauguin, Ensor). It also houses a dazzling assemblage of Art Nouveau glassware, jewelry, and furniture.

Don't expect to see this art in chronological order. Galleries are organized thematically, to show the art in context with the period's literature, opera, architecture, and photography.

• *Backtrack along the ground-floor passageway to find the...*

Magritte Museum: The exhibits take you on a chronological route through René Magritte's life and art. The museum divides his life into three sections, with one floor devoted to each. In each section, a detailed timeline (in English) puts the work you'll see in a biographical and historical context.

Magritte had his own private reserve of symbolic images. You'll see clouds, blue sky, windows, the female torso, men in bowler hats, rocks, pipes, sleigh bells, birds, turtles, and castles arranged side by side as if the arrangement means something. He heightens the mystery by making objects unnaturally large or small. People morph into animals or inanimate objects. The juxtaposition short-circuits your brain only when you try to make sense of it. Magritte's works are at once playful and disorienting...and, at times, disturbing.

▲Musical Instruments Museum (Musée des Instruments de Musique)

One of Europe's best music museums (nicknamed "MIM")

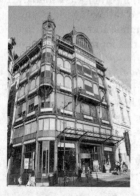

is housed in one of Brussels' most impressive Art Nouveau buildings, the beautifully renovated Old England department store. This museum has more than 1,500 instruments—from Egyptian harps, to medieval lutes, to groundbreaking harpsichords, to the Brussels-built saxophone.

Cost and Hours: €8 includes fun audioguide, Tue-Fri 9:30-17:00, Sat-Sun 10:00-17:00, closed Mon, last entry 45 minutes before closing, mandatory free coat and bag check, Rue

Montagne de la Cour 2, just downhill and toward Grand Place from the Royal Museums, tel. 02-545-0130, www.mim.be.

▲▲BELvue Museum

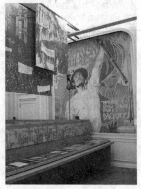

This earnest museum is the best introduction to modern Belgian history (1830-2000) you'll find in Brussels. It's chronological, self-contained, well-described in English, and spiced up with a few videos. But it's also Belgian history—so it is what it is.

Cost and Hours: €6; Tue-Fri 9:30-17:00, July-Aug until 18:00, Sat-Sun 10:00-18:00, closed Mon; audioguide-€2.50, to the right of the palace at Place des Palais 7, tel. 070-220-492, www.belvue.be.

Eating in Brussels

Brussels is known for both its high-quality, French-style cuisine and for multicultural variety. Seafood—fish, eel, shrimp, and oys-

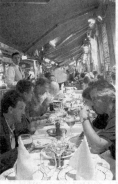

ters—is especially well-prepared here. As in France, if you ask for the *menù* (muh-noo) at a restaurant, you won't get a list of dishes; you'll get a fixed-price meal. *Menùs,* which include three or four courses, are generally a good value if you're hungry. Ask for *la carte* (lah kart) if you want to see a printed menu and order à la carte.

When it comes to choosing a restaurant, many tourists congregate on the Grand Place or at the Rue des Bouchers, "Restaurant Row." While the Grand Place is undeniably magnificent, locals suggest enjoying dessert or a drink there, but going elsewhere to eat well. For the locations of my recommended restaurants, see the map on page 908

Dining on the Grand Place

My vote for northern Europe's grandest medieval square is lined with hardworking eateries that serve predictable dishes to tourist crowds. Of course, you won't get the best quality or prices—but, after all, it's the Grand Place.

For an atmospheric cellar or a table right on the Grand Place, **La Rose Blanche** and **L'Estaminet du Kelderke** have the same formulas, with tables outside overlooking the action. L'Estaminet

Mussels in Brussels

Mussels *(moules)* are available all over town. Mostly harvested from aqua farms along the North Sea, they are available for most of the year (except from about May through mid-July, when they're brought in from Denmark). The classic Belgian preparation is *à la marinière,* cooked in white wine, onions, celery, parsley, and butter. Or, instead of wine, cooks use light Belgian beer for the stock. For a high-calorie version, try *moules à la crème,* where the stock is thickened with heavy cream.

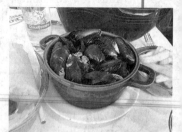

You order by the kilo (just more than 2 pounds), which is a pretty big bucket. While restaurants don't promote these as splittable, they certainly are. Your mussels come with Belgian fries (what we think of as "French fries"—dip them in mayo). To accompany your mussels, try a French white wine such as Muscadet or Chablis, or a Belgian blonde ale such as Duvel or La Chouffe. When eating mussels, you can feel a little more local by nonchalantly using an empty mussel shell as a pincher to pull the meat out of other shells. It actually works quite nicely.

du Kelderke—with its one steamy vault under the square packed with both natives and tourists—is a real Brussels fixture. It serves local specialties, including mussels (a splittable kilo bucket for €22-25; daily 12:00-24:00, no reservations taken, Grand Place 15, tel. 02-511-0956). **Brasserie L'Ommegang,** with a fancier restaurant upstairs, offers perhaps the classiest seating and best food on the square.

Lunches near the Grand Place

The super-central square dubbed the "Agora" (officially Marché aux Herbes, just between the Grand Place and Central Station) is lined with low-end eateries—Quick, Subway, Panos sandwich shop, Exki health-food store—and is especially fun on sunny days. On the other side of the Grand Place is a "restaurant row" street called Rue du Marché aux Fromages, jammed with mostly Greek and gyros places, with diners sitting elbow-to-elbow at cramped tables out front. But for something fresher and more interesting, stroll a few blocks to one of the following alternatives.

Bia Mara offers five different styles of fish-and-chips made with sustainable ingredients (plus a chicken option and a rotating special with creative international flavors). Around the corner from the Grand Place, this place serves up convenient, affordable, unique meals with a foodie emphasis. The industrial-mod interior is small, so lines can be long at peak times (€10-12 fish-and-chips, daily 12:00-14:30 & 17:30-22:30, Fri-Sun open throughout the day, Rue du Marché aux Poulets 41, tel. 02-502-0061).

C'Est Bon, C'Est Belge ("It's good, it's Belgian") is a cheery little café tucked on a side street a few blocks from the Grand Place. They serve a simple lunch menu of Belgian specials in their very tight, funhouse-floors dining room or at a few sidewalk tables. They also run a small shop selling Belgian food products (€8-12 lunches, Thu-Mon 10:30-18:00, closed Tue-Wed, Rue du Bon Secours 14, tel. 02-512-1999).

Peck 47—named for its location along "Chicken Market" street—is a mod café with artistic decor and white subway tile. They offer €5-8 breakfasts and €5 sandwiches with fresh and innovative style (Mon-Fri 7:30-17:00, Sat-Sun 11:00-18:00, Rue du Marché aux Poulets 47, tel. 02-513-0287).

Picnics: A convenient **Carrefour Express** is along the street between the Grand Place and the Bourse, near the "Is it raining?" fountain (daily 8:00-22:00, Rue au Beurre 27). **AD Delhaize** is at the intersection of Rue du Marché aux Poulets and Boulevard Anspach (Mon-Sat 9:00-20:00, Sun 9:00-18:00, Boulevard Anspach 63).

More Eateries near the Grand Place

Arcadi Café is a delightful little eatery serving daily plates (€10-15), salads, and a selection of quiche-like tortes (€7.50/slice). The interior comes with a fun, circa-1900 ambience; grab a table there, on the street, or at the end of Galeries St. Hubert (daily 7:00-23:30, 1 Rue d'Arenberg, tel. 02-511-3343).

Le Mokafé is inexpensive but feels splurgy. They dish up light café fare at the quiet end of the elegant Galeries St. Hubert, with great people-watching outdoor tables. This is also a good spot to try a Brussels waffle or to order a *café-filtre*—a rare, old-fashioned method where the coffee drips directly into your cup (€3-6 sandwiches, €7-11 salads, €8-10 pastas, €9-12 main dishes, daily 8:00-24:00, Galerie du Roi 9, tel. 02-511-7870).

La Maison des Crêpes, a little eatery a half-block south of the Bourse, looks underwhelming but serves delicious €8-10 crêpes (both savory and sweet varieties) and salads. Even though it's just a few steps away from the tourist bustle, it feels laid-back and local (good beers, fresh mint tea, sidewalk seating, daily 12:00-23:00, Rue du Midi 13, mobile 0475-957-368).

Yaki is a tempting Vietnamese and Thai noodle bar in a stately old flatiron building tucked between the Grand Place and the Rue du Marché au Charbon café/nightlife zone. Choose between the tight interior and the outdoor tables (€10-13 meals,

Sampling Belgian Beer in Brussels

Brussels is full of atmospheric cafés to savor the local brew. The places lining the Grand Place are touristy, but the setting—plush, old medieval guildhalls fronting all that cobbled wonder—is hard to beat.

All varieties of Belgian beer are available, but Brussels' most distinctive beers are *lambic*-based. Look for *lambic doux*, *lambic blanche*, *gueuze* (pronounced "kurrs"), and *faro*, as well as fruit-flavored *lambics*, such as *kriek* (cherry) and *framboise* (raspberry—*frambozen* in Dutch). These beers look and taste more like a dry, somewhat bitter cider. The brewer doesn't add yeast—the beer ferments naturally from wild yeast floating in the marshy air around Brussels.

The following places are generally open daily from about 11:00 until late.

A la Mort Subite, a few steps above the top end of the Galeries St. Hubert, is a classic old bar that has retained its 1928 decor...and its loyal customers seem to go back just about as far. The decor is simple, with wood tables, grimy yellow wallpaper, and some-other-era garland trim. A typical lunch or snack here is an omelet with a salad or a *tartine* spread with *fromage blanc* (cream cheese) or pressed meat. Eat it with one of the home-brewed, *lambic*-based beers. This is a good place to try the *kriek* beer. While their beer list is limited, they do have Chimay on tap (Rue Montagne aux Herbes Potagères 7, tel. 02-513-1318).

Le Cirio, across from the Bourse, feels a bit more upscale, with a faded yet still luxurious gilded-wood interior, booths with velvet padding, and dark tables that bear the skid marks of over a century's worth of beer glasses. The service is jaded—perhaps understandably given its touristy location (Rue de la Bourse 18-20, tel. 02-512-1395).

A la Bécasse is lower profile than Le Cirio, with less pretense

daily 12:00-23:00, Rue du Midi 52, tel. 02-503-3409).

Osteria a l'Ombra, a true Italian joint, is good for a quality bowl of pasta with a glass of fine Italian wine. A block off the Grand Place, it's pricey, but the woody bistro ambience and tasty food make it a good value. If you choose a main dish (€15-18), your choice of pasta or salad is included in the price (otherwise €10-15 pasta meals). The ground-floor seating on high stools is fine, but also consider sitting upstairs (Mon-Sat 12:00-15:00 & 18:30-23:30, closed Sun, Rue des Harengs 2, tel. 02-511-6710).

Waffles near the Grand Place

Dozens of waffle windows clog the streets surrounding the Grand Place. Most of them sell suspiciously cheap €1 waffles—but the big stack of stale waffles in the window clues you in that these are far from top-quality. Next I list a couple of good options.

and a simple wood-panel and wood-table decor that appeals to both poor students and lunching businessmen. The *lambic doux* has been served in clay jars since 1825. This place is just around the corner from Le Cirio, toward the Grand Place, hidden away at the end of a tight lane (Tabora 11, tel. 02-511-0006).

Poechenellekelder Estaminet is a great bar with lots of real character located conveniently, if oddly, right across the street from the *Manneken-Pis*. As the word *estaminet* (tavern) indicates, it's not brewery-owned, so they have a great selection of beers. Inside tables are immersed in *Pis* kitsch and puppets. Outside tables offer some fine people-watching (Rue du Chêne 5, tel. 02-511-9262).

Moeder Lambic has a modern industrial feel, with owners who are maniacs about craft beer and sell only traditional brews from independent producers. With a knowledgeable staff, this is an excellent place to start exploring the acquired tastes of *lambic, gueuze,* and *kriek*. For a snack, try the toast with *pottekaas,* a spread made with local white cheese and beer (on a square off Boulevard Anspach at Place Fontainas 8, tel. 02-503-6068).

Two tiny and extremely characteristic bars are tucked away down long entry corridors just off Rue du Marché aux Herbes. **A l'Imaige Nostre-Dame** (closed Sun, at #8) and **Au Bon Vieux Temps** (at #12) both treat fine beer with great reverence and seem to have extremely local clientele, which you're bound to meet if you grab a stool.

Delirium Tap House is a sloppy frat party with no ambience, a noisy young crowd, beer-soaked wooden floors, rock 'n' roll, and a famous variety of great Belgian beers on tap (near "Restaurant Row," not far from Chez Leon at Impasse de la Fidélité 4).

Maison Dandoy, which has been making waffles since the 19th century, is the pricey, elegant choice. You can take the waffles to go or enjoy them at a table surrounded by an upscale Parisian atmosphere (daily 9:30-19:00, just off the Grand Place at Rue Charles Buls 14, tel. 02-512-6588).

Waffle Factory, near the *Manneken-Pis*, is cheaper but still good. While it has an American fast-food ambience, it's efficient and popular—and thanks to the high turnover, you'll usually get a waffle that's grilled while you wait. Get your waffle to go, or sit upstairs to enjoy some peace and quiet (and free Wi-Fi). For a very Belgian taste treat, top your waffle with *speculoos*—a decadent spread with a peanut butter-like consistency but made with ground-up gingerbread cookies (€2-3 waffles plus toppings, open long hours daily, look for green-and-red-striped awning at corner of Rue du Lombard and Rue de l'Etuve).

Rue des Bouchers ("Restaurant Row")

Brussels' restaurant streets, two blocks north of the Grand Place, are touristy and notorious for touts who aggressively suck you in and predatory servers who greedily rip you off. If you are seduced into a meal here, order carefully, understand the prices thoroughly, and watch your wallet.

Restaurant Chez Leon is a touristy mussels factory, slamming out piles of cheap buckets since 1893. The €16 "Formula Leon" is a light meal consisting of a small bucket of mussels, fries, and a beer (daily 12:00-23:00, kids under 12 eat free, Rue des Bouchers 18, tel. 02-511-1415).

Aux Armes de Bruxelles is a venerable restaurant that has been serving reliably good food to locals in a dressy setting for generations. You'll pay for the formality (€8-23 starters, €19-57 main dishes, €22 fixed-price lunch, €40 fixed-price dinner, daily 12:00-22:45, indoor seating only, Rue des Bouchers 13, tel. 02-511-5550, www.auxarmesdebruxelles.com).

Restaurant Vincent has you enter through the kitchen to enjoy their 1905-era ambience. This place is better for meat dishes than for seafood (€15-20 starters, €20-32 main dishes, daily 12:00-14:30 & 18:30-23:30, Rue des Dominicains 8-10, tel. 02-511-2607, Michel and Jacques).

Finer Dining near Rue des Bouchers

These options, though just steps away from those listed above, are more authentic and a better value.

Restaurant de l'Ogenblik, a remarkably peaceful eddy just off the raging restaurant row, fills an early-20th-century space in the corner of an arcade. The waiters serve well-presented, near-gourmet French cuisine. This mussels-free zone has a great, split-table rack of lamb with 10 vegetables. Their sea bass with risotto and truffle oil, at €27, is a hit with return eaters. Reservations are smart (€20 first courses, €30 plates, Mon-Sat 12:00-14:30 & 19:00-24:00, closed Sun, across from Restaurant Vincent—listed earlier—at Galerie des Princes 1, tel. 02-511-6151, www.ogenblik.be, Yves).

Belga Queen Brasserie, a huge, dressy brasserie filling a palatial former bank building, is crowded with Brussels' beautiful people and visiting European diplomats. It's more expensive than most of my alternatives, but their "creative Belgian cuisine" is admirable, the service is sharp, and the experience is memorable—from the fries served in silver cones, to the double-decker platters of iced shellfish (€65/person for the Belga Queen platter), to the transparent toilets stalls, which become opaque only after you nervously lock the door (€15-25 starters, €20-30 main dishes, €30-50 fixed-price meals, daily 12:00-14:30 & 19:00-24:00, reservations smart, Rue Fosse-aux-Loups 32, tel. 02-217-2187, www.belgaqueen.be). The vault downstairs is a plush cigar and cocktail lounge.

Shopping in Brussels

The obvious temptations—available absolutely everywhere—are chocolate and lace. Other popular Brussels souvenirs include EU gear with the gold circle of stars on a blue background (flags, T-shirts, mugs, bottle openers, hats, pens, and so on) and miniature reproductions of the *Manneken-Pis*. Belgian beers are a fun, imbibable souvenir that you can enjoy at a picnic.

Souvenirs near the Grand Place

The streets immediately surrounding the Grand Place are jammed with Belgium's tackiest souvenir stands, with a few good shops mixed in. In my Grand Place Walk, I've listed some good places to pick up chocolates (page 906) and to browse for tapestries and lace (page 904).

De Biertempel, facing the TI on the street that runs below the Grand Place, not only stocks hundreds of types of Belgian beer, but an entire wall of beer glasses—each one designed to highlight the qualities of a specific beer (Rue du Marché aux Herbes 56, tel. 02-502-1906).

Fashion on Rue Antoine Dansaert

While Antwerp is the epicenter of Belgian design, Brussels has worked hard in recent years to catch up. To browse the best selection of Belgian boutiques, start by heading up Rue Antoine Dansaert (from the big Bourse building, cross Boulevard Anspach and continue straight up Rue Auguste Orts, which becomes Rue Antoine Dansaert). Along here, you'll see an eclectic array of both Belgian and international apparel. While specific designers seem to come and go, the genteel vibe persists. Window-shopping this street, you'll pass fine parks. After Place du Nouveau Marché aux Grains, the high-fashion focus downshifts, and the rest of the street feels like an emerging neighborhood with some funkier, lower-rent shops.

BRUGES & BRUSSELS

Ghent

Made terrifically wealthy by the textile trade, medieval Ghent was a powerhouse, and for a time, it was one of the biggest cities in Europe. It erected grand churches and ornate guild houses to celebrate its resident industry. But, like its rival Bruges, eventually Ghent's fortunes fell, leaving it with a well-preserved historic nucleus surrounded by a fairly drab modern shell.

Ghent doesn't ooze with cobbles and charm, as Bruges does; this is a living place—home to Belgium's biggest university. Ghent enjoys just the right amount of urban grittiness, with a welcome splash of creative hipster funkiness. It's also a browser's delight, with a wide range of characteristic little shops that aren't aimed squarely at the tourist crowds. Ghent is the kind of town that you visit for a few hours, and find yourself wishing you had a few days.

Visitors enjoy exploring the historic quarter, ogling the breathtaking Van Eyck altarpiece in the massive cathedral, touring impressive art and design museums, strolling picturesque embankments, basking in finely decorated historic gables, and prowling the revitalized Patershol restaurant quarter.

Orientation to Ghent

Although it's a midsized city (pop. 250,000), Ghent's historic core is appealingly compact—you can walk from one end to the other in about 15 minutes. The train station (with several museums nearby) is a 15-minute tram ride south of the center. Its Flemish residents call the town Gent (gutturally: *h*ent), while its French name is Gand (sounds like "gone").

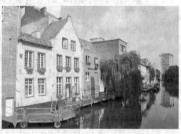

TOURIST INFORMATION
Ghent's TI is in the Old Fish Market (Oude Vismijn) building next to the Castle of the Counts (daily mid-March-mid-Oct 9:30-18:30, off-season until 16:30, tel. 09-266-5660, www.visitgent.be). Pick up a free town map and a pile of brochures (including a good self-guided walk).

ARRIVAL AT GHENT'S MAIN TRAIN STATION
Ghent's main train station, Gent-Sint-Pieters, is about a mile and a half south of the city center. As the station is undergoing an extensive renovation (through 2020), it might differ from

what's described here. In the main hall, be sure to look up at the meticulously restored frescoes celebrating great Flemish cities and regions.

It's a dull 30-minute **walk** to the city center. Instead, take the **tram:** Buy a ticket from the train station's Relay shop, at the ticket machines outside, or on board (€1.30 if you buy ticket in advance, €2 from the driver; you can also get a shareable 10-ride ticket for €10). Find the stop for tram #1: It's out the front door and 100 yards to the left, under the big, blocky, modern building on stilts. Board tram #1 in the direction of Wondelgem/Evergem (departs about every 10 minutes, 15-minute ride). Get off at the Korenmarkt stop, and continue one block straight ahead to Korenmarkt, from where you can see most of the city's landmark towers. Figure €10 for a **taxi** into town.

Sights in Ghent

Ghent is a rewarding town to simply wander and explore. Most visitors focus on the city's historic core, along a gentle bend in the river. You could have an enjoyable day simply strolling the riverbank, crisscrossing the bridges, and lingering in the city's many fine squares (the best are described below). While the city has several fine museums, churches, and other sights, I've listed only those that most warrant your limited time.

▲▲**Squares**—Of Ghent's many inviting squares, be sure to at least pass through these:

Korenmarkt (Corn Market): The historic square, next to St. Michael's Bridge (one of the town's best viewpoints), is squeezed between the palatial former post office and St. Nicholas' Church. This square flows directly into two others: **Emile-Braunplein** (watched over by a Neo-Gothic belfry) and **St. Bavo's Square** (in front of the namesake cathedral, described below).

Groentenmarkt (Vegetable Market): This tidy and atmospheric square, right on the river, is tucked alongside the medieval Butchers Hall (Groot Vleeshuis, now housing artisanal local foods).

Vrijdagmarkt (Friday Market): Watched over by a statue of local hero Jakob van Artevelde, this fine square is ringed by skinny burghers' mansions and the "House of the People" (Ons Huis), the ornately decorated headquarters for the region's socialist movement.

▲▲Cathedral of St. Bavo
(Sint-Baafskathedraal) and Ghent Altarpiece

This cathedral, the main church of Ghent, houses three of the city's art treasures: the exquisite Van Eyck *Adoration of the Mystic Lamb* altarpiece—famously known as the Ghent Altarpiece; an elaborately carved pulpit; and an altar painting by Rubens depicting

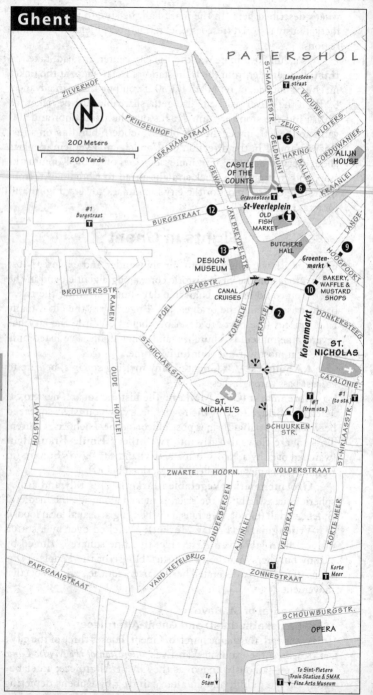

Ghent

PATERSHOL

ZILVERHOF

PRINSENHOF

ABRAHAMSTRAAT

200 Meters
200 Yards

GEWAD

ST-MAGRIETSTR.

Langesteen-
straat

VROUWE

ZEUG

GELDMUNT

HARING

BALLEN

PLOTERS.

CORDUWANIER

ALIJN
HOUSE

KRAANLEI

CASTLE
OF THE
COUNTS

Gravensteen

St-Veerleplein

OLD
FISH
MARKET

❺

❻

#1
Burgstraat

BURGSTRAAT

❶❷

JAN BREYDELSTR.

BUTCHERS
HALL

LANGE-

HOOGPOORT

❾

BROUWERSSTR.

RAMEN

DRABSTR.

POEL

DESIGN
MUSEUM

❶❸

CANAL
CRUISES

KORENLEI

GRASLEI

Groenten-
markt

BAKERY,
WAFFLE &
MUSTARD
SHOPS

❶⓿

❷

DONKERSTEEG

Korenmarkt

ST.
NICHOLAS

OUDE

HOUTLEI

ST-MICHAELSTR.

CATALONIE.

ST-NIKLAASSTR.

HOLSTRAAT

ST.
MICHAEL'S

SCHUURKEN-
STR.

❶

#1
(from stn.)

#1
(to stn.)

ZWARTE HOORN

VOLDERSTRAAT

ONDERBERGEN

AJUINLEI

VELDSTRAAT

KORTE MEER

PAPEGAAISTRAAT

VAND. KETELBRUG

ZONNESTRAAT

Korte
Meer

SCHOUWBURGSTR.

OPERA

To
Stam

To Sint-Pieters
Train Station & SMAK
Fine Arts Museum

BRUGES & BRUSSELS

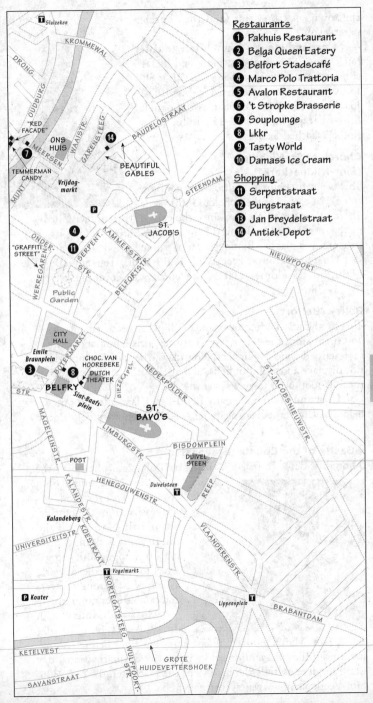

Restaurants
1. Pakhuis Restaurant
2. Belga Queen Eatery
3. Belfort Stadscafé
4. Marco Polo Trattoria
5. Avalon Restaurant
6. 't Stropke Brasserie
7. Souplounge
8. Lkkr
9. Tasty World
10. Damass Ice Cream

Shopping
11. Serpentstraat
12. Burgstraat
13. Jan Breydelstraat
14. Antiek-Depot

the town's patron saint (and the church's namesake).

Cost and Hours: Church free to enter but €4 to see original altarpiece and its facsimile; April-Oct Mon-Sat 9:30-17:00, Sun 13:00-17:00; Nov-March Mon-Sat 10:30-16:00, Sun 13:00-16:00; includes audioguide, Sint-Baafsplein, tel. 09-225-1626, www. sintbaafskathedraal.be.

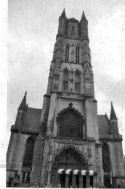

Church of St. Nicholas (Sint-Niklaaskerk)

This beautiful church, built of Tournai limestone, is a classic of the Scheldt Gothic style.
There's been a church here since the early 12th century; Ghent's merchants started building this one in the 1300s. Among its art treasures is a massive Baroque altar of painted wood.

Cost and Hours: Free, Mon 14:00-17:00, Tue-Sun 10:00-17:00, on Cataloniëstraat at the corner of Korenmarkt, tel. 09-234-2869.

Belfry (Belfort)

This combination watchtower and carillon has been keeping an eye on Ghent since the 1300s. For centuries, this landmark building safeguarded civic documents. Nowadays, the mostly empty interior displays an exhibit of bells, and an elevator whisks visitors up the 300-foot tower to views over the city.

Cost and Hours: €6, daily 10:00-18:00, last entry 30 minutes before closing, Sint-Baafsplein, tel. 09-233-3954, www.belfortgent. be.

▲Castle of the Counts (Gravensteen)

Though it dates from 1180, this fortress has morphed over the

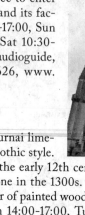

centuries, and much of it is rebuilt and restored. It's impressive from the outside, but mostly bare inside and information is skimpy. Still, it's a fun opportunity to get a feel for the medieval world as you twist through towers and ramble over ramparts.

Cost and Hours: €10, daily April-Oct 10:00-18:00, Nov-March 9:00-17:00, last entry one hour before closing, includes unhelpful audioguide with corny dramatizations, dry €1.50 guidebook tells the history of the place, tel. 09-225-9306, Sint-Veerleplein, www.gravensteengent.be.

▲Ghent Design Museum (Design Museum Gent)

This collection celebrating the Belgian knack for design is enjoyable for everyone, but worth ▲▲▲ for those interested in decorative arts of the 17th to 20th centuries. It combines a classic old building with a creaky wood interior, with a bright-white, spacious, and glassy new hall in the center. Just explore: Everything is clearly explained in English and easy to appreciate.

Cost and Hours: €8, Tue-Sun 10:00-18:00, closed Mon, Jan Breydelstraat 5, tel. 09-267-9999, www.designmuseumgent.be.

Shopping in Ghent

Ghent has an enjoyable real-world feel that makes it a fun place to browse—not for souvenirs, but for interesting, design-oriented items.

Serpentstraat

This little pedestrian street, buried deep between the cathedral and Vrijdagmarkt square, has a fun, funky collection of creative shops. **Roark,** on the corner with Onderstraat at #1B, shows off cutting-edge/retro home decor; next door is the boutique of local clothing designer **Nathalie Engels** (#1A). Zsa Zsa, with wildly colorful, smartly designed gadgets and toys (for kids and grown-ups alike), has two branches: **Petit Zsa Zsa** for children, at #5, and **Zsa Zsa Rogue** at #22. Between them, at #8, sits the **Zoot** shoe shop.

Streets near the Castle of the Counts

The busy, tram-lined **Burgstraat,** just across the bridge from the castle, isn't particularly charming, but it's an enjoyable place to window-shop several furniture and home-decor shops and art galleries. The side street **Jan Breydelstraat,** which leads to the Design Museum, has an eclectic array of clothing, linens, jewelry, design, and chocolate shops.

Antiques Mall

Antiek-Depot is a sprawling antiques mall made for browsing. It sits along a postcard-perfect gabled street just north of Vrijdagmarkt square (closed Tue, Baudelostraat 15).

Eating in Ghent

Pakhuis is a gorgeously restored, late-19th-century warehouse now filled with a classy, lively brasserie and bar. In this light, airy, two-story, glassed-in birdhouse of a restaurant, they serve up good traditional Belgian food with an emphasis on locally sourced and organic ingredients. It's tucked down a nondescript brick alley, but worth taking the few steps out of your way (€15 weekday two-course lunch menu is a great deal, otherwise €9-16 starters, €14-33 main dishes, €27-45 fixed-price meals, Mon-Sat 12:00-14:30 & 18:30-23:00, closed Sun, Schuurkenstraat 4, tel. 09-223-5555).

Belga Queen, an outpost of a similarly popular eatery in Brussels (see page 918), is the most enticing of the restaurants with seating along the embankment in the picturesque core of Ghent. The food is "Belgian-inspired international," and the trendy interior is minimalist/industrialist (three floors of seating, plus a top-floor lounge). While pricey, the place is packed with locals and visitors. Be sure to check out the bathrooms, with windows that turn opaque when you lock the doors (€18 lunches, €15-22 starters, €21-35 main dishes, €33-42 fixed-price dinners, daily 12:00-14:30 & 19:00-22:30, Graslei 10, tel. 09-280-0100).

Belfort Stadscafé occupies the basement of the sleek new market hall in the shadow of its namesake bell tower. Choose between the stylish-but-casual interior or the covered outdoor tables (€13 lunch special available Mon-Sat, otherwise €18-19 pastas, €19-24 main dishes, daily 8:00-24:00, Emile Braunplein 40, tel. 09-225-6005).

Marco Polo Trattoria is a good choice for Italian-style "slow food" (specializing in fish) at reasonable prices. It fills one long, cozy room with warm, mellow music and tables crowded by locals celebrating special occasions. Reservations are smart (€9-17 antipasti, €15-21 pastas, €8-16 pizzas, Tue-Sat 18:00-22:00, Fri also 12:00-15:00, closed Sun-Mon, Serpentstraat 11, tel. 09-225-0420).

Eateries in Patershol: For decades this former sailors' quarter was a derelict and dangerous no-man's land, where only fools and thieves dared to tread. But today it's one of Ghent's most inviting—and priciest—neighborhoods for dining. Stroll the streets and simply drop in on any place that looks good. Peek into courtyards, many of which hide restaurant and café tables.

Avalon, up the street from the Castle of the Counts, offers tasty vegetarian fare (daily 11:30-14:30, Geldmuntstraat 32); **'t Stropke** ("The Noose"), down the street from Avalon, serves Belgian and French food, with Ghent specialties, such as the creamy *waterzooi* soup (Fri-Wed 9:00-22:00, closed Thu, Kraanlei 1).

Quick Eats: **Souplounge** is basic, but cheap and good. They offer four daily soups, along with salads (daily 10:00-19:00, Zuivelbrugstraat 6). **Lkkr ("Yum"),** tucked behind the Belfry, is a small, modern shop selling sandwiches and salads (Mon-Sat 10:00-18:00, closed Sun, Botermarkt 6). **Tasty World** serves up decent €5 veggie burgers, plus a wide range of fresh fruit juices and salads (Mon-Sat 11:00-20:00, closed Sun, Hoogpoort 1).

Dessert: **Damass** is a popular ice-cream place where you can hang out and enjoy people-watching or get a cone to stroll with (at the north end of Korenmarkt, #2-C).

What If I Miss My Boat?

Remember that you can get help from the cruise line's port agent (listed on the destination information sheet distributed on the ship) and the local TI (see pages 868 and 894). If the port agent suggests a costly solution (such as a private car with a driver), you may want to consider public transit.

From the Blankenberge station, you can connect through Brussels or Antwerp by train to reach **Le Havre** (via Paris), London (with connections to **Southampton** and **Dover**), Amsterdam, Copenhagen, Warnemünde (via Berlin), and beyond.

If you need to catch a plane to your next destination, you have two options: the main Brussels Airport (sometimes called "Zaventem," tel. 0900-70000, www.brusselsairport. be), and Brussels South Charleroi Airport, used primarily by discount airlines and located about 30 miles from downtown Brussels (tel. 09-020-2490, www.charleroi-airport.com).

Local travel agents in Zeebrugge, Blankenberge, Bruges, or Brussels can help you. For more advice on what to do if you miss the boat, see page 139.

Dutch Survival Phrases

Northern Belgium speaks Dutch, but for cultural and historical reasons, the language is often called Flemish. Most people speak English, but if you learn the pleasantries and key phrases, you'll connect better with the locals. To pronounce the guttural Dutch "g" (indicated in phonetics by *h*), make a clear-your-throat sound, similar to the "ch" in the Scottish word "loch."

English	Dutch	Pronunciation
Hello.	Hallo.	**hah**-loh
Good day.	Dag.	da*h*
Good morning.	Goedemorgen.	**hoo**-deh-mor-*h*ehn
Good afternoon.	Goedemiddag.	**hoo**-deh-mid-da*h*
Good evening.	Goedenavond.	**hoo**-dehn-ah-fohnd
Do you speak English?	Spreekt u Engels?	shpraykt oo **eng**-ehls
Yes. / No.	Ja. / Nee.	yah / nay
I (don't) understand.	Ik begrijp (het niet).	ik beh-**hripe** (heht neet)
Please. (can also mean "You're welcome")	Alstublieft.	**ahl**-stoo-bleeft
Thank you.	Dank u wel.	dahnk oo vehl
I'm sorry.	Het spijt me.	heht spite meh
Excuse me.	Pardon.	**par**-dohn
(No) problem.	(Geen) probleem.	(hayn) **proh**-blaym
Good.	Goede.	**hoo**-deh
Goodbye.	Tot ziens.	toht zeens
one / two	een / twee	ayn / t'vay
three / four	drie / vier	dree / feer
five / six	vijf / zes	fife / zehs
seven / eight	zeven / acht	**zay**-fehn / aht
nine / ten	negen / tien	**nay**-hehn / teen
What does it cost?	Wat kost het?	vaht kohst heht
Is it free?	Is het vrij?	is heht fry
Is it included?	Is het inclusief?	is heht in-**kloo**-seev
Can you please help me?	Kunt u alstublieft helpen?	koont oo **ahl**-stoo-bleeft **hehl**-pehn
Where can I buy / find...?	Waar kan ik kopen / vinden...?	var kahn ik **koh**-pehn / **fin**-dehn
I'd like / We'd like...	Ik wil graag / Wij willen graag...	ik vil *h*rah / vy **vil**-lehn *h*rah
...a room.	...een kamer.	ayn **kah**-mer
...a train / bus ticket to ____.	...een trein / bus kaartje naar ____.	ayn trayn / boos **kart**-yeh nar ___
...to rent a bike.	...een fiets huren.	ayn feets **hoo**-rehn
Where is...?	Waar is...?	var is
...the train / bus station	...het trein / bus station	heht trayn / boos **staht**-see-ohn
...the tourist info office	...de VVV	deh fay fay fay
...the toilet	...het toilet	heht **twah**-leht
men / women	mannen / vrouwen	**mah**-nehn / **frow**-ehn
left / right	links / rechts	links / re*h*ts
straight ahead	rechtdoor	**re*h*t**-dor
What time does it open / close?	Hoe laat gaat het open / dicht?	hoo laht *h*aht heht **oh**-pehn / di*h*t
now / soon / later	nu / straks / later	noo / strahks / **lah**-ter
today / tomorrow	vandaag / morgen	**fahn**-da*h* / **mor**-*h*ehn

LONDON
Great Britain

Great Britain Practicalities

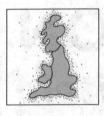

The island of Great Britain contains the countries of England, Wales, and Scotland. Hilly England—which contains all of the places in this chapter—occupies the lower two-thirds of the isle. The size of Louisiana (about 50,000 square miles), England's population is just over 56 million. England's ethnic diversity sets it apart from its fellow UK countries: Nearly one in three citizens is not associated with the Christian faith. The cradle of the Industrial Revolution, today's Britain has little heavy industry—its economic drivers are banking, insurance, and business services, plus energy production and agriculture. For the tourist, England offers a little of everything associated with Britain: castles, cathedrals, royalty, theater, and tea.

Money: 1 British pound (£1) = about $1.60. An ATM is called a cashpoint. The local VAT (value-added sales tax) rate is 20 percent; the minimum purchase eligible for a VAT refund is £30 (for details on refunds, see page 134).

Language: The native language is English.

Emergencies: Dial 999 for police, medical, or other emergencies. In case of theft or loss, see page 125.

Time Zone: Great Britain is one hour earlier than most of continental Europe, and five/eight hours ahead of the East/West Coasts of the US.

Embassies in London: The **US embassy** is at 24 Grosvenor Square (tel. 020/7499-9000, http://london.usembassy.gov). The **Canadian High Commission** is at 38 Grosvenor Square (tel. 020/7258-6600, www.unitedkingdom.gc.ca). Call ahead for passport services.

Phoning: Britain's country code is 44; to call from another country to Britain, dial the international access code (011 from the US/Canada, 00 from Europe, or + from a mobile phone), then 44, followed by the area code (without initial zero) and the local number. For calls within Britain, dial just the number if you are calling locally, and add the area code if calling long distance. To place an international call from Britain, dial 00, the code of the country you're calling (1 for US and Canada), and the phone number. For more tips, see page 1146.

Tipping: Tipping in Britain isn't as automatic as it is in the US; always check your menu or bill to see if gratuity is included. If not, tip about 10 percent. To tip a cabbie, round up a bit (if the fare is £4.50, give £5). For more tips on tipping, see page 138.

Tourist Information: www.visitbritain.com

LONDON and the PORTS of SOUTHAMPTON and DOVER

Southampton • Portsmouth • Dover •
Canterbury • London

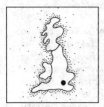

Many cruises begin, end, or call at English ports with easy access to London. While this island nation has dozens of ports, cruise lines favor two in particular: Southampton, 80 miles southwest of London; and Dover, 80 miles southeast of London (each about a 1.5-hour drive or train ride into the city).

From Southampton and Dover, most people choose to head into **London**—and for good reason. London is more than its museums and landmarks. It's the L.A., D.C., and N.Y.C. of Britain—a living, breathing, thriving organism...a coral reef of humanity. London is a city of nearly eight million separate dreams, inhabiting a place that tolerates and encourages them. Those beginning or ending their cruise in one of these ports will want to allocate ample extra time to experience London. But if your cruise only stops here for the day—even if it's a long day—you'll be very limited in what you can see in London. For this reason, some people choose to skip the trip into the big city and visit towns closer to their port, which offer an enticing taste of English culture.

In **Southampton,** you could stick around town, but there's little to see there beyond its fine SeaCity Museum. However, it's a short train ride to **Portsmouth,** a gentrified city with a wide array of maritime and nautical-themed sights.

Dover has a castle that's well worth touring, famous White Cliffs (visible from the cruise dock)...and not much else. But it's a quick train trip to **Canterbury,** an exceptionally pleasant town with one of England's biggest and best cathedrals.

All of these destinations—Southampton, Portsmouth, Dover, Canterbury, and, of course, London—are covered individually in this chapter, with "Planning Your Time" suggestions for each one.

Excursions from Southampton and Dover

Cruise-line excursions from both ports feature visits to London, as well as local destinations.

Excursions to London: There are plenty of ways to skin this cat, but most begin with an orientation **bus tour** around town; you'll zip by (and possibly have a photo-op stop) at such landmarks as the Houses of Parliament (Big Ben), Westminster Abbey, Buckingham Palace, London Eye, and the Tower of London. Some also feature a guided sightseeing visit; popular options include the **Tower of London** and a guided tour of the interior of **Buckingham Palace. Shopping tours** ("West End shopping" at Harrods and other famous department stores) are also offered. A **London On Your Own** excursion—a round-trip bus ride to Piccadilly Circus and free time in the city with no guide—runs about $100 (compared to about $65 round-trip by train from Southampton, or about $57 from Dover).

Other Excursions from Southampton: A side-trip to **Stonehenge and Salisbury** is perhaps the best choice, as it shows you Britain's iconic, mysterious, and ancient stone circle as well as a lovely midsize market town with a grand cathedral. A tour of **Windsor Castle,** the primary residence of the royal family, is another good choice. Rounding out your options are a scenic drive through the **Dorset County Countryside** (often with a stop at the dramatic ruins of **Corfe Castle**); the stately **Palace of Beaulieu,** with its nearby National Motor Museum (250 historic automobiles); and a shopping-oriented visit to the town of **Winchester,** with yet another giant cathedral.

Other Excursions from Dover: The nearby town of **Canterbury** combines charm, history, and one of England's most important cathedrals—making it the best choice here. (Canterbury is also easy to do on your own, using the information in this chapter.) Other options include a boat trip for a closer look at Dover's famous **White Cliffs** and the South Foreland Lighthouse; the adorable village of **Rye** and a scenic drive through the Kent countryside; the stout, ninth-century **Leeds Castle;** the 15th-century, timber-framed **Great Dixter** house and its delightful gardens; Henry VIII's heavily fortified **Walmer Castle,** generally combined with the enchanting village of **Sandwich;** and the village of **Chilham** (a popular filming location).

While any of these offers a pleasant look at England's inimitable charm, none of these sights can challenge the greatness of London.

The Port of Southampton

Arrival at a Glance: From the Ocean Cruise Terminal, QEII Cruise Terminal, or City Cruise Terminal, you can walk into town or hop a bus to the train station; from the Mayflower Cruise Terminal, spring for a taxi. Trains go to London (1.5 hours, 2/hour) and Portsmouth (50 minutes, hourly).

Port Overview

With 240,000 people, Southampton is a sprawling port town with a relatively compact downtown core. Everything is, to a point, walkable—though some of the cruise terminals are distant, and there's not much of interest to see en route. (For more on the town itself, see page 940.) Within Southampton's sprawling port, cruises use two dock areas, each with two terminals.

• The **Eastern Docks** consist of long piers jabbing straight out from Southampton, with two cruise terminals: **Ocean Cruise Terminal** at the near end (Berth 46/47), and **QEII Cruise Terminal** at the tip (Berth 38/39). You'll access this area through Dock Gate 4.

• The **Western Docks** hug Southampton's coastline west of downtown. Shuffled between the endless parking lots and container shipping berths are two cruise terminals: **City Cruise Terminal,** close to the town center (Berth 101); and **Mayflower Cruise Terminal,** farther out (Berth 106). You'll access this area through Dock Gate 8 (at the downtown end of the docks, close to City Cruise Terminal) or through Dock Gate 10 (farther from downtown but just south of the train station).

For details, see www.cruisesouthampton.com.

Terminal Services: Each of the four terminal buildings has similar services. You'll typically find WCs, a rack of tourist brochures and maps, a basic café, and a taxi stand out front, but none of the terminals have Wi-Fi or ATMs. There's no convenient public transportation from your ship to the port gate. You'll have to either use a taxi (most take credit cards) or walk—either to the nearest public bus stop (5-15 minutes, depending on where you arrive) or all the way into town or the train station.

Tourist Information: Neither the terminals nor the town has a TI. Your best bet for visitor information is www.discoversouthampton.co.uk.

GETTING INTO TOWN AND TO THE TRAIN STATION

The train station—with convenient connections to London, Portsmouth, and more—sits northwest of the port zone; it's

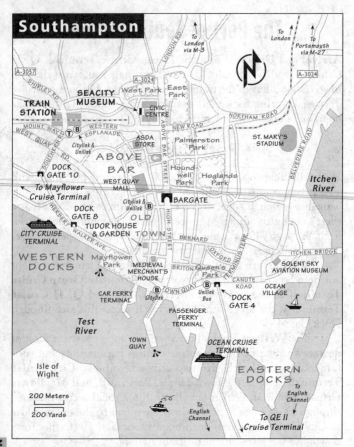

walkable, but far enough away that a taxi or bus is worth considering. Roughly between the port and the train station is the downtown core, including the underwhelming "Old Town," and above that, the street called Above Bar (because it's north of Bargate) and the Civic Centre (with the SeaCity Museum).

Depending on where you arrive, I'd consider the simplicity of a taxi. The Citylink and Unilink buses, which connect the port area to the train station, are also handy—though they don't go all the way to the cruise terminals, so you'll need to walk to reach them. It's also possible to walk all the way from your ship to the museum or to the train station (but it's not recommended from the Mayflower terminal).

By Taxi

Since Southampton is a relatively compact city, cabs are affordable —especially if you can team up with other cruisers to split the cost.

For rides within the city limits, drivers are required to use the meter. It should cost around £5-8 from any cruise terminal either to the train station or to the town center. Ask for an estimate up front, then make sure they use the meter.

If leaving the city, you can either use the meter or negotiate a fixed price. Here are some ballpark one-way figures for trips farther afield: Central London—£125; Heathrow Airport—£100; Gatwick Airport—£130; Salisbury: £45; Portsmouth: £40; Southampton Airport—£15.

If you need to call a taxi, try West Quay Cars (tel. 023/8099-9999, www.westquaycars.com).

By Bus

If your cruise line offers an affordable **shuttle bus** to downtown or the train station, consider taking it.

Southampton's **Citylink bus** is a service designed to help those arriving at the public ferry dock—called Town Quay—reach the town center and train station for just £1 (www.bluestarbus.co.uk). It runs through the city every 30 minutes, and is generally jam-packed with grungy backpackers fresh off the ferry. The city's **Unilink bus** #U1 connects the Eastern Docks with the station and town center for £2 (www.unilinkbus.co.uk). Unfortunately, neither bus goes directly to the cruise terminals, so you'll have to walk to reach them. From the City Cruise Terminal at the Western Docks, it's a 15-minute walk to the Citylink bus stop. If arriving at the Eastern Docks—Ocean Cruise or QEII Cruise Terminals—the Unilink bus stops right at the port entrance (Dock Gate 4), a 5-15 minute walk. If arriving at Mayflower Cruise Terminal, it's best to take a taxi directly to the train station.

The Citylink bus stop is at Town Quay, at the base of the passenger pier that sticks out into the bay from the end of Southampton's High Street. Board the bus at the stop in front of the Red Funnel ticket office. The bus arrives at the train station in about 10-15 minutes. To visit the SeaCity Museum, ask if the driver will let you off at the Asda supermarket (between West Quay and the train station, a short walk from the Civic Centre). The Unilink bus stops at both the train station and the Civic Centre.

On Foot

Read over your options below, then decide whether it's worth the walk...or if you should spring for a cab.

From the Eastern Docks (Dock Gate 4)

On this very long pier, it's a short five-minute walk from **Ocean Cruise Terminal,** or a long 15-minute walk from the **QEII Cruise**

LONDON

Services in Southampton

Unfortunately, there aren't many services available at the cruise terminals. For most, you'll need to head into town (or wait for London).

ATMs: You likely won't find an ATM in your terminal. To find one, your best bet is either in downtown Southampton (several banks with ATMs line High Street, the main drag) or in London (Waterloo Station, where you'll arrive, has several). Most taxi drivers take credit cards (ask before you hop in), and you can buy train tickets with credit cards—so it's relatively easy to get into London cash-free.

Internet Access: There is no Wi-Fi at the terminals. You'll find Internet terminals and free Wi-Fi at the library (located in the Civic Centre, must sign up with The Cloud service—see page 981). Otherwise, look for one of the many ubiquitous Costa Coffee shops (including one on High Street), which offer free Wi-Fi with a purchase.

Pharmacy: The biggest and handiest is Boots, on Above Bar just outside Bargate (Mon-Sat 8:00-19:00, Thu until 19:30, Sun 10:30-16:30).

Terminal, to reach Dock Gate 4. In both cases, just follow the main road to the exit. Turn left onto the busy road, where you'll see a stop for the Unilink #U1 bus (£2 to downtown or the train station, bus direction is marked *Airport*).

Or, if you feel like **walking,** continue along the road with a park on your right and parking lots on your left. At the fork, continue straight, bearing left slightly and passing the old stone tower.

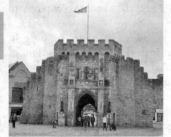

When you reach Town Quay, turn right and head up High Street, which leads in about 15 minutes up through the town center to the Civic Centre area. This shop-lined drag gives you a sense of workaday England; a few blocks to your left is the unimpressive "Old Town." Halfway up the main drag, you reach Bargate, one of the original town wall's towers. Beyond that, the street becomes "Above Bar." After a few short blocks you'll see a big, stately building with a lighthouse tower on your left—this is the Civic Centre, with the SeaCity Museum next door. To reach the train station, turn left onto Civic Centre Road (just before the Civic Centre itself), which takes you to the station in about 10 minutes.

From the Western Docks (Dock Gate 8 or 10)

The best plan here depends on which terminal you arrive at. **City Cruise Terminal** is within an easy walk of the Citylink bus stop, while **Mayflower Cruise Terminal** is much farther out, requiring a dull slog through industrial ports to reach anything.

City Cruise Terminal: This terminal is conveniently situated at the near end of the Western Docks. To get into town, exit the terminal to the right, then continue straight until you pop out at Dock Gate 8. From here, continue straight along the street (keeping the port on your right) until you reach Town Quay—about 10 minutes' walk from your ship. At Town Quay, find the **Citylink bus** stop in front of the Red Funnel ticket office (£1; bus stops in Southampton's "Old Town" and train station). It's a dreary 20-minute **walk** to the train station (turn left out of the terminal, hike through the port area to Dock Gate 10—at the roundabout, turn right to exit through the gate, continue straight up Southern Road, then turn right after the second cross-street, cutting through the park to the station).

Mayflower Cruise Terminal: The most distant of any Southampton cruise terminal, Mayflower is far enough out that a **taxi** is your best bet (the taxi stand is to the left as you exit the terminal).

TAKING THE TRAIN TO LONDON (OR ELSEWHERE)

Southampton Central Station is small and manageable, with ticket windows and ticket machines just inside the door. You can enter or exit the station from either side, but most people come and go from the southern entrance; this entrance faces the Western Docks (for those walking in) and is also the location of the Citylink bus stop to Town Quay. A walkway over the tracks connects this entrance to tracks 1 and 2, used by London-bound trains.

Trains depart at least every 30 minutes from Southampton to **London's Waterloo Station** (about 1.5 hours; additional departures require a change in Basingstoke; slower trains go to London's Victoria Station in 2.5 hours). A same-day off-peak return (round-trip) ticket to London costs about £42; a one-way ticket costs about £39. For details on arriving in London, see page 969.

For a closer and more manageable side-trip, consider **Portsmouth.** Trains leave Southampton about hourly (typically at :05 past the hour) and head directly to Portsmouth Harbour Station, within easy walking distance of the sights (50 minutes; £9.90 "single"/one-way, £10.70 "day return"/same-day round-trip). There are additional connections, with a change in Fareham or Havant, but these take longer (60-70 minutes).

LONDON

BY SHUTTLE BUS TO LONDON

Remember, many cruise lines offer a "London On Your Own" excursion, providing an unguided, round-trip bus transfer to Piccadilly Circus in London. Most lines charge about $100 for this trip—significantly more than the round-trip train ticket, but very convenient.

BY TOUR

Southampton doesn't have any tour options worth considering. For information on local tour options in London—including bus, walking, and bike tours—see "Tours in London" on page 976.

RETURNING TO YOUR SHIP

First take the train from London's Waterloo Station (or Portsmouth Harbour Station) to **Southampton Central Station** (don't get off at Southampton Airport Parkway). Exiting the station, you'll see a **taxi** stand (figure around £5-8 to your ship), and stops for the **Citylink** and **Unilink buses.** If you're feeling thrifty and have plenty of time, consider a bus—but remember that they won't take you directly to your ship. CityLink works best for the City Cruise Terminal; the Unilink #U1 bus serves the Ocean Cruise and QEII Cruise Terminals—look for buses marked *NOC* or *Dock Gate 4*. Take a cab to the Mayflower Cruise Terminal.

See page 1023 for help if you miss your boat.

Southampton

An important English port city for centuries, Southampton is best known for three ships that set sail from here and gained fame for very different reasons: the *Mayflower* in 1620, the *Titanic* in 1912, and in 1936, the *Queen Mary*—the luxurious great-grandma of the ship you arrived on. Like many port cities, Southampton was badly damaged by WWII bombs, obliterating whatever cobbled charm it once had. Today Southampton has one excellent museum (the state-of-the-art SeaCity Museum), but otherwise disappoints sightseers with a gloomy urban core, a few fragments of old city walls and towers, and an "Old Town" halfheartedly rebuilt to vaguely resemble a long-gone salty sailor's town.

PLANNING YOUR TIME

Upon arrival in Southampton, most people will want to get out. London is a 1.5-hour train ride away, and Portsmouth (with a variety of great maritime exhibits; see page 940) is just 50 minutes away. However, for those who want to stay in Southampton, there are a few ways to occupy yourself.

• **SeaCity Museum:** This well-presented museum thoughtfully tells the story of Southampton and the *Titanic*. It could occupy an attentive sightseer for two hours or longer.

• **Tudor House and Gardens:** Worth about 30 minutes, this modest museum peels back the layers of history of an old house in the town center.

There's little else to do in Southampton. The town center is nondescript, and the so-called "Old Town" near the Tudor House and Gardens is tiny and disappointing.

Sights in Southampton

An £11.50 combo-ticket covers both the museum and the house/gardens.

▲▲SeaCity Museum

This state-of-the-art facility, designed to consolidate and update various crusty old museums, features one of the best exhibits anywhere on the *Titanic*. It also has a good local history collection and well-presented temporary exhibits.

Cost and Hours: £8.50, daily 10:00-17:00, last entry at 16:00, Havelock Road, tel. 023/8083-3007, www.seacitymuseum.co.uk.

Visiting the Museum: From the ground-floor entrance level (with a gift shop, cafeteria, and temporary exhibits), head upstairs to the Grand Hall. From here, you can enter the two permanent collections.

The highlight, called **Southampton's *Titanic* Story,** explores every facet of the ill-fated ocean liner that set sail from here on April 10, 1912, and sank in the North Atlantic a few days later. Three-quarters of the *Titanic*'s 897 crew members lived in Southampton—making the global disaster a very local matter. With a smart multimedia approach, this outstanding exhibit invites you to linger over each detail.

Across the Grand Hall is the other permanent exhibit, **Southampton: Gateway to the World,** which traces the history of this shipping settlement from prehistoric and Anglo Saxon times until today. The museum's prized possession is its 23-foot-long model of the *Queen Mary*, which made its maiden voyage from Southampton in 1936.

Tudor House and Gardens

A rare surviving 520-year-old home tucked in Southampton's underwhelming and mostly reconstructed Old Town, this house offers a step back in time. Your visit begins with a 10-minute, semi-hokey audiovisual show of "ghosts" telling the building's history. Then you'll explore the various rooms, with exhibits and videos explaining how restorers have peeled back the historical layers of the place: Tudor, Georgian, Victorian, and even a WWII-era bunker. The experience is worthwhile for those with an interest in historical architecture (or anyone wanting to kill some time). But anyone can enjoy the pleasant garden (free to enter) and fine café.

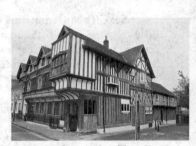

Cost and Hours: £4.75, includes audioguide, Tue-Fri 10:00-5:00, Sat-Sun 10:00-17:00, closed Mon, Bugle Street, tel. 023/8083-4242, www.tudorhouseandgarden.com.

Portsmouth

Portsmouth, the age-old home of the Royal Navy and Britain's second-busiest ferry port after Dover, is best known for its Historic

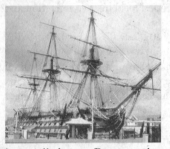

Dockyard and many nautical sights. For centuries, Britain, a maritime superpower, relied on fleets based in Portsmouth to expand and maintain its vast empire and guard against invaders. When sea power was needed, British leaders—from Henry VIII to Winston Churchill to David Cameron—have called upon Portsmouth to ready the ships. Today, the large city of Portsmouth (with about 200,000 inhabitants) has a revitalized urban core and old nautical sights that are as impressive as ever. Visiting landlubbers can tour the HMS *Victory*, which played a key role in Britain's battles with Napoleon's navy, and see what's left of the *Mary Rose*, a 16th-century warship.

PLANNING YOUR TIME

On a visit from nearby Southampton, Portsmouth can easily fill a day. Focus your time on the Historic Dockyards (allow 2-3 hours to tour all the museums and ships). With more time, explore Old Portsmouth or ascend Spinnaker Tower.

Orientation to Portsmouth

Tourist Information: The TI is inconveniently located inside the D-Day Museum in Southsea, about two miles southeast of the Portsmouth Harbour train station (daily April-Sept 10:00-17:00,

Oct-March until 16:30, tel. 023/9282-6722, www.visitportsmouth. co.uk).

Arrival by Train in Portsmouth: Trains from Southampton are described on page 937. Portsmouth has two train stations. Stay on the train until the final stop at the Portsmouth Harbour Station, conveniently located one long block from the entrance to the Historic Dockyard.

Returning to Southampton: Most of Portsmouth's sights (Historic Dockyards, Spinnaker Tower, Old Portsmouth) are within walking distance of the Portsmouth Harbour Station. From here, direct trains depart about hourly for the 50-minute trip to **Southampton Central Station** (more connections possible with changes).

Sights in Portsmouth

▲▲HISTORIC DOCKYARD

When Britannia ruled the waves, it did so from Portsmouth's Historic Dockyard. Britain's great warships, known as the "Wooden Walls of England," were all that lay between the island nation and invaders from the Continent. Today, this harbor is still the base of the Royal Navy. (If you sneak a peek beyond the guard stations, you can see the British military at work.) The shipyard offers visitors a glimpse of maritime attractions new and old. Marvel at the modern-day warships anchored on the docks, then explore the fantastic collection of historic naval memorabilia and preserved ships. The highlight is the HMS *Victory*, arguably the most important ship in British history—from its deck, Admiral Nelson defeated Napoleon's French fleet at Trafalgar, saving Britain from invasion and escargot. And don't miss the ongoing restoration of the *Mary Rose*, one of Henry VIII's favorite warships. Friendly and knowledgeable docents—many of whom were once seamen—are found throughout the complex, happily answering questions and telling tales of the sea.

Cost: You can stroll around the Dockyard to see the exteriors of the HMS *Victory* and HMS *Warrior* for free (except during special events), but going inside the attractions requires a ticket. The £28 ticket covers everything, while the £18 version gives you entry to your choice of one attraction.

Hours: The Dockyard is open daily April-Oct 10:00-18:00, Nov-March 10:00-17:30 (last tickets sold 1.5 hours before closing).

Information: Tel. 023/9283-9766, recorded info tel. 023/9298-6423, www.historicdockyard.co.uk).

Crowd-Beating Tips: To skip the line, buy tickets in advance online at www.historicdockyard.co.uk/tickets or at the Southsea TI (10 percent discount). Otherwise, you might have to wait 20-45

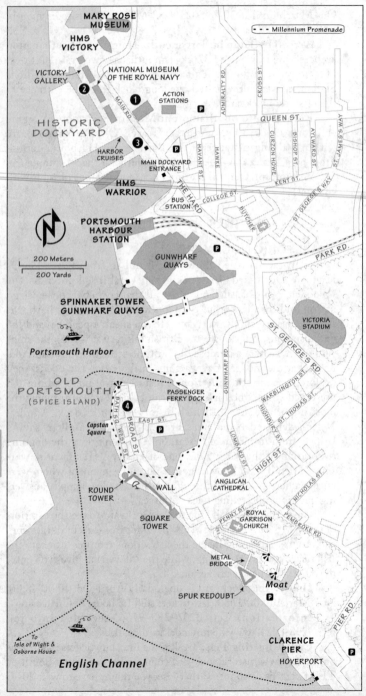

MARY ROSE MUSEUM

HMS VICTORY

VICTORY GALLERY

NATIONAL MUSEUM OF THE ROYAL NAVY

ACTION STATIONS

HISTORIC DOCKYARD

HARBOR CRUISES

MAIN DOCKYARD ENTRANCE

HMS WARRIOR

PORTSMOUTH HARBOUR STATION

200 Meters
200 Yards

GUNWHARF QUAYS

SPINNAKER TOWER
GUNWHARF QUAYS

Portsmouth Harbor

OLD PORTSMOUTH
(SPICE ISLAND)

PASSENGER FERRY DOCK

Capstan Square

EAST ST.

BROAD ST.
BATH SQ.
WEST ST.

ROUND TOWER

WALL

SQUARE TOWER

ANGLICAN CATHEDRAL

METAL BRIDGE

SPUR REDOUBT

Moat

To Isle of Wight & Osborne House

English Channel

CLARENCE PIER

HOVERPORT

Millennium Promenade

ADMIRALTY RD.
CROSS ST.
QUEEN ST.
HAVANT ST.
CURZON HOWE
HAWKE
BISHOP ST.
AYLWARD ST.
ST. JAMES'S WAY
KENT ST.
ST. GEORGE'S WAY
COLLEGE ST.
THE HARD
BUS STATION
BUTCHER
PARK RD.

VICTORIA STADIUM

ST. GEORGE'S RD.

GUNWHARF RD.

WARBLINGTON ST.

HIGHBURY ST.

ST. THOMAS ST.

LOMBARD ST.

HIGH ST.

ST. NICHOLAS ST.

PEMBROKE RD.

PENNY ST.

ROYAL GARRISON CHURCH

PIER RD.

LONDON

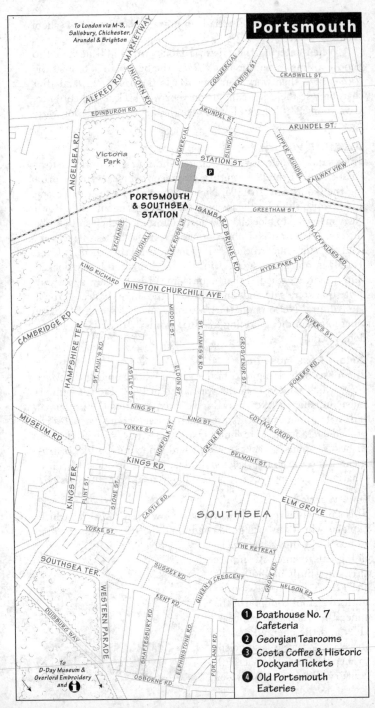

Portsmouth

To London via M-3, Salisbury, Chichester, Arundel & Brighton

CRASWELL ST.

ALFRED RD.

MARKETWAY

UNICORN RD.

COMMERCIAL

PARADISE ST.

ANGLESEA RD.

EDINBURGH RD.

ARUNDEL ST.

ARUNDEL ST.

UPPER ARUNDEL

RAILWAY VIEW

Victoria Park

COMMERCIAL

STATION ST.

SLINDON

P

PORTSMOUTH & SOUTHSEA STATION

ISAMBARD BRUNEL RD.

GREETHAM ST.

EXCHANGE

GUILDHALL

ALEC ROSE LN.

HYDE PARK RD.

BLACKFRIARS RD.

KING RICHARD

WINSTON CHURCHILL AVE.

CAMBRIDGE RD.

HAMPSHIRE TER.

ST. PAUL'S RD.

ASTLEY ST.

MIDDLE ST.

ST. JAMES'S RD.

GROSVENOR ST.

SOMERS RD.

RIVER'S ST.

KING ST.

KING ST.

GREEN RD.

COTTAGE GROVE

MUSEUM RD.

YORKE ST.

NORFOLK ST.

BELMONT ST.

KINGS TER.

FLINT ST.

STONE ST.

KINGS RD.

CASTLE RD.

SOUTHSEA

ELM GROVE

YORKE ST.

THE RETREAT

SOUTHSEA TER.

WESTERN PARADE

DUISBURG WAY

SUSSEX RD.

QUEEN'S CRESCENT

GROVE RD.

NELSON RD.

SHAFTESBURY RD.

KENT RD.

ELPHINSTONE RD.

PORTLAND RD.

OSBORNE RD.

To D-Day Museum & Overlord Embroidery and

❶ Boathouse No. 7 Cafeteria

❷ Georgian Tearooms

❸ Costa Coffee & Historic Dockyard Tickets

❹ Old Portsmouth Eateries

minutes to buy tickets, especially in July and August, when school is out.

When entering the Historic Dockyard, you'll be asked to choose a time to see the *Mary Rose*. The best plan is to visit the *Victory* first, then work your way over to the *Mary Rose,* and after that, browse the other exhibits on your way back to the entrance. Give yourself at least an hour to see the *Victory* before your *Mary Rose* appointment.

▲▲▲HMS *Victory*

This grand historic warship changed the course of world history. At the turn of the 19th century, Napoleon's forces were terrorizing the Continent. In 1805, Napoleon amassed a fleet of French and Spanish ships for the purpose of invading England. The Royal Navy managed to blockade the fleets, but some French ships broke through. Admiral Nelson, commander of the British fleet, pursued the ships aboard the HMS *Victory,* cornering them at Cape Trafalgar, off the coast of Spain. For the British, this dry-docked ship is more a cathedral than a museum. Visitors follow a one-way route that spirals up and down through the ship's six decks. You'll see Admiral Nelson's quarters, various gun decks, and the place where Nelson died, gasping his final words: "Thank God, I have done my duty."

▲Mary Rose Museum

The museum building next to the *Victory* is the home of the *Mary Rose,* which sank in 1545 and was raised in 1982. The £36 million museum, shaped like an oval jewel box, reunites the preserved hull with thousands of its previously unseen contents. All sorts of Tudor-era items were found inside the wreck, such as clothes, dishes, weapons, a backgammon board, and an oboe-like instrument. There's even the skeleton of Hatch, the ship's dog. It's a fascinating look at everyday shipboard life from almost 500 years ago.

HMS *Warrior*

This ship, while very impressive, never saw a day of battle...which explains why it's in such good condition. The *Warrior* was the first 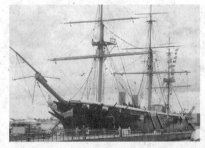 ironclad warship, a huge technological advance. Compare this ship, built in 1860, with the *Victory,* which was similar to the warships common at the time. The *Warrior* was unbeatable, and the enemy knew it. Its very existence was sufficient to keep the peace. The late 19th century didn't see many sea battles, however, and by the time warships were needed again, the *Warrior* was obsolete.

Other Sights at the Dockyards

With more time, dip into the **National Museum of the Royal Navy,** tour the **"Action Stations"** exhibit (thinly veiled propaganda for the military), and consider a 45-minute **harbor cruise** (departs about hourly during the summer).

OTHER SIGHTS IN PORTSMOUTH

Gunwharf Quays

Part of the major (and successful) makeover of Portsmouth, the bustling Gunwharf Quays (pronounced "keys") is an American-style outdoor shopping center on steroids, with restaurants, shops, and entertainment.

Hours: Mall open Mon-Sat 10:00-20:00, Sun 10:00-17:00, tel. 023/9283-6700, www.gunwharf-quays.com.

Spinnaker Tower

Out at the far end of the Gunwharf Quays shopping zone is this futuristic-looking 557-foot-tall tower, evocative of the billowing ships' sails that played such a key role in the history of this city and country. You can ride to the 330-foot-high view deck for a panorama of the port and sea beyond, or court acrophobia with a stroll across "Europe's biggest glass floor."

Cost and Hours: £9, daily 10:00-18:00, last entry 30 minutes before closing; can be crowded at midday July-Aug—smart to book ahead, reserve online for a 15 percent discount; tel. 023/9285-7520, www.spinnakertower.co.uk.

Old Portsmouth

Portsmouth's historic district—once known as "Spice Island" after the ships' precious cargo—is surprisingly quiet. For a long time, the old sea village was dilapidated and virtually empty. But successful revitalization efforts have brought a few inviting pubs and B&Bs. It's a pleasant place to stroll around and imagine how different this district was in the old days, when it was filled with salty fishermen and sailors who told tall tales and sang sea shanties in rough-and-tumble pubs.

▲D-Day Museum and Overlord Embroidery

This small museum was built to house the remarkable 272-foot long Overlord Embroidery, created to commemorate the 40th anniversary of the D-Day invasions. Its 34 appliquéd panels—stitched together over five years by a team of seamstresses—chronologically trace the years from 1940 to 1944, from the first British men receiving their call-up papers in the mail to the successful implementation of D-Day. It celebrates everyone from famous

WWII figures to unsung heroes of the home front.

Cost and Hours: £6.70, worthwhile audioguide-£0.50, daily April-Sept 10:00-17:30, Oct-March 10:00-17:00, last entry 30 minutes before closing; tel. 023/9282-6722, www.ddaymuseum.co.uk. A café is on site (open April-Sept).

Getting There: The museum is on the waterfront about two miles south of the Spinnaker Tower on the Clarence Esplanade in Southsea. From Portsmouth's Hard Interchange bus station, which is next to the train station, take First Bus Company's bus #16 or Stagecoach bus #700.

Eating in Portsmouth

AT THE HISTORIC DOCKYARD

The Historic Dockyard has an acceptable **cafeteria,** called **Boathouse No. 7,** with a play area that kids enjoy (£5-8 meals, daily 10:00-16:00). The **Georgian Tearooms** are across the pedestrian street in Storehouse #9, with good sandwich and cake offerings (daily April-Oct 10:00-17:00, shorter hours off-season). The **Costa Coffee** inside the entrance building offers surprisingly good grilled sandwiches and coffee drinks to go (daily 10:00-17:00).

IN OLD PORTSMOUTH

The Still & West Country House pub has dining in two appealing zones. Eat from the simpler and cheaper menu on the main floor, or outside on the picnic benches with fantastic views of the harbor (£7 baguette sandwiches and £8 fish-and-chips). Or head upstairs to the dining room, with a gorgeous glassed-in conservatory that offers sea views—especially enticing in cold weather (dining room open Mon-Sat 12:00-15:00 & 18:00-21:00, Sun 12:00-19:30, longer hours in the bar, 2 Bath Square, tel. 023/9282-1567).

The Spice Island Inn, at the tip of the Old Portsmouth peninsula, has terrific outdoor seating, a family-friendly dining room upstairs, and many vegetarian offerings, although service can be slow (£5-9 lunches, £7-12 dinners, food served daily 11:00-22:00, bar open longer, 1 Bath Square, tel. 023/9287-0543).

For a quick snack, visit the **Spinnaker Café,** located at the end of the old quay (£5-8 eggs, burgers, and sandwiches; breakfast served all day, daily 8:00-16:00, 96 Broad Street, tel. 023/9299-0017).

The Port of Dover

Arrival at a Glance: As it's a long walk (30 minutes or more), opt for the affordable shuttle bus or a taxi into downtown or up to the castle. From downtown, it's an easy 15-minute walk to the train station for trains to London (1.5 hours) or Canterbury (20-30 minutes).

Port Overview

Gritty, urban-feeling Dover seems bigger than its population of 30,000. The town lies between two cliffs, with Dover Castle on one side and the Western Heights on the other. While the streets stretch longingly toward the water, the core of the town is cut off from the harbor by the rumbling A-20 motorway (connecting Dover with cities to the west) and a long, eyesore apartment building.

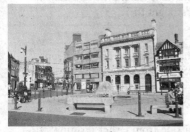

The workaday city center is anchored by Market Square and the mostly pedestrianized (but not particularly charming) main shopping drag, Cannon Street/ Biggin Street, which runs north from Market Square to the old town jail. A short five-minute walk south of Market Square, through a pedestrian underpass ("subway"), takes you to the waterfront—a pleasant pebbly beach lined with a promenade; at its western end, you can enjoy fine views of the castle and White Cliffs. But this is only worth it on a gorgeous day—views of the White Cliffs are better from out of town, and the beach is pretty tame even by British standards.

Little Dover has a huge port, and cruises put in at its far western edge—at the **Western Docks,** along the extremely long Admiralty Pier. Near the port gate at the base of the pier, Terminal 1 is a converted old railway station; farther out at the tip, Terminal 2 is a modern facility. For more info, see www.whitecliffscountry. org.uk.

Tourist Information: There's no TI at the cruise terminal, but the shuttle bus drops you near one that is inside the Dover Museum (see page 951).

GETTING INTO TOWN

The walk into town is grueling and dull. Spring instead for the reasonably priced shuttle bus or a taxi into town or to the castle.

Services in Dover

There aren't many services at the port itself, but if you make your way to Market Square (by shuttle bus or taxi), you'll find the following:

ATMs: Several ATMs are on or near Market Square and Cannon Street/Biggin Street.

Internet Access: The library, called the Dover Discovery Centre—next to the Dover Museum/TI, just off Market Square—has terminals with free Internet access (Mon-Fri 9:00-18:00, Wed until 20:00, Sat 9:00-17:00, closed Sun). Three eateries along Cannon Street/Biggin Street, up from the TI, have free Wi-Fi for customers: Heading up this street, after one short block, you'll first reach The Eight Bells pub (on the left); one long block farther, on the right, you'll pass Costa Coffee; and just beyond that, on the left, is McDonald's.

Pharmacy: The most convenient is Boots, next door to Costa Coffee, two blocks up Cannon Street/Biggin Street from Market Square (Mon-Sat 9:00-17:30, Sun 10:00-16:00).

To reach the train station, you'll either take the shuttle downtown, then walk 15 minutes; or take a taxi straight there.

By Taxi

In this small town, taxis are reasonable. For two or more people traveling together within town, taxis are the cheapest way to go. Most taxis take credit cards, as well as British pounds and US dollars. Taxis are standing by, or you can call 01304/204-040, 01304/204-420, or 01304/228-882.

Expect to pay around £8 for a ride from either terminal to downtown (Market Square), to the train station, or to the castle. The hourly rate is about £30. Licensed taxis are not allowed to charge more than the following rates (one-way); the numbers in parentheses indicate what most companies actually charge:

To Dover Castle or the train station: £8

To downtown London or Heathrow Airport: £180 (usually £140-155)

To Gatwick Airport: £150 (usually £110-115)

To Canterbury: This rate is not regulated—figure on a one-way fare of around £27-30

By Shuttle Bus

When cruise ships are in port, Classic Omnibus runs a bright-blue shuttle bus into town from the terminals (10-minute trip). There are two stops: first at Market Square (in the heart of town, next to the TI and a 15-minute walk from the train station); and then up at the castle. If you don't have British pounds, you can pay in dollars or euros (£3/€4/$5 one-way into town; add £1/€1/$1 to continue up to the castle; www.opentopbus.co.uk).

Arriving at Market Square: From the Market Square bus stop, walk straight ahead a few steps and curl around to the left into the square. The TI and Dover Museum are just to your left; down the street beyond that is the Discovery Centre/library (with Internet access). The main drag, Cannon Street—which becomes Biggin Street—begins across the square from the TI. Head up this street to find some eateries with free Wi-Fi, and eventually the train station. There are ATMs all around Market Square and along Cannon/Biggin Street.

Walking to the Dover Priory Train Station: Figure about 15 minutes from Market Square to the station. First, head up Cannon Street (directly across the square from the TI), and follow it for three blocks. Just after passing Costa Coffee and Boots pharmacy, and just before the street ahead of you becomes cobbled and traffic-free, turn left onto Priory Street. After a short block, you'll come to a big roundabout; circle around the right and use the crosswalks to go more or less straight through it. On the far side of the roundabout, continue slightly uphill on Folkestone Road; a half-block after the gas station, watch for *Dover Priory* signs on the right marking the station.

TO LONDON OR CANTERBURY BY TRAIN

From the Dover Priory train station, you can get to London or Canterbury.

To **London,** you can choose between the faster "Javelin" train (2/hour, 1.5 hours to St. Pancras Station; £39 one-way or off-peak same-day return, £71 anytime return) and the slower train (1-2/hour to Victoria Station or Charing Cross Station, each 2 hours; around £36 one-way or off-peak same-day return). When choosing which train to take, consider this: St. Pancras and Victoria Stations are both well-connected to any point in the city by Tube (subway) or bus (and St. Pancras is right next to the British Library); but Charing Cross Station is particularly handy, as it's within easy walking distance of the sights many first-timers want to see (Trafalgar Square, National Gallery, West End, Whitehall, Houses of Parliament)—so the extra time spent on that train could save you some time commuting to your sightseeing later in London. For details on arriving by train in London, see page 969.

Trains depart for **Canterbury** twice hourly; some are direct (16 minutes), while others make a few stops en route (27 minutes; for either train, fares are £8 "single"/one-way, £8.10 "day return"/same-day round trip). These trains stop at the Canterbury East Station (for arrival tips in Canterbury, see page 960).

RETURNING TO YOUR SHIP

Arriving at the Dover Priory train station, there's no direct public-transit option to the ship. You can either take a taxi directly there (about £8 without luggage), or walk 15 minutes to Market Square, then take the cruise shuttle bus from there (£3/€4/$5, described earlier). If you stick around Dover for the day, you can use this same bus, from either Market Square or the castle.

See page 1023 for help if you miss your boat.

Dover

Dover—like much of southern England—sits on a foundation of chalk. Miles of cliffs stand at attention above the beaches; the most famous are the White Cliffs of Dover. Sitting above those cliffs is the impressive Dover Castle, England's primary defensive stronghold from Roman through modern times. From the nearby port, ferries, hydrofoils, and hovercrafts shuttle people and goods back and forth across the English 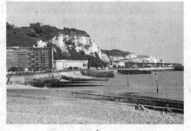 Channel. France is only 23 miles away—on a sunny day, you can see it off in the distance.

Dover's run-down town center isn't worth a second look. Focus instead on Dover's looming castle, standing guard as it has for almost a thousand years. Or take a train ride to nearby and far more charming Canterbury (described on page 960).

PLANNING YOUR TIME

London is the main attraction from here (a 1.5-hour train ride away), but those preferring to stay closer to the ship could fill the better part of a day in Dover if you linger at the castle or cliffs. Better yet, for a busy but satisfying day, make a quick trip up to Dover Castle, then ride the train just 20-30 minutes to pleasant Canterbury for the afternoon.

• **Dover Castle:** If you do both of the guided tours at the Secret Wartime Tunnels, as well as touring the Great Tower and hiking around the battlements, this could easily take 4-5 hours; if you're in a rush, do only the Operation Dynamo tour and sprint through the tower (allow 2 hours).

• **White Cliffs:** There are a number of ways to get a good look at these famous cliffs, from an easy walk out the Prince of Wales Pier, to a harbor cruise (allow an hour for either), to a trip to a viewpoint farther from town (allow 2-3 hours).

• **Canterbury:** This historic town—with a great cathedral and fine historic core—has a lot more personality than Dover. Allow 4-5 hours, including the round-trip train ride, a tour of the cathedral, and a bit of time to explore the town.

TOURIST INFORMATION

There's no TI at the cruise terminal, but the shuttle bus drops you a few steps away from the TI inside the Dover Museum, on Market Square (Mon-Sat 9:30-17:00, open Sun 10:00-13:00 April-Sept only; Market Square, tel. 01304/201-066, www.whitecliffscountry. org.uk, tic@doveruk.com).

Sights in Dover

▲▲DOVER CASTLE

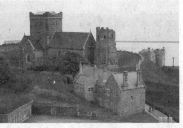

Strategically located Dover Castle—considered "the key to England" by would-be invaders—perches grandly atop the White Cliffs of Dover. English troops were garrisoned within the castle's medieval walls for almost 900 years, protecting the coast from European invaders (a record of military service rivaled only by Windsor Castle and the Tower of London). With a medieval Great Tower as its centerpiece and battlements that survey 360 degrees of windswept coast, Dover Castle has undeniable majesty. Today, the biggest invading menaces are the throngs of school kids on field trips, so it's best to arrive early. While the historic parts of the castle are unexceptional, the exhibits in the WWII-era Secret Wartime Tunnels are unique and engaging—particularly the new, powerful, well-presented tour that tells the story of Operation Dynamo, a harrowing WWII rescue operation across the English Channel.

Cost and Hours: £17.50, £45.50 family ticket; April-Sept daily 10:00-18:00, from 9:30 in Aug; Oct daily 10:00-17:00; Nov-March open Sat-Sun only 10:00-16:00; last entry one hour before closing, keep yard may close in high winds.

Information: Tel. 01304/211-067, www.english-heritage.org. uk/dovercastle.

Getting There: The easiest way to get here is by taxi or shuttle bus from the cruise port (both options explained earlier).

Avoiding Lines: Arrive early for the fewest crowds (busiest on summer bank holidays and weekends; worst around 11:30). While crowds can impede your progress throughout the site, the biggest potential headaches are lines for the two tours of the

LONDON

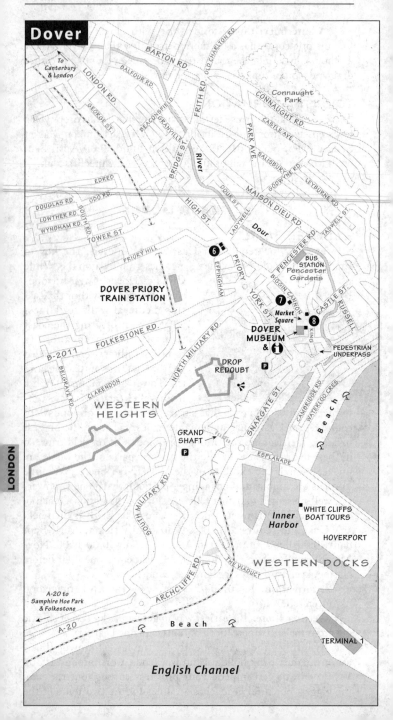

Dover

To Canterbury & London

BARTON RD

BALFOUR RD

FRITH RD

OLD CHARLTON RD

Connaught Park

CONNAUGHT RD

LONDON RD.

GEORGE ST.

BEACONSFIELD

GRANVILLE

CASTLE AVE.

PARK AVE.

SALISBURY RD.

GODWYNE RD.

LEYBURNE RD.

BRIDGE ST.

River

MAISON DIEU RD.

PENCESTER RD.

TASWELL ST.

EDRED

DOUGLAS RD.

LOWTHER RD.

SOUTH RD.

ODO RD.

HIGH ST.

DOUR ST.

LADWELL

Dour

WYNDHAM RD.

TOWER ST.

PRIORY HILL

EFFINGHAM

PRIORY RD.

6

YORK ST.

BIGGIN CANON

PENCESTER RD.

BUS STATION Pencester Gardens

CASTLE ST.

RUSSELL

DOVER PRIORY TRAIN STATION

7

Market Square

8

FOLKESTONE RD.

NORTH MILITARY RD.

DOVER MUSEUM & 1

KING

PEDESTRIAN UNDERPASS

B-2011

BELGRAVE RD.

CLAKENDON

DROP REDOUBT

P

CAMBRIDGE RD.

WATERLOO CRES.

WESTERN HEIGHTS

SNARGATE ST.

Beach

GRAND SHAFT

P

ESPLANADE

SOUTH MILITARY RD.

Inner Harbor

WHITE CLIFFS BOAT TOURS

HOVERPORT

ARCHCLIFFE RD.

THE VIADUCT

WESTERN DOCKS

A-20 to Samphire Hoe Park & Folkestone

A-20

B e a c h

TERMINAL 1

English Channel

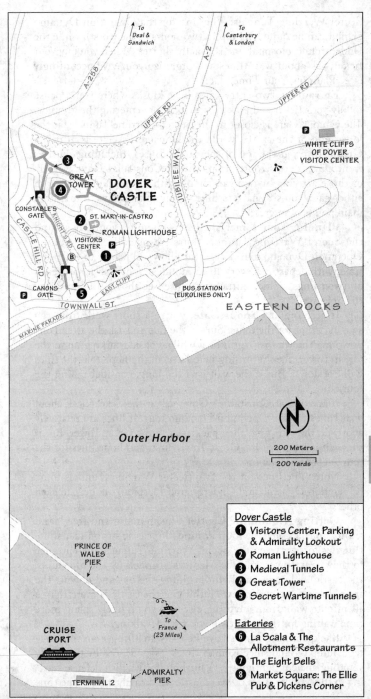

To Deal & Sandwich

To Canterbury & London

UPPER RD.

A-258

A-2

JUBILEE WAY

UPPER RD.

WHITE CLIFFS OF DOVER VISITOR CENTER

❸ GREAT TOWER

DOVER CASTLE

❹

CONSTABLE'S GATE

KNIGHT'S RD.

ST. MARY-IN-CASTRO

❷

ROMAN LIGHTHOUSE

VISITORS CENTER

CASTLE HILL RD.

Ⓑ

❶

CANONS GATE

❺

EAST CLIFF

TOWNWALL ST.

BUS STATION (EUROLINES ONLY)

EASTERN DOCKS

MARINE PARADE

Outer Harbor

N

200 Meters
200 Yards

LONDON

PRINCE OF WALES PIER

To France (23 Miles)

CRUISE PORT

TERMINAL 2

ADMIRALTY PIER

Dover Castle
❶ Visitors Center, Parking & Admiralty Lookout
❷ Roman Lighthouse
❸ Medieval Tunnels
❹ Great Tower
❺ Secret Wartime Tunnels

Eateries
❻ La Scala & The Allotment Restaurants
❼ The Eight Bells
❽ Market Square: The Ellie Pub & Dickens Corner

Secret Wartime Tunnels: The line for the Operation Dynamo exhibit can be quite long (up to two hours at the worst), while the Underground Hospital line is usually shorter. When you buy your ticket, ask about wait times and organize your visit accordingly (see "Planning Your Time," later).

Entrances: Two entry gates have kiosks where you'll pause to buy your ticket and pick up a map before entering the grounds. The Canons Gate is closer to the Secret Wartime Tunnels, at the lower end of the castle, while the Constable's Gate is near the Great Tower, at the top of the castle. Buses (including shuttles from Dover's cruise port) drop off near Constable's Gate; walkers or those arriving by taxi can choose either gate. Note that from either gate, you still have to hike uphill quite a ways to reach the main points of interest.

Planning Your Time: The key is planning your day around the Secret Wartime Tunnels tours—especially the excellent Operation Dynamo tour. Each tour allows 30 people to enter at a time, with departures every 10-15 minutes. Your decision depends on two things: Which entrance you use (see above), and how long the lines are.

If arriving at **Canons Gate,** you're a short walk from the starting point for the tours. Survey the line and ask the attendants how long the wait is. If it'll be a while, consider hiking up to the Great Tower, then returning here later, in the hope that the lines will die down. But if the wait isn't too long, consider taking the tour now.

If arriving at **Constable's Gate,** ask at the ticket kiosk about wait times for the Operation Dynamo tour. If lines are relatively short, do the tour first, then backtrack to the Great Tower. But if the wait is long, see the Great Tower first, and hope lines for the tour get shorter later on.

Note: The lines for the two Secret Wartime Tunnels tours (Operation Dynamo and Underground Hospital) are next to each other.

Getting Around the Castle: The sporadic and free "land train" does a constant loop around the castle's grounds, shuttling visitors between the Secret Wartime Tunnels, the entrance to the Great Tower, and the Medieval Tunnels (at the top end of the castle). Though handy for avoiding the ups and downs, the train doesn't run every day. Nothing at the castle is more than a 10-minute walk from anything else—so you'll likely spend more time waiting for the train than you would walking.

Background: Armies have kept a watchful eye on this strategic lump of land since Roman times (as evidenced by the partly standing ancient lighthouse). A linchpin for English defense starting in the Middle Ages, Dover Castle was heavily used in the time

Dover Castle and Operation Dynamo

It was during World War II that Dover Castle lived its most dramatic moments, most notably as the headquarters for the inspiring Operation Dynamo—a story you'll hear retold again and again on your visit here.

In the spring of 1940, in the early days of the war, a joint French-British-Dutch-Belgian attack on the Nazis was met by a shockingly aggressive German counteroffensive. While Allied forces were distracted with their eastern front, the Nazis flanked them to the west, pinning them into an ever-narrowing corner of northern France (around the port cities of Calais and Dunkerque, which Brits call Dunkirk). As the Nazis closed in, it became clear that hundreds of thousands of British and other Allied troops being squeezed against the English Channel would soon be captured—or worse. From the tunnels below Dover Castle, Admiral Sir Bertram Ramsay oversaw Operation Dynamo. In 10 days, using a variety of military and civilian ships, Ramsay staged a dramatic evacuation of 338,000 Allied soldiers from the beaches of Dunkirk (several thousand troops, both British and French, were captured).

Because so many survived the desperate circumstances, the operation has been called a "victory in defeat." And although the Allies were forced to leave northern France to Hitler, Operation Dynamo saved an untold number of lives and bolstered morale in a country just beginning the most devastating war it would ever face. This unlikely evacuation is often called the "Miracle at Dunkirk."

of Henry VIII and Elizabeth I. After a period of decline, the castle was reinvigorated during the Napoleonic Wars, and it became a central command in World War II (when naval headquarters were buried deep in the cliffside). Parts of the tunnels were also used as a hospital and triage station for injured troops. After the war, in the 1960s, the tunnels were converted into a dramatic Cold War bunker—one of 12 designated sites in the UK that would house government officials and a BBC studio in the event of nuclear war. When it became clear that even the stout cliffs of Dover couldn't be guaranteed to stand up to a nuclear attack, Dover Castle was retired from active duty in 1984.

OTHER SIGHTS IN DOVER
Dover Museum
This museum, right off the tiny main square, houses a large, impressive, and well-preserved 3,600-year-old Bronze Age boat unearthed near Dover's shoreline. The boat is displayed on the top floor along with other finds from the site, an exhibit on boat

construction techniques, and a 12-minute film. Nearby, an endearing exhibit fills one big room (the Dover History Gallery) with the story of how this small but strategically located town has shaped history—from Tudor times to the Napoleonic era to World War II. The ground floor has exhib-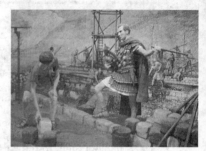
its covering the Roman and Anglo-Saxon periods.

Cost and Hours: £4; Mon-Sat 9:30-17:00, also Sun 10:00-15:00 April-Sept; tel. 01304/201-066, www.dovermuseum.co.uk.

Prince of Wales Pier

If it's a sunny day and you want a nice view of the White Cliffs and castle without heading out of town, stroll to the western end of the beachfront promenade (to the right as you face the water), then hike out along the Prince of Wales Pier for perfect panoramas back toward the city.

Cost and Hours: Free, daily June-Aug 8:00-21:00, Sept-May 8:00-19:00.

Boat Tours

The famous White Cliffs of Dover are almost impossible to appreciate from town. A 40-minute Dover White Cliffs Boat Tour around the bay gives you all the photo ops you need. It leaves from the Dover Marina—just past the western end of the waterfront promenade, near the Prince of Wales Pier.

Cost and Hours: £10; May-Aug 4-5 tours daily; Sept-April by appointment only, tel. 01303/271-388, mobile 07971/301-379, www.doverwhiteclifftours.com.

Eating in Dover

If you're touring the **castle,** consider having lunch at one of its two cafés. Other dining options in town include:

La Scala is tiny, but in a romantic way, and serves a good variety of Italian dishes (£9-11 pastas, £13-17 meat and fish dishes, open for lunch and dinner Mon-Sat, closed Sun, 19 High Street, tel. 01304/208-044).

The Allotment is trying to bring class to this small town, with an emphasis on locally sourced ingredients (in Brit-speak, an "allotment" is like a community garden). The rustic-chic interior feels a bit like an upscale deli (£3-6 breakfast dishes, £6-7 starters, £8-16 main dishes, Tue-Sat 8:30-23:00, closed Sun-Mon, 9 High Street, tel. 01304/214-467).

The Eight Bells, lively and wood-paneled, is a huge Wetherspoon chain pub that feels like a Vegas lounge (£4-7 "pub classics," bigger £6-10 meals, £8 lunch specials, daily 8:00-24:00, facing the small church at 19 Cannon Street, tel. 01304/205-030).

Lunch Eateries on Market Square: Dover's main shopping square is surrounded by places for a quick lunch. **The Ellie,** a generic, modern pub at a convenient location (right next door to the Dover Museum), spills out onto Market Square (£4 sandwiches, £6 main dishes, open daily, inviting outdoor seating on the square, tel. 01304/215-685). Across the square is the more genteel **Dickens Corner,** a comfy diner with a tearoom upstairs (£3-5 "jacket potatoes," sandwiches, and soups; open Mon-Sat, closed Sun, 7 Market Square, tel. 01304/206-692).

Canterbury

Canterbury—an easy train ride from Dover (less than 30 minutes away)—is one of England's most important religious destinations.

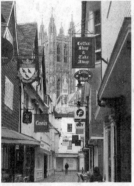

For centuries, it has welcomed hordes of pilgrims to its grand cathedral and abbey. Pleasant, walkable Canterbury, like many cities in southern England, was originally founded by the pagan Romans. Later, as Christianity became more established in England, Canterbury became its center, and the Archbishop of Canterbury emerged as one of the country's most powerful men. The famous pilgrimages to Canterbury increased in the 12th century, after the assassination of Archbishop Thomas Becket by followers of King Henry II (with whom Becket had been in a long feud). Becket was canonized as a martyr, rumors of miracles at the cathedral spread, and flocks of pilgrims showed up at its doorstep. Today, much of the medieval city—heavily bombed during World War II—exists only in fragments. Miraculously, the cathedral and surrounding streets are fairly well-preserved. Thanks to its huge student population and thriving pedestrian-and-shopper-friendly zone in the center, Canterbury is an exceptionally livable and fun-to-visit town.

LONDON

PLANNING YOUR TIME

On a quick visit to Canterbury, head straight for the cathedral, then spend the rest of your time strolling the town's pleasant pedestrian core.

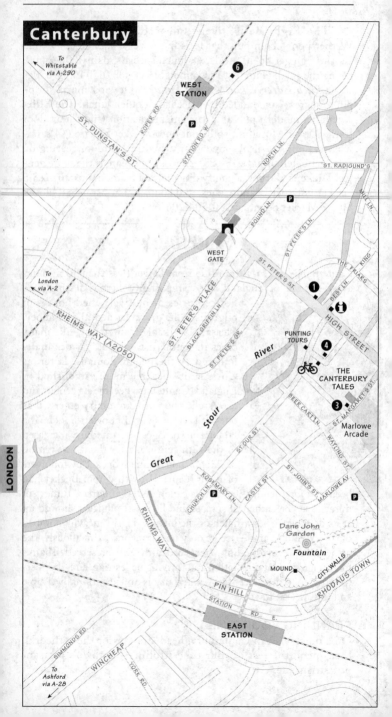

Canterbury

To Whitstable via A-290

WEST STATION

ROPER RD.

STATION RD. W.

ST. DUNSTAN'S ST.

NORTH LN.

ST. RADIGUND'S

MILL LN.

POUND LN.

ST. PETER'S LN.

THE FRIARS

KING

To London via A-2

RHEIMS WAY (A2050)

WEST GATE

ST. PETER'S ST.

ST. PETER'S PLACE

BLACK GRIFFIN LN.

ST. PETER'S GR.

River

HIGH STREET

BEST LN.

PUNTING TOURS

THE CANTERBURY TALES

ST. MARGARET'S ST.

Marlowe Arcade

Stour

BEER CART LN.

WATLING ST.

Great

ST. DUK ST.

ROSEMARY LN.

CHURCH LN.

CASTLE ST.

ST. JOHN'S ST.

MAKLOWE AV.

RHEIMS WAY

Dane John Garden

Fountain

MOUND

CITY WALLS

RHODAUS TOWN

PIN HILL

STATION   RD.   E.

EAST STATION

SIMMONDS RD.

WINCHEAP

YORK RD.

To Ashford via A-28

LONDON

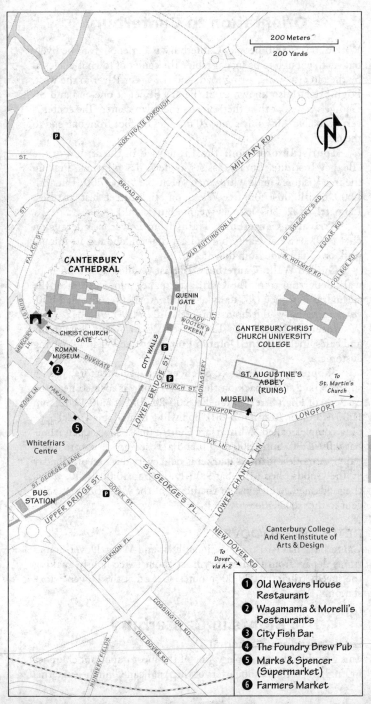

200 Meters
200 Yards

NORTHGATE BOROUGH

MILITARY RD.

BROAD ST.

ST.

ST.

ST.

PALACE ST.

OLD RUTTINGTON LN.

ST. GREGORY'S RD.

EDGAR RD.

COLLEGE RD.

N. HOLMES RD.

CANTERBURY CATHEDRAL

SUN ST.

QUENIN GATE

LADY WOOTEN'S GREEN

CANTERBURY CHRIST CHURCH UNIVERSITY COLLEGE

MERCERY LN.

CHRIST CHURCH GATE

ROMAN MUSEUM

BURGATE

❷

CITY WALLS

LOWER BRIDGE ST.

CHURCH ST.

MONASTERY ST.

ST. AUGUSTINE'S ABBEY (RUINS)

MUSEUM

LONGPORT

To St. Martin's Church

ROSE LN.

PARADE

❺

Whitefriars Centre

ST. GEORGE'S LANE

LONGPORT

IVY LN.

LOWER CHANTRY LN.

ST. GEORGE'S PL.

BUS STATION

DOVER ST.

UPPER BRIDGE ST.

VERNON PL.

NEW DOVER RD.

Canterbury College And Kent Institute of Arts & Design

To Dover via A-2

COSSINGTON RD.

OLD DOVER RD.

NUNNERY FIELDS

LONDON

❶ Old Weavers House Restaurant
❷ Wagamama & Morelli's Restaurants
❸ City Fish Bar
❹ The Foundry Brew Pub
❺ Marks & Spencer (Supermarket)
❻ Farmers Market

Orientation to Canterbury

With about 55,000 people, Canterbury is big enough to be lively but small enough to be manageable. The center of town is enclosed by the old city walls, a ring road, and the Stour River to the west. High Street (also known as St. Peter's Street at one end and St. George's Street at the other) bisects the town center. The center is very walkable—it's only about 20 minutes on foot from one end to the other.

Tourist Information: The TI, housed in the atrium of the "Beaney Institute" library, assists modern-day pilgrims. Pick up the free Visitors Guide with a map (Mon-Sat 9:00-17:00, Thu until 19:00, Sun 10:00-17:00, free Wi-Fi, on High Street, just past Best Lane, tel. 01227/862-162, www.canterbury.co.uk).

Arrival in Canterbury: Trains from Dover (see details on page 949) arrive at Canterbury's East Station, about a 10-minute walk or £5 taxi ride from downtown.

Guided Walk: Canterbury Tourist Guides offer a 1.5-hour walk departing from The Old Buttermaker pub, in front of the cathedral entrance (£7, daily at 11:00, April-Oct also at 14:00, www.canterburyguidedtours.com, tel. 01227/459-779).

Internet Access: The TI has free Wi-Fi. Many restaurants and cafés, including the **Dolphin Pub,** offer free Wi-Fi for paying customers.

Shopping: A **Marks & Spencer** department store, with a supermarket at the back on the ground floor, is located near the east end of High Street (Mon-Fri 8:00-20:00, Sat 8:00-19:00, Sun 11:00-17:00, tel. 01227/462-281). Sprawling behind it is a vast shopping complex called **Whitefriars Centre** (most shops open Mon-Sat 9:00-17:30, Sun 11:00-17:00) and a **Tesco** grocery store (open daily). A modest **farmers market** is held every day except Monday at The Goods Shed (Tue-Sat 9:00-19:00, Sun 10:00-16:00, www.thegoodsshed.co.uk), just to the north of the West Station, adjacent to the parking lot.

RETURNING TO DOVER

Canterbury has two train stations, East and West. Dover-bound trains depart from **Canterbury East** about twice hourly, making the speedy trip in just 20-30 minutes. Get off at the **Dover Priory** station.

Sights in Canterbury

▲▲▲Canterbury Cathedral

This grand landmark of piety, one of the most important churches in England, is the headquarters of the Anglican Church—in terms

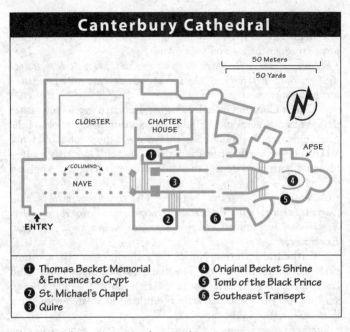

Canterbury Cathedral

50 Meters

50 Yards

CLOISTER

CHAPTER HOUSE

APSE

COLUMNS

NAVE

ENTRY

❶ Thomas Becket Memorial & Entrance to Crypt
❷ St. Michael's Chapel
❸ Quire
❹ Original Becket Shrine
❺ Tomb of the Black Prince
❻ Southeast Transept

of church administration, it's something like the English Vatican. It's been a Christian site ever since St. Augustine, the cathedral's first archbishop, broke ground in 597. In the 12th century, the cathedral became world-famous because of an infamous act: the murder of its then-archbishop, Thomas Becket. Canterbury became a prime destination for religious pilgrims, trumped in importance only by Rome and Santiago de Compostela, Spain. The dramatic real-life history of Canterbury Cathedral is the tale of two King Henrys (Henry II and Henry VIII), and of the martyred Becket.

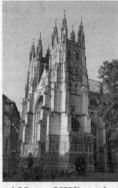

Cost and Hours: £10.50; Easter-Oct Mon-Sat 9:00-17:30, Sun 12:30-14:30; slightly shorter hours Nov-Easter; last entry 30 minutes before closing, tel. 01227/762-862, www.canterbury-cathedral.org.

Tours: Guides wearing golden sashes are posted throughout the cathedral to answer your questions. Guided £5 tours are offered Mon-Fri at 10:30, 12:00, and 14:30 (14:00 in winter); and Sat at 10:30, 12:00, and 13:30 (no tours Sun). At the shop inside the cathedral, you can rent a dry but informative £4 audioguide.

● Self-Guided Tour

Although guided tours and audioguides are available, it's simple just to wander through on your own.

• *Begin your tour in the pedestrian shopping zone just outside the cathedral grounds. Before going through the passageway (and admission area), take a moment to appreciate the...*

Christ Church Gate: This highly decorated gate is the cathedral yard's main entrance. Find the royal seals and symbols on the gate, including the Tudor rose. This rose was the symbol of Henry VIII, who—shortly after the Christ Church Gate was built—divorced both his wife and the Vatican, establishing the Anglican Church.

• *Go through the gate (where you'll buy your ticket) and walk into the courtyard that surrounds this massive, impressive church. An information booth, where you can get a free map of the building, is to your right. Examine the...*

Cathedral Exterior: Notice the cathedral's length, and how each section is distinctive. The church was already considered large in pre-pilgrim days, but in the 15th century, builders began another 100 years of construction (resulting in a patchwork effect that you'll notice in the interior).

• *Enter the church through the side door—the front doors of English cathedrals tend to be used only for special occasions—and pick up a map at the desk before you take a seat in the...*

Nave: The interior of the nave shows the inner workings of this sprawling, eclectic structure. Look around, and you'll see a church that's had many incarnations. Archaeological excavations in the early 1990s showed that the building's core is Roman. Through the ages, new sections were added on, with the biggest growth during the 1400s, when the cathedral had to be expanded to hold all of its pilgrims.

• *From here, we'll follow the route laid out by the map you picked up when you entered. Head up the left aisle. When you get to the quire (marked by a beautifully carved stone portal in the center of the nave), go down the stairs to your left. Immediately to your right is the...*

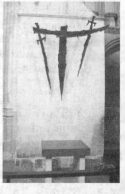

Thomas Becket Memorial: This is where Thomas Becket was martyred. You'll see a humble plaque and an overly dramatic wall sculpture of lightning-rod arrows pointing to the place where he died.

• *Continue down the stairs next to the memorial and enter the...*

Crypt: Notice the heavy stone arches. This lower section was started by the Normans, who probably built on top of St.

Thomas Becket and Canterbury Cathedral

In the 12th century, Canterbury Cathedral had already been a Christian church for more than 500 years. The king at the

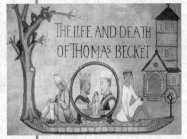

time was Henry II (who rebuilt and expanded nearby Dover Castle). Henry was looking for a new archbishop, someone who would act as a yes-man and allow him to gain control of the Church (and its followers). He found a candidate in his drinking buddy and royal chancellor: Thomas Becket (also called Thomas à Becket). In 1162, the king's friend was consecrated as archbishop.

But Becket surprised the king, and maybe even himself. Inspired by his new position—and wanting to be a true religious leader to his mighty flock—he cleaned up his act, became dedicated to the religious tenets of the Church (dressing as a monk), and refused to bow to the king's wishes. As tensions grew, Henry wondered aloud, "Will no one rid me of this turbulent priest?" Four knights took his words seriously, and assassinated Becket during vespers in the cathedral. The act shocked the medieval world. King Henry later submitted to walking barefoot through town while being flogged by priests as an act of pious penitence.

Not long after Becket's death in 1170, word spread that miracles were occurring in the cathedral, prompting the pope to canonize Becket. Soon the pilgrims came, hoping some of Becket's steadfast goodness would rub off (perhaps they also wanted to see the world—just like travelers today).

Augustine's original church. Work your way to the other (right) side of the vast crypt. The small chapel marked *Église Protestante Française* celebrates a Mass in French every Sunday at 15:00. This chapel has been used for hundreds of years by French (Huguenot) and Belgian (Walloon) Protestant communities, who fled persecution in their home countries for the more welcoming atmosphere in Protestant England.

• *Facing this chapel, turn right, walk to the end of the crypt, and climb up the stairs. At the landing, turn left to find...*

St. Michael's Chapel: Also known as the Warrior's Chapel, this was built by Lady Margaret Holland (d. 1439) to house family tombs. The chapel, which may be undergoing restoration when you visit, is also associated with the Royal East Kent Regiment ("The Buffs").

• *Head up the stairs across from the tomb, and go through the ornate stone portal we passed earlier. This will bring you into the* **quire,** *where the choir sings evensong. Walk toward the high altar, then turn left through the gate and walk with the quire on your right to the side of the church (the apse). Behind the quire, and to your right (up some steps), you'll see a candle in the center of the floor. This was the site of the...*

Original Becket Shrine: Beginning in the 12th century, hundreds of thousands of pilgrims came to this site to leave offerings. Imagine this site in the Dark Ages. You're surrounded by humble, devout pilgrims who've trudged miles upon miles to reach this spot. (Try to ignore the B.O.) Now that they've finally arrived, they're hoping to soak up just a bit of the miraculous power that's supposed to reside here.

Then came King Henry VIII, who broke away from the pope so he could marry on his own terms. In 1538, he destroyed the original altar (and lots more, including the original abbey of St. Augustine on the edge of town). Dictatorial Henry VIII—no fan of a priest who would stand up to a king—had Thomas Becket's body removed from the cathedral. Legend says that Henry had Becket's body burned and the ashes scattered, as part of his plan to drive religious pilgrims away from the site.

• *Follow the curve of the apse to the...*

Tomb of the Black Prince: This is the final resting place of the Black Prince, Edward of Woodstock (d. 1376). The Prince of Wales and the eldest son of Edward III, the Black Prince was famous for his cunning in battle and his chivalry—the original "knight in shining armor."

• *Head downstairs and make your way to the southeast transept (on your left).*

Southeast Transept: The small ship's bell standing to the left may be moved back to St. Michael's Chapel after restoration work is done there. This bell once rang from the HMS *Canterbury,* a ship that waged war against those disobedient colonists during the American Revolution. Each day at 11:00, the bell is rung and a prayer is said here to honor those who have lost their lives in battle.

The stained-glass windows in the transept are actually modern, relatively speaking, created by Hungarian-born artist and refugee Ervin Bossányi, who was commissioned by the Dean of Canterbury to replace earlier windows damaged by WWII bombs.

Our tour is finished. As you leave the cathedral, consider this: Even with all their power, wealth, and influence, two English kings were unable to successfully eradicate Thomas Becket's influence (if they had, the line to get into the cathedral would be shorter). A man of conscience—who once stood up to the most powerful ruler in England—continues to inspire visitors, nearly a thousand years after his death.

Eating in Canterbury

As a student town, Canterbury is packed with eateries—especially along the pedestrianized shopping zone.

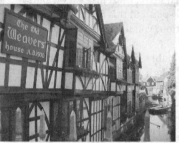

Old Weavers House serves solid English food in a pleasant, historic building next to the river. Sit inside beneath sunny walls and creaky beams, or outside on their riverside garden patio. This is the most atmospheric of my listings, and it can get very busy (£6-8 lunch specials, daily 11:30-23:00, 1 St. Peter's Street, tel. 01227/464-660).

Wagamama, part of the wildly popular British chain known for slinging tasty pan-Asian fare, has a convenient location just off the main shopping street (£8-13 main dishes, daily 11:30-22:00, 7-11 Longmarket Street, tel. 01227/454-307).

Morelli's Restaurant serves typical soups, sandwiches, and "jacket potatoes" with take-away options. You'll find it above the recommended Wagamama on Longmarket Street, with glassy indoor seating and a fine outdoor terrace (£5-7 light lunches, Mon-Sat 8:00-17:00, Sun 9:00-17:00, tel. 01227/454-307).

City Fish Bar is your quintessential British "chippie," serving several kinds of fried fish. Get yours for take-away or grab a side-walk table on this charming pedestrian street (£5-8 fish-and-chips, daily 9:00-19:00, 30 St. Margaret's Street, tel. 01227/760-873).

The Foundry Brew Pub offers up to 57 homebrews on tap (depending on the season) and serves beer-inspired dishes like steak-and-ale pie and BBQ beer ribs. Bartenders happily pour generous samples for curious customers (with the intent of selling you a pint) and explain the inspiration behind the name of their signature draft, Torpedo (£4-7 starters and salads, £9-10 meat pies, £9-14 main dishes, food served daily 12:00-18:00, Thu-Sat until 20:00, pub open until 24:00, White Horse Lane, tel. 01227/455-899).

LONDON

London

London, which has long attracted tourists, seems perpetually at your service, with an impressive slate of sights, entertainment, and eateries, all linked by a great transit system. With just a few hours here, you'll get no more than a quick splash in this teeming human tidal pool. But with a good orientation, you'll find London manageable and fun.

Blow through the city on a double-decker bus, or take a pinch-me-I'm-in-London walk through the West End. Gawk at the crown jewels at the Tower of London, hear the chimes of Big Ben, or see the Houses of Parliament in action. Cruise the Thames River, or take a spin on the London Eye. Hobnob with poets' tombstones in Westminster Abbey, or visit with Leonardo, Botticelli, and Rembrandt in the National Gallery. Whisper across the dome of St. Paul's Cathedral, or rummage through our civilization's attic at the British Museum. Sip your tea with pinky raised and clotted cream dribbling down your scone.

PLANNING YOUR TIME

The sights of London alone could easily fill a trip to Great Britain. But you only have a few hours...so you'll need to be very selective. I've clustered sights geographically and listed them roughly in the order of priority for a first-time visitor who just wants a taste.

• **Westminster:** For the best single-day visit to London, focus on the big, famous sights on and near Whitehall. Begin by ogling the Houses of Parliament, then consider dipping into **Westminster Abbey** (allow an hour). Follow my self-guided **Westminster Walk** up Whitehall for about 30 minutes—possibly poking into the **Churchill War Rooms** (history buffs will want at least an hour)—to reach Trafalgar Square. Here you can pop in to the **National Gallery** and/or the **National Portrait Gallery** (allow an hour each). Or, to get a look at nonmuseum London, stroll behind the National Gallery to explore **Leicester Square, Piccadilly Circus, Chinatown, Soho, Covent Garden,** and other bits of London's famously trendy and lively "West End" (allow an hour or more just to wander here). With time to spare, you could also hook around to see **Buckingham Palace** (from the outside; little to see inside). All told, the options noted here will more than eat up your London time (pick and choose museum and church visits carefully). But if you'd rather focus on other parts of the city, see the next few options.

• **London Eye:** While famous and relatively close to the Westminster sights mentioned above, this gigantic observation wheel is very expensive and can be time-consuming (allow 30 minutes for

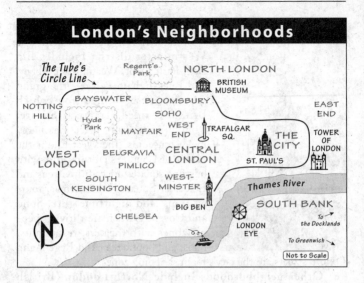

London's Neighborhoods

The Tube's Circle Line

Regent's Park

NORTH LONDON

BRITISH MUSEUM

BAYSWATER

BLOOMSBURY

NOTTING HILL

Hyde Park

SOHO

EAST END

MAYFAIR

WEST END

TRAFALGAR SQ.

THE CITY

TOWER OF LONDON

WEST LONDON

BELGRAVIA

CENTRAL LONDON

ST. PAUL'S

PIMLICO

SOUTH KENSINGTON

WEST-MINSTER

Thames River

BIG BEN

SOUTH BANK

CHELSEA

To the Docklands

LONDON EYE

To Greenwich

Not to Scale

the ride itself, but likely much more time waiting in lines).

• **British Museum:** One of the world's best collections of antiquities (from Egyptian mummies to the Rosetta Stone to the Parthenon Frieze)—but inconveniently located relative to other places on this list—this museum is worth at least two hours.

• **British Library:** This succinct collection of great works of literature can be seen in an hour, and is conveniently located next door to St. Pancras Station (with trains to Dover).

• **St. Paul's Cathedral:** It takes about an hour to tour London's biggest church and Christopher Wren's masterpiece (add another hour to climb the dome).

• **Tower of London:** London's original fortress takes about two hours to see (including an entertaining Beefeater tour).

With limited time, it may be folly to focus too tightly on any particular sight. Consider instead a **hop-on, hop-off bus tour** to get your bearings in this grand and sprawling metropolis. For suggested companies, see page 976.

Orientation to London

London is more than 600 square miles of urban jungle—a world in itself and a barrage on all the senses. On my first visit, I felt extremely small. To grasp London more comfortably, see it as the old town in the city center without the modern, congested sprawl. (Even from that perspective, it's still huge.)

The Thames River (pronounced "tems") runs roughly west to east through the city, with most of the visitor's sights on the North Bank.

On a brief visit, focus on **Central London.** This area contains Westminster and what Londoners call the West End. The 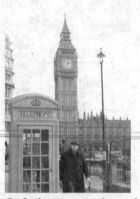Westminster district includes Big Ben, Parliament, Westminster Abbey, and Buckingham Palace—the grand government buildings from which Britain is ruled. Trafalgar Square, London's gathering place, has many major museums. The West End is the center of London's cultural life, with bustling squares: Piccadilly Circus and Leicester Square host cinemas, tourist traps, and nighttime glitz. Soho and Covent Garden are thriving people zones with theaters, restaurants, pubs, and boutiques. And Regent and Oxford streets are the city's main shopping zones.

Other neighborhoods include **North London** (British Museum, British Library, overhyped Madame Tussauds Waxworks); **"The City"** (today's modern financial district, just east of central London, with St. Paul's Cathedral and the Tower of London); **East London** (the increasingly gentrified former stomping ground of Cockney ragamuffins and Jack the Ripper); **The South Bank** (with the Tate Modern, Shakespeare's Globe, and the London Eye—all linked by a riverside walkway); and **West London** (a mostly upscale, residential, park-filled zone where the Queen hangs her crown and Kate goes to shop).

TOURIST INFORMATION

London's only publicly funded (and therefore impartial) "real" TI is the **City of London Information Centre,** inconveniently located just south of St. Paul's Cathedral. They hand out dozens of free brochures, including the *London Planner* monthly events guide. They also sell sightseeing passes, advance tickets, and skip-the-queue "Fast Track" tickets to big, crowded sights (Mon-Sat 9:30-17:30, Sun 10:00-16:00, across the busy street from St. Paul's Cathedral—around the right side as you face the main staircase, Tube: St. Paul's, www.visitthecity.co.uk). For phone inquiries, contact the more commercial **Visit London TI** (toll tel. 0870-156-6366, www.visitlondon.com).

You'll see "Tourist Information" offices elsewhere around town, but most of them are either private agencies pushing tours and tickets for big profits or are primarily focused on providing public-transit advice.

London Pass: This pricey pass, which covers many big sights and lets you skip some lines, is worthwhile only if you'll be cramming in lots of sightseeing (£47/1 day; sold at TIs, major train stations, and airports; tel. 0870-242-9988, www.londonpass.com).

ARRIVAL IN LONDON

By Train from Southampton: You'll ride to London's **Waterloo Station** (for details, see page 937). The Jubilee Promenade along the South Bank and London Eye are both a short walk from the station. Or you can hop on the Tube to get anywhere in town: As you exit the train, with the tracks to your back, the stop for the Jubilee line is to the right, and the stop for the Northern/Waterloo and Bakerloo lines are to the left.

By Train from Dover: Remember that you have the option of riding the train to three of London's stations: St. Pancras (fastest connection), Charing Cross, or Victoria (see details on page 949). All three are right in the thick of London's transit system. If arriving at **St. Pancras Station,** head down the escalator and go toward the big, glass, modern entryway nearby; you'll find an Underground (Tube) station just inside the door. Alternatively, if you want to reach the British Library or buses, first follow signs for Euston Station, then turn left and head all the way down the long main hall, and follow signs for Way Out and Euston Road. You'll pop out the station's front door along busy Euston Road. The public bus stops are on the road in front of you, and the British Library is a block to your right. If arriving at **Charing Cross Station,** you can simply exit the station, turn left along the busy street called The Strand, and you're a short walk from Trafalgar Square—right in the heart of town. From **Victoria Station,** you'll want to hop on the Tube; the Circle or District line zips you in two stops to Westminster, where you can exit the Tube station and peer up at Big Ben.

By Shuttle Bus: If you're taking an "On Your Own" shuttle bus excursion into London from your ship, it will likely drop you off at Piccadilly Circus, in the center of London's bustling West End. From this point, it's an easy 10-minute walk to Trafalgar Square, with the National Gallery and National Portrait Gallery. You can also hop on the Tube; the Piccadilly Circus Tube stop serves the Bakerloo line and the Piccadilly line.

RETURNING TO SOUTHAMPTON OR DOVER

To make it back to your ship, follow the instructions under "Getting from Central London to the Cruise Ports," on page 1026.

HELPFUL HINTS

Theft Alert: Wear your money belt. The Artful Dodger is alive and well in London. Be on guard, particularly on public transportation and in places crowded with tourists, who,

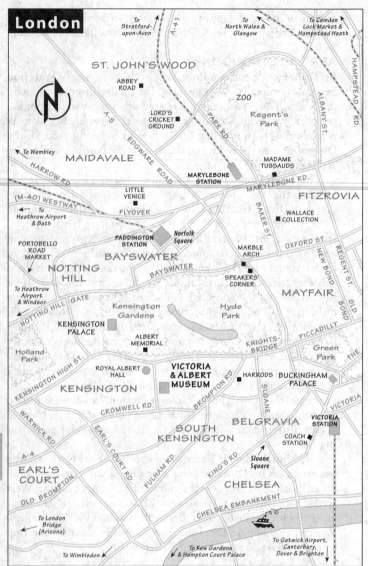

London

To Stratford-upon-Avon

To North Wales & Glasgow

To Camden Lock Market & Hampstead Heath

ST. JOHN'S WOOD

ABBEY ROAD

ZOO

Regent's Park

LORD'S CRICKET GROUND

MADAME TUSSAUDS

MARYLEBONE STATION

To Wembley

MAIDA VALE

MARYLEBONE RD.

FITZROVIA

(M-40) WESTWAY

LITTLE VENICE

To Heathrow Airport & Bath

FLYOVER

WALLACE COLLECTION

PORTOBELLO ROAD MARKET

PADDINGTON STATION

Norfolk Square

MARBLE ARCH

OXFORD ST.

NOTTING HILL

BAYSWATER

BAYSWATER

SPEAKERS' CORNER

MAYFAIR

To Heathrow Airport & Windsor

NOTTING HILL GATE

Kensington Gardens

Hyde Park

KENSINGTON PALACE

ALBERT MEMORIAL

KNIGHTS BRIDGE

PICCADILLY

Holland Park

Green Park

ROYAL ALBERT HALL

VICTORIA & ALBERT MUSEUM

HARRODS

BUCKINGHAM PALACE

KENSINGTON

CROMWELL RD.

VICTORIA

WARWICK RD.

BELGRAVIA

VICTORIA STATION

SOUTH KENSINGTON

COACH STATION

A-4

EARL'S COURT

Sloane Square

OLD BROMPTON

KING'S RD.

CHELSEA

To London Bridge (Arizona)

CHELSEA EMBANKMENT

To Kew Gardens & Hampton Court Palace

To Gatwick Airport, Canterbury, Dover & Brighton

To Wimbledon

considered naive and rich, are targeted. The Changing of the Guard scene is a favorite for thieves. And more than 7,500 purses are stolen annually at Covent Garden alone.

Pedestrian Safety: Cars drive on the left side of the road—which can be as confusing for foreign pedestrians as for foreign drivers. Before crossing a street, I always look right, look left, then look right again just to be sure. Most crosswalks are even

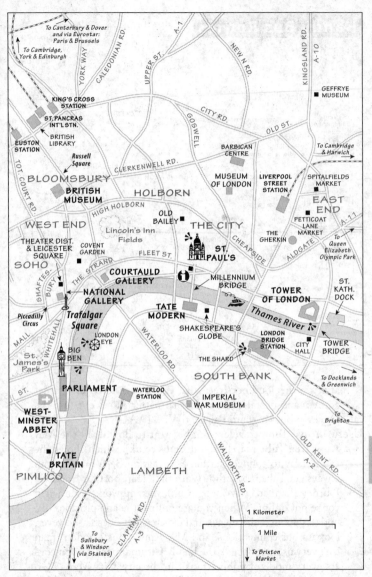

painted with instructions, reminding foreign guests to "Look right" or "Look left."

Getting Online with a Mobile Device: It's smart to get a free account with **The Cloud,** a Wi-Fi service found in many convenient spots around London, including most train stations and many museums, coffee shops, cafés, and shopping centers (though the connection can be slow). When you sign up

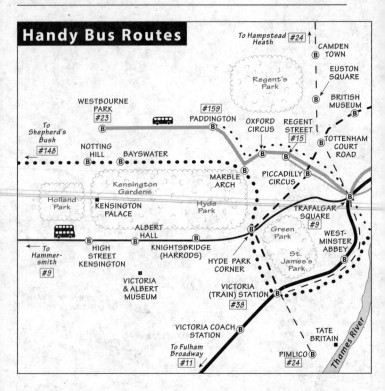

Handy Bus Routes

To Hampstead Heath #24

CAMDEN TOWN

EUSTON SQUARE

BRITISH MUSEUM

Regent's Park

WESTBOURNE PARK #23

#159

PADDINGTON

OXFORD CIRCUS

REGENT STREET #15

TOTTENHAM COURT ROAD

To Shepherd's Bush #148

NOTTING HILL

BAYSWATER

PICCADILLY CIRCUS

Kensington Gardens

MARBLE ARCH

Holland Park

KENSINGTON PALACE

Hyde Park

TRAFALGAR SQUARE #9

ALBERT HALL

Green Park

WEST-MINSTER ABBEY

To Hammersmith #9

HIGH STREET KENSINGTON

KNIGHTSBRIDGE (HARRODS)

HYDE PARK CORNER

St. James's Park

VICTORIA & ALBERT MUSEUM

VICTORIA (TRAIN) STATION #38

VICTORIA COACH STATION

TATE BRITAIN

To Fulham Broadway #11

PIMLICO #24

To Hampstead Heath #24

Thames River

at www.thecloud.net/free-wifi, you'll have to enter a street address and postal code; it doesn't matter which one (use the Queen's: Buckingham Palace, SW1A 1AA).

Useful Apps: Tube travelers might want to download the **MX Apps free Tube map** (www.mxapps.co.uk), which shows the easiest way to connect station A to station B. While you can always get Tube info online (with the "Transport for London's Journey Planner," www.tfl.gov.uk), the app works even when you're not online. When you are online, the app provides live updates about Tube delays and closures. (It doesn't, however, look up bus connections, and MX Apps' "Bus London" map isn't very useful offline.) The handy **Citymapper London** covers every mode of public transit in the city. **City Maps 2Go** lets you download searchable offline maps; their London version is quite good. **Time Out London**'s free app has reviews and listings for theater, museums, movies, and more (download the "Things to Do" version, which is updated weekly, rather than the boilerplate "Travel Guide" version).

Updates to This Book: Check www.ricksteves.com/update for updates to this book.

LONDON

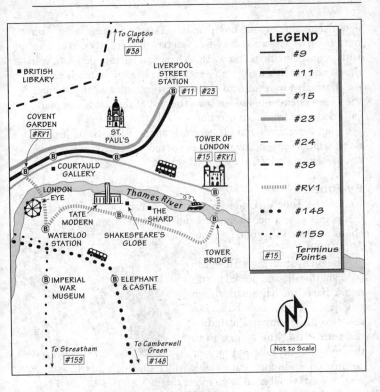

GETTING AROUND LONDON

In London, you're never more than a 10-minute walk from a stop on the Underground (the Tube). Buses are also convenient, and taxis are everywhere. For public transit info, see www.tfl.gov.uk.

Buying Tickets and Public-Transit Passes

A single ticket to ride the Tube costs a whopping £4.80. But the options explained below are much cheaper, and cover both the Tube and the bus system.

One-Day Travelcard: This pass gives unlimited travel on the Tube and buses for a day for £12. To use it, feed the Travelcard into the Tube turnstile like a paper ticket (and retrieve it), or show it to the bus driver. There's also a seven-day version (issued on an Oyster card) for £32. On a short visit where you think you'll be zipping around a lot, the One-Day Travelcard works best.

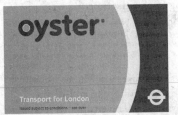

Oyster Card: This pay-as-you-go plastic debit card lets you travel at about half the price per ride of single Tube or bus tickets (the card is not shareable among companions taking the same ride). You must pay a £3 activation fee when you buy the card, then load it up with as much credit as you want. When your balance gets low, you simply add credit—or "top up"—at a ticket window or machine. To use it, simply touch the card to the turnstile/reader when you enter the Tube system or board the bus. The cost of the ride is automatically deducted from your account.

Buy Travelcards and Oyster cards at any Tube station, from a ticket window or vending machine. For more detailed info on tickets, passes, and prices, see www.tfl.gov.uk.

By Tube

Called the Tube or Underground (but never "subway"), one of this planet's great people-movers runs Monday through Saturday about 5:00-24:00, Sunday about 7:00-23:00.

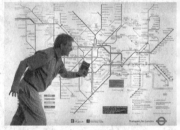

Begin by studying a Tube map (available locally and posted in stations). Each line has a name (such as Circle, Northern, or Bakerloo) and two directions (indicated by the end-of-the-line stops). Find the line that will take you to your destination, and figure out roughly which direction (north, south, east, or west) you'll need to go to get there.

In the Tube station, use your Travelcard, Oyster card, or individual ticket to pass through the turnstile. Find your train by following signs to your line and the direction it's headed (such as "Central Line: east"). Since some tracks are shared by several lines, read signs on the platform to confirm that the approaching train is going to your specific destination. Transfers to another train are free (but transferring to a bus requires a new ticket). You'll need your Oyster card, Travelcard, or ticket to pass through the exit turnstile. Save walking time by choosing the best street exit—check the maps on the walls or ask any station personnel.

Rush hours (8:00-10:00 and 16:00-19:00) can be packed and sweaty. Be prepared to walk significant distances within Tube stations and ride long escalators (stand on the right to let others pass). Delays are common; bring something to pass the time. Be wary of thieves, especially amid the jostle of boarding and leaving crowded trains. For more info on the Tube, see www.tfl.gov.uk.

By Bus

London's excellent bus system works like buses anywhere. Every bus stop has a name, and every bus is headed to one end-of-the-line stop or the other. Buses are covered by Travelcards, Oyster cards, and one-day £5 bus passes—no individual tickets are sold. The bus is easier to use if you know where you are going—carry a good London map or pick up a free bus map; the most user-friendly is in the free *Welcome to London* brochure (download it at www.tfl.gov. uk).

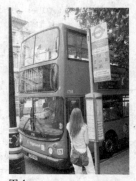

As you board, show your Travelcard or pass to the driver, or touch your Oyster card to the card reader. During bump-and-grind rush hours (8:00-10:00 and 16:00-19:00), you'll go faster by Tube.

A few bus routes handy to sights are:

Route #9: High Street Kensington to Knightsbridge (Harrods) to Hyde Park Corner to Piccadilly Circus to Trafalgar Square.

Route #11: Victoria Station to Westminster Abbey to Trafalgar Square to St. Paul's and Liverpool Street Station and the East End.

Route #15: Regent Street to Piccadilly Circus to Trafalgar Square to St. Paul's to Tower of London.

Routes #23 and #159: Paddington Station to Oxford Circus to Piccadilly Circus to Trafalgar Square; from there, #23 heads east to St. Paul's and Liverpool Street Station, while #159 heads to Westminster and the Imperial War Museum. In addition, several buses (including #6, #13, and #139) also make the corridor run between Marble Arch, Oxford Circus, Piccadilly Circus, and Trafalgar Square.

Route #24: Pimlico to Victoria Station to Westminster Abbey to Trafalgar Square to Euston Square.

Route #38: Victoria Station to Hyde Park Corner to Piccadilly Circus to British Museum.

Route #RV1 (a scenic South Bank joyride): Tower of London to Tower Bridge to Southwark Street (five-minute walk behind Tate Modern/Shakespeare's Globe) to London Eye/Waterloo Station, then over Waterloo Bridge to Aldwych and Covent Garden.

Route #148: Westminster Abbey to Victoria Station to Notting Hill and Bayswater (by way of the east end of Hyde Park and Marble Arch).

By Taxi

London is the best taxi town in Europe. Big, black cabs are everywhere, and there's no meter-cheating. They know every nook and cranny in town. I've never met a crabby London cabbie.

LONDON

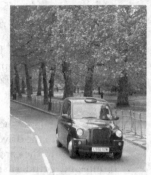

If a cab's top light is on, just wave it down—even if it's going the opposite way—or find the nearest taxi stand. Telephoning a cab will get you one in minutes, but costs about £2-3 more (tel. 0871-871-8710).

Rides start at £2.40. All extra charges are explained in writing on the cab wall. Tip a cabbie by rounding up (maximum 10 percent).

A typical daytime trip—from the Tower of London to St. Paul's—costs about £6-10. All cabs can carry five passengers, and some take six, for the same cost as a single traveler. So for a short ride, three adults in a cab travel at close to Tube prices. Avoid cabs when traffic is bad—they're slow and expensive, because the meter keeps running even at a standstill.

Tours in London

To sightsee on your own, download my series of free audio tours that illuminate some of London's top sights and neighborhoods: Westminster Walk, British Museum, British Library, St. Paul's Cathedral, and City of London Walk (see sidebar on page 50 for details).

▲▲▲Hop-On, Hop-Off Double-Decker Bus Tours

For a grand and efficient intro to London, ride through the city on an open-air bus past the main sights, while you listen to commentary. Hop on at any of the 30 stops along the two-hour loop, pay as you board, ride awhile, hop off to sightsee, then catch the next bus (10-20 minutes later) to carry on. Some routes have good live guides, while others have mediocre recorded commentary.

Several similar companies offer several different routes. Pick up their brochures or check online for the various options, extras, and discounts. **Original London Sightseeing Bus Tour** is cheapest (£29, £4 less with this book, limit four discounts per book, they'll rip off the corner of this page—raise bloody hell if they won't honor discount; also online deals, tel. 020/8877-1722, www.theoriginaltour.com). **Big Bus London Tours** tend to have more departures (£30, 30 percent discount online, tel. 020/7233-9533, www.bigbustours.com).

▲▲Walking Tours

Top-notch, highly entertaining local guides lead groups on two-hour tours through specific slices of London's past. Choose from the world of Charles Dickens, Harry Potter, the Plague,

Shakespeare, Legal London, the Beatles, the ever-popular Jack the Ripper, plus many others. To see what's available, look for brochures, check www.timeout.com/london, or contact the various companies directly. To take a walking tour, you simply show up at the announced location and pay the guide (usually cash only). Of the many companies, **London Walks** has a wide and fascinating repertoire of tours led by professional guides and actors (£9, tel. 020/7624-3978, recorded info 020/7624-9255, www.walks.com).

Private Guides

Standard rates for registered Blue Badge guides are about £150-165 for four hours, and £250 or more for nine hours (tel. 020/7611-2545, www.guidelondon.org.uk or www.britainsbestguides.org). For a personal guide who can also drive you around London (£475/day), try www.driverguidetours.com or http://seeitinstyle.synthasite.com.

Bike Tours

Though London traffic is pretty intense to navigate on your own, consider pedaling through London's pleasant parks or taking a guided bike tour. **London Bicycle Tour Company** rents to individuals (£3.50/hour, £20/day) and leads tours (£24 and up, includes bike) on three different routes (located at 1 Gabriel's Wharf on the South Bank, Tube: Waterloo, tel. 020/7928-6838, www.londonbicycle.com). **Fat Tire Bike Tours** offers two different itineraries, as well as a range of walking tours (£20-28, £2 discount with this book, mobile 078-8233-8779, www.fattirebiketourslondon.com).

▲▲Thames Cruises

Several boat companies ply the Thames, useful for either a relaxing guided cruise or for point-A-to-B travel around London. The handiest boats leave from Westminster Pier (near Big Ben) and Waterloo Pier (near the London Eye). Some helpful stops for sightseers are Bankside (Shakespeare's Globe), Blackfriars (St. Paul's), London Bridge, and Tower of London. A one-way trip within the city center costs about £10. Buy tickets at the docks. Some companies give discounts for the Tube's Travelcard and Oyster card, and for children and seniors—it's worth asking.

From **Westminster Pier,** City Cruises is handy to the Tower of London (www.citycruises.com), as is the similar Thames River Services (www.thamesriverservices.co.uk). Crown River Services has a hop-on, hop-off "Circular Cruise" route (www.crownriver.com).

From **Waterloo Pier,** Thames Clippers is more like an express commuter bus than a tour cruise, traveling fast and making all the stops along the way (£6.50 single trip, £15 all-day, www.thamesclippers.com).

Westminster Walk

Just about every visitor to London strolls along historic Whitehall from Big Ben to Trafalgar Square. This self-guided walk gives meaning to that touristy ramble (most of the sights you'll see are described in more detail later). Under London's modern traffic and big-city bustle lie 2,000 fascinating years of history. You'll get a whirlwind tour as well as a practical orientation to London. (You can download a free, extended audio version of this walk to your mobile device; see page 50.)

Start halfway across ❶ **Westminster Bridge** for that "Wow, I'm really in London!" feeling. Get a close-up view of the **Houses of Parliament** and **Big Ben.** Downstream you'll see the **London Eye.** Down the stairs to Westminster Pier are boats to the Tower of London and Greenwich (downstream) or Kew Gardens (upstream).

En route to Parliament Square, you'll pass a ❷ **statue of Boadicea,** the Celtic queen defeated by Roman invaders in A.D. 60.

For fun, call home from near Big Ben at about three minutes before the hour to let your loved one hear the bell ring. You'll find four red phone booths lining the north side of ❸ **Parliament Square** along Great George Street—also great for a phone-box-and-Big-Ben photo op.

Wave hello to Winston Churchill and Nelson Mandela in Parliament Square. To Churchill's right is **Westminster Abbey,** with its two stubby, elegant towers. The white building (flying the Union Jack) at the far end of the square houses Britain's **Supreme Court.**

Head north up Parliament Street, which turns into ❹ **Whitehall,** and walk toward Trafalgar Square. You'll see the thought-provoking ❺ **Cenotaph** in the middle of the boulevard, reminding passersby of the many Brits who died in the last century's world wars. To visit the **Churchill War Rooms,** take a left before the Cenotaph, on King Charles Street.

Continuing on Whitehall, stop at the barricaded and guarded ❻ **#10 Downing Street** to see the British "White House," home of the prime minister. Break the bobby's boredom and ask him a question. The huge building across Whitehall from Downing Street is the **Ministry of Defence** (MOD), the "British Pentagon."

Nearing Trafalgar Square, look for the 17th-century ❼ **Banqueting House** across the street and the ❽ **Horse Guards** behind the gated fence.

The column topped by Lord Nelson marks ❾ **Trafalgar Square.** The stately domed building on the far side of the square is the **National Gallery,** which has a classy café in the Sainsbury wing. To the right of the National Gallery is **St.**

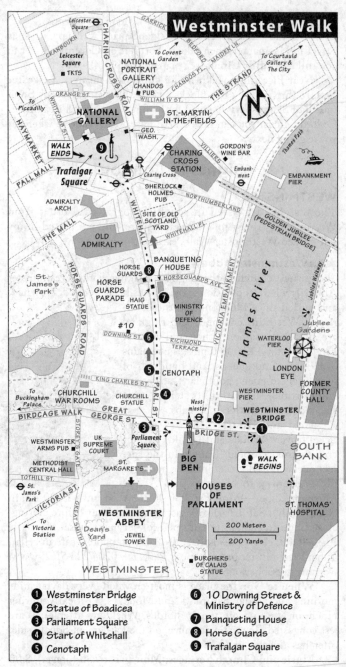

Westminster Walk

Leicester Square

CRANBOURN ST

Leicester Square

■ TKTS

ORANGE ST.

NATIONAL GALLERY

HAYMARKET

WHITCOMB ST.

CHARING CROSS ROAD

GARRICK

BEDFORD

MAIDEN LN.

To Covent Garden

NATIONAL PORTRAIT GALLERY

CHANDOS PUB

CHANDOS PL.

WILLIAM IV ST.

ST.-MARTIN-IN-THE-FIELDS

THE STRAND

To Courtauld Gallery & The City

N

WALK ENDS

GEO. WASH.

Trafalgar Square

9

PALL MALL

ADMIRALTY ARCH

THE MALL

To Piccadilly

St. James's Park

OLD ADMIRALTY

HORSE GUARDS ROAD

CHARING CROSS STATION

VILLIERS

GORDON'S WINE BAR

Embankment

Thames Path

EMBANKMENT PIER

Charing Cross

SHERLOCK HOLMES PUB

NORTHUMBERLAND

WHITEHALL

SITE OF OLD SCOTLAND YARD

WHITEHALL PL.

GOLDEN JUBILEE (PEDESTRIAN BRIDGE)

BANQUETING HOUSE

8 HORSE GUARDS

HORSEGUARDS AVE.

HORSE GUARDS PARADE

HAIG STATUE

7

MINISTRY OF DEFENCE

VICTORIA EMBANKMENT

Thames River

Jubilee Walkway

#10

DOWNING ST. **6**

RICHMOND TERRACE

5

PARL. ST.

CENOTAPH

Jubilee Gardens

WATERLOO PIER

LONDON EYE

To Buckingham Palace

KING CHARLES ST.

4

CHURCHILL WAR ROOMS

CHURCHILL STATUE

GREAT GEORGE ST.

BIRDCAGE WALK

STOREY'S GATE

WESTMINSTER ARMS PUB

UK SUPREME COURT

3

Parliament Square

West-minster

2

WESTMINSTER PIER

FORMER COUNTY HALL

BRIDGE ST.

WESTMINSTER BRIDGE

1

SOUTH BANK

METHODIST CENTRAL HALL

ST. MARGARET'S

BIG BEN

WALK BEGINS

TOTHILL ST.

St. James's Park

VICTORIA ST.

GREAT SMITH ST.

HOUSES OF PARLIAMENT

ST. THOMAS' HOSPITAL

To Victoria Station

WESTMINSTER ABBEY

Dean's Yard

JEWEL TOWER

200 Meters

200 Yards

WESTMINSTER

BURGHERS OF CALAIS STATUE

LONDON

❶ Westminster Bridge
❷ Statue of Boadicea
❸ Parliament Square
❹ Start of Whitehall
❺ Cenotaph
❻ 10 Downing Street & Ministry of Defence
❼ Banqueting House
❽ Horse Guards
❾ Trafalgar Square

Martin-in-the-Fields Church and its Café in the Crypt.

To get to Piccadilly from Trafalgar Square, walk up Cockspur Street to Haymarket, then take a short left on Coventry Street to colorful **Piccadilly Circus** (see map on page 1014).

Near Piccadilly, you'll find a number of theaters. **Leicester Square** thrives just a few blocks away. Walk through seedy **Soho** (north of Shaftesbury Avenue) for its fun pubs. From Piccadilly or Oxford Circus, you can take a taxi, bus, or the Tube to wherever you're going next.

Sights in London

WESTMINSTER

These sights are listed in roughly geographical order from Westminster Abbey to Trafalgar Square, and are linked in my self-guided Westminster Walk, earlier.

▲▲▲Westminster Abbey

The greatest church in the English-speaking world, Westminster Abbey is where the nation's royalty has been wedded, crowned, and buried since 1066. Indeed, the histories of Westminster Abbey and England are almost the same. A thousand years of English history—3,000 tombs, the remains of 29 kings and queens, and hundreds of memorials to poets, politicians, scientists, and warriors—lie within its stained-glass splendor and under its stone slabs.

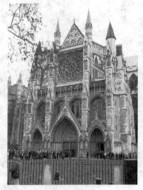

Cost and Hours: £18, £36 family ticket (covers 2 adults and 1 child), cash or credit cards accepted (line up in the correct queue to pay), ticket includes audioguide and entry to cloisters and Abbey Museum; abbey—Mon-Fri 9:30-16:30, Wed until 19:00 (main church only), Sat 9:30-14:30, last entry one hour before closing, closed Sun to sightseers but open for services; museum—daily 10:30-16:00; cloisters—daily 8:00-18:00; no photos, café in cellar, Tube: Westminster or St. James's Park, tel. 020/7222-5152, www.westminster-abbey.org.

When to Go: The place is most crowded every day at mid-morning and all day Saturdays and Mondays. Visit early, during lunch, or late to avoid tourist hordes. Weekdays after 14:30 are less congested. The main entrance, on the Parliament Square side, often has a sizable line.

Music and Church Services: Mon-Fri at 7:30 (prayer), 8:00 (communion), 12:30 (communion), 17:00 evensong (except on

LONDON

Wed, when the evening service is generally spoken—not sung); **Sat** at 8:00 (communion), 9:00 (prayer), 15:00 (evensong; May-Aug it's at 17:00); **Sun** services generally come with more music: at 8:00 (communion), 10:00 (sung Matins), 11:15 (sung Eucharist), 15:00 (evensong), 18:30 (evening service). Services are free to anyone, though visitors who haven't paid church admission aren't allowed to linger afterward.

Tours: Entertaining **guided tours** from a verger—the church equivalent of a museum docent—are offered up to five times a day in summer (£3, schedule posted both outside and inside entry, 4/day in winter, 1.5 hours).

❯ **Self-Guided Tour:** You'll have no choice but to follow the steady flow of tourists through the church, following the route laid out for the audioguide. My tour covers the Abbey's top stops.

• *Walk straight in through the north transept. Follow the crowd flow to the right and enter the spacious...*

Nave: Look down the long and narrow center aisle of the church. Lined with the praying hands of the Gothic arches, glowing with light from the stained glass, it's clear that this is more than a museum. With saints in stained glass, heroes in carved stone, and the bodies of England's greatest citizens under the floor stones, Westminster Abbey is the religious heart of England.

The king who built the Abbey was Edward the Confessor. Find him in the stained-glass windows on the left side of the nave ("left" as you face the altar). He's in the third bay from the end (marked *S: Edwardus rex...*), with his crown, scepter, and ring.

The Abbey's 10-story nave is the tallest in England. On the floor near the west entrance of the Abbey is the flower-lined Grave of the Unknown Warrior, one ordinary WWI soldier buried in soil from France with lettering made from melted-down weapons from that war. Contemplate the million-man army from the British Empire, and all those who gave their lives. Their memory is so revered that, when Kate Middleton walked up the aisle on her wedding day, by tradition she had to step around the tomb (and her wedding bouquet was later placed atop this tomb, also in accordance with tradition).

• *Walk up the nave toward the altar. This is the same route every future monarch walks on the way to being crowned. Midway up the nave, you pass through the colorful screen of an enclosure known as the...*

Choir: These elaborately carved-wood and gilded seats are where monks once chanted their services in the "quire"—as it's known in British churchspeak. Today, it's where the Abbey boys' choir sings the evensong. The "high" (main) altar, which usually has a cross and candlesticks atop it, sits on the platform up the five stairs in front of you.

• *It's on this platform—up the five steps—that the monarch is crowned.*

London at a Glance

▲▲▲Westminster Abbey Britain's finest church and the site of royal coronations and burials since 1066. **Hours:** Mon-Fri 9:30-16:30, Wed until 19:00, Sat 9:30-14:30, closed Sun to sightseers except for worship. See page 980.

▲▲▲Churchill War Rooms Underground WWII headquarters of Churchill's war effort. **Hours:** Daily 10:00-18:00. See page 986.

▲▲▲National Gallery Remarkable collection of European paintings (1250-1900), including Leonardo, Botticelli, Velázquez, Rembrandt, Turner, Van Gogh, and the Impressionists. **Hours:** Daily 10:00-18:00, Fri until 21:00. See page 988.

▲▲▲British Museum The world's greatest collection of artifacts of Western civilization, including the Rosetta Stone and the Parthenon's Elgin Marbles. **Hours:** Daily 10:00-17:30, Fri until 20:30 (selected galleries only). See page 995.

▲▲▲British Library Fascinating collection of important literary treasures of the Western world. **Hours:** Mon-Fri 9:30-18:00, Tue until 20:00, Sat 9:30-17:00, Sun 11:00-17:00. See page 999.

▲▲▲St. Paul's Cathedral The main cathedral of the Anglican Church, designed by Christopher Wren, with a climbable dome and daily evensong services. **Hours:** Mon-Sat 8:30-16:30, closed Sun except for worship. See page 1002.

▲▲▲Tower of London Historic castle, palace, and prison housing the crown jewels and a witty band of Beefeaters. **Hours:** March-Oct Tue-Sat 9:00-17:30, Sun-Mon 10:00-17:30; Nov-Feb Tue-Sat 9:00-16:30, Sun-Mon 10:00-16:30. See page 1005.

▲▲Houses of Parliament London landmark famous for Big Ben and occupied by the Houses of Lords and Commons. **Hours:**

LONDON

Coronation Spot: The area immediately before the high altar is where every English coronation since 1066 has taken place.

Royalty are also given funerals here. Princess Diana's coffin was carried to this spot for her funeral service in 1997. The "Queen Mum" (mother of Elizabeth II) had her funeral here in 2002. This is also where most of the last century's royal weddings have taken place, including the unions of Queen Elizabeth II and Prince Philip (1947), Prince Andrew and Sarah Ferguson (1986), and Prince William and Kate Middleton (2011).

• *Veer left and follow the crowd. Pause at the wooden staircase on your right.*

Always viewable from the outside; interior not worth touring on a short visit. See page 986.

▲▲**Trafalgar Square** The heart of London, where Westminster, The City, and the West End meet. **Hours:** Always open. See page 988.

▲▲**National Portrait Gallery** A *Who's Who* of British history, featuring portraits of this nation's most important historical figures. **Hours:** Daily 10:00-18:00, Thu-Fri until 21:00, first and second floors open Mon at 11:00. See page 991.

▲▲**Covent Garden** Vibrant people-watching zone with shops, cafés, street musicians, and an iron-and-glass arcade that once hosted a produce market. **Hours:** Always open. See page 992.

▲▲**Changing of the Guard at Buckingham Palace** Hour-long spectacle at Britain's royal residence. **Hours:** Generally May-July daily at 11:30, Aug-April every other day. See page 993.

▲▲**London Eye** Enormous observation wheel, dominating—and offering commanding views over—London's skyline. **Hours:** Daily April-Aug 10:00-21:00, Sept-March 10:00-20:30, later on weekends. See page 1008.

▲▲**Tate Modern** Works by Monet, Matisse, Dalí, Picasso, and Warhol displayed in a converted powerhouse. **Hours:** Daily 10:00-18:00, Fri-Sat until 22:00. See page 1010.

▲▲**Shakespeare's Globe** Timbered, thatched-roofed reconstruction of the Bard's original "wooden O." **Hours:** Theater complex, museum, and actor-led tours generally daily 9:00-17:00; in summer, morning theater tours only. Plays are also staged here. See page 1011.

LONDON

Shrine of Edward the Confessor: Step back and peek over the dark coffin of Edward I to see the tippy-top of the green-and-gold wedding-cake tomb of King Edward the Confessor—the man who built Westminster Abbey. God had told pious Edward to visit St. Peter's Basilica in Rome. But with the Normans thinking conquest, it was too dangerous for him to leave England. Instead, he built this grand church and dedicated it to St. Peter. It was finished just in time to bury Edward and to crown his foreign successor, William the Conqueror, in 1066. After Edward's death, people prayed at his tomb, and, after getting good results, Pope Alexander III canonized him. This elevated, central tomb—which lost some of its luster when Henry VIII melted down the gold coffin-case—is surrounded by the tombs of eight kings and queens.

• *At the top of the stone staircase, veer left into the private burial chapel of Queen Elizabeth I.*

Tomb of Queens Elizabeth I and Mary I: Although only one effigy is on the tomb (Elizabeth's), there are actually two queens buried beneath it, both daughters of Henry VIII (by different mothers). Bloody Mary—meek, pious, sickly, and Catholic—enforced Catholicism during her short reign (1553-1558) by burning "heretics" at the stake.

Elizabeth—strong, clever, and Protestant—steered England on an Anglican course. She holds a royal orb symbolizing that she's queen of the whole globe. When 26-year-old Elizabeth was crowned in the Abbey, her right to rule was questioned (especially by her Catholic subjects) because she was considered the bastard seed of Henry VIII's unsanctioned marriage to Anne Boleyn. But Elizabeth's long reign (1559-1603) was one of the greatest in English history, a time when England ruled the seas and Shakespeare explored human emotions. When she died, thousands turned out for her funeral in the Abbey. Elizabeth's face on the tomb, modeled after her death mask, is considered a very accurate take on this hook-nosed, imperious "Virgin Queen."

• *Continue into the ornate, flag-draped room up a few more stairs, directly behind the main altar.*

Chapel of King Henry VII (The Lady Chapel): The light from the stained-glass windows; the colorful banners overhead; and the elaborate tracery in stone, wood, and glass give this room the festive air of a medieval tournament. The prestigious Knights of the Bath meet here, under the magnificent ceiling studded with gold pendants. The ceiling—of carved stone, not plaster (1519)—is the finest English Perpendicular Gothic and fan vaulting you'll see (unless you're going to King's College Chapel in Cambridge). The ceiling was sculpted on the floor in pieces, then jigsaw-puzzled into place. It capped the Gothic period and signaled the vitality of the coming Renaissance.

• *Go to the far end of the chapel and stand at the banister in front of the modern set of stained-glass windows.*

Royal Air Force Chapel: Saints in robes and halos mingle with pilots in parachutes and bomber jackets. This tribute to WWII flyers is for those who earned their angel wings in the Battle of Britain (July-Oct 1940). A bit of bomb damage has been preserved: Look for the little glassed-over hole in the wall beneath the windows in the lower left-hand corner.

• *Exit the Chapel of Henry VII. Turn left into a side chapel with the tomb (the central one of three in the chapel).*

Tomb of Mary, Queen of Scots: The beautiful, French-educated queen (1542-1587) was held under house arrest for 19 years by Queen Elizabeth I, who considered her a threat to her sovereignty. Elizabeth got wind of an assassination plot, suspected Mary was behind it, and had her first cousin (once removed) beheaded. When Elizabeth—who was called the "Virgin Queen"—died heirless, Mary's son, James VI, King of Scots, also became King James I of England and Ireland. James buried his mum here (with her head sewn back on) in the Abbey's most sumptuous tomb.

• *Exit Mary's chapel. Continue on, until you emerge in the south transept. You're in...*

Poets' Corner: England's greatest artistic contributions are in the written word. Here the masters of arguably the world's

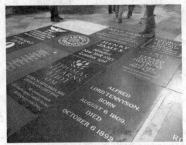

most complex and expressive language are remembered: Geoffrey Chaucer *(Canterbury Tales)*; Lord Byron; Dylan Thomas; W. H. Auden; Lewis Carroll *(Alice's Adventures in Wonderland)*; T. S. Eliot *(The Waste Land)*; Alfred, Lord Tennyson; Robert Browning; and Charles Dickens. Many writers are honored with plaques and monuments; relatively few are actually buried here. Shakespeare is commemorated by a fine statue that stands near the end of the transept, overlooking the others.

• *Exit the church (temporarily) at the south door, which leads to the...*

Cloisters and Abbey Museum: The buildings that adjoin the church housed the monks. Cloistered courtyards gave them a place to meditate on God's creations.

The small **Abbey Museum,** formerly the monks' lounge, is worth a peek for its fascinating and well-described exhibits. Look into the impressively realistic eyes of Elizabeth I,

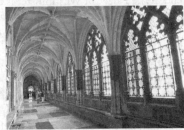

Charles II, Admiral Nelson, and a dozen others, part of a compelling series of wax-and-wood statues that, for three centuries, graced coffins during funeral processions. The once-exquisite, now-fragmented Westminster Retable, which decorated the high altar in 1270, is the oldest surviving altarpiece in England.

• *Go back into the church for the last stop.*

Coronation Chair: A gold-painted oak chair waits here under a regal canopy for the next coronation. For every English coronation since 1308 (except two), it's been moved to its spot before the high altar to receive the royal buttocks. The chair's legs rest on lions, England's symbol.

▲▲Houses of Parliament (Palace of Westminster)

This Neo-Gothic icon of London, the royal residence from 1042 to 1547, is now the meeting place of the legislative branch of government. The Houses of Parliament are located in what was once the Palace of Westminster, until it was largely destroyed by fire in 1834. The palace was rebuilt in a retro, Neo-Gothic style that recalled England's medieval Christian roots—pointed arches, stained-glass windows, spires, and saint-like stat-

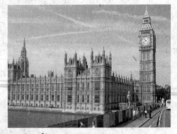

ues. At the same time, Britain was also retooling its government. Democracy was on the rise, the queen became a constitutional monarch, and Parliament emerged as the nation's ruling body. The Palace of Westminster became a symbol—a kind of cathedral—of democracy.

Like the US Capitol in Washington, DC, the complex is open to visitors (www.parliament.uk). You can view parliamentary sessions from the public galleries in either the bickering House of Commons or the sleepy House of Lords. Or you can tour the historic building on your own or with a guide (through a few closely monitored rooms). But on a quick visit to London, the views from outside are most worthwhile.

Nearby: Big Ben, the 315-foot-high clock tower at the north end of the Palace of Westminster is named for its 13-ton bell, Ben. The light above the clock is lit when Parliament is in session. The face of the clock is huge—you can actually see the minute hand moving. For a good view of it, walk halfway over Westminster Bridge.

▲▲▲Churchill War Rooms

This excellent sight offers a fascinating walk through the underground headquarters of the British government's fight against the Nazis in the darkest days of the Battle for Britain. It has two parts: the war rooms themselves, and a top-notch museum dedicated to the man who steered the war from here, Winston Churchill. For details on all the blood, sweat, toil, and tears, pick up the excellent, essential, and included audioguide at the entry, and dive in. Allow yourself 1-2 hours for this sight.

Cost and Hours: £17.50 includes audioguide (and 10 percent optional donation), £5 guidebook, daily 10:00-18:00, last entry one hour before closing; on King Charles Street, 200 yards off Whitehall, follow the signs, Tube: Westminster, tel. 020/7930-6961, www.iwm.org.uk/churchill. The museum's gift shop is great for anyone nostalgic for the 1940s.

Cabinet War Rooms: The 27-room, heavily fortified nerve center of the British war effort was used from 1939 to 1945.

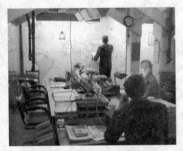

Churchill's room, the map room, and other rooms are just as they were in 1945. As you follow the one-way route, be sure to take advantage of the audioguide, which explains each room and offers first-person accounts of wartime happenings here. Be patient—it's well worth it. While the rooms are spartan, you'll see how British gentility survived even as the city was bombarded—posted signs informed those working underground what the weather was like outside, and a cheery notice reminded them to turn off the light switch to conserve electricity.

Churchill Museum: Don't bypass this museum, which occupies a large hall amid the war rooms. It dissects every aspect of the man behind the famous cigar, bowler hat, and V-for-victory sign. It's extremely well-presented and engaging, using artifacts, quotes, political cartoons, clear explanations, and high-tech interactive exhibits to bring the colorful statesman to life. You'll get a taste of Winston's wit, irascibility, work ethic, passion for painting, American ties, writing talents, and drinking habits. The exhibit shows Winston's warts as well: It questions whether his party-switching was just political opportunism, examines the basis for his opposition to Indian self-rule, and reveals him to be an intense taskmaster who worked 18-hour days and was brutal to his staffers (who deeply respected him nevertheless).

Horse Guards

The Horse Guards change daily at 11:00 (10:00 on Sun), and a colorful dismounting ceremony takes place daily at 16:00. The rest of the day, they just stand there—terrible for video cameras (at Horse Guards Parade on Whitehall, directly across from the Banqueting House, between Trafalgar Square and 10 Downing Street, Tube: Westminster, www.royal.gov.uk—search "Changing the Guard"). Buckingham Palace pageantry is canceled when it rains, but the Horse Guards change regardless of the weather.

▲Banqueting House

England's first Renaissance building (1619-1622) is still standing. Designed by Inigo Jones, built by King James I, and decorated by his son Charles I, the Banqueting House came to symbolize the Stuart kings' "divine right" management style—the belief that God himself had anointed them to rule. The house is one of the few London landmarks spared by the 1698 fire and is the only surviving part of the original Palace of Whitehall. Today it opens its doors to visitors, who enjoy a restful 15-minute audiovisual history, a 30-minute audioguide, and a look at the exquisite banqueting hall itself. As a tourist attraction, it's basically one big room, with sumptuous ceiling paintings by Peter Paul Rubens. At Charles I's request, these paintings drove home the doctrine of the legitimacy of the divine right of kings. Ironically, in 1649—divine right ignored—King Charles I was famously executed right here.

Cost and Hours: £6 includes audioguide (and 10 percent optional donation), daily 10:00-17:00, last entry at 16:30, may close for government functions—though it promises to stay open at least until 13:00 (call ahead for recorded information about closures), aristocratic WC, immediately across Whitehall from the Horse Guards, Tube: Westminster, tel. 020/3166-6150, www.hrp.org.uk.

▲▲TRAFALGAR SQUARE

London's central square—at the intersection of Westminster, The City, and the West End—is the climax of most marches and demonstrations, and a thrilling place to simply hang out. At the top of Trafalgar Square (north) sits the domed National Gallery with its grand staircase, and, to the right, the steeple of St. Martin-in-the-Fields, built in 1722, inspiring the steeple-over-the-entrance style of many town churches in New England.

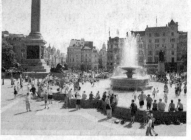

In the center of the square, Lord Horatio Nelson stands atop his 185-foot-tall fluted granite column, gazing out toward Trafalgar, where he lost his life but defeated the French fleet. Part of this 1842 memorial is made from his victims' melted-down cannons. He's surrounded by spraying fountains, giant lions, hordes of people, and—until recently—even more pigeons. A former London mayor decided that London's "flying rats" were a public nuisance and evicted Trafalgar Square's venerable seed salesmen (Tube: Charing Cross). For a map of the area, see page 1014.

▲▲▲National Gallery

Displaying an unsurpassed collection of European paintings from 1250 to 1900—including works by Leonardo, Botticelli, Velázquez, Rembrandt, Turner, Van Gogh, and the Impressionists—this is one of Europe's great galleries. You'll peruse 700 years of art—from gold-backed Madonnas to Cubist bathers. The collection is huge; following the route suggested in my self-guided tour will give you the best quick visit.

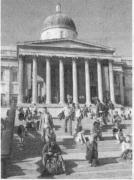

Cost and Hours: Free, but suggested donation of £4, special exhibits extra, daily 10:00-18:00, Fri until 21:00, last entry to special exhibits 45 minutes before closing; free guided tours available, no photos, on Trafalgar Square, Tube: Charing Cross or Leicester Square.

Information: Info tel. 020/7747-2885, switchboard tel. 020/7839-3321, www.nationalgallery.org.uk.

Tours: Free one-hour **overview tours** leave from the Sainsbury Wing info desk daily at 11:30 and 14:30, plus Fri at 19:00 and Sat-Sun at 16:00; excellent £3.50 **audioguides**—choose from the one-hour highlights tour, several theme tours, or a tour option that lets you dial up info on any painting in the museum; **ArtStart computer terminals** help you study any artist, style, or topic in the museum, and print out a tailor-made tour map (located in the comfy Espresso Bar on the ground floor of the main building).

Eating: Consider splitting afternoon tea at the excellent-but-pricey National Dining Rooms, on the first floor of the Sainsbury Wing. The National Café, located near the Getty Entrance, also has afternoon tea.

◆ Self-Guided Tour: Go in through the Sainsbury Entrance (in the smaller building to the left of the main entrance), and approach the collection chronologically.

Medieval and Early Renaissance: In the first rooms, you see shiny paintings of saints, angels, Madonnas, and crucifixions floating in an ethereal gold never-never land.

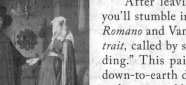

After leaving this gold-leaf peace, you'll stumble into Uccello's *Battle of San Romano* and Van Eyck's *The Arnolfini Portrait*, called by some "The Shotgun Wedding." This painting—a masterpiece of down-to-earth details—was once thought to depict a wedding ceremony forced by the lady's swelling belly. Today it's understood as a portrait of a solemn, well-dressed, well-heeled couple, the Arnolfinis of Bruges, Belgium (she likely was not pregnant—the fashion of the day was to gather up the folds of one's extremely full-skirted dress).

Renaissance: In painting, the Renaissance meant realism. Artists rediscovered the beauty of nature and the human body, expressing the optimism and confidence of this new age. Look for Botticelli's *Venus and Mars*, Michelangelo's *The Entombment*, Raphael's *Pope Julius II*, and Leonardo's *The Virgin of the Rocks*.

Hans Holbein the Younger's *The Ambassadors* depicts two well-dressed, suave men flanking a shelf full of books, globes, navigational tools, and musical instruments—objects that symbolize the secular knowledge of the Renaissance. So what's with the gray, slanting blob at the bottom? If you view the blob from the right-hand edge of the painting (get real close, right up to the frame), the blob suddenly becomes...a skull, a reminder that—despite the fine clothes, proud poses, and worldly knowledge—we will all die.

In *The Origin of the Milky Way* by Venetian Renaissance painter Tintoretto, the god Jupiter places his illegitimate son, baby Hercules, at his wife's breast. Juno says, "Wait a minute. That's not my baby!" Her milk spurts upward, becoming the Milky Way.

Northern Protestant: Greek gods and Virgin Marys are out, and home-town folks and hometown places are in. Highlights include Vermeer's *A Young Woman Standing at a Virginal* and Rembrandt's *Belshazzar's Feast*.

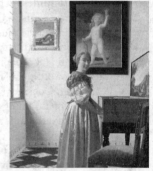

Rembrandt painted his *Self-Portrait at the Age of 63* in the year he would die. He was bankrupt, his mistress had just passed away, and he had also buried several of his children. We see a disillusioned, well-worn, but proud old genius.

Baroque: The museum's outstanding Baroque collection includes Van Dyck's *Equestrian Portrait of Charles I* and Caravaggio's *The Supper at Emmaus*. In Velázquez's *The Rokeby Venus*, Venus lounges diagonally across the canvas, admiring herself, with flaring red, white, and gray fabrics to highlight her rosy white skin and inflame our passion. This work by the king's personal court painter is a rare Spanish nude from that ultra-Catholic country.

British Romantics: The reserved British were more comfortable cavorting with nature than with the lofty gods, as seen in Constable's *The Hay Wain* and Turner's *The Fighting Téméraire*. Turner's messy, colorful style influenced the Impressionists and gives us our first glimpse into the modern art world.

Impressionism: At the end of the 19th century, a new breed of artists burst out of the stuffy confines of the studio. They donned scarves and berets and set up their canvases in farmers' fields or carried their notebooks into crowded cafés, dashing off quick sketches in order to catch a momentary...impression. Check out Impressionist and Post-Impressionist masterpieces such as Monet's *Gare St. Lazare* and *The Water-Lily Pond*, Renoir's *The Skiff*, Seurat's *Bathers at Asnières*, and Van Gogh's *Sunflowers*.

Cézanne's *Bathers* are arranged in strict triangles. Cézanne uses the Impressionist technique of building a figure with dabs of paint (though his "dabs" are often larger-sized "cube" shapes) to make solid 3-D geometrical figures in the style of the Renaissance. In the process, his cube shapes helped inspire a radical new style—Cubism—bringing art into the 20th century.

▲▲National Portrait Gallery

Put off by halls of 19th-century characters who meant nothing to me, I used to call this "as interesting as someone else's year-book." But a selective walk through this 500-year-long *Who's Who* of British history is quick and free, and puts faces on the story of England.

Some highlights: Henry VIII and wives; portraits of the "Virgin Queen" Elizabeth I, Sir Francis Drake, and Sir Walter Raleigh; the only real-life portrait of William Shakespeare; Oliver Cromwell and Charles I with his head on; portraits by Gainsborough and Reynolds; the Romantics (William Blake, Lord Byron, William Wordsworth, and company); Queen Victoria and her era; and the present royal family, including the late Princess Diana.

The collection is well-described, not huge, and in historical sequence, from the 16th century on the second floor to today's royal family on the ground floor.

Cost and Hours: Free, but suggested donation of £5, special exhibits extra; daily 10:00-18:00, Thu-Fri until 21:00, first and second floors open Mon at 11:00, last entry to special exhibits one hour before closing; audioguide-£3, floor plan-£1; entry 100 yards off Trafalgar Square (around the corner from National Gallery, opposite Church of St. Martin-in-the-Fields), Tube: Charing Cross or Leicester Square, tel. 020/7306-0055, recorded info tel. 020/7312-2463, www.npg.org.uk.

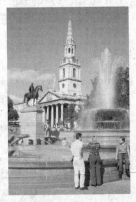

▲St. Martin-in-the-Fields

The church, built in the 1720s with a Gothic spire atop a Greek-type temple, is an oasis of peace on wild and noisy Trafalgar Square. St. Martin cared for the poor. "In the fields" was where the first church stood on this spot (in the 13th century), between Westminster and The City. Stepping inside, you still feel a compassion for the needs of the people in this neighborhood—the church serves the homeless and houses a Chinese community center. The modern east window—with grillwork bent into the shape of a warped cross—was installed in 2008 to replace one damaged in World War II.

A freestanding glass pavilion to the left of the church serves as the entrance to the church's underground areas. There you'll find the concert ticket office, a gift shop, brass-rubbing center, and the recommended support-the-church Café in the Crypt.

Cost and Hours: Free, but donations welcome; hours vary but generally Mon-Fri 8:30-13:00 & 14:00-18:00, Sat 9:30-18:00, Sun 15:30-17:00; £3.50 audioguide at shop downstairs, Tube: Charing Cross, tel. 020/7766-1100, www.smitf.org.

Music: The church is famous for its concerts. Consider a free lunchtime concert (suggested £3 donation; Mon, Tue, and Fri at 13:00).

THE WEST END AND NEARBY

▲Piccadilly Circus

Although this square is slathered with neon billboards and tacky attractions (think of it as the Times Square of London), the surrounding streets are packed with great shopping opportunities and swimming with youth on the rampage.

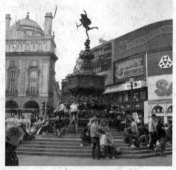

Nearby Shaftesbury Avenue and Leicester Square teem with fun-seekers, theaters, Chinese restaurants, and street singers. To the northeast is London's Chinatown and, beyond that, the funky Soho neighborhood (described next). And curling to the northwest from Piccadilly Circus is genteel Regent Street, lined with exclusive shops.

▲Soho

North of Piccadilly, seedy Soho has become trendy—with many recommended restaurants—and is well worth a gawk. It's the epicenter of London's thriving, colorful youth scene, a fun and funky *Sesame Street* of urban diversity. Although gentrifying, Soho is also London's red light district (especially near Brewer and Berwick Streets), and a center of its gay community.

▲▲Covent Garden

The centerpiece of this boutique-ish shopping district is an iron-and-glass arcade. The "Actors' Church" of St. Paul and the Royal

Opera House border the square, and theaters are nearby. The area is a people-watcher's delight, with cigarette eaters, Punch-and-Judy acts, food that's good for you (but not your wallet), trendy crafts, and row after row of boutique shops and market stalls. Better Covent Garden lunch deals can be found by walking a block or two away from the eye of this touristic hurricane (check out the places north of the Tube station, along Endell and Neal Streets).

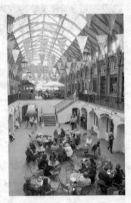

BUCKINGHAM PALACE AREA

While it's possible to enter various sights related to the palace, on a brief visit I'd just take a quick look at its famous facade. The Changing of the Guard (described below) might entice you, but planning your day around it leaves little time for other options; because you'll need to fight the crowds to secure a suitable vantage point, this is more time-consuming than it sounds.

▲▲Changing of the Guard at Buckingham Palace

This is the spectacle every visitor to London has to see at least once: stone-faced, red-coated (or in winter, gray-coated), bearskin-hatted guards changing posts with much fanfare, in an hour-long ceremony accompanied by a brass band.

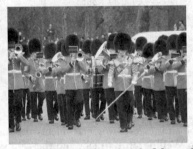

It's 11:00 at Buckingham Palace, and the on-duty guards (the "Queen's Guard") are ready to finish their shift. Nearby at St. James's Palace (a half-mile northeast), a second set of guards is also ready for a break. Meanwhile, fresh replacement guards (the "New Guard") gather for a review and inspection at Wellington Barracks, 500 yards east of the palace (on Birdcage Walk).

At 11:15, the tired St. James's guards head out to the Mall, and then take a right turn for Buckingham Palace. At 11:30, the replacement troops, led by the band, also head for Buckingham Palace. Meanwhile, a fourth group—the Horse Guard—passes by along the Mall on its way back to Hyde Park Corner from its own changing-of-the-guard ceremony on Whitehall (which just took place at Horse Guards Parade at 11:00, or 10:00 on Sun).

At 11:45, the tired and fresh guards converge on Buckingham Palace in a perfect storm of red-coat pageantry. Everyone parades

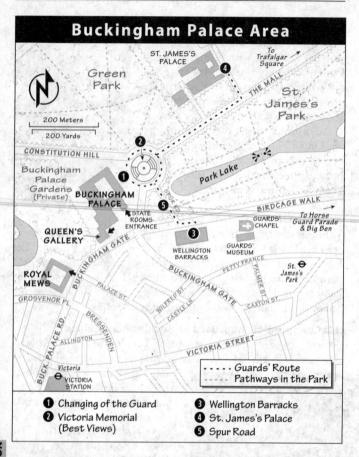

Buckingham Palace Area

ST. JAMES'S PALACE

To Trafalgar Square

Green Park

THE MALL

St. James's Park

200 Meters
200 Yards

CONSTITUTION HILL

Buckingham Palace Gardens (Private)

BUCKINGHAM PALACE

❷

❶

Park Lake

SPUR RD.

❺

BIRDCAGE WALK

STATE ROOMS ENTRANCE

GUARDS' CHAPEL

To Horse Guard Parade & Big Ben

QUEEN'S GALLERY

❸

WELLINGTON BARRACKS

GUARDS' MUSEUM

St. James's Park

BUCKINGHAM GATE

ROYAL MEWS

PETTY FRANCE

PALMER ST.

BUCKINGHAM GATE

PALACE ST.

WILFRED ST.

CASTLE LN.

CAXTON ST.

GROSVENOR PL.

BRESSENDEN

ALLINGTON

BUCK. PALACE RD.

VICTORIA STREET

Victoria

VICTORIA STATION

- - - - - Guards' Route
- - - - - Pathways in the Park

❶ Changing of the Guard
❷ Victoria Memorial (Best Views)
❸ Wellington Barracks
❹ St. James's Palace
❺ Spur Road

around, the guard changes (passing the regimental flag, or "colour") with much shouting, the band plays a happy little concert, and then they march out. At noon, two bands escort two detachments of guards away: the tired guards to Wellington Barracks and the fresh guards to St. James's Palace. As the fresh guards set up at St. James's Palace and the tired ones dress down at the barracks, the tourists disperse.

Cost and Hours: Free, daily May-July at 11:30, every other day Aug-April, no ceremony in very wet weather; exact schedule subject to change—call 020/7766-7300 for the day's plan, or check www.royal.gov.uk (search "Changing the Guard"); Buckingham Palace, Tube: Victoria, St. James's Park, or Green Park. Or hop into a big black taxi and say, "Buck House, please."

Sightseeing Strategies: Most tourists just show up and get lost in the crowds, but those who know the drill will enjoy the event more. The action takes place in stages over the course of an hour, at several different locations. The main event is in the fore-court right in front of Buckingham Palace (between Buckingham Palace and the fence) from 11:30 to 12:00. To see it close up, you'll need to get here no later than 10:30 to get a place front and center, next to the fence.

But there's plenty of pageantry elsewhere. Get out your map and strategize. You could see the guards mobilizing at Wellington Barracks or St. James's Palace (11:00-11:15). Or watch them parade with bands down The Mall and Spur Road (11:15-11:30). After the ceremony at Buckingham Palace is over (and many tourists have gotten bored and gone home), the parades march back along those same streets (12:10).

Pick one event and find a good, unobstructed place from which to view it. The key is to get either right up front along the road or fence, or find some raised elevation to stand or sit on—a balustrade or a curb—so you can see over people's heads.

If you get there too late to score a premium spot right along the fence, head for the high ground on the circular Victoria Memorial, which provides the best overall view (come before 11:00 to get a place).

You can also stroll down to St. James's Palace and wait near the corner for a great photo-op. At about 12:15, the parade marches up The Mall to the palace and performs a smaller changing ceremony—with almost no crowds. Afterward, stroll through nearby St. James's Park.

NORTH LONDON
▲▲▲British Museum

Simply put, this is the greatest chronicle of civilization...any-where. A visit here is like taking a long hike through *Encyclopedia Britannica* National Park. The

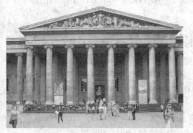

vast British Museum wraps around its Great Court (the huge entrance hall), with the most popular sections filling the ground floor: Egyptian, Assyrian, and ancient Greek, with the famous frieze sculptures from the Parthenon in Athens. The museum's stately Reading Room—famous as the place where Karl Marx hung out while formulating his ideas on communism and writing *Das Kapital*—sometimes hosts special exhibits.

Cost and Hours: Free but a £5 donation requested, special exhibits usually extra (and with timed ticket); daily 10:00-17:30, Fri until 20:30 (selected galleries only), least crowded weekday late afternoons; Great Russell Street, Tube: Tottenham Court Road.

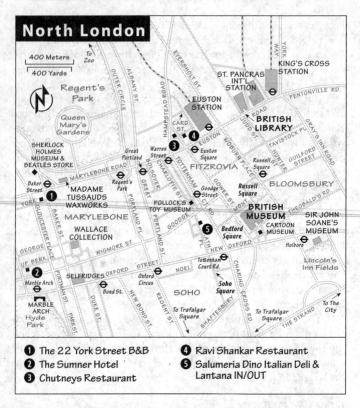

North London

400 Meters
400 Yards

To Zoo

Regent's Park

Queen Mary's Gardens

SHERLOCK HOLMES MUSEUM & BEATLES STORE

Baker Street

MADAME TUSSAUDS WAXWORKS

MARYLEBONE

WALLACE COLLECTION

Marble Arch

MARBLE ARCH Hyde Park

SELFRIDGES

Oxford Circus

Bond St.

SOHO

To Trafalgar Square

KING'S CROSS STATION

ST. PANCRAS INT'L STATION

EUSTON STATION

BRITISH LIBRARY

FITZROVIA

Euston Square

Russell Square

BLOOMSBURY

Goodge Street

Russell Square

POLLOCK'S TOY MUSEUM

Bedford Square

BRITISH MUSEUM

CARTOON MUSEUM

SIR JOHN SOANE'S MUSEUM

Holborn

Lincoln's Inn Fields

Tottenham Court Rd.

Soho Square

To Trafalgar Square

To The City

❶ The 22 York Street B&B
❷ The Sumner Hotel
❸ Chutneys Restaurant
❹ Ravi Shankar Restaurant
❺ Salumeria Dino Italian Deli & Lantana IN/OUT

Information: General info tel. 020/7323-8299, ticket desk tel. 020/7323-8181, www.britishmuseum.org. Information desks provide a basic map (£1 donation), but it's not essential for this tour. The *Visitor's Guide* (£3.50) offers 15 different tours and skimpy text.

Tours: Free 30-minute **eyeOpener tours** are led by volunteers, who focus on select rooms (daily 11:00-15:45, generally every 15 minutes). Free 45-minute **gallery talks** on specific subjects are offered Tue-Sat at 13:15; a free 20-minute highlights tour is available on Friday evening. The £5 **multimedia guide** offers dial-up audio commentary and video on 200 objects, as well as several theme tours (must leave photo ID). You can download a free Rick Steves **audio tour** of the museum's highlights (see page 50).

❍ Self-Guided Tour: From the Great Court, doorways lead to all wings. To the left are the exhibits on Egypt, Assyria, and Greece—our tour.

Egypt: Start with the Egyptian section. Egypt was one of the world's first "civilizations"—a group of people with a government, religion, art, free time, and a written language. The Egypt we think of—pyramids, mummies, pharaohs, and guys who walk funny—lasted from 3000 to 1000 B.C. with hardly any change in the government, religion, or arts. Imagine two millennia of Nixon.

The first thing you'll see in the Egypt section is the **Rosetta Stone.** When this rock was unearthed in the Egyptian desert in 1799, it was a sensation in Europe. This black slab, dating from 196 B.C., caused a quantum leap in the study of ancient history. The Rosetta Stone contains a single inscription repeated in three languages. The bottom third is plain old Greek, while the middle is medieval Egyptian. By comparing the two known languages with the one they didn't know, translators figured out the hieroglyphics. Finally, Egyptian writing could be decoded.

Next, wander past the many **statues,** including a seven-ton statue of Ramesses II with the traditional features of a pharaoh—goatee, cloth headdress, and cobra diadem on his forehead. When Moses told the king of Egypt, "Let my people go!" this was the stony-faced look he got. You'll also see the Egyptian gods as animals—these include Amun, king of the gods, as a ram, and Horus, the god of the living, as a falcon.

At the end of the hall, climb the stairs to **mummy** land (or use the elevator). To mummify a body, you first disembowel it (but leave the heart inside), then pack the cavities with pitch, and dry it with natron, a natural form of sodium carbonate (and, I believe, the active ingredient in Twinkies). Then carefully bandage it head to toe with hundreds of yards of linen strips. Let it sit 2,000 years, and...*voilà!*

The mummy was placed in a wooden coffin, which was put in a stone coffin, which was placed in a tomb. The result is that we now have Egyptian bodies that are as well preserved as Liza Minnelli.

Many of the mummies here are from the time of the Roman occupation, when fine memorial portraits painted in wax became popular. X-ray photos in the display cases tell us more about these people.

Assyria: Long before Saddam Hussein, Iraq was home to other palace-building, iron-fisted rulers—the Assyrians, who conquered their southern neighbors and dominated the Middle East for 300 years (c. 900-600 B.C.). Their strength came from a superb army (chariots, mounted cavalry, and siege engines), a policy of terrorism against enemies ("I tied their heads to tree trunks all around the city," reads a royal inscription), ethnic cleansing and mass deportations of the vanquished, and efficient administration (roads and express postal service). They have been called the "Romans of the East."

Standing guard over the Assyrian exhibit halls are two human-headed winged **lions.** These stone lions guarded an

Assyrian palace (11th-8th century B.C.). With the strength of a lion, the wings of an eagle, the brain of a man, and the beard of ZZ Top, they protected the king from evil spirits and scared the heck out of foreign ambassadors and left-wing newspaper reporters. (What has five legs and flies? Take a close look. These quintupeds, which appear complete from both the front and the side, could guard both directions at once.)

Carved into the stone between the bearded lions' loins, you can see one of civilization's most impressive achievements—writing. This wedge-shaped **(cuneiform)** script is the world's first written language, invented 5,000 years ago by the Sumerians (of southern Iraq) and passed down to their less-civilized descendants, the Assyrians.

The **Nimrud Gallery** is a mini version of the throne room and royal apartments of King Ashurnasirpal II's Northwest Palace at Nimrud (9th century B.C.). It's filled with royal propaganda reliefs, 30-ton marble bulls, and panels depicting wounded lions (lion-hunting was Assyria's sport of kings).

Greece: During their civilization's Golden Age (500-430 B.C.), the ancient Greeks set the tone for all of Western civilization to follow. Democracy, theater, literature, mathematics, philosophy, science, gyros, art, and architecture, as we know them, were virtually all invented by a single generation of Greeks in a small town of maybe 80,000 citizens.

Your walk through Greek art history starts with **pottery**, usually painted red and black and a popular export product for the sea-trading Greeks. The earliest featured geometric patterns (8th century B.C.), then a painted black silhouette on the natural orange clay, then a red figure on a black background. Later, painted vases show a culture really into partying.

The highlight is the **Parthenon Sculptures,** which graced the temple dedicated to Athena, goddess of wisdom and the patroness of Athens—the crowning glory of an enormous urban-renewal plan during Greece's Golden Age. The sculptures are also called the Elgin Marbles, named for the shrewd British ambassador who had his men hammer, chisel, and saw them off the Parthenon in the early 1800s. Though the Greek government complains about losing its marbles, the Brits feel they rescued and preserved the impressive sculptures (from about 450 B.C.). The often-bitter controversy continues.

The marble panels you see lining the walls of this large hall are part of the frieze that originally ran around the exterior of the Parthenon, under the eaves. The statues at either end of the hall once filled the Parthenon's triangular-shaped pediments, and showed the birth of Athena. The relief panels known as metopes tell the story of the struggle between human civilization and

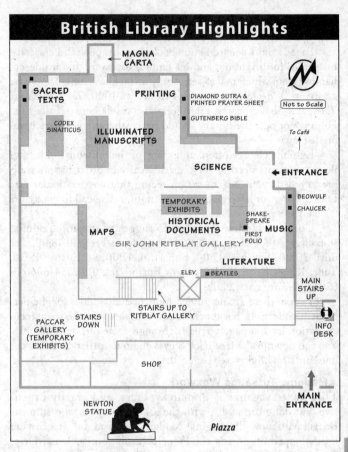

British Library Highlights

MAGNA CARTA

SACRED TEXTS

PRINTING

DIAMOND SUTRA & PRINTED PRAYER SHEET

GUTENBERG BIBLE

Not to Scale

CODEX SINAITICUS

ILLUMINATED MANUSCRIPTS

To Café

SCIENCE

ENTRANCE

BEOWULF

CHAUCER

TEMPORARY EXHIBITS

SHAKE-SPEARE

HISTORICAL DOCUMENTS

MUSIC

MAPS

FIRST FOLIO

SIR JOHN RITBLAT GALLERY

LITERATURE

ELEV.

BEATLES

MAIN STAIRS UP

STAIRS UP TO RITBLAT GALLERY

INFO DESK

PACCAR GALLERY (TEMPORARY EXHIBITS)

STAIRS DOWN

SHOP

MAIN ENTRANCE

NEWTON STATUE

Piazza

animal-like barbarism.

The Rest of the Museum: Be sure to venture upstairs to see artifacts from **Roman Britain** that surpass anything you'll see at Hadrian's Wall or elsewhere in the country. Also look for the Sutton Hoo Ship Burial artifacts from a seventh-century royal burial on the east coast of England (Room 41). A rare Michelangelo cartoon (preliminary sketch) is in Room 90 (Level 4).

Other Sights in North London
▲▲▲British Library

The British Empire built its greatest monuments out of paper; it's through literature that England made her most lasting and significant contribution to civilization and the arts. Here, in just two rooms, are the literary treasures of Western civilization, from early Bibles, to the Magna Carta, to Shakespeare's *Hamlet*, to Lewis Carroll's *Alice's Adventures in Wonderland*. You'll see the

Lindisfarne Gospels transcribed on an illuminated manuscript, as well as Beatles lyrics scrawled on the back of a greeting card.

Pages from Leonardo's notebook show his powerful curiosity, his genius for invention, and his famous backward and inside-out handwriting, which makes sense only if you know Italian and have a mirror. A *Beowulf* manuscript from A.D. 1000, *The Canterbury Tales*, and Shakespeare's First Folio also reside here. (If the First Folio is not out, the library should have other Shakespeare items on display.)

Exhibits change often, and many of the museum's old, fragile manuscripts need to "rest" periodically in order to stay well-preserved. If your heart's set on seeing that one particular rare Dickens book or letter penned by Gandhi, call ahead to make sure it's on display.

Cost and Hours: Free, but £5 suggested donation, admission charged for some special exhibits; Mon-Fri 9:30-18:00, Tue until 20:00, Sat 9:30-17:00, Sun 11:00-17:00; 96 Euston Road, Tube: King's Cross St. Pancras or Euston, tel. 019/3754-6060 or 020/7412-7676, www.bl.uk.

Tours: There are no guided tours or audioguides for the permanent collection, but touch-screen computers in the permanent collection let you page virtually through some of the rare books. You can download a free Rick Steves audio tour that describes the museum's highlights (see page 50).

▲Madame Tussauds Waxworks

This waxtravaganza is gimmicky, crass, and crazily expensive, but dang fun...a hit with the kind of tourists who skip the British Museum. The original Madame Tussaud did wax casts of heads lopped off during the French Revolution (such as Marie-Antoinette's). She took her show on the road and ended up in London in 1835. In addition to posing with all the eerily realistic wax dummies—from Barack Obama to the Beatles—you'll have the chance to tour a hokey haunted-house exhibit; learn how they created this waxy army; hop on a people-mover and cruise through a kid-pleasing "Spirit of London" time trip; and visit with Spider-Man, the Hulk, and other Marvel superheroes. A nine-minute "4-D" show features a 3-D movie heightened by wind, "back ticklers," and other special effects.

Cost: £30, up to 25 percent discount and shorter lines if you buy tickets on their website (also consider combo-deal with London Eye; see page 1009); often even bigger discount—up to 50 percent—if you get "Late Saver" tickets at the door after 17:30, but be aware that some experiences close at 18:00. Kids also get a discount of about £4, and those under 5 are free.

Hours: Mid-July-Aug and school holidays daily 9:00-19:00;

Sept-mid-July Mon-Fri 9:30-17:30, Sat-Sun 9:00-18:00; these are last entry times—place stays open roughly two hours later, Marylebone Road, Tube: Baker Street, tel. 0871-894-3000, www.madametussauds.com.

Crowd-Beating Tips: This popular attraction can be swamped with people. To avoid the ticket line, buy an Online Saver and reserve a time slot at least a day in advance. If you wait to buy tickets at the attraction, you'll discover that the ticket-buying line is often halfway down the block, and once inside it continues to twist endlessly (believe the posted signs about the wait—an hour or more is not unusual at busy times). If you buy your tickets at the door, try to arrive after 15:00—a smart move even with advance tickets, as the crowds inside thin out later in the day.

▲Sir John Soane's Museum

Architects love this quirky place, as do fans of interior decor, eclectic knickknacks, and Back Door sights. Tour this furnished home on a bird-chirping square and see 19th-century chairs, lamps, wood-paneled nooks and crannies, sculptures, and stained-glass skylights. (Some sections may be closed for restoration through 2015, but the main part of the house will be open.) As professor of architecture at the Royal Academy, Soane created his home to be a place of learning, cramming it floor to ceiling with ancient relics, curios, and famous paintings, including several excellent Canalettos and Hogarth's series on *The Rake's Progress* (which is hidden behind a panel in the Picture Room and opened randomly at the museum's discretion, usually twice an hour). In 1833, just before his death, Soane established his house as a museum, stipulating that it be kept as nearly as possible in the state he left it. If he visited today, he'd be entirely satisfied by the diligence with which the staff safeguards his treasures. You'll leave wishing you'd known the man.

Cost and Hours: Free, but donations much appreciated; Tue-Sat 10:00-17:00, open and candlelit the first Tue of the month 18:00-21:00, closed Sun-Mon, last entry 30 minutes before closing, long entry lines on Sat; guidebook-£5, guided tour-£10—includes guidebook—Tue and Fri 11:30, Wed and Thu 3:30; 13 Lincoln's Inn Fields, quarter-mile southeast of British Museum, Tube: Holborn, tel. 020/7405-2107, www.soane.org.

THE CITY

When Londoners say "The City," they mean the one-square-mile business center in East London that 2,000 years ago was Roman Londinium. The outline of the Roman city walls can still be seen in the arc of roads from Blackfriars Bridge to Tower Bridge. Within The City are 23 churches designed by Sir Christopher

Wren, mostly just ornamentation around St. Paul's Cathedral. Today, while home to only 7,000 residents, The City thrives with nearly 300,000 office workers coming and going daily. It's a fascinating district to wander on weekdays, but since almost nobody actually lives there, it's dull in the evenings and on Saturday and Sunday.

For a walking tour, you can download a free Rick Steves **audio tour** of The City, which peels back the many layers of history in this oldest part of London (see page 50). For a general map of the area, see page 970.

▲▲▲St. Paul's Cathedral

Sir Christopher Wren's most famous church is the great St. Paul's, its elaborate interior capped by a 365-foot dome. There's been a church on this spot since 604.

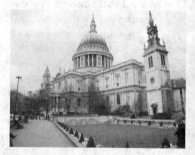

After the Great Fire of 1666 destroyed the old cathedral, Wren created this Baroque masterpiece. Since World War II, St. Paul's has been Britain's symbol of resilience. Despite 57 nights of bombing, the Nazis failed to destroy the cathedral, thanks to St. Paul's volunteer fire watchmen, who stayed on the dome.

Cost and Hours: £16, includes church entry, dome climb, crypt, tour, and audioguide; Mon-Sat 8:30-16:30, last entry for sightseeing 16:00 (dome opens at 9:30, last entry at 16:15), closed Sun except for worship; sometimes closed for special events, no photos, café and restaurant in crypt, Tube: St. Paul's, recorded info tel. 020/7236-4128, reception tel. 020/7246-8350, www.stpauls.co.uk.

Music and Church Services: If interested, check the website for worship times the day of your visit. Communion is generally Mon-Sat at 8:00 and 12:30. On Sunday, services are held at 8:00, 10:15 (Matins), 11:30 (sung Eucharist), 15:15 (evensong), and 18:00. The rest of the week, evensong is at 17:00 Tue-Sat (not Mon). If you come 20 minutes early for evensong worship (under the dome), you may be able to grab a big wooden stall in the choir, next to the singers. On some Sundays, there's a free organ recital at 16:45.

Tours: Guided 1.5-hour tours are offered Mon-Sat at 10:00, 11:00, 13:00, and 14:00 (confirm schedule at church or call 020/7246-8357). Free 20-minute introductory talks are offered throughout the day. The audioguide (included in admission) contains video clips that show the church in action. You can also download a free Rick Steves audio tour of St. Paul's (see page 50).

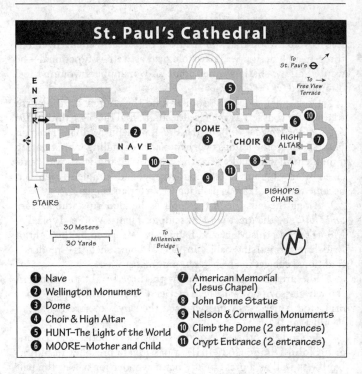

St. Paul's Cathedral

To St. Paul's ⊖

To → Free View Terrace

E N T E R →

⑤

⑪

⑥ ⑩

DOME ③

① ② **N A V E** ⑩

CHOIR ④ **HIGH ALTAR** ⑦

⑧

⑨ ⑪

STAIRS

BISHOP'S CHAIR

30 Meters
30 Yards

To Millennium Bridge

Ⓝ

① Nave
② Wellington Monument
③ Dome
④ Choir & High Altar
⑤ HUNT–The Light of the World
⑥ MOORE–Mother and Child

⑦ American Memorial (Jesus Chapel)
⑧ John Donne Statue
⑨ Nelson & Cornwallis Monuments
⑩ Climb the Dome (2 entrances)
⑪ Crypt Entrance (2 entrances)

❂ Self-Guided Tour: Even now, as skyscrapers encroach, the 365-foot-high dome of St. Paul's rises majestically above the rooftops of the neighborhood. The tall dome is set on classical columns, capped with a lantern, topped by a six-foot ball, and iced with a cross. As the first Anglican cathedral built in London after the Reformation, it is Baroque: St. Peter's in Rome filtered through clear-eyed English reason. Often the site of historic funerals (Queen Victoria and Winston Churchill), St. Paul's most famous ceremony was a wedding—when Prince Charles married Lady Diana Spencer in 1981.

Go inside. This big church feels big. At 515 feet long and 250 feet wide, it's Europe's fourth largest, after Rome (St. Peter's), Sevilla, and Milan. The spaciousness is accentuated by the relative lack of decoration. The simple, cream-colored ceiling and the clear glass in the windows light everything evenly. Wren wanted this: a simple, open church with nothing to hide. Unfortunately, only this entrance area keeps his original vision—the rest was encrusted with 19th-century Victorian ornamentation.

The **dome** you see from here, painted with scenes from the life of St. Paul, is only the innermost of three. From the painted interior of the first dome, look up through the opening to see the light-filled lantern of the second dome. Finally, the whole thing is covered on the outside by the third and final dome, the shell of lead-covered wood that you see from the street. Wren's ingenious three-in-one design was psychological as well as functional—he wanted a low, shallow inner dome so worshippers wouldn't feel diminished.

Do a quick clockwise spin around the church. In the north transept (to your left as you face the altar), find the big painting *The Light of the World* (1904), by the Pre-Raphaelite William Holman Hunt. Inspired by Hunt's own experience of finding Christ during a moment of spiritual crisis, the crowd-pleasing work was criticized by art highbrows for being "syrupy" and "simple"—even as it became the most famous painting in Victorian England.

Along the left side of the choir is the modern statue *Mother and Child*, by the great modern sculptor Henry Moore. Typical of Moore's work, this Mary and Baby Jesus—inspired by the sight of British moms nursing babies in WWII bomb shelters—renders a traditional subject in an abstract, minimalist way.

The area behind the altar, with three bright and modern stained-glass windows, is the **American Memorial Chapel**—honoring the Americans who sacrificed their lives to save Britain in World War II.

Around the other side of the choir is a shrouded statue honoring **John Donne** (1621-1631), a passionate preacher in old St. Paul's, as well as a great poet ("never wonder for whom the bell tolls—it tolls for thee"). In the south transept are monuments to military greats **Horatio Nelson,** who fought Napoleon, and **Charles Cornwallis,** who was finished off by George Washington at Yorktown.

Climbing the Dome: The 528-step climb is worthwhile, and each level (or gallery) offers something different. First you get to the Whispering Gallery (257 steps, with views of the church interior). Whisper sweet nothings into the wall, and your partner (and anyone else) standing far away can hear you. After another set of stairs, you're at the Stone Gallery, with views of London. Finally a long, tight, metal staircase takes you to the very top of the cupola, the Golden Gallery. Once at the top, you emerge to stunning unobstructed views of the city.

The Crypt: The crypt is a world of historic bones and interesting cathedral models. Many legends are buried here—Horatio Nelson, who wore down Napoleon; the Duke of Wellington, who finished Napoleon off; and even Wren himself. Wren's actual tomb is marked by a simple black slab with no statue, though he considered the church itself to be his legacy. Back up in the nave, on the floor directly under the dome, is Christopher Wren's name and epitaph (written in Latin): "Reader, if you seek his monument, look around you."

▲Museum of London

This museum tells the fascinating story of London, taking you on a walk from its pre-Roman beginnings to the present. It features London's distinguished citizens through history—from Neanderthals, to Romans, to Elizabethans, to Victorians, to Mods, to today. The displays are chronological, spacious, and informative without being overwhelming. Scale models and costumes help you visualize everyday life in the city at different periods. There are enough whiz-bang multimedia displays (including the Plague and the Great Fire) to spice up otherwise humdrum artifacts. This regular stop for the local school kids gives the best overview of London history in town.

Cost and Hours: Free, daily 10:00-18:00, galleries shut down 30 minutes before closing, see the day's events board for special talks and tours, café, £1 lockers, 150 London Wall at Aldersgate Street, Tube: Barbican or St. Paul's plus a five-minute walk, tel. 020/7001-9844, www.museumoflondon.org.uk.

The Monument

Wren's 202-foot-tall tribute to London's 1666 Great Fire was recently restored. Climb the 331 steps inside the column for a monumental view of The City.

Cost and Hours: £3, £10.50 combo-ticket with Tower Bridge, daily 9:30-18:00, until 17:30 Oct-March, last entry 30 minutes before closing, junction of Monument Street and Fish Street Hill, Tube: Monument, tel. 020/7626-2717, www.themonument.info.

▲▲▲Tower of London

The Tower has served as a castle in wartime, a king's residence in peacetime, and, most notoriously, as the prison and execution site

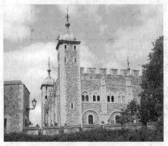

of rebels. You can see the crown jewels, take a witty Beefeater tour, and ponder the executioner's block that dispensed with Anne Boleyn, Sir Thomas More, and troublesome heirs to the throne.

Cost and Hours: £22, family-£57 (prices include a 10 percent optional donation); March-Oct Tue-Sat 9:00-17:30, Sun-Mon 10:00-17:30; Nov-Feb Tue-Sat 9:00-16:30, Sun-Mon 10:00-16:30; last entry 30 minutes before closing; free Beefeater tours available, skippable audioguide-£4, Tube: Tower Hill, switchboard tel. 0844-482-7777, www.hrp.org.uk.

Advance Tickets: To avoid the long ticket-buying lines at the Tower, buy your ticket at the Trader's Gate gift shop, located down the steps from the Tower Hill Tube stop (tickets here are

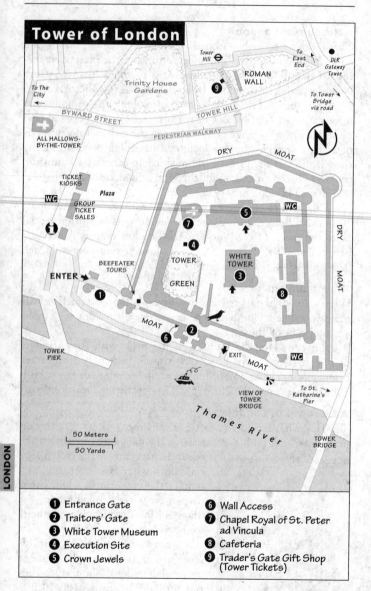

Tower of London

- Tower Hill
- Trinity House Gardens
- ROMAN WALL
- To East End
- DLR Gateway Tower
- To The City
- To Tower Bridge via road
- BYWARD STREET
- TOWER HILL
- PEDESTRIAN WALKWAY
- ALL HALLOWS-BY-THE-TOWER
- DRY MOAT
- TICKET KIOSKS
- Plaza
- WC
- GROUP TICKET SALES
- BEEFEATER TOURS
- ENTER
- TOWER GREEN
- WHITE TOWER
- DRY MOAT
- MOAT
- EXIT MOAT
- TOWER PIER
- VIEW OF TOWER BRIDGE
- To St. Katharine's Pier
- Thames River
- TOWER BRIDGE
- 50 Meters
- 50 Yards

1 Entrance Gate
2 Traitors' Gate
3 White Tower Museum
4 Execution Site
5 Crown Jewels
6 Wall Access
7 Chapel Royal of St. Peter ad Vincula
8 Cafeteria
9 Trader's Gate Gift Shop (Tower Tickets)

LONDON

generally slightly cheaper than at the gate). Tickets are also sold at various locations (such as travel agencies) throughout London. You can also buy tickets, with credit card only, at the Tower Welcome Centre to the left of the normal ticket lines—though on busy days, it can be crowded here as well. It's easy to book online (www.hrp.org.uk, £1 discount, no fee) or by phone (tel. 0844-482-7799 within UK or tel. 011-44-20-3166-6000 from the US; £2 fee), then pick up your tickets at the Tower.

More Crowd-Beating Tips: It's most crowded in summer, on weekends (especially Sundays), and during school holidays. Any time of year, the line for the crown jewels—the best on earth—can be just as long as the line for tickets. For fewer crowds, arrive before 10:00 and go straight for the jewels. Alternatively, arrive in the afternoon, tour the rest of the Tower first, and see the jewels an hour before closing time, when crowds die down.

Yeoman Warder (Beefeater) Tours: Today, while the Tower's military purpose is history, it's still home to the Beefeaters—the 35 Yeoman Warders and their families. (The original duty of the Yeoman Warders was to guard the Tower, its prisoners, and the jewels.) The free, worthwhile, one-hour Beefeater tours leave every 30 minutes from inside the gate (first tour Tue-Sat at 10:00, Sun-Mon at 10:30, last one at 15:30—or 14:30 in Nov-Feb). The boisterous Beefeaters are great entertainers, whose historical talks include lots of bloody anecdotes and corny jokes.

Sunday Worship: On Sunday morning, visitors are welcome on the grounds for free to worship in the Chapel Royal of St. Peter ad Vincula. You get in without the lines, but you can only see the chapel—no sightseeing (9:15 Communion or 11:00 service with fine choral music, meet at west gate 30 minutes early, dress for church, may be closed for ceremonies—call ahead; phone number listed earlier).

Visiting the Tower: William I, still getting used to his new title of "the Conqueror," built the stone "White Tower" (1077-1097) to keep the Londoners in line. Standing high above the rest of old London, the White Tower provided a gleaming reminder of the monarch's absolute power over his subjects. If you made the wrong move here, you could be feasting on roast boar in the banqueting hall one night and chained to the walls of the prison the next. The Tower also served as an effective lookout for seeing invaders coming up the Thames.

This square, 90-foot-tall tower was the original structure that gave this castle complex of 20 towers its name. William's successors enlarged the complex to its present 18-acre size. Because of the security it provided, the Tower of London served over the centuries as a royal residence, the Royal Mint, the Royal Jewel House, and, most famously, as the prison and execution site of those who dared oppose the Crown.

You'll find more bloody history per square inch in this original tower of power than anywhere else in Britain. Inside the White Tower is a museum with exhibits re-creating medieval life and chronicling the torture and executions that took place here. In the Royal Armory, you'll see some suits of armor of Henry VIII—slender in his youth (c. 1515), heavy-set by 1540—with his bigger-is-better codpiece. On the top floor, see the Tower's actual execution ax and chopping block.

The actual **execution site,** however, in the middle of the Tower Green, looks just like a lawn. It was here that enemies of the crown would kneel before the king for the final time. With their hands tied behind their backs, they would say a final prayer, then lay their heads on a block, and—*shlit*—the blade would slice through their necks, their heads tumbling to the ground. Tower Green was the most prestigious execution site at the Tower. Henry VIII axed a couple of his ex-wives here (divorced readers can insert their own joke), including Anne Boleyn and his fifth wife, teenage Catherine Howard.

The Tower's hard stone and glittering **crown jewels** represent the ultimate power of the monarch. The Sovereign's Scepter is encrusted with the world's largest cut diamond—the 530-carat Star of Africa, beefy as a quarter-pounder. The Crown of the Queen Mother (Elizabeth II's famous mum, who died in 2002) has the 106-carat Koh-I-Noor diamond glittering on the front (considered unlucky for male rulers, it only adorns the crown of the king's wife). The Imperial State Crown is what the Queen wears for official functions such as the State Opening of Parliament. Among its 3,733 jewels are Queen Elizabeth I's former earrings (the hanging pearls, top center), a stunning 13th-century ruby look-alike in the center, and Edward the Confessor's ring (the blue sapphire on top, in the center of the Maltese cross of diamonds).

The Tower was defended by state-of-the-art **walls** and fortifications in the 13th century. Walking along them offers a good look at the walls, along with a fine view of the famous Tower Bridge, with its twin towers and blue spans.

Nearby: The iconic **Tower Bridge** (often mistakenly called London Bridge) was recently painted and restored. The hydraulically powered drawbridge was built in 1894 to accommodate the growing East End. While fully modern, its design was a retro Neo-Gothic look.

SOUTH BANK

The South Bank of the Thames is a thriving arts and cultural center, tied together by the riverfront Jubilee Walkway.

▲▲London Eye

This giant Ferris wheel, towering above London opposite Big Ben, is one of the world's highest observa-

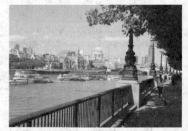

tional wheels and London's answer to the Eiffel Tower. Riding it

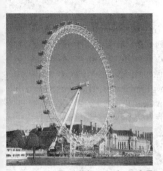 is a memorable experience, even though London doesn't have much of a skyline, and the price is borderline outrageous. Whether you ride or not, the wheel is a sight to behold.

The experience starts with a brief (four-minute) and engaging show combining a 3-D movie with wind and water effects. Then it's time to spin around the Eye. Designed like a giant bicycle wheel, it's a pan-European undertaking: British steel and Dutch engineering, with Czech, German, French, and Italian mechanical parts. It's also very "green," running extremely efficiently and virtually silently. Twenty-five people ride in each of its 32 air-conditioned capsules (representing the boroughs of London) for the 30-minute rotation (you go around only once). From the top of this 443-foot-high wheel—the second-highest public viewpoint in the city—even Big Ben looks small.

Cost: £20, family ticket available, about 10 percent cheaper if bought online. Buy tickets in advance at www.londoneye.com, by calling 0870-500-0600, or in person at the box office (in the corner of the County Hall building nearest the Eye). A combo-ticket that also covers Madame Tussauds Waxworks is cheaper online.

Hours: Daily April-Aug 10:00-21:00, Sept-March 10:00-20:30, these are last-ascent times, open later on weekends, closed Dec 25 and a few days in Jan for annual maintenance, Tube: Waterloo or Westminster. Thames boats come and go from Waterloo Pier at the foot of the wheel.

Crowd-Beating Tips: The London Eye is busiest between 11:00 and 17:00, especially on weekends year-round and every day in July and August. You might have to wait up to 30 minutes to buy your ticket, then another 30-45 minutes to board your capsule—it's best to call ahead or go online to prebook your ticket during these times. To retrieve your ticket at the sight, punch your confirmation code into the machine in the ticket office (or pick it up in the short "Groups and Ticket Collection" line at desk #5). Even if you prereserve, you still have to wait a bit to board the wheel. You can pay an extra £10 for a Fast Track ticket that lets you jump the queue, but it's probably not worth the expense.

By the Eye: The area next to the London Eye has developed a cotton-candy ambience of kitschy, kid-friendly attractions. There's an aquarium, game arcade, and London Film Museum dedicated to movies filmed in London, from *Harry Potter* to *Star Wars* (not to be confused with the far superior British Film Institute, a.k.a. the BFI Southbank, just to the east).

▲▲Imperial War Museum

This impressive museum covers the wars of the last century—from World War I biplanes, to the rise of fascism, to Montgomery's Africa campaign tank, to the Cold War, the Cuban Missile Crisis, the Troubles in Northern Ireland, the wars in Iraq and Afghanistan, and terrorism. Rather than glorify war, the museum encourages an understanding of the history of modern warfare and the wartime experience, including the effect it has on the everyday lives of people back home. The museum's coverage never neglects the human side of one of civilization's more uncivilized, persistent traits.

Cost and Hours: Free, daily 10:00-18:00, special exhibits extra, audioguide-£3.50, guided tours usually Sat-Sun at 11:30 and 13:30—confirm at info desk, Tube: Lambeth North or Elephant and Castle; buses #3, #12, and #159 come here from Westminster area; tel. 020/7416-5000, www.iwm.org.uk.

Visiting the Museum: Allow plenty of time, as this powerful museum—with lots of artifacts and video clips—can be engrossing. The highlights are the new WWI galleries (renovated to commemorate the 100-year anniversary of that conflict) and the WWII area, the "Secret War" section, and the Holocaust exhibit. War wonks love the place, as do general history buffs who enjoy patiently reading displays. For the rest, there are enough interactive experiences and multimedia exhibits and submarines for the kids to climb in to keep it interesting.

The museum (which sits in an inviting park equipped with an equally inviting café) is housed in what had been the Royal Bethlam Hospital. Also known as "the Bedlam asylum," the place was so wild that it gave the world a new word for chaos. Back in Victorian times, locals—without reality shows and YouTube—paid admission to visit the asylum on weekends for entertainment.

▲▲Tate Modern

Dedicated in the spring of 2000, the striking museum across the river from St. Paul's opened the new century with art from the previous one. Its powerhouse collection of Monet, Matisse, Dalí, Picasso, Warhol, and much more is displayed in a converted powerhouse.

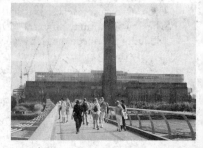

The permanent collection is on levels 2 through 4. Paintings are arranged according to theme, not chronologically or by artist. Paintings by Picasso, for example, are scattered all over the building. Don't just come to see the Old Masters of modernism. Push your mental envelope with more recent works by Pollock, Miró, Bacon, Picabia, Beuys, Twombly, and others.

Of equal interest are the many temporary exhibits featuring cutting-edge art. Each year, the main hall features a different monumental installation by a prominent artist—always one of the highlights of the art world. The Tate is constructing a new wing to the south, which will double the museum's exhibition space. The new wing is opening bit by bit and, once it's finished, the permanent exhibits will likely be rearranged, with some pieces moving to the new section.

Cost and Hours: Free, but £4 donation appreciated, fee for special exhibitions, open daily 10:00-18:00, Fri-Sat until 22:00, last entry to special exhibits 45 minutes before closing, especially crowded on weekend days (crowds thin out on Fri and Sat evenings), free 45-minute guided tours offered about four times daily, videoguide-£4, view restaurant on top floor, cross the Millennium Bridge from St. Paul's; Tube: Southwark, London Bridge, St. Paul's, or Mansion House plus a 10-15-minute walk; tel. 020/7887-8888, www.tate.org.uk.

▲▲Shakespeare's Globe

This replica of the original Globe Theatre was built, half-timbered and thatched, as it was in Shakespeare's time. (This is the first

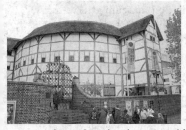

thatched roof constructed in London since they were outlawed after the Great Fire of 1666.) The Globe originally accommodated 2,200 seated and another 1,000 standing. Today, slightly smaller and leaving space for reasonable aisles, the theater holds 800 seated and 600 groundlings. Its promoters brag that the theater melds "the three A's"—actors, audience, and architecture—with each contributing to the play. The working theater hosts authentic performances of Shakespeare's plays with actors in period costumes, modern interpretations of his works, and some works by other playwrights. For details on attending a play, see page 1030.

The Globe complex has four parts: the Globe theater itself, the box office, a museum (called the Exhibition), and the new Sam Wanamaker Playhouse. This indoor Jacobean theater, which is attached to the back of the Globe complex, allows performances to continue through the winter. The horseshoe-shaped venue, seating fewer than 350, uses authentic candle-lighting for period performances. The repertoire focuses less on Shakespeare and more on the work of his contemporaries (Jonson, Marlow, Fletcher), as well as concerts. (For details on getting tickets, see page 1030.)

Cost: £13.50 ticket (good all day) includes Exhibition, audioguide, and 40-minute tour of the Globe; when theater is in use, you can tour the Exhibition only for £10.

Hours: The complex is open daily 9:00-17:00. Tours start every 30 minutes; during Globe theater season (late April-early Oct), last tour Mon at 17:00, Tue-Sat at 12:30, Sun at 11:30; located on the South Bank directly across Thames over Southwark Bridge from St. Paul's, Tube: Mansion House or London Bridge plus a 10-minute walk; tel. 020/7902-1400, box office tel. 020/7401-9919, www.shakespearesglobe.com.

Visiting the Globe: You browse on your own in the **Exhibition** (with the included audioguide) through displays of Elizabethan-era costumes and makeup, music, script-printing, and special effects (the displays change). There are early folios and objects that were dug up on site. Videos and scale models help put Shakespearean theater within the context of the times. (The Globe opened one year after England mastered the seas by defeating the Spanish Armada. The debut play was Shakespeare's *Julius Caesar*.) You'll also learn how they built the replica in modern times, using Elizabethan materials and techniques. Take advantage of the touch screens to delve into specific topics.

You must **tour the theater** at the time stamped on your ticket, but you can come back to the Exhibition museum afterward. A guide (usually an actor) leads you into the theater to see the stage and the various seating areas for the different classes of people. You take a seat and learn how the new Globe is similar to the old Globe (open-air performances, standing-room by the stage, no curtain) and how it's different (female actors today, lights for night performances, concrete floor). It's not a backstage tour—you don't see dressing rooms or costume shops or sit in on rehearsals—but the guides are energetic, theatrical, and knowledgeable, bringing the Elizabethan period to life.

Eating: The Swan at the Globe café offers a sit-down restaurant (for lunch and dinner, reservations recommended, tel. 020/7928-9444), a drinks-and-plates bar, and a sandwich-and-coffee cart (daily 9:00-closing, depending on performance times).

Shopping in London

London is great for shoppers—and thanks to the high prices, perhaps even better for window-shoppers. In the 1960s, London set the tone for Mod clothing, and it's been a major fashion capital ever since.

British clothing sizes are different from those in the US. For example, a woman's size 10 dress (US) is a UK size 14, and a size 8 woman's shoe (US) is a UK size 5½.

Most stores are open Monday through Saturday from roughly 10:00 to 18:00, and many close Sundays. Large department stores stay open until 20:00 or 21:00. For one-stop shopping for essential items, try large chain stores such as Marks & Spencer (www.marksandspencer.com).

West End High Fashion

You'll find big-name fashion stores along Regent Street (between Oxford Circus and Piccadilly), old-fashioned gentlemen's stores on Jermyn Street, bookstores along Charing Cross Road, and more boutiques around Covent Garden.

Harrods and "Harvey Nick's"

Near Hyde Park, you'll find London's most famous and touristy department store, **Harrods.** With more than four acres of retail space covering seven floors, it has everything from elephants to toothbrushes, from artisan cheese to a £10,000 toy car (Mon-Sat 10:00-20:00, Sun 11:30-18:00, Brompton Road, Tube: Knightsbridge, tel. 020/7730-1234, www.harrods.com).

A few blocks away is **Harvey Nichols.** Once Princess Diana's favorite (and now serving Kate Middleton), "Harvey Nick's" remains *the* department store du jour (Mon–Sat 10:00–20:00, Sun 12:00–18:00, near Harrods, 109–125 Knightsbridge, Tube: Knightsbridge, tel. 020/7235-5000, www.harveynichols.com).

Street Markets

London's weekend flea markets are legendary. **Covent Garden's** daily market is handy to other sightseeing (produce stalls open daily 10:30–18:00, tel. 020-7420-5856, www.coventgardenlondonuk.com). **Portobello Road Market** is the classic London street market. On Fridays and Saturdays (9:00-19:00), this funky-yet-quaint Notting Hill street of pastel-painted houses and offbeat antiques shops is enlivened even more with 2,000 additional stalls (on Sundays everything is closed, Tube: Notting Hill Gate, tel. 020/7229-8354, www.portobelloroad.co.uk). **Camden Lock Market** in north London is a huge, trendy, youth-oriented arts-and-crafts festival. It runs daily 10:00–18:00, but is busiest on weekends (Tube: Camden Town, 020/7485-7963, www.camdenlockmarket.com).

LONDON

Eating in London

With "modern English" cuisine on the rise, London's sheer variety of foods—from every corner of its former empire and beyond—is astonishing. You'll be amazed at the number of hopping,

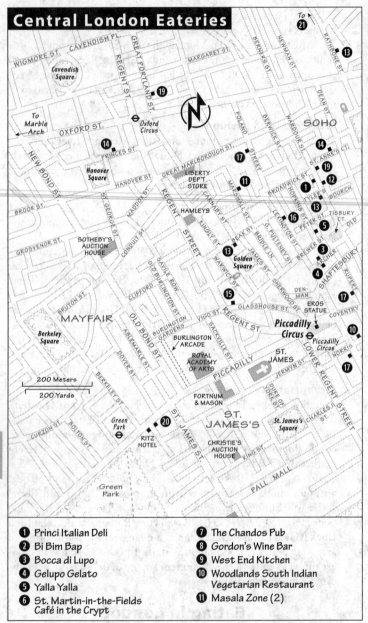

Central London Eateries

1. Princi Italian Deli
2. Bi Bim Bap
3. Bocca di Lupo
4. Gelupo Gelato
5. Yalla Yalla
6. St. Martin-in-the-Fields Café in the Crypt
7. The Chandos Pub
8. Gordon's Wine Bar
9. West End Kitchen
10. Woodlands South Indian Vegetarian Restaurant
11. Masala Zone (2)

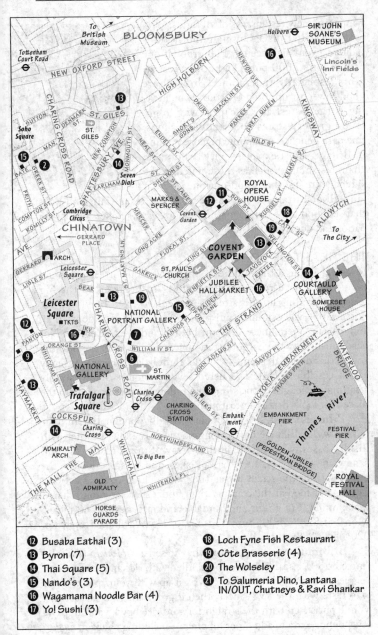

⑫	Busaba Eathai (3)	⑱	Loch Fyne Fish Restaurant
⑬	Byron (7)	⑲	Côte Brasserie (4)
⑭	Thai Square (5)	⑳	The Wolseley
⑮	Nando's (3)	㉑	To Salumeria Dino, Lantana
⑯	Wagamama Noodle Bar (4)		IN/OUT, Chutneys & Ravi Shankar
⑰	Yo! Sushi (3)		

happening new restaurants of all kinds.

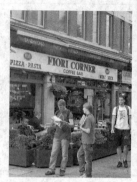

I've listed places by neighborhood—handy to your sightseeing. Pub grub (at one of London's 7,000 pubs) and ethnic restaurants (especially Indian and Chinese) are good low-cost options. Of course, picnicking is the fastest and cheapest way to go. Good grocery stores and sandwich shops, fine park benches, and polite pigeons abound in Britain's most expensive city. Affordable chain restaurants (such as those noted in the sidebar) are another good option. London (and all of Britain) is smoke-free. Expect restaurants and pubs that sell food to be non-smoking indoors, with smokers occupying patios and doorways outside.

THE HEART OF SOHO

Running through the middle of Soho, Wardour Street is ground zero for creative restaurateurs hoping to break in to the big leagues. Strolling up this street—particularly from Brewer Street northward—you can take your pick from a world of options: Thai, Indonesian, Vietnamese, Italian, French and even...English. Not yet tarnished by the corporatization creeping in from areas to the south, this drag still seems to hit the right balance between trendy and accessible. While I've listed several choices below, simply strolling the length of the street and following your appetite to the place that looks best is a great plan.

Princi is a vast, bright, efficient, wildly popular Italian deli/bakery with Milanese flair. Along one wall is a long counter with display cases offering a tempting array of pizza rustica, panini sandwiches, focaccia, a few pasta dishes, and desserts (look in the window from the street to see their wood-fired oven in action). Order your food at the counter, then find a space at a long shared table; or get it to go for an affordable and fast meal (£7-13 meals, Mon-Sat 8:00-24:00, Sun 8:30-22:00, 135 Wardour Street, tel. 020/7478-8888).

Bi Bim Bap is named for what it sells: *bibimbap* (literally "mixed rice"), a scalding stone bowl filled with rice and thinly sliced veggies, topped with a fried egg. Mix it up with your spoon, flavor it to taste with the two sauces, then dig in with your chopsticks. While purists go with the straightforward rice bowl, you can pay a few pounds extra to add other toppings—including chicken, *bulgogi* (marinated beef strips), and mushrooms. Though the food is traditional Korean, the stylish, colorful interior lets you know you're in Soho (£7-10 meals, Mon-Fri 12:00-15:00 & 18:00-23:00, Sat 12:00-23:00, closed Sun, 11 Greek Street, tel. 020/7287-3434).

LONDON

Bocca di Lupo, a pricey and popular splurge, serves small portions of classic regional Italian food. Dressy and a bit snooty, it's a place where you're glad you made a reservation. The counter seating, on cushy stools with a view into the open kitchen, is particularly memorable (Mon-Sat 12:30-15:00 & 17:30-23:00, Sun 12:30-15:30 & 17:30-21:30, 12 Archer Street, tel. 020/7734-2223, www.boccadilupo.com).

Gelupo, Bocca di Lupo's sister gelateria across the street, has a wide array of ever-changing but always creative and delicious dessert favorites—ranging from popular standbys like the incredibly rich chocolate sorbet to fresh-mint *stracciatella* to hay (yes, hay). A £3 sampler cup or cone gets you two flavors (and little taster spoons are generously offered to help you choose). Everything is homemade, and the white subway-tile interior feels clean and bright. They also have espresso drinks and—at lunchtime—£5-6 deli sandwiches (daily 12:00 until late, 7 Archer Street, tel. 020/7287-5555).

Yalla Yalla is a hole-in-the-wall serving up high-quality Beirut street food—hummus, baba ghanoush, tabbouleh, and *shawarmas*. Stylish as you'd expect for Soho, it's tucked down a seedy alley across from a sex shop. Eat in the cramped and cozy interior or at one of the few outdoor tables, or get your food to go (£3-4 sandwiches, £4-6 *meze*, £8 *mezes* platter available until 17:00, £10-15 bigger dishes, Mon-Sat 10:00-23:00, Sun 10:00-22:00, 1 Green's Court—just north of Brewer Street, tel. 020/7287-7663).

And for Dessert: In addition to the outstanding gelato at **Gelupo** and the treats at **Princi** (both described earlier), several other places along Wardour Street boast window displays that tickle the sweet tooth. In just a couple of blocks, you'll see pastry shops, a *crêperie*, and a Hummingbird cupcake shop.

Soho Chain Restaurants: **Byron** (particularly appealing industrial-mod branch at 97-99 Wardour Street), **Busaba Eathai** (106 Wardour Street), **Thai Square** (27-28 St. Anne's Court, plus one near Trafalgar Square at 21-24 Cockspur Street), **Wagamama** (10A Lexington Street), **Masala Zone** (9 Marshall Street), **Côte** (124-126 Wardour Street), and **Nando's** (10 Frith Street). For descriptions, see page 1018.

NEAR TRAFALGAR SQUARE

These traditional places, all of which provide a more "jolly olde" experience than high cuisine, are within about 100 yards of Trafalgar Square.

St. Martin-in-the-Fields Café in the Crypt is just right for a tasty meal on a monk's budget—maybe even on a monk's tomb. You'll dine sitting on somebody's gravestone in an ancient crypt. Their enticing buffet line is kept stocked all day, serving

London Chain Restaurants

I know—you're going to London to enjoy characteristic little hole-in-the-wall pubs, so mass-produced food is the furthest thing from your mind. But several excellent chains can be a nice break from pub grub. Each of these places has multiple branches throughout London—keep an eye out for the ones that sound good to you.

Carry-Out Chains

While the following places might have some seating, they're best as an easy place to grab some prepackaged food on the run.

Major supermarket chains have smaller, offshoot branches that specialize in sandwiches, salads, and other prepared foods to go. These can be a picnicker's dream come true. Some shops are stand-alone, while others are located inside a larger store. The most prevalent—and best—is **M&S Simply Food** (an offshoot of the Marks & Spencer department-store chain; there's one in every major train station). **Sainsbury's Local** grocery stores also offer some decent prepared food; **Tesco Express** and **Tesco Metro** run a distant third.

Some "cheap and cheery" chains, such as **Pret à Manger, Eat, Apostrophe,** and **Pod** provide office workers with good, healthful sandwiches, salads, and pastries to go. Among these, Eat has a reputation for slightly higher quality...and higher prices.

West Cornwall Pasty Company and **Cornish Bakehouse** sell a variety of these traditional savory pies for around £3—as do many smaller, independent bakeries.

Sit-Down Chains

Most branches of the chains listed here open daily no later than noon (several at 8:00 or 9:00), and close sometime between 22:00 and midnight. Occasionally a place may close on Sundays or in the afternoon between lunch and dinner, but these are rare exceptions.

Busaba Eathai is a hit with Londoners for its snappy (sometimes rushed) service, boisterous ambience, and good, inexpensive Thai cuisine. Wedge yourself at one of the 16-person hardwood tables or at a two-person table by the window—with everyone in the queue staring at your noodles (£7-12 meals, www.busaba.com).

Wagamama Noodle Bar, serving up pan-Asian cuisine (udon noodles, fried rice, and curry dishes), is a noisy, organic slurpathon. Portions are huge and splittable. While the quality has gone downhill a bit as they've expanded, this remains a reliable choice with reasonable prices (£8-12 main dishes big enough for light eaters to share, good veggie options, www.wagamama.com).

Masala Zone, serving accessible Indian food, makes a predictable, good alternative to the many one-off, hole-in-the-wall Indian joints around town (£8-12 meals, www.masalazone.com). Locations include Soho, Covent Garden, Bayswater, and in the Selfridges department store on Oxford Street.

Côte Brasserie is a contemporary French chain serving good-value French cuisine in reliably pleasant settings, and at the right prices (£9-14 main dishes, early dinner specials, www.cote-restaurants.co.uk).

Byron, an upscale hamburger chain with hip interiors, is worth seeking out if you need a burger fix. While British burgers aren't exactly like American ones—they tend to be a bit overcooked by our standards—Byron's burgers are your best bet (£7-10 burgers, www.byronhamburgers.com). **Gourmet Burger Kitchen (GBK)** provides a cheaper alternative, serving burgers that are, if not quite gourmet, very good. Choices range from a simple cheeseburger to more elaborate options, such as Jamaican. Choose a table and order at the counter—they'll bring the food to you (£7-11 burgers).

Loch Fyne Fish Restaurant is part of a Scottish chain that raises its own oysters and mussels. Its branches offer an inviting, lively atmosphere with a fine fishy energy and no pretense (£10-18 main dishes, two- and three-course specials often available before 19:00, www.lochfyne-restaurants.com).

Nando's is understandably popular as a casual, affordable place to get flame-broiled chicken with a range of Portuguese and South African flavors (£10 meals, www.nandos.co.uk).

At **Yo! Sushi,** sushi dishes trundle past on a conveyor belt. Color-coded plates tell you how much each dish costs (£1.90-5), and a picture-filled menu explains what you're eating. For £1.50, you get unlimited green tea (water for £1.05). Snag a bar stool and grab dishes as they rattle by (www.yosushi.com).

Ask and **Pizza Express** serve quality pasta and pizza in a pleasant, sit-down atmosphere that's family-friendly. **Jamie's Italian** (from celebrity chef Jamie Oliver) is hipper and pricier, and feels more upmarket.

breakfast, lunch, and dinner (£7-10 cafeteria plates, hearty traditional desserts, free jugs of water). They also serve a restful cream tea (£6, daily 14:00-18:00). You'll find the café directly under the St. Martin-in-the-Fields Church, facing Trafalgar Square—enter through the glass pavilion next to the church (Mon-Tue 8:00-20:00, Wed 8:00-22:30, Thu-Sat 8:00-21:00, Sun 11:00-18:00, profits go to the church, Tube: Charing Cross, tel. 020/7766-1158 or 020/7766-1100).

The Chandos Pub's Opera Room floats amazingly apart from the tacky crush of tourism around Trafalgar Square. Look for it opposite the National Portrait Gallery (corner of William IV Street and St. Martin's Lane) and climb the stairs (to the left or right of the pub entrance) to the Opera Room. This is a fine Trafalgar rendezvous point and wonderfully local pub. They serve £5 sandwiches and a better-than-average range of traditional pub meals for under £10—meat pies and fish-and-chips are their specialty. The ground-floor pub is stuffed with regulars and offers snugs (private booths) and more serious beer drinking. To eat on that level, you have to order upstairs and carry it down. Chandos proudly serves the local Samuel Smith beer at £3 a pint (kitchen open daily 11:00-19:00, Fri and Sun until 18:00, order and pay at the bar, 29 St. Martin's Lane, Tube: Leicester Square, tel. 020/7836-1401).

Gordon's Wine Bar is really a Back Door eatery—you have to enter through its leafy patio just past its locked street entrance. This candlelit 15th-century wine cellar is filled with dusty old bottles, faded British memorabilia, and nine-to-fivers. At the "English rustic" buffet, choose a hot meal or cold meat dish with a salad (figure around £7-8/dish); the £10 cheese plate comes with two cheeses, bread, and a pickle. Then step up to the wine bar and consider the many varieties of wine and port available by the glass (this place is passionate about port). The low carbon-crusted vaulting deeper in the back seems to intensify the Hogarth-painting atmosphere. Although it's crowded, you can normally corral two chairs and grab the corner of a table. The crowd often spills out onto the patio, and on hot days a chef cooks at a barbecue for a long line of tables (arrive before 17:00 to get a seat, Mon-Sat 11:00-23:00, Sun 12:00-22:00, 2 blocks from Trafalgar Square, bottom of Villiers Street at #47, Tube: Embankment, tel. 020/7930-1408, manager Gerard Menan).

NEAR PICCADILLY

Hungry and broke in the theater district? Head for Panton Street (off Haymarket, two blocks southeast of Piccadilly Circus), where several hardworking little places compete, all seeming to offer a three-course meal for about £9. Peruse the entire block (vegetarian, Pizza Express, Moroccan, Chinese, and diners) before making your choice.

The **West End Kitchen** serves up Italian (£7-10 pizzas, £9-17 meals, daily 11:45-22:30, 5 Panton Street, tel. 020/7839-4241). The **Woodlands South Indian Vegetarian Restaurant** offers an impressive £19 *thali* combination plate (otherwise £7 main courses, daily 12:00-22:45, 37 Panton Street, tel. 020/7839-7258).

Good Chains near Piccadilly: **Busaba Eathai** (35 Panton Street), **Wagamama** (another in Leicester Square at 14 Irving Street), **Byron** (11 Haymarket, but enter around the corner on Whitcomb Street), and **Nando's** (46 Glasshouse Street). For descriptions, see page 1018.

NEAR THE BRITISH MUSEUM

Salumeria Dino serves up hearty sandwiches, pasta, and Italian coffee. Dino, a native of Naples, has run his little shop for more than 30 years and has managed to create a classic Italian deli that's so authentic, you'll walk out singing "O Sole Mio" (£3-5 sandwiches, £1 takeaway cappuccinos, Mon-Fri 9:00-18:00, closed Sat-Sun, 15 Charlotte Place, see map on page 1006, tel. 020/7580-3938).

Lantana OUT, next door to Salumeria Dino, is an Australian coffee shop that sells modern soups, sandwiches, and salads at their takeaway window (£3-7 meals, pricier sit-down café—**Lantana IN** serving £8-10 meals—next door, Mon-Fri 7:30-15:00, café also open Sat-Sun 9:00-17:00, 13 Charlotte Place, see map on page 996, tel. 020/7637-3347).

Nearby Chains: Several recommended chain restaurants are a short walk from the museum, including **Busaba Eathai** (22 Store Street), **Wagamama** (4 Streatham Street and near Holborn Tube stop at 123 Kingsway), **Côte** (5 Charlotte Street), **Byron** (6 Store Street, with another at 6 Rathbone Place), and **Nando's** (9-10 Southampton Place).

NEAR ST. PAUL'S CATHEDRAL

De Gustibus Sandwiches is where an artisan bakery meets the public, offering fresh, you-design-it sandwiches, salads, and soups. Communication can be difficult, but it's worth the effort. Just one block below St. Paul's, it has simple seating or take-out picnic sacks for lugging to one of the great nearby parks (£4-8 sandwiches, £6 hot dishes, Mon-Fri 7:00-17:00, closed Sat-Sun, from church steps follow signs to youth hostel a block downhill, 53-55 Carter Lane, tel. 020/7236-0056; another outlet is inside the Borough Market in Southwark).

NEAR THE BRITISH LIBRARY

Drummond Street (running just west of Euston Station—see map on page 996) is famous for cheap and good Indian vegetarian food (£5-10 dishes, £7 lunch buffets). For a good *thali* (combo plate) consider **Chutneys** (124 Drummond, tel. 020/7388-0604) and **Ravi Shankar** (133-135 Drummond, tel. 020/7388-6458, both open long hours daily).

Taking Tea in London

TEA TERMS

The cheapest "tea" on the menu is generally a "cream tea"; the most expensive is the "champagne tea." **Cream tea** is simply a pot of tea and a homemade scone or two with jam and thick clotted cream. (For maximum pinkie-waving taste per calorie, slice your scone thin like a miniature loaf of bread.) **Afternoon tea**—what many Americans would call "high tea"—generally is a cream tea plus a tier of three plates holding small finger foods (such as cucumber sandwiches) and an assortment of small pastries. **Champagne tea** includes all of the goodies, plus a glass of bubbly. **High tea** to the English generally means a more substantial late-afternoon or early-evening meal, often served with meat or eggs.

Tearooms, which often also serve appealing light meals, are usually open for lunch and close about 17:00, just before dinner. At all the places listed below, it's perfectly acceptable for two people to order one afternoon tea and one cream tea (at about £5) and share the afternoon tea's goodies.

PLACES TO SIP TEA

The Wolseley serves a good afternoon tea between their meal service. Split one with your companion and enjoy two light meals at a great price in classic elegance (£11 cream tea, £24 afternoon tea, served Mon-Fri 15:00-18:30, Sat 15:30-17:30, Sun 15:30-18:30, reservations smart, 160 Piccadilly, tel. 020/7499-6996, www. thewolseley.com).

The **Fortnum & Mason** department store offers tea at several different restaurants within its walls. You can "Take Tea in the Parlour" for £18 (including ice-cream cakes; Mon-Sat 10:00-20:00, Sun 11:30-18:00), or try the all-out "Gallery Tea" for £26 (daily 15:00-18:00). But the pièce de resistance is their Diamond Jubilee Tea Salon, named in honor of the Queen's 60th year on the throne. At these royal prices, consider it dinner (£40-44, Mon-Sat 12:00-21:00, Sun 12:00-20:00, dress up a bit—no shorts, "children must be behaved," 181 Piccadilly—see map on page 1014, smart to reserve online or by phone at least a week in advance, tel. 0845-602-5694, www.fortnumandmason.com).

Other Places Serving Good Tea: The **National Dining Rooms**, within the National Gallery on Trafalgar Square, offers a £7 cream tea and £17.50 afternoon tea with a great view (served 14:30-17:00, in Sainsbury Wing of National Gallery, Tube: Charing Cross

What If I Miss My Boat?

Remember that you can get help from the cruise line's port agent (listed on the destination information sheet distributed on the ship) and the local TI (see page 968). If the port agent suggests a costly solution (such as a private car with a driver), you may want to consider public transit.

You'll very likely find that your best option is to **fly.** London has several airports, and many low-cost, no-frills carriers are based here, offering frequent and cheap (sometimes even last-minute) flights to just about anywhere. Check www.skyscanner.com for options. For information on London's airports, see "Airport Connections," later.

Overland, it could be more complicated to reach your next destination. The fast option is to head back to London and hop the speedy Eurostar ("Chunnel") train under the English Channel to Paris (then 2 hours by train to **Le Havre**) or Brussels (then 1.5 hours by train to **Zeebrugge,** 2 hours by express or 3.5 hours by local train to **Amsterdam**). For points west or north (such as **Copenhagen** or **Berlin/Warnemünde**), you'll probably find it's best to Chunnel to Brussels and connect from there.

To reach **Le Havre,** you could consider the ferry connections across the English Channel from Portsmouth, such as those offered by Brittany Ferries (www.brittany-ferries.co.uk).

Local **travel agents** in London, Southampton, or Dover can help you. For more advice on what to do if you miss the boat, see page 139.

or Leicester Square, tel. 020/7747-2525, www.peytonandbyrne.co.uk). **The National Café,** at the other end of the building, is a bit cheaper (£16.50 afternoon tea served 14:30-17:30). **The Café at Sotheby's,** on the ground floor of the auction giant's headquarters, gives shoppers a break from fashionable New Bond Street (£9-25, tea served Mon-Fri only 15:00-16:45, reservations smart, 34-35 New Bond Street—see map on page 1014, Tube: Bond Street or Oxford Circus, tel. 020/7293-5077, www.sothebys.com/cafe).

Cheaper Options: **John Lewis'** mod third-floor brasserie serves a nice afternoon tea from 15:30 (£10, on Oxford Street one block west of the Bond Street Tube station, tel. 020/7629-7711, www.johnlewis.com). Many museums and bookstores have cafés serving afternoon tea goodies à la carte, where you can put together a spread for less than £10—**Waterstones'** fifth-floor café and the **Victoria and Albert Museum** café are two of the best. **Teapod,** a modern place near the Tower Bridge, serves cream tea for £5.50 and afternoon tea for £13.50 (Mon-Fri 8:00-18:00, Sat-Sun 9:30-18:30, 31 Shad Thames, tel. 020/7407-0000).

Starting or Ending Your Cruise in London

If your cruise begins and/or ends in London, you'll want plenty of extra time here; for most travelers, two days is a bare minimum. For a longer visit here, pick up my *Rick Steves London* guidebook; for other destinations in the country, see *Rick Steves England* or *Rick Steves Great Britain*.

Airport Connections

London has six airports. Most tourists arrive at **Heathrow** or **Gatwick** airport, although flights from elsewhere in Europe may land at **Stansted, Luton, Southend,** or **London City** airport.

To get from any airport to your cruise port (or vice versa), you'll have to connect through London. I've given specific directions for each airport below, followed by tips for continuing on to Southampton or Dover. For a list of hotels in London, see the end of this chapter.

Some cruise lines offer convenient **shuttle bus service** directly from the airport to the cruise port; check with your cruise line for details.

HEATHROW AIRPORT

One of the world's busiest airports, Heathrow has five terminals, T-1 through T-5. Each terminal has all the necessary travelers' services (info desks, ATMs, shops, eateries, etc.). T-1, T-2, and T-3 are connected and walkable, while T-4 and T-5 are separate and farther away. You can travel between terminals on free trains and buses, but it can be time-consuming—plan ahead if you'll need to change terminals. For airport and flight information, call 0844-335-1801 or visit www.heathrowairport.com (airport code: LHR).

Getting from Heathrow to London

To get between Heathrow and London (14 miles away), you have several options:

Taxi: The one-hour trip costs £45-75 to west and central London, for up to four people. Just get in the queue outside the terminal.

Tube: For £5.50, the Tube takes you from any Heathrow terminal to downtown London in 50-60 minutes on the Piccadilly Line (6/hour). If you plan to use the Tube for transport in London, consider buying a Travelcard covering Zone 1-2 (central London) and paying a small supplement for the Heathrow-to-London

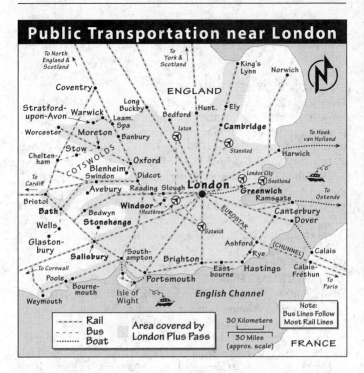

Public Transportation near London

To North England & Scotland

To York & Scotland

King's Lynn · Norwich

Coventry

ENGLAND

Stratford-upon-Avon · Warwick
Long Buckby · Bedford · Hunt. · Ely
Leam. Spa
Worcester · Moreton · Banbury
Luton · Cambridge

To Hoek van Holland

Cheltenham · Stow
COTSWOLDS
Blenheim · Oxford
Swindon · Didcot
Stansted · Harwich

To Cardiff
Avebury · Reading · Slough · London
London City · Southend

Bristol
Bath · Bedwyn · Windsor
Heathrow
Greenwich · Ramsgate

To Ostende

Wells
Stonehenge
EUROSTAR
Canterbury · Dover

Glastonbury
Salisbury · Southampton · Brighton
Gatwick
Ashford · Rye
(CHUNNEL) · Calais

To Cornwall
Poole · Bournemouth
Isle of Wight
Portsmouth
East-bourne · Hastings
Calais-Fréthun

To Paris

Weymouth

English Channel

—— Rail
- - - Bus
········ Boat

Area covered by London Plus Pass

30 Kilometers

30 Miles (approx. scale)

Note: Bus Lines Follow Most Rail Lines

FRANCE

portion, or a pay-as-you-go Oyster card. For details on these passes, see page 973.

Train: From terminals T-1/T-2/T-3, the **Heathrow Connect** train goes to Paddington Station (£10 one-way, 2/hour Mon-Sat, 1-2/hour Sun, 40 minutes, tel. 0845-678-6975, www.heathrowconnect.com). From T-1/T-2/T-3 and T-5, the **Heathrow Express** goes to Paddington (£21 one-way, £34 round-trip, 4/hour, 15-21 minutes, tel. 0845-600-1515, www.heathrowexpress.co.uk).

Bus: There's a central bus station outside terminals T-1/T-2/T-3. National Express buses go to Victoria Coach Station near the Victoria train and Tube station (£6-9, 1-2/hour, 45-75 minutes, tel. 0871-781-8181, www.nationalexpress.com).

Heathrow Shuttle: These share-the-ride shuttle vans work like those at home, carrying passengers directly to or from their hotel (£18/person, book at least 24 hours in advance, tel. 0845-257-8068, www.heathrowshuttle.com).

From London to Heathrow: To get to Heathrow from central London, your transportation options are the same as above. Here are a few tips: Confirm with your airline in advance which terminal your flight will use, to avoid having to transfer between terminals. If arriving by Tube, note that not every Piccadilly Line train stops at every terminal. Before boarding, make sure your train is going to the terminal you want. A taxi arranged through your hotel can often be cheaper (£40) than from Heathrow to London.

LONDON'S OTHER AIRPORTS

Gatwick is London's second-biggest airport (tel. 0844-892-0322, www.gatwickairport.com, airport code: LGW). To get from Gatwick into London, **Gatwick Express trains** shuttle conveniently to Victoria Station (£20 one-way, £35 round-trip, 4/hour, 30 minutes, tel. 0845-850-1530, www.gatwickexpress.com).

London's other, lesser airports are **Stansted Airport** (tel. 0844-335-1803, www.stanstedairport.com), **Luton Airport** (tel. 01582/405-100, www.london-luton.co.uk), **London City Airport** (tel. 020/7646-0088, www.londoncityairport.com), and **Southend Airport** (tel. 01702/608-100, www.southendairport.com).

GETTING FROM CENTRAL LONDON TO THE CRUISE PORTS

Even if you're coming directly from any of London's airports, you'll need to transfer through London to reach either Southampton or Dover (unless your cruise line offers **shuttle service** from the airport to your ship). For either port, also ask your cruise line whether they're offering a shuttle from the train station in Southampton or Dover to your ship. Compare it to the taxi cost to decide if it's right for you.

To Southampton

To reach Southampton's cruise ports, bus, Tube, or taxi to London Waterloo train station, where trains depart to Southampton Central (about £39 "single"/one-way, 2-3/hour, 1.5 hours; a few more options with a change in Basingstoke; a few slow trains go from London Victoria in 2.5 hours). Don't get off at "Southampton Airport Parkway"—stay on until "Southampton Central."

Exiting the station in Southampton, you'll find a row of **taxis** ready to take you to your ship. Figure around £5, but it shouldn't be more than £7-8 (£1 extra on Sun)—ask for an estimate first, then insist on the meter.

If you're packing light and feeling thrifty and energetic, you could take advantage of the **Citylink** or **Unilink buses** that depart from the curb just outside the station; however, note that they do not take you all the way to your ship—you'll still have to walk between 5 and 15 minutes, depending on where your ship is. For the Mayflower Cruise Terminal, take a taxi. For details on these buses, see page 935.

To Dover

Trains head to Dover from various London stations. The fastest connection is on the "Javelin" train from St. Pancras Station (£39 "single"/one-way, 2/hour, 1.5 hours). Slower trains to Dover leave from Victoria or Charing Cross Stations (for either one: around £36 "single"/one-way, 1-2/hour, 2 hours).

If you're staying near Victoria or Charing Cross Stations, you might as well take the train from there; but all other things being equal, I'd take the faster connection from St. Pancras Station.

Arriving at Dover Priory Station, your best bet is to pay £8 for a **taxi** to your ship. While it's possible to walk 15 minutes to Market Square to catch a **shuttle bus** to your ship, two people can take a taxi for about the same price. There's no public bus from the station to the cruise port.

Hotels in London

London is an expensive city for lodging. Cheaper rooms are relatively dumpy. Don't expect £130 cheeriness in a £70 room. For

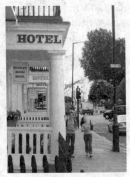

£70, you'll get a double with breakfast in a safe, cramped, and dreary place with minimal service and the bathroom down the hall. For £90, you'll get a basic, clean, reasonably cheery double with a private bath in a usually cramped, cracked-plaster building, or a soulless but comfortable room without breakfast in a huge Motel 6-type place. My London splurges, at £160-290, are spacious, thoughtfully appointed places good for entertaining or romancing.

Looking for Hotel Deals Online: Given London's high hotel prices, using the Internet can help you score a deal. Various websites list rooms in high-rise, three- and four-star business hotels. You'll give up the charm and warmth of a family-run establishment, and breakfast probably won't be included, but you might find that the price is right. Start by browsing the websites of several chains to get a sense of typical rates and online deals. Midrange chains to consider include Premier Inn, Travelodge, Ibis, Jurys Inn, and the stripped-down easyHotel. Pricier London hotel chains include Millennium/Copthorne, Thistle, Intercontinental/Holiday Inn, Radisson Hilton, and Red Carnation.

VICTORIA STATION NEIGHBORHOOD

The streets behind Victoria Station teem with little, moderately priced-for-London B&Bs. It's a safe, surprisingly tidy, and decent

LONDON

area without a hint of the trashy, touristy glitz of the streets in front of the station. For locations please see individual hotel websites.

$$$ Lime Tree Hotel, enthusiastically run by Charlotte and Matt, is a gem, with 25 spacious, stylish, comfortable, thoughtfully decorated rooms, a helpful staff, and a fun-loving breakfast room (Sb-£110, Db-£165, larger superior Db-£195, Tb-£205, family room-£225, usually cheaper Jan-Feb, guest computer and Wi-Fi, small lounge opens onto quiet garden, 135 Ebury Street, tel. 020/7730-8191, www.limetreehotel.co.uk, info@limetreehotel.co.uk, Alex manages the office).

$$ Luna Simone Hotel rents 36 fresh, spacious, remodeled rooms with modern bathrooms. It's a smartly managed place, run for more than 40 years by twins Peter and Bernard—and Bernard's son Mark—and they still seem to enjoy their work (Sb-£80, Db-£115, Tb-£140, Qb-£170, ask for a discount with cash and this book, guest computer and Wi-Fi, at 47 Belgrave Road near the corner of Charlwood Street, handy bus #24 to Victoria Station and Trafalgar Square stops out front, tel. 020/7834-5897, www.lunasimonehotel.com, stay@lunasimonehotel.com).

$ Cherry Court Hotel, run by the friendly and industrious Patel family, rents 12 very small but bright and well-designed rooms in a central location. Considering London's sky-high prices, this is a fine budget choice (Sb-£60, Db-£75, Tb-£110, Quint/b family room-£135, ask for Rick Steves prices with this book, 5 percent fee to pay with credit card, fruit-basket breakfast in room, aircon, guest computer and Wi-Fi, laundry, peaceful garden patio, 23 Hugh Street, tel. 020/7828-2840, www.cherrycourthotel.co.uk, info@cherrycourthotel.co.uk, daughter Neha answers emails and offers informed restaurant advice).

SOUTH KENSINGTON

To stay on a quiet street so classy it doesn't allow hotel signs, surrounded by trendy shops and colorful restaurants, call "South Ken" your London home. Shoppers like being a short walk from Harrods and the designer shops of King's Road and Chelsea. When I splurge, I splurge here. For locations please see individual hotel websites.

$$$ Aster House, well-run by friendly and accommodating Simon and Leonie Tan, has a cheerful lobby, lounge, and breakfast room. Its 13 rooms are comfy and quiet, with TV, phone, and air-conditioning. Enjoy breakfast or just lounging in the whisper-elegant Orangery, a glassy greenhouse. Simon and Leonie offer free loaner mobile phones to their guests (Sb-£135, Db-£200, bigger Db-£250 or £295, does not include 20 percent VAT, ask about Rick Steves discount for multiple nights and cash, check website for specials, pay guest computer, Wi-Fi, 3 Sumner Place, tel.

020/7581-5888, www.asterhouse.com, asterhouse@gmail.com).

$$$ Number Sixteen, for well-heeled travelers, packs over-the-top class into its 41 artfully imagined rooms, plush designer-chic lounges, and tranquil garden. It's in a labyrinthine building, with boldly modern decor—perfect for an urban honeymoon (Sb-from £180, "superior" Db-from £294—but soft, ask for discounted "seasonal rates," especially on weekends and in Aug—subject to availability, larger "luxury" Db-£330, breakfast buffet in the conservatory-£19 continental or £20 full English, elevator, guest computer and Wi-Fi, 16 Sumner Place, tel. 020/7589-5232, US tel. 800-553-6674, www.numbersixteenhotel.co.uk, sixteen@firmdale.com).

ELSEWHERE IN CENTRAL LONDON

For locations, please see the map on page 996.

$$$ The 22 York Street B&B offers a casual alternative in the city center, renting 10 traditional, hardwood, comfortable rooms, each named for a notable London landmark (Sb-£120, Db-£150, Tb-£180, guest computer and Wi-Fi, inviting lounge; near Marylebone/Baker Street: from Baker Street Tube station, walk 2 blocks down Baker Street and take a right to 22 York Street—since there's no sign, just look for #22; tel. 020/7224-2990, www.22yorkstreet.co.uk, mc@22yorkstreet.co.uk, energetically run by Liz and Michael Callis).

$$$ The Sumner Hotel rents 19 rooms in a 19th-century Georgian townhouse sporting a lounge decorated with fancy modern Italian furniture and large contemporary rooms. This swanky place packs in all the amenities and is conveniently located north of Hyde Park and near Oxford Street, a busy shopping destination—with a convenient Marks & Spencer within walking distance (queen Db-£193, king Db-£213, "deluxe" Db-£229, mention this book for Rick Steves rates, can be cheaper off-season, extra bed-£60, air-con, elevator, Wi-Fi, 54 Upper Berkeley Street, a block and a half off Edgware Road, Tube: Marble Arch, tel. 020/7723-2244, www.thesumner.com, reservations@thesumner.com).

Entertainment in London

NIGHTLIFE

London bubbles with top-notch entertainment seven days a week: plays, movie premieres, concerts, Gilbert and Sullivan, tango lessons, stand-up comedy, Baha'i meetings, walking tours, shopping, museums open late, and the endlessly entertaining pub scene. Perhaps your best entertainment is just to take the Tube to Leicester Square on a pleasant evening, and explore the bustling

LONDON

West End. The two best sources for what's on are www.timeout.com/london and the TI's free monthly *London Planner*.

THEATER (A.K.A. "THEATRE")

London's theater scene rivals Broadway's in quality and usually beats it in price. Choose from Shakespeare, glitzy musicals, sex farces, serious chamber drama, cutting-edge fringe, revivals starring movie celebs, and more. London does it all well. To see what's showing, pick up the *Official London Theatre Guide* (free at hotels and box offices) or check www.officiallondontheatre.co.uk. Tickets range from about £25 to £120. Buy in person from the theater box office (no booking fee), or order by phone (some charge a booking fee) or online from the theater's website (£3 booking fee). The famous TKTS booth at Leicester Square sells discounted tickets for top-price seats to shows on the push list (Mon-Sat 9:00–19:00, Sun 11:00–16:30, check the day's list of available shows at www.tkts.co.uk). Other ticket agencies, located in offices around London, can be convenient but generally charge a 25 percent fee above the face value. Most theaters are found in the West End, between Piccadilly and Covent Garden, especially along Shaftesbury Avenue. **Shakespeare's Globe** (on the South Bank) presents a full repertoire May through September in a thatched, open-air replica of the Bard's original theater. The £5 "groundling" tickets—standing-room at the foot of the stage—are most fun (tel. 020/7401-9919, www.shakespeareglobe.com).

PARIS
France

France Practicalities

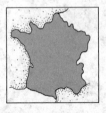

France is Europe's most diverse, tasty, and, in many ways, most exciting country to explore. It's a complex cultural bouillabaisse—and a day in port at Le Havre lets you get an enticing taste. France is a big country by European standards, but it's only about the size of Texas. Bordering eight countries, France has three impressive mountain ranges (the Alps, Pyrenees, and Massif Central), two very different coastlines (Atlantic and Mediterranean), cosmopolitan cities (including Paris), charming villages (such as Honfleur), and romantic castles. The majority of its population of nearly 66 million people is Roman Catholic, and virtually everyone speaks French.

Money: 1 euro (€) = about $1.10. An ATM is called a *distributeur*. The local VAT (value-added sales tax) rate is 20 percent; the minimum purchase eligible for a VAT refund is €175 (for details on refunds, see page 134).

Language: The native language is French. For useful phrases, see page 1141.

Emergencies: In case of any emergency, dial 112; to summon an ambulance, dial 15. In case of theft or loss, see page 125.

Time Zone: France is on Central European Time (the same as most of the Continent, one hour ahead of Great Britain, and six/nine hours ahead of the East/West Coasts of the US).

Embassies in Paris: The **US embassy** is at 4 Avenue Gabriel (tel. 01 43 12 22 22, http://france.usembassy.gov). The **Canadian embassy** is at 35 Avenue Montaigne (tel. 01 44 43 29 00, www.amb-canada.fr). Call ahead for passport services.

Phoning: France's country code is 33; to call from another country to France, dial the international access code (011 from the US/Canada, 00 from Europe, or + from a mobile phone), then 33, followed by the local number (drop the initial zero). For local calls within France, just dial the number as it appears in this book—whether you're calling from across the street or across the country. To place an international call from France, dial 00, the code of the country you're calling (1 for US and Canada), and the phone number. For more tips, see page 1146.

Tipping: Restaurant prices already include a tip, and most French people never leave anything extra, but for special service, it's kind to tip up to 5 percent. To tip a cabbie, round up a bit (if the fare is €13, pay €14). For more tips on tipping, see page 138.

Tourist Information: http://us.rendezvousenfrance.com

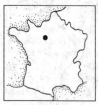

PARIS
and the PORT of LE HAVRE

Le Havre • Paris • Honfleur • D-Day Beaches • Rouen

Paris—the City of Light—offers sweeping boulevards, chatty crêpe stands, chic boutiques, and world-class art galleries. Sip decaf with deconstructionists at a sidewalk café, then step into an Impressionist painting in a tree-lined park. Climb Notre-Dame and rub shoulders with the gargoyles. Cruise the Seine, zip to the top of the Eiffel Tower, or saunter down Avenue des Champs-Elysées. Master the Louvre and Orsay museums.

To reach Paris from the port city of Le Havre, it's about a 2.5-hour train ride each way. If you'd rather stick closer to your ship, consider these alternatives: the harbor town of Honfleur (30 minutes by bus); the historic D-Day beaches (an hour or so to the west); and the pleasant small city of Rouen (one hour by train).

PLANNING YOUR TIME

Most visitors arriving at Le Havre will zip into Paris. While the round-trip is time-consuming, if this is your one chance to experience the City of Light, it's hard to resist. On the other hand, several good, easier-to-visit options sit much closer to Le Havre—worth considering for those who've already been to Paris (or want to save it for a longer visit).

Here are your basic options:

• **Paris:** With just a few hours in Paris, you'll need to be selective—but if that's all the time you have, you can still see a lot. For details, see page 1045.

• **Honfleur:** An easy (though relatively infrequent) bus ride from Le Havre, this sleepy, colorful port town that inspired the Impressionists can fill a lazy day.

• **D-Day Beaches:** The historic beaches of the WWII Allied

Excursions from Le Havre

If you're heading into Paris, consider doing it on your own, by train. If skipping Paris, there's no shortage of fascinating destinations accessible from Le Havre.

In and near Paris: The basic excursion option is a bus-and-riverboat tour of the city, with fleeting glimpses of the Arc de Triomphe, Champs-Elysées, Opéra Garnier, Louvre, Ile de la Cité with Notre-Dame Cathedral, Latin Quarter, and Hôtel des Invalides. Some tours include a guided tour of the **Louvre;** on others, you'll get about three hours of free time. For more independence, the cruise lines' **Paris On Your Own** excursion—a round-trip bus ride with no guiding—is pricier than a round-trip train ticket but saves you the hassle and stress of getting there and back.

Just outside Paris, the sumptuous **Palace of Versailles** (with its sprawling gardens and famously opulent Hall of Mirrors) is best seen by excursion, as the public-transit connection from Le Havre to Versailles is a hassle.

Between Paris and Normandy: The city of **Rouen** has a charming old town, a church honoring Joan of Arc (who was burned here), and a cathedral that was famously painted 30 different times by Claude Monet as a way to study how light clings to surfaces. Rouen is easy to reach by train from Le Havre; excursions to Rouen may include the enchanting lily-pad gardens at **Giverny,** built by Monet to be his muse.

In Normandy: The region of Normandy bursts with sights both related and unrelated to D-Day. Because it's hard to

invasion, west of Le Havre, are best visited with a guide.

• **Rouen:** About halfway to Paris on the train line, this city (with a cobbled old town and historic ties to Joan of Arc) is worth a day.

• **More Normandy:** With a driver or on an excursion, you can reach other points in Normandy—such as **Caen** (top-notch D-Day Museum), **Bayeux** (historic tapestry), and the evocative pilgrim town of **Mont St-Michel.** Another popular choice for art and garden lovers is **Giverny,** whose water lily ponds inspired Monet. (For details on all of these, see the sidebar above.) I wouldn't recommend any of these by public transit.

The Port of Le Havre

Arrival at a Glance: Ride a cruise-line shuttle bus or walk about 35 minutes from the port to the train/bus station; from there, connect to Paris (2.5 hours by train), Rouen (1 hour by train), or Honfleur (30 minutes by bus).

efficiently link the destinations (especially the D-Day beaches) using public transportation, a guided excursion (or a privately arranged guide) can be a smart choice.

Le Havre itself may be offered as a tour, but you might as well see it on your own using the tips in this chapter. Adorable **Honfleur,** with its colorful harbor and historic ties to Impressionist painters such as Boudin and Monet, is the nearest attraction to Le Havre (just a 30-minute drive; also doable by public bus). Trips to the so-called **Alabaster Coast** north of Le Havre (including the chalky cliffs at Etrétat—which inspired several Impressionists, and the salty fishing harbor of Fécamp) are pretty but lack the impact of other options.

The **D-Day beaches,** where the Allies came ashore on June 6, 1944, are farther away but well worth touring. Excursions often include some beaches, the **American Cemetery, Arromanches** (the tiny seafront town that became the staging area for the invasion), and the **Longues-sur-Mer** gun battery. The city of **Caen** has the definitive museum about Operation Overlord.

A few more-distant sights eat up lots of transit time, and are only occasionally offered as an excursion. Bayeux, just beyond the D-Day beaches, houses the famous **Bayeux Tapestry,** a remarkable, intricately woven medieval masterwork detailing another invasion—the Battle of Hastings in 1066. The famous castaway abbey at **Mont St-Michel,** connected to the mainland only by a tenuous causeway, is understandably touristy.

Port Overview

Le Havre's cruise port is located at Pointe de Floride, which is flanked by two piers: Roger Meunier Pier and Pierre Callet Pier. Both feed into a spacious, modern terminal building with Internet access, car rental, bike rental, a gift shop, and WCs. Port information: www.cruiselehavre.com.

Tourist Information: There's a TI right at the **cruise terminal.** Pick up a map of the city, info on local and regional sights, and current train and bus schedules. You can also rent bicycles here (€6/5 hours, €10/day, requires ID or €200 credit-card deposit). The main TI in Le Havre (described later), rents bikes for less.

GETTING INTO LE HAVRE AND TO THE TRAIN/BUS STATION

Le Havre's cruise port is about a mile and a half from the train station (to the northeast) or downtown (due north). While you can walk through industrial port areas into town (figure about 35 minutes), most cruise lines offer a shuttle bus. (Shuttle bus drop-off

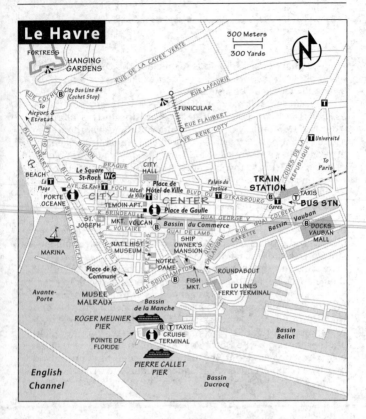

points vary by company.) Taxis are also readily available at the port (charging €8 to most points in town). Once in Le Havre, you can hop a train to Paris or Rouen, or a bus to Honfleur.

Step 1: From the Cruise Port to Downtown Le Havre

To make the short trip from your ship to downtown Le Havre, you can either take the shuttle bus, walk, or pay for a taxi. The first two options are outlined in detail below.

By Cruise-Line Shuttle Bus

Most cruise ships provide a shuttle bus (sometimes free, sometimes for a fee) that takes you to different stops in Le Havre. I've listed tips for each one. For the train/bus station, get off either at the station itself or at Les Docks; for in-town sightseeing, consider Quai de Southampton or Place Général de Gaulle.

Train/Bus Station: Ideally, your shuttle bus will drop you here—with easy connections to Paris, Rouen, Honfleur, and elsewhere.

Les Docks: This giant complex houses performance space,

Services near the Port of Le Havre

ATMs: While there are no ATMs at the terminal, you'll find one inside the train/bus station and another across the street. If you're walking from the port into the city center, the nearest ATM is at the post office on the left-hand side of Rue de Paris, just up the street from Quai de Southampton (directly across the harbor from the cruise terminal).

Internet Access: You can get online at the Internet stations in the terminal building (pay for access code at souvenir shop); there's no Wi-Fi at the terminal.

Pharmacy: The nearest pharmacy to the port is at 27 Rue du Général Faidherbe, one block up from the first roundabout as you leave the port area (toward downtown). Several more are downtown (including one on Rue de Paris, across from Notre-Dame Cathedral). French pharmacies are generally open Monday-Friday 9:00-12:30 and 14:30-19:30, Saturday 9:00-12:30, and are closed Sunday.

Car Rental: The terminal's **Rent-A-Car** agency often runs out of cars by midmorning, making it smart to book ahead (tel. 02 35 41 76 76, www.rentacar.fr, le_havre@rentacar.fr). Lining the nearby Quai de Southampton, across the harbor from the cruise port, are **Europcar** (at #51, tel. 02 35 25 21 95, www.europcar.fr) and **National/Citer** (at #91, tel. 02 35 21 30 81, www.citer.fr). All are closed on Sunday.

Other Services: The TIs at the terminal and on Boulevard Clemenceau rent **bikes.** The TIs also have information about **aquatic activities** such as kayaking, fishing, or sailing.

Tramway: Le Havre's sleek **tram** zips silently through the city center (from the train station west to City Hall, the inviting Square St-Roch, and Porte Océane near the TI and beach). While it's not useful for getting into town from the port, the tram can be handy for sightseers who stick around Le Havre. For details, ask at the TI.

the Docks Vauban shopping mall, a movie theater, restaurants, and a supermarket. The train/bus station is an easy five-minute walk from here, across the harbor canal to the north: Cross the water on the skinny Passerelle Hubert Raoul Duval footbridge, continue straight through a few crosswalks, and you'll arrive on the bus station side of the train/bus station.

Quai de Southampton: This embankment hemming in the northern edge of the port area is a convenient stop if you are heading to the **Malraux Museum** (a fine Impressionist museum). Other nearby sights include the Baroque-style **Cathédrale de Notre Dame du Havre,** the **Ship Owner's Mansion,** and the **Natural History Museum** (housed in the former Palace of Justice). Also nearby are the post office (with ATM) and a couple of rental-car offices.

PARIS

Place Général de Gaulle: This square—right in the heart of town—is graced by the proud, yet solemn, Monument Aux Morts (erected in 1924 to honor WWI casualties). Across the street, you'll see the big, white, tub-shaped Le Volcan, dubbed *le pot de yaourt* ("the yogurt pot") by locals. It's the city's cultural center for music, theater, dance, and cinema. Most sightseeing is south and west of here; the **market** is just one block west on Rue Voltaire.

By Foot

Walking into town takes about 35 minutes (25 minutes to the roundabout at the port's edge, another 10 minutes to the town center or train/bus station): Turn right out of the terminal, look left for the *centre-ville* sign, and follow it. Green pedestrian-area stripes guide you along the length of the pier. After the second bridge, turn left, continuing to follow signs for *centre-ville* (and passing the LD Lines ferry terminal on your right). Eventually, you'll come to the roundabout; from here, important places around town are well-marked. To get to the **city center,** bear left through the roundabout. To get to the **train/bus station,** bear right through the roundabout onto Quai Casimir Delavigne, staying on the right side of the street (along the water). Turn right onto Rue André Carette, which becomes Quai Colbert (follow signs for *gares*). Finally, turn left on the wide Cours de la République; after a block, the train station is on your right (the ugly concrete box marked *Gare du Havre/SNCF*), with the bus station just behind it.

Step 2: From Le Havre's Train/Bus Station to Paris, Rouen, Honfleur, or Other Points

From the train/bus station, you can make your way to anywhere in northern France. The train station *(gare)* and bus station *(gare routière)* are conveniently located side by side. (Facing the front entrance of the train station, the bus station is directly to the right of and behind the train station.)

Train Connections: For regional trips (to Rouen or Caen, for example), you may be able to buy tickets from the yellow machines (may accept American credit cards). To buy a ticket to destinations farther afield—such as Paris—or if you prefer speaking with a human or paying cash, you can buy tickets at the *guichets* (ticket windows). Before boarding the train, validate your ticket at the slender yellow ticket puncher near the doors leading to the train tracks. If you're tight on time, you can hop on the train and buy a ticket from the conductor on board—but find him before he finds you (to avoid a hefty fine).

Trains leave about every 1-2 hours for **Paris** (arriving at St. Lazare station, 2.5 hours); all of these also stop in **Rouen** (station called "Rouen-Rive-Droite," 1 hour). A few Paris connections require a change in Rouen, and fast TGV trains require an advance reservation). Be aware that on weekends there are fewer trains. For schedules, see the French rail website at www.sncf.com.

Bus Connections: From Le Havre's bus station, buses #20, #39, and #50 go over the Normandy Bridge to **Honfleur** (4-6/day Mon-Sat, 2/day on Sun, 30 minutes, www.busverts.fr). Bus #39 continues on to **Caen** (1-2/day, 1.5 hours total; otherwise you can reach Caen by a slower train connection via Rouen).

For tips on what to do when you arrive in Paris, see page 1045. For Rouen, see page 1129; for Honfleur, see page 1115.

OTHER OPTIONS

In addition to the options explained above, consider these ways to reach downtown Le Havre, Paris, or elsewhere.

By Taxi

Taxis wait to the right as you exit the cruise terminal. A ride to anywhere in the Le Havre city center (including to the train/bus station) costs about €8. Taxis waiting at the cruise port or train station offer "discovery tours," with some commentary en route, for the following round-trip rates (these are approximate prices for up to 4 people): Around Le Havre (1.5 hours)—€60; Etrétat (3 hours)—€125; Honfleur (3 hours)—€125; Rouen (6 hours)— €280; Giverny (6 hours)—€340; Normandy (8 hours)—€320; Versailles (8 hours)—€395; D-Day Beaches (8 hours)—€450; Mont St-Michel (10 hours)—€460; Paris (10 hours)—€460

While most cabbies speak a bit of English, some are more fluent than others; if you're paying for a tour, feel free to chat with several drivers to assess their language abilities before choosing. Note: These cabbies may provide information, but they're not trained guides. Most drivers belong to **Radio Taxi Le Havre** (tel. 02 35 25 81 00, www.radiotaxi-lehavre.com).

By Cruise-Line Shuttle Bus to Paris

Most cruise lines offer a Paris On Your Own excursion, which consists of an unnarrated bus ride to a designated point in Paris (generally near Place de la Concorde, between the Champs-Elysées and the Louvre), then back again at an appointed time. While the price is hefty compared to public transit (typically $110-130, compared with about $85 for the round-trip train), some cruisers appreciate the efficiency and the lack of stress about making it back to the ship on time. For tips on arriving via shuttle bus in Paris, see page 1048.

By Tour

The Le Havre TI can help you arrange a private guide in town.

PARIS

Normandy Sightseeing Tours can pick you up at the ship, and offers a variety of tours, including Paris, Bayeux/Caen, Mont St-Michel, various D-Day itineraries, Monet-themed tours, and more (tel. 02 31 51 70 52, www.normandy-sightseeing-tours.com). For other tour options for the D-Day beaches, see page 1124.

For information on local tour options in Paris—including local guides for hire, walking tours, and bus tours on the Seine—see page 1058.

RETURNING TO YOUR SHIP

If you're returning from **Paris** to Le Havre, be sure to leave plenty of time. Trains leave Paris' St. Lazare Station for Le Havre about every two hours and take about 2.5 hours (confirm and double-check the departure time of your return train before you head out), plus the time it takes to get back to your ship from the Le Havre train station. To get to St. Lazare from central Paris, hop a taxi, ride the Métro (line 14/purple stops near Notre-Dame, but many other lines also reach the station), or take bus #24 (which stops at Notre-Dame, the Orsay, and Place de la Concorde); either way, get off at the stop called "Gare Saint-Lazare."

Shuttle-bus excursions from your cruise line will tell you when and where to meet them for the trip back; most use Place de la Concorde.

Back at the **Le Havre** train/bus station, the easiest choice is to spring for a **taxi** (€8; you'll find them at the bus station end of the complex), or ride your cruise line's **shuttle bus** back to your ship (catch the bus where you got off earlier).

If you prefer to **walk,** allow about 35 minutes: Leaving the train station, turn left and head toward the water on Cours de la République. Go straight across to the water side of Quai Colbert, turn right, and follow the street (with the water on your left) as it becomes Rue André Carette. Turn left at Quai Casimir Delavigne; at the roundabout, bear left to continue toward the port (passing the LD Lines ferry terminal). After crossing the bridge, turn right and look for green stripes on the ground—these mark the pedestrian route back to the terminal.

For information on Le Havre's **bus and tram systems,** see www.transports-lia.fr (French only).

If you have time to kill before heading back, see the options described under "Sights in Le Havre," later.

See page 1139 for help if you miss your boat.

PARIS

Le Havre

A city of 180,000, Le Havre is France's second-biggest port (after Marseille), and the primary French port on the Atlantic. Its name (pronounced "luh ahv") means, simply, "The Port." Situated at the mouth of the Seine River (which also flows through Paris), Le Havre faces the English Channel and the British Isles. Its sprawling port area—harboring industrial, leisure, and cruise ships—stretches along the northern bank of the Seine.

Le Havre is proud of its connection to the Impressionist painters who found inspiration in this part of France, and nine panels scattered around town show Impressionist depictions of real-world locations (ask the TI for a pamphlet identifying these). Fittingly, the city's best sight is the fine Impressionist collection at the Malraux Museum. Le Havre was bombed to bits in World War II, and rebuilt (by local hero Auguste Perret) in an old-meets-modern style that lacks charm. But the city is a useful springboard for northern France and Paris.

PLANNING YOUR TIME

A full day in port is more than you need to fully experience Le Havre, and allows you to see it at a relaxed pace. If you decide to stick around, visit the Malraux Museum, dip into your choice of other museums, visit St. Joseph Church, browse the market, consider a stroll through the Hanging Gardens, or relax at the beach. Any of these activities can take as little or as long as you like.

TOURIST INFORMATION

The full-service **main TI** is at the western edge of town, between the marina and the beach (daily July-Aug 9:00-19:00, Sept-June 9:30-12:30 & 14:00-18:30; Wi-Fi and Internet access—free for up to 20 minutes, get code from desk; 186 Boulevard Clemenceau, tel. 02 32 74 04 04, www.le-havre-tourism.com). Another TI is **downtown,** a block straight ahead from the City Hall park at 181 Rue de Paris (tel. 02 35 22 31 22). There's also a TI at the port.

Sights in Le Havre

Cruisers who skip the trip to Paris find that Le Havre has several worthwhile sights of its own. While none of these can match the thrills of Paris, if you're in the mood to stick around town, here are some ideas to fill your day.

▲Malraux Museum (a.k.a. "MuMa")

Named for the former Minister of Culture, André Malraux, this delightfully airy and modern space is home to a superb

PARIS

Le Havre Experiences for Cruisers

To experience the city like a local, stop by **Les Halles Centrales** indoor market, featuring stalls selling fresh produce, fresh-made deli foods, baked goods, regional specialties, and more (one block west of Le Volcan on Rue Voltaire, Mon-Sat 8:30-19:30, Sun 9:00-13:00). On Sunday mornings, Les Halles Centrales' parking lot hosts a farmers market.

Bring your freshly purchased picnic on a 10-minute walk north to **Le Square St-Roch** (at the corner of Avenue Foch and Rue Raoul Dufy)—a serene oasis in the middle of the city—where you can park yourself on a bench or a patch of grass, enjoy your lunch, and watch as families, workers on break, wise grandmothers, and couples in love go by. This park is dappled with wistful willows that tickle a petite pond, flamboyant flowers, humble statues, and play areas for children. WCs are available on the east end, not far from the entrance.

For a more competitive experience, try your hand at *pétanque*, the French cousin to American horseshoes and Italian *bocce*. The best place is at the small, gravelly square called **Place de la Commune** (near the Malraux Museum, on the corner of Boulevard François I and Rue Jeanne d'Arc). In the afternoons, you'll often find crusty old fishermen and their not-yet-crusty descendants playing this traditional French game. Don't be shy—ask if you can join in for a round or two.

collection of works by Impressionist biggies who lived and worked in Normandy: Monet, Renoir, Degas, Manet, Courbet, Cézanne, Camille Corot, and others. It also boasts the world's largest collection of works by Eugène Boudin, Monet's mentor. While it may not quite live up to its billing as the "finest Impressionist collection in France outside Paris," it's certainly worthwhile for art lovers. It lacks the wall-to-wall crowds of Paris' Musée d'Orsay, creating a wonderful opportunity to get up close and personal with quality examples of late 19th- and early 20th-century artwork. Beyond the Impressionists, the collection spans five centuries, from the 16th century up to modern works by Matisse and Pierre Bonnard. Take a break and enjoy sea views in their restaurant or tea room.

Cost and Hours: €5, Wed-Mon 11:00-18:00, Sat-Sun until 19:00, closed Tue, 2 Boulevard Clemenceau, tel. 02 35 19 62 62, www.muma-lehavre.fr.

St. Joseph Church

Built in the 1950s, this church serves as a memorial to the 5,000 Le Havre civilians who died during World War II. Its 350-foot-tall octagonal tower (which resembles a Chicago skyscraper more than a steeple) is *the* dominant structure on Le Havre's skyline. The stark, somber, Neo-Gothic interior is worth a quick visit only to appreciate its Greek-cross floor plan and to peer up inside the tower. On a sunny day, the whimsical play of light through its 13,000 panels of stained glass is delightful.

Cost and Hours: Free, daily 9:00-17:30 except during services, at corner of Boulevard François I and Rue Louis Brindeau.

Ship Owner's Mansion (La Maison de l'Armateur)

This historic building offers a glimpse into the 18th-century lifestyle of a wealthy Le Havre citizen. Five stories of furnishings, artwork, and collectibles evoke life in this port city from 1750 to 1870. The rooms are arranged around an octagonal, vertical space reminiscent of the St. Joseph Church tower.

Cost and Hours: €5, includes obligatory guided tour in French (English pamphlet provided); Wed 14:00-18:00, Thu-Mon 11:00-12:30 & 13:30-18:00, closed Tue; 3 Quai de l'Ile, tel. 02 35 19 09 85.

Témoin Apartment (L'Appartement Témoin Perret)

At the 1947 World's Fair, architect and urban planner André Perret presented a "show flat" to illustrate his vision for how Le Havre could be rebuilt after having been pummeled by WWII bombs. Today, this replica of that apartment is still smartly decorated with period furniture, appliances, knickknacks, and products. It's cute but skippable—particularly since the required guided tours are only in French.

Cost and Hours: €3, includes obligatory tour in French; Wed and Sat-Sun at 14:00, 15:00, 16:00, and 17:00; additional tour departures mid-June-mid-Sept, 181 Rue de Paris, tel. 02 35 22 31 22.

▲Hanging Gardens (Les Jardins Suspendus)

For nature enthusiasts who need a break from shipboard life, this fine park—about two miles north of the port—is the place. The grass-topped walls of a former fortress enclose a massive complex, with splendid city and beach views that invite you to wander and explore. Inside the fort are more gardens, along with extensive greenhouses that feature plants from five continents. The gardens are popular with picnickers and often host special events.

Cost and Hours: Free, €1 to enter greenhouses, April-Sept daily 10:30-20:00, shorter hours off-season, Rue du Fort, tel. 02 35 19 45 45.

Getting There: It's easiest by taxi (€8 each way from the port), but prearrange a pickup to avoid getting stranded. You can also take bus #3 (to Cochet or A. Copieux).

Beach

On a sunny day, relax at Le Havre's pebbly beach (at the western edge of town, just north of the main TI). Bring your flip-flops (better than going barefoot on pebbles) and find your own patch of beach (the tempting cabanas are usually rented monthly or yearly). While working on your tan, enjoy the view of dozens of sailboats gliding across the water. The boardwalk offers all types of tasty treats, plus activities and services including bike rentals, water equipment rentals, volleyball, *pétanque*, WCs, and showers (most open April-Sept). You can get there by taxi or tram.

NEAR LE HAVRE
▲Normandy Bridge (Pont de Normandie)
The 1.25-mile-long Normandy Bridge is the longest cable-stayed bridge in the Western world. This is a key piece of European expressway that links the Atlantic ports from Belgium to Spain. Consider visiting the bridge's free Exhibition Hall (under toll-booth on Le Havre side, daily 8:00-19:00). The Seine finishes its winding 500-mile journey here, dropping only 1,500 feet from its source, 450 miles away. The river flows so slowly that, in certain places, a stiff breeze can send it flowing upstream.

▲Etrétat
France's answer to the White Cliffs of Dover, these chalky cliffs soar high above a calm, crescent beach. Walking trails lead hikers from the small seaside resort of Etrétat along a vertiginous route with sensational views (and crowds of hikers in summer and on weekends). You'll recognize these cliffs—and the arches and stone spire that decorate them—from countless Impressionist paintings, including several at the Eugène Boudin Museum in Honfleur. The small, Coney Island-like town holds plenty of cafés and a **TI** (Place Maurice Guillard, tel. 02 35 27 05 21, www.etretat.net).

Getting There: Etrétat is north of Le Havre. To get here by car, cross the Normandy Bridge and follow A-29, then exit at *sortie Etrétat*. Buses serve Etrétat from Le Havre's *gare routière*, adjacent to the train station (5/day, 1 hour, www.keolis-seine-maritime.com).

Paris

Paris has been a beacon of culture for centuries. As a world capital of art, fashion, food, literature, and ideas, it stands as a symbol of all the fine things human civilization can offer. Come prepared to celebrate this, rather than judge our cultural differences, and you'll capture the romance and *joie de vivre* that this city exudes.

PLANNING YOUR TIME

Of course, "seeing" Paris in just a few hours is in-Seine. But if that's all the time you have, here are your most likely choices:

• **Historic Paris Walk:** My self-guided stroll orients you to the city's core (Ile de la Cité, Notre-Dame, Latin Quarter, Sainte-Chapelle) in about four hours.

• **Louvre:** While art lovers could spend all day at one of the world's great museums, a targeted visit can take two hours. You can tack on a visit to the nearby **Orangerie** (a misty world of Monet's water lilies) in about an hour.

• **Orsay:** This sumptuous collection of Impressionist art can be seen succinctly in two hours.

• **Eiffel Tower:** If you reserve ahead to avoid the long line (see page 1093), you can zip to the top of Paris' most iconic structure, and back down, in two hours; to save time, do only the first level.

• **Arc de Triomphe and Champs-Elysées:** On a quick visit, you can stroll down Paris' finest boulevard in about an hour (or even less, if you only do the more interesting upper half, to Rond Pont). Add an hour to ascend to the top of the Arc de Triomphe.

• **Other Museums and Sights:** With a special interest, consider some of Paris' other excellent museums, including Rodin, Picasso, Army Museum/Napoleon's Tomb, Marmottan Museum, Cluny Museum, and more. The Montmartre neighborhood (surrounding Sacré-Cœur basilica) and the Luxembourg Garden are also fine places to explore. Any of these destinations can take at least an hour or two.

On a brief visit, you'll need to be very selective. Choose just two or three options, and take geography and public-transit connections into account to be as efficient as possible. The best first-time visit plan may be the Historic Paris Walk, followed by a visit to the Louvre or Orsay.

Orientation to Paris

Central Paris (population 2.2 million) is circled by a ring-road and split in half by the Seine River, which runs east to west. If you were on a boat floating downstream, the Right Bank (Rive Droite)

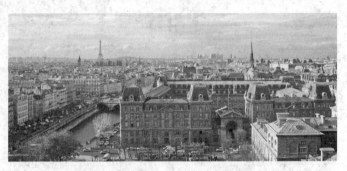

would be on your right, and the Left Bank (Rive Gauche) on your left. The bull's-eye on your map is Notre-Dame, on an island in the middle of the Seine.

Twenty arrondissements (administrative districts) spiral out from the center, like an escargot shell. The city is speckled with Métro stops, and most Parisians locate addresses by the closest stop. So in Parisian jargon, the Eiffel Tower is on *la Rive Gauche* (the Left Bank) in the *7ème* (7th arrondissement), zip code 75007, Mo: Trocadéro (the nearest Métro stop).

As you're tracking down addresses, these words and pronunciations will help: Métro (may-troh), *place*

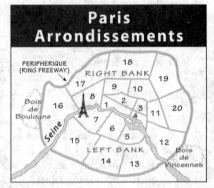

(plahs; square), *rue* (roo; road), *avenue* (ah-vuh-noo), *boulevard* (boo-luh-var), and *pont* (pohn; bridge).

TOURIST INFORMATION

Paris' TIs can provide useful information but may have long lines. They offer free city maps and, for those who ask, themed booklets on eating, shopping, or walking in Paris (also available online—go to http://en.parisinfo.com and click on "Practical Paris," then "Our Paris Cityguides"). TIs sell Museum Passes and individual tickets to sights (see "Sightseeing Strategies" on page 1064).

Paris has several TI locations, including **Pyramides** (daily May-Oct 9:00-19:00, Nov-April 10:00-19:00, 25 Rue des Pyramides—at Pyramides Métro stop between the Louvre and Opéra), **Gare du Nord** (daily 8:00-18:00), **Gare de Lyon** (Mon-Sat 8:00-18:00, closed Sun), and two in **Montmartre** (21 Place du Tertre, daily 10:00-18:00, covers only Montmartre sights and doesn't sell Museum Passes, tel. 01 42 62 21 21; and at the Anvers Métro stop, full-service office,

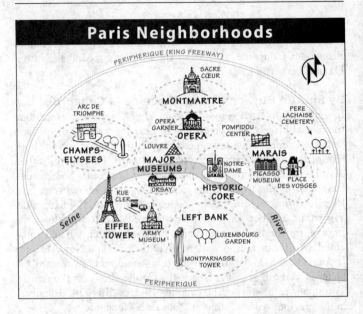

Paris Neighborhoods

daily 10:00-18:00). In summer, TI kiosks may pop up in the squares in front of Notre-Dame and Hôtel de Ville. The official website for Paris' TIs is www.parisinfo.com.

Pariscope: The weekly €0.50 *Pariscope* magazine (or one of its clones, available at any newsstand) lists museum hours, art exhibits, concerts, festivals, plays, movies, and nightclubs. Smart sightseers rely on this for the latest listings.

Helpful Websites: These websites come highly recommended for local information on events, restaurants, and other happenings: www.gogoparis.com, www.secretsofparis.com, www.bonjourparis.com, and www.parisbymouth.com.

ARRIVAL IN PARIS
By Train at St. Lazare Station (Gare St. Lazare)

All trains from Le Havre arrive and depart at this compact station, about a mile north of the river. Trains are one floor above street level. Trains to and from Le Havre use tracks 23-27; from here, it's a long, well-signed walk from the tracks to the Métro. The ticket office is near track 27; train information offices *(accueil)* are scattered about the station. St. Lazare Station also has a three-floor shopping mall.

To head straight to Notre-Dame to begin my self-guided Historic Paris Walk, your best bet is to either take the Métro (faster, but it's a longer walk to Notre-Dame) or the bus (which drops you closer to the cathedral). Take the **Métro** line 14 (purple) south (direction: Olympiades), and ride three stops to Châtelet;

this stop is three short blocks north of the river and Ile de la Cité. **Bus #24** departs from in front of the station and goes to Madeleine, Place de la Concorde, the Orsay, the Louvre, St. Michel, Notre-Dame, and beyond.

By Shuttle Bus, on or near Place de la Concorde

If you arrive in Paris via an On Your Own shuttle-bus excursion, the bus will likely drop you off on or near the square called Place de la Concorde, which is wedged between the Louvre and the bottom of the grand Champs-Elysées boulevard. From here, it's an easy 15- to 20-minute **walk** to either the Louvre or (just across the river) the Orsay. From the nearby Concorde **Métro** stop, line 1 (yellow) makes things easier: Ride it in direction: Château de Vincennes, and hop off at the second stop, Palais Royal-Musée du Louvre, for the Louvre's entrance; a few stops later, Châtelet and Hôtel de Ville are a short walk north of the river and Notre-Dame. If you ride this Métro line in the opposite direction, toward La Défense, you can get off at Charles de Gaulle-Etoile for the Arc de Triomphe, at the start of the Champs-Elysées. **Bus #24,** described in the previous section, stops at Place de la Concorde.

HELPFUL HINTS

Theft Alert: Thieves thrive near famous monuments and on Métro and RER lines that serve airports and high-profile tourist sights. Beware of pickpockets working busy lines (e.g., at ticket windows at train stations). Pay attention when it's your turn and your back is to the crowd: Keep your bag closed and firmly gripped in front of you. Look out for groups of young girls who swarm around you (be very firm—even forceful—and walk away). Smartphones are a thief magnet anytime, so be aware whenever you're using it or holding it up to take a picture.

In general, it's smart to wear a money belt, put your wallet in your front pocket, loop your day bag over your shoulders, and keep a tight hold on your purse or shopping bag. Muggings are rare, but they do occur. If you're out late, avoid the dark riverfront embankments and any place where the lighting is dim and pedestrian activity is minimal.

Paris has taken action to combat crime by stationing police at monuments, on streets, and on the Métro, and installing security cameras at key sights. You'll go through quick and reassuring airport-like security checks at many major attractions.

Tourist Scams: Be aware of the latest tricks, such as the "found ring" scam (i.e., a con artist pretends to find a ring on the ground that he proclaims is "pure gold" and offers to sell it to you) or the "friendship bracelet" scam (a vendor asks you to help with a demo, makes a bracelet on your arm that you can't easily take off, and then asks you to pay for it).

Distractions by a stranger—often a "salesman," someone asking you to sign a petition, or someone posing as a deaf person to show you a small note to read—can all be tricks that function as a smokescreen for theft. As you try to wriggle away from the pushy stranger, an accomplice picks your pocket.

To all these scammers, simply say "no" firmly (without smiling or apologizing) and step away purposefully. For reports from my readers on the latest scams, go to https://community.ricksteves.com/travel-forum/tourist-scams.

Pedestrian Safety: Parisian drivers are notorious for ignoring pedestrians. Look both ways (many streets are one-way), and be careful of seemingly quiet bus/taxi lanes. Don't assume you have the right of way, even in a crosswalk. When crossing a street, keep your pace constant and don't stop suddenly. By law, drivers are allowed to miss pedestrians by up to just one meter—a little more than three feet (1.5 meters in the countryside). Drivers calculate your speed so they won't hit you, provided you don't alter your route or pace.

Watch out for bicyclists and electric cars. These popular and silent "vehicles" may come at you from unexpected places and directions. Cyclists ride in specially marked bike lanes on wide sidewalks and also have a right to use lanes reserved for buses and taxis. Bikes commonly go against traffic, as many bike paths are on one-way streets. Always look both ways. Paris' popular and cheap short-term electric-car rental program (Autolib') has put many of these small, silent machines on the streets—be careful.

Busy Parisian sidewalks are much like freeways, so conduct yourself as if you were a foot-fueled-car: Stick to your lane, look to the left before passing a slow-moving pedestrian, and if you need to stop, look for a safe place to pull over.

Medical Help: The American Hospital, established by a group of American expat doctors, has English-speaking staff (63 Boulevard Victor Hugo, in Neuilly suburb, Mo: Porte Maillot, then bus #82, tel. 01 46 41 25 25, www.american-hospital.org).

Avoiding Lines at Sights: Lines at Paris' major sights can be long. The Paris Museum Pass, which covers most sights in the city and allows you to skip ticket lines, is sold at museums and monuments, as well as TIs and FNAC stores (no surcharge). For cruisers, the Museum Pass may not be worth the cost, but there are other ways to save time in line, such as buying tickets in advance at certain sights. For information on all of these options, see page 1064.

PARIS

Free Wi-Fi: You'll find free wireless hotspots at many of Paris' cafés (with a purchase) and at more than 200 public hotspots (including parks, squares, museums, and so on). In a Parisian café, Wi-Fi works just like at home—you order something, then ask the waiter for the Wi-Fi ("wee-fee") password (*"mot de passe"*; moh duh pahs).

Most public parks offer free Wi-Fi (look for purple *Zone Wi-Fi* signs). The one-time registration process is easy: Select the Wi-Fi network (usually called "Paris_WIFI" plus a number), enter your name and email address, check the *"j'accepte"* box, and click *"Me connecter."* You get two hours per connection. Some convenient hotspots include the park alongside Notre-Dame, Square Viviani (also near Notre-Dame), Place des Vosges (Marais), Champ de Mars park (100 yards south of the Eiffel Tower along Allée Thomy-Thierry), Esplanade des Invalides (along Rue Paul at the north end), the St. Jacques Tower (Mo: Chatelet), and hundreds more.

The Orange network also has many hotspots and offers a free two-hour pass. If you come across one, click "Select Your Pass" to register.

Public WCs: Most public toilets are free. If it's a pay toilet, the price will be clearly indicated. If the toilet is free but there's an attendant, it's polite (but not necessary) to leave a tip of €0.20-0.50. Booth-like toilets on the sidewalks provide both relief and a memory (don't leave small children inside unattended). The restrooms in museums are free and the best you'll find. Bold travelers can walk into any sidewalk café like they own the place and find the toilet downstairs or in the back. Or do as the locals do—order a shot of espresso *(un café)* while standing at the café bar (then use the WC with a clear conscience). Keep toilet paper or tissues with you, as some WCs are poorly stocked.

Tobacco Stands *(Tabacs):* These little kiosks—usually just a counter inside a café—are handy and very local. Most sell public-transit tickets, cards for parking meters, postage stamps (though not all sell international postage—to mail something home, use two domestic stamps, or go to a post office), prepaid phone cards, and...oh yeah, cigarettes. To find one of these kiosks, just look for a *Tabac* sign and the red cylinder-shaped symbol above certain cafés. A *tabac* can be a godsend for avoiding long ticket lines at the Métro, especially at the end of the month when ticket booths get crowded with locals buying next month's pass.

Updates to This Book: For updates to this book, check www.ricksteves.com/update.

PARIS

GETTING AROUND PARIS

Paris is easy to navigate. Your basic choices are Métro (in-city subway), RER (suburban rail tied into the Métro system), public bus, and taxi. (Also consider the hop-on, hop-off bus and boat tours, described under "Tours in Paris," later.)

You can buy tickets and passes at Métro stations and at many *tabacs*. Staffed ticket windows in stations are gradually being phased out in favor of ticket machines, so expect some stations to have only machines and an information desk. Machines accept coins or small bills of €20 or less (none takes American credit cards unless you have a chip-and-PIN card). If a ticket machine is out of order or if you're out of change, buy tickets at a *tabac*.

Public-Transit Tickets: The Métro, RER, and buses all work on the same tickets. You can make as many transfers as you need on a single ticket, except when transferring between the Métro/RER system and the bus system, which requires using an additional ticket. A **single ticket** costs €1.70. If planning to use multiple tickets, buy a *carnet* (kar-nay) of 10 tickets for €13.70 (cheaper for ages 4-10). *Carnets* can be shared among travelers. Kids under four ride free. A handy one-day bus/Métro pass (called **Mobilis**) is available for €6.80.

By Métro

In Paris, you're never more than a 10-minute walk from a Métro station. Europe's best subway system allows you to hop from sight to sight quickly and cheaply (runs Sun-Thu 5:30-24:30, Fri-Sat 5:30-2:00 in the morning, www.ratp.fr). Learn to use it.

Using the Métro System: To get to your destination, determine the closest "Mo" stop and which line or lines will get you

there. The lines are color-coded and numbered, and you can tell their direction by their end-of-the-line stops. For example, the La Défense/Château de Vincennes line, also known as line 1 (yellow), runs between La Défense, on its west end, and Vincennes on its east end. Once in the Métro station, you'll see the color-coded line numbers and/or blue-and-white signs directing you to the train going in your direction (e.g., *direction: La Défense*). Insert your ticket in the automatic turnstile, reclaim your ticket, pass through, and keep it until you exit the system (some stations require you to pass your ticket through a turnstile to exit). The smallest stations are unstaffed and have ticket machines (coins are essential). Be warned that fare inspectors regularly check for

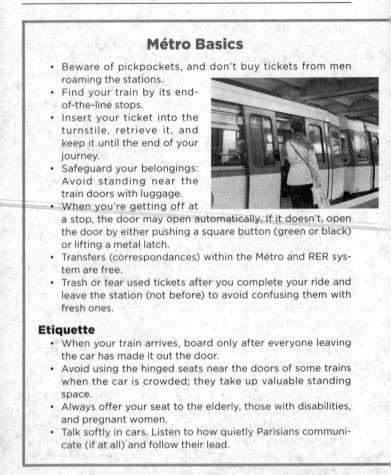

Métro Basics

- Beware of pickpockets, and don't buy tickets from men roaming the stations.
- Find your train by its end-of-the-line stops.
- Insert your ticket into the turnstile, retrieve it, and keep it until the end of your journey.
- Safeguard your belongings: Avoid standing near the train doors with luggage.
- When you're getting off at a stop, the door may open automatically. If it doesn't, open the door by either pushing a square button (green or black) or lifting a metal latch.
- Transfers (correspondances) within the Métro and RER system are free.
- Trash or tear used tickets after you complete your ride and leave the station (not before) to avoid confusing them with fresh ones.

Etiquette

- When your train arrives, board only after everyone leaving the car has made it out the door.
- Avoid using the hinged seats near the doors of some trains when the car is crowded; they take up valuable standing space.
- Always offer your seat to the elderly, those with disabilities, and pregnant women.
- Talk softly in cars. Listen to how quietly Parisians communicate (if at all) and follow their lead.

cheaters and accept absolutely no excuses—keep that ticket or pay a minimum fine of €45.

Be prepared to walk significant distances within Métro stations (especially when you transfer). Transfers are free and can be made wherever lines cross, provided you do so within 1.5 hours. When you transfer, follow the appropriately colored line number and end-of-the-line stop to find your next train, or look for orange *correspondance* (connection) signs that lead to your next line.

When you reach your destination, look for the blue-and-white *sortie* signs pointing you to the exit. Before leaving the station, check the helpful *plan du quartier* (map of the neighborhood) to get your bearings. At stops with several *sorties*, you can save time by choosing the best exit.

After you finish the entire ride and exit onto the street, toss or tear your used ticket so you don't confuse it with unused tickets.

- When standing, hold on to the bar with one hand, leaving room for others while stabilizing yourself so you don't tumble or step on neighboring toes.
- If you find yourself blocking the door at a stop, step out of the car to let others off, then get back on.
- Métro doors close automatically. Don't try to hold open the door for late-boarding passengers.
- On escalators and stairs, keep to the right and pass on the left.
- When leaving a station, hold the door for the person behind you.

Key Words for the Métro and RER

French	Pronounced	English
direction	dee-rek-see-ohn	direction
ligne	leen-yuh	line
correspondance	kor-res-pohn-dahns	connection/transfer
sortie	sor-tee	exit
carnet	kar-nay	discounted set of 10 tickets
Pardon, madame/ monsieur.	par-dohn, mah-dahm/mes-yur	Excuse me, ma'am/ sir.
Je descends.	juh day-sahn	I'm getting off.
Rendez-moi mon porte-monnaie!	rahn-day-mwah mohn port-moh-nay	Give me back my wallet!

Métro Resources: Métro maps are free at Métro stations and included on freebie Paris maps available around town. Several good online tools can also help you navigate the public-transit system. The website Metro.paris provides an interactive map of Paris' sights and Métro lines, with a trip-planning feature and information about each sight and station's history (www.metro.paris). The free RATP mobile app (in English, download at www.ratp.fr) and the more user-friendly Kemtro app ($2, www.kemtro.com) can estimate Métro travel times, help you locate the best station exit, and tell you when the next bus will arrive, among other things. Just be careful when using your smartphone in any crowded area, as it can attract thieves.

Beware of Pickpockets: Thieves dig the Métro and RER. Be on guard. If your pocket is picked as you pass through a turnstile, you end up stuck on the wrong side (after the turnstile bar

PARIS

has closed behind you) while the thief gets away. Stand away from Métro doors to avoid being a target for a theft-and-run just before the doors close. Any jostling or commotion—especially when boarding or leaving trains—is likely the sign of a thief or a team of thieves in action. Make any fare inspector show proof of identity (ask locals for help if you're not certain). Keep your bag close, and never show anyone your wallet.

By RER

The RER (Réseau Express Régionale; air-ay-air) is the suburban arm of the Métro, serving outlying destinations such as Versailles, Disneyland Paris, and the airports. These routes are indicated by thick lines on your subway map and identified by the letters A, B, C, and so on.

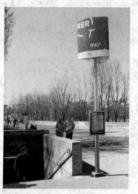

On a short visit from Le Havre, you're unlikely to use the RER for distant locations, but you may use it to zip between points in town. Within the city center, the RER works like the Métro and can be speedier if it serves your destination directly, because it makes fewer stops. Métro tickets are good on the RER when traveling in the city center. You can transfer between the Métro and RER systems with the same ticket. But to travel outside the city (to Versailles, for example), you'll need a separate, more expensive ticket. Unlike the Métro, not every train stops at every station along the way; check the sign or screen over the platform to see if your destination is listed as a stop (*"toutes les gares"* means it makes all stops along the way), or confirm with a local before you board. For RER trains, you may need to insert your ticket in a turnstile to exit the system.

By City Bus

Buses require less walking and fewer stairways than the Métro, and you can see Paris unfold as you travel. Bus stops are everywhere, and every stop comes with all the information you need: a good city bus map, route maps showing exactly where each bus that uses this stop goes, a frequency

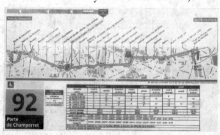

PARIS

chart and schedule, and a *plan du quartier* map of the immediate neighborhood (www.ratp.fr). Bus-system maps are also available in any Métro station (and in the €6.50 *Paris Pratique* map book sold at newsstands).

Using the Bus System: Buses use the same tickets and passes as the Métro and RER. One Zone 1 ticket buys you a bus ride

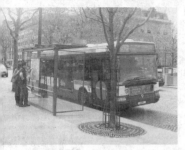

anywhere in central Paris within the freeway ring road *(le périphérique)*. Use your Métro ticket or buy one on board for €0.30 more, though note that tickets bought on board are *sans correspondance*, which means you can't use them to transfer to another bus.

Board your bus through the front door. (Families with strollers can use any doors—the ones in the center of the bus are wider. To open the middle or back doors on long buses, push the green button located by those doors.) Validate your ticket in the machine and reclaim it. Keep track of what stop is coming up next by following the onboard diagram or listening to recorded announcements. When you're ready to get off, push the red button to signal you want a stop, then exit through the central or rear door. Even if you're not certain you've figured out the system, do some joyriding.

More Bus Tips: Avoid rush hour (Mon-Fri 8:00-9:30 & 17:30-19:30), when buses are jammed and traffic doesn't move. Not all city buses are air-conditioned, so they can become rolling greenhouses on summer days. *Carnet* ticket holders—but not those buying individual tickets on the bus—can transfer from one bus to another on the same ticket (within 1.5 hours, revalidate your ticket on the next bus), but you can't do a round-trip or hop on and off on the same line. You can use the same ticket to transfer between buses and tramlines, but you can't transfer between the bus and Métro/RER systems (it'll take two tickets).

By Taxi

Parisian taxis are reasonable, especially for couples and families. The meters are tamper-proof. Fares and supplements (described in English on the rear windows) are straightforward and tightly regulated.

A taxi can fit three people comfortably. Cabbies are legally required to accept four passengers, though they don't always like it. If you have five in your group, you can book a larger taxi in advance, or try your luck at a taxi stand. Beyond three passengers, expect to pay €3 extra per person.

Rates: All Parisian taxis start with €2.60 on the meter and

Scenic Buses for Tourists

Of Paris' many bus routes, these are some of the most scenic. They provide a great, cheap, and convenient introduction to the city.

Bus #69 crosses the city east-west, passing these great sights and neighborhoods: Eiffel Tower, Rue Cler, Les Invalides (Army Museum and Napoleon's Tomb), Louvre Museum, Ile de la Cité, Ile St. Louis, Hôtel de Ville, Pompidou Center, Marais, Bastille, and Père Lachaise.

Bus #87 also links the Marais and Rue Cler areas, but stays mostly on the Left Bank, connecting the Eiffel Tower, St. Sulpice Church, Luxembourg Garden, St. Germain-des-Prés, the Latin Quarter, the Bastille, and Gare de Lyon.

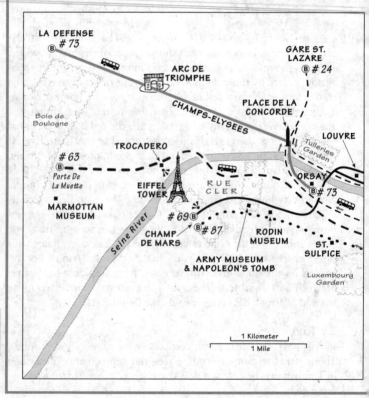

Bus #24 runs east-west along the Seine riverbank from Gare St. Lazare to Madeleine, Place de la Concorde, Orsay Museum, the Louvre, St. Michel, Notre-Dame, and Jardin des Plantes, all the way to Bercy Village (cafés and shops).

Bus #63 is another good east-west route, connecting the Marmottan Museum, Trocadéro (Eiffel Tower), Pont de l'Alma, Orsay Museum, St. Sulpice Church, Luxembourg Garden, Latin Quarter/Panthéon, and Gare de Lyon.

Bus #73 is one of Paris' most scenic lines, starting at the Orsay Museum and running westbound around Place de la Concorde, then up the Champs-Elysées, around the Arc de Triomphe, and down Avenue Charles de Gaulle to La Défense.

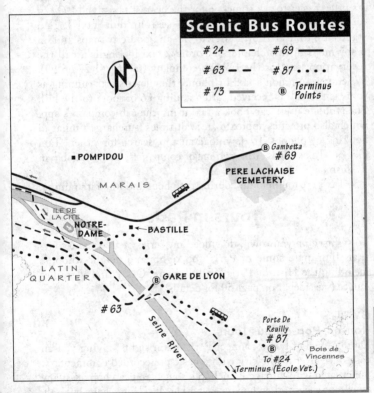

Scenic Bus Routes

# 24 – – –	# 69 ——
# 63 – –	# 87 ••••
# 73 ▬▬▬	Ⓑ Terminus Points

■ POMPIDOU

MARAIS

Ⓑ Gambetta #69

PERE LACHAISE CEMETERY

ILE DE LA CITÉ

NOTRE-DAME

■ BASTILLE

LATIN QUARTER

Ⓑ GARE DE LYON

63

Seine River

Porte De Reuilly #87

Ⓑ

To #24 Terminus (École Vet.)

Bois de Vincennes

have a minimum charge of €6.86. A 20-minute ride (e.g., Bastille to the Eiffel Tower) costs about €20 (versus about €1.40/person to get anywhere in town using a *carnet* ticket on the Métro or bus). Drivers charge higher rates at rush hour, at night, all day Sunday, and for extra passengers. Each piece of luggage that goes in the trunk is €1 extra (no fee for the first bag; charge won't appear on the meter, but it is legitimate). To tip, round up to the next euro (at least €0.50). The A, B, or C lights on a taxi's rooftop sign correspond to hourly rates, which vary with the time of day and day of the week (for example, the A rate of €32/hour applies Mon-Sat 10:00-17:00). Tired travelers need not bother with these mostly subtle differences in fares—if you need a cab, take it.

How to Catch *un Taxi:* You can try waving down a taxi, but it's often easier to ask someone for the nearest taxi stand (*"Où est une station de taxi?";* oo ay ewn stah-see-ohn duh "taxi"). Taxi stands are indicated by a circled "T" on good city maps and on many maps in this chapter. To order a taxi in English, call the reservation line for the G7 cab company (tel. 01 41 27 66 99). When you summon a taxi by phone, the meter starts running as soon as the call is received, often adding €6 or more to the bill. Smartphone users can book a taxi using the cab company's app, which also provides approximate wait times (surcharge similar to booking by phone). To download an app, search for either "Taxi G7" or "Taxis Bleus" (the two major companies, both available in English).

Taxis are tough to find during rush hour and when it's raining.

Tours in Paris

To sightsee on your own, download my series of free audio tours that illuminate some of Paris' top sights and neighborhoods, including the Historic Paris Walk, Louvre, Orsay, and Versailles Palace (see sidebar on page 50 for details).

BY BUS
Hop-on, Hop-off Bus Tours

Double-decker buses connect Paris' main sights, giving you an easy once-over of the city with a basic prerecorded commentary, punctuated with vintage French folk songs. You can hop off at any stop, tour a sight, then hop on a later bus. It's dang scenic, but only if you get a top-deck seat and the weather's decent—otherwise, the trip may not be worth it. Because of traffic and stops, these buses can be dreadfully slow. (Busy sightseers will do better using the Métro to connect sights.) On the plus side, because the buses move so slowly, you have time to read my sight descriptions, making this a decent orientation tour.

Of the several different hop-on, hop-off bus companies, **L'OpenTour** is best. They offer frequent service on four routes covering all of central Paris. You can even transfer between routes with one ticket. Look up the various routes and stops either on their website or by picking up a brochure (available at any TI or on one of their bright yellow buses). Their Paris Grand Tour (green route) offers the best introduction and most frequent buses (every 10 minutes). Other routes run a bit less frequently (every 15-30 minutes). You can catch the bus at just about any major sight, such as the Eiffel Tower (look for the Open Bus icon on public transit bus shelters and signs). Buy your tickets from the driver (1 day-€32, 2 days-€36, 3 days-€40, kids 4-11-€16 for 1 or 2 days, allow 2 hours per route, tel. 01 42 66 56 56, www.parislopentour.com). A combo-ticket also covers the Batobus boats, described later (1 day-€41, 2 days-€45, 3 days-€49, kids 4-11-€20 for 2 or 3 days).

Big Bus Paris runs a fleet of buses around Paris on a route with just 10 stops and recorded narration (1 day-€29, 2 days-€33, kids 4-12-€16, 10 percent cheaper if you book online, tel. 01 53 95 39 53, www.bigbustours.com).

Paris' cheapest "bus tour" is simply to hop on **city bus #69** and enjoy the sights as they roll by (see sidebar on page 1056).

BY BOAT
Seine Cruises

Several companies run one-hour boat cruises on the Seine. While best at night, these can also be enjoyable during the daytime. Some offer discounts for early online bookings.

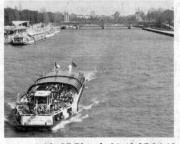

Bateaux-Mouches, the oldest boat company in Paris, departs from Pont de l'Alma's right bank and has the biggest open-top, double-decker boats (higher up means better views). But this company caters to tour groups, making their boats jammed and noisy (€12.50, kids 4-12-€5.50, tel. 01 42 25 96 10, www.bateaux-mouches.fr).

Bateaux Parisiens has smaller covered boats with handheld audioguides, fewer crowds, and only one deck. It leaves from right in front of the Eiffel Tower (€13, kids 3-12-€5, tel. 01 76 64 14 45, www.bateauxparisiens.com).

Vedettes du Pont Neuf offers essentially the same one-hour tour as the other companies, but starts and ends at Pont Neuf. The boats feature a live guide whose delivery (in English and French) is as stiff as a recorded narration—and as hard to understand, given the quality of their sound system (€14, ask about discount

PARIS

if you book direct with this book, discounts for online bookings, kids 4-12 pay €7, tip requested, tel. 01 46 33 98 38, www.vedettesdupontneuf.com).

Hop-on, Hop-off Boat Tour

Batobus allows you to get on and off as often as you like at any of eight popular stops along the Seine. The boats, which make a continuous circuit, stop in this order: Eiffel Tower, Orsay Museum, St. Germain-des-Prés, Notre-Dame, Jardin des Plantes, Hôtel de Ville, the Louvre, and Pont Alexandre III, near the Champs-Elysées (1 day-€15, 45 minutes one-way, 1.5-hour round-trip, www.batobus.com). If you use this for getting around—sort of a scenic, floating alternative to the Métro—it can be worthwhile, but if you just want a guided boat tour, the Seine cruises described earlier are a better choice.

ON FOOT
Walking Tours

Paris Walks offers a variety of two-hour walks, led by British and American guides. Tours are thoughtfully prepared and entertaining. Don't hesitate to stand close to the guide to hear (€12-15, generally 2/day—morning and afternoon, private tours available, family guides and Louvre tours are a specialty, call 01 48 09 21 40 for schedule in English or check printable online schedule at www.paris-walks.com). Tours focus on the Marais (4/week), Montmartre (3/week), medieval Latin Quarter (Mon), Ile de la Cité/Notre-Dame (Mon), the "Two Islands" (Ile de la Cité and Ile St. Louis, Wed), the Revolution (Tue), and Hemingway's Paris (Fri). Call a day or two ahead to hear the current schedule and starting point. Most tours don't require reservations, but specialty tours—such as the Louvre, fashion, or chocolate tours—require advance reservations and prepayment with credit card (deposits aren't refundable).

Context Travel offers "intellectual by design" walking tours geared for serious learners. The tours are led by docents (historians, architects, and academics) and cover both museums and specific neighborhoods. They range from traditional topics such as French art history in the Louvre and the Gothic architecture of Notre-Dame to more thematic explorations like immigration and the changing face of Paris, jazz in the Latin Quarter, and the history of the baguette. It's best to book in advance—groups are limited to six participants and can fill up fast (€60-100/person, admission to sights extra, generally 3 hours, tel. 09 75 18 04 15, US tel. 800-691-6036, www.contexttravel.com).

Classic Walks' lowbrow, lighter-on-information but high-on-fun walking tours are run by Fat Tire Bike Tours. Their 3.5-hour

Classic Walk covers most major sights (€20, usually at 10:00—see website for days of week; meet at their office at 24 Rue Edgar Faure, Mo: Dupleix, tel. 01 56 58 10 54, http://paris.classicwalks.com). They also offer neighborhood walks of Montmartre, the Marais, and the Latin Quarter, as well as themed walks on the French Revolution (€20, tours run several times a week—see website for details). The company promises a €2 discount on all walks with this book (two-discount maximum per book).

Easy Pass (also operated by Fat Tire Bike) offers skip-the-line interior tours of major sights, including the Louvre, Notre-Dame Tower, Eiffel Tower, Orsay, Sainte-Chapelle, and the Picasso Museum (€40-85/person, includes entry and guided tour). Reservations are required and can be made on their website, by phone, or in person at their Easy Pass office near the Eiffel Tower (daily 9:00-18:00, longer hours in high season, 36 Avenue de la Bourdonnais, Mo: Ecole Militaire, tel. 01 56 58 10 54, http://paris.easypasstours.com). They also offer a skip-the-line Eiffel Tower pass without an interior tour for €40—handy if you weren't able to get advance tickets directly from the Eiffel Tower website.

Local Guides

For many, Paris merits hiring a Parisian as a personal guide. **Thierry Gauduchon** is a terrific guide and a gifted teacher (€230/half-day, €450/day, tel. 06 19 07 30 77, tgauduchon@gmail.com). **Sylvie Moreau** also leads good tours in Paris (€200 for 3 hours, €320 for 7 hours, tel. 01 46 07 96 28, mobile 06 87 02 80 67, sylvie.ja.moreau@gmail.com). **Arnaud Servignat** is a fine guide who has taught me much about Paris (private tours starting at €190, also does car tours of the countryside around Paris for a little more, mobile 06 68 80 29 05, www.french-guide.com, arnotour@me.com). **Elisabeth Van Hest** is another likable and very capable guide (€200/half-day, tel. 01 43 41 47 31, mobile 06 77 80 19 89, elisa.guide@gmail.com). **Sylviane Ceneray** is gentle and knowledgeable (€200/half-day, tel. 06 84 48 02 44, www.paris-asyoulikeit.com).

Food Tours

Dig deeper into Paris' food scene on a culinary walking tour. Visit markets, shop at specialty stores, and sample food at locals' favorite eateries.

Friendly Canadian **Rosa Jackson** designs personalized "Edible Paris" itineraries based on your interests and three-hour "food-guru" tours of Paris led by her or one of her two colleagues (unguided itineraries from €125, guided tours—€300 for 1 person, €150/person for 2-3 people, €100/person for 4-6 people, mobile 06 81 67 41 22, www.edible-paris.com, rosa@rosajackson.com).

Paris By Mouth offers more casual and frequent small

Paris at a Glance

▲▲▲**Notre-Dame Cathedral** Paris' most beloved church, with towers and gargoyles. **Hours:** Cathedral—daily 7:45-18:45, Sun until 19:30; Tower—daily April-Sept 10:00-18:30, Fri-Sat until 23:00 in July-Aug, Oct-March 10:00-17:30. See page 1068.

▲▲▲**Sainte-Chapelle** Gothic cathedral with peerless stained glass. **Hours:** Daily March-Oct 9:30-18:00, Wed until 21:30 mid-May-mid-Sept, Nov-Feb 9:00-17:00. See page 1073.

▲▲▲**Louvre** Europe's oldest and greatest museum, starring *Mona Lisa* and *Venus de Milo*. **Hours:** Wed-Mon 9:00-18:00, Wed and Fri until 21:45, closed Tue. See page 1079.

▲▲▲**Orsay Museum** Europe's greatest Impressionist collection. **Hours:** Tue-Sun 9:30-18:00, Thu until 21:45, closed Mon. See page 1086.

▲▲▲**Eiffel Tower** Paris' soaring exclamation point. **Hours:** Daily mid-June-Aug 9:00-24:45, Sept-mid-June 9:30-23:45. See page 1092.

▲▲▲**Champs-Elysées** Paris' grand boulevard. **Hours:** Always open. See page 1098.

▲▲**Orangerie Museum** Monet's water lilies, plus works by Utrillo, Cézanne, Renoir, Matisse, and Picasso, in a lovely setting. **Hours:** Wed-Mon 9:00-18:00, closed Tue. See page 1092.

▲▲**Rue Cler** Ultimate Parisian market street. **Hours:** Stores open Tue-Sat 8:30-13:00 & 15:00-19:30, Sun 8:30-12:00, dead on Mon. See page 1096.

▲▲**Army Museum and Napoleon's Tomb** The emperor's imposing tomb, flanked by museums of France's wars. **Hours:** Daily 10:00-18:00, July-Aug until 19:00, Nov-March until 17:00; tomb

PARIS

group tours, with a maximum of seven foodies per group. Tours are organized by location or flavor and led by local food writers (€95/3 hours, includes tastings, www.parisbymouth.com, tasteparisbymouth@gmail.com).

ON WHEELS
Bike Tours

A bike tour is a fun way to see Paris. Two companies—Bike About Tours and Fat Tire Bike Tours—offer tours and bike maps of Paris, and give good advice on cycling routes in the city. Their tour

plus WWI and WWII wings open Tue until 21:00 April-Sept; museum (except for tomb) closed first Mon of month Oct-June; Charles de Gaulle exhibit closed Mon year-round. See page 1096.

▲▲**Rodin Museum** Works by the greatest sculptor since Michelangelo, with many statues in a peaceful garden. **Hours:** Tue-Sun 10:00-17:45, Wed until 20:45, closed Mon. See page 1097.

▲▲**Marmottan Museum** Untouristy art museum focusing on Monet. **Hours:** Tue-Sun 10:00-18:00, Thu until 20:00, closed Mon. See page 1097.

▲▲**Cluny Museum** Medieval art with unicorn tapestries. **Hours:** Wed-Mon 9:15-17:45, closed Tue. See page 1098.

▲▲**Arc de Triomphe** Triumphal arch with viewpoint, marking start of Champs-Elysées. **Hours:** Interior—daily April-Sept 10:00-23:00, Oct-March 10:00-22:30. See page 1100.

▲▲**Picasso Museum** World's largest collection of Picasso's works. **Hours:** Tue-Fri 11:30-18:00, Sat-Sun 9:30-18:00, until 21:00 third Fri of month, closed Mon. See page 1102.

▲▲**Pompidou Center** Modern art in colorful building with city views. **Hours:** Wed-Mon 11:00-21:00, closed Tue. See page 1102.

▲▲**Sacré-Cœur and Montmartre** White basilica atop Montmartre with spectacular views. **Hours:** Daily 6:00-22:30; dome climb daily May-Sept 9:00-19:00, Oct-April 9:00-17:00. See page 1103.

▲**Carnavalet Museum** Paris' history wrapped up in a 16th-century mansion. **Hours:** Tue-Sun 10:00-18:00, closed Mon. See page 1101.

routes cover different areas of the city, so avid cyclists could do both without much repetition.

Run by Christian (American) and Paul (New Zealander), **Bike About Tours** offers easygoing tours with a focus on the eastern half of the city. Their four-hour tours run daily year-round at 10:00 (also at 15:00 June-Sept). You'll meet at the statue of Charlemagne in front of Notre-Dame, then walk to the nearby rental office to get bikes. The tour includes a good back-street visit of the Marais, Rive Gauche outdoor sculpture park, Ile de la Cité, heart of the Latin Quarter (with a lunch break), Louvre,

Les Halles, and Pompidou Center. Group tours have a 12-person maximum—reserve online to guarantee a spot, or show up and take your chances (€30, €5 discount with this book, maximum 2 discounts per book, includes helmets upon request, private tours available, tel. 06 18 80 84 92, www.bikeabouttours.com).

Run by a gang of young anglophone expats, **Fat Tire Bike Tours** offers an extensive program of bike, Segway, and walking tours (see Classic Walks listing, earlier). Their young guides run four-hour bike tours of Paris (adults-€32, kids-€30, show this book to get a €4 discount per person, maximum 2 discounts per book, reservations recommended but not required—you can also just show up, especially in off-season). Kid-sized bikes are available, as are tandem attachments that hook on to a parent's bike. On the day tour, you'll pedal with a pack of 10-20 riders, mostly in parks and along bike lanes, with a lunch stop in the Tuileries Garden (tours leave daily rain or shine at 11:00, April-Oct also at 15:00). Tours meet at the exit of the Dupleix Métro station near the Eiffel Tower; from there you'll walk to the nearby Fat Tire office to pick up bikes (helmets available upon request at no extra charge, tel. 01 56 58 10 54, http://paris.fattirebiketours.com).

Sightseeing Strategies

If you plan ahead, you can avoid many of the lines that tourists suffer through in Paris.

PARIS MUSEUM PASS

This sightseeing pass admits you to many of Paris' most popular sights (€42 for a 2-day pass, no 1-day version). The pass covers most recommended Paris sights except the Eiffel Tower, Picasso Museum, Marmottan Museum, Notre-Dame Treasury, and Sacré-Cœur's dome. Most importantly, the pass lets you skip ticket-buying lines at most sights. If you're in town for just a few hours, you'll have to sightsee like crazy to get your money's worth. Still, it might be worth the price of purchase just to skip long lines (but keep in mind you can also prebuy line-skipping tickets for a few individual sights—described next). Add up the costs of the sights you'll realistically have time to visit during your day in town, compare that with the cost of the pass, weigh the likelihood that you'll waste time standing in ticket lines, and decide. The pass is sold at participating sights, FNAC department stores, and TIs. Avoid buying the pass at a major museum (such as the Louvre), where supply can be spotty and lines long. For more info, visit www.parismuseumpass.com or call 01 44 61 96 60.

To use your pass at sights, look for signs designating the entrance for prereserved ticket holders. If it's not obvious, boldly walk to the front of the ticket line (after going through security if necessary), hold up your pass, and ask the ticket taker: *"Entrez, pass?"* (ahn-tray pahs). You'll either be allowed to enter at that point, or you'll be directed to a special entrance. Don't be shy—some places (Orsay Museum and the Arc de Triomphe, in particular) have long lines in which passholders wait needlessly.

OTHER TICKET-BUYING OPTIONS

For some sights, you can **buy tickets online** at their official website. This is essential at the Eiffel Tower, which isn't covered by the Museum Pass and is plagued by long lines in peak season (note that you must choose an entry time when booking). You can also book tickets online for the Orsay, Rodin Museum, and Picasso Museum.

TIs and FNAC department stores sell individual *"coupe-file"* **tickets** (pronounced "koop-feel") for some sights, which allow you to use the Museum Pass entrance (worth the trouble only for the most important sights where lines are longest). TIs sell these tickets for no extra fee, but FNACs add a surcharge of 10-20 percent. FNAC stores are everywhere, even on the Champs-Elysées. Despite the surcharges and often-long lines to buy them, getting *coupe-file* tickets can still be a good idea.

Fat Tire Bike Tours offers **Easy Pass** skip-the-line tickets or tours of major sights, including the Louvre, Notre-Dame Tower, Eiffel Tower, Orsay, Sainte-Chapelle, and Picasso Museum (for details, see page 1061 or visit http://paris.easypasstours.com).

Some sights, such as the Louvre, have **ticket-vending machines** that save time in line. Note that these only accept cash (usually no bills larger than €20) or chip-and-PIN cards. At certain sights, including the Louvre and Orsay, **nearby shops** sell tickets, allowing you to avoid the main ticket lines (for details, see the Louvre and Orsay Museum listings).

Historic Paris Walk

PARIS

This information is distilled from the Historic Paris Walk chapter in *Rick Steves Paris*, by Rick Steves, Steve Smith, and Gene Openshaw. You can download a free Rick Steves audio version of this walk; see page 50.

• *You'll start where the city did—on the Ile de la Cité, the island in the Seine River and the physical and historic bull's-eye of your Paris map. The closest Métro stops are Cité, Hôtel de Ville, and St. Michel, each a short walk away.*

Allow four hours to do justice to this three-mile self-guided walk, beginning at the Notre-Dame Cathedral and ending at Pont Neuf; just follow the dotted line on the "Historic Paris Walk" map.

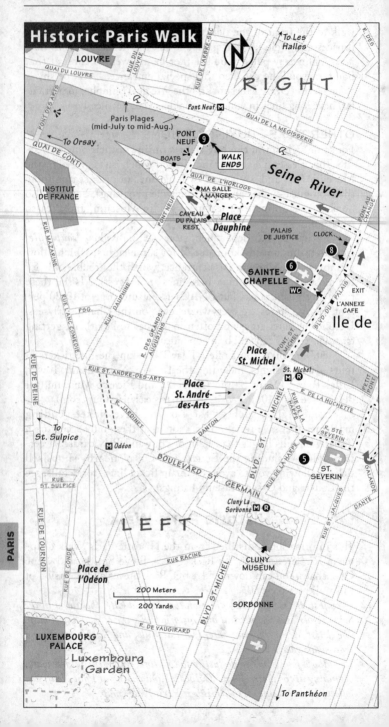

Historic Paris Walk

LOUVRE

QUAI DU LOUVRE

R. DU LOUVRE

R. DE L'ARBRE-SEC

R. DES

To Les Halles

RIGHT

QUAI DE LA MEGISSERIE

Pont Neuf Ⓜ

Paris Plages (mid-July to mid-Aug.)

To Orsay

QUAI DE CONTI

BOATS

PONT NEUF ❾

WALK ENDS

QUAI DE L'HORLOGE

Seine River

INSTITUT DE FRANCE

PONT NEUF

MA SALLE À MANGER

CAVEAU DU PALAIS REST.

Place Dauphine

PALAIS DE JUSTICE

CLOCK

PONT AU CHANGE

❽

RUE MAZARINE

RUE DAUPHINE

PSG

SAINTE-CHAPELLE ❻

WC

EXIT

L'ANNEXE CAFE

Ile de

RUE ANC. COMEDIE

RUE DES GRANDS-AUGUSTINS

BLVD. DU PALAIS

Place St. Michel

RUE ST. ANDRE-DES-ARTS

Place St. André-des-Arts

St. Michel Ⓜ Ⓡ

R. DE LA HUCHETTE

RUE DE SEINE

R. JARDINET

R. DANTON

PONT ST. MICHEL

BLVD. ST. MICHEL

R. DE LA HARPE

R. STE. SEVERIN

PETIT PONT

To St. Sulpice

Ⓜ Odéon

BOULEVARD ST. GERMAIN

❺

ST. SEVERIN

RUE ST. JACQUES

DANTE

GALANDE

RUE ST. SULPICE

Cluny La Sorbonne Ⓜ Ⓡ

LEFT

RUE RACINE

CLUNY MUSEUM

RUE DE CONDE

RUE DE TOURNON

Place de l'Odéon

200 Meters

200 Yards

SORBONNE

BLVD. ST. MICHEL

LUXEMBOURG PALACE

Luxembourg Garden

R. DE VAUGIRARD

To Panthéon

PARIS

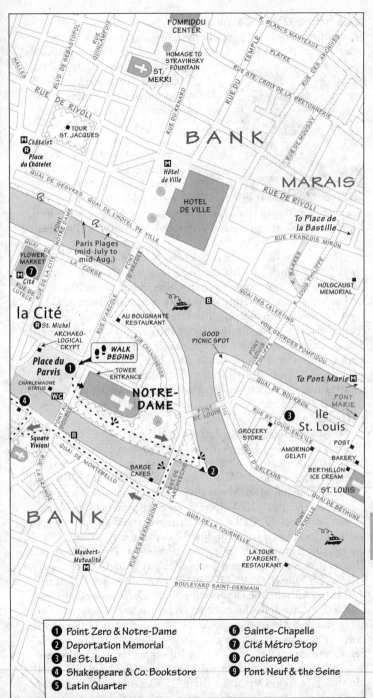

POMPIDOU CENTER

HOMAGE TO STRAVINSKY FOUNTAIN

ST. MERRI

R. BLANCS MANTEAUX

PLATRE

RUE DES ARCHIVES

RUE DU TEMPLE

RUE STE. CROIX DE LA BRETONNERIE

RUE DU RENARD

HALLES

RUE BLVD. DE SEBASTOPOL

RUE QUINCAMPOIX

RUE DE RIVOLI

TOUR ST. JACQUES

M Châtelet

R Place du Châtelet

BANK

RUE DE MOUSSY

Hôtel de Ville

M

QUAI DE GESVRES

QUAI DE L'HOTEL DE VILLE

HOTEL DE VILLE

MARAIS

RUE DE RIVOLI

To Place de la Bastille →

RUE FRANÇOIS MIRON

Paris Plages (mid-July to mid-Aug.)

QUAI DE LA CORSE

PONT NOTRE-DAME

PONT D'ARCOLE

R. BARRES

R. LOUIS PHILIPPE

FLOWER MARKET

M **7** Cité

RUE DE LUTECE

QUAI DES CELESTINS

VOIE GEORGES POMPIDOU

HOLOCAUST MEMORIAL

la Cité

R St. Michel

ARCHAEO-LOGICAL CRYPT

RUE D'ARCOLE

AU BOUGNANTE RESTAURANT

RUE CHANOINESSE

GOOD PICNIC SPOT

PONT LOUIS PHILIPPE

To Pont Marie **M**

Place du Parvis **1**

WALK BEGINS

TOWER ENTRANCE

NOTRE-DAME

QUAI DE BOURBON

PONT MARIE

CHARLEMAGNE STATUE

WC

4

PONT AU DOUBLE

RUE ST. LOUIS-EN-L'ILE

Ile St. Louis **3**

Square Viviani

B

QUAI DE MONTEBELLO

BARGE CAFES

PONT ST. LOUIS

PONT DE L'ARCHEVECHE

GROCERY STORE

QUAI D'ORLEANS

2

POST

AMORINO GELATI

BAKERY

BERTHILLON ICE CREAM

ST. LOUIS

RUE LA GRANGE

BANK

RUE DES BERNARDINS

QUAI DE LA TOURNELLE

PONT TOURNELLE

QUAI DE BETHUNE

Maubert-Mutualité **M**

LA TOUR D'ARGENT RESTAURANT

BOULEVARD SAINT-GERMAIN

PARIS

1 Point Zero & Notre-Dame
2 Deportation Memorial
3 Ile St. Louis
4 Shakespeare & Co. Bookstore
5 Latin Quarter

6 Sainte-Chapelle
7 Cité Métro Stop
8 Conciergerie
9 Pont Neuf & the Seine

▲▲▲Notre-Dame Cathedral

For centuries, the main figure in the Christian pantheon has been Mary, the mother of Jesus. Catholics petition her in times of trou-

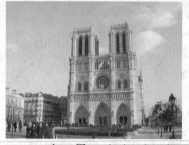

ble to gain comfort, and to ask her to convince God to be compassionate with them. The church is dedicated to "Our Lady" *(Notre Dame)*, and there she is, cradling God, right in the heart of the facade (circular window in the center), surrounded by the halo of the rose window. Though the church is massive and imposing, it has always stood for the grace and compassion of Mary, the "mother of God."

Imagine the faith of the people who built this cathedral. They broke ground in 1163 with the hope that someday their great-great-great-great-great-great grandchildren might attend the dedication Mass, which finally took place two centuries later, in 1345. Look up the 200-foot-tall bell towers and imagine a tiny medieval community mustering the money and energy for construction. Master masons supervised, but the people did much of the grunt work themselves for free—hauling the huge stones from distant quarries, digging a 30-foot-deep trench to lay the foundation, and treading like rats on a wheel designed to lift the stones up, one by one. This kind of backbreaking, arduous manual labor created the real hunchbacks of Notre-Dame.

Cost and Hours: Cathedral—free, daily 7:45-18:45, Sun until 19:30; **Treasury**—€4, not covered by Museum Pass, Mon-Fri 9:30-18:00, Sat 9:30-18:30, Sun 13:30-18:40; audioguide-€5, free English tours—normally Wed-Thu at 14:00, Sat-Sun at 14:30.

The cathedral hosts **Masses** several times daily (early morning, noon, evening), plus Vespers at 17:45. The international Mass is held Sun at 11:30. Call or check the website for a full schedule. On Good Friday and the first Friday of the month at 15:00, the (physically underwhelming) relic known as Jesus' **Crown of Thorns** (Couronne d'Epines) goes on display (Mo: Cité, Hôtel de Ville, or St. Michel; tel. 01 42 34 56 10, www.notredamedeparis.fr).

Tower Climb: The entrance for Notre-Dame's tower climb is outside the cathedral, along the left side. You can hike to the top of the facade between the towers and then to the top of the south tower (400 steps total) for a gargoyle's-eye view of the cathedral, Seine, and city (€8.50, covered by Museum Pass but no bypass line for passholders; daily April-Sept 10:00-18:30, Fri-Sat until 23:00 in July-Aug, Oct-March 10:00-17:30, last entry 45 minutes before closing; tel. 01 53 10 07 00, http://notre-dame-de-paris. monuments-nationaux.fr).

❷ Self-Guided Tour

"Walk this way" toward the front of the cathedral, and view it from the bronze plaque on the ground marked "Point Zero" (30 yards from the central doorway). You're standing at the center of France, the point from which all distances are measured.

Facade: Look at the left doorway, and to the left of the door, find the statue with his head in his hands. The man with the misplaced head is **St. Denis,** the city's first bishop and patron saint. He stands among statues of other early Christians who helped turn pagan Paris into Christian Paris. Sometime in the third century, Denis came here from Italy to convert the Parisii. He settled here on the Ile de la Cité, back when there was a Roman temple on this spot and Christianity was suspect. Denis proved so successful at winning converts that the Romans' pagan priests got worried. Denis was beheaded as a warning to those forsaking the Roman gods. But those early Christians were hard to keep down. The man who would become St. Denis got up, tucked his head under his arm, headed north, paused at a fountain to wash it off, and continued until he found just the right place to meet his maker: Montmartre. The Parisians were convinced by this miracle, Christianity gained ground, and a church soon replaced the pagan temple.

Medieval art was OK if it embellished the house of God and told biblical stories. For a fine example, move as close as you can get to the **base of the central column** (at the foot of Mary, about where the head of St. Denis could spit if he were really good). Working around from the left, find God telling a barely created Eve, "Have fun, but no apples." Next, the sexiest serpent I've ever makes apples à la mode. Finally, Adam and Eve, now ashamed of their nakedness, are expelled by an angel. This is a tiny example in a church covered with meaning.

Above the arches is a row of 28 statues, known as the **Kings of Judah.** In the days of the French Revolution (1789-1799), these biblical kings were mistaken for the hated French kings, and Notre-Dame represented the oppressive Catholic hierarchy. The citizens stormed the church, crying, "Off with their heads!" Plop—they lopped off the crowned heads of these kings with glee, creating a row of St. Denises that weren't repaired for decades.

Notre-Dame Interior: Enter the church at the right doorway (the line moves quickly). Be careful: Pickpockets attend church here religiously.

Notre-Dame has the typical basilica floor plan shared by so many Catholic churches: a long central **nave** lined with columns and flanked by side aisles. It's designed in the shape of a cross, with the altar placed where the crossbeam intersects. The church can hold up to 10,000 faithful, and it's probably buzzing with visitors now, just as it was 600 years ago. The quiet, deserted churches we see elsewhere are in stark contrast to the busy, center-of-life places they were in the Middle Ages.

Just past the altar is the so-called choir, the area enclosed with carved-wood walls, where more intimate services can be held in this spacious building. Looking past the altar to the far end of the choir (under the cross), you'll see a fine **17th-century *pietà***, flanked by two kneeling kings: Louis XIII (1601-1643, not so famous) and his son Louis XIV (1638-1715, very famous, also known as the Sun King, who ruled gloriously and flamboyantly from Versailles).

In the right transept, a statue of **Joan of Arc** (Jeanne d'Arc, 1412-1431), dressed in armor and praying, honors the French teen-ager who rallied her country's soldiers to try to drive English invaders from Paris. Join the statue in gazing up to the blue-and-purple, **rose-shaped window** in the opposite transept—with teeny green Mary and baby Jesus in the center—the only one of the three rose windows still with its original medieval glass.

The back side of the choir walls feature **scenes of the resurrected Jesus** (c. 1350) appearing to his followers, starting with Mary Magdalene. Their starry robes still gleam, thanks to a 19th-century renovation. The niches below these carvings mark the tombs of centuries of archbishops. Just ahead on the right is the **Treasury.** It contains lavish robes, golden reliquaries, and the humble tunic of King (and St.) Louis IX, but it probably isn't worth the entry fee.

Notre-Dame Side View: Back outside, alongside the church you'll notice the **flying buttresses.** These 50-foot stone "beams" that stick out of the church were the key to the complex Gothic architecture. The pointed arches we saw inside cause the weight of the roof to push outward rather than downward. The "flying" buttresses support the roof by pushing back inward.

Picture Quasimodo (the fictional hunchback) limping around along the railed balcony at the base of the roof among the **"gargoyles."** These grotesque beasts sticking out from pillars and buttresses represent souls caught between heaven and earth. They also function as rainspouts (from the same French root word as "gargle") when there are no evil spirits to battle.

The Neo-Gothic 300-foot **spire** is a product of the 1860 reconstruction of the dilapidated old church. Victor Hugo's book *The Hunchback of Notre-Dame* (1831) inspired a young architecture student named Eugène-Emmanuel Viollet-le-Duc to dedicate his career to a major renovation in Gothic style. Find Viollet-le-Duc at the base of the spire among the green apostles and evangelists (visible as you approach the back end of the church). The apostles look outward, blessing the city, while the architect (at top) looks up the spire, marveling at his fine work.

Nearby: The **Paris Archaeological Crypt** is an intriguing 20-minute stop. View Roman ruins from Emperor Augustus' reign (when this island became ground zero in Paris), trace the street plan of the medieval village, and see diagrams of how early Paris grew. It's all thoughtfully explained in English (pick up the floor plan with some background info) and well-presented with videos and touchscreens (€7, covered by Museum Pass, Tue-Sun 10:00-18:00, closed Mon, last entry 30 minutes before closing, enter 100 yards in front of cathedral, tel. 01 55 42 50 10, www.crypte.paris. fr).

• *Behind Notre-Dame, cross the street and enter through the iron gate into the park at the tip of the island. Look for the stairs and head down to reach the...*

▲Deportation Memorial
(Mémorial de la Déportation)

This memorial to the 200,000 French victims of the Nazi concentration camps (1940-1945) draws you into their experience. France was quickly overrun by Nazi Germany, and Paris spent the war years under Nazi occupation. Jews and dissidents were rounded up and deported—many never returned.

Cost and Hours: Free, April-Sept Tue-Sun 10:00-12:30 & 13:30-18:45, Oct-March Tue-Sun 10:00-12:00 & 13:30-17:00 (lunch closure times can vary), closed Mon year-round, may randomly close at other times; at the east tip of the island named Ile de la Cité, behind Notre-Dame and near Ile St. Louis (Mo: Cité); mobile 06 14 67 54 98.

Visiting the Memorial: As you descend the steps, the city around you disappears. Surrounded by walls, you have become a prisoner. Your only freedom is your view of the sky and the tiny glimpse of the river below. Enter the dark, single-file chamber up ahead. Inside, the circular plaque in the floor reads, "They went to the end of the earth and did not return."

The hallway stretching in front of you is lined with 200,000 lighted crystals, one for each French citizen who died. Flickering at the far end is the eternal flame of hope. The tomb of the unknown deportee lies at your feet. Above, the inscription reads, "Dedicated to the living memory of the 200,000 French deportees shrouded by the night and the fog, exterminated in the Nazi concentration camps." The side rooms are filled with triangles—reminiscent of the identification patches inmates were forced to wear—each bearing the name of a concentration camp. Above the exit as you leave is the message you'll find at many other Holocaust sites: "Forgive, but never forget."

• Back on street level, look across the river (north) to the island called...

Ile St. Louis

If Ile de la Cité is a tugboat laden with the history of Paris, it's towing this classy little residential dinghy, laden only with high-rent apartments, boutiques, characteristic restaurants, and famous ice-cream shops.

Ile St. Louis wasn't developed until much later than Ile de la Cité (17th century). What was a swampy mess is now harmonious Parisian architecture and one of Paris' most exclusive neighborhoods. Consider taking a brief detour across the pedestrian bridge, Pont St. Louis. It connects the two islands, leading right to Rue St. Louis-en-l'Ile. This spine of the island is lined with appealing shops, reasonably priced restaurants, and a handy grocery. A short stroll takes you to the famous Berthillon ice-cream parlor at #31, which is still family-owned. The ice cream is famous not just because it's good, but because it's made right here on the island. Gelato lovers can comparison-shop by also sampling the (mass-produced-but-who's-complaining) Amorino Gelati at 47 Rue St. Louis-en-l'Ile. This walk is about as peaceful and romantic as Paris gets. When you're finished exploring, loop back to the pedestrian bridge along the park-like quays (walk north to the river and turn left).

*• From the Deportation Memorial, cross the bridge to the Left Bank. Turn right after crossing the bridge and walk along the river, toward the front end of Notre-Dame. Stairs detour down to the riverbank if you need a place to picnic. This side view of the church from across the river is one of Europe's great sights and is best from river level. At times, you may find **barges** housing restaurants with great cathedral views docked here.*

*After passing the Pont au Double (the bridge leading to the facade of Notre-Dame), cross the street on your left and find **Shakespeare and Company**, an atmospheric reincarnation of the original 1920s bookshop and a good spot to page through books (37 Rue de la Bûcherie). Before returning to the island, walk a block behind Shakespeare and Company, and take a spin through...*

▲The Latin Quarter

This area's touristy fame relates to its intriguing, artsy, bohemian character. This was perhaps Europe's leading university district in the Middle Ages, when Latin was the language of higher education. The neighborhood's main boulevards (St. Michel and St. Germain) are lined with cafés—once the haunts of great poets and philosophers, now the hangouts of tired tourists. Though still youthful and artsy, much of this area has become a tourist ghetto filled with cheap North African eateries. Exploring a few blocks up or downriver from here gives you a better chance of feeling the pulse of what survives of Paris' classic Left Bank.

Walking along Rue St. Séverin, you can still see the shadow of the medieval sewer system. The street slopes into a central channel of bricks. In the days before plumbing and toilets, when people still went to the river or neighborhood wells for their water, flushing meant throwing it out the window. At certain times of day, maids on the fourth floor would holler, *"Garde de l'eau!"* ("Watch out for the water!") and heave it into the streets, where it would eventually wash down into the Seine.

Consider a visit to the **Cluny Museum** for its medieval art and unicorn tapestries (see page 1098). The **Sorbonne**—the University of Paris' humanities department—is also nearby; visitors can ogle at the famous dome, but they are not allowed to enter the building (two blocks south of the river on Boulevard St. Michel).

Don't miss **Place St. Michel.** This square (facing Pont St. Michel) is the traditional core of the Left Bank's artsy, liberal, hippie, bohemian district of poets, philosophers, and winos. In less commercial times, Place St. Michel was a gathering point for the city's malcontents and misfits. In 1830, 1848, and again in 1871, the citizens took the streets from the government troops, set up barricades *Les Miz*-style, and fought against royalist oppression. During World War II, the locals rose up against their Nazi oppressors (read the plaques under the dragons at the foot of the St. Michel fountain). Even today, whenever there's a student demonstration, it starts here.

• *From Place St. Michel, look across the river and find the prickly steeple of the Sainte-Chapelle church. Head toward it. Cross the river on Pont St. Michel and continue north along the Boulevard du Palais. On your left, you'll see the doorway to Sainte-Chapelle (usually with a line of people).*

Security is strict at the Sainte-Chapelle complex because this is more than a tourist attraction: France's Supreme Court meets to the right of Sainte-Chapelle in the Palais de Justice. Expect a long wait. First comes the security line (all sharp objects and glass are confiscated). No one can skip this line. Security lines are shortest first thing in the mornings and on weekends (when the courts are closed), and longest around 13:00-14:00 (when staff takes lunch). Once past security, you'll enter the courtyard outside Sainte-Chapelle, where you'll find WCs and the ticket-buying line—those with combo-tickets (purchased at the Conciergerie) or Museum Passes can skip this lineup. (L'Annexe Café, across the street from the main entry, sells cheap coffee to go—perfect for sipping while you wait in the security line.)

▲▲▲Sainte-Chapelle

This triumph of Gothic church architecture is a cathedral of glass like no other. It was speedily built between 1242 and 1248 for King

Louis IX—the only French king who is now a saint—to house the supposed Crown of Thorns. Its architectural harmony is due to the fact that it was completed under the direction of one architect and in only six years—unheard of in Gothic times. In contrast, Notre-Dame took over 200 years.

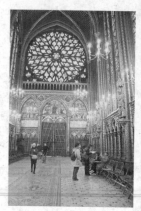

Cost and Hours: €8.50, €12.50 combo-ticket with Conciergerie, free for those under age 18, covered by Museum Pass; daily March-Oct 9:30-18:00, Wed until 21:30 mid-May-mid-Sept, Nov-Feb 9:00-17:00; last entry 30 minutes before closing, audioguide-€4.50 (€6 for two), 4 Boulevard du Palais, Mo: Cité, tel. 01 53 40 60 80, http://sainte-chapelle.monuments-nationaux.fr.

Visiting the Church: Though the inside is beautiful, the exterior is basically functional. The muscular buttresses hold up the stone roof, so the walls are essentially there to display stained glass. The lacy spire is Neo-Gothic—added in the 19th century. Inside, the layout clearly shows an *ancien régime* approach to worship. The low-ceilinged basement was for staff and other common folks—worshipping under a sky filled with painted fleurs-de-lis, a symbol of the king. Royal Christians worshipped upstairs. The paint job, a 19th-century restoration, helps you imagine how grand this small, painted, jeweled chapel was. (Imagine Notre-Dame painted like this.) Each capital is playfully carved with a different plant's leaves.

Climb the spiral staircase to the Chapelle Haute. Fill the place with choral music, crank up the sunshine, face the top of the altar, and really believe that the Crown of Thorns is there, and this becomes one awesome space.

Fiat lux. "Let there be light." From the first page of the Bible, it's clear: Light is divine. Light shines through stained glass like God's grace shining down to earth. Gothic architects used their new technology to turn dark stone buildings into lanterns of light. The glory of Gothic shines brighter here than in any other church.

There are 15 separate panels of **stained glass** (6,500 square

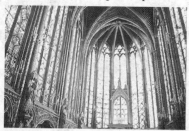

feet—two thirds of it 13th-century original), with more than 1,100 different scenes, mostly from the Bible. These cover the entire Christian history of the world, from the Creation in Genesis (first window on the left, as you

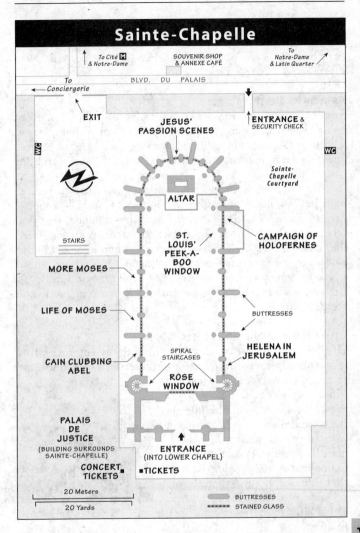

Sainte-Chapelle

To Cité Ⓜ & Notre-Dame

SOUVENIR SHOP & ANNEXE CAFÉ

To Notre-Dame & Latin Quarter

To Conciergerie

BLVD. DU PALAIS

EXIT

JESUS' PASSION SCENES

ENTRANCE & SECURITY CHECK

WC

WC

Sainte-Chapelle Courtyard

ALTAR

STAIRS

ST. LOUIS' PEEK-A-BOO WINDOW

CAMPAIGN OF HOLOFERNES

MORE MOSES

LIFE OF MOSES

BUTTRESSES

CAIN CLUBBING ABEL

SPIRAL STAIRCASES

HELENA IN JERUSALEM

ROSE WINDOW

PALAIS DE JUSTICE (BUILDING SURROUNDS SAINTE-CHAPELLE)

ENTRANCE (INTO LOWER CHAPEL)

CONCERT TICKETS

TICKETS

20 Meters

20 Yards

BUTTRESSES

STAINED GLASS

PARIS

face the altar), to the coming of Christ (over the altar), to the end of the world (the round "rose"-shaped window at the rear of the church). Each individual scene is interesting, and the whole effect is overwhelming. If you can't read much into the individual windows, you're not alone. (For some tutoring, a little book with color photos is on sale downstairs with the postcards.)

The **altar** was raised up high to better display the Crown of Thorns, the relic around which this chapel was built. The supposed crown cost King Louis more than three times as much as this church. Today, it is kept by the Notre-Dame Treasury (though it's occasionally brought out for display).

• *Exit Sainte-Chapelle. Back outside, as you walk around the church exterior, look down to see the foundation and take note of how much Paris has risen in the 750 years since Sainte-Chapelle was built. Next door to Sainte-Chapelle is the...*

Palais de Justice

Sainte-Chapelle sits within a huge complex of buildings that has housed the local government since ancient Roman times. It was the site of the original Gothic palace of the early kings of France. The only surviving medieval parts are Sainte-Chapelle and the Conciergerie prison.

Most of the site is now covered by the giant Palais de Justice, built in 1776, home of the French Supreme Court. The motto *Liberté, Egalité, Fraternité* over the doors is a reminder that this was also the headquarters of the Revolutionary government. Here they doled out justice, condemning many to imprisonment in the Conciergerie downstairs—or to the guillotine.

• *Now pass through the big iron gate to the noisy Boulevard du Palais. Cross the street to the wide, pedestrian-only Rue de Lutèce and walk about halfway down.*

Cité "Metropolitain" Métro Stop

Of the 141 original early-20th-century subway entrances, this is one of only a few survivors—now preserved as a national art treasure. (New York's Museum of Modern Art even exhibits one.) It marks Paris at its peak in 1900—on the cutting edge of Modernism, but with an eye for beauty. The curvy, plantlike ironwork is a textbook example of Art Nouveau, the style that rebelled against the erector-set squareness of the Industrial Age. 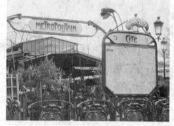 Other similar Métro stations in Paris are Abbesses and Porte Dauphine.

The flower and plant market on Place Louis Lépine is a pleasant detour. On Sundays this square flutters with a busy bird market.

• *Pause here to admire the view. Sainte-Chapelle is a pearl in an ugly architectural oyster. Double back to the Palais de Justice, turn right onto Boulevard du Palais, and enter the Conciergerie. It's free with the Museum Pass; passholders can sidestep the bottleneck created by the ticket-buying line.*

▲Conciergerie

Though pretty barren inside, this former prison echoes with

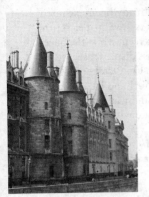

history. Positioned next to the courthouse, the Conciergerie was the gloomy prison famous as the last stop for 2,780 victims of the guillotine, including France's last *ancien régime* queen, Marie-Antoinette. Before then, kings had used the building to torture and execute failed assassins. (One of its towers along the river was called "The Babbler," named for the pain-induced sounds that leaked from it.) When the Revolution (1789) toppled the king, the building kept its same function, but without torture. The progressive Revolutionaries proudly unveiled a modern and more humane way to execute people—the guillotine. The Conciergerie was the epicenter of the Reign of Terror—the year-long period of the Revolution (1793-94) during which Revolutionary fervor spiraled out of control and thousands were killed. It was here at the Conciergerie that "enemies of the Revolution" were imprisoned, tried, sentenced, and marched off to Place de la Concorde for decapitation.

Cost and Hours: €8.50, €12.50 combo-ticket with Sainte-Chapelle, covered by Museum Pass, daily 9:30-18:00, last entry 30 minutes before closing, 2 Boulevard du Palais, Mo: Cité, tel. 01 53 40 60 80, http://conciergerie.monuments-nationaux.fr.

Visiting the Conciergerie: Pick up a free map and breeze through the one-way circuit. It's well-described in English. See the spacious, low-ceilinged Hall of Men-at-Arms (Room 1), originally a guards' dining room, with four large fireplaces (look up the chimneys). During the Reign of Terror, this large hall served as a holding tank for the poorest prisoners. Then they were taken upstairs (in an area not open to visitors), where the Revolutionary tribunals grilled scared prisoners on their political correctness. Continue to the raised area at the far end of the room (Room 4, today's bookstore). In Revolutionary days, this was notorious as the walkway of the executioner, who was known affectionately as "Monsieur de Paris."

Upstairs is a memorial room with the names of the 2,780 citizens condemned to death by the guillotine, including ex-King Louis XVI, Charlotte Corday (who murdered the Revolutionary writer Jean-Paul Marat in his bathtub), and—oh, the irony—Maximilien de Robespierre, the head of the Revolution, the man who sent so many to the guillotine.

Just past the courtyard is a re-creation of Marie-Antoinette's cell. On August 12, 1793, the queen was brought here to be tried for her supposed crimes against the people. Imagine the queen spending her last days—separated from her 10-year-old son and now widowed because the king had already been executed. Mannequins, period furniture, and the real cell wallpaper set the scene. The guard stands modestly behind a screen, while the queen psyches herself up with a crucifix. In the glass display case, see her actual crucifix, rug, and small water pitcher. On October 16, 1793, the queen was awakened at 4:00 in the morning and led away. She walked the corridor, stepped onto the cart, and was slowly carried to Place de la Concorde, where she had a date with "Monsieur de Paris."

• *Back outside, turn left on Boulevard du Palais. On the corner is the city's oldest public clock. The mechanism of the present clock is from 1334, and even though the case is Baroque, it keeps on ticking.*

Turn left onto Quai de l'Horloge and walk along the river, past "The Babbler" tower. The bridge up ahead is the Pont Neuf, where we'll end this walk. At the first corner, veer left into a sleepy triangular square called Place Dauphine. It's amazing to find such coziness in the heart of Paris. From the equestrian statue of Henry IV, turn right onto Pont Neuf. Pause at the little nook halfway across.

Pont Neuf and the Seine

This "new bridge" is now Paris' oldest. Built during Henry IV's reign (about 1600), its arches span the widest part of the river.

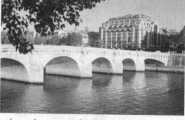

Unlike other bridges, this one never had houses or buildings growing on it. The turrets were originally for vendors and street entertainers. In the days of Henry IV, who promised his peasants "a chicken in every pot every Sunday," this would have been a lively scene. From the bridge, look downstream (west) to see the next bridge, the pedestrian-only Pont des Arts. Ahead on the Right Bank is the long Louvre museum. Beyond that, on the Left Bank, is the Orsay. And what's that tall black tower in the distance?

• *Our walk is finished. From here, you can tour the Seine by boat (the departure point for Seine River cruises offered by Vedettes du Pont Neuf is through the park at the end of the island—see page 1059), continue to the Louvre, or (if it's summer) head to the...*

▲Paris Plages (Paris Beaches)

The Riviera it's not, but this string of fanciful faux beaches—assembled in summer along a one-mile stretch of the Right Bank of the Seine—is a fun place to stroll, play, and people-watch on a sunny day. Each summer, the Paris city government closes the embankment's highway and trucks in potted palm trees, hammocks, lounge chairs, and 2,000 tons of sand to create colorful urban beaches. You'll also find "beach cafés," climbing walls, prefab pools, trampolines, *boules,* a library, beach volleyball, badminton, and Frisbee areas in three zones: sandy, grassy, and wood-tiled. (Other less-central areas of town, such as Bassin de la Vilette, have their own *plages*.)

Cost and Hours: Free, mid-July–mid-Aug daily 8:00-24:00, no beach off-season; on Right Bank of Seine, just north of Ile de la Cité, between Pont des Arts and Pont de Sully; for information, go to www.paris.fr, click on "English," then "Visit," then "Highlights."

Sights in Paris

Paris has some of Europe's—arguably the world's—best sightseeing. Cruisers in town for just a few hours are spoiled for choice: You'll need to be picky and quick to hit a few highlights from the many options listed here.

MAJOR MUSEUMS NEIGHBORHOOD

Paris' grandest park, the Tuileries Garden, was once the private property of kings and queens. Today it links the Louvre, Orangerie, and Orsay museums. And across from the Louvre are the tranquil, historic courtyards of the Palais Royal.

▲▲▲Louvre (Musée du Louvre)

This is Europe's oldest, biggest, greatest, and second-most-crowded museum (after the Vatican). Housed in a U-shaped, 16th-century

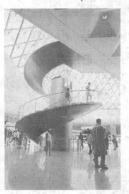

palace (accentuated by a 20th-century glass pyramid), the Louvre is Paris' top museum and one of its key landmarks. It's home to *Mona Lisa, Venus de Milo,* and hall after hall of Greek and Roman masterpieces, medieval jewels, Michelangelo statues, and paintings by the greatest artists from the Renaissance to the Romantics (mid-1800s).

Touring the Louvre can be overwhelming, so be selective. Focus on the Denon wing (south, along the river), with Greek sculptures, Italian paintings (by Raphael and da Vinci), and—of course—French paintings (Neoclassical and Romantic), and the adjoining Sully wing, with Egyptian artifacts and more French paintings. For extra credit, tackle the Richelieu wing (north, away from the river), displaying works from ancient Mesopotamia (today's Iraq), as well as French, Dutch, and Northern art.

PARIS

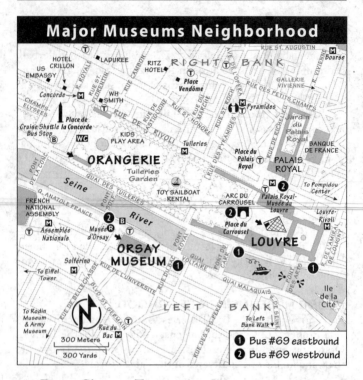

Major Museums Neighborhood

❶ Bus #69 eastbound
❷ Bus #69 westbound

Expect Changes: The sprawling Louvre is constantly shuffling its deck. Rooms close, and pieces can be on loan or in restoration. During your visit, a renovation of the pyramid entry may temporarily affect locations of the bag check, guided tour meeting point, and even the entrance itself. Be flexible. If you don't find the artwork you're looking for, ask the nearest guard for its new location.

Cost and Hours: €12, free on first Sun of month Oct-March, covered by Museum Pass, tickets good all day, reentry allowed; Wed-Mon 9:00-18:00, Wed and Fri until 21:45 (except on holidays), closed Tue, galleries start shutting 30 minutes before closing, last entry 45 minutes before closing; tel. 01 40 20 53 17, recorded info tel. 01 40 20 51 51, www.louvre.fr. Crowds can be miserably bad on Sun, Mon (the worst day), Wed, and in the morning.

Buying Tickets: Self-serve ticket machines located under the pyramid may be faster to use than the ticket windows (machines accept euro bills, coins, and chip-and-PIN Visa cards). A shop in the underground mall sells tickets to the Louvre, Orsay, and Versailles, plus Museum Passes, for no extra charge (cash only). To find it from the Carrousel du Louvre entrance off Rue de Rivoli (described under "Getting In," next page), turn right after the last

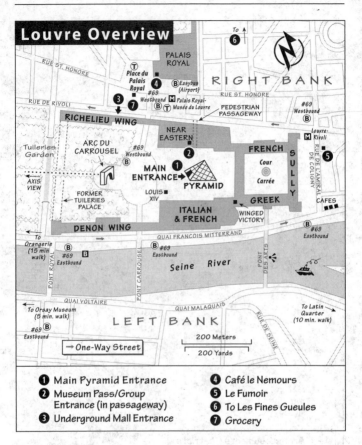

Louvre Overview

RIGHT BANK

PALAIS ROYAL

RUE ST. HONORE

Place du Palais Royal

Easypass (Airport)

RUE ST. HONORE

#69 Westbound

RUE DE RIVOLI

Palais Royal-Musée du Louvre

PEDESTRIAN PASSAGEWAY

#69 Westbound

Louvre-Rivoli

RICHELIEU WING

NEAR EASTERN

FRENCH

RUE DE L'AMIRAL DE COLIGNY

Tuileries Garden

ARC DU CARROUSEL

#69 Westbound

MAIN ENTRANCE

PYRAMID

Cour Carrée

SULLY

AXIS VIEW

FORMER TUILERIES PALACE

LOUIS XIV

ITALIAN & FRENCH

GREEK

WINGED VICTORY

CAFES

DENON WING

QUAI FRANCOIS MITTERRAND

#69 Eastbound

To Orangerie (15 min. walk)

#69 Eastbound

#69 Eastbound

PONT ROYAL

PONT CARROUSEL

Seine River

PONT DES ARTS

QUAI VOLTAIRE

QUAI MALAQUAIS

RUE DE SEINE

To Orsay Museum (5 min. walk)

LEFT BANK

To Latin Quarter (10 min. walk)

#69 Eastbound

200 Meters

200 Yards

→ One-Way Street

❶ Main Pyramid Entrance
❷ Museum Pass/Group Entrance (in passageway)
❸ Underground Mall Entrance
❹ Café le Nemours
❺ Le Fumoir
❻ To Les Fines Gueules
❼ Grocery

escalator down onto Allée de France, and follow *Museum Pass* signs.

Getting There: It's at the Palais Royal-Musée du Louvre Métro stop. (The old Louvre Métro stop, called Louvre-Rivoli, is farther from the entrance.) Bus #69 also runs past the Louvre.

Getting In: There is no grander entry than through the main entrance at the **pyramid** in the central courtyard, but lines (for security reasons) can be long. Expect some changes during the pyramid's renovation in 2015. Museum Pass holders can use the **group entrance** in the pedestrian passageway (labeled *Pavilion Richelieu*) between the pyramid and Rue de Rivoli. It's under the arches, a few steps north of the pyramid; find the uniformed guard at the security checkpoint entrance, at the down escalator.

Anyone can enter the Louvre from its less-crowded **underground entrance,** accessed through the Carrousel du Louvre shopping mall. Enter the mall at 99 Rue de Rivoli (the door with the red awning) or directly from the Métro stop Palais Royal-Musée

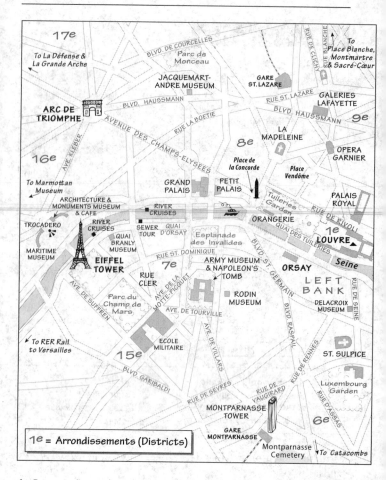

1e = Arrondissements (Districts)

du Louvre (stepping off the train, take the exit to *Musée du Louvre-Le Carrousel du Louvre*). Once inside the underground mall, continue toward the inverted pyramid next to the Louvre's security entrance. Museum Pass holders can skip to the head of the security line.

Tours: Ninety-minute English-language **guided tours** leave twice daily (except the first Sun of the month Oct-March) from the *Accueil des Groupes* area, under the pyramid (normally at 11:00 and 14:00, possibly more often in summer; €12 plus your entry ticket, tour tel. 01 40 20 52 63). **Videoguides** (€5) provide commentary on about 700 masterpieces. Or you can

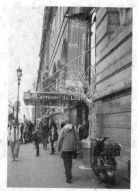

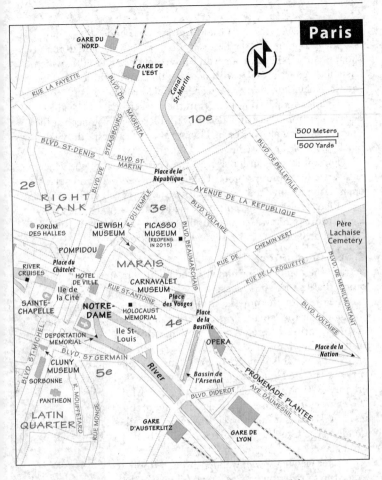

download a free Rick Steves **audio tour** (see page 50).

Baggage Check: The free *bagagerie* is under the pyramid, behind the Richelieu wing escalator (look for the *visiteurs individuels* sign). Bigger bags must be checked (though they won't take very large bags), and you can also check small bags to lighten your load. The baggage-claim clerk might ask you in French, "Does your bag contain anything of value?" You can't check cameras, money, passports, or other valuables.

Services: WCs are located under the pyramid, behind the escalators to the Denon and Richelieu wings. Once you're in the galleries, WCs are scarce.

Cuisine Art: The Louvre has several cafés. The best is **Café Mollien,** located near the end of our tour (€6 sandwiches, on terrace overlooking pyramid, closes at 18:00). A reasonably priced self-service lunch **cafeteria** is up the escalator from the pyramid in the Richelieu wing. **Le Grand Louvre Café** under the pyramid is a pricier option. For the best selection, walk to the underground shopping mall, the **Carrousel du Louvre** (daily 8:30-23:00), which has a food court upstairs with decent-value, multiethnic fast-food eateries, including—*quelle horreur*—a McDonald's.

Picnics are painting-perfect in the adjacent Palais Royal gardens (enter from Place du Palais Royal). Pick up all you need at the Franprix market at 165 Rue St-Honoré and take a fresh-air break a block north of the museum.

For a fine, elegant lunch near the Louvre, head to the venerable **Café le Nemours** (good €10-13 *croque monsieur* and salads, open daily; leaving the Louvre, cross Rue de Rivoli and veer left to 2 Place Colette, adjacent to Comédie Française) or the classy **Le Fumoir** (€22 two-course lunch *menu*, open daily, 6 Rue de l'Amiral de Coligny, near Louvre-Rivoli Métro stop).

❖ Self-Guided Tour

Start in the Denon Wing and visit the highlights, in the following order (thanks to Gene Openshaw for his help writing this tour).

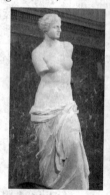

Begin with the pre-classical **Greek statues,** then look for the famous *Venus de Milo (Aphrodite)* statue (pictured here). You'll find her not far from another famous statue, the *Winged Victory of Samothrace.* This goddess of love (late 2nd century B.C.) created a sensation when she was discovered in 1820 on the Greek island of Melos. Most "Greek" statues are actually later Roman copies, but *Venus* is a rare Greek original. She, like Golden Age Greeks, epitomizes stability, beauty, and balance.

After viewing *Venus,* wander through Room 6 to see the **Parthenon friezes** (stone fragments that once decorated the exterior of the greatest Athenian temple, dating from mid-5th century B.C.). A left turn into Room 22 takes you on a detour through some **Roman works,** including mosaics from the ancient city of Antioch, Etruscan sarcophagi, and Roman portrait busts.

Later Greek art was Hellenistic, adding motion and drama. For a good example, see the exciting *Winged Victory of Samothrace* (*Victoire de Samothrace,* c. 190 B.C., on the landing). This statue of a woman with wings, poised on the prow of a ship, once stood on a hilltop to commemorate a naval victory. This is the *Venus de Milo* gone Hellenistic.

The Italian collection—including the *Mona Lisa*—is scattered throughout the rooms of the long Grand Gallery, to the right (as you face her) of *Winged Victory* (look for **two Botticelli frescoes** as you enter). In painting, the Renaissance (1400-1600) meant realism, and for the Italians, realism was spelled "3-D." Painters were inspired by the realism and balanced beauty of Greek sculpture. Painting a 3-D world on a 2-D surface is tough, and after a millennium of Dark Ages, artists were rusty. Living in a religious age, they painted mostly altarpieces full of saints, angels, Madonnas-and-bambinos, and crucifixes floating in an ethereal gold-leaf heaven. Gradually, though, they brought these otherworldly scenes down to earth.

Two masters of the Italian High Renaissance (1500-1600) were Raphael (see his ***La Belle Jardinière***, showing the Madonna, Child, and John the Baptist) and Leonardo da Vinci. The Louvre has the greatest collection of Leonardos in the world—five of them, including the exquisite *Virgin and Child with St. Anne;* the neighboring *Virgin of the Rocks;* and the androgynous *John the Baptist.*

But his most famous, of course, is the ***Mona Lisa*** (*La Joconde* in French), located in the Salle des Etats, midway down the Grand Gallery, on the right. After several years

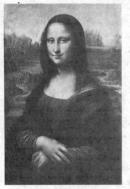

and a €5 million renovation, Mona is alone behind glass on her own false wall. Leonardo was already an old man when François I invited him to France. Determined to pack light, he took only a few paintings with him. One was a portrait of Lisa del Giocondo, the wife of a wealthy Florentine merchant. When Leonardo arrived, François immediately fell in love with the painting, making it the centerpiece of the small collection of Italian masterpieces that would, in three centuries, become the Louvre museum. He called it *La Gioconda* (*La Joconde* in French)—a play on both her last name and the Italian word for "happiness." We know it as the *Mona Lisa*—a contraction of the Italian for "my lady Lisa." Warning: François was impressed, but *Mona* may disappoint you. She's smaller than you'd expect, darker, engulfed in a huge room, and hidden behind a glaring pane of glass.

The huge canvas opposite *Mona* is Paolo Veronese's ***The Marriage at Cana,*** showing the Renaissance love of beautiful things gone hog-wild. Venetian artists like Veronese painted the good life of rich, happy-go-lucky Venetian merchants.

Now for something **Neoclassical.** Exit behind *Mona Lisa* and turn right into the Salle Daru to find *The Coronation of Emperor Napoleon* by Jacques-Louis David. Neoclassicism, once the rage in France (1780-1850), usually features Greek subjects, patriotic sentiment, and a clean, simple style. After Napoleon quickly conquered most of Europe, he insisted on being made emperor (not merely king) of this "New Rome." He staged an elaborate coronation ceremony in Paris, and rather than let the pope crown him, he crowned himself. The setting was Notre-Dame Cathedral, with Greek columns and Roman arches thrown in for effect. Napoleon's mom was also added, since she couldn't make it to the ceremony. A key on the frame describes who's who in the picture.

The **Romantic** collection, in an adjacent room (Salle Mollien), has works by Théodore Géricault (*The Raft of the Medusa*—one of my favorites) and Eugène Delacroix *(Liberty Leading the People).* Romanticism, with an emphasis on motion and emotion, is the flip side of cool, balanced Neoclassicism, though they both flourished in the early 1800s.

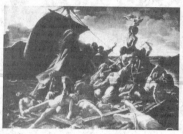

Delacroix's *Liberty,* commemorating the stirrings of democracy in France, is also an appropriate tribute to the Louvre, the first museum ever opened to the common rabble of humanity. The good things in life don't belong only to a small, wealthy part of society, but to everyone. The motto of France is *Liberté, Egalité, Fraternité*—liberty, equality, and the brotherhood of all.

Exit the room at the far end (past Café Mollien) and go downstairs, where you'll bump into the bum of a large, twisting male nude looking like he's just waking up after a thousand-year nap. The two *Slaves* (1513-1515) by Michelangelo are a fitting end to this museum—works that bridge the ancient and modern worlds. Michelangelo, like his fellow Renaissance artists, learned from the Greeks. The perfect anatomy, twisting poses, and idealized faces appear as if they could have been created 2,000 years earlier. Michelangelo said that his purpose was to carve away the marble to reveal the figures God put inside. The *Rebellious Slave,* fighting against his bondage, shows the agony of that process and the ecstasy of the result.

Although this makes for a good first tour, there's so much more. After a break (or on a second visit), consider a stroll through a few rooms of the Richelieu wing, which contain some of the Louvre's most ancient pieces. Bible students, amateur archaeologists, and Iraq War vets may find the collection especially interesting.

▲▲▲Orsay Museum (Musée d'Orsay)

The Musée d'Orsay (mew-zay dor-say) houses French art of the 1800s and early 1900s (specifically, 1848-1914), picking up where the Louvre's art collection leaves off. For us, that means

Impressionism, the art of sun-dappled fields, bright colors, and crowded Parisian cafés. The Orsay houses the best general collection anywhere of Manet, Monet, Renoir, Degas, Van Gogh, Cézanne, and Gauguin.

Cost and Hours: €11, €8.50 Tue-Wed and Fri-Sun after 16:30 and Thu after 18:15, free on first Sun of month and often right

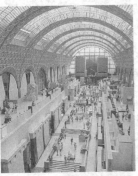

when the ticket booth stops selling tickets (Tue-Wed and Fri-Sun at 17:00, Thu at 21:00; they won't let you in much after that), covered by Museum Pass, tickets valid all day, combo-ticket with Orangerie Museum (€16) or Rodin Museum (€15); open Tue-Sun 9:30-18:00, Thu until 21:45, closed Mon, Impressionist galleries start shutting 45 minutes before closing, last entry one hour before closing (45 minutes before on Thu); tel. 01 40 49 48 14, www.musee-orsay.fr.

Avoiding Lines: The ticket-buying line can be long, but you can skip it with a Museum Pass or an advance ticket. Advance tickets can be purchased online and printed at home (for a small surcharge), or you can buy them in person at FNAC department stores and TIs (see www.musee-orsay.fr). You can also buy tickets and Museum Passes (no markup) at the newspaper kiosk just outside the Orsay (on the steps below the passholder entry—Entrance C), allowing you to skip the ticket-buying line at the museum itself. If you're planning to visit either the Orangerie or the Rodin (and you don't have a Museum Pass), consider starting at one of those museums instead (both of which have shorter lines than the Orsay) and buying an Orsay combo-ticket.

Getting There: The museum, at 1 Rue de la Légion d'Honneur, sits above the RER-C stop called Musée d'Orsay; the nearest Métro stop is Solférino, three blocks southeast of the Orsay. Bus #69 also stops at the Orsay. From the Louvre, it's a lovely 15-minute walk through the Tuileries Garden and across the pedestrian bridge to the Orsay.

Getting In: As you face the entrance, passholders and ticket holders enter on the right (Entrance C). Ticket purchasers enter on the left (Entrance A). Security checks slow down all entrances.

Tours: Audioguides cost €5. English **guided tours** usually run daily at 11:30 (€6/1.5 hours, none on Sun, tours may also run at 14:30—inquire when you arrive). Or you can download a free Rick Steves **audio tour** (see page 50).

Cuisine Art: The snazzy Le Restaurant is on the second floor, with affordable tea and coffee served daily except Thursday from 14:45 (€18 *plats du jour*, Tue-Sun 11:45-17:45, Thu 9:30-14:45

& 19:00-21:00). A simple café is on the main floor (far end), and a convenient-if-pricier one is on the fifth floor beyond the Impressionist galleries (€10-15 quiche or *croque monsieur*-type plates). Outside, behind the museum, a number of classy eateries line Rue du Bac.

◯ Self-Guided Tour

This former train station, the Gare d'Orsay, barely escaped the wrecking ball in the 1970s, when the French realized it'd be a great place to house the enormous collections of 19th-century art scattered throughout the city.

The ground floor (level 0) houses early 19th-century art, mainly conservative art of the Academy and Salon, plus Realism. On the top floor (not visible from here) is the core of the collection—the Impressionist rooms. If you're pressed for time, go directly there. Remember that the museum rotates its large collection often, so find the latest arrangement on your current Orsay map, and be ready to go with the flow.

Conservative Art to Realism

In the Orsay's first few rooms, you're surrounded by visions of idealized beauty—nude women in languid poses, Greek mythological figures, and anatomically perfect statues. This was the art adored by French academics and the middle-class *(bourgeois)* public.

Alexandre Cabanel's *The Birth of Venus* (*La Naissance de Vénus*, 1863; Room 3) and **Edouard Manet**'s *Olympia* (1863; Room 14) offer two opposing visions of Venus. Cabanel's Venus is a perfect fantasy, an orgasm of beauty. Manet's nude is a Realist's take on the traditional Venus. Manet doesn't gloss over anything. The pose is classic, but the sharp outlines and harsh, contrasting colors are new and shocking. Manet replaced soft-core porn with hard-core art.

Jean-François Millet's *The Gleaners* (*Les Glaneuses*, 1867) shows us three gleaners, the poor women who pick up the meager leftovers after a field has already been harvested for the wealthy. Here he captures the innate dignity of these stocky, tanned women who bend their backs quietly in a large field for their small reward. This is "Realism" in two senses. It's painted "realistically," not prettified. And it's the "real" world—not the fantasy world of Greek myth, but the harsh life of the working poor.

Impressionism

The Impressionist collection is scattered randomly through Rooms 29-36, on the top floor. You'll see Monet hanging next to Renoir, Manet sprinkled among Pissarro, and a few Degas here and a few Degas there. Shadows dance and the displays mingle. Where they're hung is a lot like their brushwork...delightfully sloppy.

In **Edouard Manet**'s *Luncheon on the Grass* (*Le Déjeuner sur l'Herbe*, 1863), you can see that a new revolutionary movement was starting to bud—Impressionism. Notice the background: the messy brushwork of trees and leaves, the play of light on the pond, and the light that filters through the trees onto the woman who stoops in the haze. Also note the strong contrast of colors (white skin, black clothes, green grass).

Edgar Degas blends classical lines and Realist subjects with Impressionist color, spontaneity, and everyday scenes from urban Paris. He loved the unposed "snapshot" effect, catching his models off guard. Dance students, women at work, and café scenes are approached from odd angles that aren't always ideal but make the scenes seem more real. He gives us the backstage view of life. For instance, a dance rehearsal lets Degas capture a behind-the-scenes look at bored, tired, restless dancers (*The Dance Class, La Classe de Danse*, c. 1873-1875). In the painting *In a Café (Dans un Café*, 1875-1876), a weary lady of the evening meets morning with a last, lonely, nail-in-the-coffin drink in the glaring light of a four-in-the-morning café. The pale green drink at the center of the composition is the toxic substance absinthe, which fueled many artists and burned out many more.

Claude Monet, the father of Impressionism, is known for his series of paintings on a single subject. For example, you may see several canvases of the cathedral in Rouen. In 1893, Monet went to Rouen, rented a room across from the cathedral, set up his easel... and waited. He wanted to catch "a series of differing impressions" of the cathedral facade at various times of day and year. He often had several canvases going at once. In all, he did 30 paintings of the cathedral, and each is unique. The time-lapse series shows the sun passing slowly across the sky, creating different-colored light and shadows. The labels next to the art describe the conditions: in gray weather, in the morning, morning sun, full sunlight, and so on.

One of Monet's favorite places to paint was the garden he landscaped at his home in Giverny, west of Paris. The Japanese bridge and the water lilies floating in the pond were his two favorite subjects. As Monet aged and his eyesight failed, he made bigger canvases of smaller subjects. The final water lilies are monumental smudges of thick paint surrounded by paint-splotched clouds that are reflected on the surface of the pond.

Pierre-Auguste Renoir started out as a painter of landscapes, along with Monet, but later veered from the Impressionist's philosophy and painted images that were unabashedly "pretty."

Renoir's best-known work is *Dance at the Moulin de la Galette* (*Bal du Moulin de la Galette*, 1876). On Sunday afternoons, working-class folk would dress up and head for the fields on Butte Montmartre (near Sacré-Cœur basilica) to dance, drink, and eat little crêpes (galettes) till dark. Renoir liked to go there to paint the common Parisians living and loving in the afternoon sun. The sunlight filtering through the trees creates a kaleidoscope of colors, like the 19th-century equivalent of a mirror ball throwing darts of light onto the dancers. The painting glows with bright colors. Even the shadows on the ground, which should be gray or black, are colored a warm blue. Like a photographer who uses a slow shutter speed to show motion, Renoir paints a waltzing blur.

Post-Impressionism

Post-Impressionism—the style that employs Impressionism's bright colors while branching out in new directions—is scattered all around the museum. You'll get a taste of the style with Cézanne, on the top floor, with much more on level 2.

Paul Cézanne brought Impressionism into the 20th century. Bowls of fruit, landscapes, and a few portraits were Cézanne's passion (see *The Card Players, Les Joueurs de Cartes, 1890-1895*). Where the Impressionists built a figure out of a mosaic of individual brushstrokes, Cézanne used blocks of paint to create a more solid, geometrical shape. These chunks are like little "cubes." It's no coincidence that his experiments in reducing forms to their geometric basics inspired the...Cubists. Because of his style (not the content), he is often called the first Modern painter.

Like Michelangelo, Beethoven, Rembrandt, Wayne Newton, and a select handful of others, **Vincent van Gogh** put so much of himself into his work that art and life became one. In the Orsay's collection of paintings (level 2), you'll see both Van Gogh's painting style and his life unfold.

Encouraged by his art-dealer brother, Van Gogh moved to Paris, and *voilà!* The color! He met Monet, drank with Gauguin and Toulouse-Lautrec, and soaked up the Impressionist style. (For example, see how he might build a bristling brown beard using thick strokes of red, yellow, and green side by side.)

But the social life of Paris became too much for the solitary Van Gogh, and he moved to the south of France. At first, in the glow of the bright spring sunshine, he had a period of incredible creativity and happiness. He was overwhelmed by the bright colors, landscape vistas, and common people. It was an Impressionist's dream (see *Midday, La Méridienne, 1889-90*).

But being alone in a strange country began to wear on him. An ugly man, he found it hard to get a date. A painting of his rented bedroom in Arles shows a cramped, bare-bones place (*Van Gogh's Room at Arles, La Chambre de Van Gogh à Arles, 1889*). He invited his friend Gauguin to join him, but after two months together arguing passionately about art, nerves got raw. Van Gogh threatened Gauguin with a razor, which drove his friend back to

Paris. In crazed despair, Van Gogh cut off a piece of his own ear.

The people of Arles realized they had a madman on their hands and convinced Vincent to seek help at a mental hospital. The paintings he finished in the peace of the hospital are more meditative—there are fewer bright landscapes and more closed-in scenes with deeper, almost surreal colors.

His final self-portrait shows a man engulfed in a confused background of brushstrokes that swirl and rave (*Self-Portrait, Portrait de l'Artiste,* 1889). But in the midst of this rippling sea of mystery floats a still, detached island of a face. Perhaps his troubled eyes know that in only a few months, he'll take a pistol and put a bullet through his chest.

Nearby are the paintings of **Paul Gauguin,** who got the travel bug early in childhood and grew up wanting to be a sailor. Instead, he became a stockbroker. At the age of 35, he got fed up with it all, quit his job, abandoned his wife (her stern portrait bust may be nearby) and family, and took refuge in his art.

Gauguin traveled to the South Seas in search of the exotic, finally settling on Tahiti. There he found his Garden of Eden. Gauguin's best-known works capture an idyllic Tahitian landscape peopled by exotic women engaged in simple tasks and making music (*Arearea,* 1892). The native girls lounge placidly in unselfconscious innocence (so different from Cabanel's seductive, melodramatic *Venus*). The style is intentionally "primitive," collapsing the three-dimensional landscape into a two-dimensional pattern of bright colors. Gauguin intended that this simple style carry a deep undercurrent of symbolic meaning. He wanted to communicate to his "civilized" colleagues back home that he'd found the paradise he'd always envisioned.

French Sculpture

The open-air mezzanine of level 2 is lined with statues. Stroll the mezzanine, enjoying the works of great French sculptors, including **Auguste Rodin.**

Born of working-class roots and largely self-taught, Rodin combined classical solidity with Impressionist surfaces to become the greatest sculptor since Michelangelo. Like his statue, *The Walking Man* (*L'Homme Qui Marche,* c. 1900), Rodin had one foot in the past, while the other stepped into the future. This muscular, forcefully striding man could be a symbol of Renaissance Man with his classical power. With no mouth or hands, he speaks with his body. But get close and look at the statue's surface. This rough, "unfinished" look reflects light in the same way the rough Impressionist brushwork does, making the statue come alive, never quite at rest in the viewer's eye. Rodin created this statue in a flash of inspiration. He took two unfinished statues—torso and

PARIS

legs—and plunked them together at the waist. You can still see the seam.

Rodin's sculptures capture the groundbreaking spirit of much of the art in the Orsay Museum. With a stable base of 19th-century stone, he launched art into the 20th century.

▲▲Orangerie Museum (Musée de l'Orangerie)

Step out of the tree-lined, sun-dappled Impressionist painting that is the Tuileries Garden, and into the Orangerie (oh-rahn-zheh-ree), a little bijou of select 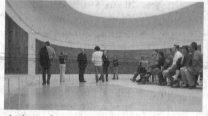 works by Claude Monet and his contemporaries. Start with the museum's claim to fame—Monet's water lilies. These eight mammoth-scale paintings are displayed exactly as Monet intended them—surrounding you in oval-shaped rooms—so you feel as though you're immersed in his garden at Giverny.

Cost and Hours: €8, €5 after 17:00, free for those under age 18, €16 combo-ticket with Orsay Museum, covered by Museum Pass; Wed-Mon 9:00-18:00, closed Tue, galleries shut down 15 minutes before closing time; audioguide-€5, English guided tours usually Mon and Thu at 14:30 and Sat at 11:00, located in Tuileries Garden near Place de la Concorde (Mo: Concorde or scenic bus #24), 15-minute stroll from the Orsay, tel. 01 44 77 80 07, www.musee-orangerie.fr.

EIFFEL TOWER AND NEARBY
▲▲▲Eiffel Tower (La Tour Eiffel)

It's crowded, expensive, and there are probably better views in Paris, but visiting this 1,000-foot-tall ornament is worth the trouble. Visitors to Paris may find *Mona Lisa* to be less than expected,

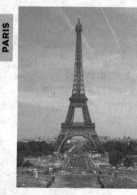

but the Eiffel Tower rarely disappoints, even in an era of skyscrapers. This is a once-in-a-lifetime, I've-been-there experience. Making the trip gives you membership in the exclusive society of the quarter of a billion other humans who have made the Eiffel Tower the most visited monument in the modern world.

Cost and Hours: €15 all the way to the top, €9 for just the two lower levels, €5 to skip the elevator line and climb the stairs to the first or second level (€4

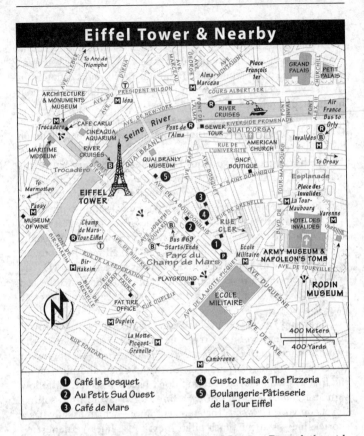

Eiffel Tower & Nearby

1 Café le Bosquet
2 Au Petit Sud Ouest
3 Café de Mars
4 Gusto Italia & The Pizzeria
5 Boulangerie-Pâtisserie de la Tour Eiffel

if you're under age 25), not covered by Museum Pass; daily mid-June-Aug 9:00-24:45, Sept-mid-June 9:30-23:45; cafés and great view restaurants, Mo: Bir-Hakeim or Trocadéro, RER: Champ de Mars-Tour Eiffel (all stops about a 10-minute walk away).

Reservations: Frankly, you'd be crazy to show up without a reservation. At www.toureiffel.paris, you can book an entry time (for example, June 12 at 16:30) and skip the initial entry line (the longest)—at no extra cost. Time slots can fill up months in advance (especially if visiting from April through September). Online ticket sales open up about three months before any given date (at 8:30 Paris time)—and can sell out for that day within hours. Be sure of your date, as reservations are nonrefundable. If there are no reservation slots available, try the website again about a week before your visit—last-minute spots occasionally open up, especially for tickets up to the second level only.

The website is easy, but here are a few tips: When you "Choose a ticket," make sure you select "Lift entrance ticket with access to the summit" if you'd like to go all the way to the top. Then select your date, the number of people in your party, and the time slot (available times show up in green). You must create an account, with a 10-digit mobile phone number as your login. (If you don't have one, make up a number, if you must, but make a note of it in case you need to log in again.) Enter the 10 numbers without hyphens, parentheses, or country codes.

After paying with a credit card, you can print your tickets. Follow the printing specifications carefully (white paper, blank on both sides, etc.).

Other Tips for Avoiding Lines: Crowds overwhelm this place much of the year, with one- to two-hour waits to get in (unless it's rainy, when lines can evaporate). Weekends and holidays are worst, but prepare for ridiculous crowds almost any time.

You can bypass some (but not all) lines if you have a reservation at either of the tower's view restaurants, or you can hike the stairs (shorter lines). When you buy tickets on-site, all members of your party must be with you. To get reduced fares for kids, bring ID.

You can buy a reservation time (almost right up to the last minute) for €40 (or a €59 guided tour) through Fat Tire Bikes (see page 1061).

Getting In: If you have a reservation, arrive at the tower 10 minutes before your entry time, and look for either of the two entrances marked *Visiteurs avec Reservation* (Visitors with Reservation), where attendants scan your ticket and put you on the first available elevator. If you don't have a reservation, follow signs for *Individuels* or *Visiteurs sans Tickets* (avoid lines selling tickets only for *Groupes*). The stairs entrance—which usually has a shorter line—is at the south pillar (next to Le Jules Verne restaurant entrance).

Pickpockets: Beware. Street thieves plunder awestruck visitors gawking below the tower. And tourists in crowded elevators are like fish in a barrel for predatory pickpockets. *En garde.* There's a police station at the Jules Verne pillar.

Security Check: Bags larger than 19 by 8 by 12 inches are not allowed, but there is no baggage check. All bags are subject to a security search. No knives, glass bottles, or cans are permitted.

Services: Free WCs are at the base of the tower, behind the east pillar. Inside the tower itself, WCs are on all levels, but they're small, with long lines.

Visiting the Tower

The first visitor to the Paris World's Fair in 1889 walked beneath the "arch" formed by the newly built Eiffel Tower and entered the fairgrounds. This event celebrated both the centennial of the French Revolution and France's position as a global superpower. Bridge builder Gustave Eiffel (1832-1923) won the contest to build the fair's centerpiece by beating out rival proposals such as a giant guillotine.

Delicate and graceful when seen from afar, the Eiffel Tower is massive—even a bit scary—close up. You don't appreciate its size until you walk toward it; like a mountain, it seems so close but takes forever to reach.

The tower, including its antenna, stands 1,063 feet tall, or slightly higher than the 77-story Chrysler Building in New York. Its four support pillars straddle an area of 3.5 acres. Despite the tower's 7,300 tons of metal and 60 tons of paint, it is so well-engineered that it weighs no more per square inch at its base than a linebacker on tiptoes.

There are three observation platforms, at roughly 200, 400, and 900 feet. To get to the top, you need to change elevators at the second level. Note: Some elevators stop on the first level going up. If yours does, don't get off. It's more efficient to see the first floor on the way down. For the hardy, stairs lead from the ground level up to the first and second levels—and rarely have a long line. It's 360 stairs to the first level and another 360 to the second.

If you want to see the entire tower, from top to bottom, then see it...from top to bottom. Ride the elevator to the second level, then immediately line up for the elevator to the top. Enjoy the views on top, then ride back down to the second level. Frolic there for a while and take in some more views. When you're ready, head to the first level by taking the stairs (no line and can take as little as 5 minutes) or lining up for the elevator (but before boarding, ask if the elevator will stop on the first level—some don't). Explore the shops and exhibits on the first level and have a snack. To leave, you can line up for the elevator, but it's quickest and most memorable to take the stairs back down.

The Top: The top level, called *le sommet*, is tiny. (It can close temporarily without warning when it reaches capacity.) You'll find wind and grand, sweeping views. The city lies before you (pick out sights with the help of the panoramic maps). On a good day, you can see for 40 miles. Do a 360-degree tour of Paris. Feeling proud you made it this high? You can celebrate your accomplishment with a glass of champagne from the bar.

Second Level: The second level has the best views because you're closer to the sights, and the monuments are more recognizable. (While the best views are up the short stairway, on the platform without the wire-cage barriers, at busy times much of that zone is taken up by people waiting for the elevator to the top.) The second level has souvenir shops, public telephones to call home, and a small stand-up café. The world-class Le Jules Verne restaurant is on this level, but you won't see it; access is by a private elevator.

First Level: The first level has more great views, all well-described by the tower's panoramic displays. After a recent remodel, this level now boasts a breathtaking glass floor, new eateries, and cinematic presentations about the tower's construction, paint job, place in pop culture, and more. Exhibits all around the first level explore the impact of weather on the tower—how the sun warms the metal, causing the top to expand and lean about five inches away from the sun, or how the tower oscillates slightly in the wind. Because of its lacy design, even the strongest of winds can't blow the tower down, but only cause it to sway back and forth a few inches. In fact, Eiffel designed the tower primarily with wind resistance in mind, wanting a structure seemingly "molded by the action of the wind itself."

After Your Visit: Descend back to earth. From here, consider catching the Bateaux Parisiens boat for a Seine cruise (see page 1059) or visiting one of the following nearby sights: the Rue Cler market street (see below), Army Museum and Napoleon's Tomb (see below), or Rodin Museum (page 1097). For tips on where to eat nearby, see page 1108.

Near the Eiffel Tower
▲▲Rue Cler

Paris is changing quickly, but a stroll down this market street introduces you to a thriving, traditional Parisian neighborhood and offers insights into the local culture. Although this is a wealthy district, Rue Cler retains a workaday charm still found in most neighborhoods throughout Paris. The street—traffic-free since 1984—is lined with the essential shops—wine, cheese, chocolate, bread—as well as a bank and a post office (market generally open Tue-Sat 8:30-13:00 & 15:00-19:30, Sun 8:30-12:00, dead on Mon). For those learning the fine art of living Parisian-style, Rue Cler provides an excellent classroom. And if you want to assemble the ultimate French picnic, there's no better place.

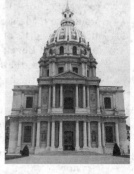

▲▲Army Museum and Napoleon's Tomb (Musée de l'Armée)

The Hôtel des Invalides—a former veterans' hospital topped by a golden dome—houses Napoleon's over-the-top-ornate tomb, as well as Europe's greatest military museum. Visiting the Army Museum's different sections, you can watch the art of war unfold from stone axes to Axis powers.

Cost and Hours: €9.50, €7.50 after 16:00, free for military personnel in uniform, free for kids but they must wait in line for ticket, covered by Museum Pass, temporary exhibits are extra; daily 10:00-18:00, July-Aug until 19:00, Nov-March until 17:00, tomb plus WWI and WWII wings open Tue until 21:00 April-Sept, museum (except for tomb) closed first Mon of month Oct-June, Charles de Gaulle exhibit closed Mon year-round, last tickets sold 30 minutes before closing; videoguide-€6, cafeteria, tel. 01 44 42 38 77 or 08 10 11 33 99, www.musee-armee.fr.

Getting There: The Hôtel des Invalides is at 129 Rue de Grenelle, a 10-minute walk from Rue Cler (Mo: La Tour Maubourg, Varenne, or Invalides). You can also take bus #69 (from the Marais and Rue Cler) or bus #87 (from Rue Cler and Luxembourg Garden area).

▲▲Rodin Museum (Musée Rodin)

This user-friendly museum is filled with passionate works by the greatest sculptor since Michelangelo. 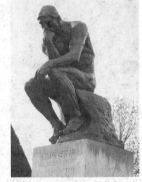 You'll see *The Kiss, The Thinker, The Gates of Hell,* and many more. (Due to ongoing renovations extending into 2015, some rooms may be closed.)

Cost and Hours: €6-9 (depending on temporary exhibits), free for those under age 18, free on first Sun of the month, €2 for garden only (possibly Paris' best deal, as several important works are on display there), €15 combo-ticket with Orsay Museum, both museum and garden covered by Museum Pass; Tue-Sun 10:00-17:45, Wed until 20:45, closed Mon; gardens close at 18:00, Oct-March at 17:00; last entry 30 minutes before closing; audioguide-€6, mandatory baggage check, self-service café in garden, near the Army Museum and Napoleon's Tomb at 79 Rue de Varenne, Mo: Varenne, tel. 01 44 18 61 10, www.musee-rodin.fr.

▲▲Marmottan Museum (Musée Marmottan Monet)

This intimate, less-touristed mansion on the southwest fringe of urban Paris has the best collection of works by the father of Impressionism, Claude Monet (1840–1926). Fiercely independent and dedicated to his craft, Monet gave courage to the other Impressionists in the face of harsh criticism.

Cost and Hours: €10, not covered by Museum Pass, Tue-Sun 10:00-18:00, Thu until 20:00, closed Mon, last entry 30 minutes before closing, audioguide-€3, 2 Rue Louis-Boilly, Mo: La Muette, tel. 01 44 96 50 33, www.marmottan.fr.

LEFT BANK

Opposite Notre-Dame, on the left bank of the Seine, is the Latin Quarter. (For more information on this neighborhood, see my Historic Paris Walk, earlier.)

▲▲Cluny Museum
(Musée National du Moyen Age)

The Cluny is a treasure trove of Middle Ages *(Moyen Age)* art. Located on the site of a Roman bathhouse, it offers close-up looks

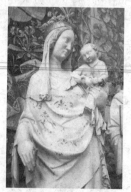

at stained glass, Notre-Dame carvings, fine goldsmithing and jewelry, and rooms of tapestries. The highlights are several original stained-glass windows from Sainte-Chapelle and the exquisite Lady and the Unicorn series of six tapestries: A delicate, as-medieval-as-can-be noble lady introduces a delighted unicorn to the senses of taste, hearing, sight, smell, and touch.

Cost and Hours: €8, free on first Sun of month, covered by Museum Pass; Wed-Mon 9:15-17:45, closed Tue, ticket office closes at 17:15; ticket includes audioguide though passholders must pay €1; near corner of Boulevards St. Michel and St. Germain at 6 Place Paul Painlevé; Mo: Cluny-La Sorbonne, St. Michel, or Odéon; tel. 01 53 73 78 16, www.musee-moyenage.fr.

▲Luxembourg Garden (Jardin du Luxembourg)

Paris' most beautiful, interesting, and enjoyable garden/park/rec-reational area, le Jardin du Luxembourg, is a great place to watch

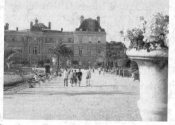

Parisians at rest and play. This 60-acre garden, dotted with fountains and statues, is the property of the French Senate, which meets here in the Luxembourg Palace. Although it seems like something out of an espionage thriller, it's a fact that France's secret service *(Générale de la Sécurité Extérieure)* is "secretly" headquartered beneath Luxembourg Garden. (Don't tell anyone.)

Cost and Hours: Free, daily dawn until dusk, Mo: Odéon, RER: Luxembourg.

CHAMPS-ELYSEES AND NEARBY
▲▲▲Champs-Elysées

This famous boulevard is Paris' backbone, with its greatest concentration of traffic. From the Arc de Triomphe down Avenue

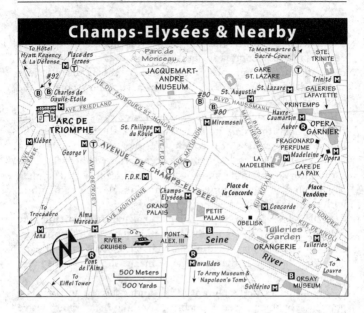

Champs-Elysées & Nearby

To Hôtel Hyatt Regency & La Défense

Place des Ternes

#92

Parc de Monceau

JACQUEMART-ANDRE MUSEUM

To Montmartre & Sacré-Coeur

STE. TRINITE

Trinité

GARE ST. LAZARE

St. Augustin   St. Lazare

GALERIES LAFAYETTE

PRINTEMPS

#80

BLVD. HAUSSMANN

Charles de Gaulle-Etoile

AVE. FRIEDLAND

RUE DU FAUBOURG ST-HONORE

#80

Miromesnil

Havre-Caumartin

Auber

OPERA GARNIER

ARC DE TRIOMPHE

St. Philippe du Roule

AVE DE MESSINE

FRAGONARD PERFUME

Madeleine

Opéra

Kléber

George V

LA MADELEINE

CAFE DE LA PAIX

AVENUE DE CHAMPS-ELYSEES

AVE. MATIGNON

AVE. GEORGE V

AVE KLEBER

F.D.R.

RUE ROYALE

Place de la Concorde

Place Vendôme

RUE ST. HONORE

To Trocadéro

Alma Marceau

AVE. MONTAIGNE

AVE GEORGE V

Champs-Elysées

GRAND PALAIS

PETIT PALAIS

Concorde

OBELISK

RUE DE RIVOLI

Tuileries Garden

Iéna

RIVER CRUISES

PONT-ALEX. III

Seine

ORANGERIE

Tuileries

Pont de l'Alma

To Eiffel Tower

500 Meters

500 Yards

Invalides

To Army Museum & Napoleon's Tomb

River

Solférino

ORSAY MUSEUM

To Louvre

des Champs-Elysées, all of France seems to converge on Place de la Concorde, the city's largest square. And though the Champs-Elysées has become as international as it is Parisian, a walk here is still a must.

● Self-Guided Walk

In 1667, Louis XIV opened the first section of the street as a short extension of the Tuileries Garden. This year is considered the birth of Paris as a grand city. The Champs-Elysées soon became *the* place to cruise in your carriage. One hundred years later, the café scene arrived. From the 1920s until the 1960s, this boulevard was pure elegance; Parisians actually dressed up to come here. It was mainly residences, rich hotels, and cafés.

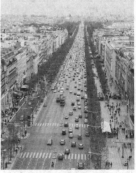

To reach the top of the Champs-Elysées, take the Métro to the **Arc de Triomphe** (Mo: Charles de Gaulle-Etoile), then saunter down the grand boulevard (Métro stops every few blocks, including George V and Franklin D. Roosevelt). If you plan to tour the Arc de Triomphe (see next listing), do it before starting this walk.

Fancy car dealerships include **Peugeot,** at #136 (showing off its futuristic concept cars, often alongside the classic models), and

Mercedes-Benz, a block down at #118, where you can pick up a Mercedes bag and perfume to go with your new car. In the 19th century this was an area for horse stables; today, it's the district of garages, limo companies, and car dealerships. If you're serious about selling cars in France, you must have a showroom on the Champs-Elysées.

Next to Mercedes is the famous **Lido,** Paris' largest cabaret (and a multiplex cinema). You can walk all the way into the lobby, passing videos of the show. Paris still offers the kind of burlesque-type spectacles that have been performed here since the 19th century, combining music, comedy, and scantily clad women. Moviegoing on the Champs-Elysées provides another kind of fun, with theaters showing the very latest releases.

The flagship store of leather-bag maker **Louis Vuitton** may be the largest single-brand luxury store in the world. Step inside. The store insists on providing enough salespeople to treat each customer royally—if there's a line, it means shoppers have overwhelmed the place.

Fouquet's café-restaurant (#99), under the red awning, is a popular spot among French celebrities, serving the most expensive shot of espresso I've found in downtown Paris (€10). Opened in 1899 as a coachman's bistro, Fouquet's gained fame as the hangout of France's WWI biplane fighter pilots—those who weren't shot down by Germany's infamous "Red Baron." It also served as James Joyce's dining room.

Since the early 1900s, Fouquet's has been a favorite of French celebrities. The golden plaques at the entrance honor winners of France's Oscar-like film awards, the Césars (one is cut into the ground at the end of the carpet). There are plaques for Gérard Depardieu, Catherine Deneuve, Yves Montand, Roman Polanski, Juliette Binoche, and several famous Americans (but not Jerry Lewis). More recent winners are shown on the floor just inside.

From posh cafés to stylish shops, monumental sidewalks to glimmering showrooms, the Champs-Elysées is Paris at its most Parisian.

On or near the Champs-Elysées
▲▲Arc de Triomphe
Napoleon had the magnificent Arc de Triomphe commissioned to commemorate his victory at the battle of Austerlitz. There's no triumphal arch bigger (165 feet high, 130 feet wide). And, with 12 converging boulevards, there's no traffic circle more thrilling to experience—either from behind the wheel or on foot (take the underpass).

The foot of the arch is a stage on which the last two centuries of Parisian history have played out—from the funeral of

Napoleon to the goose-stepping arrival of the Nazis to the triumphant return of Charles de Gaulle after the Allied liberation. Examine the carvings on the pillars, featuring a mighty Napoleon and excitable Lady Liberty. Pay your respects at the Tomb of the Unknown Soldier. Then climb the 284 steps to the observation deck up top, with sweeping sky-

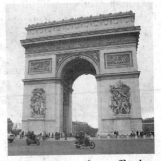

line panoramas and a mesmerizing view down onto the traffic that swirls around the arch.

Cost and Hours: Outside and at the base—free, always viewable; steps to rooftop—€9.50, free for those under age 18, free on first Sun of month Oct-March, covered by Museum Pass; daily April-Sept 10:00-23:00, Oct-March 10:00-22:30, last entry 45 minutes before closing; Place Charles de Gaulle, use underpass to reach arch, Mo: Charles de Gaulle-Etoile, tel. 01 55 37 73 77, http://arc-de-triomphe.monuments-nationaux.fr.

Avoiding Lines: You can bypass the slooow ticket line if you have a Museum Pass (though if you have kids, you'll need to line up to get the free tickets for children). Expect another line (that you can't skip) at the entrance to the stairway up the arch.

THE MARAIS

The Marais extends along the Right Bank of the Seine, from the Bastille to the Pompidou Center. The main east-west axis is formed by Rue St. Antoine, Rue des Rosiers (the heart of Paris' Jewish community), and Rue Ste. Croix de la Bretonnerie. The centerpiece of the neighborhood is the stately Place des Vosges. Helpful Métro stops are Bastille, St-Paul, and Hôtel de Ville. For restaurant recommendations in this neighborhood, see page 1110.

▲Place des Vosges

Henry IV built this centerpiece of the Marais in 1605 and called it "Place Royal." As he'd hoped, it turned the Marais into Paris' most exclusive neighborhood. Walk to the center, where Louis XIII, on horseback, gestures, "Look at this wonderful square my dad built."

▲Carnavalet Museum (Musée Carnavalet)

At the Carnavalet Museum, French history unfolds in a series of stills—like a Ken Burns documentary, except you have to walk. The Revolution is the highlight, but you get a good overview of everything—from Louis XIV-period rooms to Napoleon to the belle époque.

Cost and Hours: Free, fee for some temporary (but optional) exhibits, Tue-Sun 10:00-18:00, closed Mon; avoid lunchtime (11:45-14:30), when many rooms may be closed; audioguide-€5, 23 Rue de Sévigné (entrance is off Rue des Francs-Bourgeois), Mo: St-Paul, tel. 01 44 59 58 58, www.carnavalet.paris.fr.

▲▲Picasso Museum (Musée Picasso)

Whatever you think about Picasso the man, as an artist he was unmatched in the 20th century for his daring and productivity. The Picasso Museum has over 400 pieces, showing the whole range of the artist's long life and many styles. The women he loved and the global events he lived through appear in his canvases, filtered through his own emotional lens. You don't have to admire Picasso's lifestyle or like his modern painting style. But a visit here might make you appreciate the sheer vitality and creativity of this hardworking and unique man.

Cost and Hours: €11, extra charge for special exhibits, covered by Museum Pass, free on first Sun of month and for those under age 18 with ID; Tue-Fri 11:30-18:00, Sat-Sun 9:30-18:00, until 21:00 third Fri of month, last entry 45 minutes before closing; timed-entry tickets available from museum website, 5 Rue de Thorigny, Mo: St-Paul or Chemin Vert, tel. 01 42 71 25 21, www.musee-picasso.fr.

▲▲Pompidou Center (Centre Pompidou)

One of Europe's greatest collections of far-out modern art is housed in the Musée National d'Art Moderne, on the fourth and fifth floors of this colorful exhibition hall. The building itself is "exoskeletal" (like Notre-Dame or a crab), with its functional parts—the pipes, heating ducts, and escalator—on the outside, and the meaty art inside. It's the epitome of Modern architecture, where "form follows function." Created ahead of its time, the 20th-century art in this collection is still waiting for the world to catch up.

Cost and Hours: €13, free on first Sun of month, Museum Pass covers permanent collection and view escalators (but not temporary exhibits), €3 Panorama Ticket lets you ride to the sixth floor for the view (doesn't include museum entry); Wed-Mon 11:00-21:00, closed Tue, ticket counters close at 20:00; audioguide-€5 (rent on ground floor), café on mezzanine, pricey view restaurant on level 6, Mo: Rambuteau or Hôtel de Ville, tel. 01 44 78 12 33, www.centrepompidou.fr.

MONTMARTRE

Paris' highest hill, topped by Sacré-Cœur Basilica, is best known as the home of cabaret nightlife and bohemian artists. Struggling painters, poets, dreamers, and drunkards came here for cheap rent, untaxed booze, rustic landscapes, and views of the underwear of high-kicking cancan girls at the Moulin Rouge. These days, the hill is equal parts charm and kitsch—still vaguely village-like but mobbed with tourists and pickpockets on sunny weekends. Come for a bit of history, a getaway from Paris' noisy boulevards, and the view.

▲▲Sacré-Cœur

You'll spot Sacré-Cœur, the Byzantine-looking white basilica atop Montmartre, from most viewpoints in Paris. Though only 130 years old, it's impressive and iconic, with a climbable dome. The exterior, with its onion domes and bleached-bone pallor, looks ancient, but was finished only a century ago by Parisians humiliated by German invaders.

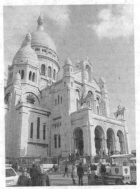

Cost and Hours: Church—free, daily 6:00-22:30, last entry at 22:15; dome—€6, not covered by Museum Pass, daily May-Sept 9:00-19:00, Oct-April 9:00-17:00; tel. 01 53 41 89 00, www.sacre-coeur-montmartre.com.

Getting There: You have several options. You can take the Métro to the Anvers stop (to avoid the stairs up to Sacré-Cœur, buy one more Métro ticket and ride up on the funicular). Alternatively, from Place Pigalle, you can take the "Montmartrobus," a city bus that drops you right by Sacré-Cœur (Funiculaire stop, costs one Métro ticket, 4/hour). A taxi from the Seine or the Bastille saves time and avoids sweat (about €15, €20 at night).

The Heart of Montmartre

Montmartre's main square **(Place du Tertre),** one block from the church, was once the haunt of Henri de Toulouse-Lautrec and the original bohemians. Today, it's crawling with tourists and unoriginal bohemians (best on a weekday or early on weekend mornings). From the main square, head up Rue des Saules to find Paris' lone vineyard and the **Montmartre Museum** (open daily). Return uphill, then follow Rue Lepic down to the old windmill, **Moulin de la Galette,** which once pressed monks' grapes and farmers' grain, and crushed gypsum rocks into powdery plaster of Paris (there were once 30 windmills on Montmartre). When the gypsum mines closed (c. 1850) and the vineyards sprouted apartments, this windmill turned into the ceremonial centerpiece of a popular outdoor dance hall. Farther down Rue Lepic, you'll pass near the former homes of **Toulouse-Lautrec** (at Rue Tourlaque—look for

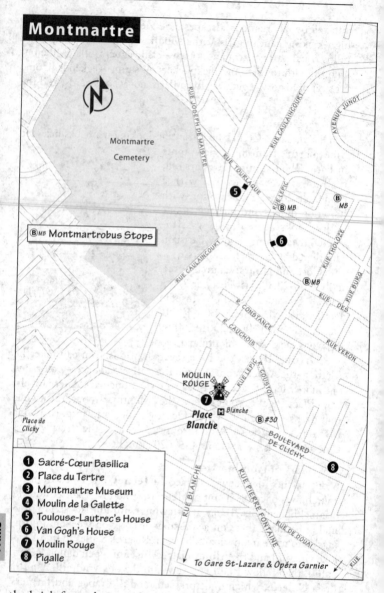

Montmartre

Montmartre Cemetery

Ⓑᴹᴮ Montmartrobus Stops

MOULIN ROUGE

Place Blanche

Ⓜ Blanche

Ⓑ #30

Place de Clichy

❶ Sacré-Cœur Basilica
❷ Place du Tertre
❸ Montmartre Museum
❹ Moulin de la Galette
❺ Toulouse-Lautrec's House
❻ Van Gogh's House
❼ Moulin Rouge
❽ Pigalle

To Gare St-Lazare & Opéra Garnier

the brick-framed art-studio windows under the heavy mansard roof) and **Vincent van Gogh** (54 Rue Lepic).

Pigalle

Paris' red light district, the infamous "Pig Alley," is at the foot of Butte Montmartre. *Ooh la la.* It's more racy than dangerous. Walk from Place Pigalle to Place Blanche, teasing desperate barkers and

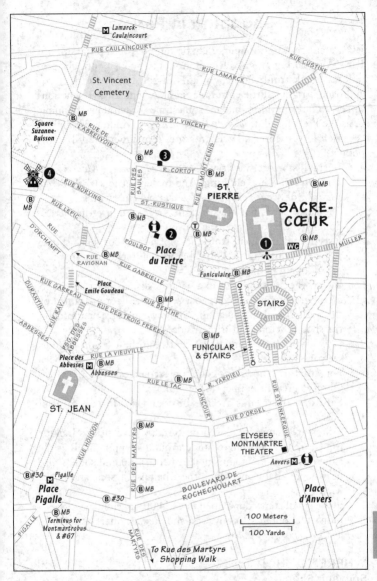

fast-talking temptresses. In bars, a €150 bottle of (what would otherwise be) cheap champagne comes with a friend. Stick to the bigger streets, hang on to your wallet, and exercise good judgment. Cancan can cost a fortune, as can con artists in topless bars. After dark, tour guides make big bucks by bringing their groups to touristy nightclubs like the famous Moulin Rouge (Mo: Pigalle or Abbesses).

Shopping in Paris

Even staunch anti-shoppers may be tempted to indulge in chic Paris. Wandering among elegant and outrageous boutiques provides a break from the heavy halls of the Louvre and, if you approach it right, a little cultural enlightenment. Even if you don't intend to buy anything, budget some time for window-shopping, or as the French call it, *faire du lèche-vitrines* ("window-licking").

Before you enter a Parisian store, remember the following points:

- In small stores, always say, *"Bonjour, Madame* or *Mademoiselle* or *Monsieur"* when entering. And remember to say *"Au revoir, Madame* or *Mademoiselle* or *Monsieur"* when leaving.
- The customer is not always right. In fact, figure the clerk is doing you a favor by waiting on you.
- Except in department stores, it's not normal for the customer to handle clothing. Ask first before you pick up an item: *"Je peux?"* (zhuh puh), meaning, "Can I?"
- By law the price of items in a window display must be visible, often written on a slip of paper set on the floor or framed on the wall. This gives you an idea of how expensive or affordable the shop is before venturing inside.
- For clothing size comparisons between the US and Europe, see page 133.
- Forget returns (and don't count on exchanges).
- Observe French shoppers. Then imitate.
- Saturday afternoons are *très* busy and not for the faint of heart.
- Stores are generally closed on Sunday. Exceptions include the Carrousel du Louvre (underground shopping mall at the Louvre with a Printemps department store) and some shops near Sèvres-Babylone, along the Champs-Elysées, and in the Marais.
- Some small stores don't open until 14:00 on Mondays.
- Don't feel obliged to buy. If a shopkeeper offers assistance, just say, *"Je regarde, merci."*

WHERE TO SHOP
Souvenir Shops

Avoid souvenir carts in front of famous monuments. You can find cheaper gifts around the Pompidou Center, on the streets of Montmartre, and in some department stores. The riverfront stalls near Notre-Dame sell a variety of used books, old posters and postcards, magazines, refrigerator magnets, and other tourist paraphernalia in the most romantic setting. You'll find better deals at the souvenir shops that line Rue d'Arcole between

Notre-Dame and Hôtel de Ville and on Rue de Rivoli, across from the Louvre.

Department Stores (Les Grands Magasins)

Parisian department stores begin with their showy perfume sections, almost always central on the ground floor, and worth a visit to see how much space is devoted to pricey, smelly water. Helpful information desks are usually located at the main entrances near the perfume section (with floor plans in English). Stores generally have affordable restaurants (some with view terraces) and a good selection of fairly priced souvenirs and toys. Shop at these great Parisian department stores: Galeries Lafayette (Mo: Chaussée d'Antin–La Fayette, Havre-Caumartin, or Opéra), Printemps (next door to Galeries Lafayette), and Bon Marché (Mo: Sèvres-Babylone). Opening hours are customarily Monday through Saturday from 10:00 to 19:00. Some are open later on Thursdays, and all are jammed on Saturdays and closed on Sundays (except in December). The Printemps (pran-tom) store in the Carrousel du Louvre is an exception—it's open every day.

Open-Air Markets

Several traffic-free street markets overflow with flowers, produce, fish vendors, and butchers, illustrating how most Parisians shopped before there were supermarkets and department stores. Shops are open daily except Sunday afternoons, Monday, and lunchtime throughout the week (13:00-15:00).

Rue Cler—a wonderful place to sleep and dine as well as shop—is like a refined street market, serving an upscale neighborhood near the Eiffel Tower (Mo: Ecole Militaire).

Rue Montorgueil is a thriving and locally popular café-lined street. Ten blocks from the Louvre and five blocks from the Pompidou Center, Rue Montorgueil (mohn-tor-goo-ee) is famous as the last vestige of the once-massive Les Halles market (just north of St. Eustache Church, Mo: Etienne Marcel).

Rue Mouffetard, originally built by the Romans, is a happening market street by day and does double-duty as restaurant row at night. Hiding several blocks behind the Panthéon, it starts at Place Contrescarpe and ends below at St. Médard Church (Mo: Censier Daubenton). The upper stretch is pedestrian and touristic; the bottom stretch is purely Parisian.

Rue des Martyrs, at the base of Butte Montmartre and Sacré-Coeur, offers an authentic, less-touristy market street serving village Paris (Mo: Pigalle).

PARIS

Eating in Paris

Although Paris is famous for its cuisine, I've focused my recommendations on eateries convenient to your sightseeing, listed by neighborhood. These places are

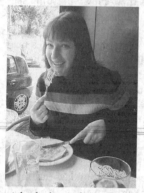

(mostly) authentically local, but—for the most part—fast and functional rather than haute cuisine. Below you'll find suggestions near the Eiffel Tower and in the historic core of Paris, near Notre-Dame. For eateries near the Louvre, see page 1083; for choices near the Orsay, see page 1087.

To save piles of euros, go to a bakery for takeout, or stop at a café for lunch. Cafés and brasseries are happy to serve a *plat du jour* (garnished plate of the day, about €13-18) or a chef-like salad (about €10-13). To save even more, consider picnics (tasty takeout dishes available at charcuteries).

Most restaurants I've listed have set-price *menus* between €20 and €35. In most cases, the few extra euros you pay are well-spent, and open up a variety of better choices. A service charge is included in the prices (so little or no tipping is expected, although it's polite to round up). Before choosing a seat outside, remember that smokers love outdoor tables.

NEAR THE EIFFEL TOWER

For locations, see the map on page 1093.

$$ Café le Bosquet is a contemporary Parisian brasserie where you'll dine for a decent price inside or outside on a broad sidewalk. Come here for standard café fare—salad, French onion soup, *steak-frites,* or a *plat du jour.* Lanky owner "Jeff" offers a three-course meal for €22, and *plats* from €13 to €19. The escargots are tasty, the house wine is quite good, and the beer is cheap for Paris (closed Sun, free Wi-Fi, corner of Rue du Champ de Mars and Avenue Bosquet, 46 Avenue Bosquet, tel. 01 45 51 38 13, www.bosquetparis.com).

$$ Au Petit Sud Ouest comes wrapped in stone walls and wood beams, making it a cozy place to sample cuisine from southwestern France. Duck, goose, foie gras, *cassoulet,* and truffles are all on *la carte.* Tables come with toasters to heat your bread—it enhances the flavors of the foie gras (*salade* with foie gras-€12, *plats*-€15, *cassoulet*-€16, closed Sun-Mon, 46 Avenue de la Bourdonnais, tel. 01 45 55 59 59, www.au-petit-sud-ouest.fr, managed by friendly Chantal).

Good Picnic Spots

Paris is picnic-friendly. Almost any park will do. Many have benches or grassy areas, though some lawns are off-limits—obey the signs. Parks generally close at dusk, so plan your sunset picnics carefully. Here are some especially scenic areas located near major sights:

Palais Royal: Escape to a peaceful courtyard full of relaxing locals across from the Louvre (Mo: Palais Royal-Musée du Louvre). The nearby Louvre courtyard surrounding the pyramid is less tranquil, but very handy.

Place des Vosges: Relax in an exquisite grassy courtyard in the Marais, surrounded by royal buildings (Mo: Bastille).

Square du Vert-Galant: For great river views, try this little triangular park on the west tip of Ile de la Cité. It's next to the statue of King Henry IV (Mo: Pont Neuf).

Pont des Arts: Munch from a perch on this pedestrian bridge over the Seine (near the Louvre)—it's equipped with benches (Mo: Pont Neuf).

Along the Seine: A grassy parkway runs along the left bank of the Seine between Les Invalides and Pont de l'Alma (Mo: Invalides, near Rue Cler).

Tuileries Garden: Have an Impressionist "Luncheon on the Grass" nestled between the Orsay and Orangerie museums (Mo: Tuileries).

Luxembourg Garden: The classic Paris picnic spot is this expansive Left Bank park (Mo: Odéon).

Les Invalides: Take a break from the Army Museum and Napoleon's Tomb in the gardens behind the complex (Mo: Varenne).

Champ de Mars: The long grassy strip below the Eiffel Tower has breathtaking views of this Paris icon. However, you must eat along the sides of the park, as the central lawn is off-limits (Mo: Ecole Militaire).

Pompidou Center: There's no grass, but the people-watching is unbeatable; try the area by the *Homage to Stravinsky* fountains (Mo: Rambuteau or Hôtel de Ville).

$$ Café de Mars is a cool place for a fine-quality, reasonably priced meal. It's also comfortable for single diners thanks to a convivial counter (closed Sun, 11 Rue Augereau, tel. 01 45 50 10 90, www.cafedemars.com).

$ Gusto Italia serves up tasty, good-value Italian cuisine in two minuscule places across from each other, each with a few tables outside. Arrive early or plan to wait (€12 salads, €14 pasta, daily, 199 Rue de Grenelle, tel. 01 45 55 00 43).

$ Boulangerie-Pâtisserie de la Tour Eiffel sells inexpensive salads, quiches, and sandwiches, and other traditional café fare. Enjoy the views of the Eiffel Tower (daily, outdoor and indoor seating, one block southeast of the tower at 21 Avenue de la Bourdonnais, tel. 01 47 05 59 81).

$ The Pizzeria is kid-friendly and cheap (closed Sun, eat in or take out, 28 Rue Augereau, tel. 01 45 55 45 16).

IN THE HISTORIC CORE

Eating options abound as you spiral out in any direction from the historic center of Paris. The lively, colorful Marais is just north-east of Notre-Dame, across the river. I've focused on two parts of this neighborhood: in the heart of the Marais and near Hôtel de Ville (a bit closer to Notre-Dame). Another option is the island of Ile St. Louis. This romantic and peaceful neighborhood, just a few minutes behind Notre-Dame (across the bridge), is littered with promising and surprisingly reasonable possibilities. Cruise the island's main street for a variety of options, and sample Paris' best ice cream. For locations, see the map on page 1112.

Another option (not covered here) is to head south of the river, into the Latin Quarter, where the dense streets are loaded with touristy but quick crêperies and falafel joints.

In the Heart of the Marais

These are closest to the St-Paul Métro stop.

On Place du Marché Ste. Catherine: This small, romantic square, just off Rue St. Antoine, is an international food festival cloaked in extremely Parisian, leafy-square ambience. On a balmy evening, this is a neighborhood favorite, with a handful of res-taurants offering mediocre cuisine (you're here for the setting). It's also kid-friendly: Most places serve French hamburgers, and kids can dance around the square while parents breathe. Study the square, and you'll find three French bistros with similar features and menus: **$ Le Marché, Chez Joséphine,** and **Au Bistrot de la Place** (all open daily with €20-32 *menus* on weekdays, must order *à la carte* on weekends, tight seating on flimsy chairs indoors and out, Chez Joséphine has best chairs).

Several hardworking **$ Asian fast-food eateries,** great for an €8 meal, line Rue St. Antoine.

On Rue des Rosiers in the Jewish Quarter: These places line up along the same street in the heart of the Jewish Quarter.

$$ Chez Marianne is a neighborhood fixture that blends delicious Jewish cuisine with Parisian *élan* and wonderful atmo-sphere. Choose from several indoor zones with a cluttered wine shop/deli feeling, or sit outside. You'll select from two dozen *Zakouski* elements to assemble your €14-18 *plat*. Vegetarians will find great options (€12 falafel sandwich—half that if you order it to go, long hours daily, corner of Rue des Rosiers and Rue des Hospitalières-St-Gervais, tel. 01 42 72 18 86). For takeout, pay inside first and get a ticket before you order outside.

$ Le Loir dans la Théière ("The Dormouse in the Teapot") is a cozy, mellow teahouse offering a welcoming ambience for tired travelers (laptops and smartphones are not welcome). It's ideal for lunch and popular for weekend brunch. They offer a daily assortment of creatively filled quiches, and bake up an impressive array of homemade desserts that are proudly displayed in the dining room (€10-14 *plats*, daily 9:00-19:00, 3 Rue des Rosiers, tel. 01 42 72 90 61).

$ L'As du Falafel rules the falafel scene in the Jewish quarter. Monsieur Isaac, the "Ace of Falafel" here since 1979, brags, "I've got the biggest pita on the street...and I fill it up." (Apparently it's Lenny Kravitz's favorite, too.) Your inexpensive meal comes on plastic plates; the €8 "special falafel" is the big hit (€5.50 to go), but many enjoy his lighter chicken version *(poulet grillé)* or the tasty and massive *assiette de falafel* (€10). Wash it down with a cold Maccabee beer. Their takeout service draws a constant crowd (long hours most days except closed Fri evening and all day Sat, air-con, 34 Rue des Rosiers, tel. 01 48 87 63 60).

$ La Droguerie, a hole-in-the-wall crêpe stand a few blocks farther down Rue des Rosiers, has a lighthearted owner. It's a good budget option if falafels don't work for you, but cheap does. Eat as you walk or grab a stool (€5 savory crêpes, daily 12:00-22:00, 56 Rue des Rosiers).

Near Hôtel de Ville

To reach these eateries, use the Hôtel de Ville Métro stop.

$$ Au Bourguignon du Marais is a handsome wine bar/bistro for Burgundy lovers, where excellent wines (Burgundian only, available by the glass) blend with a good selection of well-designed dishes and efficient service. The *œufs en meurette* are mouthwatering, and the *bœuf bourguignon* could feed two (€11-14 starters, €20-30 *plats*, closed Sun-Mon, pleasing indoor and outdoor seating, 52 Rue François Miron, tel. 01 48 87 15 40, run by helpful Mattieu).

$ L'Ebouillanté is a breezy café, romantically situated near the river on a broad, cobbled pedestrian lane behind a church. With great outdoor seating and an artsy, cozy interior, it's perfect for an inexpensive and relaxing tea, snack, or lunch—or for dinner on a warm evening. Their *bricks*—paper-thin Tunisian-inspired pancakes stuffed with what you would typically find in an omelet—come with a small salad (€15 *bricks*, €13-16 *plats* and big salads, Tue-Sun 12:00-21:30, closed Mon, closes earlier in winter, a block off the river at 6 Rue des Barres, tel. 01 42 71 09 69).

$ Pizza Sant'Antonio is bustling and cheap, serving up €11 pizzas and salads on a fun Marais square (daily, barely off Rue de Rivoli at 1 Rue de la Verrerie, tel. 01 42 77 78 47).

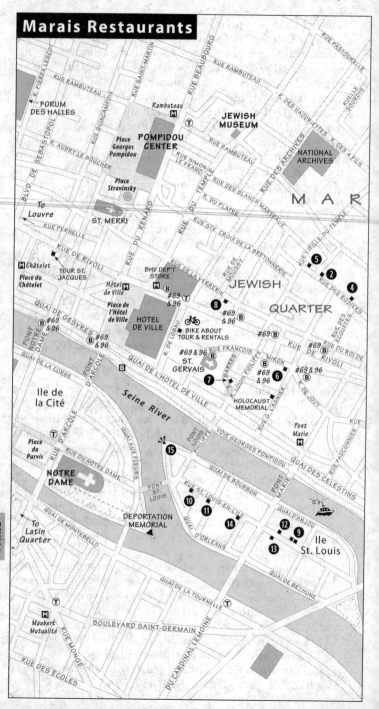

Marais Restaurants

FORUM DES HALLES

JEWISH MUSEUM

NATIONAL ARCHIVES

Rambuteau

Place Georges Pompidou

POMPIDOU CENTER

Place Stravinsky

M A R

To Louvre

ST. MERRI

RUE DE RIVOLI

Châtelet

Place du Châtelet

TOUR ST. JACQUES

BHV DEP'T STORE

JEWISH

Hôtel de Ville

QUARTER

Place de l'Hôtel de Ville

HOTEL DE VILLE

#69 & 96

8

#69 & 96

BIKE ABOUT TOUR & RENTALS

#69 B

QUAI DE GESVRES

#69 & 96

#69 & 96

#69 & 96

ST. GERVAIS

RUE FRANÇOIS

#69 MIRON

6

#69 & 96

7

HOLOCAUST MEMORIAL

Ile de la Cité

Seine River

QUAI DE L'HOTEL DE VILLE

Pont Marie

Place du Parvis

15

NOTRE DAME

DEPORTATION MEMORIAL

QUAI DE BOURBON

10

RUE ST. LOUIS-EN-L'ILE

11

14

QUAI D'ANJOU

12

9

To Latin Quarter

QUAI D'ORLEANS

13

Ile St. Louis

QUAI DE BETHUNE

QUAI DE LA TOURNELLE

Maubert Mutualité

BOULEVARD SAINT-GERMAIN

RUE DES ECOLES

PARIS

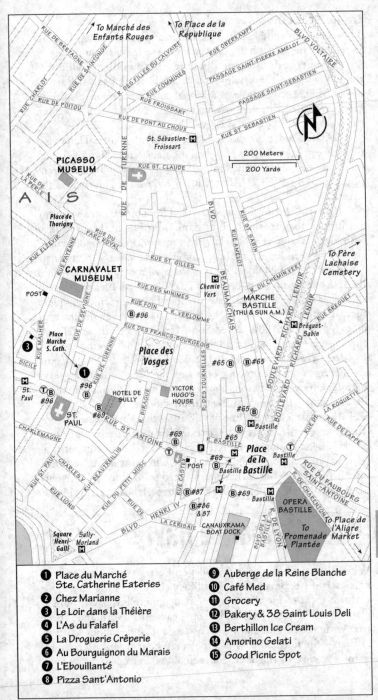

1. Place du Marché Ste. Catherine Eateries
2. Chez Marianne
3. Le Loir dans la Théière
4. L'As du Falafel
5. La Droguerie Crêperie
6. Au Bourguignon du Marais
7. L'Ebouillanté
8. Pizza Sant'Antonio
9. Auberge de la Reine Blanche
10. Café Med
11. Grocery
12. Bakery & 38 Saint Louis Deli
13. Berthillon Ice Cream
14. Amorino Gelati
15. Good Picnic Spot

On Ile St. Louis

These recommended spots line the island's main drag, Rue St. Louis-en-l'Ile (to get here, use the Pont Marie Métro stop).

$ Auberge de la Reine Blanche welcomes diners willing to rub elbows with their neighbors under heaving beams. Earnest owner Michel serves basic, traditional cuisine at reasonable prices. His giant salad can be a beefy meal all by itself (€21-27 *menus*, closed Wed, 30 Rue St. Louis-en-l'Ile, tel. 01 46 33 07 87).

$ Café Med, near the pedestrian bridge to Notre-Dame, is a tiny, cheery *crêperie* with good-value salads, crêpes, and €11 *plats* (€14 and €20 *menus,* daily, limited wine list, 77 Rue St. Louis-en-l'Ile, tel. 01 43 29 73 17). Two similar *crêperies* are just across the street.

Riverside Picnic for Impoverished Romantics: During sunny lunchtimes, the *quai* on the Left Bank side of Ile St. Louis is lined with locals who have more class than money, spreading out tablecloths and even lighting candles for elegant picnics. And tourists can enjoy the same budget meal. A handy grocery store at #67 on Ile St. Louis' main drag (open until 22:00, closed Tue) has tabouli and other simple, cheap takeaway dishes for your picnicking pleasure. The bakery a few blocks down at #40 serves quiche and pizza (open until 20:00, closed Sun-Mon), and a gourmet deli and cheese shop—aptly named **38 Saint Louis**—can be found at #38.

Ice-Cream Dessert: Half the people strolling Ile St. Louis are licking an ice-cream cone because this is the home of *les glaces Berthillon* (now sold throughout Paris though still made here on Ile St. Louis). The original **Berthillon** shop, at 31 Rue St. Louis-en-l'Ile, is marked by the line of salivating customers (closed Mon-Tue). For a less famous but satisfying treat, the Italian gelato a block away at **Amorino Gelati** is giving Berthillon competition (no line, bigger portions, easier to see what you want, and they offer little tastes—Berthillon doesn't need to, 47 Rue St. Louis-en-l'Ile, tel. 01 44 07 48 08). Having some of each is not a bad thing.

Near Le Havre

While Paris is the big draw for most cruisers, several other options lie closer to Le Havre. The most likely choices are the charming seafront town of Honfleur (a quick 30-minute bus ride from Le Havre), the historic WWII D-Day beaches of Normandy (best seen with a local guide or on an excursion), and—about halfway to Paris—the fine cathedral at Rouen (an hour from Le Havre by train). I've covered the basics for each of these next.

Honfleur

Gazing at its cozy harbor lined with skinny, soaring houses, it's easy to overlook the historic importance of Honfleur (ohn-flur).

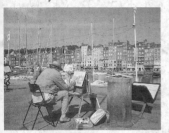

For more than a thousand years, sailors have enjoyed this port's ideal location, where the Seine River greets the English Channel. The town was also a favorite of 19th-century Impressionists who were captivated by Honfleur's unusual light—the result of its river-meets-sea setting. Eugène Boudin (boo-dahn) lived and painted in Honfleur, drawing Monet and other creative types from Paris. In some ways, modern art was born in the fine light of idyllic little Honfleur.

Honfleur escaped the bombs of World War II, and today it offers a romantic port enclosed on three sides by sprawling outdoor cafés. Long eclipsed by the gargantuan port of Le Havre just across the Seine, Honfleur happily uses its past as a bar stool...and sits on it.

Orientation to Honfleur

All of Honfleur's appealing lanes and activities are within a short stroll of its old port (Vieux Bassin). The Seine River flows just east of the center, the hills of the Côte de Grâce form its western limit, and Rue de la République slices north-south through the center to the port. Honfleur has two can't-miss sights—the harbor and Ste. Catherine Church—and a handful of other intriguing monuments. But really, the town itself is its best sight.

TOURIST INFORMATION

The TI is in the glassy public library *(Mediathèque)* on Quai le Paulmier, two blocks from the Vieux Bassin toward Le Havre (July-Aug Mon-Sat 9:30-19:00, Sun 10:00-17:00; Sept-June Mon-Sat 9:30-12:30 & 14:00-18:30, Sun 10:00-12:30 & 14:00-17:00 except closed Sun afternoon Oct-Easter; free WCs inside, pay Internet access, tel. 02 31 89 23 30, www.ot-honfleur.fr).

ARRIVAL IN HONFLEUR

By Bus from Le Havre: Get off at the small bus station *(gare routière),* and confirm your departure at the helpful information counter. To reach the TI and old town, turn right as you exit the station and walk five minutes up Quai le Paulmier.

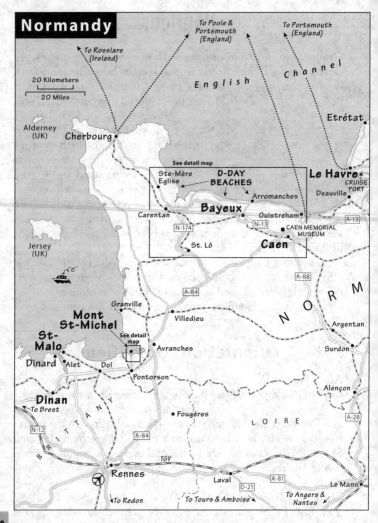

Normandy

20 Kilometers
20 Miles

To Rosslare
(Ireland)

To Poole &
Portsmouth
(England)

To Portsmouth
(England)

English Channel

Etrétat

Alderney
(UK)

Cherbourg

See detail map

Ste-Mère
Eglise

**D-DAY
BEACHES**

Le Havre

CRUISE
PORT

Arromanches

Deauville

Carentan

Bayeux

Ouistreham

A-13

N-174

N-13

CAEN MEMORIAL
MUSEUM

St. Lô

Caen

Jersey
(UK)

A-88

Granville

Mont
St-Michel

Villedieu

N O R M

Argentan

St-
Malo

See detail
map

Avranches

Surdon

Dinard

Alet

Dol

Pontorson

Alençon

Dinan
To Brest

Fougères

L O I R E

A-28

N-12

A-84

B R I T T A N Y

TGV

Rennes

Laval

A-81

D-21

To Angers &
Nantes

Le Mans

To Redon

To Tours & Amboise

RETURNING TO LE HAVRE

Buses run sporadically from Honfleur to Le Havre (roughly 4-6/
day Mon-Sat, 2/day on Sun, 30 minutes, www.busverts.fr). As this
service is relatively infrequent, be sure to double-check your connection locally.

HELPFUL HINTS

Grocery Store: There's a grocery store near the TI with long hours
(daily July-Aug, closed Mon off-season, 16 Quai le Paulmier).

Regional Products with Panache: Visit **Produits Regionaux
Gribouille** for any Norman delicacy you can dream up. Say

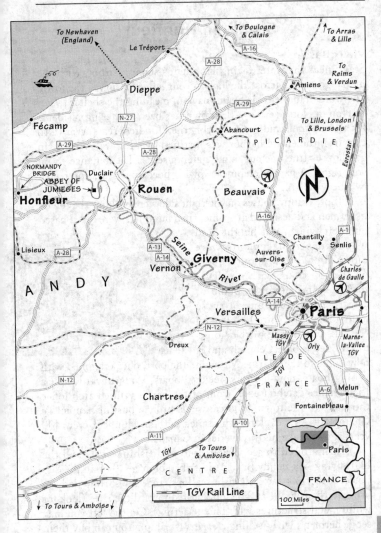

bonjour to Monsieur Gribouille (gree-boo-ee), and watch your head—his egg-beater collection hangs from above (Thu-Tue 9:30-13:00 & 14:00-19:00, closed Wed, 16 Rue de l'Homme de Bois, tel. 02 31 89 29 54).

Internet Access: Free Wi-Fi is available at the recommended **Travel Coffee Shop** and at several other cafés in town. Ask the TI for a list of cafés with computer terminals and Wi-Fi.

Taxi: Call mobile 06 18 18 38 38.

Sights in Honfleur

Vieux Bassin

Stand near the water facing Honfleur's square harbor, with the merry-go-round across the lock to your left, and survey the town. The word "Honfleur" is Scandinavian, meaning the shelter *(fleur)* of Hon (a Norse settler). This town has been sheltering residents for about a thousand years. During the Hundred Years' War (14th century), the entire harbor was fortified by a big wall with twin gatehouses (the one surviving gatehouse, La Lieutenance, is on your right). A narrow channel allowing boats to pass was protected by a heavy chain.

Those skinny houses on the right side were built for the town's fishermen and designed at a time when buildings were taxed based on their width, not height (and when knee replacements were unheard of). How about a room on the top floor, with no eleva-tor? Imagine moving a piano or a refrigerator into one of these units today. The spire halfway up the left side of the port belongs to Honfleur's oldest church and is

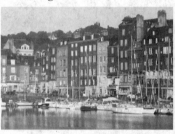

now home to the Marine Museum. The port, once crammed with fishing boats, now harbors sleek sailboats. Walk toward the La Lieutenance gatehouse. In front of the barrel-vaulted arch (once the entry to the town), you can see a bronze bust of Samuel de Champlain—the explorer who sailed with an Honfleur crew 400 years ago to make his discoveries in Canada.

Turn around to see various tour and fishing boats and the high-flying Normandy Bridge (described on page 1044) in the dis-tance. Fisherfolk catch flatfish, scallops, and tiny shrimp daily to bring to the Marché au Poisson, located toward the river (look for white metal structures with blue lettering). On the left you may see fishermen's wives selling *crevettes* (shrimp). You can buy them *cuites* (cooked) or *vivantes* (alive and wiggly). They are happy to let you sample one (rip off the cute little head and tail, and pop the middle into your mouth—*délicieuse!*), or buy a cupful to go for a few euros (daily in season).

You'll probably see artists sitting at easels around the har-bor, as Boudin and Monet did. Many consider Honfleur the birth-place of 19th-century Impressionism. This was a time when people began to revere, not fear, the out-of-doors, and started to climb mountains "because they were there." Pretty towns like Honfleur and the nearby coast made perfect subjects to paint—and still are—thanks to what locals called the "unusual luminosity" of the region. And with the advent of trains in the late 1800s, artists could travel to the best light like never before. Artists would set up easels along the harbor to catch the light playing on the line of buildings, slate shingles, timbers, geraniums, clouds, and reflections in the water. Monet came here to visit the artist Boudin, a hometown boy, and the battle cry of the Impressionists—"Out of the studio and into the light!"—was born.

▲▲Ste. Catherine Church (Eglise Ste. Catherine)

The unusual wood-shingled exterior suggests that this church has a different story to tell than most. Walk inside. You'd swear that if it were turned over, it would float—the legacy of a community of sailors and fishermen, with loads of talented boat-builders and nary a cathedral architect.

The church's bell tower was built away from the church to avoid placing too much stress on the wooden church's roof, and to help minimize fire hazards. Go inside to appreciate the ancient wood framing and to see a good 15-minute video describing the bell tower's history. The highlights of the tiny museum inside are two wooden sculptures from the bows of two Louis XIII ships.

Cost and Hours: Church—free, daily July-Aug 9:00-18:30, Sept-June 9:00-17:15; bell tower—€2, free with ticket to the Eugène Boudin Museum, April-Sept Wed-Mon 10:00-12:00 & 14:00-18:00; closed Oct-March and Tue year-round.

Boat Excursions

Boat trips in and around Honfleur depart from various docks between Hôtel le Cheval Blanc and the opposite end of the outer port (Easter-Oct usually about 11:00-17:00). The tour boat *Calypso* takes good 45-minute spins around Honfleur's harbor (€6, mobile 06 71 64 50 46).

Museums and Galleries

Honfleur-born landscape painter Eugène Boudin ignited this city's artistic tradition, which still burns today. The town is a popular haunt of artists, many of whom display their works in Honfleur's many art galleries (the best ones are along the streets between Ste. Catherine Church and the port). As you walk around the town visiting the museums, take time to enjoy today's art, too.

A €10.10 **museum pass** covers all of the museums described next and pays for itself with visits to just the Boudin and Satie museums (pass sold at TI and participating museums).

▲Eugène Boudin Museum

This pleasing little museum has three interesting floors with many paintings of Honfleur and the surrounding countryside. The first floor displays Norman folk costumes, the second floor has

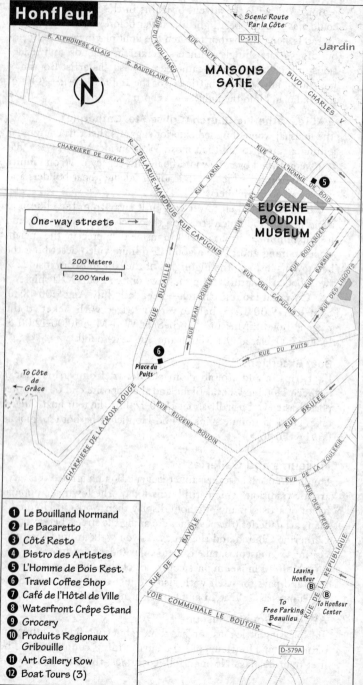

Honfleur

Scenic Route
Par la Côte

D-513

Jardin

R. ALPHONESE ALLAIS

R. BAUDELAIRE

RUE DU TROULMIARD

RUE HAUTE

MAISONS
SATIE

BLVD. CHARLES V

CHARRIERE DE GRACE

R. L. DELARUE-MARDRUS

RUE DE L'HOMME DE BOIS

RUE VARIN

❺

EUGENE
BOUDIN
MUSEUM

One-way streets →

RUE CAPUCINS

RUE ALBERT

RUE BOULANGER

RUE BARBEL

RUE DES LINGOTS

200 Meters
200 Yards

RUE BUCAILLE

RUE JEAN DOUBLET

RUE DES CAPUCINS

RUE DU PUITS

❻

Place du
Puits

To Côte
de ←
Grâce

CHARRIERE DE LA CROIX ROUGE

RUE EUGENE BOUDIN

RUE BRULEE

RUE DE LA FOULERIE

RUE DES PRES

RUE DE LA BAVOLE

RUE DE LA REPUBLIQUE

Leaving
Honfleur
Ⓑ   Ⓑ
To   To Honfleur
Free Parking   Center
Beaulieu

VOIE COMMUNALE LE BOUTOIR

D-579A

❶ Le Bouilland Normand
❷ Le Bacaretto
❸ Côté Resto
❹ Bistro des Artistes
❺ L'Homme de Bois Rest.
❻ Travel Coffee Shop
❼ Café de l'Hôtel de Ville
❽ Waterfront Crêpe Stand
❾ Grocery
❿ Produits Regionaux
   Gribouille
⓫ Art Gallery Row
⓬ Boat Tours (3)

PARIS

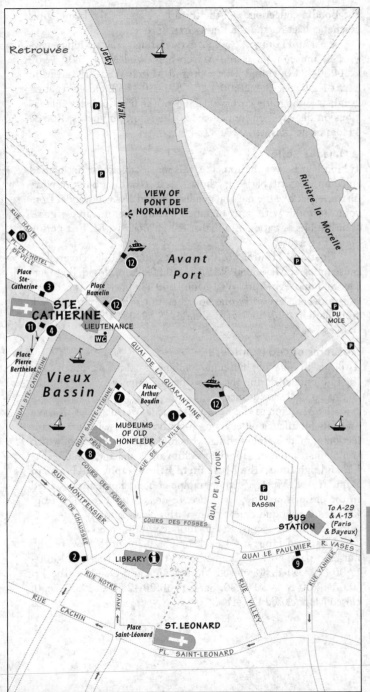

Retrouvée

Jetty Walk

P

P

VIEW OF
PONT DE
NORMANDIE

Avant
Port

Rivière la Morelle

P

RUE HAUTE

◆ 10

PL. DE L'HOTEL
DE VILLE

Place Ste-
Catherine

❸

Place
Hamelin

P
DU
MOLE

❶❷

**STE.
CATHERINE**

❶❷

✚

P

❶❶ ❹

LIEUTENANCE

WC

QUAI DE LA QUARANTAINE

Place
Pierre
Berthelot

*Vieux
Bassin*

QUAI STE-CATHERINE

❼

Place
Arthur
Boudin

❶

❶❷

MUSEUMS OF
OLD HONFLEUR

QUAI SAINTE-ETIENNE

◆ ❽

RUE DE LA VILLE

QUAI DE LA TOUR

P
DU
BASSIN

RUE MONTPENSIER

COURS DES FOSSES

RUE DE CHAUSSEE

COURS DES FOSSES

**BUS
STATION**

To A-29
& A-13
(Paris
& Bayeux)

PARIS

R. VASES

QUAI LE PAULMIER

❾

◆ ❷

LIBRARY ℹ

RUE NOTRE DAME

RUE VANNIER

RUE VILLEY

RUE CACHIN

Place
Saint-Léonard

ST. LEONARD

✚

PL. SAINT-LEONARD

the Boudin collection, and the third floor houses the Hambourg/ Rachet collection and the Katia Granoff room.

Cost and Hours: €6.50, €2 extra during special exhibits, covered by museum pass; mid-March-Sept Wed-Mon 10:00-12:00 & 14:00-18:00, closed Tue; Oct-mid-March Wed-Fri and Mon 14:30-17:30, Sat-Sun 10:00-12:00 & 14:30-17:30, closed Tue; €2 English audioguide covers selected works (no English explanations on display—but none needed); elevator, no photos, Rue de l'Homme de Bois, tel. 02 31 89 54 00.

▲Maisons Satie

If Honfleur is over-the-top cute, this remarkable museum, housed in composer Erik Satie's birthplace, is a refreshing burst of witty charm—just like the musical genius it honors. As you wander from room to room with your included audioguide, infrared signals transmit bits of Satie's minimalist music, along with a first-person story (in English).

Cost and Hours: €6.10, includes audioguide, covered by museum pass; May-Sept Wed-Mon 10:00-19:00, closed Tue; Oct-Dec and mid-Feb-April Wed-Mon 11:00-18:00, closed Tue; closed Jan-mid-Feb; last entry one hour before closing, 5-minute walk from harbor at 67 Boulevard Charles V, tel. 02 31 89 11 11, www. musees-honfleur.fr.

Museums of Old Honfleur

Two side-by-side folk museums combine to paint a picture of daily life in Honfleur during the time when its ships were king and the city had global significance.

The **Museum of the Sea** (Musée de la Marine) faces the port and fills Honfleur's oldest church (15th century) with a cool collection of models from fishing boats to naval ships (many of which were constructed in Honfleur's shipyards), marine paraphernalia, and paintings. The **Museum of Ethnography and Norman Popular Art** (Musée d'Ethnographie et d'Art Populaire), located in the old prison and courthouse, re-creates typical rooms from Honfleur's past and crams them with objects of daily life—costumes, furniture, looms, and an antique printing press.

Cost and Hours: €4 each or €5.20 for both, covered by museum pass; both museums open April-Sept Tue-Sun 10:00-12:00 & 14:00-18:30, closed Mon; March and Oct-Nov Tue-Fri 10:00-12:00 & 14:30-17:30, Sat-Sun 10:00-12:00 & 14:00-17:30, closed Mon; closed Dec-Feb.

Eating in Honfleur

Eat seafood or cream sauces here. It's a tough choice between the irresistible waterfront tables of the many look-alike places lining the harbor and the eateries with good reputations elsewhere in town.

Le Bouilland Normand hides a block off the port on a pleasing square and offers a true Norman experience at reasonable prices. Claire and chef-hubbie Bruno provide quality *Normand* cuisine and enjoy serving travelers. Daily specials complement the classic offerings (€22-30 *menus*, closed Wed, dine inside or out, 7 Rue de la Ville, tel. 02 31 89 02 41, www.aubouillonnormand.fr).

Le Bacaretto wine bar-café is run by laid-back Hervé, the antithesis of a wine snob. This relaxed and tiny wine-soaked place offers a fine selection of wines by the glass for good prices and a small but appealing assortment of appetizers and *plats du jour* that can make a full meal (closed Wed-Thu, 44 Rue de la Chaussée, tel. 02 31 14 83 11).

Côté Resto saddles up on the left side of Ste. Catherine Church and serves a top selection of seafood in a classy setting. The value is excellent for those in search of a special meal (€24 two-course *menu*, €30 three-course *menu*, great selection, closed Thu, 8 Place Ste. Catherine, tel. 02 31 89 31 33, www.cote-resto-honfleur.com).

Bistro des Artistes is a two-woman operation and the joy of locals (call ahead for a window table). Hardworking Anne-Marie cooks from a select repertoire upstairs while her server takes care of business in the pleasant little dining room. Portions are huge and very homemade; order only one course and maybe a dessert (€18-26 *plats*, closed Wed, 30 Place Berthelot, tel. 02 31 89 95 90).

L'Homme de Bois combines way-cozy ambience with authentic Norman cuisine and good prices (€23 three-course *menu* with few choices, €26 *menu* gives more choices, daily, a few outside tables, 30 Rue de l'Homme de Bois, tel. 02 31 89 75 27).

Travel Coffee Shop is an ideal breakfast or lunch option for travelers wanting conversation—in either English or French—and good food at very fair prices (May-Sept 8:00-17:00, closed Wed, April and Oct-Nov Sat-Sun only, closed Dec-March, 6 Place du Puits).

Of the harborfront options, **Café de l'Hôtel de Ville** owns the best afternoon sun exposure (and charges for it) and looks across to Honfleur's soaring homes (open daily July-Aug, closed Tue off-season, Place de l'Hôtel de Ville, tel. 02 31 89 07 29).

Dessert: Honfleur is ice-cream crazy, with gelato and traditional ice-cream shops on every corner. If you need a Ben & Jerry's ice-cream fix or a scrumptious dessert crêpe, find the **waterfront stand** at the southeast corner of the Vieux Bassin.

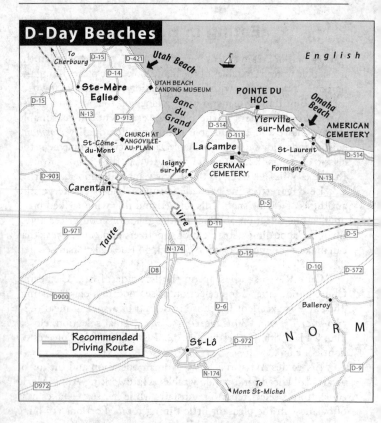

D-Day Beaches

The 54 miles of Atlantic coast north of Bayeux—stretching from Utah Beach on the west to Sword Beach on the east—are littered with WWII museums, monuments, cemeteries, and battle remains left in tribute to the courage of the British, Canadian, and American armies that successfully carried out the largest military operation in history: D-Day. (It's called *Jour J* in French—the letters "D" and "J" come from the first letter for the word "day" in either English or French.) It was on these serene beaches, at the crack of dawn on June 6, 1944, that the Allies finally gained a foothold in France, and Nazi Europe was doomed to crumble.

The most famous D-Day sights lie significantly west of Le Havre; for example, Omaha Beach is about a 1.5-hour drive from your cruise port (in good traffic). Other sights are closer—Caen, with its exceptional museum, is about an hour from Le Havre—but still far enough to make it challenging and rushed to see in a short day in port. Many of the best D-Day guides are based

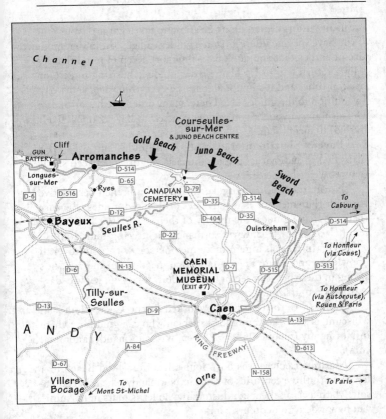

closer to the beaches, making it a long journey for them to come meet your ship, then take you back later. All of this makes visiting the D-Day beaches more expensive and less efficient than it could be (ideally, save it for another trip when you can really give it some time). However, if this is your one chance to see this historic sliver of French coastline, and you don't mind splurging on a guide or an excursion to do it efficiently, a D-Day side-trip is worth considering.

GETTING AROUND THE D-DAY BEACHES

By Guided Tour: An army of small companies offers all-day excursions to the D-Day beaches. Most are based in or near Bayeux, about 75 miles west of Le Havre, and prefer not to do tours from Le Havre's cruise port. However, the companies and guides listed here are willing to make the trip...for a price. Because they pick up and drop off in Le Havre, they are popular with cruisers (and other day-trippers). Book your tour as far in advance as possible (three months is best), or pray for a last-minute cancellation.

Request extra time at the American Cemetery to see the

excellent visitors center. Don't be afraid to take charge of your tour if you have specific interests (some guides can get lost in the minutiae of battles that you don't have time for). Keep in mind that it's a long return trip to Le Havre, your guide is hustling to get you back in time, and it's impossible to see everything in a short day. In addition to the guides listed here, many others are happy to do a D-Day tour for you...*if* you can get yourself to Bayeux (most likely by taxi) to meet them.

Bayeux Shuttle offers well-trained guides and uses GPS maps tied to audiovisual presentations as you drive between sights (www.bayeuxshuttle.com).

Normandy Sightseeing Tours delivers a French perspective through the voices of its small fleet of licensed guides. Because there are many guides, the quality of their teaching is less consistent (tel. 02 31 51 70 52, www.normandy-sightseeing-tours.com).

Sylvain Kast is a genuinely nice person with good overall knowledge and many French family connections to the war; he's strong in the American sector (mobile 06 17 44 04 46, www.d-day-experience-tours.com).

Vanessa Letourneur, who worked at the Caen Memorial Museum, is a low-key and likable person who can guide anywhere in Normandy (mobile 06 98 95 89 45, www.normandypanorama.com).

Mathias Leclere was born four miles from Juno Beach to a family with three centuries of roots in Normandy—he is part of its soil. Mathias is a self-taught historian who leads tours in his minivan (www.ddayguidedtours.com).

On Your Own: Though guided tours teach important history lessons, **renting a car** can be a good and less expensive way to visit the beaches, particularly for three or more people (for rental suggestions in Le Havre, see page 1037). Park in monitored locations at the sites, since break-ins are a problem—particularly at the American Cemetery—and consider hiring a guide to join you. Of course, be sure to leave yourself plenty of time to make it back to Le Havre to drop off your car and get back to your ship.

For small groups, hiring a **taxi for the day** is cheaper than taking a tour (see rates on page 1039), but you don't get the full history lesson.

D-Day Sights

With one day, you'll only have time to visit a few D-Day locations. From Le Havre, it takes longer to reach the American sector, which is west of Arromanches, with sights scattered between Omaha and Utah beaches. The British and Canadian sectors (east of Arromanches) are closer to Le Havre, but have been overbuilt with resorts, making it harder to envision the events of June 1944. For more information on visiting the D-Day beaches, www.normandiememoire. com is a useful resource.

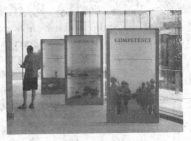

West of Arromanches

The small town of **Arromanches** was ground zero for the D-Day invasion. Almost overnight, it sprouted the immense harbor, Port Winston, which gave the Allies a foothold in Normandy, allowing them to begin their victorious push to Berlin and end World War II. You'll find a view over the site of that gigantic makeshift harbor, a good museum, an evocative beach and bluff, and a touristy-but-fun little town that offers a pleasant cocktail of war memories, cotton candy, and beachfront trinket shops. From here, you'll find the following sights (listed roughly from east to west):

Longues-sur-Mer Gun Battery: Four German casemates (three with guns intact)—built to guard against seaborne attacks—hunker down at the end of a country road. This battery—with the only original coastal artillery guns remaining in place in the D-Day region—was a critical link in Hitler's Atlantic Wall defense, which consisted of more than 15,000 structures stretching from Norway to the Pyrenees. Today visitors can see the bunkers at this strategic site.

WWII Normandy American Cemetery and Memorial: Crowning a bluff just above Omaha Beach and the eye of the D-Day storm, 9,387 brilliant white-marble crosses and Stars of David glow in memory of Americans who gave their lives to free Europe on the beaches below.

Vierville-sur-Mer and Omaha Beach: Omaha Beach witnessed by far the most intense battles of any along the D-Day beaches. The hills above were heavily fortified, and a single German machine gun could fire 1,200 rounds a minute. The highest casualty rates in Normandy occurred at Omaha Beach, nicknamed "Bloody Omaha." Here you'll find a museum and a chance to walk on the beach where anywhere from 2,500 to 4,800 Americans were killed and wounded, making way for some 34,000 to land on the beach by day's end.

Pointe du Hoc: The intense bombing of the beaches by Allied forces is best experienced here, where US Army Rangers scaled impossibly steep cliffs to disable a German gun battery. Pointe du

Hoc's bomb-cratered, lunar-like landscape and remaining bunkers make it one of the most evocative of the D-Day sites.

German Military Cemetery: To ponder German losses, visit this somber, thought-provoking resting place of 21,000 German soldiers. Compared to the American Cemetery, which symbolizes hope and victory, this one is a clear symbol of defeat and despair. A small visitors center gives more information on this and other German war cemeteries.

Utah Beach Landing Museum: Built around the remains of a concrete German bunker, this museum—the best one located on the D-Day beaches—nestles in the sand dunes on Utah Beach, with floors above and below sea level. For the Allied landings to succeed, many coordinated tasks had to be accomplished: Paratroopers had to be dropped inland, the resistance had to disable bridges and cut communications, bombers had to deliver payloads on target and on time, the infantry had to land safely on the beaches, and supplies had to follow the infantry closely. This thorough yet manageable museum pieces those many parts together in a series of fascinating exhibits and displays.

Church at Angoville-au-Plain: At this simple Romanesque church, two American medics (Kenneth Moore and Robert Wright) treated German and American wounded while battles raged only steps away.

Ste-Mère Eglise: Made famous by the film *The Longest Day*, this village was the first to be liberated by the Americans. The area around Ste-Mère Eglise was the center of action for American paratroopers, whose objective was to land behind enemy lines in support of the American landing at Utah Beach. It was around this village that many paratroopers, facing terrible weather and heavy anti-aircraft fire, landed off-target—including one who dangled from the town's church steeple for two hours. Today, the village greets travelers with flag-draped streets, that famous church, and a museum honoring the paratroopers.

East of Arromanches

Juno Beach Centre: Located on the beachfront in the Canadian sector, this facility is dedicated to teaching travelers about the vital role Canadian forces played in the invasion.

Canadian Cemetery: This small, touching cemetery makes a modest statement when compared with other, more grandiose cemeteries in this area. To me, it captures the understated nature of

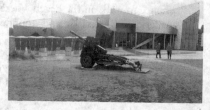

Canadians perfectly.

Caen Memorial Museum: Caen, the modern capital of lower Normandy, has the most thorough WWII museum in France. Located at the site of an important German headquarters during World War II, its official name is "The Caen Memorial: Center for the History for Peace" *(Le Mémorial de Caen: La Cité de l'Histoire pour la Paix)*. With two video presentations and numerous exhibits on the lead-up to World War II, coverage of the war in both Europe and the Pacific, accounts of the Holocaust and Nazi-occupied France, the Cold War aftermath, and more, it effectively puts the Battle of Normandy into a broader context.

Rouen

This 2,000-year-old city mixes Gothic architecture, half-timbered houses, and contemporary bustle like no other place in France.

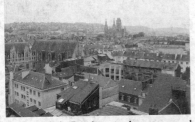

Busy Rouen (roo-ahn) is France's fifth-largest port and Europe's biggest food exporter (mostly wheat and grain).

Rouen was a regional capital during Roman times, and France's second-largest city in medieval times (with 40,000 residents—only Paris had more). In the ninth century, the Normans made the town their capital. William the Conqueror called it home before moving to England. Rouen walked a political tightrope between England and France for centuries, and was an English base during the Hundred Years' War. Joan of Arc was burned here (in 1431).

Rouen's historic wealth was built on its wool industry and trade—for centuries, it was the last bridge across the Seine River before the Atlantic. In April of 1944, as America and Britain weakened German control of Normandy prior to the D-Day landings, Allied bombers destroyed 50 percent of Rouen. And though the industrial suburbs were devastated, most of the historic core survived, keeping Rouen a pedestrian haven.

Rouen is right along the main Paris-bound train line, just an hour from Le Havre. If you've been to Paris before (or prefer to save it for another trip), and you want a dose of a smaller—yet lively—French city, Rouen is a good choice.

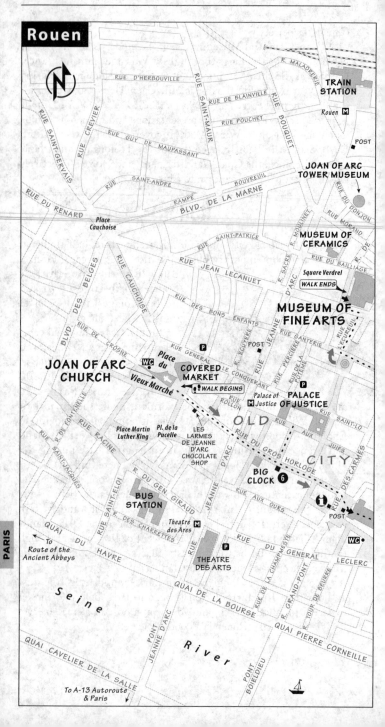

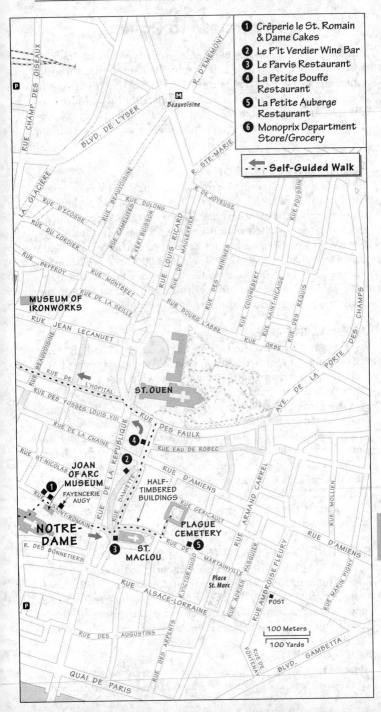

1 Crêperie le St. Romain & Dame Cakes
2 Le P'it Verdier Wine Bar
3 Le Parvis Restaurant
4 La Petite Bouffe Restaurant
5 La Petite Auberge Restaurant
6 Monoprix Department Store/Grocery

- - - - Self-Guided Walk

PARIS

Orientation to Rouen

Although Paris embraces the Seine, Rouen ignores it. The area we're most interested in is bounded by the river to the south, the Museum of Fine Arts (Esplanade Marcel Duchamp) to the north, Rue de la République to the east, and Place du Vieux Marché to the west. It's a 20-minute walk from the train station to the Notre-Dame Cathedral or TI. Everything else of interest is within a 10-minute walk of the cathedral or TI.

TOURIST INFORMATION

Pick up the English map with information on Rouen's museums at the TI, which faces the cathedral. The TI also has €5 audioguide tours covering the cathedral and Rouen's historic center, though this book's self-guided walk is enough for most. They also have free Wi-Fi (for 30 minutes) and a loaner tablet (May-Sept Mon-Sat 9:00-19:00, Sun 9:30-12:30 & 14:00-18:00; Oct-April Mon-Sat 9:30-12:30 & 13:30-18:00, closed Sun; 25 Place de la Cathédrale, tel. 02 32 08 32 40, www.rouentourisme.com). A small office in the TI changes money (closed during lunch year-round).

ARRIVAL IN ROUEN

By Train from Le Havre: Get off at the station called "Rouen-Rive-Droite." From here, Rue Jeanne d'Arc cuts straight down from Rouen's train station through the town center to the Seine River. **Walk** from the station down Rue Jeanne d'Arc toward Rue du Gros Horloge—a busy pedestrian mall in the medieval center (and near the starting point of my self-guided walk).

Rouen's **subway** (Métrobus) whisks travelers from under the train station to the Palais de Justice in one stop (€1.50 for 1 hour; descend and buy tickets from machines one level underground, then validate ticket on subway two levels down; subway direction: Technopôle or Georges Braque).

Taxis (to the right as you exit station) will take you to various points in town for about €8.

RETURNING TO LE HAVRE

Trains head back to Le Havre about hourly and take around an hour. To reach the train station from downtown Rouen, head straight up Rue Jeanne d'Arc from Rue du Gros Horloge (the main shopping street). For a quicker return, take the subway in direction: Boulingrin and get off at Gare-Rue Verte.

HELPFUL HINTS

Closed Days: Most of Rouen's museums are closed on Tuesday, and many sights also close midday (12:00-14:00). The cathedral doesn't open until 14:00 on Monday and is closed during Mass (usually Tue-Sat at 10:00, July-Aug also at 18:00; Sun and holidays at 8:30, 10:00, and 12:00). The Joan of Arc Church is closed Friday and Sunday mornings, and during Mass.

Supermarket: Small grocery shops are scattered about the city, and a big **Monoprix** is on Rue du Gros Horloge (groceries at the back, Mon-Sat 8:30-21:00, closed Sun).

Internet Access: The TI offers 30 minutes of free Wi-Fi and has a loaner tablet. Rouen is riddled with Wi-Fi cafés; several are within a few blocks of the train station on Rue Jeanne d'Arc.

Taxi: Call **Les Taxi Blancs** at 02 35 61 20 50 or 02 35 88 50 50.

Rouen Walk

On this 1.5-hour self-guided walk, you'll see the essential Rouen sights and experience its pedestrian-friendly streets filled with half-timbered buildings. Remember that many sights are closed midday (12:00-14:00). This walk is designed for day-trippers coming by train.

From Place du Vieux Marché, you'll walk the length of Rue du Gros Horloge to Notre-Dame Cathedral. From there, walk four blocks to the plague cemetery (Aître St. Maclou), loop up to the church of St. Ouen, and return along Rue de l'Hôpital ending at the Museum of Fine Arts (a 5-minute walk to the train station). The map on page 1130 highlights the route.

• *From the train station, walk down Rue Jeanne d'Arc and turn right on Rue du Guillaume le Conquérant (notice the Gothic Palace of Justice building across Rue Jeanne d'Arc—we'll get to that later). This takes you to the back door of our starting point...*

Place du Vieux Marché

• *Stand near the entrance of the striking Joan of Arc Church.*

Surrounded by half-timbered buildings, this old market square houses a cute, covered produce and fish market, a park commemorating Joan of Arc's burning, and a modern church named after her. Find the tall aluminum cross, planted in a small garden near the church entry. This marks the spot where Rouen publicly punished and executed people. The pillories stood here, and during the Revolution, the town's guillotine made 800 people "a foot shorter at the top." In 1431, Joan of Arc—only 19 years old—was burned right here. Joan had rallied French soldiers to drive out English invaders but was sentenced to death for being a witch and a heretic. Find her flaming statue facing the cross. As the flames engulfed her, an English soldier said, "Oh my God, we've killed a saint." (Nearly 500 years later, Joan was canonized, and the soldier was proved right.)

PARIS

▲▲Joan of Arc Church (Eglise Jeanne d'Arc)

This modern church is a tribute to the young woman who was canonized in 1920 and later became the patron saint of France. The church, completed in 1979, feels Scandinavian inside and out—another reminder of Normandy's Nordic roots. Sumptuous 16th-century windows, salvaged from a church lost during World War II, were worked into the soft architectural lines (the €0.50 English pamphlet provides some background and describes the stained-glass scenes). The pointed, stake-like support columns to the right seem fitting for a church dedicated to Joan of Arc. Similar to modern churches designed by the 20th-century architect Le Corbusier, this is an uplifting place to be, with a ship's-hull vaulting and sweeping wood ceiling that sail over curved pews and a wall of glass below. Make time to savor this unusual place.

Cost and Hours: Free; Mon-Thu and Sat 10:00-12:00 & 14:00-18:00, Fri and Sun 14:00-17:30; closed during Mass. A public WC is 30 yards straight ahead from the church doors.

• *Turn left out of the church and step over the ruins of a 15th-century church that once stood on this spot (destroyed during the French Revolution). Leave the square and join the busy pedestrian street, Rue du Gros Horloge—the town's main shopping street since Roman times. A block up on your right (at #163) is Rouen's most famous chocolate shop...*

Les Larmes de Jeanne d'Arc

The chocolate-makers of Les Larmes de Jeanne d'Arc would love to tempt you with their chocolate-covered almond "tears *(larmes)* of Joan of Arc." Although you must resist touching the chocolate fountain (which may be near the back), you are welcome to taste a tear (delicious). The first one is free; a small bag costs about €9 (Mon-Sat 9:15-19:15, closed Sun).

• *Your route continues past a medieval McDonald's and across busy Rue Jeanne d'Arc to the...*

▲Big Clock (Gros Horloge)

This impressive, circa-1528 Renaissance clock, le Gros Horloge (groh or-lohzh), decorates the former City Hall. Is something missing? Not really. In the 16th century, an hour hand offered sufficient precision; minute hands became necessary only in a later, faster-paced age. The lamb at the end of the hour hand is a reminder that wool rules—it was the source of Rouen's wealth. The town medallion features a sacrificial lamb, which has both religious and commercial significance (center, below the clock). The silver orb above the clock makes one revolution in 29 days. The clock's artistic highlight fills the underside of the arch (walk underneath and stretch your back), with the "Good Shepherd" and loads of sheep.

Bell Tower Panorama: To see the inner workings of the clock and an extraordinary panorama over Rouen (including a stirring view of the cathedral), climb the clock tower's 100 steps. You'll tour several rooms with the help of a friendly audioguide and learn about life in Rouen when the tower was built. The big bells at the top weigh 1 to 2 tons each and ring on the hour—a deafening experience if you're in the tower. Don't miss the 360-degree view outside from the very top.

Cost and Hours: €6, includes audioguide; April-Oct Tue-Sun 10:00-12:00 & 13:00-19:00; Nov-March Tue-Sun 14:00-18:00; closed Mon year-round, last entry one hour before closing.
• *Walk under le Gros Horloge, then take a one-block detour left on Rue Thouret to see the...*

Palace of Justice (Palais de Justice)

Years of cleaning have removed the grime that once covered this fabulously flamboyantly Gothic building, the former home of Normandy's *parlement* and the largest civil Gothic building in France. The result is striking; think of this as you visit Rouen's other Gothic structures; some are awaiting baths of their own. Pockmarks on the side of the building that faces Rue Jeanne d'Arc are leftovers from bombings during the Normandy invasion. Look for the English-language plaques on the iron fence—they provide some history and describe the damage and tedious repair process.
• *Double back and continue up Rue du Gros Horloge. In a block you'll see a stone plaque dedicated to Cavelier de la Salle (high on the left), who explored the mouth of the Mississippi River, claimed the state of Louisiana for France, and was assassinated in Texas in 1687. Soon you'll reach...*

▲▲Notre-Dame Cathedral (Cathédrale Notre-Dame)

This cathedral is a landmark of art history. You're seeing essentially what Claude Monet saw as he painted 30 different studies of this frilly Gothic facade at various times of the day. Using the physical

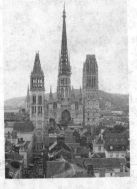

building only as a rack upon which to hang light, mist, dusk, and shadows, Monet was capturing "impressions." One of the results is in Rouen's Museum of Fine Arts; four others are at the Orsay Museum in Paris. Find the plaque showing two of these paintings (in the corner of the square, about 30 paces to your right if you were exiting the TI). The interior has chapels in a range of architectural styles, and stone tombs dating from when Rouen was the Norman capital (including one that holds the heart of Richard the Lionhearted).

Cost and Hours: Free, Tue-Sun 8:00-19:00, Mon 14:00-19:00; closed during Mass Tue-Sat at 10:00, July-Aug also at 18:00, Sun and holidays at 8:30, 10:30, and 12:00; also closed Nov-March daily 12:00-14:00.

• *From this courtyard, a gate deposits you on a traffic-free street. Turn right and walk along...*

Rue St. Romain

This appealing street is lined with half-timbered buildings. In a short distance, you can look up through an opening above the entrance to the new Joan of Arc Museum, and gaze back at the cathedral's prickly spire. Made of cast iron in the late 1800s—about the same time Gustave Eiffel was building his tower in Paris—the spire is, at 490 feet, the tallest in France. You can also see the former location of the missing smaller (green) spire—downed in a violent 1999 storm that blew the spire off the roof and sent it crashing to the cathedral floor.

Along the street find the new **Joan of Arc Museum** (L'Historical Jeanne d'Arc), which should be open by the time you visit. This long-overdue museum highlights the mystical person whose fiery death brought such notoriety to Rouen. It's housed in what was once the archbishop's palace next to the cathedral. Check with the TI for the cost and opening hours.

• *Farther down the street, find a shop that shows off a traditional art form in action.*

At **Fayencerie Augy** (at #26), Monsieur Augy and his staff welcome shoppers to browse his studio/gallery/shop and see Rouen's clay "china" being made the traditional way. First, the clay is molded and fired. Then it's dipped in white enamel, dried, lovingly hand-painted, and fired a second time. Rouen was the first city in France to make faience, earthenware with colored glazes. In the 1700s, the town had 18 factories churning out the popular product (Mon-Sat 9:00-19:00, closed Sun, 26 Rue St. Romain, VAT tax refunds nearly pay for the shipping, www.fayencerie-augy.com).

• *Continue along Rue St. Romain, which (after crossing Rue de la République) leads to the fancy...*

St. Maclou Church

This church's unique, bowed facade is textbook Flamboyant Gothic. Its recent cleaning revealed a brilliant white facade. Notice the flame-like tracery decorating its gable. Because this was built at the very end of the Gothic age—and construction took many years—the doors are from the next age: the Renaissance (c. 1550). Study the graphic Last Judgment above the doors; it was designed when Rouen was riddled with the Black Plague. The bright and airy interior is worth a quick peek.

Cost and Hours: Free, Fri-Mon 10:00-12:00 & 14:00-17:30, closed Tue-Thu.

• *Leaving the church, turn right, and then take another right (giving the little boys on the corner wall a wide berth). Wander past a fine wall of half-timbered buildings fronting Rue Martainville, to the end of St. Maclou Church.*

Half-Timbered Buildings

Because the local stone—a chalky limestone from the cliffs of the Seine River—was of poor quality (your thumbnail is stronger), and because local oak was plentiful, half-timbered buildings became a Rouen specialty from the 14th through 19th century. Cantilevered floors were standard until the early 1500s. These top-heavy designs made sense: City land was limited, property taxes were based on ground-floor square footage, and the cantilevering minimized unsupported spans on upper floors. The oak beams provided the structural skeleton of the building, which was then filled in with a mix of clay, straw, pebbles...or whatever was available.

• *A block farther down on the left, at 186 Rue Martainville, a covered lane leads to the...*

Plague Cemetery (Aître St. Maclou)

During the great plagues of the Middle Ages, as many as two-thirds of the people in this parish died. For the decimated community, dealing with the corpses was an overwhelming task. This half-timbered courtyard (c. 1520) was a mass grave, an ossuary where the bodies were "processed." Bodies would be dumped into the grave (where the well is now) and drenched in liquid lime to help speed decomposition. Later, the bones would be stacked in alcoves above the colonnades that line this courtyard. Notice the ghoulish carvings (c. 1560s) of gravediggers' tools, skulls, crossbones, and characters doing the "dance of death." In this *danse macabre*, Death, the great equalizer, grabs people of all social classes. The place is now an art school. Peek in on the young artists. As you leave, spy the dried black cat (died c. 1520, in tiny glass case to the left of the door). To overcome evil, it was buried during the building's construction.

Cost and Hours: Free, daily mid-March-Oct 8:00-19:00, Nov-mid-March 8:00-18:00.

Nearby: Farther down Rue Martainville, at Place St. Marc, a colorful market blooms Sunday until about 12:30 and all day Tuesday, Friday, and Saturday. If it's not market day, you can double back to the cathedral and Rue du Gros Horloge, or continue with me to explore more of Rouen and find the Museum of Fine Arts (back toward the train station).

• To reach the museum, turn right upon leaving the boneyard, then right again at the little boys (onto Rue Damiette), and hike up antique row to the vertical St. Ouen Church (a 7th-century abbey turned church in the 15th century, fine park behind). Turn left at the church on Rue des Faulx (an English-language bookstore, ABC Books, is two blocks to the right) and cross the busy street (the horseman you see to the right is a short-yet-majestic Napoleon Bonaparte who welcomes visitors to Rouen's city hall).

Continue down Rue de l'Hôpital's traffic-free lane, which becomes Rue Ganterie (admire the Gothic fountain at Rue Beauvoisine). A right at the modern square on Rue de l'Ecureuil leads you to the **Museum of Fine Arts** and the **Museum of Ironworks** (both described next). This is the end of our tour. The tower where Joan of Arc was imprisoned is a few blocks uphill, on the way back to the train station.

Sights in Rouen

▲Museum of Fine Arts (Musée des Beaux-Arts)

Paintings from many periods are beautifully displayed in this overlooked two-floor museum, including works by Caravaggio, Peter Paul Rubens, Paolo Veronese, Jan Steen, Velázquez, Théodore Géricault, Jean-Auguste-Dominique Ingres, Eugène Delacroix, and several Impressionists. With its reasonable entry fee and calm interior, this museum is worth a short visit for the Impressionists and a surgical hit of a few other key artists. The museum café is good for a peaceful break from the action outside.

Cost and Hours: €5, occasional temporary exhibitions cost extra, €8 combo-ticket includes ironworks and ceramics museums; open Wed-Mon 10:00-18:00, 15th-17th-century rooms closed 13:00-14:00, closed Tue; a few blocks below train station at 26 bis Rue Jean Lecanuet, tel. 02 35 71 28 40.

Museum of Ironworks (Musée le Secq des Tournelles, a.k.a. Musée de la Ferronnerie)

This deconsecrated church houses iron objects, many of them more than 1,500 years old. Locks, chests, keys, tools, thimbles, coffee grinders, corkscrews, and flatware from centuries ago—virtually anything made of iron is on display. You can duck into the entry area for a glimpse of a medieval iron scene without passing through the turnstile.

Cost and Hours: €3, €8 combo-ticket includes fine arts and ceramics museums, no English explanations—bring a French/English dictionary, Wed-Mon 14:00-18:00, closed Tue, behind Museum of Fine Arts, 2 Rue Jacques Villon, tel. 02 35 88 42 92.

What If I Miss My Boat?

Remember that you can get help from the cruise line's port agent (listed on the destination information sheet distributed on the ship) and the local TI (see page 1046). If the port agent suggests a costly solution (such as a private car with a driver), you may want to consider public transit.

For destinations on the Continent, your best bet is to ride the train to Paris, where you can connect to **Zeebrugge** (via Brussels), **Amsterdam, Warnemünde** (via Berlin), **Copenhagen,** and beyond.

To reach the ports for **London** (Southampton or Dover), consider an overnight ferry, several of which leave from Normandy. From Caen, Brittany Ferries runs to Portsmouth (tel. 0871-244-0744, www.brittany-ferries.co.uk). And from Dieppe, DFDS Seaways goes to Newhaven (tel. 0800-650-100, www.dfdsseaways.co.uk).

If you need to catch a **plane** to your next destination, your best bet is to head to one of Paris' two main airports (allow at least 3-4 hours by train from Le Havre, with a connection in Paris): Charles de Gaulle or Orly (these share a website: www.adp.fr). Slightly closer to Le Havre, at the northern edge of Paris, is Beauvais Airport, used predominantly by budget carriers (www.aeroportbeauvais.com).

Local **travel agents** in Le Havre or Paris can help you. For more advice on what to do if you miss the boat, see page 139.

Eating in Rouen

You can eat well in Rouen at fair prices. Because you're in Normandy, *crêperies* abound. To find the best eating action, prowl the streets between the St. Maclou and St. Ouen churches (Rues Martainville and Damiette) for *crêperies*, wine bars, international cuisine, and traditional restaurants.

Crêperie le St. Romain, between the cathedral and St. Maclou Church, is an excellent budget option. It's run by gentle Mr. Pegis, who serves filling €9-11 crêpes with small salads and offers many good options in a warm setting (tables in the rear are best). The hearty *gatiflette* is delicious (lunch Tue-Sat, dinner Thu-Sat, closed Sun-Mon, 52 Rue St. Romain, tel. 02 35 88 90 36).

Dame Cakes is ideal if it's lunchtime or teatime and you need a Jane Austen fix. The decor is from another, more precious era, and the baked goods are out of this world. Locals adore the tables in the back garden, while tourists eat up the cathedral view from the first-floor room (€12-15 salads and *plats*, garden terrace in back, Mon-Sat 11:00-18:00, closed Sun, 70 Rue St. Romain, tel. 02 35 07 49 31).

Le P'it Verdier is a lively wine bar-café where locals gather for

PARIS

a glass of wine and appetizers in the thick of restaurant row (closed Sun-Mon, 13 Rue Père Adam, tel. 02 35 36 34 43).

Le Parvis, which faces St. Maclou Church, is a good bet for a fine homemade Norman meal. There's comfortable seating inside and out (€25 two-course *menu*, €30 three-course *menu*, ask about their Bouillabaisse Normand, closed Sun-Mon, 7 Place Barthlémy, tel. 02 35 15 28 80).

La Petite Bouffe is a young-at-heart, appealing, cheery place with tall windows and good prices (€20 three-course *menus,* great choices, inside dining only, closed Sun, 1 Rue des Boucheries St-Ouen, tel. 02 35 98 13 14).

La Petite Auberge, a block off Rue Damiette, is the most traditional place I list. It has an Old World interior, reasonable prices, and it's also open on Sunday (*menus* from €22, closed Mon, 164 Rue Martainville, tel. 02 35 70 80 18).

French Survival Phrases

When using the phonetics, try to nasalize the n sound.

English	French	Pronunciation
Good day.	Bonjour.	bohn-zhoor
Mrs. / Mr.	Madame / Monsieur	mah-dahm / muhs-yur
Do you speak English?	Parlez-vous anglais?	par-lay-voo ahn-glay
Yes. / No.	Oui. / Non.	wee / nohn
I understand.	Je comprends.	zhuh kohn-prahn
I don't understand.	Je ne comprends pas.	zhuh nuh kohn-prahn pah
Please.	S'il vous plaît.	see voo play
Thank you.	Merci.	mehr-see
I'm sorry.	Désolé.	day-zoh-lay
Excuse me.	Pardon.	par-dohn
(No) problem.	(Pas de) problème.	(pah duh) proh-blehm
It's good.	C'est bon.	say bohn
Goodbye.	Au revoir.	oh vwahr
one / two	un / deux	uhn / duh
three / four	trois / quatre	twah / kah-truh
five / six	cinq / six	sank / sees
seven / eight	sept / huit	seht / weet
nine / ten	neuf / dix	nuhf / dees
How much is it?	Combien?	kohn-bee-an
Write it?	Ecrivez?	ay-kree-vay
Is it free?	C'est gratuit?	say grah-twee
Included?	Inclus?	an-klew
Where can I buy / find...?	Où puis-je acheter / trouver...?	oo pwee-zhuh ah-shuh-tay / troo-vay
I'd like / We'd like...	Je voudrais / Nous voudrions...	zhuh voo-dray / noo voo-dree-ohn
...a room.	...une chambre.	ewn shahn-bruh
...a ticket to ___.	...un billet pour ___.	uhn bee-yay poor ___
Is it possible?	C'est possible?	say poh-see-bluh
Where is...?	Où est...?	oo ay
...the train station	...la gare	lah gar
...the bus station	...la gare routière	lah gar root-yehr
...tourist information	...l'office du tourisme	loh-fees dew too-reez-muh
Where are the toilets?	Où sont les toilettes?	oo sohn lay twah-leht
men	hommes	ohm
women	dames	dahm
left / right	à gauche / à droite	ah gohsh / ah dwaht
straight	tout droit	too dwah
When does this open / close?	Ça ouvre / ferme à quelle heure?	sah oo-vruh / fehrm ah kehl ur
At what time?	À quelle heure?	ah kehl ur
Just a moment.	Un moment.	uhn moh-mahn
now / soon / later	maintenant / bientôt / plus tard	man-tuh-nahn / bee-an-toh / plew tar
today / tomorrow	aujourd'hui / demain	oh-zhoor-dwee / duh-man

APPENDIX

Contents

Tourist Information

TOURIST INFORMATION OFFICES

Before your trip, scan the websites of national tourist offices for the countries you'll be visiting, or contact them to briefly describe your trip and request information. Some will mail you a general-interest brochure, and you can often download other brochures free of charge. For websites, see the **Practicalities** section that precedes each port destination.

In Europe, a good first stop in a new town is the official tourist information office (abbreviated **TI** in this book). TIs are usually good places to get a city map and information on public transit (including bus and train schedules), walking tours, and special events. But be wary of the travel agencies or special information services that masquerade as TIs but serve fancy hotels and tour companies. They're in the business of selling things you don't need.

European Calling Chart

Just smile and dial, using this key:
AC = Area Code, LN = Local Number.

European Country	Calling long distance within ...	Calling from the US or Canada to ...	Calling from a European country to ...
Austria	AC + LN	011 + 43 + AC (without initial zero) + LN	00 + 43 + AC (without initial zero) + LN
Belgium	LN	011 + 32 + LN (without initial zero)	00 + 32 + LN (without initial zero)
Bosnia-Herzegovina	AC + LN	011 + 387 + AC (without initial zero) + LN	00 + 387 + AC (without initial zero) + LN
Croatia	AC + LN	011 + 385 + AC (without initial zero) + LN	00 + 385 + AC (without initial zero) + LN
Czech Republic	LN	011 + 420 + LN	00 + 420 + LN
Denmark	LN	011 + 45 + LN	00 + 45 + LN
Estonia	LN	011 + 372 + LN	00 + 372 + LN
Finland	AC + LN	011 + 358 + AC (without initial zero) + LN	00 + 358 + AC (without initial zero) + LN
France	LN	011 + 33 + LN (without initial zero)	00 + 33 + LN (without initial zero)
Germany	AC + LN	011 + 49 + AC (without initial zero) + LN	00 + 49 + AC (without initial zero) + LN
Gibraltar	LN	011 + 350 + LN	00 + 350 + LN
Great Britain & N. Ireland	AC + LN	011 + 44 + AC (without initial zero) + LN	00 + 44 + AC (without initial zero) + LN
Greece	LN	011 + 30 + LN	00 + 30 + LN
Hungary	06 + AC + LN	011 + 36 + AC + LN	00 + 36 + AC + LN
Ireland	AC + LN	011 + 353 + AC (without initial zero) + LN	00 + 353 + AC (without initial zero) + LN
Italy	LN	011 + 39 + LN	00 + 39 + LN

European Country	Calling long distance within ...	Calling from the US or Canada to ...	Calling from a European country to ...
Latvia	LN	011 + 371 + LN	00 + 371 + LN
Montenegro	AC + LN	011 + 382 + AC (without initial zero) + LN	00 + 382 + AC (without initial zero) + LN
Morocco	LN	011 + 212 + LN (without initial zero)	00 + 212 + LN (without initial zero)
Netherlands	AC + LN	011 + 31 + AC (without initial zero) + LN	00 + 31 + AC (without initial zero) + LN
Norway	LN	011 + 47 + LN	00 + 47 + LN
Poland	LN	011 + 48 + LN	00 + 48 + LN
Portugal	LN	011 + 351 + LN	00 + 351 + LN
Russia	8 + AC + LN	011 + 7 + AC + LN	00 + 7 + AC + LN
Slovakia	AC + LN	011 + 421 + AC (without initial zero) + LN	00 + 421 + AC (without initial zero) + LN
Slovenia	AC + LN	011 + 386 + AC (without initial zero) + LN	00 + 386 + AC (without initial zero) + LN
Spain	LN	011 + 34 + LN	00 + 34 + LN
Sweden	AC + LN	011 + 46 + AC (without initial zero) + LN	00 + 46 + AC (without initial zero) + LN
Switzerland	LN	011 + 41 + LN (without initial zero)	00 + 41 + LN (without initial zero)
Turkey	AC (if there's no initial zero, add one) + LN	011 + 90 + AC (without initial zero) + LN	00 + 90 + AC (without initial zero) + LN

- The instructions above apply whether you're calling to or from a European landline or mobile phone.
- If calling from any mobile phone, you can replace the international access code with "+" (press and hold 0 to insert it).
- The international access code is 011 if you're calling from the US or Canada.
- To call the US or Canada from Europe, dial 00, then 1 (country code for US and Canada), then the area code and number. In short, 00 + 1 + AC + LN = Hi, Mom!

Communicating

"How can I stay connected in Europe?"—by phone and online—may be the most common question I hear from travelers. Smart travelers use the telephone or the Web to get tourist information, reserve restaurants, confirm tour times, and phone home. For the details on your options—both from a cruise ship and in port—see page 87.

For emergency telephone numbers and dialing advice, see the Practicalities sections earlier in this book. For more in-depth information on dialing, see www.ricksteves.com/phoning.

HOW TO DIAL

Many Americans are intimidated by dialing European phone numbers. You needn't be. It's simple, once you break the code. The European calling chart on page 1144 will walk you through it.

No matter where you're calling from, to dial internationally you must first dial the international access code of the place you're calling from (to "get out" of the domestic phone system), and then the country code of the place you're trying to reach.

The US and Canada have the same international access code: 011. Most European countries use the same international access code: 00. The exceptions are Russia (where you dial 8 to get an international line) and Finland (where you dial 999 or another 900 number, depending on the phone service you're using). You might see a + in front of a European number; that's a reminder to dial the access code of the place you're calling from. If you're calling from a mobile phone, you can simply insert a "+" before the number—no additional access code required.

Transportation

While in port, you're likely to use public transportation to get around (and, in some cases, to get to) the cities you're here to see.

TAXIS

Taxis are underrated, scenic time-savers that zip you effortlessly from the cruise terminal to any sight in town, or between sights. Especially for couples and small groups who value their time, a taxi ride can be a good investment. Unfortunately, many predatory taxi drivers prey on cruisers who are in town just for the day by charging them inflated fares for short rides. Prepare yourself by reading the "Taxi Tips" on page 122.

CITY TRANSIT

Shrink and tame big cities by mastering their subway, bus, and tram systems. Europe's public-transit systems are so good that many Europeans go through life never learning to drive. With a map, anyone can decipher the code to cheap and easy urban transportation.

Subway Basics

Most of Europe's big cities are blessed with excellent subway systems, often linked effortlessly with suburban trains. Learning a city's network of underground trains is a key to efficient sightseeing. European subways go by many names, but "Metro" is the most common term. In Scandinavia, these systems often start with "T" (*T-bane* in Oslo and *T-bana* in Stockholm, for example). In some cities—such as Copenhagen and Berlin—the network also includes suburban trains, often marked with "S."

Plan your route. Figure out your route before you enter the station so you can march confidently to the correct train. Get a good subway map (often included on free city maps, or ask for one at the station) and consult it often. In the stations, maps are usually posted prominently. A typical subway map is a spaghetti-like tangle of intersecting, colorful lines. Individual lines are color-coded, numbered, and/or lettered; their end points are also indicated. These end points—while probably places you will never go—are important, since they tell you which direction the train is moving and appear (usually) as the name listed on the front of the train. Figure out the line you need, the end point of the direction you want to go, and (if necessary) where to transfer to another line.

Validate your ticket. You may need to insert your ticket into a slot in the turnstile (then retrieve it) in order to validate it. If you have an all-day or multiday ticket, you may only need to validate it the first time you use it, or not at all (ask when you buy it).

Get off at the right place. Once on the train, follow along with each stop on your map (some people count stops). Sometimes the driver or an automated voice announces the upcoming stop—but don't count on this cue, as a foreign name spoken by a native speaker over a crackly loudspeaker can be difficult to understand. As you pull into each station, its name will be posted prominently on the platform or along the wall.

Transfer. Changing from one subway line to another can be as easy as walking a few steps away to an adjacent platform—or a bewildering wander via a labyrinth of stairs and long passageways. Fortunately, most subway systems are clearly signed—just follow along (or ask a local for help).

Exit the station. When you arrive at your destination station, follow exit signs up to the main ticketing area, where you'll usually

APPENDIX

find a posted map of the surrounding neighborhood to help you get your bearings. Individual exits are signposted by street name or nearby landmarks. Bigger stations have multiple exits. Choosing the right exit will help you avoid extra walking and having to cross busy streets.

Bus and Tram Basics

Getting around town on the city bus or tram system has some advantages over subways. Buses or trams are often a better bet for shorter distances. Some buses go where the subway can't. Since you're not underground, it's easier to stay oriented and get the lay of the land.

Plan your route. Tourist maps often indicate bus and tram lines and stops. If yours doesn't, ask for a specific bus map at the TI. Many bus and tram stops have timetables and route maps posted.

Validate your ticket. Tickets are checked on European buses and trams in a variety of ways. Usually you enter at the front of the bus or tram and show your ticket to the driver, or validate it by sticking it in a time-stamp box. In some cases, you buy your ticket directly from the driver; other times, you'll buy your ticket at a kiosk or machine near the stop.

TRAINS

If you venture beyond your port city, European trains generally go where you need them to go and are fast, frequent, and affordable. "Point-to-point" or buy-as-you-go tickets can be your best bet for short travel distances anywhere. (If you're doing a substantial amount of pre- or post-cruise travel on your own, a rail pass can be a good value.) You can buy train tickets either from home, or once you get to Europe. If your travel plans are set, and you don't want to risk a specific train journey selling out, it can be smart to get your tickets before your trip. For details on buying tickets on European websites and complete rail pass information, see www.ricksteves.com/rail. To study ahead on the Web, check www.bahn.com (Germany's excellent Europe-wide timetable).

If you want to be more flexible, you can keep your options open by buying tickets in Europe. Nearly every station has old-fashioned ticket windows staffed by human beings, usually marked by long lines. Bridge any communication gap by writing out your plan: destination city, date (European-style: day/month/year), time (if you want to reserve a specific train), number of people, and first or second class.

To get tickets faster, savvy travelers figure out how to use ticket machines: Choose English, follow the step-by-step instructions, and swipe your credit card (though you may need to know your PIN, and some machines don't accept American cards—see page 130). Some machines accept cash. It's often possible to buy tickets on board the train, but expect to pay an additional fee for the convenience.

Seat reservations guarantee you a place to sit on the train, and can be optional or required depending on the route and train. Reservations are required for any train marked with an "R" in the schedule. Note that seat reservations are already included with many tickets, especially for the fastest trains (such as France's TGV). But for many trains (local, regional, interregional, and many EuroCity and InterCity trains), reservations are not necessary and not worth the trouble and expense unless you're traveling during a busy holiday period.

Be aware that many cities have more than one train station. Ask for help and pay attention. Making your way through stations and onto trains is largely a matter of asking questions, letting people help you, and assuming things are logical. I always ask someone on the platform if the train is going where I think it is (point to the train or track and ask, *"Pah-ree?"*).

BUSES

In most countries, trains are faster, more comfortable, and have more extensive schedules than buses. Bus trips are usually less expensive than trains, but often take longer. Use buses mainly to pick up where Europe's great train system leaves off.

Resources

RESOURCES FROM RICK STEVES

Books: *Rick Steves Northern European Cruise Ports* is one of many books in my series on European travel, which includes another

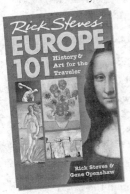

cruise book, *Mediterranean Cruise Ports*, along with many country guidebooks, city guidebooks (Paris, London, Amsterdam, etc.), Snapshot Guides (excerpted chapters from my country guides), Pocket Guides (full-color little books on big cities), and my budget-travel skills handbook, *Rick Steves Europe Through the Back Door*. Most of my titles are available as ebooks. My phrase books—for French, Spanish, German, Italian, and Portuguese—are practical and budget-oriented. My other books include *Europe 101* (a crash course on art and history designed for travelers) and *Travel as a Political Act* (a travelogue sprinkled with tips for bringing home a global perspective). A

Begin Your Trip at
www.RickSteves.com

My **website** is *the* place to plan your trip and explore Europe. You'll find thousands of fun articles, videos, photos, and radio interviews on European destinations; money-saving tips for planning your dream trip; monthly travel news; my travel talks and travel blog; my latest guidebook updates (www.ricksteves.com/update); and my free Rick Steves Audio Europe app. You can also follow me on Facebook and Twitter.

Our **Travel Forum** is an immense, yet well-groomed collection of message boards, where our travel-savvy community answers questions and shares their personal travel experiences (www.ricksteves.com/forums).

Our online Travel Store offers travel bags and accessories that I've designed specifically to help you travel smarter and lighter. These include my popular bags (roll-aboard and rucksack versions), money belts, totes, toiletries kits, adapters, other accessories, and a wide selection of guidebooks, planning maps, and DVDs.

Want to travel with greater efficiency and less stress? We organize **tours** with more than three dozen itineraries and more than 800 departures reaching the best destinations in this book...and beyond. Many of our tours begin or end at the major ports of embarkation (Copenhagen, Stockholm, Amsterdam, and London). Tours such as Scandinavia in 14 Days, Belgium and Holland in 11 Days, or England in 14 Days are great ways to extend your European adventure before or after a cruise. You'll enjoy great guides, a fun bunch of travel partners (with small groups of 24 to 28 travelers), and plenty of room to spread out in a big, comfy bus when touring between towns. You'll find European adventures to fit every vacation length. For all the details, and to get our Tour Catalog and a free Rick Steves Tour Experience DVD (filmed on location during an actual tour), visit www.ricksteves.com or call us at 425/608-4217.

more complete list of my titles appears near the end of this book.

Video: My public television series, *Rick Steves' Europe*, covers European destinations in 100 shows. To watch full episodes online for free, see www.ricksteves.com/tv. Or to raise your travel I.Q. with video versions of our popular classes, including a talk on northern European cruise ports, see www.ricksteves.com/travel-talks.

Audio: My weekly public radio show, *Travel with Rick Steves*, features interviews with travel experts from around the world. I've also produced free, self-guided **audio tours** of the top sights in Paris, London, Amsterdam, Berlin, and other great cities. All of

APPENDIX

this audio content is available for free at Rick Steves Audio Europe, an extensive online library organized by destination. Choose whatever interests you, and download it for free via the Rick Steves Audio Europe smartphone app, www.ricksteves.com/audioeurope, iTunes, or Google Play.

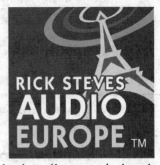

More Resources

If you're like most travelers, this book is all you need, though there's a staggering array of websites, guidebooks, and other useful resources for people interested in cruising. For a summary of good websites to peruse to help you choose your cruise, see page 34. For reviews of various cruise lines and ships, refer to my list on page 18.

Beyond the guidebook format, look for the well-written history of the cruise industry, *Devils on the Deep Blue Sea* (by Kristoffer Garin). A variety of tell-all type books offer behind-the-scenes intrigue from a life working on cruise ships. More titillating than well-written, these are good vacation reads to enjoy poolside. They include *Cruise Confidential* (by Brian David Bruns) and *The Truth about Cruise Ships* (by Jay Herring).

Holidays

The following list will alert you to times when days in port might coincide with a holiday. While holidays can close sights and bring crowds, they can also occasion festivals, parades, and merrymaking. Your best source for general information is the TI in each town—it's worth a quick look at their websites to turn up possible holiday closures and/or special events.

Jan 1	New Year's Day
Jan 6	Epiphany
March/April	Easter weekend (Good Friday-Easter Monday): March 25-28, 2016; April 14-17, 2017
May 1	Labor Day
May	Ascension: May 5, 2016; May 25, 2017
May/June	Pentecost and Whitmonday: May 15-16, 2016; June 4-5, 2017
May/June	Corpus Christi: May 26, 2016; June 15, 2017
Aug 15	Assumption
Nov 1	All Saint's Day

Nov 11	Armistice Day/St. Martin's Day
Dec 25	Christmas Day
Dec 26	Boxing Day
Dec 31	New Year's Eve

Note that many of the above holidays are Catholic and Protestant dates; in Orthodox countries (such as Russia and certain communities in Estonia, Latvia, and Finland), the dates for these holidays can differ.

Conversions and Climate

NUMBERS AND STUMBLERS

- Europeans write a few of their numbers differently than we do. 1 = 1, 4 = 4, 7 = 7.
- In Europe, dates appear as day/month/year, so Christmas 2016 is 25/12/16.
- Commas are decimal points and decimals are commas. A dollar and a half is $1,50, one thousand is 1.000, and there are 5.280 feet in a mile.
- When counting with fingers, start with your thumb. If you hold up your first finger to request one item, you'll probably get two.
- What Americans call the second floor of a building is the first floor in Europe.
- On escalators and moving sidewalks, Europeans keep the left "lane" open for passing. Keep to the right.

METRIC CONVERSIONS

A kilogram is 2.2 pounds, and 1 liter is about a quart, or almost four to a gallon. A kilometer is six-tenths of a mile. I figure kilometers to miles by cutting them in half and adding back 10 percent of the original (120 km: 60 + 12 = 72 miles, 300 km: 150 + 30 = 180 miles).

1 foot = 0.3 meter	1 square yard = 0.8 square meter
1 yard = 0.9 meter	1 square mile = 2.6 square kilometers
1 mile = 1.6 kilometers	1 ounce = 28 grams
1 centimeter = 0.4 inch	1 quart = 0.95 liter
1 meter = 39.4 inches	1 kilogram = 2.2 pounds
1 kilometer = 0.62 mile	32°F = 0°C

IMPERIAL WEIGHTS AND MEASURES

Britain hasn't completely gone metric. Driving distances and speed limits are measured in miles. Beer is sold as pints (though milk can be measured in pints or liters), and a person's weight is measured in

stone (a 168-pound person weighs 12 stone).
1 stone = 14 pounds
1 British pint = 1.2 US pints
1 imperial gallon = 1.2 US gallons or about 4.5 liters

CLOTHING SIZES

For US-to-European clothing size conversions, see page 133.

CLIMATE

First line, average daily high; second line, average daily low; third line, average days without rain. For more detailed weather statistics for European destinations (and the rest of the world), check www.wunderground.com.

	J	F	M	A	M	J	J	A	S	O	N	D
DENMARK												
Copenhagen												
	37°	37°	42°	51°	60°	66°	70°	69°	64°	55°	46°	41°
	29°	28°	31°	37°	45°	51°	56°	56°	51°	44°	38°	33°
	14	15	19	18	20	18	17	16	14	14	11	12
SWEDEN												
Stockholm												
	30°	30°	37°	47°	58°	67°	71°	68°	60°	49°	40°	35°
	26°	25°	29°	37°	45°	53°	57°	56°	50°	43°	37°	32°
	15	14	21	19	20	17	18	17	16	16	14	14
FINLAND												
Helsinki												
	26°	25°	32°	44°	56°	66°	71°	68°	59°	47°	37°	31°
	17°	15°	20°	30°	40°	49°	55°	53°	46°	37°	30°	23°
	11	10	17	17	19	17	17	16	16	13	11	11
RUSSIA												
St. Petersburg												
	29°	28°	37°	50°	60°	69°	74°	71°	60°	48°	35°	30°
	18°	15°	22°	32°	40°	49°	55°	52°	44°	36°	26°	20°
	10	11	15	15	16	13	15	15	14	09	10	11
ESTONIA												
Tallinn												
	25°	25°	32°	45°	57°	66°	68°	66°	59°	50°	37°	30°
	14°	12°	19°	32°	41°	50°	54°	52°	48°	39°	30°	19°
	12	12	18	19	19	20	18	16	14	14	12	12
LATVIA												
Rīga												
	33°	33°	40°	53°	62°	69°	74°	72°	62°	51°	39°	33°
	26°	24°	28°	36°	44°	51°	56°	56°	47°	40°	32°	26°
	12	12	15	16	17	15	16	15	15	12	11	12

	J	F	M	A	M	J	J	A	S	O	N	D

POLAND
Gdańsk

	J	F	M	A	M	J	J	A	S	O	N	D
	35°	36°	42°	52°	62°	67°	71°	71°	62°	53°	41°	35°
	27°	27°	30°	35°	43°	49°	54°	54°	47°	41°	33°	28°
	30	27	30	29	30	30	30	30	29	29	29	29

GERMANY
Berlin

	J	F	M	A	M	J	J	A	S	O	N	D
	35°	37°	46°	56°	66°	72°	75°	74°	68°	56°	45°	38°
	26°	26°	31°	39°	47°	53°	57°	56°	50°	42°	36°	29°
	14	13	19	17	19	17	17	17	18	17	14	16

NORWAY
Oslo

	J	F	M	A	M	J	J	A	S	O	N	D
	28°	30°	39°	50°	61°	68°	72°	70°	60°	48°	38°	32°
	19°	19°	25°	34°	43°	50°	55°	53°	46°	38°	31°	25°
	16	16	22	19	21	17	16	17	16	17	14	14

THE NETHERLANDS
Amsterdam

	J	F	M	A	M	J	J	A	S	O	N	D
	41°	42°	49°	55°	64°	70°	72°	71°	66°	56°	48°	41°
	30°	31°	35°	40°	45°	52°	55°	55°	51°	43°	37°	33°
	8	9	16	14	16	16	14	12	11	11	10	9

BELGIUM
Brussels

	J	F	M	A	M	J	J	A	S	O	N	D
	41°	44°	51°	58°	65°	71°	73°	72°	69°	60°	48°	42°
	30°	32°	34°	40°	45°	53°	55°	55°	52°	45°	38°	32°
	9	11	14	12	15	15	13	12	15	13	10	11

GREAT BRITAIN
London

	J	F	M	A	M	J	J	A	S	O	N	D
	43°	44°	50°	56°	62°	69°	71°	71°	65°	58°	50°	45°
	36°	36°	38°	42°	47°	53°	56°	56°	52°	46°	42°	38°
	16	15	20	18	19	19	19	20	17	18	15	16

FRANCE
Paris

	J	F	M	A	M	J	J	A	S	O	N	D
	43°	45°	54°	60°	68°	73°	76°	75°	70°	60°	50°	44°
	34°	34°	39°	43°	49°	55°	58°	58°	53°	46°	40°	36°
	14	14	19	17	19	18	19	18	17	18	15	15

FAHRENHEIT AND CELSIUS CONVERSION

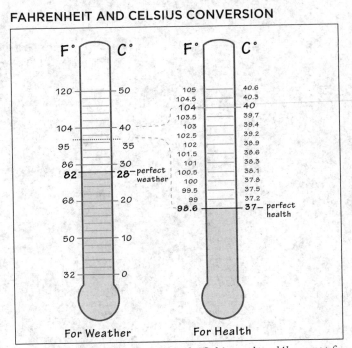

Europe takes its temperature using the Celsius scale, while we opt for Fahrenheit. For a rough conversion from Celsius to Fahrenheit, double the number and add 30. For weather, remember that 28°C is 82°F—perfect. For health, 37°C is just right.

INDEX

INDEX

INDEX

MAP INDEX

MAP INDEX

Explore Europe

At ricksteves.com you can browse through thousands of articles, videos, photos and radio interviews, plus find a wealth of money-saving travel tips for planning your dream trip. And with our mobile-friendly website, you can easily access all this great travel information anywhere you go.

TV Shows

Preview the places you'll visit by watching entire half-hour episodes of Rick Steves' Europe (choose from all 100 shows) on-demand, for free.

your travel dreams into affordable reality

Radio Interviews

Enjoy ready access to Rick's vast library of radio interviews covering travel

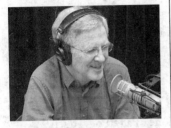

tips and cultural insights that relate specifically to your Europe travel plans.

Travel Forums

Learn, ask, share! Our online community of savvy travelers is a great resource for first-time travelers to Europe, as well as seasoned pros. You'll find forums on each country, plus travel tips and restaurant/hotel reviews. You can even ask one of our well-traveled staff to chime in with an opinion.

Travel News

Subscribe to our free Travel News e-newsletter, and get monthly updates from Rick on what's happening in Europe.

Rick's Free Travel App

Get your FREE **Rick Steves Audio Europe**™ app to enjoy…

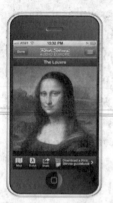

- Dozens of self-guided tours of Europe's top museums, sights and historic walks
- Hundreds of tracks filled with cultural insights and sightseeing tips from Rick's radio interviews
- All organized into handy geographic playlists
- For iPhone, iPad, iPod Touch, Android

With Rick whispering in your ear, Europe gets even better.

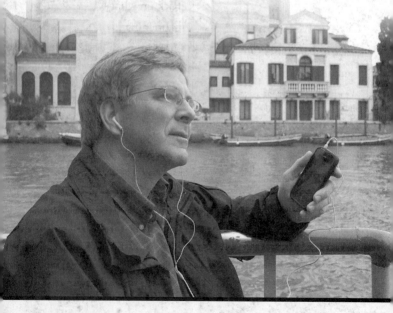

Find out more at ricksteves.com

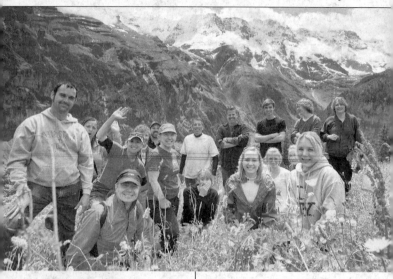

Experience maximum Europe

Save time and energy

This guidebook is your independent-travel toolkit. But for all it delivers, it's still up to you to devote the time and energy it takes to manage the preparation and logistics that are essential for a happy trip. If that's a hassle, there's a solution.

Rick Steves Tours

A Rick Steves tour takes you to Europe's most interesting places with great

with minimum stress

guides and small groups of 28 or less. We follow Rick's favorite itineraries, ride in comfy buses, stay in family-run hotels, and bring you intimately close to the Europe you've traveled so far to see. Most importantly, we take away the logistical headaches so you can focus on the fun.

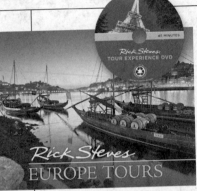

customers—along with us on 40 different itineraries, from Ireland to Italy to Istanbul. Is a Rick Steves tour the right fit for your travel dreams? Find out at ricksteves.com, where you can also get Rick's latest tour catalog and free Tour Experience DVD.

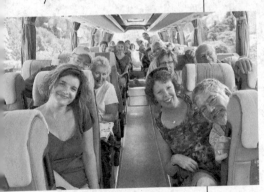

Join the fun

This year we'll take 18,000 free-spirited travelers— nearly half of them repeat

Europe is best experienced with happy travel partners. We hope you can join us.

Credits

CONTRIBUTORS

Gene Openshaw

Gene is the co-author of a dozen Rick Steves books. For this book, he wrote material on Europe's art, history, and contemporary culture. When not traveling, Gene enjoys composing music, recovering from his 1973 trip to Europe with Rick, and living everyday life with his daughter.

Steve Smith

Steve manages tour guides for Rick Steves' Europe tour program and has been researching guidebooks with Rick for over two decades. Fluent in French, he's lived in France on several occasions, starting when he was just seven. Steve owns a restored farmhouse in rural Burgundy where he hangs his beret in research season. Steve's wife, Karen Lewis Smith, who's an expert on French cuisine and wine, provides invaluable contributions to his books.

ACKNOWLEDGMENTS

This book would not have been possible without the help of our cruising friends. Special thanks to Todd and Carla Hoover, cruisers extraordinaire, and to Sheri Smith at Elizabeth Holmes Travel (www.elizabethholmes.com). Applause for Vanessa Bloy at Windstar Cruises, Paul Allen and John Primeau at Holland America Line, Courtney Recht at Norwegian Cruise Line, and Melissa Rubin at Oceania Cruises. And high fives for Ben Curtis, Sheryl Harris, Paul and Bev Hoerlein, Jenn Schutte, Lisa Friend, and Noelle Kenney.